Instructional
Course Lectures

Volume 48 1999

American Academy
of Orthopaedic Surgeons

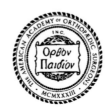

Instructional Course Lectures

Volume 48 1999
including index for 1997, 1998, and 1999

Edited by
Joseph D. Zuckerman, MD
Professor and Chairman
Department of Orthopaedic Surgery
New York University-Hospital for Joint Diseases
New York, New York

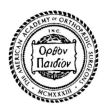

American Academy
of Orthopaedic Surgeons
6300 North River Road
Rosemont, IL 60018

American Academy of Orthopaedic Surgeons®
Instructional Course Lectures
Volume 48

Vice President, Educational Programs: Mark W. Wieting
Director, Department of Publications: Marilyn L. Fox, PhD
Senior Editor: Bruce A. Davis
Senior Editor: Joan Abern
Associate Senior Editor: Lisa Moore
Production Manager: Loraine Edwalds
Assistant Production Managers: Sophie Tosta,
      David Stanley
Production Assistants: Geraldine Dubberke, Jana Ronayne,
      Vanessa Villarreal

The material presented in *Instructional Course Lectures Volume 48* has been made available by the American Academy of Orthopaedic Surgeons® for educational purposes only. This material is not intended to present the only, or necessarily best, methods or procedures for the medical situations discussed, but rather is intended to represent an approach, view, statement, or opinion of the author(s) or producer(s), which may be helpful to others who face similar situations.

Some drugs and medical devices demonstrated in Academy courses or described in Academy print or electronic publications have not been cleared by the Food and Drug Administration (FDA) or have been cleared by the FDA for specific purposes only. The FDA has stated that it is the responsibility of the physician to determine the FDA status of each drug or device he or she wishes to use in clinical practice.

At the time of this writing, bone screws placed posteriorly into vertebral elements have been cleared for use in this specific manner by the Food and Drug Administration (FDA) to provide immobilization and stabilization as an adjunct to fusion in the treatment of the following acute and chronic instability or deformities of the thoracic, lumbar and sacral spine: degenerative spondylolisthesis with objective evidence of neurological impairment; fracture; dislocation; scoliosis; kyphosis; spinal tumor and failed previous fusion (pseudoarthrosis). In addition, anterior vertebral body screws (cervical, thoracic, and lumbar) are Class II devices and can be used as labeled in vertebral bodies.

Furthermore, any statements about commercial products are solely the opinion(s) of the author(s) and do not represent an Academy endorsement or evaluation of these products. These statements may not be used in advertising or for any commercial purpose.

ISBN 0-89203-212-x

Contributors

Albert J. Aboulafia, MD, Assistant Professor, Department of Orthopaedics, Emory University School of Medicine, Atlanta Veterans Administration Hospital, Atlanta, Georgia

Zoe Agnidis, MSc, PT, Research Clinician, Department of Surgery, Clinical Research Office, Mount Sinai Hospital, Toronto, Ontario, Canada

Behrooz A. Akbarnia, MD, Clinical Associate Professor of Orthopaedic Surgery, University of California, San Diego, Medical Director, San Diego Center for Spinal Disorders, San Diego, California

Todd J. Albert, MD, Associate Professor of Orthopaedics, Co-Director of Reconstructive Spinal Surgery and Spinal Fellowship Program, Rothman Institute, Thomas Jefferson University, Philadelphia, Pennsylvania

Peter C. Amadio, MD, Professor of Orthopaedics and Consultant in Hand and Orthopaedic Surgery, Division of Hand Surgery, Mayo Medical Center, Rochester, Minnesota

Annunziato Amendola, MD, FRCSC, Associate Professor of Orthopaedic Surgery, Department of Surgery, University of Western Ontario, London, Ontario, Canada

Deborah J. Ammeen, BS, Research Associate, Anderson Orthopaedic Research Institute, Alexandria, Virginia

Ram Aribindi, MD, FRCSC, Clinical Instructor, Department of Orthopaedic Surgery, Rush Presbyterian St. Luke's Medical Center, Chicago, Illinois

John V. Banta, MD, Director of Orthopaedics, Newington Department of Pediatric Orthopaedics, Connecticut Children's Medical Center, Hartford, Connecticut

Mark Barba, MD, Private Practice, Carlson Orthopaedics, Rockford, Illinois

Robert L. Barrack, MD, Professor of Orthopaedic Surgery, Director of Adult Reconstructive Surgery, Department of Orthopaedic Surgery, Tulane University School of Medicine, New Orleans, Louisiana

Christopher P. Beauchamp, MD, Assistant Professor of Orthopaedics, Mayo Graduate School of Medicine, Mayo Clinic, Scottsdale, Arizona

Richard A. Berger, MD, PhD, Assistant Professor, Departments of Orthopaedic Surgery and Anatomy, Division of Hand Surgery, Mayo Clinic, Rochester, Minnesota

John A. Bergfeld, MD, Professor and Head Section of Sports Medicine, Department of Orthopaedics, The Cleveland Clinic, Cleveland, Ohio

William S. Bolling, MD, Resident, General Surgery, Department of Surgery, Mayo Clinic, Scottsdale, Arizona

John H. Bowker, MD, Professor and Head, Division of Foot and Ankle Surgery, Department of Orthopaedics and Rehabilitation, University of Miami School of Medicine, Miami, Florida

James W. Brodsky, MD, Clinical Associate Professor, University of Texas Southwestern Medical Center, Director, Foot and Ankle Surgery Fellowship, Baylor University Medical Center, Dallas, Texas

Joseph A. Buckwalter, MD, Professor of Orthopaedic Surgery, Department of Orthopaedic Surgery, University of Iowa, Iowa City, Iowa

Pieter Buma, PhD, Department of Orthopaedics, Orthopaedic Research Laboratory, Academic Hospital Nijmegen, Nijmegen, The Netherlands

David G. Campbell, BM, BS, FRACS (Orth), Former Fellow, Department of Orthopaedics, University of British Columbia, Vancouver, British Columbia, Canada

Daniel A. Capen, MD, Associate Clinical Professor, University of Southern California, Los Angeles, California Neuro-Trauma Service, Rancho Los Amigos Medical Center, Downey, California

Arnold I. Caplan, PhD, Professor of Biology, Case Western Reserve University, Cleveland, Ohio

William L. Cats-Baril, PhD, Professor, School of Business, University of Vermont, Burlington, Vermont, Data Harbor, Chicago, Illinois

Brian Cho, Research Student, Mount Sinai Hospital, Orthopaedic Surgery, Toronto, Ontario, Canada

Michael G. Ciccotti, MD, Associate Professor, Director of Sports Medicine, Department of Orthopaedic Surgery, Rothman Institute at Thomas Jefferson University, Philadelphia, Pennsylvania

Robert H. Cofield, MD, Professor of Orthopaedics, Mayo Medical School, Chair, Department of Orthopaedics, Mayo Clinic, Rochester, Minnesota

Stephen F. Conti, MD, Chief, Division of Foot and Ankle Surgery, Department of Orthopaedic Surgery, University of Pittsburgh School of Medicine, Pittsburgh, Pennsylvnia

Jerome M. Cotler, MD, The Everett J. and Marian Gordon Professor, Department of Orthopaedic Surgery, Jefferson Medical College of Thomas Jefferson University, Philadelphia, Pennsylvania

Edward V. Craig, MD, Professor of Clinical Orthopaedics, Hospital for Special Surgery, Cornell Medical College, New York, New York

Haemish A. Crawford, MBCLB, FRACS, Clinical and Research Fellow, Fowler-Kennedy Sports Medicine Clinic, University of Western Ontario, London, Ontario, Canada

Randall W. Culp, MD, Associate Professor of Orthopaedic, Hand, and Microsurgery, Jefferson Medical College of Thomas Jefferson University, The Philadelphia Hand Center, PC, King of Prussia, Pennsylvania

Andrei Czitrom, MD, FRCSC, Associate Professor, Department of Orthopaedics, Southwest University, Dallas, Texas

James C. Drennan, MD, Professor, Department of Orthopaedics and Pediatrics, University of New Mexico School of Medicine, Albuquerque, New Mexico

Denis S. Drummond, MD, Emeritus Chief of Orthopaedics Professor of Orthopaedic Surgery, Department of Orthopaedics, The Children's Hospital of Philadelphia, Philadelphia, Pennsylvania

Clive P. Duncan, MB, MSc, FRCSC, Professor and Head, Department of Orthopaedics, Faculty of Medicine, The University of British Columbia, Vancouver, British Columbia, Canada

Paul Duwelius, MD, Associate Professor, Department of Orthopaedics and Rehabilitation, Oregon Health Sciences University, Portland, Oregon

Scott F. Dye, MD, Associate Clinical Professor of Orthopaedic Surgery, University of California, San Francisco, San Francisco, California

Roger H. Emerson, Jr, MD, Senior Associate, Texas Center for Joint Replacement, Presbyterian Hospital of Plano, Plano, Texas

Sanford E. Emery, MD, Associate Professor, Department of Orthopaedics, University Hospitals of Cleveland, Case Western Reserve University, Cleveland, Ohio

C. Anderson Engh, Jr, MD, Trustee and Senior Technical Advisor, Anderson Orthopaedic Research Institute, Alexandria, Virginia

Charles Engh, Sr, MD, Medical Director, Director of Hip Research, Anderson Orthopaedic Research Institute, Alexandria, Virginia

Charles A. Engh, MD, Massachusetts General Hospital, Harvard Medical School, Boston, Massachusetts

Gerard A. Engh, MD, Director, Knee Research, Anderson Orthopaedic Research Institute, Alexandria, Viriginia Associate Clinical Professor, Division of Orthopaedic Surgery, University of Maryland School of Medicine, Baltimore, Maryland

Roger W. Evans, PhD, Head, Section of Health Services Evaluation, Department of Health Sciences Research, Mayo Clinic, Rochester, Minnesota

Ronney L. Ferguson, MD, Chief of Staff, Shriners Hospitals for Children, Spokane, Spokane, Washington

Larry D. Field, MD, Co-Director, Upper Extremity Service, Mississippi Sports Medicine and Orthopaedic Center, Jackson, Mississippi

Donald C. Fithian, MD, Assistant Clinical Professor, Department of Orthopaedic Surgery, University of California, San Diego, Southern California Kaiser Permanente, San Diego, California

Timothy C. Fitzgibbons, MD, Assistant Clinical Professor, Department of Orthopaedics, Creighton University School of Medicine, Omaha, Nebraska

Adam E. Flanders, MD, Associate Professor of Radiology, Department of Radiology/Neuroradiology, Thomas Jefferson University Hospital, Philadelphia, Pennsylvania

Peter J. Fowler, MD, FACSC, Professor and Chief of Sports Medicine, Department of Orthopaedics, University Hospital, London, Ontario, Canada

Carol Frey, MD, Director, Orthopaedic Foot and Ankle Center, Orthopaedic Hospital, Manhattan Beach, California

Freddie H. Fu, MD, David Silver Professor and Chairman, Department of Orthopaedic Surgery, Head Team Physician, Athletic Department, University of Pittsburgh, Pittsburgh, Pennsylvania

Donald S. Garbuz, MD, FRCSC, Orthopaedic Surgeon, Vancouver Hospital, Vancouver, British Columbia, Canada

Jean W.M. Gardeniers, MD, PhD, Department of Orthopaedics, Academic Hospital Nijmegen, Nijmegen, The Netherlands

William B. Geissler, MD, Associate Professor and Division Head of Upper Extremity Surgery, Chief, Section of Arthroscopic Surgery and Sports Medicine, Department of Orthopaedic Surgery, University of Mississippi Medical Center, Jackson, Mississippi

Thomas J. Gill, MD, Instructor in Orthopedic Surgery, Department of Orthopedic Surgery, Massachusetts General Hospital, Boston, Massachusetts

Jan Gillquist, MD, PhD, Professor of Sports Medicine, Department of Neuroscience and Locomotion, Faculty of Health Sciences, Linköping University, Linköping, Sweden

Victor M. Goldberg, MD, Charles H. Herndon Professor and Chairman, Department of Orthopaedics, University Hospitals of Cleveland, Case Western Reserve University, Cleveland, Ohio

Frank A. Gottschalk, MD, Associate Professor, Department of Orthopaedic Surgery, University of Texas Southwestern Medical Center, Dallas, Texas

Walter B. Greene, MD, Chairman and J. Vernon Luck Professor of Orthopaedic Surgery, Department of Orthopaedic Surgery, University of Missouri, Columbia, Missouri

Allan E. Gross, MD, FRCSC, Professor of Surgery, University of Toronto, Head, Division of Orthopaedic Surgery, Mount Sinai Hospital, Toronto, Ontario, Canada

Douglas P. Hanel, MD, Associate Professor, Department of Orthopaedics, University of Washington Medical Center/Harborview Medical Center, Seattle, Washington

Arlen D. Hanssen, MD, Associate Professor of Orthopedics, Mayo Medical School, Mayo Clinic, Rochester, Minnesota

Robert H. Haralson, III, MD, Assistant Clinical Professor, University of Tennessee, Center for the Health Sciences, Southeastern Orthopaedics, Maryville, Tennessee

Christopher D. Harner, MD, Associate Professor and Chief, Section of Sports Medicine, Department of Orthopaedic Surgery, University of Pittsburgh, Pittsburgh, Pennsylvania

Richard J. Hawkins, MD, FRCSC, Clinical Professor, Department of Orthopaedics, University of Colorado, Team Physician, Denver Broncos, Orthopaedic Consultant, Steadman Hawkins Clinic, Vail, Colorado

William C. Head, MD, Senior Associate, Texas Center for Joint Replacement, Presbyterian Hospital of Plano, Plano, Texas

Robert E. Hunter, MD, Clinical Associate Professor, Department of Orthopaedic Surgery, University of Colorado, Aspen Foundation for Sports Medicine, Education and Research, Aspen, Colorado

Carol R. Hutchinson, MD, FRCSC, MEd, Assistant Professor of Orthopaedic Surgery, University of Toronto, Mount Sinai Hospital, Toronto, Ontario, Canada

Frank W. Jobe, MD, Clinical Professor, Department of Orthopaedics, University of Southern California School of Medicine, Associate, Kerlan-Jobe Orthopaedic Clinic, Centinela Hospital Medical Center, Inglewood, California

Norman A. Johanson, MD, Associate Professor, Department of Orthopaedic Surgery, Temple University School of Medicine, Philadelphia, Pennsylvania

Jeffrey E. Johnson, MD, Associate Professor, Chief, Foot and Ankle Service, Department of Orthopaedic Surgery, Washington University School of Medicine, St. Louis, Missouri

Morton L. Kasdan, MD, FACS, Clinical Professor, Department of Plastic and Reconstructive Surgery, University of Louisville School of Medicine, Louisville, Kentucky

E. Michael Keating, MD, Orthopaedic Surgeon, The Center for Hip and Knee Surgery, Mooresville, Indiana

Robert M. Kerry, MB, BCh, FRCS (Orth), Fellow, Department of Orthopaedics, University of British Columbia, Vancouver, British Columbia, Canada

Scott E. Kilpatrick, MD, Assistant Professor of Pathology and Laboratory Medicine, Department of Pathology, University of North Carolina at Chapel Hill, Chapel Hill, North Carolina

Harold B. Kitaoka, MD, Department of Orthopaedics, Mayo Clinic, Rochester, Minnesota

Kenneth A. Krackow, MD, Professor Full Time Faculty, State University of New York at Buffalo, Department Head, Orthopaedic Surgery, The Buffalo General Hospital, Buffalo, New York

John Kronick, MD, Assistant Professor, Department of Orthopaedic Surgery, Wayne State University, Detroit, Michigan

Paul F. Lachiewicz, MD, Professor, Department of Orthopaedics, University of North Carolina at Chapel Hill, Chapel Hill, North Carolina

Floris P.J.G. Lafeber, PhD, Department of Rheumatology and Clinical Immunology, University Medical Centre of Utrecht, Utrecht, The Netherlands

G. Douglas Letson, MD, Clinical Professor, University of South Florida, Department of Orthopaedic Oncology, Moffitt Cancer Center, Tampa, Florida

Mark I. Loebenberg, MD, Fellow, Shoulder Service, Department of Orthopaedic Surgery, New York University-Hospital for Joint Diseases, New York, New York

Steven C. Ludwig, MD, Resident, Department of Orthopaedic Surgery, Rothman Institute, Thomas Jefferson University, Philadelphia, Pennsylvania

William J. Maloney, MD, Associate Professor, Chief, Orthopaedic Surgery, Barnes-Jewish Hospital, Department of Orthopaedic Surgery, Washington University Medical School, St. Louis, Missouri

Bassam A. Masri, MD, FRCSC, Clinical Associate Professor and Head, Division of Reconstructive Orthopaedics, University of British Columbia, Vancouver, British Columbia, Canada

Joel M. Matta, MD, Clinical Professor, Department of Orthopaedics, University of Southern California, Los Angeles, California

James P. McAuley, MD, Senior Technical Advisor, Anderson Orthopaedic Research Institute, Alexandria, Virginia

Richard E. McCarthy, MD, Clinical Associate Professor, University of Arkansas for Medical Sciences, Arkansas Spine Center, Little Rock, Arkansas

William C. McGarvey, MD, Clinical Instructor, Orthopaedic Surgery, University of Texas, Houston, Houston, Texas

Mark D. Miller, MD, Lt Col, USAF, MC, Clinical Associate Professor and Chief of Sports Medicine, Department of Orthopaedics, Wilford Hall USAF Medical Center, Lackland Air Force Base, Texas

Tom Minas, MD, FRCSC, MS, Department of Orthopaedic Surgery, Brigham and Women's Hospital, Boston, Massachusetts

Berton R. Moed, MD, Professor of Orthopaedic Surgery, Wayne State University, Chief, Department of Orthopaedic Surgery, Detroit Receiving Hospital, Detroit, Michigan

Elsayed Morsi Z. Mohamed, MD, MBBCH, MS (Orth), Consultant and Lecturer of Orthopaedic Surgery, Department of Orthopaedic Surgery, Faculty of Medicine, Menoufyia University, Menoufyia, Egypt

Michael A. Mont, MD, Associate Professor, Department of Orthopaedic Surgery, The Johns Hopkins Medical Institutions, Baltimore, Maryland

William K. Montgomery, MD, Junior Associate, Texas Center for Joint Replacement, Presbyterian Hospital of Plano, Plano, Texas

Bernard F. Morrey, MD, Emeritus Chairman, Professor of Orthopaedics, Mayo Clinic, Rochester, Minnesota

Michael J. Moskal, MD, Fellow, Upper Extremity Sports Medicine, Mississippi Sports Medicine and Orthopaedic Center, Jackson, Mississippi

Mark S. Myerson, MD, Director, Foot and Ankle Services, Union Memorial Hospital, Baltimore, Maryland

Paul Nourbash, MD, Clinical Instructor, Department of Orthopaedic Surgery, Rush Presbyterian St. Luke's and Central DuPage Hospital, Chicago, Illinois

Frank R. Noyes, MD, Professor and Chief of Sports Medicine, Department of Orthopaedics, Cincinnati Sports Medicine and Orthopaedic Center, Cincinnati, Ohio

Steven Olson, MD, Associate Professor and Chief, Orthopaedic Trauma Service, University of California, Davis, Sacramento, California

Robert F. Ostrum, MD, Associate Director of Orthopaedic Trauma, Clinical Associate Professor of Orthopaedic Surgery, Ohio State University, Grant Medical Center, Columbus, Ohio

Wayne G. Paprosky, MD, Associate Professor, Department of Orthopaedic Surgery, Rush Presbyterian St. Luke's Medical Center, Chicago, Illinois

Paul F. Partington, MB, BS, FRCS (Orth), Clinical Fellow, Department of Orthopaedic Surgery, London Health Sciences Centre, University Campus, London, Ontario, Canada

Walter J. Pedowitz, MD, Associate Clinical Professor, Department of Orthopaedic Surgery, College of Physicians and Surgeons, Columbia University, Columbia, New York

Clayton R. Perry, MD, Associate Clinical Professor, Department of Orthopaedic Surgery, St. Louis University School of Medicine, U.S. Center of Sports Medicine, St. Louis, Missouri

Robert K. Peterson, MD, Fellow in Sports Medicine, Mississippi Sports Medicine and Orthopaedic Center, Jackson, Mississippi

Matthew J. Phillips, MD, Assistant Clinical Professor of Orthopaedic Surgery, Department of Orthopaedic Surgery, State University of New York, Buffalo, Buffalo, New York

Michael S. Pinzur, MD, Professor of Orthopaedic Surgery, Loyola University Stritch School of Medicine, Department of Orthopaedic Surgery and Rehabilitation, Loyola University Medical Center, Maywood, Illinois

Ann Marie Plate, MD, Fellow, Hand Service, Department of Orthopaedic Surgery, New York University-Hospital for Joint Diseases, New York, New York

James A. Rand, MD, Consultant in Orthopaedics, Chair, Department of Orthopaedics, Mayo Clinic, Scottsdale, Arizona

Glenn R. Rechtine, MD, Professor, Department of Orthopaedics, University of Texas Southwestern Medical Center, Dallas, Texas

B. Stephens Richards, MD, Associate Professor, Department of Orthopaedic Surgery, University of Texas Southwestern, Texas Scottish Rite Hospital for Children, Dallas, Texas

E. Greer Richardson, MD, Professor of Orthopaedic Surgery, University of Tennessee, Campbell Clinic, Memphis, Tennessee

Charles A. Rockwood, Jr, MD, Professor and Chairman Emeritus, Department of Orthopaedics, University of Texas Medical School and Health Science Center, San Antonio, Texas

Cecil H. Rorabeck, MD, FRCSC, Professor and Chair, Department of Orthopaedic Surgery, London Health Sciences Centre, University Campus, London, Ontario, Canada

Harry E. Rubash, MD, Chief, Orthopaedic Surgery, Massachusetts General Hospital, Harvard Medical School, Boston, Massachusetts

Charles L. Saltzman, MD, Associate Professor, Departments of Orthopaedic Surgery and Biomedical Engineering, University of Iowa, Iowa City, Iowa

Felix H. Savoie III, MD, Co-Director, Upper Extremity Service, Mississippi Sports Medicine and Orthopaedic Center, Jackson, Mississippi

Robert C. Schenck, Jr, MD, Associate Professor and Deputy Chairman, Department of Orthopaedics, University of Texas Health Science Center, San Antonio, San Antonio, Texas

B. Willem Schreurs, MD, PhD, Department of Orthopaedics, Academic Hospital Nijmegen, Nijmegen, The Netherlands

Todd D. Sekundiak, Assistant Professor, University of Manitoba, St. Boniface Hospital, Winnipeg, Canada

Barry P. Simmons, MD, Department of Orthopaedic Surgery, Brigham and Women's Hospital, Boston, Massachusetts

Raj K. Sinha, MD, PhD, Assistant Professor, Department of Orthopaedic Surgery, University of Medicine and Dentistry of New Jersey, Newark, New Jersey

Thomas J.J.H. Slooff, MD, PhD, Professor of Orthopaedics, University Hospital St. Badboud, Nijmegen, The Netherlands

Douglas G. Smith, MD, Associate Professor, Department of Orthopaedics, University of Washington and Harborview Medical Center, Seattle, Washington

Dempsey Springfield, MD, Professor and Chair, Leni and Peter W. May Department of Orthopaedics, Mount Sinai Medical Center, New York, New York

Michael J. Stuart, MD, Associate Professor, Department of Orthopaedic Surgery, Mayo Clinic, Rochester, Minnesota

Steven A. Stuchin, MD, Associate Professor of Clinical Orthopaedics, New York University-Hospital for Joint Diseases, Orthopaedic Institute, New York, New York

Marc F. Swiontkowski, MD, Professor and Chair, Department of Orthopaedic Surgery, University of Minnesota Medical School, Minneapolis, Minnesota

David C. Templeman, MD, Assistant Professor, Department of Orthopaedic Surgery, University of Minnesota Medical School, Minneapolis, Minnesota

Thomas E. Trumble, MD, Professor, Hand and Microvascular Surgery, University of Washington, Seattle, Washington

Alexander R. Vaccaro, MD, Associate Professor, Department of Orthopaedic Surgery, Thomas Jefferson University, Philadelphia, Pennsylvania

C. Niek van Dijk, MD
Amsterdam, The Netherlands

Peter M. van Roermund, PhD, Orthopaedics, University Medical Centre of Utrecht, Utrecht, The Netherlands

Michael I. Vender, MD, Hand Surgery Associates, SC, Arlington Heights, Illinois

William G. Ward, Sr, MD, Associate Professor, Department of Orthopaedic Surgery, Wake Forest University Baptist Medical Center, Winston-Salem, North Carolina

Russell F. Warren, MD, Surgeon in Chief, Hospital for Special Surgery, Professor of Surgery, Orthopaedics, Cornell Medical College, New York, New York

Leo A. Whiteside, MD, Director, Biomechanical Research Laboratory, Director, Missouri Bone and Joint Center, Barnes-Jewish West County Hospital, St. Louis, Missouri

Edward M. Wojtys, MD, Professor of Surgery, University of Michigan Medical School, Medsport, Ann Arbor, Michigan

Natalie Wong, MD, Department of Orthopaedic Surgery, University of Toronto, Toronto, Ontario, Canada

Isadore G. Yablon, MD, Professor and Chairman Emeritus, Boston University, School of Medicine, Boston, Massachusetts

Robert J. Zehr, MD, Head, Section of Orthopaedic Oncology, Department of Orthopaedic Surgery, The Cleveland Clinic Foundation, Cleveland, Ohio

Joseph D. Zuckerman, MD, Professor and Chairman, Department of Orthopaedic Surgery, New York University-Hospital for Joint Diseases, New York, New York

Preface

The Instructional Course Lectures first became a part of the Annual Meeting of the American Academy of Orthopaedic Surgeons in 1942. The goal was to provide those members who were attending the meeting with practical and up-to-date information provided by recognized authorities. The Instructional Course Lectures were quickly recognized as an invaluable educational resource by those attending the meeting. This led, in part, to the decision to publish selected Instructional Course Lectures on an annual basis. The first volume devoted to the Instructional Course Lectures, published in 1943, was entitled "Lectures on Peace and War—Orthopaedic Surgery" and was edited by James E.M. Thomson, MD. The current volume, published in 1999, is Volume 48 of what has become one of the most popular textbook series in orthopaedic surgery.

The Instructional Course Lectures remain one of the most popular educational offerings at the Annual Meeting. Up until 1993, Instructional Course Lectures were offered between 8:00 a.m. and 10:00 a.m. each morning of the Annual Meeting. With this schedule, each year over 15,000 registrants attended the Instructional Course Lectures. Since 1994, the Instructional Course Lectures have been offered during the entire day of each day of the meeting. Since that time, more than 160 instructional courses have been offered at each meeting, with an average annual attendance of over 28,000.

The Instructional Course Lectures are the responsibility of the Instructional Course Lectures Committee. I was honored to be able to serve as Chairman of this committee during the 1998 meeting in New Orleans. I applaud the efforts of the members of the committee—S. Terry Canale, Dill Cannon, Henry Cowell, Richard Gelberman, Doug Pritchard, and Franklin Sim—for their hard work and dedication to this effort. Although the committee membership changes each year, the true constant in the Instructional Course Lectures program has been the American Academy of Orthopaedic Surgeons staff. Kathie Niesen has been responsible for coordinating the Instructional Course Lectures since 1986. Assisted by Lynn Mondack, they have provided the foundation upon which this program has been built.

Volume 48 represents Instructional Course Lectures selected from those printed at the 1998 Annual Meeting. In choosing the topics for inclusion, I reviewed Volumes 45, 46, and 47 so that information from those volumes would not be repeated. I am very pleased to say that all Instructional Course Lectures faculty who were invited to participate in this volume agreed to do so. They are responsible for the 80 chapters in this volume.

Volume 48 does represent an important change from previous volumes. For the first time, a CD-ROM component has been developed, which includes 11 demonstrations of surgical procedures that are described in the text. It is our hope that this will be the first step in expanding the Instructional Course Lectures Volume into a multimedia educational experience.

Volume 48 represents the efforts of many people. Those that deserve special recognition are Marilyn Fox, PhD, Director of the Department of Publications for the American Academy of Orthopaedic Surgeons, Bruce Davis, Senior Editor, and, particularly, Sophie Tosta, Assistant Production Manager. Ms Tosta has dedicated her efforts to address every detail of the editorial process from the time the manuscript was submitted until it was approved for final printing. In addition, the CD-ROM component in this volume would not have been possible without the efforts of Howard Mevis, Director of the Department of Electronic Media, Evaluation, and Course Operations, and Reid Stanton, Manager of Electronic Media.

It is my hope that this volume provides the readers with important useful information that will assist in the care of their patients. This has always been, and will remain, the goal of the Instructional Course Lectures.

Joseph D. Zuckerman, MD
New York, New York

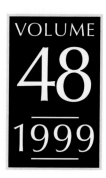

Dedication

This volume
is dedicated to

Clement B. Sledge, MD
and
Victor Frankel, MD, PhD

In recognition of all they have
contributed to their students,
residents, fellows, faculty,
and to the specialty of
Orthopaedic
Surgery.

Contents

Section 7 Shoulder and Elbow

Section 8 Spine

Section 9 Fractures and Dislocations

SECTION

1

Hip: Adult Reconstruction

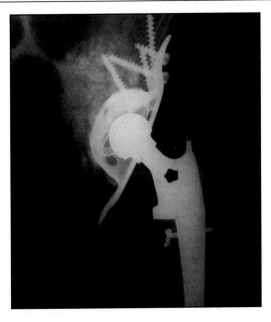

Surgical Approaches for Revision Total Hip Replacement Surgery: The Anterior Trochanteric Slide and the Extended Conventional Osteotomy

C. Anderson Engh, Jr, MD
James P. McAuley, MD
Charles Engh, Sr, MD

Introduction

Revision total hip arthroplasty is complex and demanding, requiring surgeons to have a clear preoperative plan. That plan should include the revision diagnosis, the surgical approach, and the choice of instruments, bone grafts, and implants to carry out the plan. Unfortunately, the nature of revision total hip arthroplasty is such that unexpected findings and complications can arise. Surgeons must be prepared to handle any situation that occurs intraoperatively. Often the unexpected problems encountered require a more extensive procedure with greater exposure than was originally planned.

The nature of revision hip surgery has affected our choice of approaches. All revisions are performed with a posterior approach because the exposure can easily be extended proximally or distally. Proximally, the approach can be converted to a triradiate exposure of the entire ilium and anterior column. However, the most common extensile measure is the performance of a trochanteric osteotomy. In most cases, the osteotomy is part of the planned surgical exposure, but occasionally it is needed to address unexpected intraoperative findings.

Of the 4 types of osteotomy we use for revision surgery, the most common is the extended trochanteric slide.[1] We also use the simple trochanteric slide popularized by the senior author.[2] The third osteotomy is the conventional trochanteric osteotomy, and the fourth osteotomy is a modification of the conventional osteotomy, called an extended conventional osteotomy because a portion of the lateral femoral shaft is included with the greater trochanter (Fig. 1).

Two factors dictate the type of osteotomy chosen: what needs to be exposed and the bone quality of the patient's greater trochanter. When the greater trochanter is compromised with osteolysis or osteopenia and a conventional osteotomy is performed, the trochanteric fragment may be inadequate for wire fixation. In this situation, extending the osteotomy distally to include several inches of the lateral femoral shaft ensures that there will be an adequate amount of lateral bone for secure fixation. Proximal medial bone loss is also an indication for extending the length of a trochanteric osteotomy. The trochanteric fragment must be fixed to strong medial bone. If medial bone is not present, the wires or cables will contact the medial prosthesis and cable fretting or wire breakage will occur. In this situation the osteotomy is extended into the diaphysis so that medial bone is available for wire or cable fixation of the osteotomy.

Where bone stock is not a concern but increased exposure is needed, the choice of osteotomy is based on the required exposure. The anterior trochanteric slide exposes the metaphysis of the femur to the level of the lesser trochanter. It also improves the exposure of the hip capsule and anterior acetabular rim. A conventional trochanteric osteotomy yields the same femoral exposure but greatly improves exposure of the acetabulum, anterior wall, and ilium.

Femoral exposure is increased when the osteotomy is extended to the femoral diaphysis. This femoral exposure is especially helpful with cement removal. The additional bone with an extended osteotomy also allows a stronger repair with the potential for a lower nonunion rate.

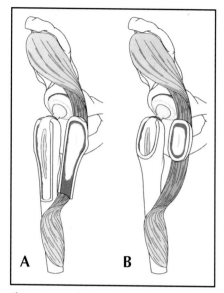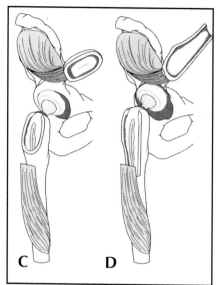

Fig. 1 Four trochanteric osteotomies used for revision total hip arthroplasty: **A,** Extended slide; **B,** Anterior slide; **C,** Conventional; **D,** Extended conventional.

The extended trochanteric slide gives acetabular exposure comparable to that of the simple anterior trochanteric slide with improved femoral exposure. Maximum exposure of the femur and acetabulum is obtained with the extended conventional osteotomy. The removal of the vastus from the trochanteric fragment allows the trochanter and the abductors to be flipped cephalad, exposing the ilium.

This article focuses on our preferred basic surgical approach, and on 2 of the 4 types of femoral osteotomies we use. Our description is limited to the anterior trochanteric slide and the extended type of conventional osteotomy, because the extended anterior slide is described separately by another author, and the conventional Charnley type trochanteric osteotomy is already well known. The indications, technique, and method of repair for the trochanteric slide and extended femoral osteotomies are presented. Finally, a postoperative rehabilitation program based on such factors as the stability of the new components, the

adequacy of osteotomy repair, and hip joint stability is discussed.

Revision Surgical Approach

Our standard approach is posterolateral. The patient is placed on the operating room table in the lateral decubitus position with the pelvis stabilized by 3 or 4 padded clamps. If the previous approach was posterolateral or direct lateral, this incision is reopened. If a new incision is necessary, it is placed halfway between the anterior and posterior borders of the greater trochanter to allow more anterior exposure, rather than over the posterior border of the greater trochanter as in primary procedures. The upper half of the incision is parallel to the underlying fibers of the gluteus maximus, and the lower half extends longitudinally toward the knee. The iliotibial band is identified and incised from distal to the midpoint of the greater trochanter, and the fibers of the gluteus maximus are separated to expose the greater trochanter. The insertion of the gluteus maximus into the femur is routinely released and the

sciatic nerve exposed. If the gluteus maximus tendon is not released, the sciatic nerve is predisposed to constriction when the femur is retracted anteriorly for acetabular exposure.

If the femoral component is retained, anterior displacement of the femur to expose the acetabulum is more difficult but is facilitated by complete division of the anterior capsule. A bone hook is positioned around the femur just distal to the lesser trochanter and the femur is lifted upward to expose the anterior capsule. An instrument is directed into the iliopsoas tendon sheath. The position of the instrument defines the plane between the iliopsoas tendon and the anterior capsule, and the capsule is divided from inside out, starting distally at the lesser trochanter. This technique is illustrated in Figure 2.

Once the anterior capsule has been divided, a retractor can be placed over the anterior rim of the acetabulum, thereby displacing the femur anteriorly and exposing the acetabulum. This approach is adequate for most uncomplicated revisions, such as the removal of a worn polyethylene liner from a modular porous-coated cup or the revision of a loose acetabular cup with minimal bone stock damage. Trochanteric osteotomies are used for more complex cases.

Anterior Trochanteric Slide

Indications Femoral indications for the anterior trochanteric slide include the removal of a well-fixed, proximally porous-coated prosthesis and the removal of a failed endoprosthesis with bone growth through its fenestrations. The anterior trochanteric slide exposes the anterior and posterior bone implant interfaces of proximally porous-coated or fenestrated endoprostheses. The displacement of the greater trochanter makes it possi-

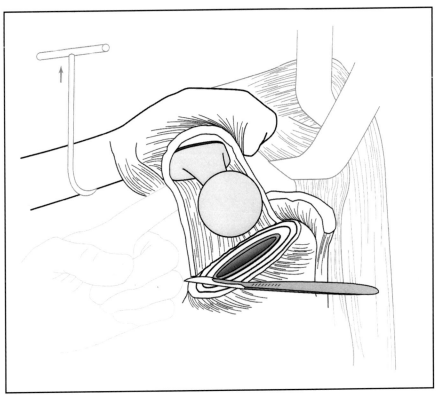

Fig. 2 An instrument or finger is placed in the iliopsoas sheath while the femur is lifted out of the wound. The capsule can be divided with a knife or electrocautery.

ble to direct a thin osteotome along the anterior and posterior femoral component just beneath the collar, thereby allowing bone-ingrown areas to be disrupted (Fig. 3).

Acetabular indications for the anterior trochanteric slide include acetabular protrusio cases that can not be easily dislocated as well as some acetabular revision cases with femoral component retention. When dislocation of the hip is difficult, displacement of the trochanter exposes the gluteus minimus and the hip capsule beneath it. It is then possible to remove acetabular rim osteophytes to facilitate dislocation (Fig. 4). Because the trochanteric fragment is small, it can be displaced anteriorly without disrupting the femoral bone-cement or bone-prosthesis interface, thereby facilitating revision of the acetabular compo-

nent without removing a stable femoral component.

The small size of the fragment does, however, limit the indications. Two situations demonstrate how the trochanteric slide can be problematic. If the revision of the acetabular component results in leg lengthening, the small fragment may not reach healthy femoral bone for reattachment. The second situation involves the absence of medial bone for securing wires or cables. In such situations, the trochanteric osteotomy must be extended distally so that a secure trochanter reattachment is possible.

Technique The anterior trochanteric slide requires more exposure of the greater trochanter than does a routine posterolateral approach. For this osteotomy, the incision is extended approximately 2 inches distally. After the iliotibial band has been

split, the posterior border of the vastus lateralis muscle is identified and elevated from the lateral femoral shaft up to the flare of the greater trochanter. A Bennet retractor is then placed around the femur beneath the vastus muscle to expose the trochanteric flare. Complete exposure of the gluteus medius is required to mobilize the osteotomy anteriorly. The femur is externally rotated and the anterior border of the gluteus medius identified. Next, the plane between the gluteus medius and the gluteus minimus muscle is developed and a blunt instrument placed in the interval. The distal margin of the osteotomy is just below the insertion of the vastus lateralis, where the femoral shaft begins to flare laterally, forming the greater trochanter. The superior margin is lateral to the piriformis fossa between the insertions of the gluteus medius and the gluteus minimus. With the femur internally rotated, the osteotomy is performed with a reciprocating saw, leaving the attachments of the medius proximally and the lateralis distally (Fig. 5). Once the osteotomy is complete, any anterior capsule attached to the anterior trochanteric fragment is divided, allowing the osteotomy fragment to be separated from the femur, elevated, and displaced anteriorly. It can be held in the new position by the anterior blade of a self-retaining retractor.

The trochanteric fragment is reattached with 18-gauge monofilament wires or cables placed below the lesser trochanter or through a drill hole in the lesser trochanter. Four holes drilled in the greater trochanter for the wires control the position of the osteotomy fragment. Tightening the wires or cables compresses the trochanteric fragment against the femur as shown in Figure 6. When a failed femoral component has been replaced by a larger implant, the later-

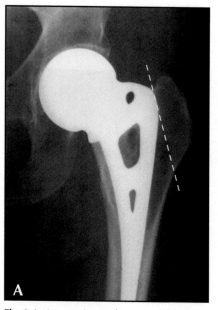
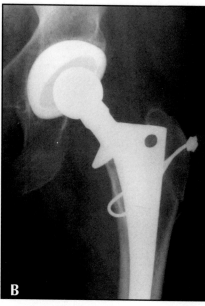

Fig. 3 A, An anterior trochanteric slide allows access to bone that has bridged the fenestrations of this implant. **B,** The osteotomy is repaired with a single wire or cable.

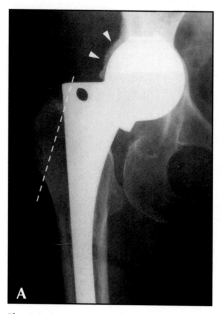
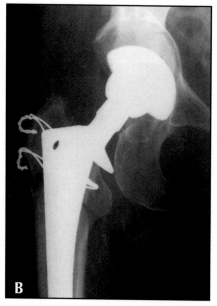

Fig. 4 A, An anterior trochanteric slide allows access to the superior osteophytes that prevented hip dislocation. Arrows mark rim osteophytes. **B,** With the osteotomy, the hip was dislocated and a complete revision performed.

secured, it is essential to check the range of motion of the hip with the trochanteric fragment repositioned to ensure that the trochanter does not abut the pelvis and cause instability. If such impingement occurs, a portion of the greater trochanter is removed or the drill holes repositioned to adjust the position of the reattached greater trochanter. **(CD–1.1)**

Extended Conventional Trochanteric Osteotomy

Indications Extensive acetabular bone stock damage is a major challenge in revision hip surgery. Since the extent of this damage often cannot be appreciated preoperatively, successful revision requires the surgeon to be adaptable both in surgical approaches and in methods of reconstruction. Converting a posterolateral approach to the extended conventional osteotomy is an excellent method for improving acetabular exposure, because it allows extensive exposure of the entire acetabular rim, the ischium below, and the ilium above. A common indication for this type of osteotomy is a Paprosky type 3B acetabular defect.[3] Our preference for the reconstruction of this type of acetabular deficiency is a metal antiprotrusio cage fixed with large cancellous screws to the ilium and ischium. This type of acetabular defect and this method of reconstruction are illustrated in Figure 7. Difficult acetabular revisions in which excessive leg lengthening can occur are also indications for this osteotomy.

A potential contraindication to this osteotomy is the case in which the surgeon plans to retain a well-fixed femoral component. Although the longer trochanteric osteotomy facilitates trochanteric reattachment, it can also disrupt fixation of a proximally porous-coated or cemented femoral component. This possibility must be

al shoulder of the new device may prevent adequate trochanteric reattachment. If this occurs, bone or cement should be removed from within the osteotomy fragment so that bone surfaces can be reopposed. The

trochanteric fragment may also be advanced distally to improve hip stability. In such cases, the position of the drill holes in the greater trochanter is altered so that the trochanter is drawn distally. Before the wires or cables are

taken into account when an extended conventional osteotomy is considered for an isolated acetabular revision.

Technique Converting the basic posterolateral approach to this type of osteotomy requires distal lengthening of the skin incision. The distal margin of the osteotomy begins on the lateral femoral shaft approximately 5 cm distal to the trochanter. This part of the femur is exposed by dividing the vastus origin on the greater trochanter and stripping the vastus from the lateral femur. The proximal margin of the osteotomy exits the greater trochanter between the gluteus medius and the superior hip capsule. With the hip in an internally rotated position, the posterior border of the medius is identified. The hip is then externally rotated and the anterior border of the medius identified. A blunt instrument, placed beneath the gluteus medius from anterior to posterior, defines the interval between the medius and the hip capsule (Fig. 8). The diaphyseal portion of the osteotomy includes the lateral half of the periosteal surface but only the lateral third of the endosteal surface of the femur. To perform the osteotomy, the surgeon angles the anterior and posterior longitudinal cuts toward each other with a reciprocating saw. The distal transverse cut is completed with a saw or a high-speed burr. With the osteotomy completed, the trochanteric fragment and attached gluteus medius are elevated as needed off the remaining hip capsule and the ilium. The trochanteric fragment with the medius can then be rotated and retracted cephalad. Care must be taken not to injure the inferior gluteal nerve.

The osteotomy is repaired with 2 wires or cables. The upper wire is placed through a drill hole on the

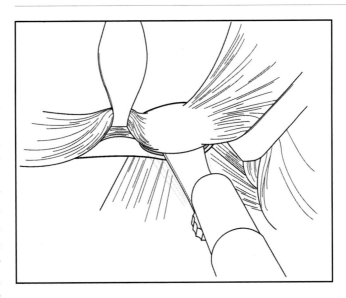

Fig. 5 With the vastus lateralis exposed distally and the gluteus medius exposed proximally, the osteotomy includes their insertions and the lateral aspect of the greater trochanter.

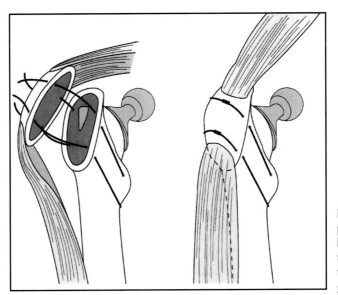

Fig. 6 Wires are placed through or below the lesser trochanter and through holes in the greater trochanter.

lesser trochanter and through 2 holes in the greater trochanter. The distal wire is placed beneath the lesser trochanter and around the distal portion of the osteotomy fragment (Fig. 9). With the revision components in place, it may be necessary to contour the osteotomy fragment with a saw or high-speed burr. If apposition of the osteotomy site is still not obtained, 1 or 2 cortical strut grafts can be added across the osteotomy site beneath the wires or cables. **(CD–1.2)**

Postoperative Rehabilitation

Postoperative rehabilitation varies depending on hip stability, the fixation of the new components, and the strength of the trochanteric reattachment. Limitations on range of motion are determined intraoperatively. The hip range of motion is recorded and positions of hip-joint instability noted. The fixation strength of the components is more difficult to quantify, and can be estimated by evaluating the force required for insertion and by the postoperative radiographic appearance

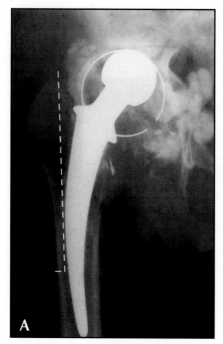
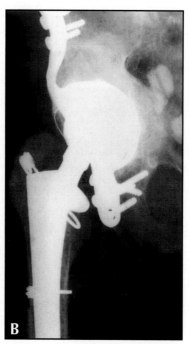

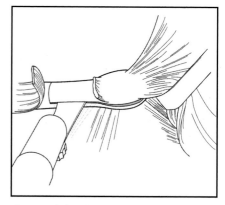

Fig. 8 With the gluteus medius exposed and the vastus lateralis stripped distally, the trochanteric osteotomy is extended to the femoral diaphysis.

Fig. 7 A, An extended conventional osteotomy provided the maximum exposure of the acetabulum and femur in this complex revision. **B,** Extending the osteotomy distally and flipping it cephalad increased exposure of the ilium, allowing placement of an antiprotrusio cage.

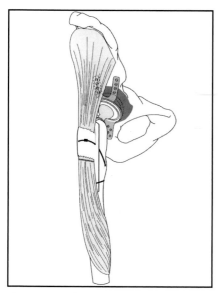

Fig. 9 Repair of the osteotomy involves wire fixation of the trochanteric region and the diaphyseal extension combined with suture of the vastus lateralis.

of the implants. The fixation strength of the reattached trochanter is evaluated visually by stressing the trochanter with slight adduction, and by putting the hip through a range of motion. If no motion is visible at the osteotomy site, the reattached trochanter is considered stable.

Under optimum circumstances, patients are allowed to bear full weight on the operated-on hip at 3 months. Passive range of motion, with the exception of adduction, is allowed within the recorded limits of hip stability. Hip flexion and hip adduction strengthening exercises are not allowed for 6 weeks. A brace is used if the strength of the osteotomy repair is tenuous, or if hip stability or patient compliance are concerns. Morbidly obese patients are not braced. Trochanteric osteotomy patients are reevaluated at 6 weeks postoperatively. If radiographs suggest trochanteric migration or fracture, we consider prompt reoperation, because delayed reattachment of a nonunited trochanter is usually unsuccessful.

In conclusion, the standard posterior lateral approach will allow adequate exposure for most uncomplicated revisions. It is essential for surgeons to be able to increase surgical exposure as the revision dictates. The osteotomy indications, techniques, and rehabilitation described will increase the surgeon's ability to deal optimally with complex revision procedures or intraoperative complications.

References

1. Younger TI, Bradford MS, Magnus RE, Paprosky WG: Extended proximal femoral osteotomy: A new technique for femoral revision arthroplasty. *J Arthroplasty* 1995;10:329–338.

2. Glassman AH, Engh CA, Bobyn JD: A technique of extensile exposure for total hip arthroplasty. *J Arthroplasty* 1987;2:11–21.

3. Paprosky WG, Perona PG, Lawrence JM: Acetabular defect classification and surgical reconstruction in revision arthroplasty: A 6-year follow-up evaluation. *J Arthroplasty* 1994;9:33–44.

Reference to Video

Engh CA Jr, Engh CA: *Surgical Approaches for Revision Total Hip Replacement.* Alexandria, VA, Anderson Orthopaedic Research Institute, 1997.

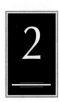

The Vascularized Scaphoid Window for Access to the Femoral Canal in Revision Total Hip Arthroplasty

Robert M. Kerry, MD, FRCS (Orth)

Bassam A. Masri, MD, FRCSC

Donald S. Garbuz, MD, FRCSC

Clive P. Duncan, MD, FRCSC

Introduction

Removal of the distally fixed broken or intact femoral prosthesis and cement from the femoral canal can be a daunting task, and a number of techniques have been suggested to facilitate this difficult and often risky procedure. Removal of all distal cement from the femoral canal, particularly with a long-stem component or a long cement tail, involves a substantial risk of canal perforation and may be impossible if the cement extends below the apex of the anterior femoral bow. A cortical perforation presents a risk of later femoral fracture, particularly if it is unrecognized at the time of surgery.[1] The most widely used techniques in such a situation are the creation of controlled perforations or windows or the use of a very extended trochanteric osteotomy. In many cases, it is possible and prudent to disregard the distal cement mantle. However, when dealing with infection, the cement must be removed and done so with minimal devascularization of bone.

Options

Femoral Windows

Several techniques have been described to create controlled femoral windows. As early as 1970, Müller[2] described a 1-cm by 20-cm anterior gutter for the removal of the femoral cement mantle after elevation of the vastus lateralis from the lateral intermuscular septum. Nelson and Weber[3] described a laterally situated rectangular window approximately 2-cm wide and 6-cm long created through a muscle-splitting incision in the vastus lateralis.

Moreland and associates[4] described a 10-mm by 4-mm anterior window to allow access for a tungsten carbide punch for removal of broken femoral stems. Tyer and associates[5] described a rectangular window involving a musculo-osseous flap based on the vastus lateralis extending below the distal extent of the original prosthesis with a view to fixation of the new implant beyond the end of the window. Shepherd and Turnbull[6] advocated a 1-cm by 2-cm window on the anterior surface of the femur between 3.2-mm drill holes and replacement without fixation. They reported early healing and good results.

Sydney and Mallory[7] also advocated serial 9-mm perforations to guide instruments and to afford access for a tungsten carbide punch for removal of broken stems or other instruments and for the removal of cement. They described a 1-cm by 20-cm anterior

reported 9 postoperative fractures out of 219 cases using this technique. Klein and Rubash[8] reported the results of a 2-cm by 5-cm window in 21 cases. The window was created between drill holes in the manner described by Shepherd, with complete detachment of the "windowpane" from all soft tissue, followed by fixation with cerclage wires. The mean healing time reported for the window was 17 weeks, and no postoperative fractures were encountered. Although the use of such windows has been well documented, there is no consensus as to the optimal technique.

Extended Femoral Osteotomy

An alternative technique is to extend a trochanteric osteotomy distally along the femoral shaft, thereby giving good exposure of the hip joint and femoral canal. Variations of the so-called trochanteric slide have been described by Mercati and associates[9] and English[10] and popularized by Glassman and associates.[11] This approach provides the advantage of the digastric and opposing pull of the vastus lateralis and the hip abductors but affords limited access to the length of the femoral canal. Peters and associates[12] reported an extended

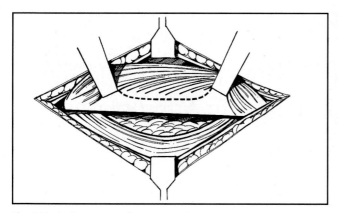

Fig. 1 Limited exposure of osteotomy site.

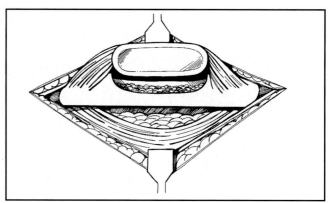

Fig. 2 Elevation of myo-osseous flap.

version of this osteotomy, giving superior access to the canal. Younger and associates[13] reported the results in 20 cases of an extended osteotomy of the greater trochanter that included about one third of the cortical diameter of the femur. This osteotomy is hinged anteriorly about an intact musculoperiosteal sleeve, and the blood supply of the osteotomy fragment is maintained by virtue of an intact muscle attachment to the osteotomy fragment. Healing was predictable and was observed by 3 months at most. Migration of the osteotomy fragment by more than 2 mm was not observed. The reported advantages of this osteotomy include the ease of component and cement extraction, as well as the superior visualization of the distal femoral canal, which allows more accurate preparation of the distal femur and eliminates varus placement of the revision implant.

Such osteotomies have the added advantage of allowing anterolateral, posterior, or combined approaches to the hip joint itself, providing a utilitarian approach in many circumstances. Nevertheless, although the potential for access to the femoral canal that an extended form of this approach affords may be desirable, violation of the greater trochanter

may be contraindicated or undesired, for example, in patients with severe proximal osteolysis.

Although we do not claim originality, we describe a technique that we believe incorporates the advantages of many of the techniques described above without mandatory detachment of the greater trochanter. It affords excellent access to the femoral canal, maintains good soft-tissue attachment and viability of the "windowpane," allows rapid healing, and minimizes the risk of fracture caused by stress risers. It is of singular value when access to the distal canal is required for the removal of foreign material in the management of infection.

Surgical Technique

Preoperative planning allows identification of the optimal site for the proposed osteotomy, taking into consideration the length of the prosthesis and any associated cement tail. Planning also must take account of the need for an adequate bypass of the window with the revision prosthesis.

A lateral incision curving 30° posteriorly proximal to the greater trochanter allows a choice of approaches to the hip joint: usually either the approach described by Harding,[14] the modification of this

popularized by Head and associates,[15] a trochanteric slide,[11] or the posterior approach to the hip. If the prosthesis cannot be removed with ease, assistance can be provided from below, through the proposed osteotomy.

The incision is extended distally along the lateral aspect of the femoral shaft in an extensile fashion far enough to extend beyond the distal extent of the proposed osteotomy. The femoral shaft proximal and distal to the proposed osteotomy is exposed extraperiosteally, and narrow retractors are placed around the femur at these sites (Fig. 1). The vastus lateralis is elevated from the lateral intermuscular septum and femoral cortex for a width of only 1 cm, in order to expose the lateral aspect of the femur. This limited exposure maintains the muscular attachments and blood supply of the proposed osteotomized fragment, thereby optimizing its healing potential.

Using an oscillating saw with a thin and narrow blade, a scaphoid osteotomy is then created through both cortices of the femur from laterally to medially, leaving smooth, rounded margins proximally and distally so as to minimize stress risers. This osteotomy allows the elevation of the anterior cortex of the femur as a myo-osseous flap (Fig. 2). Great care should be taken to avoid stripping muscle from the elevated fragment. If there is concern regarding fracture of the femoral shaft during instrumentation, precautionary cerclage wires can be passed above and below the osteotomy site. Occasionally, the prosthesis is firmly fixed and the bone stock between the lateral margin of the prosthesis and femoral cortex is too thin for an adequately thick and strong windowpane. In this situation, the anterolateral portion of the osteotomy can be created with a saw and the medial portion by serial localized transmuscular osteotomies without significant further muscular stripping. The window can then be elevated, while maintaining its muscular attachments and blood supply, to give excellent exposure of the femoral canal (Fig. 3) for instrumentation both through the window and from above.

Following completion of the instrumentation, the cortical window is replaced and secured with one or more cerclage wires. A reimplanted component should bypass the window by at least two cortical diameters, and weightbearing should be protected for 12 weeks. If for any reason use of a long-stem implant is undesirable, the window may be bypassed with an anterolaterally placed cortical onlay allograft strut, but this can be done only in the absence of infection.

Conclusion

This technique combines the advantages of many previously described techniques, while avoiding many of the disadvantages. It affords a choice of approach to the hip joint, as dictated by other surgical considerations, and provides excellent exposure of the femoral canal over whatever length is required for safe implant and cement removal. It permits almost all reconstructive possibilities and is designed to minimize the risk of complications, most notably nonunion of the window and fracture through it.

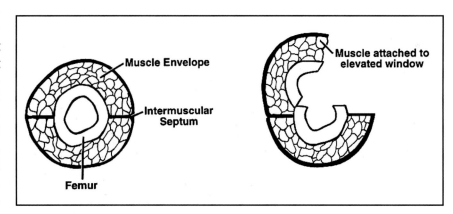

Fig. 3 Preservation of muscle attachment and blood supply.

References

1. Brooks DB, Burstein AH, Frankel VU: The biomechanics of torsional fractures: The stress concentration effect of a drill hole. *J Bone Joint Surg* 1970;52A:507–514.

2. Müller ME: Total hip prostheses. *Clin Orthop* 1970;72:46–68.

3. Nelson CL, Weber MJ: Technique of windowing the femoral shaft for removal of bone cement. *Clin Orthop* 1981;154:336–337.

4. Moreland JR, Marder R, Anspach WE Jr: The window technique for the removal of broken femoral stems in total hip replacement. *Clin Orthop* 1986;212:245–249.

5. Tyer HD, Huckstep RL, Stalley PD: Intraluminal allograft restoration of the upper femur in failed total hip arthroplasty. *Clin Orthop* 1987;224:26–32.

6. Shepherd BD, Turnbull A: The fate of femoral windows in revision joint arthroplasty. *J Bone Joint Surg* 1989;71A:716–718.

7. Sydney SV, Mallory TH: Controlled perforation: A safe method of cement removal from the femoral canal. *Clin Orthop* 1990;253:168–172.

8. Klein AH, Rubash BE: Femoral windows in revision total hip arthroplasty. *Clin Orthop* 1993;291:164–170.

9. Mercati E, Guary A, Myquel C, Bourgeon A: A postero-external approach to the hip joint: Value of the formation of a digastric muscle. *J Chir (Paris)* 1972;103:499–504.

10. English TA: The trochanteric approach to the hip for prosthetic replacement. *J Bone Joint Surg* 1975;57A:1128–1133.

11. Glassman AH, Engh CA, Bobyn JD: A technique of extensile exposure for total hip arthroplasty. *J Arthroplasty* 1987;2:11–21.

12. Peters PC Jr, Head WC, Emerson RH Jr: An extended trochanteric osteotomy for revision total hip replacement. *J Bone Joint Surg* 1993;75B:158–159.

13. Younger TI, Bradford MS, Magnus RE, Paprosky WG: Extended proximal femoral osteotomy: A new technique for femoral revision arthroplasty. *J Arthroplasty* 1995;10:329–338.

14. Hardinge K: The direct lateral approach to the hip. *J Bone Joint Surg* 1982;64B:17–19.

15. Head WC, Mallory TH, Berklacich FM, Dennis DA, Emerson RH Jr, Wapner KL: Extensile exposure of the hip for revision arthroplasty. *J Arthroplasty* 1987;2:265–273.

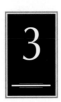

Vastus Slide and Controlled Perforations

William C. Head, MD
William K. Montgomery, MD
Roger H. Emerson, Jr, MD

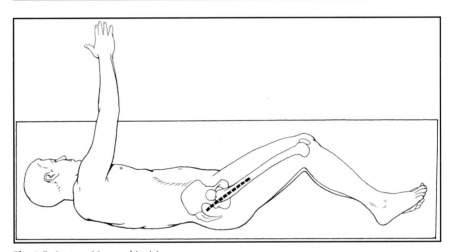

Fig. 1 Patient position and incision.

An increasing number of revision total hip arthroplasties continue to be performed. It has long been recognized that this surgery is more challenging and has a higher potential for complications. Acrylic cement removal from the femur remains one of the most challenging and difficult aspects of the operation. Various surgical approaches and techniques have been described, ranging from external guides to intraoperative fluoroscopy.[1–3] We favor a wide extensile exposure for hip revision.[4] A vastus slide affords ready access to the femur. Controlled perforations offer a safe, expedient method for cement removal.[5]

The patient is placed in the lateral decubitus position, using well-padded bracing posts (Fig. 1). The ipsilateral arm is supported on a Mayo stand, while the contralateral arm is supported on a padded arm board. Special attention is taken to ensure the patient is rigidly held in a straight lateral position. Leg length and femoral offset are assessed prior to surgery. During the surgery, the superior poles of the patellae are used as guides to leg length. The down leg patella can easily be palpated through the drapes and compared to the up or operated-on extremity.

An incision for revision surgery must afford extensile access to both the femur and the acetabulum. The incision must be one that can be extended proximally and distally, and provide anterior to posterior access to the hip joint. The incision should allow for sciatic nerve exploration when indicated, and follow anatomic planes to avoid potential for neurovascular injury. The vastus slide technique provides a viable muscle cuff to place over the revision hip construct.

The utilitarian revision incision begins 10 to 15 cm superior and slightly posterior to the greater trochanter, and is carried distally over the greater trochanter and along the lateral aspect of the femur. The incision should be carried distally several centimeters below the area of the femur requiring cement removal or reconstruction. Although every attempt is made to follow previous incisions, previous incisions are not allowed to compromise our revision technique.

The incision traverses skin, subcutaneous tissue, gluteus maximus fascia, and the iliotibial band. The fibers of the gluteus maximus are bluntly separated to expose the underlying abductor musculature. At this point, the abductor musculature, the greater

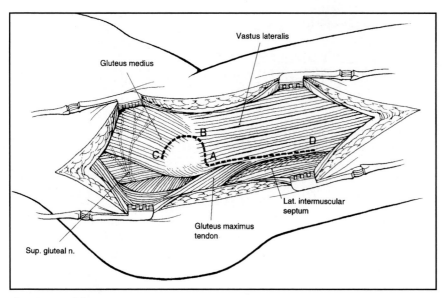

Fig. 2 Vastus slide exposure.

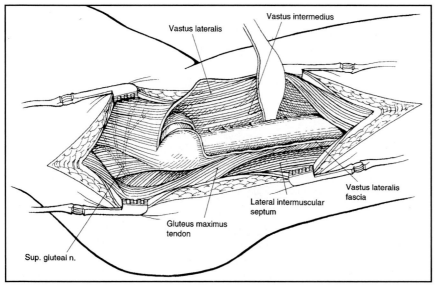

Fig. 3 Reflected vastus slide.

eralis and vastus intermedius can be reflected off the femur to the level of the knee, if necessary. Distal exposure is determined by the length of the femoral reconstruction or cement removal. The exposure and the reflection of the vastus lateralis and vastus intermedius musculature is facilitated by placing tension on the muscle cuff. A Cushing retractor or Cobra is placed anteriorly under the vastus lateralis and over the surface of the femur. Frequently, several retractors will be required as the exposure proceeds distally. A small fascia cuff of vastus lateralis is maintained just anterior to the intermuscular septum, which allows for a ready repair at the time of closure (Figs. 3 and 4). After the distal vastus slide is established, the attention is turned to the proximal limb of the lazy "Z" shaped incision, which corresponds to the reflection of the anterior portion of the gluteus medius and gluteus minimus musculature from the greater trochanter (lines B to C in Figure 2). The incision extends around the anterior margin of the greater trochanter and ends proximal at the superior mid portion of the greater trochanter. A cuff of tendinous tissue is preserved for closure (Fig. 3). Care is taken not to violate the substance of the abductor musculature. The abductor muscles are innervated by the superior gluteal nerve, which transverses from the sciatic notch and continues anteriorly. The location of the nerve is between the gluteus medius and gluteus minimus muscle, 4 to 5 cm above the greater trochanter.[6] This surgical exposure avoids risk to the nerve.

As the leg is rotated externally, the anterior portion of the abductor musculature along with the vastus intermedius and lateralis musculature are reflected anteriorly, exposing the hip capsule. A complete anterior cap-

trochanter, the vastus lateralis, the gluteus maximus tendon, and the lateral intermuscular septum occupy the surgical field. The lateral intermuscular septum remains intact at all times as a barrier for sciatic nerve protection.

The slide technique to the gluteus medius and vastus lateralis is done through a lazy "Z" shaped incision (Fig. 2). The vertical limb, A to B, and the distal limb, A to D, are first devel-

oped in a subperiosteal fashion. The vastus lateralis tubercule is palpated superior and just anterior to the broad tendinous insertion of the gluteus maximus. Periosteal dissection is begun and carried distally, reflecting the vastus lateralis and vastus intermedius off the femur. As the vastus lateralis is swept anteriorly off the intermuscular septum, the perforating vessels are ligated. The vastus lat-

sulectomy is performed, followed by dislocation of the hip. The femoral head is removed and a medial release is performed to the level of the lesser trochanter to allow mobilization of the femur. An external rotation contracture can be addressed by posterior capsular release and, if necessary, release of the short external rotators. During acetabular reconstruction, the femur is left in a side-lying position.

For cement removal, the femur is mobilized and externally rotated out of the incision. The knee is flexed and the leg is dropped off the table into a sterile bag (Fig. 5). The proximal lateral cement must be removed prior to removal of the femoral component. Should cement not be removed, the risk of trochanteric fracture increases, especially when removing a prosthesis with a lateral shoulder. After the prosthesis is removed, the primary method for removing the cement is a Midas-Rex pneumatic cutting tool. Using the high speed burr, along with various osteotomes, chisels, and, at times, ultrasonic equipment, removal of the cement proceeds distally until visualization of the femoral canal becomes impaired, either by narrowing of the femoral diameter or femoral boring. At this point, which is usually 5 to 7 cm from the proximal femoral margin, a round 7-mm perforation is placed in the anterior border of the femur and carried through the cortex and adherent cement, and into the medullary canal (Fig. 5). This is done with a Midas-Rex burr. Routinely, two portals are required for a primary implant. Additional portals are placed depending on the length of the cement mantle. Portals are placed at least 5 cm apart, and the distal portal is placed at least 2.5 cm proximal to the tip of the revision prosthesis. Controlled perforation portals allow the Midas-Rex burr to be viewed as it passes down the

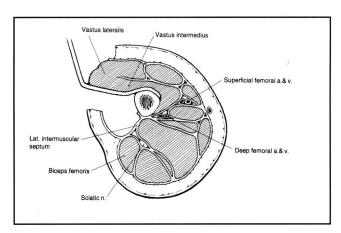

Fig. 4 Cross-section of reflected vastus lateralis and intermedius.

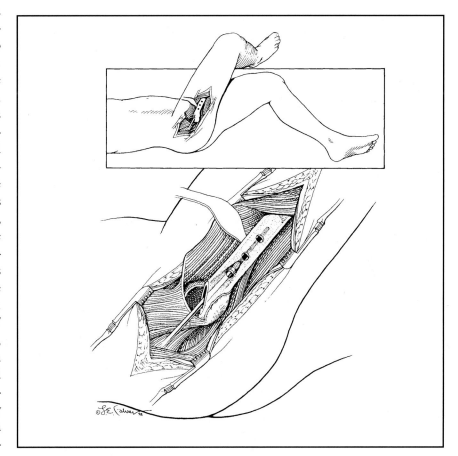

Fig. 5 Femoral controlled perforations.

femur, and these perforations assist in centralizing the burr. The Midas-Rex burr can be centralized not only in the medial to lateral planes, but also in the anterior to posterior planes. These portals allow the use of irrigation to remove cement debris generated by the high speed burr. The controlled portals allow for direct visualization of the femoral canal to assist in ensuring the complete removal of cement from the femur.

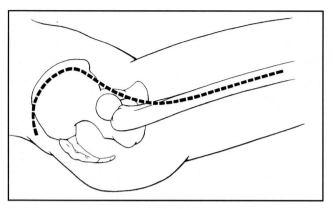

Fig. 6 Skin incision, Smith-Peterson vastus slide technique.

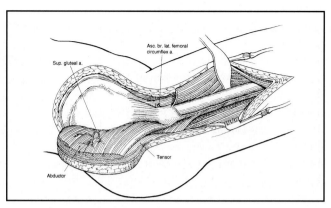

Fig. 7 Deep incision, Smith-Peterson vastus slide.

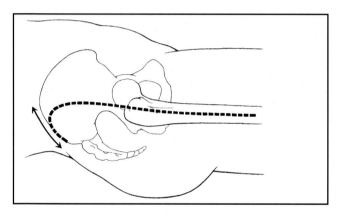

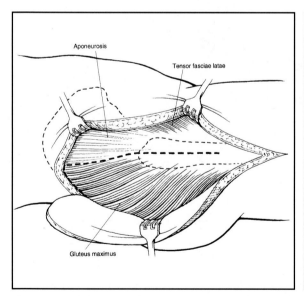

Fig. 9 Proximal dissection of the extensile Henry approach.

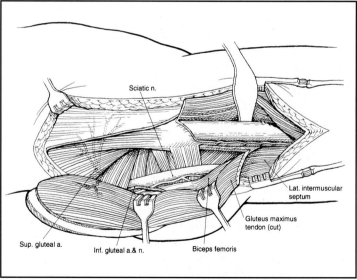

Fig. 8 Skin incision, Henry approach and vastus slide.

Fig. 10 Deep exposure, extensile Henry approach and vastus slide.

This technique allows the surgeon complete access to the femur, and preserves the muscle cuff as an intact unit for closing over this revision construct. Through this exposure, routine acetabular revision can be accomplished. If an extensive acetabular reconstruction is required, this technique can be combined with the proximal limb of

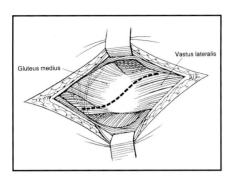

Fig. 11 Hardinge incision.

the Smith-Peterson[7] approach (Figs. 6 and 7) or the acetabular approach described by Henry[8] (Fig. 8).

The upper portion of the Smith-Peterson approach allows the tensor fascia, the femoral musculature, and the abductor muscles to be swept posteriorly off the ilium. This affords wide acetabular exposure. The nerve and blood supply are preserved. This is a technique used for bulk acetabular grafts, and, at times, protrusio rings or cages.

Whenever wide posterior exposure is required, the upper limb of the Henry exposure is combined with the vastus slide (Figs. 9 and 10). This is useful for sciatic nerve exposure or application of a posterior column plate. This technique, along with a trochanteric osteotomy, affords total access to the hip.

The vastus slide differs from the Hardinge approach in that the substance of the abductor musculature is not invaded[9] (Fig. 11). This approach does not compromise the blood supply of the femur, in that the medial and posterior muscle attachments are maintained. All reconstructive hip procedures can be accomplished using these surgical techniques.

References

1. Müller ME: Total hip prostheses. *Clin Orthop* 1970;72:46–68.

2. Razzano CD: Removal of methylmethacrylate in failed total hip arthroplasties: An improved technique. *Clin Orthop* 1977;126:181–182.

3. Turner RH, Emerson RH Jr: Femoral revision total hip arthroplasty, in Turner RH, Scheller AD Jr (eds): *Revision Total Hip Arthroplasty*. Orlando, FL, Grune & Stratton, 1982, pp 75–106.

4. Head WC, Mallory TH, Berklacich FM, Dennis DA, Emerson RH Jr, Wapner KL: Extensile exposure of the hip for revision arthroplasty. *J Arthroplasty* 1987;2:265–273.

5. Dennis DA, Dingman CA, Meglan DA, O'Leary JF, Mallory TH, Berme N: Femoral cement removal in revision total hip arthroplasty: A biomechanical analysis. *Clin Orthop* 1987;220:142–147.

6. Foster DE, Hunter JR: The direct lateral approach to the hip for arthroplasty: Advantages and complications. *Orthopedics* 1987;10:274–280.

7. Smith-Petersen MN: Approach to and exposure of the hip joint for mold arthroplasty. *J Bone Joint Surg* 1949;31A:40–46.

8. Henry AK: *Exposure of the Long Bones and Surgical Methods*, ed 2. Edinburgh, Scotland, Churchill-Livingstone, 1966.

9. Hardinge K: The direct lateral approach to the hip. *J Bone Joint Surg* 1982;64B:17–19.

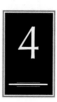

Extended Proximal Femoral Osteotomy

Ram Aribindi, MD, FRCSC
Wayne Paprosky, MD, FACS
Paul Nourbash, MD
John Kronick, MD
. Mark Barba, MD

Most primary hip arthroplasties and many revisions can be performed without the use of any trochanteric osteotomy. However, the use of an extended proximal femoral osteotomy has made femoral revision arthroplasty a less daunting task, and quite often a routine procedure.

Working proximally to remove distal cement or disrupt ingrowth surfaces of porous coated stems can damage the existing bone stock and cause perforations of the cortex, leading to fractures.[1] Although cortical windows can be used, they weaken the remaining bone stock[2] and require the use of longer stems to bypass the distal lesions created. The extended proximal femoral osteotomy provides relatively easy access to the interface surface, which may be bone or fibrous ingrowth with cementless stems or cement in cemented stems.[3,4] It greatly facilitates exposure, implant removal, correction of deformity, and implantation of revision components.[3] Other advantages of the osteotomy include predictable healing of the osteotomized fragment, proper tensioning of the abductors with distal advancement, decreased inadvertent cortical perforations, neutral reaming of the femoral canal, decreased surgical time, and enhanced exposure of the acetabulum.[3,5] The osteotomy readily permits the addition of cortical strut grafts to augment fixation of the greater trochanter and supplement host bone.

Results of femoral revisions with extensively porous coated implants have been superior to those obtained with cemented implants.[6–14] Since 1992, we have routinely performed femoral revisions with the use of extended proximal femoral osteotomies and implantation of extensively porous coated femoral components.

Indications

The extended proximal femoral osteotomy is indicated for the removal of well-fixed cemented and cementless implants, as well as removal of cement in patients with a loose femoral component in a well-fixed cement mantle. It is an absolute indication in patients with femoral component loosening and subsequent varus remodeling of the proximal femur, found in 30% of patients at time of revision.[15] The osteotomy diminishes the risk of an inadvertent fracture of the often compromised greater trochanter, especially upon removal of a failed femoral compo-

nent from its subsided or migrated position. The osteotomy enhances the exposure of the acetabulum, a difficult undertaking in the revision setting because of multiple surgeries, severe migration of the acetabular component, or heterotopic ossification.

The extended proximal femoral osteotomy can also be used in the primary setting when a proximal femoral deformity interferes with straight reaming of the femoral canal, such as in patients with various dysplasias, previous corrective osteotomies, or malunions.

Preoperative Planning

An anteroposterior (AP) view of the pelvis, and AP lateral views of the hip/femur are needed for preoperative planning. Clinical examination and the AP view of the pelvis are used to evaluate leg lengths. The AP view can also be used to judge anatomic offset by comparing with the opposite side.

Templates are used to estimate the length and diameter of the stem that will obtain a scratch fit over 4 to 6 cm of cortical bone. The lateral view is used to determine if a straight or curved stem is appropriate. The template must be neutrally aligned within the femoral canal. If the template cannot be aligned neutrally secondary

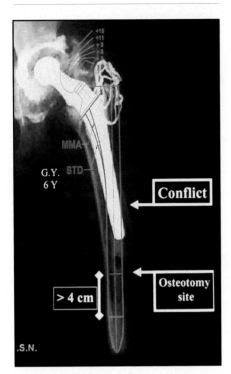

Fig. 1 Varus remodeling of the proximal femur in a patient with aseptic loosening of the femoral component results in a "conflict," easily seen with a superimposed template. The site of the conflict and the proposed osteotomy site are marked.

to contact with proximal bone, a "conflict" is present (Fig. 1). This is often the result of varus deformity of the proximal femur secondary to remodeling, present in 30% of cases at time of revision.[15] The apex of the deformity is usually at the tip of the old stem. Less frequently, the proximal femur is remodeled into valgus. In some instances the conflict may arise from a previously osteotomized trochanter, trochanteric overgrowth, malunion, or a previous corrective osteotomy. Conflicts can be managed with an extended proximal femoral osteotomy. The osteotomy may need to be completed medially in the rare case of a valgus proximal femur, or in case of a malunion or previous osteotomy.

When an osteotomy is indicated, the level of the transverse limb is marked on the radiographs. The level of the osteotomy is a compromise between access to the canal and preservation of fixation surface (Fig. 1). The osteotomy must resolve any "conflict" to allow neutral reaming of the canal. The transverse limb of the osteotomy is marked on the film and the distance from a fixed landmark, such as the vastus ridge, is measured. This will serve as an intraoperative reference.

Technique
Exposure
A standard posterior approach has been widely used in both the primary and the revision settings. The incision is centered over the tip of the greater trochanter and is extended distally as necessary to complete the distant extent of the osteotomy. The tensor fascia lata and the fascia of the gluteus maximus are incised in line with the skin incision. The pseudocapsule and the short external rotators are raised as a single flap. The insertion of the gluteus maximum tendon is routinely released to relieve undue tension on the soft tissues posteriorly and to mobilize the proximal femur. When possible, the hip is then dislocated. However, dislocation may be difficult in cases with severe protrusio or heterotopic ossification. In such circumstances, an extended proximal femoral osteotomy is performed prior to dislocation.

After thoroughly clearing the introitus of the femur of granuloma, scar, and bone, a loose prosthesis can be removed. However, on extraction of the implant, impingement of the shoulder of the prosthesis against the trochanter can lead to an inadvertent fracture. To avoid this complication, the region surrounding the shoulder of the prosthesis must be thoroughly cleared of any cement or bone that may cause impingement. If a stem cannot be extracted safely then an episiotomy or an extended proximal femoral osteotomy is performed prior to removal of the prosthesis. An episiotomy consists of only the longitudinal limb of the extended proximal femoral osteotomy.

Osteotomy
The osteotomy can be performed at 1 of 3 times during the procedure: prior to dislocation of the hip, after dislocation but prior to removal of the femoral component, or after dislocation and removal of the femoral component. The osteotomy is performed prior to dislocation if there is difficulty with dislocation because of stiffness, subsidence of the femoral component, bony overgrowth, or heterotopic ossification. On occasion, the osteotomy is required to aid in the removal of the femoral component. However, the osteotomy is much easier to perform with the hip dislocated and the femoral component removed.

The osteotomy is performed with the hip in extension and internal rotation such that the posterior aspect of the femur is facing the ceiling. The vastus lateralis is elevated from the posterolateral femur along the linea aspera to the distal extent of the osteotomy (Fig. 2, A). The proposed osteotomy site is marked by an electrocautery, along the exposed posterior surface of the femur, just anterolateral to the linea aspera. Distally, the transverse limb of the osteotomy is marked using measurements made from preoperative templating or by using the removed prosthesis as a guide. An oscillating saw is then used to make the longitudinal arm of the osteotomy, which is one third of the femoral circumference, along the posterolateral aspect of the proximal femur, as the osteotomized fragment (Fig. 2, B and C). This longitudinal

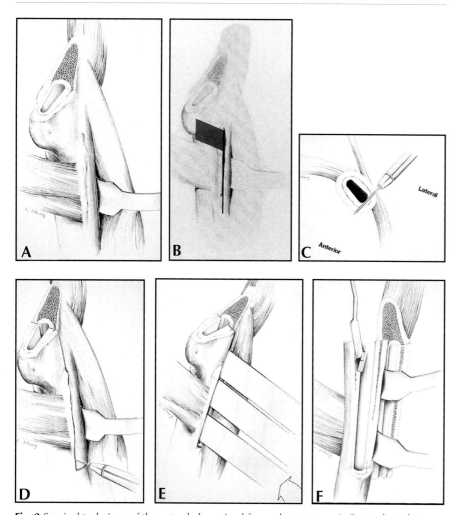

Fig. 2 Surgical technique of the extended proximal femoral osteotomy. **A,** Posterolateral view of the femur, with a Bennet retractor holding the vastus lateralis anteriorly. **B,** After marking the osteotomy site, an oscillating saw is used to make the longitudinal limb of the osteotomy. The saw is oriented perpendicular to the anteversion of the hip. **C,** Cross section of the proximal femur. The saw is directed from posterolateral to anterolateral to perforate the anterior cortex. The osteotomized fragment should encompass the posterolateral third of the proximal femur. **D,** Proximally, at the level of the vastus tubercle, the osteotomy is angled medially to incorporate all of the greater trochanter. Distally, transverse limb of the osteotomy is made with a pencil burr to avoid stress risers. **E,** Wide Lambotte osteotomes are passed from posterior to anterior to gently lever open the osteotomy site, after the tight pseudocapsule from the anterior aspect of the greater trochanter is released. **F,** The osteotomy fragment is retracted anteriorly. The cement from the proximal femur is removed with offset osteotomes and high speed burrs. The osteotomy allows direct access to the distal cement plug. (Figures 2A and 2C through 2F are reproduced with permission from Younger TI, Bradford MS, Magnus RE, Paprosky WG: Extended proximal femoral osteotomy: A new technique for femoral revision arthroplasty. *J Arthroplasty* 1995;10:329–338.)

The blade of an oscillating saw can notch the femur and create a stress riser. A pencil burr can be used to create smooth, rounded edges that diminish the risk of fracture at time of implantation. Multiple wide Lambotte osteotomes are passed across the osteotomy site from posterior to anterior to gently lever open the osteotomy anteriorly (Fig. 2, *E*). The gluteus medius, minimus, and vastus lateralis remain attached to the osteotomized portion of the bone. To avoid an inadvertent fracture of the greater trochanter it is important to release the tight pseudocapsule from the anterior aspect of the greater trochanter prior to levering open the osteotomy site. Release of this scar tissue anteriorly greatly facilitates the exposure of the acetabulum.

If an extended proximal femoral osteotomy is performed after removal of the femoral component, the proximal cement from the intact two thirds of the femur and the trochanter can be cleared under direct vision with the use of offset osteotomes and high-speed burrs (Fig. 2, *F*). The osteotomy allows direct access to the distal cement and plug. A high-speed barrel burr is used to remove cement for 1 cm past the distal extent of the osteotomy. The remaining cement within the canal is removed by drilling the cement column with progressively larger drills and by the use of cement taps. The surgeon must ensure that the drill is centrally aligned within the canal.

If an osteotomy is required prior to removal of the implant, such as with well-fixed, fully coated, cementless stems (Fig. 3, *A*), and highly textured or precoated cemented stems, the posterolateral cortex is sectioned as described above, but the anterior aspect of the osteotomy is completed by carefully levering on the os-

limb of the osteotomy is oriented perpendicular to the anteversion of the hip. Proximally, at the level of the vastus tubercle, the osteotomy is angled medially to incorporate all of

the greater trochanter with the osteotomized fragment. Distally, the transverse limb of the osteotomy is made with a high-speed pencil burr rather than an oscillating saw (Fig. 2, *D*).

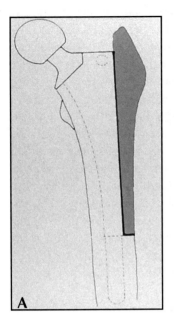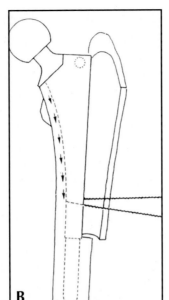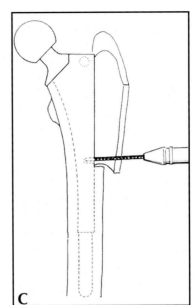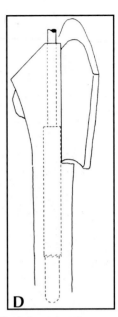

Fig. 3 Extended proximal femoral osteotomy for cementless implants. **A,** The posterolateral cortex is sectioned as described above, but the anterior aspect of the osteotomy is completed by carefully levering on the wide osteotomes and creating a greenstick fracture anteriorly. **B,** Lateral surface of the stem is exposed and there is direct access to the anterior and posterior surfaces of the stem. A Gigli saw is passed around the medial aspect of the stem and directed distally. **C,** Metal cutting burr is used to section the implant where its profile becomes cylindrical. **D,** Trephines are passed over the distal stem to remove it.

teotomes and creating a greenstick fracture anteriorly. Proximally, a pencil burr is used to start the osteotomy on the anterior femur. Caution must be exercised so as not to create an unwanted fracture plane. It is important to release the tight anterior pseudocapsule prior to the creation of a greenstick fracture. Upon completion of the osteotomy, the lateral surface of the stem is exposed and there is direct access to the anterior and posterior surfaces of the stem. For removal of a well-fixed, fully coated stem, a Gigli saw is passed around the medial aspect of the stem and is directed distally to the level where the stem profile is cylindrical (Fig. 3, *B*). A metal cutting burr is used to section the implant at this level (Fig. 3, *C*). The distal end of the stem is then removed by passing appropriately sized trephines over the distal stem (Fig. 3, *D*). To remove a well-fixed cemented stem, the technique is

nearly identical. Often, access to the cement column laterally allows explantation. If this is not adequate, the stem may be sectioned and the distal aspect trephined.

Canal Preparation

A bony pedestal is often encountered in revisions of cementless femoral components. A retained pedestal makes neutral reaming of the canal impossible. To avoid eccentric reaming and diminish the chance of perforation, the pedestal should be removed. Long drills are used to perforate the pedestal, and then reverse hooks are used to remove it from the canal. If the pedestal is solid, a barrel-shaped, high-speed burr is used to diminish its size. Appreciation of the pedestal is essential in preoperative planning and can dictate a more distal osteotomy level at the expense of a longer revision stem.

Reaming can begin once the

cement and plug or neocortex and pedestal have been removed. A clear canal will keep the reaming central and neutrally aligned. Solid reamers are used with straight stems, and flexible reamers are used with curved stems. The length of reaming is dictated by the length of the revision stem necessary to obtain stability and restore proper biomechanics of the hip. Only the length necessary for fixation is reamed. In general, this is usually 4 to 6 cm distal to the transverse limb of the osteotomy. Reaming should be performed in neutral alignment to avoid perforations and diminish the risk of fracture. Neutral positioning of the reamer within the canal may be assured if a Charnley T-handled awl inserts freely into the diaphysis without proximal obstruction. Sequential reaming is then performed in 0.5-mm increments until good endosteal cortical contact is obtained. Usually, the femoral canal is underreamed by 0.5 mm. But, how much reaming is enough? Templating provides an estimate of the size of the canal. It is usually accurate to plus or minus 1 size. The adequacy of reaming can often be gauged by the feedback obtained while reaming. If the reamer labors through the strong bone then it is easy to know when to stop; however, in patients with diminished bone quality, it can be difficult to tell how much reaming is enough. In these cases, a T-handle reamer of the same size as the prosthesis is inserted into the prepared canal. If rotational stability is achieved with 4 to 5 cm of the reamer remaining proud, then a prosthesis of this diameter is chosen. If rotational stability is not achieved, then the bone should be reamed for the next larger size. If more than 5 cm of the reamer is proud then the introitus is reamed line to line to prevent fracture on insertion of the prosthesis. After reaming, a broach is used as a trial to determine version and length. Preparation of the medial endosteal femur with a barrel burr may be necessary prior to seating the broach. If the proximal femur is in valgus then the medial limb of the osteotomy may require completion at the level of the introitus to avoid an uncontrolled fracture. If the proximal femur is too tight to allow seating of the broach, then modified medial aspect (MMA) broaches can be used with the Solution (Depuy, Warsaw, IN) system. These implants have reduced proximal profiles to accommodate narrow metaphyses.

Trial Reduction

Trial reduction is one of the key steps in revision total hip surgery. Trials permit alteration of the positions of components to obtain optimum stability. A broach sized to fit snugly in the canal is chosen to provide reason-able stability for trials. The broach stem should typically be sized 0.5 mm less than the last reamer to allow for adjustments. With a trial in place, the hip is put through a range of motion, and the stability is assessed. If the hip is unstable, then neck length, version, prosthesis height, head size, position of the osteotomized trochanter, and soft-tissue and bony impingement need evaluation.

Management of Instability
Version

In the assessment of instability, component version should be evaluated initially. The revision setting often dictates more acetabular and femoral anteversion than the primary setting. Though the individual requirements may vary, the combined femoral and acetabular version can approach 55°. The version of the components is evaluated with the Aufranc test. The hip is flexed until it is perpendicular to the opening of the acetabular component. The angle between the long axis of the body and the thigh is the acetabular anteversion. The leg is then rotated internally until the flat surface of the stem is parallel to the face of the socket. The degree of internal rotation of the leg is equal to the anteversion of the stem. These 2 angles are added to give the combined version.

Impingement

During range of motion, the sources of impingement should be assessed. Impingement may result from contact of the trunnion with the periphery of the cup. This condition may be managed by modifying component position or by using a larger diameter femoral head. On occasion, the anterior femur at the level of the calcar can act as a fulcrum against the anterior soft tissues, the remaining pseudocapsule, and the pelvis. If excision of the anterior pseudocapsule is insufficient to relieve the impingement, then the anterior trochanteric bone must be thinned. Less commonly, the hip may dislocate anteriorly with impingement in extension and external rotation. This can often be resolved by adjusting the position of the osteotomized fragment or by thinning the posterior, impinging bone on the femur. With the hip in extension and external rotation, a finger-breadth of space should be present between the posterior aspect of the femur and the posterior pelvis.

Limb Length

Limb-length inequalities must be discussed with the patient prior to surgery. In revision surgery, often with poor quality bone and soft tissue, stability rather than length is of prime importance. Limb lengthening is a common and annoying necessity in these procedures.

With trial reductions the tension of the abductors is assessed. Tension can be increased by placing the stem proud, increasing neck length, or by advancing the osteotomy fragment. The addition of neck length has the advantage of gaining femoral offset, but also has the disadvantage of adding a skirted head that can impinge and cause dislocation. The length is likely to be adequate if the hip is stable in the 90° position and in the "sleeping position": 45° of flexion, 20° of adduction, and 15° of internal rotation. The osteotomized fragment must be provisionally fixed to accurately assess stability.

Head Size

Usually 28-mm heads are used, but 32-mm heads can be used for added stability. The larger head size increases the arc of motion prior to the neck impinging on the lip of the cup. Thus,

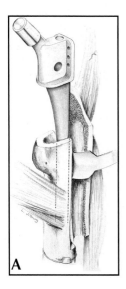 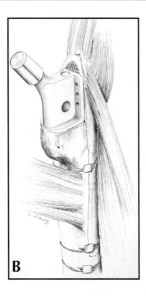

Fig. 4 Implantation. **A,** Prophylactic cerclage wire is placed slighty distal to the distal extent of the osteotomy to prevent any propagation of fractures. **B,** Upon insertion of the prosthesis, cerclage wires are used to reapproximate the osteotomy site. Strut grafts may be added to augment fixation of the osteotomized fragment and supplement host bone.

there is often a need for larger, skirted heads. The larger head size can be useful in the elderly, in whom polyethylene thickness is not as important.

Implantation

Prophylactic wiring of the shaft just distal to the osteotomy site is performed prior to implanting the stem (Fig. 4, *A*). With trials, the position of the components is established. The diameter of the femoral component should be measured with a hole gauge before implantation. Because of manufacturing tolerances or sharpening of reamers, a significant mismatch may exist between the actual diameter of the canal that is reamed and the diameter of any given implant. Ideally, the femoral canal should be underreamed by 0.5 mm to obtain a good scratch fit. If the mismatch is large, then the canal is reamed line to line for some distance or, if necessary, an alternate component is selected.

Once the revision prosthesis is inserted, the osteotomy fragment is shaped with a burr to fit over the lateral shoulder of the prosthesis. Multiple cables are used to secure the osteotomy fragment (Fig. 4, *B*). Abductor laxity can be addressed by shortening of the osteotomy fragment and distal advancement. Strut grafts may be used to augment fixation of the trochanteric fragment and supplement host bone. Before crimping the cables, the hip is placed through range of motion to allow fine tuning of the osteotomy fragment position.

Postoperative Management

All revision patients are prescribed an off-the-shelf abduction orthosis that is set at 30° of abduction with a flexion stop of 70°. The brace is worn daily for 8 weeks. Patients are allowed 30% weightbearing on the affected extremity for the first 8 weeks unless major structural allografting of the acetabulum has been performed. Only touchdown weightbearing is permitted for 3 months in such cases. The postoperative regimen for revisions performed with extended proximal femoral osteotomy has remained unchanged from revisions performed without an osteotomy.

Materials and Methods

From 1992 to 1996, 142 consecutive hip revisions were performed with the use of an extended proximal femoral osteotomy and insertion of an extensively porous-coated, canal-filling, cobalt-chrome stem (Solution, Depuy, Warsaw, IN). Twenty patients had insufficient follow-up and thus are excluded from the present review. Of the remaining 122 revisions, 83 were in women and 39 in men. The average age at time of surgery was 63.8 (26 to 84) years. The indications for revision were aseptic loosening (114), component failure (4), recurrent dislocation (2), femoral fracture (1), and second stage reimplantation for infection (1).

Results

The extended proximal femoral osteotomy gave easy access to the distal bone-cement or bone-prosthesis interface in all cases. The procedure allowed neutral reaming of the femoral canal and implantation of the revision component in proper alignment (Fig. 5, *A* and *B*). Varus remodeling of the proximal femur secondary to loosening was handled relatively easily with the use of the osteotomy (Fig. 6). The average time from the beginning of the osteotomy procedure to the complete removal of the prosthesis and cement was 35 minutes. The average surgical time for cases without a major acetabular allograft was 3 hours, 40 minutes. The mean blood loss was approximately 1,400 cc.

With a minimum follow-up of 1 year, average 2.6 years, there were no nonunions of the osteotomized fragment and no cases of proximal migration of the greater trochanteric fragment greater than 2 mm. Radiographic union of the osteotomy site was noted in all cases by 3 months. Fixation of the stem with bone ingrowth was noted in 112 of 122 hips (92%), stable fibrous fixation was seen in 9 hips (7%), and 1 stem (1%) was unstable and was subsequently revised.

Postoperatively, dislocations were noted in 13 of 122 patients (10.6%). Six of these 12 patients had Paprosky type IIIB acetabular defects with deficient or absent abductor mass. Three hips required revision for recurrent dislocation. Two patients (1.6%) developed superficial infections that were cleared with administration of oral antibiotics, and 1 required resection arthroplasty for deep infection.

Six patients (5%) required reoperations. Of these, 3 underwent revision for recurrent dislocations, 1 for drainage of a hematoma, 1 required resection arthroplasty for infection, and 1 was revised for aseptic loosening. Two patients developed peroneal nerve palsies, which resolved on follow-up.

Intraoperatively, there were 25 iatrogenic fractures (20%): 7 occurred during cement removal, 6 upon insertion of an extensively porous coated implant; 4 were osteotomized fragments fractured during cabling; 3 were perforations that occurred during attempts to pass instruments through the pedestal or to remove the cement plug; 3 were noted at the junction of the osteotomy and the diaphysis prior to implantation of the prosthesis; and 2 calcar fractures were noted on trial reduction. Strut grafts were used to augment fixation in 2 fractures. The remaining fractures were treated with the addition of cables to prevent propagation of the nondisplaced fractures. None of the fractures required a change in the length or diameter of the revision implant. All of the fractures healed uneventfully.

Discussion

Extended proximal femoral osteotomy is an efficient, safe, reliable technique in revision hip arthroplasty. Its advantages include easier access to the

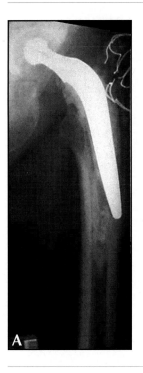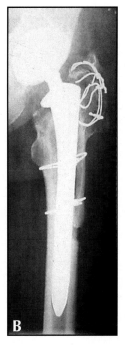

Fig. 5 A, Loosening of a cemented stem with near complete perforation of the lateral cortex distally. **B,** Neutral alignment of a canal filling extensively porous coated stem. The osteotomy is clearly visible.

fixation surface of the failed prosthesis without compromising the remaining bone stock, alteration of proximal bone deformities to allow neutral reaming of the femoral canal, predictable healing of the osteotomized fragment, proper tensioning of the abductors with distal advancement, decreased inadvertent cortical perforations, decreased surgical time, and enhanced exposure of the acetabulum. Complications such as eccentric reaming, femoral perforations, and fractures are lower in femoral revisions with extensively porous coated implants performed with osteotomy than without.[16]

In patients undergoing revisions with extensively porous coated implants, the ability to achieve fixation of the revision stem with bone ingrowth is greater (92%) in patients who have had an extended proximal femoral osteotomy than those without (81%).[10] Because the osteotomy allows neutral reaming of the femoral

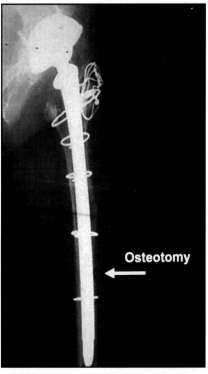

Fig. 6 Postoperative view of the patient shown in Figure 1. The revision stem is in neutral alignment and the proximal deformity has been corrected.

canal it can improve the ability to fill the canal and achieve fixation with bone ingrowth. It is this ability to fill the canal that leads to the reliable results seen with extensively porous coated implants.[6–10] Because the incidence and severity of thigh pain is more correlated with stable fibrous fixation than bone ingrowth fixation,[6–10] thigh pain should be diminished in patients undergoing femoral revision with the use of an extended proximal femoral osteotomy.

The single aseptic failure seen in this series is in a patient with extensive femoral metadiaphyseal damage with thin cortices and widened canal, a type IV defect.[10] This patient was successfully revised with impaction allografting. Although there were 25 intraoperative fractures (20%), these were mostly proximal and did not affect the axial and torsional stability of the implant. The junctional fractures (3) or perforations (3) were managed with prophylactic cerclage wires placed distally. They did not affect the length or diameter of the implanted stem.

The extended proximal femoral osteotomy has increased the speed and safety of femoral revision surgery and has become the technique of choice for removal of well-bonded distal cement bone interface, well-fixed, cementless stems, and for correction of proximal bone deformities in the revision setting.

References

1. Harris WH: Revision surgery for failed, nonseptic total hip arthroplasty: The femoral side. *Clin Orthop* 1982;170:8–20.

2. Shepherd BD, Turnbull A: The fate of femoral windows in revision joint arthroplasty. *J Bone Joint Surg* 1989;71A:716–718.

3. Younger TI, Bradford MS, Magnus RE, Paprosky WG: Extended proximal femoral osteotomy: A new technique for femoral revision arthroplasty. *J Arthroplasty* 1995; 10:329–338.

4. Cameron HU: Use of a distal trochanteric osteotomy in hip revision. *Contemp Orthop* 1991;23:235–238.

5. Kronick JL, Sekundiak TD, Paprosky WG: Complications in revision total hip arthroplasty with the extended proximal femoral osteotomy. Proceedings of the American Academy of Orthopaedic Surgeons 64th Annual Meeting, San Francisco, CA. Rosemont, IL, American Academy of Orthopaedic Surgeons, 1997, p 270.

6. Lawrence JM, Engh CA, Macalino GE: Revision total hip arthroplasty: Long-term results without cement. *Orthop Clin North Am* 1993;24:635–644.

7. Moreland JR, Bernstein ML: Femoral revision hip arthroplasty with uncemented, porous-coated stems. *Clin Orthop* 1995;319:141–150.

8. Paprosky WG, Krishnamurthy A: Five to 14-year follow-up on cementless femoral revisions. *Orthopedics* 1996;19:765–768.

9. Krishnamurthy AB, MacDonald SJ, Paprosky WG: 5- to 13-year follow-up study on cementless femoral components in revision surgery. *J Arthroplasty* 1997;12:839–847.

10. Aribindi R, Barba M, Solomon MI, Arp P, Paprosky W: Bypass fixation. *Orthop Clin North Am* 1998;29:319–329.

11. Kavanagh BF, Ilstrup DM, Fitzgerald RH Jr: Revision total hip arthroplasty. *J Bone Joint Surg* 1985;67A:517–526.

12. Pellicci PM, Wilson PD Jr, Sledge CB, et al: Long-term results of revision total hip replacement: A follow-up report. *J Bone Joint Surg* 1985;67A:513–516.

13. Katz RP, Callaghan JJ, Sullivan PM, Johnston RC: Results of cemented femoral revision total hip arthroplasty using improved cementing techniques. *Clin Orthop* 1995;319:178–183.

14. Mulroy WF, Harris WH: Revision total hip arthroplasty with use of so-called second-generation cementing techniques for aseptic loosening of the femoral component: A fifteen-year-average follow-up study. *J Bone Joint Surg* 1996;78A:325–330.

15. Kronick JL, Sekundiak TD, Paprosky WG, Kanai H: Proximal femoral deformity secondary to loosening and osteolysis: The effect on reimplantation. Proceedings of the American Academy of Orthopaedic Surgeons 64th Annual Meeting, San Francisco, CA. Rosemont, IL, American Academy of Orthopaedic Surgeons, 1997, p 392.

16. Egan KJ, Di Cesare PE: Intraoperative complications of revision hip arthroplasty using a fully porous-coated straight cobalt-chrome femoral stem. *J Arthroplasty* 1995;10(suppl):S45–S51.

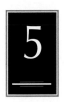

Retroperitoneal Exposure in Revision Total Hip Arthroplasty

Cecil H. Rorabeck, MD, FRCSC
Paul F. Partington, MB, BS, FRCS(Orth)

Introduction

All total hip arthroplasties will eventually fail. As revision surgery expands we have learned to deal with ever more complex and difficult revisions. A small proportion of revision surgery requires not only extensive exposure of the hip by standard arthroplasty approaches, but also exposure of the acetabulum from the *inside* of the pelvis, via a retroperitoneal approach.

This approach has been used since 1796, in vascular surgery of the iliac vessels.[1] It is now important that all hip arthroplasty and revision surgeons have an understanding of the approach and indications for its use.[2]

In this chapter, vascular injuries arising from total hip arthroplasty (THA) and revision will be reviewed, together with their causes. We will describe how to identify patients who should be considered for this additional retroperitoneal exposure, how they should be investigated, and how this access is obtained.

Vascular Injuries in Total Hip Arthroplasty

Many important viscera and neurovascular structures are located close to the hip joint. Injuries to most of them have been documented during primary and revision hip arthroplasty.

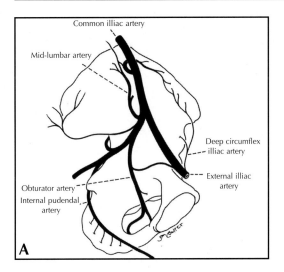

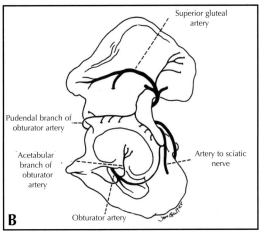

Fig. 1 A, The principal blood vessels within the inner aspect of the pelvis. **B,** The principal blood vessels along the outer aspect of the pelvis. (Reproduced with permission from Mears DC, Rubash HE: *Pelvic and Acetabular Fractures.* Thorofare, NJ, Slack, 1986, pp 38–39.)

Major vascular injury is rare, with an estimated incidence of 0.25%.[2] It has, however, the potential for immediate threat to life[3–5] and limb,[2,6–8] and complex late complications.[7,9–12]

A review of the literature shows a predominance of female patients have vascular injuries. This would be

Table 1
Instances of vascular injury during revision total hip arthroplasty (THA)

Reference	Patient Sex and Age (yrs)*	Side	Surgical Approach	Acetabular Diagnosis	Implant	Vascular Event	Management	Outcome
Nachbur et al[2]	M, 54	Left		Progressive protrusio of revision acetabulum	Cemented support ring with polyethylene cup	External iliac artery lacerated by adherent cement upon cup removal	Urgent clamping of external iliac artery	Limb salvage
Bergqvist et al[13]	F, 65	Right		Septic loosening with acetabular protrusio	Cemented all polyethylene	Hemorrhage from undiagnosed external iliac artery pseudo-aneurysm	Urgent external iliac artery ligation and femoral-femoral crossover graft	
	M, 70	Right	Posterolateral	Infected THA, no protrusio	Cemented all polyethylene	Internal iliac artery hemorrhage on cup mobilization	Urgent ligation of branch of internal iliac artery	Good
Reiley et al[7]	F, 84	Right	Posterolateral	Septic loosening with acetabular protrusio	Cemented all polyethylene	Hemorrhage from undiagnosed external iliac artery erosion caused by acetabular component	Urgent end-to-end anastomosis of external iliac artery	Hip remained as excision arthroplasty
Gruen et al[3]		Left		Aseptic loosening with protrusio	Uncemented screw-in cup	Hemorrhage from undiagnosed external iliac artery erosion caused by acetabular component		Died
Shoenfeld et al[8]	M, 78	Left	Lateral	Aseptic loosening with protrusio	Cemented all polyethylene	External iliac vein completely avulsed by adherent cement upon cup removal	Via an urgent retroperitoneal approach, external iliac vein ligated; femoral-femoral venous bypass; revision abandoned	Hip revised 1 year later; bypass graft occluded; chronic limb edema
	M, 67	Left	Lateral	Aseptic loosening of revision THA	Cemented all polyethylene	External iliac vein lacerated by adherent cement at the time of cup mobilization; subsequent external iliac artery thrombosis	Urgent retroperitoneal exploration and vein repair; revision abandoned	Re-exploration and hip revision 5 months later; elective femoral-femoral arterial bypass for severe claudication

*M, male; F, female

expected from the demographics of the arthroplasty population, as more females than males undergo THA.[13] More surprisingly, a greater number of operations are left-sided with vascular complications, totaling around 75% of all cases.[8,13] This is said to be related to the more leftward lateral position of the aortic bifurcation and

the left iliac artery.[13] Most of the injuries reported are arterial, although in extraction of implants from the acetabulum, venous injury is a greater problem.[8,14] Injuries of the external iliac and femoral vessels are the most common.[2,4,5,7–10,12–15]

A review of the vascular anatomy makes it clear why the iliac vessels are

injured in acetabular surgery (Fig. 1). The external iliac artery is the anterior division of the common iliac artery, after its bifurcation at the level of the L5-S1 vertebral disk. The external iliac artery runs obliquely down the medial border of the psoas major muscle, anterior and lateral to the external iliac vein, and is separated from the anterior column of the pelvis by the psoas. The amount of interposed psoas decreases distally as the tendinous portion starts opposite the anterosuperior corner of the acetabulum. The external iliac vein accompanies the artery. Proximally the vein lies medial and posterior to the artery, distally it is opposite the anterior superior quadrant of the acetabulum. The vein runs medial and inferior to the artery along the medial border of the psoas. This proximity makes the iliac, particularly the external iliac, vessels vulnerable to injury at revision surgery. Significant complications have been recorded, but rarely, from other vessels, such as the circumflex femoral, gluteal, and obturator arteries.[2,4,13]

Mechanisms of injuries have been examined by Nachbur and associates[2] and Aust and associates.[4] They found that vessels, in particular the common femoral artery and its branches, are at risk from penetration by sharp anterior retractors. This was the most common mechanism of injury. Patients who have severe degenerative osteoarthritis fall into the age group of those at risk of development of atherosclerosis. Retraction of femoral vessels caused fractures of atherosclerotic plaques and secondary thrombotic occlusion. These researchers also documented thermal injury occurring from extravasated cement curing close to major vessels. The external iliac vessels were at risk during acetabular preparation for cementing, and again at the time of acetabular removal for revision.

Use of blunt-tipped retractors, particularly anteriorly, is advised. Retraction of the potentially atherosclerotic vessels should not be excessive. Keyholes for acetabular cementing should be carefully prepared, avoiding penetration of the medial acetabular cortex. If the cortex is

	Risk Factor*
Clinical	Tender pelvic pain
	Pelvic pain
	Pelvic bruit
	Lower limb ischemia
Radiologic	Severe medial protrusio of the acetabular prosthesis on plain radiography
	Intrapelvic cement on plain radiography or computed tomography
Other	Infection associated with acetabular protrusio

Table 2
Risk factors predisposing to iliac vascular involvement or injury in revision total hip arthroplasty (THA)

*These findings are indications for angiography and consideration of retroperitoneal exposure at revision

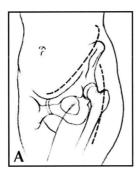

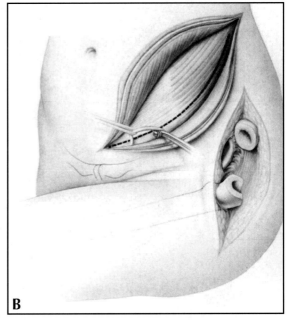

Fig. 2 A, After removal of the femoral component through a lateral incision, an oblique, lower lateral quadrant, abdominal incision is made. **B,** The external oblique muscle is incised so that the internal oblique and transversus abdominis muscles are exposed. If wide exposure is required, then the epigastic (hypogastic) vessels should be identified and divided when encountered medially. (Reproduced with permission from Eftekhar NS, Nercessian O: Intrapelvic migration of total hip prostheses: Operative treatment. *J Bone Joint Surg* 1989;71A:1480–1486.)

breached, it should be plugged prior to cementing, to prevent medial cement extravasation. Cement that extrudes anteriorly, toward the femoral vessels, should be carefully removed prior to curing. As hip arthroplasty entered the cementless era, an additional mechanism of vascular injury was encountered. Acetabular screw penetration medially caused vessel lacerations and pseudoaneurysm.[16–19] Taking care to place screws posteriorly, whenever possible, can reduce the chance of this injury.[18,19]

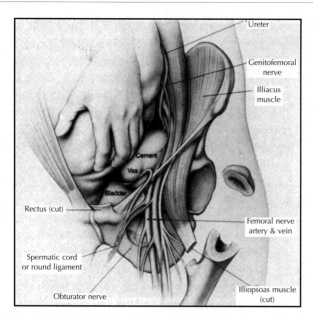

Fig. 3 After splitting or dividing the internal oblique and transversus muscles, the peritoneum and contents are retracted medially, exposing the iliopsoas and the overlying ureter and neurovascular structures. The acetabular component and cement are identified. (Reproduced with permission from Eftekhar NS, Nercessian O: Intrapelvic migration of total hip prostheses: Operative treatment. *J Bone Joint Surg* 1989;71A:1480–1486.)

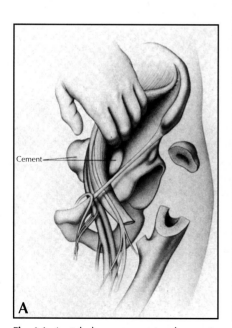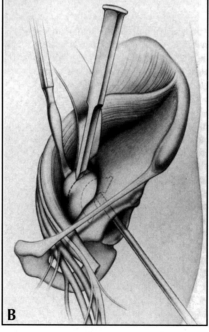

Fig. 4 A, Acetabular component and cement can be accessed either medial or lateral to the iliopsoas muscle. B, If necessary, the iliacus can be detached from the ilium and retracted medially with the neurovascular bundle. (Reproduced with permission from Eftekhar NS, Nercessian O: Intrapelvic migration of total hip prostheses: Operative treatment. *J Bone Joint Surg* 1989;71A:1480–1486.)

Revision surgery increases the risk of vascular injury, totaling 39% of Shoenfeld and associates'[8] series of 68 cases. In revision acetabular surgery, the external iliac vessels are most at risk, particularly at the time of component extraction.[16]

Consequences of vascular injuries are varied, with a 7% mortality and 15% amputation rate reported in the review of 68 cases.[8] Vascular surgery was required in all reported cases. Injuries most commonly cause thromboembolic complications, leading to distal ischemia and vessel lacerations with hemorrhage.[2,4,7,8,10,13,14,20] Additionally, pseudoaneurisms and, more rarely, arteriovenous fistulae develop.[4,9,12,21] These occasionally present many years after hip surgery.[2] Vessels can also be injured when cement extravasation occurs, or by medial migration (protrusio) of a failed acetabulum.[10,11,21,22]

Thus, revision acetabular surgery, when the iliac vessels are near cement or are damaged by a migrated prosthesis, can be fraught with difficulties. If only a lateral approach is made for acetabular removal, very severe hemorrhage or vessel injury can occur. Vascular injury may either go unrecognized or be impossible to control. Table 1 illustrates the point, with some cases in which use of a standard hip approach encountered vascular difficulties, necessitating repositioning and emergent vascular surgery. Most of these problems could have been prevented if potential vascular difficulties were identified preoperatively, and appropriately investigated.

Which Patients are at Risk in Revision THA?

al-Salman and associates[5] have identified a number of factors that can help identify patients who are at risk of iliac vessel involvement in revision THA. All are indications for further investigation. They noted the clinical signs of a tender pelvic mass, pelvic pain, or the presence of a pelvic bruit as clinical signs of vascular involvement. Radiologic factors of concern were severe medial protrusion of the acetabular prosthesis on plain radiographs, or intrapelvic cement on plain film or CT examination. Eftekhar and Nercessian[23] and Giacchetto and Gallagher[9] agree that severe protrusio should be investigated, with a view to retroperitoneal exposure at revision THA surgery.

Infection seems to be strongly associated with risk of vascular injury, either because it changes the tissue properties and obscures tissue planes or because it can cause acetabular failure and medial migration.[7,13,20] Although infection alone is not an indication for special investigations, additional care should be taken to avoid vascular injury in any infected THA. If infection is present with protrusio, the patient can be regarded as at high risk and definitely investigated further. Signs of lower limb ischemia following acetabular migration, which has obvious significance, should also be considered a risk factor.[9] We have added these 2 factors to those of al-Salman and associates,[5] and they are summarized in Table 2. Once the patients are identified, further investigation is warranted, with a view to retroperitoneal exposure of the iliac vessels to protect them from injury, or for vascular repair prior to hip revision surgery.

Preoperative Investigations

Several methods have been used to investigate patients prior to surgery. Most advocate arterial angiography.[4,5,9,15,16,20,21,24] Angiography will show the extent of vasculature involvement in cement or periacetabular fibrosis, or demonstrate a defect

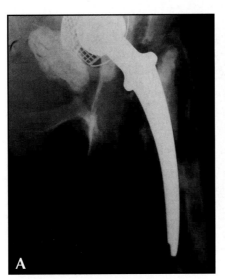 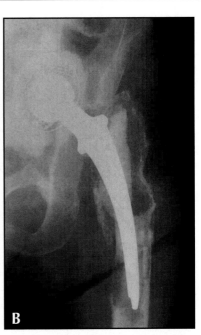

Fig. 5 A, and **B,** A 78-year-old female patient, 11 years after left cemented revision total hip arthroplasty presents with pain on ambulation and progressive shortening of her left leg. On examination, peripheral vascular status is normal. The acetabular component and cement are palpable abdominally in the left lower quadrant. Deep infection was excluded.

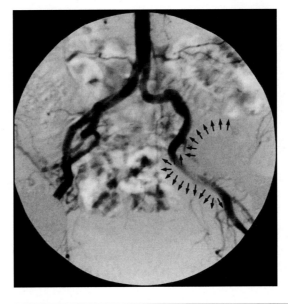

Fig. 6 Digital subtraction angiography demonstrates medial deviation of the left external iliac artery, which is closely related to the acetabular component and cement (outlined by arrows).

or pseudoaneurysm if the vessels have been eroded by implant or cement.[5,15] Venography is not usually necessary unless there is clinical evidence of venous occlusion preoperatively,[22] because the iliac veins are so close to the arteries at the acetabu-

lum.[5] Only rarely is the external iliac vein involved in isolation.[18]

Computed tomography (CT), particularly contrast enhanced, is useful to outline intrapelvic radiolucent cement[5] and vascular anatomy.[23] It is advocated by some as the only

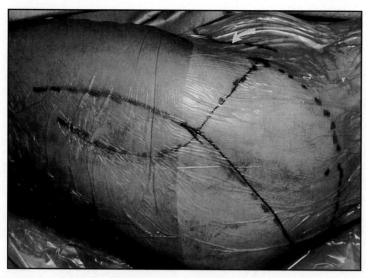

Fig. 7 Patient positioned in lateral position for surgery. This is a view from above the operating table of the lateral left hip. Previous anterolateral and posterolateral approach scars are marked. The position of the iliac crest is shown with a dotted line. The proposed retroperitoneal approach incision is marked anteriorly (arrow).

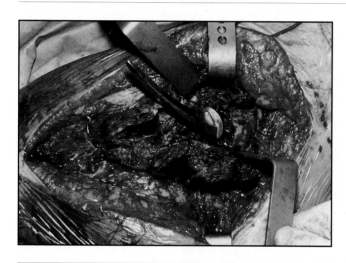

Fig. 8 Through a direct lateral approach, the femoral component is exposed and carefully extracted.

proach for removal of the femoral component. This is followed sometime later by joint reconstruction.[18,23,24] More recently, a single-stage procedure has been advocated.[5,6,24]

Providing infection is excluded, our preference is for a single procedure with 2 approaches, 1 to the medial side of the pelvis through a retroperitoneal route and a simultaneous lateral approach to the hip. Vascular surgery and revision surgery are completed during the same operation.

Surgical Technique

In these cases, preoperative planning should be done in collaboration with a vascular surgeon regarding the extent of vascular surgery that might be required. Vascular prosthetic grafts should be available, together with the revision THA armamentarium.

Following induction of general anesthesia and urinary catheterization, the patient is positioned in a lateral decubitus position with the affected hip uppermost. The position is maintained by using a vacuum bead bag. Additionally, heavy tape is used to secure the contralateral leg and the upper thorax to the operating table. This position gives good surgical access to both the lower lateral abdomen and to the hip. We have not yet found it necessary to change the position of the patient during the procedure for access to the hip or for retroperitoneal exposure, but this may be required, particularly if the vascular surgery is to be extensive.[6] With previous incisions marked, the patient is prepped from the level of the nipples inferiorly, from the midline posteriorly to beyond the umbilicus anteriorly. The limb is free draped, as for standard revision surgery.

Through our standard extended lateral approach, the femoral components and cement are carefully extract-

additional investigation required routinely.[6] Three-dimensional CT has been suggested as an elegant method of demonstrating vascular anatomy,[3] but it does not seem to be in widespread use for these revision patients. Magnetic resonance imaging (MRI) is also said to be informative.[24] Digital subtraction angiography is our investigation of choice. Delayed images can additionally outline the course of the ureter and its relationship to the acetabular com-

ponents. Positive findings are strong indications for retroperitoneal exposure to the acetabulum and iliac vessels, to prevent the catastrophes that can occur when the vessels are unprotected.

Timing of Surgery

Earlier literature suggests a 2-stage procedure with a retroperitoneal approach to explore the vessels and remove cement and/or the acetabular component, with a standard hip ap-

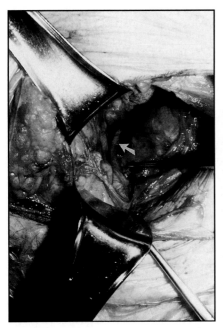

Fig. 9 The retroperitoneal exposure is made through a muscle-splitting incision. External iliac vessels (arrow) are exposed, mobilized, and protected. The acetabular component was then carefully removed through the lateral approach.

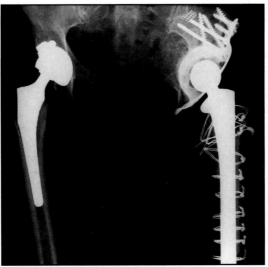

Fig. 10 Acetabular reconstruction was performed with a posterior wall structural allograft (femoral head), with 2 further morcellized allograft femoral heads, protrusio cage, and cemented cup. The femur required a proximal femoral allograft and a long, distally fixed, uncemented prosthesis. Radiograph at 6 months after surgery. Patient is pain free and walking with a cane.

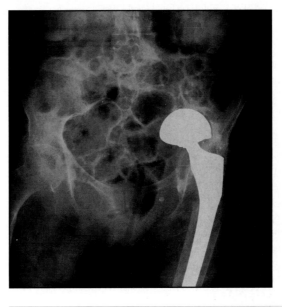

Fig. 11 Eighty-four-year-old female patient 8 years following left uncemented primary total hip arthroplasty presents with increasing hip pain. Her clinical vascular status is normal.

ed. On occasion it may be necessary to delay femoral component removal in the case of gross protrusio until the acetabulum has been mobilized, because access to the hip joint can be difficult under these circumstances.

Prior to acetabular mobilization, the retroperitoneal approach is performed. Depending on the preoperative angiography and planning, the extent of exposure is varied according to the patient. Standard exposure is similar to the Rutherford-Morrison approach, as applied to vascular and renal transplantation surgery. An oblique skin incision is made in the lower lateral quadrant, approximately 1 to 2 cm above the inguinal ligament, extending from the level of the iliac crest towards the pubic symphysis (Fig. 2). The external oblique aponeurosis is incised in line with the skin incision, in the line of its fibers,

and the internal oblique and transversus abdominus muscles are exposed. If a larger exposure is required, the inferior epigastric (hypogastric) vessels may be involved in the medial part of the incision where they cross the rectus, and these vessels should be ligated and divided. The internal oblique and transversus muscles are divided, after separating them from the underlying anterior peritoneum, in the line of the skin incision. The lateral cutaneous nerve of the thigh, which has a relatively superficial

course, should be protected.

If angiography demonstrates normal vessels without any evidence of pseudoaneurysm, sufficient access may be obtained from a muscle-splitting incision similar to the McBurney incision for appendectomy. In this case, internal oblique and transverse muscles are split in the line of their fibers, perpendicular to the overlying externus muscle, rather than cut. This muscle-dividing incision can be extended if additional access is required.

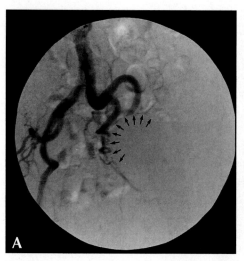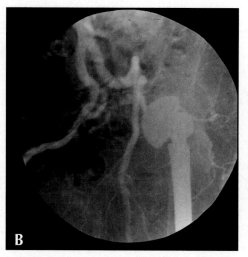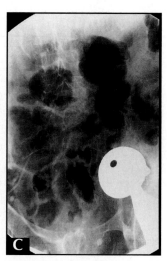

Fig. 12 Arteriography confirms the left external iliac artery proximity and distortion. **A,** Anteroposterior view. **B,** Oblique lateral view. **C,** Late films show the left ureter (arrows) also to be displaced by the migrated component.

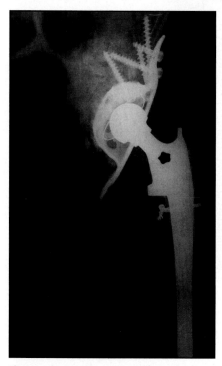

Fig. 13 After reconstruction, achieved through simultaneous lateral and retroperitoneal approaches. Acetabulum again extracted through a lateral approach; no vascular problems were encountered.

The posterior peritoneum and the acetabular contents are then reflected medially, by blunt finger dissection, from the underlying ureter, neu-rovascular structures, and psoas (Fig. 3). This may be all that is required to give access to the acetabulum and cement, medial to the iliopsoas, as it was in the 2 illustrative cases. It may be necessary, however, to detach the iliacus from the ilium to gain additional access, carefully retracting the iliopsoas and femoral nerve medially (Fig. 4). Indeed, this route of exposure has been advocated for use directly, by modifying the exposures of the medial pelvis performed in pediatric hip surgery.[24] If preoperative planning has anticipated that the femoral vessels will require exposure, the incision can be extended through a longitudinal rather than medial extension if necessary.

The external iliac vessels should be identified, mobilized, and protected. They should be repaired or bypassed if already damaged by implant or cement. Consideration should be given to ligation of the lateral branches of the iliac artery to prevent their avulsion during implant or cement extraction.[6] The acetabular component and cement can then be safely removed, often conveniently through the retroperitoneal exposure. Petrera and associates,[6] who repositioned the patient for a retroperitoneal approach, described bringing silicone vascular loops through the wound, which is then temporarily closed over a saline-soaked pack. Vascular control, if necessary, is then gained by tensioning the loops. We have found that good access is obtained in a fixed lateral position and, like others,[5] the abdominal wound need not be closed until the end of the revision procedure. If opened, the periacetabular scar tissue on the medial wall of the pelvis should then be closed to prevent herniation and to provide some support to the acetabular reconstruction.[5]

Retroperitoneal access to the acetabulum performed by the orthopaedic surgeon has been described.[24] Our policy, in agreement with Petrera and associates,[6] is to have the vascular surgeon carry out the abdominal part of the procedure. Reiley and associates[7] cautioned that vascular injuries associated with intrapelvic protrusion of components are difficult problems, even when a vascular surgeon is in consultation.

Hip reconstruction then proceeds, monitoring the vessels if and when necessary.[25] The abdominal wound is closed in layers, usually without a drain, if no vascular reconstruction has been undertaken. Good postoperative analgesia for this incision can be achieved with regional infusion of the subcostal and intercostal nerves, because the incision is in an internervous plane. The abdominal wound tends to heal well with good cosmetic results,[6] but in 1 series of retroperitoneal exposures for vascular surgery, there was a 7% incisional hernia rate and a 23% incidence of fascial and muscle weakness.[26] It is important to avoid damaging the intercostal and subcostal nerves during both opening and closure of the wound, to avoid denervating and weakening the muscles. A muscle-splitting incision has fewer wound complications.[26] Prolonged postoperative wound pain has been reported, and lumbosacral plexus injury can cause pain in the groin, testicle, and thigh. Underlying the thin fascial membrane anterior to the psoas lies the lumbosacral plexus, and the origin of the genitofemoral, iliohypogastric, and ilioinguinal nerves. In retroperitoneal dissection around the iliac vessels, these can be injured directly by traction or indirectly by ischemia or fibrosis.[26] To minimize this complication, it is essential to use proper planes of dissection, meticulously control bleeding, and avoid traction injuries. It is easy to see how the origin of some of this pain could be wrongly attributed to the hip.

Postoperatively, fluids and diet should be cautiously introduced until normal bowel function returns, because paralytic ileus is a common complication. A nasogastric tube is occasionally required.[23,24] Deep vein thrombosis is common following this degree of surgery (3 of 8 cases in 1 series),[5] and adequate prophylaxis

should be instituted. We routinely administer warfarin to our patients postoperatively until the time of hospital discharge, with Doppler ultrasound examination of the femoral and calf veins on the fifth postoperative day.

Conclusion

Many authors who documented iliac vascular injuries in revision THA conclude that they could have been prevented by appropriate investigation prior to surgery, with retroperitoneal access to the vessels at the time of acetabular revision.[2,4,7–9,13] Reiley and associates,[7] in 1984, described 1 case in which preoperative angiography and subsequent abdominal exposure *was* used to retrieve intrapelvic acetabular components. The femoral component were removed through the same abdominal incision. In this case, the postoperative course was complicated by external iliac artery thrombosis, ultimately resulting in below knee amputation. A number of successful later series are now published in which the retroperitoneal approach to the acetabulum was used without significant vascular complications.[5,6,23,24] In a total of 44 patients in the 4 papers, there were no deaths or amputations, and the revision was completed successfully in all. This is in sharp contrast to the cases illustrated in Table 1.

We encourage a low threshold for investigation prior to acetabular revision surgery if the pelvis has been encroached by cement or a migrating prosthesis, particularly in the presence of infection. Preoperative planning should consider angiography and, if necessary, collaboration with a vascular surgeon for retroperitoneal exposure of the iliac vessels and acetabulum at the time of revision surgery. Two of our cases are illustrated (Figs. 5 through 13).

References

1. Abernethy J (ed): *Surgical Observations.* London, England, TN Longman & O Rees, 1804, pp 209–231.

2. Nachbur B, Meyer RP, Verkkala K, Zürcher R: The mechanisms of severe arterial injury in surgery of the hip joint. *Clin Orthop* 1979;141:122–133.

3. Gruen GS, Mears DC, Cooperstein LA: Three-dimensional angio-computed tomography: New technique for imaging the acetabulum and adjacent vessels in a patient with acetabular protrusio. *J Arthroplasty* 1989;4:353–360.

4. Aust JC, Bredenberg CE, Murray DG: Mechanisms of arterial injuries associated with total hip replacement. *Arch Surg* 1981;116:345–349.

5. al-Salman M, Taylor DC, Beauchamp CP, Duncan CP: Prevention of vascular injuries in revision total hip replacement. *Can J Surg* 1992;35:261–264.

6. Petrera P, Trakru S, Mehta S, Steed D, Towers JD, Rubash HE: Revision total hip arthroplasty with a retroperitoneal approach to the iliac vessels. *J Arthroplasty* 1996;11:704–708.

7. Reiley MA, Bond D, Branick RI, Wilson EH: Vascular complications following total hip arthroplasty: A review of the literature and a report of two cases. *Clin Orthop* 1984;186:23–28.

8. Shoenfeld NA, Stuchin SA, Pearl R, Haveson S: The management of vascular injuries associated with total hip arthroplasty. *J Vasc Surg* 1990;11:549–555.

9. Giacchetto J, Gallagher JJ: False aneurysm of the common femoral artery secondary to migration of a threaded acetabular component: A case report and review of the literature. *Clin Orthop* 1988;231:91–96.

10. Heyes FL, Aukland A: Occlusion of the common femoral artery complicating total hip arthroplasty. *J Bone Joint Surg* 1985;67B:533–535.

11. Korovesis P, Siablis D, Salonikidis P, Sdougos G: Abdominal-hip joint fistula: Complicated revision of total hip arthroplasty for false aneurysm of external iliac artery. A case report. *Clin Orthop* 1988;231:71–75.

12. Mallory TH, Jaffe SL, Eberle RW: False aneurysm of the common femoral artery after total hip arthroplasty: A case report. *Clin Orthop* 1997;338:105–108.

13. Bergqvist D, Carlsson AS, Ericson BF: Vascular complications after total hip arthroplasty. *Acta Orthop Scand* 1983;54:157–163.

14. Fiddian NJ, Sudlow RA, Browett JP: Ruptured femoral vein: A complication of the use of gentamicin beads in an infected excision arthroplasty of the hip. *J Bone Joint Surg* 1984;66B:493–494.

15. Mody BS: Pseudoaneurysm of external iliac artery and compression of external

iliac vein after total hip arthroplasty: Case report. *J Arthroplasty* 1994;9:95–98.

16. Wasielewski RC, Cooperstein LA, Kruger MP, Rubash HE: Acetabular anatomy and the transacetabular fixation of screws in total hip arthroplasty. *J Bone Joint Surg* 1990;72A:501–508.

17. Kirkpatrick JS, Callaghan JJ, Vandemark RM, Goldner RD: The relationship of the intrapelvic vasculature to the acetabulum: Implications in screw-fixation acetabular components. *Clin Orthop* 1990;258: 183–190.

18. Keating EM, Ritter MA, Faris PM: Structures at risk from medially placed acetabular screws. *J Bone Joint Surg* 1990;72A:509–511.

19. Wasielewski RC, Crossett LS, Rubash HE: Neural and vascular injury in total hip arthroplasty. *Orthop Clin North Am* 1992;23:219–235.

20. Hopkins NF, Vanhegan JA, Jamieson CW: Iliac aneurysm after total hip arthroplasty: Surgical management. *J Bone Joint Surg* 1983;65B:359–361.

21. Woolson ST, Maloney WJ, Tanner JB: External iliac arteriovenous fistula following total hip arthroplasty: A case report. *J Arthroplasty* 1989;4:281–284.

22. Middleton RG, Reilly DT, Jessop J: Occlusion of the external iliac vein by cement. *J Arthroplasty* 1996;11:346–347.

23. Eftekhar NS, Nercessian O: Intrapelvic migration of total hip prostheses: Operative treatment. *J Bone Joint Surg* 1989;71A:1480–1486.

24. Grigoris P, Roberts P, McMinn DJ, Villar RN: A technique for removing an intrapelvic acetabular cup. *J Bone Joint Surg* 1993;75B:25–27.

25. Head WC: Prevention of intraoperative vascular complications in revision total hip-replacement arthroplasty: A case report. *J Bone Joint Surg* 1984;66A:458–459.

26. Honig MP, Mason RA, Giron F: Wound complications of the retroperitoneal approach to the aorta and iliac vessels. *J Vasc Surg* 1992;15:28–33.

A New Classification System for the Management of Acetabular Osteolysis After Total Hip Arthroplasty

Harry E. Rubash, MD
Raj K. Sinha, MD, PhD
Wayne Paprosky, MD
Charles A. Engh, MD
William J. Maloney, MD

Introduction

Periprosthetic osteolysis currently appears to be one of the most challenging problems that occurs after total hip arthroplasty. With increased awareness of this insidious process, joint replacement surgeons now have the ability to diagnose it with increasing accuracy and frequency.[1,2] In addition, considerable research efforts have provided an insight into the pathophysiologic mechanisms as well as the material concerns that lead to the development of osteolysis. This increased knowledge and understanding has helped institute improved methods of manufacture and implantation that will reduce the incidence of osteolysis in the future. Nevertheless, components implanted within the last 10 years continue to develop osteolysis at increasing rates, and will continue to pose surgical challenges.

The purpose of this chapter is to focus on acetabular osteolysis after implantation of cementless sockets. The original descriptions of this process were alarming, and the lesions often were mistaken for neoplasms.[3–5] Several early reports advocated complete removal of the components with revision and bone grafting if neces-

sary.[3–5] However, through careful systematic study and increased experience at many centers, specific indications for observation, surgical intervention, and revision have been developed. The authors propose a new classification system for acetabular osteolysis around uncemented cups, and a treatment rationale based on current understanding and preliminary results.

Pathophysiology

Briefly, the osteoclastic bone resorption of osteolysis is particle-induced, macrophase-mediated, and cytokine-propagated.[1] The proposed cycle of events occurs as follows. Normal wear in a low-friction arthroplasty leads to the production of billions of particles yearly.[6] The most abundant and probably most biologically noxious particle is that of ultra-high molecular weight polyethylene (UHMWPE),[7–9] which is used to make the acetabular liner. Initially, the wear mechanism is adhesive,[6] but as increased numbers of metal and polymeric particles are generated, third-body wear predominates.[10] There are several potential sources for wear, including the irregularities in the articular surfaces of the

femoral head and the polyethylene liner, and the incongruencies between the liner and the metal shell.[2] Additional sources include metallic particles produced by fretting, abrasion, and corrosion products that form at morse taper and screw-shell junctions. Eventually, clearance capabilities of the particles by the reticuloendothelial system are overcome, and the particles accumulate in large numbers and are distributed throughout the "effective joint space."[11–13] Like most foreign bodies, the particles are ingested by local macrophages, which secrete a variety of cellular mediators and cytokines. These mediators include interleukins (IL-1a and IL-6), tumor necrosis factor-alpha (TNF-α), prostaglandin E_2 (PGE$_2$), and others.[14–23] The mediators then stimulate osteoclasts to proliferate and actively resorb bone.[22,24] In severe cases, bone loss progresses to the point where the components ultimately become unstable.

An important concept to understand is that of the particle generator. This term refers to sources and causes of abnormal amounts of wear in a total hip arthroplasty. As mentioned above, a certain amount of wear is

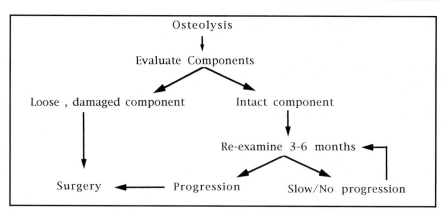

Fig. 1 Treatment algorithm for patients presenting with osteolysis. (Reproduced with permission from Rubash HE, Sinha RK, Maloney WJ, Paprosky W: Osteolysis: Surgical treatment, in Cannon WD (ed): *Instructional Course Lectures 47*. Rosemont, IL, American Academy of Orthopaedic Surgeons, 1998, pp 321–329.)

predictable even in well-functioning total hip replacements. However, excessive and accelerated wear occurs under certain conditions. Particle generators include: incongruous acetabular liner-shell interfaces;[25-27] thin polyethylene liners (< 8 mm), which are more susceptible to damage or fracture;[28] abraded polyethylene liners;[10] inferior quality polyethylene (certain batches with high numbers of asperities);[29] shelf-aged liners, which have oxidized;[30] machined polyethylene, which has inferior wear characteristics;[31,32] gamma-irradiated polyethylene, which oxidizes rapidly;[33] burnished femoral heads or implant surfaces;[34] titanium femoral heads;[35] 32-mm femoral heads;[36] damaged morse tapers on the femoral components;[37] loose or damaged porous coatings;[38] and broken cerclage wires or cable.[39] When surgical intervention is necessary, removal of the particle generators is an important part of the procedure.[2]

A general approach to the management of newly diagnosed osteolysis is outlined in Figure 1. If the components are stable and undamaged, and the osteolysis is focal, the patient can be observed initially. Serial radio-graphic examinations should be performed at 3- to 6-month intervals. If the osteolysis is documented to progress in size or extent, then surgical intervention should be considered. The appropriate surgical treatment depends upon the status of the cementless cup, as detailed below.

Classification

Figure 2 outlines the new classification scheme for cementless sockets with osteolysis. The cups can be divided into types I, II, and III. In type I cups, the osteolysis is focal, located usually at the periarticular margins or adjacent to screws and screwholes. However, the cup itself is stable and ingrown, without radio-lucencies at the implant-bone interface. Review of serial radiographs from the time of implantation to the initial appearance of the lytic lesion can be helpful in confirming whether the cup is stable or has migrated. However, though the metal shell may be stable, the polyethylene liner is worn, often visibly as detected on radiographs by the eccentric position of the femoral head within the cup. In these cases, with documented progression of the osteolysis requiring surgical treatment, type I shells can be retained because they are ingrown, are stable, and have functional locking mechanisms.

On the other hand, type II sockets must be removed. Although the radiographic appearance may be similar to that of a type I cup, at the time of surgery, type II cups are those that are found to be nonfunctional. For example, there may be excessive backsided wear of the shell, usually as a result of fracture of the polyethylene liner, or the locking mechanism may be broken (Fig. 3). In addition, nonmodular cups with excessive wear or burnishing of the polyethylene liner can be classified as type II. In both cases, the entire acetabular component must be revised.

Type III cups are those that have become unstable secondary to osteolysis. In most cases, loosening of the cup is obvious, as demonstrated by superior or medial migration of the component with change in orientation. However, in certain cases of linear osteolysis, the cup collapses into the osteolytic defect, and its stability cannot be determined on plain radiographs. However, computed tomography (CT) scans clearly show the line of demarcation between the osteolytic defect in the acetabular bone and the loose cup. All type III cups require revision.

Surgical Treatment and Preliminary Results
Type I Acetabular Components
For most type I cups with documented progression of the osteolysis, surgical treatment is required. At the time of surgery, modular femoral heads should be removed to improve exposure of the acetabulum. In addition, examine the morse taper to determine whether excessive fretting corrosion has occurred. If the morse taper is undamaged, then the femoral

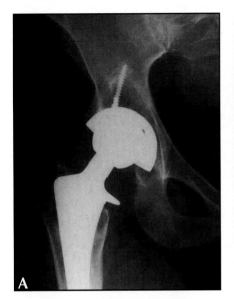

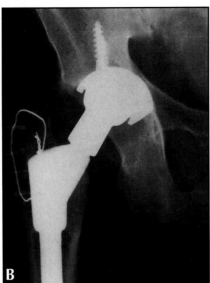

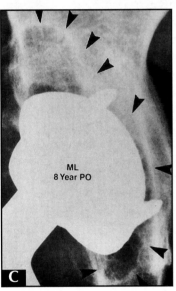

Fig. 2 Classification of acetabular osteolysis around uncemented components. **A,** Type I. Stable, functional: ingrown shell, worn polyethylene, focal lesion. **B,** Type II. Stable, damaged: nonfunctional shell due to excessive wear, broken locking mechanism, or nonmodular component. **C,** Type III. Unstable: Loosened component which has collapsed into osteolytic lesion.

component can be retained, provided that it is stable. Otherwise, the femoral component should generally be revised as well.

To facilitate exposure to the acetabular component, excise all scar and fibrous tissue carefully to allow visualization of the entire bony rim of the acetabulum. Subsequently, any overhanging osteophytes should be carefully osteotomized or rongeured to permit circumferential access to the liner-shell interface. In order to remove the liner, several techniques may be employed. If the manufacturer makes a specific device for removal of the liner, this device should be available. If this device is not available, backup methods are necessary. In shells that use tines for locking the liner in place, use a quarter-inch osteotome to gently pry the liner out of place. For ring-lock or cold-flow interference fit liners, carefully drill a 3.2-mm hole through the liner toward the shell (in a location where there is no screw hole). Then, insert a 4.5-mm cancellous screw through the drill hole into the liner. As the screw contacts the shell, it gently lifts the plastic liner away from the shell.

Once the liner has been removed, assess the locking mechanism to ensure that it was not damaged during liner extraction. If the locking mechanism is functional, test the shell for stability. A predictable method is to compress the shell with a ball or blunt impactor and look for fluid expressed from the interface. In addition, firmly grasp the cup rim with pliers or its concave surface through 2 screw holes with a Kocher clamp in order to twist or pull the cup out of its bony bed.

If the cup is stable, determine whether the osteolytic lesion is easily accessible. If the lesion is adjacent to a screw, carefully remove the screw. If there is no excessive bleeding, the cavity can be curetted and packed with morcellized bone graft (allo- or autograft, as available). If the lesion is not easily accessible, attempts to gain access unnecessarily may compromise stability of the cup, and therefore should be avoided. Note that although no graft can be placed in this scenario, it may not affect the eventual outcome.

The next step is reimplantation of a revision component. Insert a new modular 28- or 26-mm liner into the shell in order to maximize polyethylene thickness. Use trial femoral heads to determine the appropriate neck length needed for adequate stability. We routinely replace the femoral head, even though it may appear to be reusable. Adherence to these principles allows for uncomplicated revision of type I cups.

Type II Acetabular Components

For type II cups, exposure to the component and removal of the liner proceeds as for type I cups. Assessment of the metal shell is the next crucial step.

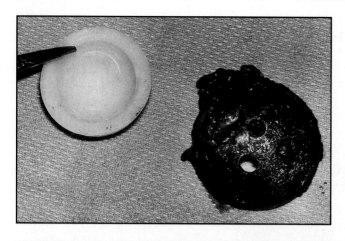

Fig. 3 Example of Type II cup. The retrieved specimen has extensive polyethylene wear and a broken polyethylene insert.

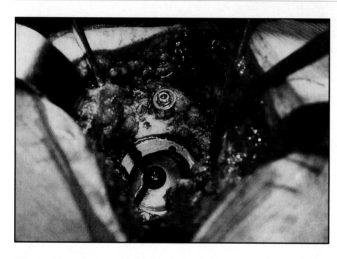

Fig. 4 Example of an acetabular component that has been sectioned prior to removal.

graft also may be necessary. In addition, pelvic discontinuity may occur and pelvic reconstruction plates or antiprotrusio cages should be available as well. After implantation of the new cup, the procedure can be completed as described above.

Type III Acetabular Components
Type III cups are unstable, and require removal. Often, in these cases, the radiograph does not show the full magnitude of the lesion, and the surgeon can rely on a computed tomogram to delineate the size and location of the defects. Although the component may be loose, it may not be easily removed. Often, as the cup migrates medially, the diameter of the mouth of the acetabulum will be smaller than that of the component. Removal of the overhanging osteophyte, as described above, opens up the mouth to expose the entire cup. In addition, dense fibrous tissue develops between the cup and the underlying bone bed. Development of the interface between the fibrous tissue and the bone may prevent unnecessary bone loss during component extraction. Once the component is removed, use hemispherical reamers to further open up the mouth in order to facilitate placement of a new porous-ingrowth shell. Adherence to meticulous techniques as described above for extraction of an ingrown cup will facilitate quick and simple removal of the loose cup. Reconstruction of osteolytic defects proceeds in a similar fashion as described above.

Particle Generators
Regarding the particle generators, several important concepts should be borne in mind. Generally, titanium monoblock femoral stems with burnished heads or stems with damaged morse tapers should be removed,

If the locking mechanism is broken, if there is excessive back-sided wear of the shell, or if the cup is known to have a poor clinical track record, then it must be removed. Once this determination has been made, removal must be performed carefully to avoid penetration of the medial wall of the pelvis. The interface between the shell and the bony bed of the acetabulum must be clearly visualized by removing capsule, scar, and overhanging osteophytes. Specially shaped acetabular osteotomes are then used to disrupt the interface. Proceed sequentially from lateral to medial around the hemisphere of the cup. Generally, a cup cannot be removed until the interface is disrupted circumferentially for 180°, as well as all the way over to the medial quadrilateral plate. When the cup abuts the medial wall of the pelvis, the use of space-occupying tools such as gouges and osteotomes is precluded in order to prevent penetration and possible damage to underlying vessels and pelvic viscera. In this situation, the metal shell may need to be sectioned into 3 or more pieces using a metal-cutting burr and then removed piecemeal (Fig. 4). Attention to these details, along with careful preoperative preparation, helps the surgeon remove the component safely.

Once the component is extracted, curette all osteolytic membrane and pack the defects with morcellized graft. If there are significant rim defects that may compromise stability of the revision cup, then bulk allo-

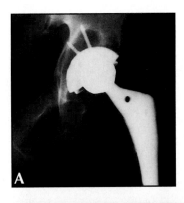

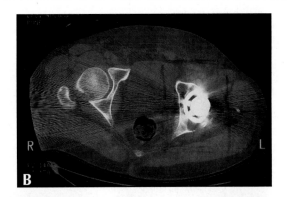

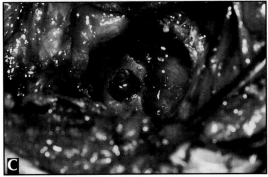

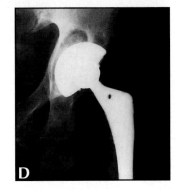

Fig. 5 Case report of a 46-year-old man with a loosened acetabular component and pelvic osteolysis. **A,** Preoperative radiograph. **B,** CT scan of the loosened component that had collapsed into an osteolytic defect. **C,** Defect seen intraoperatively. **D,** Six-month follow-up radiographs showing a stable component and allograft incorporation.

especially in young, active patients. In extenuating circumstances, such as elderly or medically unstable patients, damaged stems may be retained when removal of a well-fixed stem may prolong operative time or cause excessive blood loss. A tap-out/tap-in technique can be used to remove a damaged stem with a good cement column, and then a smaller stem can be recemented.[40] In addition, modular titanium heads should be replaced with cobalt-chrome heads because of superior wear characteristics. Likewise, 32-mm heads should be downsized to 28- or 26-mm heads, because the latter have been shown to result in smaller amounts of volumetric polyethylene wear. Polyethylene liners a minimum of 8 mm thick should be used, as thin liners are susceptible to fracture and accelerated wear. Damaged screws should be removed in well-fixed cups to eliminate fretting and corrosion products after the revision. Thus, exchange of the parti-

cle generators is a crucial part of the revision procedure.

Case

The patient is a 46-year-old man who underwent a primary total hip arthroplasty at age 41 secondary for end-stage osteonecrosis. At 5.5 years postoperatively, the patient was seen in the office for the gradual onset of progressive groin pain. As part of a routine evaluation, radiographs were obtained, which revealed moderate wear of the polyethylene liner without evidence of radiolucency at the implant-bone interface (Fig. 5, A). A CT scan was then obtained to further evaluate the extent of the pelvic lysis (Fig. 5, B). The CT scan demonstrated a circumferential radiolucency around the cup at the implant-bone interface with a sclerotic margin of bone, suggesting that the component was loose and had collapsed into an osteolytic defect. At revision surgery, the acetabular component was found to be loose and

osteolytic defects were noted in the dome of the acetabulum with extension into the anterior and posterior columns (Fig. 5, C). The osteolytic defects were packed with morcellized femoral head allograft, and the cup was revised to a 60-mm porous ingrowth component. The patient has done well and at 6-month postoperative follow-up has no pain and has been advanced to weightbearing as tolerated with a cane. Radiographs obtained at this time show incorporation of the allograft with the acetabular component in excellent position and without change from the initial postoperative films (Fig. 5, D).

Preliminary Results

These principles have been instituted in several centers. It appears that removal of the particle generators is essential to arrest the osteolytic process in type I cups, as the use of bone graft does not necessarily determine whether the lesion will heal.[41,42]

However, at intermediate follow-up, there have been only rare cases of progression of the lesions after removal of the particle generators. Thus, preliminary results are encouraging that the approach outlined here will be safe and effective. Further study and review of collective experiences will help to refine the treatment approach for osteolysis in the future.

References

1. Sinha RK, Shanbhag A, Maloney WJ, Hasselman CT, Rubash HE: Osteolysis: Cause and effect, in Cannon WD (ed): *Instructional Course Lectures 47*. Rosemont, IL, American Academy of Orthopaedic Surgeons, 1998, pp 307–320.

2. Rubash HE, Sinha RK, Maloney WJ, Paprosky W: Osteolysis: Surgical treatment, in Cannon WD (ed): *Instructional Course Lectures 47*. Rosemont, IL, American Academy of Orthopaedic Surgeons, 1998, pp 321–329.

3. Jasty MJ, Floyd WE III, Schiller AL, Goldring SR, Harris WH: Localized osteolysis in stable, non-septic total hip replacement. *J Bone Joint Surg* 1986;68A:912–919.

4. Santavirta S, Konttinen YT, Bergroth V, Eskola A, Tallroth K, Lindholm TS: Aggressive granulomatous lesions associated with hip arthroplasty: Immunopathological studies. *J Bone Joint Surg* 1990;72A:252–258.

5. Santavirta S, Hoikka V, Eskola A, Konttinen YT, Paavillainen T, Tallroth K: Aggressive granulomatous lesions in cementless total hip arthroplasty. *J Bone Joint Surg* 1990;72B:980–984.

6. Amstutz HC, Campbell P, Kossovsky N, Clarke IC: Mechanism and clinical significance of wear debris-induced osteolysis. *Clin Orthop* 1992;276:7–18.

7. Willert HG, Bertram H, Buchhorn GH: Osteolysis in alloarthroplasty of the hip: The role of ultra-high molecular weight polyethylene wear particles. *Clin Orthop* 1990;258:95–107.

8. Howie DW: Tissue response in relation to type of wear particles around failed hip arthroplasties. *J Arthroplasty* 1990;5:337–348.

9. Gelb H, Schumacher HR, Cuckler J, Ducheyne P, Baker DG: In vivo inflammatory response to polymethylmethacrylate particulate debris: Effect of size, morphology, and surface area. *J Orthop Res* 1994;12:83–92.

10. McKellop HA, Campbell P, Park S-H, et al: The origin of submicron polyethylene wear debris in total hip arthroplasty. *Clin Orthop* 1995;311:3–20.

11. Willert HG, Semlitsch M: Reactions of the articular capsule to wear products of artificial joint prostheses. *J Biomed Mater Res* 1977;11:157–164.

12. Schmalzried TP, Harris WH: The Harris-Galante porous-coated acetabular component with screw fixation: Radiographic analysis of eighty-three primary hip replacements at a minimum of five years. *J Bone Joint Surg* 1992; 74A:1130–1139.

13. Schmalzried TP, Jasty M, Harris WH: Periprosthetic bone loss in total hip arthroplasty: Polyethylene wear debris and the concept of the effective joint space. *J Bone Joint Surg* 1992; 74A:849–863.

14. Thornhill TS, Ozuna RM, Shortkroff S, Keller K, Sledge CB, Spector M: Biochemical and histological evaluation of the synovial-like tissue around failed (loose) total joint replacement prostheses in human subjects and a canine model. *Biomaterials* 1990;11:69–72.

15. Haynes DR, Rogers SD, Hay S, Pearcy MJ, Howie DW: The differences in toxicity and release of bone-resorbing mediators induced by titanium and cobalt-chromium-alloy wear particles. *J Bone Joint Surg* 1993;75A:825–834.

16. Jiranek WA, Machado M, Jasty M, et al: Production of cytokines around loosened cemented acetabular components: Analysis with immunohistochemical techniques and in situ hybridization. *J Bone Joint Surg* 1993;75A:863–879.

17. Kim KJ, Rubash HE, Wilson SC, D'Antonio JA, McClain EJ: A histological and biochemical comparison of the interface tissues in cementless and cemented hip prosthesis. *Clin Orthop* 1993;287:142–152.

18. Chiba J, Rubash HE, Kim KJ, Iwaki Y: The characterization of cytokines in the interface tissue obtained from failed cementless total hip arthroplasty with and without femoral osteolysis. *Clin Orthop* 1994;300:304–312.

19. Shanbhag AS, Jacobs JJ, Black J, Galante JO, Glant TT: Cellular mediators secreted by interfacial membranes obtained at revision total hip arthroplasty. *J Arthroplasty* 1995;10:498–506.

20. Dorr LD, Bloebaum R, Emmanual J, Meldrum R: Histologic, biochemical, and ion analysis of tissue and fluids retrieved during total hip arthroplasty. *Clin Orthop* 1990;261:82–95.

21. Schindler R, Mancilla J, Endres S, Ghorbani R, Clark SC, Dinarello CA: Correlations and interactions in the production of interleukin-6 (IL-6), IL-1, and tumor necrosis factor (TNF) in human blood mononuclear cells: IL-6 suppresses IL-1 and TNF. *Blood* 1990;75:40–47.

22. Horowitz SM, Gautsch TL, Frondoza CG, Riley L Jr: Macrophage exposure to polymethyl methacrylate leads to mediator release and injury. *J Orthop Res* 1991;9:406–413.

23. Blaine TA, Rosier RN, Puzas JE, et al: Increased levels of tumor necrosis factor-alpha and interleukin-6 protein and messenger RNA in human peripheral blood monocytes due to titanium particles. *J Bone Joint Surg* 1996;78A:1181–1192.

24. Glant TT, Jacobs JJ: Response of three murine macrophage populations to particulate debris: Bone resorption in organ cultures. *J Orthop Res* 1994;12:720–731.

25. Maloney WJ, Smith RL: Periprosthetic osteolysis in total hip arthroplasty: The role of particulate wear debris, in Pritchard DJ (ed): *Instructional Course Lectures 45*. Rosemont, IL, American Academy of Orthopaedic Surgeons, 1996, pp 171–182.

26. Chen PC, Mead EH, Pinto JG, Colwell CW Jr: Polyethylene wear debris in modular acetabular prostheses. *Clin Orthop* 1995;317:44–56.

27. Callaghan JJ, Kim YS, Brown TD, Pedersen DR, Johnston RC: Concerns and improvements with cementless metal-backed acetabular components. *Clin Orthop* 1995;311:76–84.

28. Bartel DL, Bicknell VL, Wright TM: The effect of conformity, thickness, and material on stresses in ultra-high-molecular weight components for total joint replacement. *J Bone Joint Surg* 1986;68A:1041–1051.

29. Li S, Chang JD, Barrena EG, Furman BD, Wright TM, Salvati E: Nonconsolidated polyethylene particles and oxidation in Charnley acetabular cups. *Clin Orthop* 1995;319:54–63.

30. Rimnac CM, Klein RW, Betts F, Wright TM: Post-irradiation aging of ultra-high molecular weight polyethylene. *J Bone Joint Surg* 1994; 76A:1052–1056.

31. Bankston AB, Cates H, Ritter MA, Keating EM, Faris PM: Polyethylene wear in total hip arthroplasty. *Clin Orthop* 1995;317:7–13.

32. Bankston AB, Keating EM, Ranawat C, Faris PM, Ritter MA: Comparison of polyethylene wear in machined versus molded polyethylene. *Clin Orthop* 1995;317:37–43.

33. Sutula LC, Collier JP, Saum KA, et al: Impact of gamma sterilization on clinical performance of polyethylene in the hip. *Clin Orthop* 1995; 319:28–40.

34. Dowson D, Taheri S, Wallbridge NC: The role of counterface imperfections in the wear of polyethylene. *Wear* 1987;119:277–293.

35. McKellop HA, Sarmiento A, Schwinn CP, Ebramzadeh E: In vivo wear of titanium-alloy hip prostheses. *J Bone Joint Surg* 1990;72A: 512–517.

36. Livermore J, Ilstrup D, Morrey B: Effect of femoral head size on wear of the polyethylene acetabular component. *J Bone Joint Surg* 1990; 72A:518–528.

37. Jacobs JJ, Skipor AK, Doorn PF, et al: Cobalt and chromium concentrations in patients with metal on metal total hip replacements. *Clin Orthop* 1996;329(suppl):S256–S263.

38. Sychterz CJ, Moon KH, Hashimoto Y, Terefenko KM, Engh CA Jr, Bauer TW: Wear of polyethylene cups in total hip arthroplasty: A study of specimens retrieved post mortem. *J Bone Joint Surg* 1996;78A:1193–2000.

39. Silverton CD, Jacobs JJ, Rosenberg AG, Kull L, Conley A, Galante JO: Complications of a cable grip system. *J Arthroplasty* 1996;11: 400–404.

40. Nabors ED, Liebelt R, Mattingly DA, Bierbaum BE: Removal and reinsertion of cemented femoral components during acetabular revision. *J Arthroplasty* 1996;11:146–152.

41. Maloney WJ, Herzwurm P, Paprosky W, Rubash HE, Engh CA: Treatment of pelvic osteolysis associated with a stable acetabular component inserted without cement as part of a total hip replacement. *J Bone Joint Surg* 1997; 79A:1628–1634.

42. Hozack WJ, Bicalho PS, Eng K: Treatment of femoral osteolysis with cementless total hip revision. *J Arthroplasty* 1996;11:668–672.

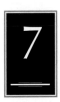

Acetabular Bone Loss During Revision Total Hip Replacement: Preoperative Investigation and Planning

David G. Campbell, BM, BS, FRACS (Orth)
Bassam A. Masri, MD, FRCSC
Donald S. Garbuz, MD, FRCSC
Clive P. Duncan, MD, FRCSC

Despite the excellent outcome after total hip arthroplasty,[1] the number of hips that require revision has increased dramatically because of the increased prevalence of hip replacements, younger age at initial procedure, and the aging population. Indeed, revision total hip arthroplasty may be the largest iatrogenic orthopaedic problem of the late twentieth century. These failed arthroplasties present many challenges, not only in intraoperative technique, but also in preoperative planning and decision making and in postoperative care. Many factors have to be considered, such as the patient's general health and older age, techniques for the safe exposure and extraction of the existing implants, and methods of bone stock augmentation and implant fixation that allow a stable and durable reconstruction.

When planning a revision hip procedure, it is useful to consider the acetabular and femoral components independently, while keeping in mind the interaction between the 2 components in terms of leg length and hip joint stability. It is not uncommon to encounter cases in which only one component is loose, while the other is solidly fixed and

does not require revision. Long-term studies on cemented arthroplasties have clearly shown a higher failure rate for cemented acetabular components, compared with femoral components, especially if the components have been in place for more than 10 years.[2,3] Although cementless components have been introduced to address this problem, some cementless designs have been plagued with a high rate of aseptic loosening and osteolysis, leading to catastrophic failure and revision procedures.[4]

Although aseptic loosening of the acetabular component may cause marked symptoms that alert the patient and the surgeon to the potential need for revision, many other patients have silent loosening, migration, and osteolysis, which only become symptomatic when the degree of bone loss is so substantial that a very complex revision procedure is necessary. In Charnley's series, 12- to 15-year results noted that 25% of the acetabulae had a significant bone-cement lucency or migration, often with no deterioration of clinical outcome.[5] This problem is not restricted to cemented implants, bone loss having been seen with cementless acetabular components as well.[4,6,7] The purpose

of this review is to outline the factors to be considered in the preoperative investigation and planning for revision of the acetabular component, with particular reference to the nature of bone stock deficiency within the remaining acetabular fossa.

General Considerations

Prior to acetabular revision, it is useful to consider a preoperative plan (Outline 1) that includes an assessment of general and specific patient factors, presence or absence of sepsis, extent of bone deficiency, and the potential strategies for reconstruction. The preoperative plan should include a plan for adequate exposure, implant removal, management of the bone deficiency, and fixation of the revision implants to achieve a stable and durable reconstruction.

Patient Factors

Most patients who require revision arthroplasty are a decade or more older than their age at the primary operation. Consequently, the medical health and physiologic reserve of these patients is often diminished. The revision procedure often involves more lengthy and complicated surgery, with a higher degree of blood loss than the primary procedure and a subsequent greater risk of perioperative morbidity. Patients undergoing revision procedures often require a more prolonged period of convalescence and rehabilitation and a longer period of protected weightbearing.

The risk of local complications, with reference to the affected hip, is also increased following revision procedures. The risk of dislocation is, on average, 2 or more times greater than that after a primary procedure.[8,9] The patient's physical and mental ability to comply with hip replacement precautions to prevent dislocation must also be considered, and the operation modified accordingly.

Preoperative assessment of the patient's general health should include both his or her fitness for surgery and for postoperative rehabilitation. Balance and strength in the upper extremities must be considered because of the need for protected weightbearing after most revision procedures.

Documentation of the neurovascular status is required because of the increased occurrence of nerve palsies following revision hip arthroplasty. Sciatic nerve palsy, which occurs in approximately 0.7% to 1% of primary hip arthroplasties, is approximately 3 times more frequent in revision arthroplasty.[10-12] Special techniques to reduce the incidence of nerve palsy should therefore be incorporated into the preoperative plan. Fortunately, vascular injury to the limb is rare after both primary and revision arthroplasty, but it is more frequent after revision.

Physical examination of the hip will influence the reconstructive plan. Previous skin incisions will suggest which approaches have been used in the past. We favor the use of a previous incision, whenever possible, to decrease the risk of wound edge necrosis, although, unlike in the knee, this is a rare complication. The hip range of motion is frequently overlooked in the presence of a painful or unstable prosthetic hip, but it is an important indicator of heterotopic bone formation and joint contracture. Extensive acetabular bone loss is often associated both with shortening of the limb and with decreased femoral offset, as the femur migrates medially, causing a short and stiff joint. A hip with very limited movement is often difficult to mobilize unless an extensive soft-tissue release is performed. In these cases, a specialized approach that affords wide exposure of the pelvis and femur, if necessary, should be considered. Intraoperative lengthening of a stiff hip may also prove problematic unless extensive releases are used. Conversely, hypermobile prosthetic joints are relatively easy to expose but the associated instability will require techniques to improve the stability of the joint, such as lengthening of the limb when appropriate, increasing femoral offset, or performing a trochanteric advance-

ment. Abductor strength is also important for stability after a revision procedure, because poor abductor strength increases the risk of postoperative dislocation. In addition, Morrey[8] has outlined factors associated with an increased incidence of hip dislocation after total hip arthroplasty, including female sex, revision surgery, posterior approach, mobile hips, decreased femoral offset, and, most importantly, acetabular orientation. Initial diagnosis, height and weight, component head size, or length inequality were not associated with an increased incidence of instability.

Preoperative Investigations to Rule Out Infection

Severe loss of bone stock, particularly within a relatively short period of time after total hip arthroplasty, should raise the index of suspicion for underlying occult infection. A detailed review of the diagnosis of infection following total hip arthroplasty is beyond the scope of this chapter; however, such a review has been published elsewhere.[13] A careful history and physical examination should precede any tests for the diagnosis of infection. A high index of suspicion is essential, particularly when the patient complains of a persistently painful arthroplasty, despite unremarkable radiographs. The patient should be carefully questioned regarding any wound-healing complications, early infections, or prolonged administration of antibiotics after surgery. Delays in discharge from the hospital also suggest a significant early complication. Questions regarding recent infections, such as skin infections or ulcerations, urinary tract infections, dental infections, or manipulations can also be revealing.

The rational use of preoperative investigation in a sequential fashion will allow the correct diagnosis of infection in the majority of cases. The initial tests should be an erythrocyte sedimentation rate (ESR) and a C-reactive protein (CRP). If both tests are normal, and the history and physical examination are not suggestive of infection, no further tests are necessary.[14,15] If the ESR and/or CRP are elevated, further tests are indicated. A hip joint aspiration, with the patient off all antibiotics for at least 4 weeks, should be performed. If the aspiration is negative, and the index of suspicion remains high, the aspiration is repeated, perhaps with the guidance of arthrography or ultrasound. If it remains negative, and the index of suspicion for infection remains high, ancillary tests such as another repeat hip aspiration, or a sequential technetium-indium nuclear scan may be considered. If all these tests are negative, the surgeon may resort to a frozen section at the time of revision arthroplasty to help distinguish between aseptic loosening and infection.[15-17] If the frozen section is negative, the surgeon can then proceed with a revision total hip arthroplasty. Intraoperative tissue cultures are obtained in all patients as confirmatory tests.

Evaluation of Acetabular Bone Loss

Anatomy and Radiologic Evaluation of the Acetabulum

Because of the complex 3-dimensional anatomy of the acetabulum, it is difficult to evaluate and quantify the degree of acetabular bone loss without having a clear understanding of the complex anatomy of the acetabulum as well as the spatial distribution of remaining bone stock about a prosthetic acetabular component. Furthermore, it is difficult to derive accurate information about the 3-dimensional bone loss from 2-dimensional radiographic images of the acetabulum without a precise understanding of the various radiographic landmarks. Nevertheless, an understanding of the surgical and mechanical anatomy of the acetabulum is simplified by the concepts of biomechanical columns described by Judet and associates.[18] Although these concepts were initially developed for the study of acetabular fractures, they can be applied with ease to the evaluation of the acetabulum in revision total hip arthroplasty.

The hemipelvis can be thought of as an inverted "Y", with the limbs of the letter "Y" representing the anterior and posterior columns straddling the acetabulum. The acetabulum can be divided into 4 regions: the roof and superior rim, the posterior column and posterior rim, the anterior column and anterior rim, and the medial wall.

Prior to hip arthroplasty, the acetabular cavity consists of the central nonarticular acetabular fossa (the floor of the acetabulum) surrounded by the semilunar articular surface. The acetabular fossa is continuous with an anteroinferior gap in the articular surface (the acetabular notch), which defines the inferior border of the acetabular cavity. The acetabular notch is radiologically defined by the inferior segment of the tear drop and the posterosuperior margin of the obturator foramen; it is surgically defined by the transverse acetabular ligament.

The posterior column extends from the ischium to the iliac wing and provides the primary support for the acetabulum. Radiographically, the ilioischial line (Köhler's line) demarcates the posterior column on the anteroposterior and iliac oblique radiographs, but it is best seen on the iliac oblique radiographs described by Judet.[18] The anterior column extends from the superior pubic ramus to the iliac wing. Radiographically, it is seen best on the obturator oblique view.[18] It is best demarcated by the iliopectineal line, which is also best seen on the obturator oblique view,[18] but it can also be seen on an anteroposterior (AP) view as well. The junction between the anterior and posterior columns is the roof, or dome of the acetabulum. This is the important weightbearing surface of the acetabulum. The lateral-most projection of the roof is the superior rim of the acetabulum, which is often deficient in cases of acetabular dysplasia. The medial wall of the acetabulum consists primarily of the quadrilateral plate, which separates the hip joint from the pelvic cavity. Radiographically, this is seen as the medial limb of the teardrop shadow.[19]

Correlation of the geometrically complex acetabular anatomy with preoperative imaging requires an understanding of the radiographic landmarks. Radiographs superimpose cortical and cancellous bone of variable thickness and density to produce summated radiologic images.[20] The common linear and regional summations within the acetabulum include the acetabular roof, the tear drop, and the ilioischial line.

The acetabular roof appears as a prominent curved line because of the summation of a broad area of iliac bone, including the dense subchondral bone and the adjacent trabecular bone. Its radiologic appearance resembles an eyebrow, hence its French description, *sourcil*.[21] The portion of the acetabular roof imaged varies with patient positioning and X-ray projection. The teardrop was originally named the *Tranenfigur* (tear figure) by Köhler and was also referred to as the "U figure" by Letournel and Judet.[22] This U-shaped structure is the summation of the anterior and medial portions of the acetabular fossa. The lateral limb of the tear drop represents the external cortex of the acetabular fossa, as it continues into the acetabular roof, whereas the medial limb represents the anterior flat part of the quadrilateral plate (interior of the acetabular wall), and the inferior segment of the tear drop represents the acetabular notch.

The ilioischial line is formed by the summation of radiodensities from approximately the posterior four fifths of the quadrilateral plate and the posterior medial portion of the subjacent ischium.[18,20] The radiographic image of this region is derived from the surface that is tangential to the x-ray beam, and it varies with patient positioning. The ilioischial line usually overlies the tear figure but this relationship varies with as little as 10° of horizontal obliquity from the true anteroposterior radiograph.[23,24] Consequently, the acetabular tear figure is a more constant reference of the medial acetabular wall.

Assessment of Bone Deficiency
The majority of acetabular revisions are adequately imaged preoperatively with plain radiographs, including anteroposterior and Judet's oblique views. The initial radiographic assessment involves an assessment of the type and interface stability of the existing component. Some acetabular components may be associated with a characteristic lytic pattern. The traditional Charnley acetabular cementing technique involves 3 cement holes, and a subsequent defect can be reliably predicted in the ischium, pubis, and superior dome at these sites when the cement is removed. Loose cementless acetabular components tend to displace into an attitude of retroversion, with superior migration and destruction of the anterior col-

umn to a greater extent than the posterior column.

The failure of acetabular components usually leads to progressive bone deficiency in a somewhat predictable manner. The vectors of force on loose acetabular components result in a superior, posterior, and medial force. However, the direction of maximal bone lysis is additionally influenced by the type of component and quality of host bone. The net result of hip forces and susceptibility to bone lysis is migration of the component in the direction of maximal bone deficiency and relative sparing of the remaining supporting structures.[25] Superior migration indicates a deficiency of the acetabular dome. Superolateral migration indicates an additional deficiency of the lateral roof but probable sparing of the medial wall, which has prevented medial migration. Superomedial migration indicates a deficiency of the dome and medial wall but probable sparing of the lateral acetabular rim. Medial migration usually spares the acetabular roof.

Migration from the original acetabular position indicates bone lysis in the direction of failure but prior radiographs often are unavailable. If initial radiographs are unavailable for comparison, our next preferred reference is the anatomically normal contralateral hip. Superior migration from the original or ideal acetabular position is measured from the inferior border of the tear drop.[26] If there is severe medial wall lysis with obliteration of the tear drop, the superior-medial border of the obturator foramen (the obturator line) is an alternative reference point and lies within 5 mm of the teardrop line.[26] Medial or lateral migration is measured from the medial border of the tear drop, if present, or from the ilioischial line.[27]

In the absence of a normal contralateral hip, the radiologic anatomy

can be used to determine the ideal acetabular position (and migration from this) even in the presence of previously abnormal anatomy (such as hip dysplasia) or severe osteolysis. The acetabular position is determined by Ranawat's method[28] using the intersection of Shenton's line and the ilioischial line, and measuring the true pelvic height. Ranawat defined the inferior-medial acetabulum by measuring 5 mm medial to the intersection of these 2 lines. The acetabular height is one fifth of the height of the pelvis measured at this point. These measures can be used to determine the true inferior and superior location of the acetabulum.

Careful study of the oblique radiographs usually demonstrates the acetabular anatomy sufficiently to characterize the bone deficiency and the remaining support for the new cup. The posterior column and anterior rim are best seen on the iliac oblique views and the anterior column and posterior rim are seen on the obturator oblique views. Particular attention should be paid to the integrity of the acetabular roof, the posterior column, and the medial wall, because they are important contributors to the stability of the cup and are common sites of bone deficiency.[29,30] The roof is seen on the AP radiograph and the obturator oblique radiograph, where the anterior and posterior columns converge (Fig. 1). Posterior column deficiencies may be seen on the iliac oblique radiograph and by a break in the ilioischial line on the AP radiograph. If there is a defect in the ilioischial line combined with a deficiency of the anterior column, the surgeon should suspect a discontinuity of the pelvis. Medial wall deficiencies should be suspected when there is a deficiency of the tear drop, but they may be obscured by an overlying metal-backed cup.

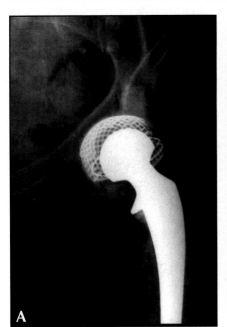 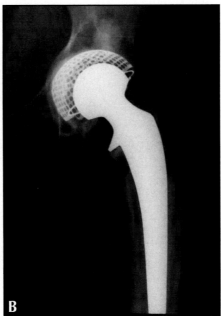 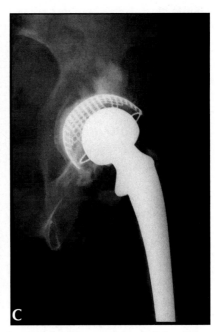

Fig. 1 A, Obturator oblique view. **B,** Anteroposterior view. **C,** Iliac oblique view. In this case, there is minimal deficiency of the medial wall, but there is an intact rim of bone medially. Because of the large keying hole in the ilium superiorly, a cavitary defect within the superior portion of the acetabulum will result following removal of the implant.

Additional imaging techniques are occasionally necessary. We rarely use additional imaging modalities such as computed tomography (CT) to demonstrate the anatomy further, although others have reported the benefits of such techniques.[31-33] CT has been used to define the medial wall, but radiographic scatter from a metal-backed cup may limit its utility. If a customized acetabular implant or a double cup is being considered, a scan may be very useful to help define the anatomy and assist in the manufacture of preoperative foam models of the defect.[34-36] CT can also accurately characterize discrete periacetabular deficiencies, such as isolated lytic lesions associated with fixation screw holes and fixation screws.

When an intrapelvic acetabular component is to be removed, we strongly recommend the use of angiography to define the relationship of the component to the iliac

vessels.[37] Gruen and associates[38] have described a new technique for imaging both the acetabulum and adjacent vessels with 3-dimensional angio-computed tomography, but we have no experience with this technique.

In summary, careful review of the anteroposterior and Judet views of the pelvis allows the surgeon to make a careful assessment of the bone stock deficiency preoperatively. Despite our best efforts, however, this assessment may not be entirely accurate, and the surgeon has to be prepared to deal with more severe bone defects at the actual time of surgery. In order to standardize the nomenclature of bone loss within the acetabulum, classifications systems to describe the degree of bone loss have evolved.

Classification of Acetabular Bone Deficiency

Numerous classification systems have been recommended to date.[25,39-45] The American Academy of Orthopaedic

Surgeons (AAOS) currently recommends the descriptive classification of D'Antonio.[31] The original AAOS classification system[40] was simplified by Engh and Glassman.[41,42] Chandler and Penenberg[39] proposed a very comprehensive classification system for acetabular bone loss. Paprosky and associates[25,43] presented a different classification system based on the various reconstructive strategies that are available. Finally, Gross and associates[44,45] proposed a classification system based on the type of bone graft needed for the reconstruction.

The American Academy of Orthopaedic Surgeons Classification

In 1989, the American Academy of Orthopaedic Surgeons (AAOS) Committee on the Hip proposed a classification system for acetabular deficiencies in total hip arthroplasty.[40] A simplified modification of the original classification has since been adopted (Table 1).[31]

Table 1
The American Academy of Orthopaedic Surgeons classification system for acetabular deficiencies in total hip arthroplasty[31]

Type	Defect
Type I	Segmental deficiencies
A	Peripheral
B	Medial
Type II	Cavitary deficiencies
A	Peripheral
B	Central
Type III	Combined deficiencies
Type IV	Pelvic discontinuity
Type V	Arthrodesis

Table 2
The Engh and Glassman classification of acetabular bone loss

Type	Bone Loss
Type I - mild	Minimal - Both rim and cavity are intact
Type II - moderate	Rim deficient, cavity intact
Type III - severe*	Both rim and cavity deficient

*Protrusio acetabuli and pelvic discontinuity are subcategories of type III bone loss [42,43]

Two basic categories are used in this system: segmental and cavitary bone loss. Segmental deficiency is defined as any complete loss of bone in the supporting hemispheric structure of the acetabulum, whereas a cavitary deficiency is defined as a localized volumetric loss of bone that does not disrupt the acetabular rim. In this system, the rim includes the medial wall. Either segmental or cavitary deficiencies may be peripheral or medial. Although the initial classification[40] subdivided peripheral segmental or cavitary deficiencies into superior, anterior, or posterior, this geographic distinction has been omitted from the current classification system.[31] If the medial wall is absent, in whole or in part, this is by definition a central segmental deficiency. However, if the medial wall is thin and medialized, but still intact, as in protrusio acetabuli; it is a central cavitary deficiency. Examples of peripheral deficiencies include cases of congenital dislocation of the hip in which the superior portion of the acetabulum is deficient. If the rim is deficient, it is a segmental deficiency. If the rim is intact, but there is a contained defect within the dome, it is a pure peripheral cavitary deficiency. If a large portion of the dome of the acetabulum is deficient, in addition

to the rim, it is both a segmental and cavitary deficiency. This third type of deficiency combines segmental and cavitary defects. The fourth type of deficiency is pelvic discontinuity. In this type, bone loss extends from the anterior to the posterior column and separates the superior and inferior portions of the acetabulum. In this catastrophic deficiency, reconstruction should not be attempted until the stability of the pelvis is restored by appropriate fixation. The last type of deficiency, or arthrodesis, is mentioned for completeness, although technically it is not a deficiency. It is included in this system because of the technical difficulties that are encountered during reconstruction.

Engh and Glassman Modification of the AAOS Classification

The original AAOS classification was modified by Engh and Glassman.[41,42] The modified classification system is simpler and consists of three categories (Table 2). Type I damage is mild. The acetabular rim and cavity are intact. This type is seen in cases with minor dysplasia or in revision arthroplasty with minimal bone loss. In type II, or moderate damage, the rim is deficient but the cavity is intact. This type is the same as segmental deficiency in the AAOS classification system. Type III damage, in which both the rim and cavity are

deficient, is the most severe type of bone loss in this classification system. Protrusio acetabuli with an intra-pelvic component and pelvic discontinuity are subcategories of type III damage.

Chandler and Penenberg Classification

Chandler and Penenberg[39] outlined their classification of acetabular bone loss based on the anatomic division of the acetabulum into a superior wall, anterior and posterior columns, and a medial wall. They further subdivided the anterior and posterior columns into a corresponding rim peripherally and an intra-acetabular portion more centrally. The different subtypes are shown in Outline 2.

Of the rim defects, superior rim defects were the deficiency most commonly encountered.[39] These defects are often seen in primary total hip arthroplasty, particularly in cases of developmental dysplasia. The significance of these defects is that the walls of the ilium converge acutely within 1 to 2 cm of the roof of the acetabulum. The pelvis is quite thin at that level and may not accommodate an acetabular component. Combined rim defects (eg, superior and posterior) were most commonly the result of a failed previous arthroplasty.

Intra-acetabular defects affect the bone stock of the anterior and posterior columns and the dome of the acetabulum without affecting the hemispheric rim of the acetabulum. Isolated intra-acetabular defects are rare.[39] These defects are commonly seen in association with a rim or medial wall defect. The most common cause of isolated intra-acetabular defects is previous surgery, with osteolysis around the keying hole of a cemented component or around the screw of a cementless shell.

Protrusio acetabuli signifies medial migration of the center of rotation of the hip joint. It is commonly seen in revision surgery, caused by medial migration of a hemiarthroplasty, a bipolar component, or a cemented or cementless cup. There may or may not be perforation of the medial wall.

Isolated perforation of the medial acetabular wall is uncommon, except as a technical error; however, it may be seen in combination with other deficiencies. The significance of this deficiency is the communication between the hip joint and the pelvic cavity, particularly if cement is to be used for the cup fixation.

Combined deficiencies are subdivided into six subtypes, depending on the pattern of bone loss, and are combinations of the isolated deficiencies described above (Outline 2). The combined deficiencies are most often encountered in revision surgery for failed total hip arthroplasty.

Paprosky Classification

The Paprosky classification system[25,43] is somewhat different from the above 3 systems. This system is designed to assess failed total hip replacements. The main parameters that are assessed are: (1) the degree of superior migration of the cup–whether it is greater than 2 cm or not; (2) lysis of the ischium, which is indicative of posterior column bone loss; (3) the integrity of Köhler's line,[46] which determines the ability of the anteromedial portion of acetabular bone to support a prosthesis; and (4) the presence or absence of a teardrop[19] indicating whether the inferomedial part of the acetabulum is able to allow the osteointegration of a porous-coated acetabular component, particularly if a structural allograft is used superiorly. There are 3 broad classes of acetabular defects in this classification system (Table 3).

A type I defect has an intact rim with no lysis or cup migration. There

is some bone loss with some lytic lesions without compromise of the integrity of the acetabular fossa. Because of the minimal bone loss, the acetabulum is capable of supporting a standard porous-coated acetabular component, with or without a small amount of morcellized bone graft.

A type II defect has superior and/or medial bone loss. The anterior and posterior columns are intact, and there is minimal lysis of the ischium. There are 3 subtypes in this classification system. In types IIA and IIB, there is superior migration of the cup that does not exceed 2 cm, and in addition to the intact anterior and posterior columns, Köhler's line and the teardrop are also intact. The migration in type IIA defects is superior, because the superior rim is intact and the dome is cavitated; whereas in type IIB defects, migration is superolateral because of loss of the superior rim as well as the dome. Because superior migration is under 2 cm, and because of the intact anterior, posterior, and medial bone stock, the acetabular bone stock in this type of defect is capable of supporting an acetabular component, without any need for structural bone grafting. In type IIC defects, there is loss of the teardrop as well, suggest-

Table 3

The Paprosky classification system for acetabular bone loss in revision total hip replacement[25,44]

Type	Defect
Type I	Supportive rim no bone lysis or migration
Type II	Distorted hemisphere with intact supportive columns less than 2 cm superomedial or lateral migration
Type IIA	Superomedial
Type IIB	Superolateral (no superior dome)
Type IIC	Medial only
Type III	Superior migration greater than 2 cm and severe ischial and medial osteolysis
Type IIIA	Köhler's line intact, 30% to 60% of component supported by graft (bone loss 10 o'clock to 2 o'clock)
Type IIIB	Köhler's line not intact, more than 60% of component supported by graft (bone loss 9 o'clock to 5 o'clock)

ing loss of the medial wall. In such cases, the component may migrate medially as well.

A type III defect has more than 2 cm of superior migration, as well as severe ischial and medial osteolysis. Because of this degree of bone loss, the acetabular rim is incapable of supporting a standard acetabular component at the anatomic hip cen-

Table 4
The classification system for acetabular deficiencies in total hip arthroplasty as proposed by Gross et al[45,46]

Type	Deficiency
Type I	Contained
Type II	Noncontained
Type IIA	Shelf/minor column < 50% of cup coverage
Type IIB	Major column > 50% loss of cup contact loss of 1 or both columns

ter without bone grafting. Type III defects have been subdivided into type IIIA and type IIIB defects. In type IIIA defects, there is bone loss from the 10 o'clock to the 2 o'clock positions, and Köhler's line remains intact, suggesting that the medial wall of the acetabulum is intact. In type IIIB defects, there is bone loss from the 9 o'clock to the 5 o'clock positions, and Köhler's line is not intact, suggesting that a significant portion of the revised acetabular component will be in contact with structural bone graft, and therefore bone ingrowth cannot be relied on. In this case, a cemented cup should be used instead.

Gross Classification

Gross and associates classified acetabular defects based on the type and size of bone graft needed for the reconstruction (Table 4).[44,45] This simple classification system has 3 types. One contained and 2 noncontained. Type I is a contained cavitary defect within the medial wall of the acetabulum, with no loss affecting the acetabular walls and columns. The 2 noncontained defects are type 2a, a shelf (minor column) defect, in which bone loss affects a part of the acetabular rim and its associated wall or column. Less than 50% of the acetabulum is defective. Type 2b is an acetab-

ular (major column) defect. This major type of bone loss, affects one or both columns, and it involves at least 50% of the acetabulum.

Preoperative Planning vis-à-vis Acetabular Bone Loss

Although accurate preoperative templating and planning are essential parts of a revision procedure, it is important to be aware of the limitations of assessing the bone deficiency preoperatively. The bone deficiency classification systems detailed above describe the intraoperative deficiency after removal of the failed component. Frequently, the bone deficiency encountered after component removal is more extensive than suggested by preoperative imaging,[47] and we recommend that the surgical plan include a strategy to manage an unexpectedly larger deficiency. Furthermore, an experienced surgeon will always anticipate the potential complications that can occur while removing the old components or while preparing the acetabulum to accept the new components. A complete preoperative plan always includes a fall-back position in case the unexpected occurs.

Following the radiographic assessment of bone deficiency, the degree of bone loss is classified and the reconstruction is planned with reference to 5 important questions: (1) Is there sufficient host bone to allow a standard acetabular component to achieve stability and restore the center of rotation, with or without morcellized bone grafting but without structural grafting? (2) Is there a segmental acetabular deficiency that will require augmentation with structural allograft, or can a high hip center be accepted? (3) Is the bone loss so severe that stable cup support and fixation will not be achieved by a simple segmental bone graft alone?

(4) Is there pelvic discontinuity? (5) What is the best surgical approach for this procedure?

When a large cavitary defect is encountered, it may be necessary to use a component of larger size. Overlying the radiographs with templates will approximate the component size required and indicate the need for an oversized component. Allograft or autograft from reamings may be needed to fill small deficiencies, such as cement keying holes. Figure 1 demonstrates a failed component that will be associated with a medial cavitary defect and superior cavitary deficiency of the acetabular roof. The obturator oblique radiographs demonstrate sufficient support for a hemispheric cup and the AP radiographs suggest a component of standard size will suffice. This case contrasts with that of Figure 2, which is also a cavitary defect with a smaller segmental deficiency of the acetabular floor. This defect is classified as an AAOS type III, Paprosky type IIA, and Gross type 1. The reconstruction can be achieved by a cementless hemispheric component, but of larger than standard size (so-called jumbo cup), while accepting a higher hip center.

Segmental deficiencies of the medial wall vary in complexity. Some deficiencies can largely be ignored and reconstructed with nonsupportive medial grafting (Fig. 3) if there is sufficient peripheral cup support. If there is insufficient peripheral stability at the time of trial fitting of the component, the surgeon should be prepared to substitute for the medial wall with a reconstruction cage or similar device. This defect is classified as an AAOS type III, Paprosky type 2A, and Gross type 1. Unfortunately, the bone deficiency classifications do not address the nature of reconstruction required, hence the need to plan

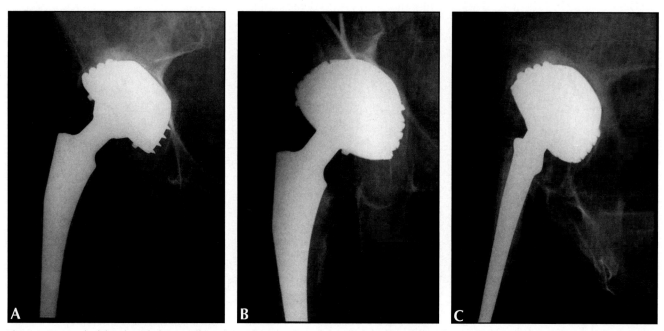

Fig. 2 A, Removal of this threaded cup will result in a large cavitary defect and small medial wall segmental deficiency. The reconstruction will require oversized components to accommodate the increased acetabular volume. The center of rotation of the hip joint will be raised by no more than 2 cm. The obturator oblique view (**B**) shows more destruction of the anterior column than the posterior column, as seen on the iliac oblique view (**C**).

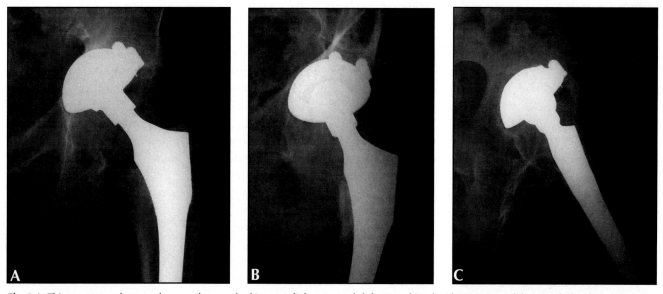

Fig. 3 A, This overreamed cementless cup has resulted in a medial segmental defect combined with cavitation of the acetabular dome. The extent of bone loss in the medial wall of the acetabulum is more extensive than in Figure 2. The remainder of the acetabular anatomy is relatively preserved. The reconstruction can be performed with a larger cementless cup and morcellized medial graft. The Judet views show more destruction of the anterior column (**B**) than the posterior column (**C**).

for both options. Figure 4 demonstrates a more severe medial deficiency with a diverging defect that will not adequately support a hemispheric press fit cup. This defect will predictably require a formal reconstruction of the medial wall with either morcellized or structural allograft and a reconstruction cage.

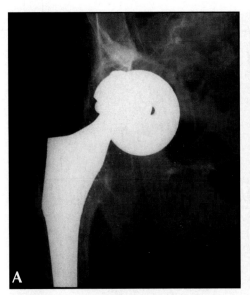 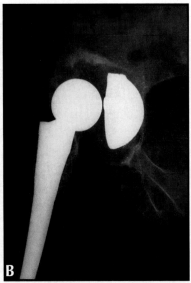 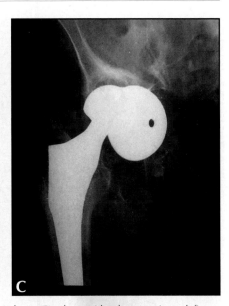

Fig. 4 In this case, there is severe destruction of the anterior column (**A**) as well as the posterior column (**B**), along with a large cavitary deficiency of the acetabular roof (**C**). This creates a massive divergent medial wall defect. Unlike the smaller segmental deficiency in Figure 3, this deficiency requires a reconstruction of the medial wall, probably using a reconstruction cage.

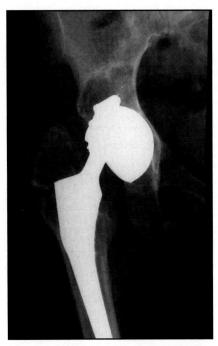

Fig. 5 Periprosthetic bone lysis has resulted in a large superior segmental defect and inadequate acetabular roof. The reconstructive options include a superior segmental graft such as a figure-of-7 graft, impacted or supported morcellized allograft, a custom implant such as an oblong cup, or accepting a high hip center.

Superior dome deficiencies may be evident on the AP or the obturator oblique radiographs. We find the obturator oblique film of great value in determining the remaining support from the acetabular dome (Fig. 1, *A*). The acetabular dome is magnified on the radiograph as the affected side of the pelvis is rotated toward the X-ray beam, and a deficiency seen on this view should be analyzed very carefully. This deficiency may result from periarticular osteolysis or from a previous deficiency, such as hip dysplasia, resulting in a high hip center.

Several reconstructive options are available for a superior dome deficiency (Fig. 5) including acceptance of a high hip center, bulk allograft reconstruction, impaction allografting, and customized components, such as oblong cups. The choice of reconstruction is controversial and all options will require careful planning and measurement of the ideal height of hip center. We find it useful to template the intended components on the radiographs and mea-

sure the height of the hip center. Alternatively, the components are templated at the true center of rotation, and the reconstruction of the remaining deficiency is planned. Surgeons using custom implants may require further studies, such as CT.

Inadequate columns represent the most severe bone deficiency and should be recognized preoperatively, because a complex reconstruction with specialized equipment such as allograft and internal fixation will be needed. This deficiency (Fig. 6) will be suspected when the acetabulum has migrated superiorly a considerable distance, such as the type 3 deficiencies of Paprosky and associates.[25,43] Close examination of the posterior column on the iliac oblique radiograph and inspection of ischial lysis and the ilioischial line on the AP radiograph will suggest this deficiency. Lysis of the tear drop, ilioischial line, and anterior column will determine the amount of host bone remaining for support of the new components. These deficiencies require preopera-

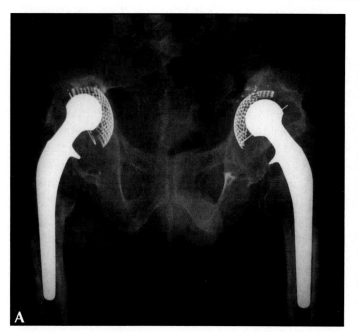
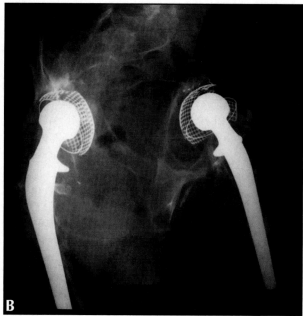

Fig. 6 Both hips show substantial acetabular bone stock deficiency. The anteroposterior view (**A**) shows superior and medial migration of the acetabular component. There is a possibly a fracture in the anterior column (**B**), with a very thin posterior column. The possibility of pelvic dissociation exits, and internal fixation of the pelvis may be required.

tive planning to determine the height of hip center and the reconstructive hardware and grafting required. Careful evaluation of both columns may suggest the presence of, or potential for, the most severe deficiency, a discontinuity, which will require stabilization of the posterior column. Our intraoperative protocol includes stabilization of discontinuities, grafting of deficiencies, and restoration of the hip center. During templating it is important to determine the true hip center and the size of the components available, particularly when considering a reconstruction cage with limited size availability. The use of a large cage may obviate the need for structural grafting, provided there is contact between the reconstruction cage and the dome of the acetabulum. If such contact is not possible, bone stock can be augmented with a bulk allograft. Similarly, severe column deficiencies require a considerable volume of structural allograft bone, in addition

to the reconstruction cages and adequate internal fixation.

Prior to embarking on a revision hip arthroplasty, the surgeon should carefully consider if it can be adequately managed by one of the standard approaches used in primary hip arthroplasty. If not, consideration should be given to an extended exposure. In addition, the necessity to proceed to one of the dedicated revision approaches should be recognized.

The particular design of the acetabular component does not usually influence the surgical approach, because good circumferential visualization is required for the removal of both cemented and uncemented designs. More extensive exposure of the outer table of the ilium is required if a reconstruction cage with a prominent flange is to be removed or inserted, or if allograft reconstruction of a superolateral or posterior column deficiency is necessary.

When revising a hip arthroplasty

for recurrent dislocation, the surgeon needs to consider the soft-tissue anatomy, which contributes to the stability of the joint. The direction of instability should be determined from history and physical examination, as well as from an intraoperative examination under anesthesia, which will help to determine whether preservation of the anterior or the posterior soft-tissue envelope is more important during exposure.

Not uncommonly, it is necessary to revise an acetabular component in the presence of a solidly fixed cemented or bioingrown femoral stem. The femoral component can generally be preserved in these situations unless a nonmodular component shows evidence of damage to the surface of the femoral head. Exposure of the acetabulum in this situation can be facilitated in a number of ways. Firstly, the femoral head may be removed if the component is modular and the less bulky neck can be retracted more easily while taking care to protect the Morse taper from damage. Secondly, if the stem is lying within an intact cement mantle, it may be removed and reimplanted into the same mantle following successful revision of the acetabular side.[48,49] Finally, the intact femoral component can be retracted anteriorly or posteriorly after adequate mobilization of the proximal femur. Placing the femoral head in a soft-tissue pocket anterior to the acetabulum may further facilitate exposure.[50]

Total acetabular allografts and stabilization of hemipelvic discontinuity require wide exposure of the acetabulum, posterior column, ischium, and the outer table of the ilium. The abductors need generous mobilization, now conveniently achieved by a trochanteric osteotomy or one of its modifications: trochanteric slide or the extended trochanteric osteotomy. Rarely, even more extensive exposure of the acetabulum may be favored for massive acetabular allografts, management of pelvic discontinuity, or tumor resections. The triradiate approach[51] or a double-incision approach (posterior and ilioinguinal) may be necessary in such circumstances.

The removal of an intrapelvic acetabular component or infected intrapelvic cement via any of the conventional approaches to the hip is associated with risk of serious injury to pelvic contents.[52,53] The sigmoid colon or cecum, rectum, bladder, and iliac vessels are the principal structures at risk in any penetration of the floor of the true acetabulum.[54] The risk of injury to these structures by traction on the prosthesis or cement is increased by the intense fibrous reaction they can provoke. Preoperative angiography of the iliac vessels is advisable when the protrusio is substantial and there is a possibility that the vessels lying interposed between the acetabular component and the pelvis. Eftekhar and Nercessian[55] reported 4 such cases, in which the intrapelvic components were removed under direct vision using the lateral 2 windows of a modified ilioinguinal approach. Prior to this, the femoral components were removed via a separate transtrochanteric approach. Petrera and associates[56] have described their experience in 23 patients with an initial retroperitoneal approach to the iliac vessels, which is closed, and followed by a revision hip arthroplasty in a standard manner. Grigoris and associates[57] reported 9 cases in which the intrapelvic cup was removed by subperiosteal mobilization of iliacus from the inner table of the pelvis. However, they recommended that a retroperitoneal approach should be used if the preoperative angiogram revealed a false aneurysm or if the cement mass to be removed is particularly large.

In general, anterolateral approaches to the hip should be reserved for simple revisions. These approaches are nonextensile, as they cannot be converted to a trochanteric osteotomy without compromising the blood supply of the trochanteric fragment and jeopardizing the reattachment of the abductors. If a trochanteric osteotomy is likely to be necessary, it should be performed before the anterior two thirds of the abductors have been unnecessarily detached. For this reason, the posterior approach is certainly more versatile, because it allows ready extension of the exposure to a classic trochanteric osteotomy or a trochanteric slide if wider exposure is required.

Of the commonly used surgical approaches, the widest exposure of the acetabulum is provided by a classical trochanteric osteotomy with proximal retraction of the trochanteric fragment and the attached abductor muscles. This is particular-ly appropriate when the femur has been medialized as a result of migration of the acetabular component into the pelvis. Particular attention should be paid to the sciatic nerve in these instances, because the medial migration of the femur can render it very superficial. Trochanteric osteotomy also provides the widest exposure of the superolateral rim of the acetabulum when this is required for the purpose of placing a reconstruction cage or a bulk allograft. Similar exposure can be achieved using the trochanteric slide.[58,59]

We favor the trochanteric slide in most instances in which a trochanteric osteotomy would be considered. This approach affords particularly good access when there is close approximation of the proximal femur to the acetabulum, such as severe protrusio, or when there is marked preoperative stiffness. It should be considered for stiff hips with poor femoral bone stock because of the risk of periprosthetic femoral fracture at the time of dislocation. The comprehensive acetabular exposure is particularly helpful when total or superior acetabular allografts are required, to allow fixation of acetabular cages or plating of the posterior column. Dynamizing the hip by advancement of the trochanteric fragment can be used to advantage when substantial limb shortening is anticipated. Cases in which instability may be a problem, such as isolated revision of the acetabular component when a solid monolithic femoral component does not require revision, may also benefit from this approach. Finally, attachment of the abductor mechanism to proximal femoral allografts is greatly facilitated by this approach.

If wide exposure of the proximal femur and its medullary canal are required, the recently popularized extended trochanteric osteotomy has all the advantages of the other 2 osteotomy techniques, with the added advantage of rapid access to the femoral canal.[60]

Conclusions

With adequate preoperative planning, the surgeon should have an assessment of the preoperative deficiencies associated with acetabular revision, including general patient factors and anatomic deficiencies that will require attention during the reconstruction. It is imperative to have a comprehensive assessment of these factors, particularly the nature of the periacetabular bone deficiency, which may require specialized techniques and resources. Many centers will not routinely have sufficient resources to manage the larger bone deficiencies, hence the importance of predicting these cases preoperatively.

References

1. Rorabeck CH, Bourne RB, Laupacis A, et al: A double-blind study of 250 cases comparing cemented with cementless total hip arthroplasty: Cost effectiveness and its impact on health-related quality of life. *Clin Orthop* 1994;298: 156–164.

2. Schulte KR, Callaghan JJ, Kelley SS, Johnston RC: The outcome of Charnley total hip arthroplasty with cement after a minimum twenty-year follow-up: The results of one surgeon. *J Bone Joint Surg* 1993;75A:961–975.

3. Kavanagh BF, Dewitz MA, Ilstrup DM, Stauffer RN, Coventry MB: Charnley total hip arthroplasty with cement: Fifteen-year results. *J Bone Joint Surg* 1989;71A:1496–1503.

4. Berry DJ, Barnes CL, Scott RD, Cabanela ME, Poss R: Catastrophic failure of the polyethylene liner of uncemented acetabular components. *J Bone Joint Surg* 1994;76B:575–578.

5. Charnley J (ed): *Low Friction Arthroplasty of the Hip: Theory and Practice.* Berlin, Germany, Springer-Verlag, 1979.

6. Berman AT, Avolio A Jr, DelGallo W: Acetabular osteolysis in total hip arthroplasty: Prevention and treatment. *Orthopedics* 1994;17: 963–965.

7. Cooper RA, McAllister CM, Borden LS, Bauer TW: Polyethylene debris-induced osteolysis and loosening in uncemented total hip arthroplasty: A cause of late failure. *J Arthroplasty* 1992;7:285–290.

8. Morrey BF: Dislocation, in Morrey BF, An KN (eds): *Reconstructive Surgery of the Joints.* New York, NY, Churchill Livingstone, 1996, vol 2, pp 1247–1260.

9. Williams JF, Gottesman MJ, Mallory TH: Dislocation after total hip arthroplasty: Treatment with an above-knee hip spica cast. *Clin Orthop* 1982;171:53–58.

10. Schmalzried TP, Amstutz HC, Dorey FJ: Nerve palsy associated with total hip replacement: Risk factors and prognosis. *J Bone Joint Surg* 1991;73A:1074–1080.

11. Solheim LF, Hagen R: Femoral and sciatic neuropathies after total hip arthroplasty. *Acta Orthop Scand* 1980;51:531–534.

12. Weber ER, Daube JR, Coventry MB: Peripheral neuropathies associated with total hip arthroplasty. *J Bone Joint Surg* 1976;58A:66–69.

13. Spangehl MJ, Younger ASE, Masri BA, Duncan CP: Diagnosis of infection following total hip arthroplasty. *J Bone Joint Surg* 1997;79A: 1578–1588.

14. Barrack RL, Harris WH: The value of aspiration of the hip joint before revision total hip arthroplasty. *J Bone Joint Surg* 1993;75A:66–76.

15. Spangehl MJ, Duncan CP, O'Connell JX, Masri BA: Prospective analysis of preoperative and intraoperative studies for the diagnosis of infection in 210 consecutive revision total hip arthroplasties. Presented at the 64th Annual Meeting of the American Academy of Orthopaedic Surgeons, San Francisco. Rosemont, IL, American Academy of Orthopaedic Surgeons, 1997, p 197.

16. Feldman DS, Lonner JH, Desai P, Zuckerman JD: The role of intraoperative frozen sections in revision total joint arthroplasty. *J Bone Joint Surg* 1995;77A:1807–1813.

17. Lonner JH, Desai P, Dicesare PE, Steiner G, Zuckerman JD: The reliability of analysis of intraoperative frozen sections for identifying active infection during revision hip or knee arthroplasty. *J Bone Joint Surg* 1996;78A: 1553–1558.

18. Judet R, Judet J, Letournel E: Fractures of the acetabulum: Classification and surgical approaches for open reduction: Preliminary report. *J Bone Joint Surg* 1964;46A:1615–1646.

19. Bowerman JW, Sena JM, Chang R: The teardrop shadow of the pelvis: Anatomy and clinical significance. *Radiology* 1982;143:659–662.

20. Pitt MJ, Lund PJ, Speer DP: Imaging of the pelvis and hip. *Orthop Clin North Am* 1990;21:545–559.

21. Pauwels F (ed): *Biomechanics of the Normal and Diseased Hip: Theoretical Foundation, Technique, and Results of Treatment. An Atlas.* Berlin, Germany, Springer-Verlag, 1976.

22. Letournel E, Judet R, Elson RA: *Fractures of the Acetabulum.* Berlin, Germany, Springer-Verlag, 1981.

23. Armbuster TG, Guerra J Jr, Resnick D, et al: The adult hip: An anatomic study. Part I: The bony landmarks. *Radiology* 1978;128:1–10.

24. Goodman SB, Adler SJ, Fyhrie DP, Schurman DJ: The acetabular teardrop and its relevance to acetabular migration. *Clin Orthop* 1988;236:199–204.

25. Paprosky WG, Perona PG, Lawrence JM: Acetabular defect classification and surgical reconstruction in revision arthroplasty: A 6-year follow-up evaluation. *J Arthroplasty* 1994;9:33–44.

26. Massin P, Schmidt L, Engh CA: Evaluation of cementless acetabular component migration: An experimental study. *J Arthroplasty* 1989;4:245–251.

27. Hubbard MJ: The measurement of progression in protrusio acetabuli. *Am J Roentgenol Radium Ther Nucl Med* 1969;106:506–508.

28. Ranawat CS, Dorr LD, Inglis AE: Total hip arthroplasty in protrusio acetabuli of rheumatoid arthritis. *J Bone Joint Surg* 1980;62A:1059–1065.

29. Perona PG, Lawrence J, Paprosky WG, Patwardhan AG, Sartori M: Acetabular micromotion as a measure of initial implant stability in primary hip arthroplasty: An in vitro comparison of different methods of initial acetabular component fixation. *J Arthroplasty* 1992;7:537–547.

30. Vasu R, Carter DR, Harris WH: Stress distributions in the acetabular region: I. Before and after total joint replacement. *J Biomech* 1982;15:155–164.

31. D'Antonio JA: Periprosthetic bone loss of the acetabulum: Classification and management. *Orthop Clin North Am* 1992;23:279–290.

32. Horne G: Preoperative assessment of the acetabulum. *Orthop Clin North Am* 1993;24:655–661.

33. Robertson DD, Magid D, Poss R, Fishman EK, Broker AF, Sledge CB: Enhanced computed tomographic techniques for the evaluation of total hip arthroplasty. *J Arthroplasty* 1989;4:271–276.

34. Stiehl JB: Acetabular allograft reconstruction in total hip arthroplasty. Part II: Surgical approach and aftercare. *Orthop Rev* 1991;20:425–432.

35. Bargar WL: Preoperative planning in revision total hip replacement surgery. *Orthop Rev* 1990;(suppl):16–22.

36. Sutherland CJ: Treatment of type III acetabular deficiencies in revision total hip arthroplasty without structural bone-graft. *J Arthroplasty* 1996;11:91–98.

37. al-Salman M, Taylor DC, Beauchamp CP, Duncan CP: Prevention of vascular injuries in revision total hip replacement. *Can J Surg* 1992;35:261–264.

38. Gruen GS, Mears DC, Cooperstein LA: Three-dimensional angio-computed tomography: New technique for imaging the acetabulum and adjacent vessels in a patient with acetabular protrusio. *J Arthroplasty* 1989;4: 353–360.

39. Chandler HP, Penenberg BL (eds): *Bone Stock Deficiency in Total Hip Replacement: Classification and Management.* Thorofare, NJ, Slack Inc, 1989.

40. D'Antonio JA, Capello WN, Borden LS, et al: Classification and management of acetabular abnormalities in total hip arthroplasty. *Clin Orthop* 1989;243:126–137.

41. Engh CA, Glassman AH: Cementless revision of failed total hip replacement. *Orthop Rev Suppl* 1990;23–28.

42. Engh CA, Glassman AH: Cementless revision of failed total hip replacement: An update, in Tullos HS (ed): *Instructional Course Lectures XL*. Park Ridge, IL, American Academy of Orthopaedic Surgeons, 1991, pp 189–197.

43. Paprosky WG, Magnus RE: Principles of bone grafting in revision total hip arthroplasty: Acetabular technique. *Clin Orthop* 1994;298: 147–155.

44. Gross AE, Allan DG, Catre M, Garbuz DS, Stockley I: Bone grafts in hip replacement surgery: The pelvic side. *Orthop Clin North Am* 1993;24:679–695.

45. Garbuz D, Morsi E, Mohamed N, Gross AE: Classification and reconstruction in revision acetabular arthroplasty with bone stock deficiency. *Clin Orthop* 1996;324:98–107.

46. DeOrio JK, Blasser KE: Indications and patient selection, in Morrey BF (ed): *Joint Replacement Arthroplasty*. New York, NY, Churchill Livingstone, 1991, pp 547–559.

47. Jerosch J, Steinbeck J, Fuchs S, Kirchhoff C: Radiologic evaluation of acetabular defects on acetabular loosening of hip alloarthroplasty. *Unfallchirurg* 1996;99:727–733.

48. McCallum JD III, Hozack WJ: Recementing a femoral component into a stable cement mantle using ultrasonic tools. *Clin Orthop* 1995; 319:232–237.

49. Lieberman JR, Moeckel BH, Evans BG, Salvati EA, Ranawat CS: Cement-within-cement revision hip arthroplasty. *J Bone Joint Surg* 1993; 75B:869–871.

50. Neil MJ, Solomon MI: A technique of revision of failed acetabular components leaving the femoral component in situ. *J Arthroplasty* 1996; 11:482–483.

51. Stiehl JB, Harlow M, Hackbarth D: Extensile triradiate approach for complex acetabular reconstruction in total hip arthroplasty. *Clin Orthop* 1993;294:162–169.

52. Roberts JA, Loudon JR: Vesico-acetabular fistula. *J Bone Joint Surg* 1987;69B:150–151.

53. Slater RN, Edge AJ, Salman A: Delayed arterial injury after hip replacement. *J Bone Joint Surg* 1989;71B:699.

54. Feeney M, Masterson E, Keogh P, Quinlan W: Risk of pelvic injury from femoral neck guidewires. *Arch Orthop Trauma Surg* 1997;116: 227–228.

55. Eftekhar NS, Nercessian O: Intrapelvic migration of total hip prostheses: Operative treatment. *J Bone Joint Surg* 1989;71A:1480–1486.

56. Petrera P, Trakru S, Mehta S, Steed D, Towers JD, Rubash HE: Revision total hip arthroplasty with a retroperitoneal approach to the iliac vessels. *J Arthroplasty* 1996;11:704–708.

57. Grigoris P, Roberts P, McMinn DJ, Villar RN: A technique for removing an intrapelvic acetabular cup. *J Bone Joint Surg* 1993;75B: 25–27.

58. Mercati E, Guary A, Myquel C, Bourgeon A: A postero-external approach to the hip joint: Value of the formation of a digastric muscle. *J Chir* (Paris) 1972;103:499–504.

59. Glassman AH, Engh CA, Bobyn JD: A technique of extensile exposure for total hip arthroplasty. *J Arthroplasty* 1987;2:11–21.

60. Younger TI, Bradford MS, Magnus RE, Paprosky WG: Extended proximal femoral osteotomy: A new technique for femoral revision arthroplasty. *J Arthroplasty* 1995;10: 329–338.

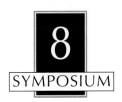

Revision Arthroplasty of the Acetabulum in Association With Loss of Bone Stock

Allan E. Gross, MD, FRCSC
Clive P. Duncan, MD, MSC, FRCSC
Donald Garbuz, MD, FRCSC
Elsayed Morsi Z. Mohamed, MBBCH, MS

The goals of revision arthroplasty of the hip are to relieve pain and to improve function. These goals can be accomplished by insertion of a new implant with stable fixation of the interface and restoration (or at least near restoration) of the anatomy.

Stable fixation may be achieved with use of components inserted either with cement[1,2] or without cement.[3,4] However, marked osteolysis caused by wear debris, abrasion, or inflammation may make this task extremely difficult.[5–13]

If there is no loss of bone stock, the anatomy may be restored by simply inserting a new implant. If there is loss of bone stock on either the acetabular or the femoral side, however, the deficit should be categorized as either contained or uncontained and should be dealt with accordingly.

Contained, or cavitary, defects are more easily dealt with because the skeleton, while weakened, is basically intact. A contained defect of the acetabulum is one in which the anterior and posterior columns and the peripheral supporting bone for the acetabular component are intact. A pelvis with a contained defect can support an implant with a little help.

This help may be biologic (in the form of a bone graft) or it may involve modification of the implant. Impaction grafting with use of morcellized bone is a biological alternative.[14] Large cups and asymmetrical cups that are designed to make contact with host bone, with no or minimum use of morcellized bone, are examples of modified implants that may be used to treat a cavitary defect.[15]

Uncontained, or segmental, defects are more of a challenge. Small and even moderate defects can be dealt with by placing the implant against host bone without structural grafting but perhaps with some compromise of the normal anatomic relationships. Placement of a cup in a high hip-center position without cement allows the cup to make contact with host bone, thereby facilitating biologic fixation by bone ingrowth.[16–18]

If the patient has a large segmental defect and there is no possibility of placing the implant against host bone or of restoring nearly normal anatomy, then the use of a structural bone graft may be indicated. This technique, if successful, restores bone stock and anatomic relationships and, if failure occurs, revision surgery

may be less challenging.[19,20]

Revision of the acetabular side of a total hip arthroplasty requires that considerable resources, including a variety of implants and banked bone, be available to the treating orthopaedic surgeon; that the surgeon be well versed in the use of comprehensive surgical exposures that allow access to the anterior and posterior aspects of the pelvis and femur; and that he or she be aware of and be able to treat the various complications that can occur in association with revision surgery.[21] Some defects are not amenable to any kind of reconstruction and are best treated with arthrodesis[22] or excision arthroplasty.[23,24]

Revision arthroplasty of the hip on the acetabular side is one of the most controversial procedures in orthopaedic surgery, partly because a wide variety of implants and techniques is available and partly because certain issues regarding bone grafting, particularly the use of structural allografts, remain unresolved. In certain situations, however, the restoration of bone stock is necessary. The purpose of this chapter is to describe the principles, surgical techniques, and results of the use of allograft bone, in morcellized and structural form, for the restoration of bone stock in revision arthroplasty of the hip on the acetabular side.

Principles of Bone Grafting

The spectrum of opinion regarding the treatment of bone defects on the acetabular side of an arthroplasty has ranged from recommendations to avoid the use of bone graft whenever possible[17,25] to suggestions that morcellized bone only[14] or complex structural grafts[26] be used. In some situations, bone stock must be restored because the loss of bone is too extensive for alternatives such as the use of a high hip center or the insertion of either a so-called jumbo cup or an asymmetrical cup. Posterior column defects and pelvic discontinuity with associated loss of bone stock are examples of such situations. Also, patients who are likely to need additional revision operations should have restoration of bone stock in order to facilitate another arthroplasty, should one be necessary.[26]

There is broad agreement that the use of structural grafts on the acetabular side may be associated with a guarded long-term prognosis and should be avoided if possible.[16,20,21,25–27] Rates of failure as high as 47% (14 of 30 hips) have been reported at 10 years.[16] However, there are situations in which bulk allograft must be used. If used properly, bulk allograft can provide a successful clinical result without the need for a revision for at least 5 years and can supply bone stock for additional procedures.[27]

Bone grafts can be classified as heterogenous grafts (bone from another species), allografts (bone from the same species), and autogenous grafts (bone from another part of the anatomy of the same individual). Because of the quantity and quality of bone that often is needed for revision operations, an allograft is usually more practical than an autogenous graft. There are, however, certain advantages and disadvantages associated with each type of graft.

Autogenous grafts have the advantages of being nonimmunogenic and, even more importantly, of being best able to induce new bone formation by the host. Their main disadvantages are that the supply of available bone is limited and that the strength, shape, and form of the graft usually cannot duplicate those of the bone that originally was present at the site of the deficit.

Allografts, in contrast, are available in large quantity, can have very good initial strength, and can be shaped to fit almost any deficit. However, they are expensive, immunogenic,[28–30] and not as effective as autogenous grafts for inducing new-bone formation.[28,29,31] Allograft bone can be further classified as morcellized or structural, depending on how it is used.

Morcellized bone (fragments of cancellous bone ranging from 5 to 10 mm in diameter) is used as a filler scaffold in contained defects. It can undergo revascularization and remodeling, and it strengthens with time. If morcellized bone is used with a cup that is designed to be inserted without cement, at least 50% of the cup should make contact with host bone and screws probably will be necessary for fixation.[15] If it is not possible for at least 50% of the cup to make contact with host bone, then a roof-reinforcement ring and a cup that is designed to be inserted with cement,[20] or, alternatively, the technique of cementing into impacted bone,[14] should be used.

The term simulated structural graft is used when bone from another anatomic region is shaped to fit the deficit. For example, the distal aspect of a femur can be sculpted to duplicate an acetabulum. The condyles can be reamed to accept an acetabular cup, and the metaphysis can provide bone for internal fixation to the ilium. Alternatively, a femoral head from either a male donor or a premenopausal female donor can be sculpted to the desired shape.

The term anatomic structural graft is used when the bone is from the same anatomic part as that being duplicated. For example, an acetabular allograft can be used, in whole or in part, to replace an acetabular defect. We have found anatomic grafts easier to shape than simulated grafts. Theoretically, an anatomic graft is better able to withstand the biomechanical forces subsequently placed on it. We prefer to use an anatomic graft, but, if one is not available, then a simulated graft is acceptable.

The advantages of structural grafts include the potential to restore the anatomy and to provide structural support for the implant. The disadvantage of these grafts is that revascularization and remodeling can lead to resorption, collapse, or both; in other words, the grafts weaken with time.

A structural graft is indicated for the treatment of an uncontained defect when it is necessary to restore the anatomy and the limb length and to provide bone support for the implant. However, if the anatomy and the limb length are acceptable and adequate bone stock is available, we prefer to use an alternative method, such as placement of the cup at a high hip center.[17] If a high hip center is used, lateralization of the implant should be avoided and there should be enough bone stock to allow the component to be seated, with or without cement, against healthy host bone.[16,17] The limb-length discrepancy must be compensated for with use of a long-neck femoral component, and impingement of the femoral neck against the ischium must be avoided.[17]

A structural allograft may fail because of resorption or fragmentation.[27] It is therefore important to use an implant that extends from host bone to host bone, thereby bridging and protecting the graft. It also is important to use strong bone. Allograft bone that is obtained from the femoral head of a postmenopausal woman should be used in morcellized form only. For structural grafting of the acetabulum, it has been our custom to use acetabular allografts because they are strong and can be readily sculpted to fit segmental defects in this area. These grafts are fixed with cancellous bone screws, and, if they support more than 50% of the cup, they are protected with a reconstruction ring. Alternatives to the use of a whole acetabular allograft include excision arthroplasty[24] and the insertion of a custom implant.

When a structural allograft is employed, it is important to use morcellized autogenous graft, which usually is available in the surgical field, for bone grafting of the host bone-allograft junctions because allograft bone has poor bone-induction properties.[31]

If an infection is suspected, it must be ruled out before allograft reconstruction and revision arthroplasty is performed. Technetium, gallium, or indium scanning as well as aspiration of the hip may be helpful for this purpose.[32–34] If, at the time of surgery, the findings on gross examination, gram-staining, or frozen-section analysis lead to a suspicion of infection, the reconstruction should be carried out in 2 stages to avoid bone-grafting into an infected site.

Classification of Bone Defects

It is important to have a functional, relatively simple system for the clas-

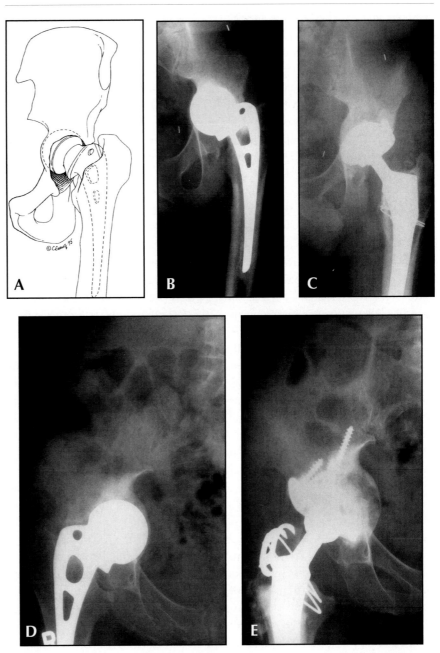

Fig. 1 Type I: Contained cavitary defect. **A,** Drawing illustrates a contained cavitary defect. (Copyright © C. Chang, 1995) **B,** Contained cavitary defect in a 30-year-old man with a superomedial protrusion 5 years after a Moore arthroplasty performed for avascular necrosis. **C,** Eleven years post revision arthroplasty with an uncemented porous coated cup and morcellized allograft bone. **D,** Contained protrusion defect in a 65-year-old female 10 years after a Moore arthroplasty done for a fracture. **E,** Four years after revision arthroplasty with morcellized allograft bone, a roof reinforcement ring and a cemented cup.

sification of bone defects associated with loose hip implants. Although more complicated systems have been described in the literature,[35,36] we have classified acetabular defects as

follows. Type-I, or cavitary, defects are contained; that is, the acetabular walls and columns are intact (Fig. 1). A central defect, even if it involves more than 50% of the acetabulum, may be considered contained as long as the acetabular rim and columns are intact and there is enough bone for the fixation of a cup or ring. Type-II, or segmental, defects are uncontained; that is, they involve structural bone loss. Type-II defects can be classified further as type-IIA defects (those involving less than 50% of the acetabulum) and type-IIB defects (those involving at least 50% of the acetabulum). Type-IIA defects involve loss of part of the rim and the corresponding structural wall (Fig. 2), and type-IIB defects involve loss of one column or both with an associated defect of the corresponding wall or walls, with or without pelvic discontinuity (Fig. 3).

These defects usually can be classified on the basis of plain radiographs. However, the final decision regarding treatment depends on the intraoperative findings after the cement and membrane have been excised. Therefore, an inventory of morcellized and structural bone should be available at the time of surgery.

Surgical Technique

Approach

A contained defect of the acetabulum can be reconstructed through any conventional approach, often without the need for a trochanteric osteotomy. For a structural defect, we prefer to have access to the anterior and posterior columns; therefore, we use a transtrochanteric approach (a so-called trochanteric slide).[37] This type of osteotomy preserves more stability than does a transverse trochanteric osteotomy because the trochanter remains in continuity with the abductor and vastus lateralis muscles and tendons, making trochanteric migration unlikely. If more exposure is needed, the trochanteric slide can be converted to a transverse osteotomy by releasing the vastus lateralis. In our

experience, the prevalence of non-union and trochanteric migration associated with the classic transverse osteotomy was unacceptably high (25%; 32 of 130 hips).[38]

A Steinmann pin is inserted into the iliac crest, and the distance between the pin and a fixed point on the resected trochanteric bed is measured as a reference for limb length. The sciatic nerve should be identified, particularly if limb-lengthening of more than 3 cm is anticipated.

The acetabulum is prepared after the hip has been dislocated. After the acetabular component and the cement have been removed, the interface membrane is gently excised. The defect then is defined by means of visualization, palpation, and the insertion of a trial cup. After the defect has been classified as cavitary or segmental, the decision is made as to which types of reconstruction and bone graft are to be used. Much of this decision-making can be done preoperatively on the basis of the radiographic findings, but the final decision is based on the intraoperative findings.

Preparation of the Graft

The allograft bone, which has been deep-frozen and irradiated at a dose of 2.5 Mrad (25,000 Gy), is not unwrapped until infection in the host joint has been ruled out and the bone defect has been classified. After the graft has been unwrapped and specimens have been obtained for culture, the graft is thawed in a warm, 50% Betadine (povidone-iodine) solution. After the bone has thawed, it is prepared on a separate table. If morcellized bone is needed, morcellization may be carried out manually with use of rongeurs or with use of a bone mill that does not make the bone too mushy. Alternatively, previously prepared morcellized bone can be

obtained from some bone banks in freeze-dried or deep-frozen form. The pieces should be approximately 3 to 5 mm in diameter.

A structural allograft can be prepared from an acetabulum, a femoral head (from either a male donor or a premenopausal female donor), or the distal part of a femur.

The allograft bone is rinsed with a mixture of one third 3% hydrogen peroxide and two thirds normal saline solution and then is rinsed with bacitracin (30,000 units in 1,000 ml of normal saline solution) before it is placed into the acetabular bed. This is our preferred mixture of cleansing solutions, although we have no data to support this combination. As the allograft bone is dead and irradiated, these solutions have no negative effect of which we are aware.

Type-I Defects

To treat type-I defects (Fig. 1), morcellized bone is compacted into the cavitary defect with use of reamers in the reverse mode. A porous-coated acetabular implant that is designed to be inserted without cement can be used if it is possible for at least 50% of the cup to make contact with host bone. Screws usually are needed for fixation.

If it is not possible for at least 50% of the cup to make contact with bleeding host bone, we use a roof-reinforcement ring of the Müller design (Sulzer, Bern, Switzerland), which is impacted superomedially and is held with 2 or 3 cancellous bone screws that are directed into the dome. The cup then is cemented into the ring. It is important that the rim of the ring be in contact with host bone superolaterally and inferiorly or it will not be stable and will loosen, possibly leading to breakage of the screws. If the ring is sitting completely on morcellized bone inferiorly, then a reconstruction

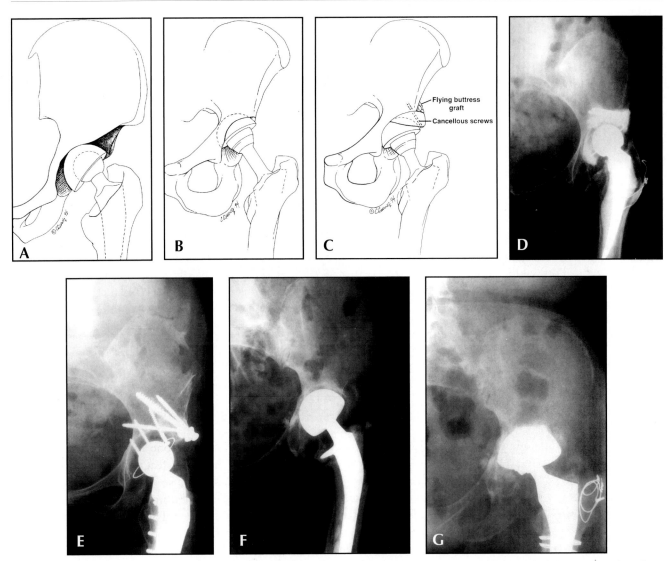

Fig. 2 Type IIA defect: Structural minor column. **A,** Drawing illustrates minor column defect. **B,** Drawing illustrates high hip center with socket placed high in order to place cup completely against host bone in the management of the minor column defect. **C,** Drawing illustrates the use of a structural minor column allograft fixed by 2 cancellous screws. Flying buttress graft is cancellous autograft bone placed between structural allograft and ilium. (Copyright © C. Chang) **D,** Fifty-year-old female with minor column defect 10 years after a cemented total hip arthroplasty. **E,** Nine years post revision arthroplasty with an uncemented cup and a minor column defect. **F,** Seventy-year-old female 8 years following a bipolar arthroplasty with a minor column defect. **G,** Seven years post revision with an uncemented cup placed high against host bone with no graft. Her bone stock was adequate and leg lengths were not a problem.

ring that provides support from the ilium superiorly to the ischium inferiorly should be used.

Type-IIA Defects

A structural acetabular allograft is used for the treatment of type-IIA segmental defects (Fig. 2), which involve less than 50% of the acetabu-lum. The size and shape of the graft are determined with a trial cup in place. A minor column allograft, also termed a shelf graft, which supports less than 50% of the cup, is fixed with two 4.5-mm cancellous bone screws. Because at least 50% of the cup will be in contact with host bone, the cup can be inserted either with or without cement. If the cup is inserted without cement, screws probably will be required. A so-called flying-buttress graft consisting of autogenous mor-cellized cancellous bone is placed between the proximal surface of the structural allograft and the ilium (Fig. 2,C). If possible, the cut surface of the allograft should not be placed in con-

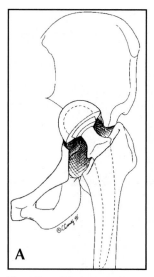 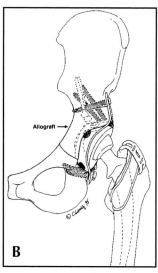 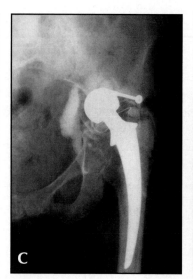 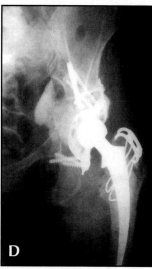

Fig. 3 Type IIB: Structural major column defect. **A,** Drawing illustrating segmental bone loss involving more than 50% of acetabulum with a pelvic discontinuity. **B,** Drawing illustrating reconstruction with major column allograft involving more than 50% of acetabulum. The graft is held with 2 cancellous screws and protected by a reconstruction ring that goes from host bone (ilium) to host bone (ischium). (Copyright © C. Chang, 1995) **C,** Major column defect with pelvic discontinuity 10 years post cemented total hip replacement. **D,** Four years post revision arthroplasty with major column graft fixed with 2 cancellous screws and protected by reconstruction ring fixed to host ilium and ischium bridging the graft. (Reproduced with permission from Garbuz D, Morsi E, Mohamed N, Gross AE: Classification and reconstruction in revision arthroplasty with bone stock deficiency. *Clin Orthop* 1996;323:98–107.)

tact with host soft tissue in order to minimize resorption.

Type-IIB Defects

Type-IIB segmental defects (Fig. 3), which involve at least 50% of the acetabulum, may be associated with pelvic discontinuity. Most commonly, these defects are posterior and superior. An acetabular allograft involving at least 50% of the acetabulum is fashioned to fit the defect and is fixed with two 6.5-mm cancellous bone screws that are directed into residual host bone, usually superoposteriorly. Any associated cavitary defects are filled with morcellized bone. A Burch-Schneider reconstruction ring (Sulzer) that extends from the ilium to the ischium is used to protect the graft; 2 or 3 cancellous bone screws are inserted for fixation at both sites. If fixation of the screws to the ischium is not adequate, then that part of the ring can simply be buttressed against or

slotted into the ischium. Because less than 50% of the cup will be in contact with host bone, the cup must be inserted with cement. The surgeon should try to make contact between at least 50% of the cup and host bone so that a minor column or shelf graft (rather than a major column graft) can be used, for reasons that will be discussed later, in the Results section of this chapter.

Morcellized bone and a roof-reinforcement ring are used for cavitary defects only. A reconstruction ring that spans the defect from the ilium to the ischium is used for segmental defects that involve at least 50% of the acetabulum. In the latter situation, we prefer to use a well fixed structural graft rather than morcellized bone because a structural graft will be load-sharing. If morcellized bone is used, it will not be load-sharing until it remodels. During the remodeling period, therefore, the

ring will bear the entire load; theoretically, this situation could cause the ring to fatigue and break. **(CD–8.1)**

Overview

In summary, cavitary defects are treated with impacted, morcellized allograft bone. If at least 50% of the cup will be in contact with host bone, the cup can be inserted without cement, usually with screw fixation. Otherwise, a roof-reinforcement ring should be used and the cup should be inserted with cement. If a segmental defect cannot be treated by placement of the cup at a high hip center, a structural allograft is used. We attempt to make contact between at least 50% of the cup and host bone so that a minor column or shelf graft can be used. If it is not possible for at least 50% of the cup to make contact with host bone, a major column graft is used. Under these circumstances, the graft should be protected with a reconstruction ring and the cup should be inserted with cement.

Results

Between January 1, 1982, and January 1, 1997, 502 hips were revised using allograft bone at Mount Sinai Hospital, University of Toronto. Of the 502, 418 hips had a revision involving the acetabulum. Of these, 244 of the hips were revised with use of morcellized allograft bone; 67, with use of a minor column allograft; and 107, with use of a major column allograft.

Eleven (4.5%) of the 244 hips that were revised with use of morcellized allograft bone had a repeat revision by January 1, 1997. Seven hips had a repeat revision because of recurrent dislocations and 4, because of loosening of the cup. Fifty-one of the 244 hips were studied after a minimum duration of follow-up of 5 years (average, 6.8 years); the rate of success in that study was 90%.[39] Success was defined as an increase of at least 20 points in the modified Harris hip score, a stable cup (no migration of the cup or fractures of the cement), and no need for an additional operation on the acetabular side. Four hips needed an additional operation on the acetabular side.

Six (9%) of the 67 hips that were revised with use of a minor column allograft had a repeat revision by January 1, 1997. Twenty-nine of the 67 hips were studied after a minimum duration of follow-up of 5 years (average, 7.1 years); the rate of success, as already defined, was 86%.[40] Four patients needed an additional operation on the acetabular side. Three patients had marked resorption of the graft, and two of them needed an additional operation because of loosening of the cup. One patient had an excision arthroplasty because of loosening of the cup. Another patient

had exploration of the joint because of pain, but the graft was intact and the cup was solidly fixed.

Thirty (28%) of the 107 hips that were revised with use of a major column allograft had a repeat revision by January 1, 1997. Ten of these 30 hips had an excision arthroplasty, and the other 20 were revised successfully. The reasons for the excision arthroplasties included loosening of the cup (3 hips), infection (3 hips), dislocation (2 hips), fracture (1 hip), and nonunion (1 hip). The reasons for the other 20 revisions included loosening of the cup (14 hips), dislocation (5 hips), and sciatic-nerve injury (1 hip). Thirty-three of the 107 hips were studied after a minimum duration of follow-up of 5 years (average, 7.1 years); 18 (55%) had a successful result.[41] In that study, success was defined as an increase of at least 20 points in the hip score; a stable cup and a united, structurally intact allograft; and no need for additional surgery related to the acetabulum. Six hips had additional surgery because of loosening of the cup, but the graft was intact and united. One hip had additional surgery for exploration of a sciatic-nerve injury. These 7 hips were considered to have had a partially successful result because no additional bone-grafting was necessary. Eight other hips needed additional surgery because of failure of the graft. The overall success rate was therefore 76% (25 of 33 hips).

In the 502 hips that had a femoral or acetabular revision with restoration of bone stock, complications included 2 deaths related to the operation, 4 vascular and 9 nerve injuries, 41 dislocations (prevalence, 8.2%), and 12 infections (prevalence, 2.4%).

Discussion

Revision arthroplasty of the hip on the acetabular side is a controversial

topic among orthopaedic surgeons. A variety of solutions has been proposed. Although there is agreement that a stable interface must be achieved, the indications for restoration of bone stock, particularly with use of structural allografts, continue to be debated.

The use of morcellized allograft bone for the treatment of cavitary defects is well accepted, and the results have been universally good.[42–47] Morcellized allograft bone can be used in conjunction with cups inserted with or without cement as well as cups inserted with cement and a ring. Heekin and associates,[42] in a retrieval study of 3 cups that had been inserted without cement in conjunction with morcellized allograft bone, reported excellent remodeling and incorporation after an average duration of follow-up of 51 months. Silverton and associates[44,45] also investigated the use of morcellized allograft bone in conjunction with cups that were inserted without cement; those authors reported excellent clinical and radiographic results and a rate of revision of 11% (13 of 115 hips) after an average duration of follow-up of 100 months. Slooff and associates,[46] in a study on the use of impacted allograft bone in conjunction with cups that were inserted with cement, reported excellent clinical and radiographic results for 78 (89%) of 88 hips after an average duration of follow-up of 70 months.[46] At our center, the use of impacted allograft bone and a roof-reinforcement ring in conjunction with a cup inserted with cement yielded a successful result for 15 of 16 hips after an average duration of follow-up of 7 years.[39]

The use of a structural graft is more of a challenge, and mixed results have been reported in the literature.[16,19,36,41] Shinar and Harris[48] reported a rate of failure of more than 60% in a study of 70 structural grafts that had been followed for an average of 16.5 years. Such results have led to the need for alternative solutions. A high hip center allows for contact between the host bone and the acetabular component, making it possible for bone to grow into a cup that has been inserted without cement. This technique produced acceptable intermediate-term results at 40 months in the study by Schutzer and Harris,[18] and it certainly is preferable to the use of a structural graft under some conditions. In order for the technique to be successful, the cup should not be lateralized, contact must be made with healthy bleeding bone, and limb length must be correctable with use of a long-neck or calcar-replacement femoral component.

Under certain circumstances, however, the use of a structural graft is indicated. In younger patients, for example, bone stock should be restored because of the potential for additional revision operations; therefore, if such a patient has a defect that is not contained, a structural graft should be used. Ideally, the graft should support less than 50% of the cup, because the results are much worse when a structural graft supports more than 50% of the cup.[39] There are occasions, however, when the graft must support more than 50% of the cup; in such situations, the prognosis is more guarded.[41]

A structural graft also is indicated when alternatives such as the use of a high hip center or a so-called jumbo cup are not technically possible. This is more likely to be the case when the patient has a posterior column defect or a defect that is associated with pelvic discontinuity.

Our experience with the use of allograft bone for revision arthroplasty of the hip has taught us that, in

order to optimize the result, a number of principles should be adhered to. Cavitary defects should be treated with morcellized bone. If at least 50% of the cup will be in contact with host bone, then the cup can be inserted without cement; otherwise, it should be inserted with cement and a roof-reinforcement ring should be used. If a structural graft is necessary, at least 50% of the cup should make contact with host bone. If less than 50% of the cup will make contact with host bone, the cup should be cemented to the allograft and the allograft should be protected with an internal fixation device that extends from the ilium to the ischium.

The adherence to good surgical principles and the use of good-quality bone from accredited banks have improved the results of restoration of bone stock with allograft bone on the acetabular side. The results associated with the use of morcellized bone[39] and minor column structural grafts[40] have been encouraging and reproducible. These types of grafts are used widely. The use of major column grafts, which support more than 50% of the acetabular component, is more controversial, and the prognosis is more guarded.[41] In some situations, however, the only alternative to the use of such a graft is an excision arthroplasty. In tertiary-care centers that specialize in revision or tumor procedures, the results have been encouraging, although the use of these grafts is still associated with a high rate of repeat revision.[41] Improvements in implants designed to be used as fixation devices for allografts should yield even better results.[41] The quality of the allograft tissue is also important. Optimally, female donors should be less than 55 years old and male donors, less than 60 years old, especially when a structural graft is needed. Allograft bone

that is obtained from the femoral head of a postmenopausal woman should be used in morcellized form only.

Transmission of disease is a potential hazard associated with the use of allograft bone. There are documented instances of transmission of hepatitis C, hepatitis B, and the human immunodeficiency virus through the use of bone allografts.[49,50] Deep-freezing alone does not notably decrease the risk. Radiation, administered at a dose of 2.5 Mrad (25,000 Gy), eliminates all bacteria as well as hepatitis B and C and markedly decreases the bioburden of the human immunodeficiency virus.[49,51,52] A dose of at least 3.0 megarad (30,000 gray) is needed to completely eliminate the DNA of the virus;[51,52] however, such a dose would substantially weaken the bone.[53] It is therefore imperative that strict screening procedures be adhered to and that the bone bank be accredited.[54,55]

Properly screened blood carries a one in 493,000 risk of transmission of the human immunodeficiency virus,[56] whereas properly screened deep-frozen bone that has not been irradiated carries a one in 1,667,600 risk of transmission of the human immunodeficiency virus.[57] Radiation administered at a dose of 2.5 Mrad (25,000 Gy) decreases the risk further but does not eliminate it completely. Antigen tests that narrow the window period for viral detection, and the use of secondary sterilization, have notably decreased the risk of transmission of disease.

Most large tissue banks offer the surgeon a choice of deep-frozen, deep-frozen and irradiated, and freeze-dried bone. Bone used in structural grafts is most commonly deep-frozen or deep-frozen and irradiated. A combination of processing and freeze-drying reduces or eliminates viable organisms but decreases the torsional and bending strength of bone;[58] therefore, we do not use freeze-dried bone for structural grafts.

Allograft bone has limited bone-induction properties.[31] These bone-induction properties are decreased further by irradiation.[53]

In conclusion, restoration of bone stock in revision arthroplasty of the acetabulum remains a challenging problem. The use of morcellized bone for the treatment of cavitary defects and the use of structural grafts that support less than 50% of the cup have provided reproducible, encouraging results. Structural grafts that support more than 50% of the cup are associated with a more guarded prognosis, but in some situations there is no alternative to their use. It is therefore imperative that surgeons who perform arthroplasty develop techniques to improve the performance of these large grafts rather than abandon their use. Better-quality bone and improved internal fixation devices have yielded encouraging results at some tertiary-care centers, but more research in these areas is required. Transmission of disease is a cause for concern throughout the entire field of transplantation, but it is of particular concern in the field of orthopaedic surgery, where the problems usually are not life-threatening but, rather, quality-of-life threatening.

References

1. Estok DM II, Harris WH: Long-term results of cemented femoral revision surgery using second-generation techniques: An average 11.7-year follow-up evaluation. *Clin Orthop* 1994;299:190–202.

2. Strömberg CN, Herberts PG, Hultmark PN: Cemented acetabular revisions, in Galante JO, Rosenberg AG, Callaghan JJ (eds): *Total Hip Revision Surgery*. New York, NY, Raven Press, 1995, pp 311–315.

3. Engh CA Sr, Macalino GE: Clinical results of cementless revision surgery: Are we doing better using extensively porous-coated stems?, in Galante JO, Rosenberg AG, Callaghan JJ (eds): *Total Hip Revision Surgery*. New York, NY, Raven Press, 1995, pp 295–303.

4. Jasty M, Harris WH: Cementless acetabular revisions, in Galante JO, Rosenberg AG, Callaghan JJ (eds): *Total Hip Revision Surgery*. New York, NY, Raven Press, 1995, pp 317–323.

5. Freeman MA, Bradley GW, Revell PA: Observations upon the interface between bone and polymethylmethacrylate cement. *J Bone Joint Surg* 1982;64B:489–493.

6. Goldring SR, Jasty M, Roelke MS, Rourke CM, Bringhurst FR, Harris WH: Formation of a synovial-like membrane at the bone-cement interface: Its role in bone resorption and implant loosening after total hip replacement. *Arthritis Rheumatol* 1986;29:836–842.

7. Goldring SR, Schiller AL, Roelke M, Rourke CM, O'Neil DA, Harris WH: The synovial-like membrane at the bone-cement interface in loose total hip replacements and its proposed role in bone lysis. *J Bone Joint Surg* 1983;65A:575–584.

8. Goodman SB, Schatzker J, Sumner-Smith G, Fornasier VL, Goften N, Hunt C: The effect of polymethylmethacrylate on bone: An experimental study. *Arch Orthop Trauma Surg* 1985;104:50–154.

9. Howie D, Oakeshott R, Manthy B, Vernon-Roberts B: Abstract: Bone resorption in the presence of polyethylene wear particles. *J Bone Joint Surg* 1987;69B:165.

10. Jasty MJ, Floyd WE III, Schiller AL, Goldring SR, Harris WH: Localized osteolysis in stable, non-septic total hip replacement. *J Bone Joint Surg* 1986;68A:912–919.

11. Linder L, Lindberg L, Carlsson A: Aseptic loosening of hip prostheses: A histologic and enzyme histochemical study. *Clin Orthop* 1983;175:93–104.

12. Pazzaglia UE, Ceciliani L, Wilkinson MJ, Dell'Orbo C: Involvement of metal particles in loosening of metal-plastic total hip prostheses. *Arch Orthop Trauma Surg* 1985;104:164–174.

13. Revell PA, Weightman B, Freeman MA, Roberts BV: The production and biology of polyethylene wear debris. *Arch Orthop Trauma Surg* 1978;91:167–181.

14. Slooff TJ, Schimmel JW, Buma P: Cemented fixation with bone grafts. *Orthop Clin North Am* 1993;24:667–677.

15. Tanzer M, Drucker D, Jasty M, McDonald M, Harris WH: Revision of the acetabular component with an uncemented Harris-Galante porous-coated prosthesis. *J Bone Joint Surg* 1992;74A:987–994.

16. Kwong LM, Jasty M, Harris WH: High failure rate of bulk femoral head allografts in total hip acetabular reconstructions at 10 years. *J Arthroplasty* 1993;8:341–346.

17. Russotti GM, Harris WH: Proximal placement of the acetabular component in total hip arthroplasty: A long-term follow-up study. *J Bone Joint Surg* 1991;73A:587–592.

18. Schutzer SF, Harris WH: High placement of porous-coated acetabular components in complex total hip arthroplasty. *J Arthroplasty* 1994;9:359–367.

19. Brick GW, Tsahakis PJ, Sledge CB: Solid allograft reconstruction of acetabular deficiencies, in Galante JO, Rosenberg AG, Callaghan JJ (eds): *Total Hip Revision Surgery*. New York, NY, Raven Press, 1995, pp 325–333.

20. Gross AE: Reconstruction of the acetabulum, in Galante JO, Rosenberg AG, Callaghan JJ (eds): *Total Hip Revision Surgery*. New York, NY, Raven Press, 1995, pp 335–345.

21. Allan DG, Lavoie G, Gross AE: Abstract: Complications of small fragment allograft reconstruction in revision total hip arthroplasty, in Brown KLB (ed): *Complications of Limb Salvage: Prevention, Management and Outcome*. Montreal, Canada, ISOLS, 1991, pp 285–286.

22. Kostuik J, Alexander D: Arthrodesis for failed arthroplasty of the hip. *Clin Orthop* 1984;188:173–182.

23. Grauer JD, Amstutz HC, O'Carroll PF, Dorey FJ: Resection arthroplasty of the hip. *J Bone Joint Surg* 1989;71A:669–678.

24. Harris WH, White RE Jr: Resection arthroplasty for nonseptic failure of total hip arthroplasty. *Clin Orthop* 1982;171:62–67.

25. Jasty M, Harris WH: Salvage total hip reconstruction in patients with major acetabular bone deficiency using structural femoral head allografts. *J Bone Joint Surg* 1990;72B:63–67.

26. Oakeshott RD, Morgan DA, Zukor DJ, Rudan JF, Brooks PJ, Gross AE: Revision total hip arthroplasty with osseous allograft reconstruction: A clinical and roentgenographic analysis. *Clin Orthop* 1987;225:37–61.

27. Gross AE: Revision arthroplasty of the hip using allograft bone, in Czitrom AA, Gross AE (eds): *Allografts in Orthopaedic Practice*. Baltimore, MD, Williams & Wilkins, 1992, pp 147–173.

28. Czitrom AA: Immunology of bone and cartilage allografts, in Czitrom AA, Gross AE (eds): *Allografts in Orthopaedic Practice*. Baltimore, MD, Williams & Wilkins, 1992, pp 15–25.

29. Czitrom AA, Gross AE, Langer F, Sim FH: Bone banks and allografts in community practice, in Bassett FH III (ed): *Instructional Course Lectures XXXVII*. Park Ridge, IL, American Academy of Orthopaedic Surgeons, 1988, pp 13–24.

30. Langer F, Czitrom A, Pritzker KP, Gross AE: The immunogenicity of fresh and frozen allogeneic bone. *J Bone Joint Surg* 1975;57A:215–220.

31. Goldberg VM, Stevenson S: Biology of bone and cartilage allografts, in Czitrom AA, Gross AE (eds): *Allografts in Orthopaedic Practice.* Baltimore, MD, Williams & Wilkins, 1992, pp 1–13.

32. Barrack RL, Harris WH: The value of aspiration of the hip joint before revision total hip arthroplasty. *J Bone Joint Surg* 1993;75A:66–76.

33. Gristina AG, Kolkin J: Total joint replacement and sepsis. *J Bone Joint Surg* 1983;65A:128–134.

34. Johnson JA, Christie MJ, Sandler MP, Parks PF Jr, Homra L, Kaye JJ: Detection of occult infection following total joint arthroplasty using sequential technetium-99m HDP bone scintigraphy and indium-111 WBC imaging. *J Nucl Med* 1988;29:1347–1353.

35. D'Antonio JA, Capello WN, Borden LS, et al: Classification and management of acetabular abnormalities in total hip arthroplasty. *Clin Orthop* 1989;243:126–137.

36. Paprosky WG, Perona PG, Lawrence JM: Acetabular defect classification and surgical reconstruction in revision arthroplasty: A 6-year follow-up evaluation. *J Arthroplasty* 1994;9:33–44.

37. Glassman AH, Engh CA, Bobyn JD: A technique of extensile exposure for total hip arthroplasty. *J Arthroplasty* 1987;2:11–21.

38. Gross AE, Hutchison CR, Alexeeff M, Mahomed N, Leitch K, Morsi E: Proximal femoral allografts for reconstruction of bone stock in revision arthroplasty of the hip. *Clin Orthop* 1995;319:151–158.

39. Gargbuz D, Morsi E, Mohamed N, Gross AE: Classification and reconstruction in revision acetabular arthroplasty with bone stock deficiency. *Clin Orthop* 1996;324:98–107.

40. Morsi E, Garbuz D, Gross AE: Revision total hip arthroplasty with shelf bulk allografts: A long-term follow-up study. *J Arthroplasty* 1996;11:86–90.

41. Garbuz D, Morsi E, Gross AE: Revision of the acetabular component of a total hip arthroplasty with a massive structural allograft: Study with a minimum five-year follow-up. *J Bone Joint Surg* 1996;78A:693–697.

42. Heekin RD, Engh CA, Vinh T: Morselized allograft in acetabular reconstruction: A postmortem retrieval analysis. *Clin Orthop* 1995;319:184–190.

43. Padgett DE, Kull L, Rozenberg A, Sumner DR, Galante JO: Revision of the acetabular component without cement after total hip arthroplasty: Three to six-year follow-up. *J Bone Joint Surg* 1993;75A:663–673.

44. Silverton CD, Rosenberg AG, Sheinkop MB, Kull LR, Galante JO: Revision total hip arthroplasty using a cementless acetabular component: Technique and results. *Clin Orthop* 1995;319:201–208.

45. Silverton CD, Rosenberg AG, Sheinkop MB, Kull LR, Galante JO: Revision of the acetabular component without cement after total hip arthroplasty: A follow-up note regarding results at seven to eleven years. *J Bone Joint Surg* 1996;78A:1366–1370.

46. Sloof TJ, Buma P, Schreurs BW, Schimmel JW, Huiskes R, Gardeniers J: Acetabular and femoral reconstruction with impacted graft and cement. *Clin Orthop* 1996;324:108–115.

47. Woolson ST, Adamson GJ: Acetabular revision using a bone-ingrowth total hip component in patients who have acetabular bone stock deficiency. *J Arthroplasty* 1996;11:661–667.

48. Shinar AA, Harris WH: Bulk structural autogenous grafts and allografts for reconstruction of the acetabulum in total hip arthroplasty: Sixteen-year average follow-up. *J Bone Joint Surg* 1997;79A:159–168.

49. Conrad EU, Gretch DR, Obermeyer KR, et al: Transmission of the hepatitis-C virus by tissue transplantation. *J Bone Joint Surg* 1995;77A:214–224.

50. Tomford WW: Transmission of disease through transplantation of musculoskeletal allografts. *J Bone Joint Surg* 1995;77A:1742–1754.

51. Campbell DG, Li P, Stephenson AJ, Oakeshott RD: Sterilization of HIV by gamma irradiation: A bone allograft model. *Int Orthop* 1994;18:172–176.

52. Fideler BM, Vangsness CT Jr, Moore T, Li Z, Rasheed S: Effects of gamma irradiation on the human immunodeficiency virus: A study in frozen human bone-patellar ligament-bone grafts obtained from infected cadavera. *J Bone Joint Surg* 1994;76A:1032–1035.

53. Eastlund T: Infectious hazards of bone allograft transplantation: Reducing the risk, in Czitrom AA, Winkler H (eds): *Orthopaedic Allograft Surgery.* Wien, Germany, Springer, 1996, pp 11–28.

54. Jacobs NJ: Establishing a surgical bone bank, in Fawcett KJ, Barr AR (eds): *Tissue Banking.* Arlington, VA, American Association of Blood Banks, 1987, pp 67–96.

55. Mowe JC (ed): *Standards for Tissue Banking.* Arlington, VA, American Association of Tissue Banks, 1984.

56. Schreiber GB, Busch MP, Kleinman SH, Korelitz JJ: The risk of transfusion-transmitted viral infections. *N Engl J Med* 1996;334:1685–1690.

57. Buck BE, Malinin TI, Brown MD: Bone transplantation and human immunodeficiency virus: An estimate of risk of acquired immunodeficiency syndrome (AIDS). *Clin Orthop* 1989;240:129–136.

58. Pelker RR, Friedlaender GE, Markham TC: Biomechanical properties of bone allografts. *Clin Orthop* 1983;174:54–57.

Reference to Video

Gross AE, Toronto, Ontario, Canada, Mt. Sinai Hospital, 1998.

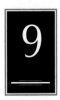

Total Acetabular Allografts

Wayne G. Paprosky, MD
Todd D. Sekundiak, MD, FRCSC

With the overall success of total joint arthroplasty, its prevalence is also increasing. This has meant that hip arthroplasties are present in a patient population with a wide age distribution—including patients who are ultimately placing greater demands on the arthroplasty because of increased activity levels over time. With the advent of improved techniques of insertion and quality of product, wear is now the most common cause of failure.[1-3] Wear and the associated osteolytic process can lead to massive bone loss. Because this process precedes actual loosening of the components, severe difficulty with the revision procedure can be encountered.

The revision procedure is also affected by other factors such as infection, instability, periprosthetic and prosthetic fractures, and component incompatibility.[1-3] Despite a multitude of techniques described for acetabular arthroplasty revision, the best results to date have been obtained with press-fit porous ingrowth implants, irrespective of the mode of failure.[1-12] More important than the mode of failure is the amount of bone loss that occurs with failure and with removal of the components. The amount of bone loss determines the type of acetabular reconstruction that will be required.

For severe acetabular defects, attempts at acetabular reconstruction have included the use of bilobed components, threaded cups, bipolar stems, cemented cups, and porous ingrowth cups.[1-12] Universally, these procedures have led to poor results in severe acetabular defects because there is not enough host bone to support the implant. Acetabular bone grafting has been used to augment these components in the revision setting and results are favorable if the proper component and acetabular defect is selected. Acetabular bone graft serves multiple functions. It aids in providing initial stability for the acetabular component and in the long term can restore bone stock that will hopefully prolong the survivability of the component.

Autogenous bone graft is advantageous because it promotes improved osteoinductive potential and decreased risk of disease transmission.[13] Unfortunately, the amount of autogenous graft available for the acetabular revision procedure is minimal and is usually a nonviable option. Allogeneic bone or bone substitutes are left as an alternative. Morcellized graft acts to fill the voids in contained cavitary defects and will aid in supporting the component and restoring bone stock.[14] Bulk grafts are used to reconstruct deficient rims or columns, to give support to the component, and to restore bone stock.[15]

The surgeon must then decide which mode of reconstruction should be chosen for each acetabular revision defect. The surgeon must not only be accountable to the patient but also to the institution to ensure the best result and at the same time incurring the least amount of risk and cost. Several factors must be considered when planning the revision. Most importantly, the surgeon must first be able to recognize what type of acetabular defect is present so that the appropriate treatment algorithm can be applied to the patient.

The use of an acetabular defect classification system, in the preoperative setting, allows the surgeon to overcome these hurdles. The classification system should be simple so that it can be applicable to all cases. It should act as a guide to the options of reconstruction, and correlate with verifiable clinical results. The classification system of the American Academy of Orthopaedic Surgeons[16] does not provide a framework for treatment options or reproducibility. Presently, we continue to support a classification system that can be used by assessing an anteroposterior radiograph of the pelvis[17] (Table 1).

Because the use of specialized radiographs or computed tomography (CT) scans is cumbersome and difficult to evaluate, the anteroposterior (AP) radiograph of the pelvis is used

Table 1
Acetabular defect classification

Defect Type	Superior Migration[*]	Ischial Lysis[†]	Medial Migration[§]	Teardrop Lysis[¶]
I	Insignificant	None	None	None
IIA	Insignificant	Mild	Grade I	Mild
IIB	Insignificant to significant	Mild	Grade II	Mild
IIC	Insignificant	Mild	Grade III	Moderate to severe
IIIA	Significant	Moderate	Grade II+ or III	Moderate
IIIB	Significant	Severe	Grade III+	Severe

[*]Insignificant = < 3 cm above superior transverse obturator line; Significant = > 3 cm above superior transverse obturator line

[†]Mild = 0 to 7 mm below superior transverse obturator line; Moderate = 7 to 14 mm below obturator line; Severe = > 15-mm lysis

[§]Grade I = lateral to Kohler's line; Grade II = migration to Kohler's line; Grade II+ = medial expansion of Kohler's line into pelvis; Grade III = migration into pelvis with violation of Kohler's line; Grade III+ = marked migration into pelvis

[¶]Mild = minimal loss of the lateral border; Moderate = complete loss of lateral border; Severe = loss of lateral and medial borders

and analyzed according to 4 criteria: hip center migration, degree of ischial lysis, presence of teardrop destruction, and extent of Kohler's line disruption. These criteria are quantitated to determine the structural integrity of the acetabular walls and columns. By knowing the extent and location of bone loss, the type of acetabular reconstruction can be determined.

With less severe acetabular defects, porous acetabular components function well. Morcellized or structural grafts are used only to augment host bone stock and are of indeterminate benefit. These defects, by definition, have at least 70% host bone remaining once the index component has been removed and preparation of the acetabulum has been completed. These are classified as type I or type II acetabular defects according to the classification using the radiographic approach. At an average 6.6-year follow-up of 125 subjects in the study series, there was no loosening of acetabular revision with these types of defects. Other authors report similar results.[1,18,19] Their function rivals a primary hip replacement and can almost be treated as such.

The more severe acetabular defects, those that have less than 70% of the host bone remaining, are classified as type IIIA defects. Attempts at press-fitting a porous-coated implant in this situation is possible but does involve some difficulty. The use of a structural allograft is recommended to reconstruct the deficient rim or column.[20] This will aid in maintaining the position and promote the fixation of the acetabular component to the host bone. When less than 50% of the host acetabulum remains, attempts at obtaining fixation with a porous-coated implant will be met with high failure rates.[21,22] For these type IIIB defects, it is accepted that there is not enough host bone to gain fixation of the implant to the host bone. An acetabular transplant allograft is recommended to restore bone and provide a fixation point for the component to be inserted. These defects are the most severe and the most difficult to manage.[22-24] Fortunately, they comprise a small number of revision procedures.

Reconstruction cages or antiprotrusio rings are now allowing more options to the surgeon. The cages have been used for a host of different defects and their variable constructions have determined when and where they can be used. If the rings are to be used in a type IIIB defect, then it must span the defect and allow for adequate fixation proximal and distal to the defect. The Muller reinforcement ring (Sulzer Orthopedics Ltd, Baar, Switzerland) cannot fulfill these requirements, whereas a Burch-Schnieder cage (Sulzer Orthopedics Ltd, Baar, Switzerland), DePuy antiprotrusio cage (DePuy, Warsaw, IN), or GAP cup (Osteonics Corp, Allendale, NJ) can span the defect present within the acetabulum and gain fixation in the remaining host bone (Fig. 1). If these cages are considered in a type III defect, it is essential that the defect be changed into a contained defect by using structural allograft to recreate deficient rims. Relying on the cage to support the entire load of the hip will lead to early failure of the cage.[25-29]

Preoperative Planning

The type IIIB acetabular defect is determined preoperatively so that proper planning can be undertaken to ensure success at the time of the procedure. On an anteroposterior radiograph of the pelvis, the 4 previously mentioned criteria are assessed to extrapolate that at least 50% of the host acetabulum is missing. This compels the surgeon to use an acetabular transplant for reconstruction. Recognition of the defect is critical so that the surgeon can be prepared for the surgery and so the revision can be done in a setting where experience with these reconstructions is prevalent.

Hip center migration is measured from a horizontal line drawn through the most superior extent of the obturator foramen on the AP radiograph. If this line measures over 3 cm, then the normal hip center has migrated at least 2 cm from its normal position. This indicates that the confluence of the anterior and posterior columns is in jeopardy with lack of superior bone to support the component. Ischial lysis is assessed by the distance the lysis has extended into the body of the ischium, as measured from the same superior transverse obturator line. If this lysis is severe or greater than 15 mm below this line, then the posteroinferior column will also be jeopardized and nonsupportive to component fixation. The anteroinferior column is assessed by regarding the extent of teardrop lysis on the radiograph. With both its lateral and medial margins being disrupted, this part of the acetabulum will also be nonsupportive. Finally, if Kohler's line is violated to a grade III or III+, indicating that the component has migrated into the pelvis with no intervening bony shell, then a type IIIB defect is present and an acetabular transplant is indicated (Fig. 2).

A caveat must be given to assessing these radiographic criteria when acetabular components are well fixed. Commonly, the acetabular defect is underestimated for a component that is well fixed, as the bone destroyed with removal instruments and with removal of the component cannot be estimated. It is essential for the surgeon to plan the removal technique and estimate the anticipated of bone loss so the appropriate reconstruction and equipment can be available. Final acetabular defects are assessed after removal of components. A large acetabular cup that is ingrown can easily lead to progression of a preoperative type II defect to a type IIIB defect if haste in removal precedes proper technique.

Each of the 4 radiographic criteria represents a separate section in the acetabulum, and by combining their degree of involvement, the acetabular

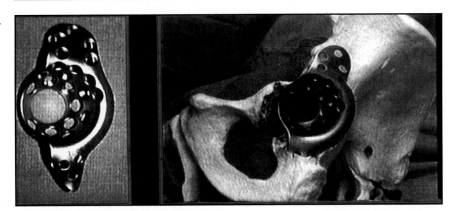

Fig. 1 DePuy antiprotrusio cage. The proximal and distal extensions on the cage allow for fixation into the remaining host bone in the ilium and ischium. If fixation is not possible in the ischium, impaling the extension into the ischial body provides adequate stability.

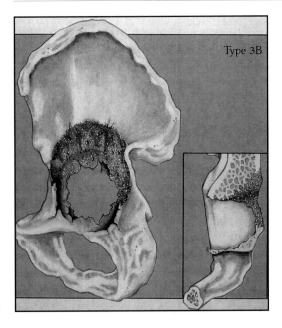

Type 3B

Fig. 2 A type IIIB acetabular defect with complete medial bone loss, loss of bone at the superior confluence of the anterior and posterior columns, and loss of the anterior and posterior inferior rims.

defect can be classified and visualized. It is essential to understand that these disruptions occur via a degenerative and not a traumatic process. These criteria, therefore, should not be applied in the traumatic setting. However, before consideration is given to reconstructing the acetabulum, the surgeon must exclude the existence of a pelvic discontinuity once the components, debris, and ectatic bone are removed. A pelvic discontinuity exists when the ilium and superior portion of the acetabulum are separated from the pubis, ischium, and the inferior portion of the acetabulum. Because the majority of bone loss occurs insidiously, a pelvic discontinuity can exist without it being overtly apparent before or during surgery. Irrespective of the type of acetabular defect, the association of a pelvic discontinuity mandates that this condition first be stabilized before further reconstruction can be considered.

With severe medial migration of the component or adherent bone cement, the condition of the intrapelvic structures must be assessed. Presently, there are no concrete recommendations as to when or how to investigate the position of the components relative to the iliac vessels, pelvic nerves, or ureter. A preoperative CT scan with arterial infusion has been employed to assess the pelvic structures. Narrow cuts of 1 to 2 mm are required with the appropriate software to subtract the metal components. Conventional angiography or intravenous pyelogram can also be entertained when there is significant concern. If suspicion is raised, an adjunctive retroperitoneal approach is required at the time of revision to aid in removal of the components.

If the defect has been determined to be a type IIIB, then the appropriate graft is selected. It should be obtained with the guidelines recommended by the Musculoskeletal Council of the American Association of Tissue Banks.[30] An ipsilateral pelvis of a young male is chosen for fit and its structural integrity. One is cautioned not to grossly mismatch the size of the graft to the host because the bulk of the graft may preclude insertion or fail to span the defect. Morcellized allograft is also recommended for impaction at the host-graft junction. Any remaining cavitary defects are also impacted with graft. Large fragment screw sets and a reconstruction plate are also required for fixation of the graft and for possible repair of pelvic discontinuity. Antiprotrusio cages, such as the Burch-Schnieder or DePuy, have also been used to fix the graft to the host. As with any revision procedure, the appropriate revision instrumentation and any removal instrumentation specific to the prosthesis to be extracted are also required.

Surgical Technique

The procedure is performed in the lateral position with a standard posterolateral approach. The proximal extent of the incision is directed to the posterior-superior iliac spine and distally along the lateral aspect of the femur. Other authors have recommended a triradiate approach to gain access to the pubic ramus, but we have found this unnecessary.[31] Visualization of the acetabular rim (both anteriorly and posteriorly), the iliac wing, pubis, and ischium is possible with this approach. Exposure is essential and an extended trochanteric osteotomy is considered solely for access to the acetabulum if visualization is compromised.[32] With debridement and removal of components, white cell counts on fluid, Gram stains on fluid, and pathologic frozen sections on suspicious tissues are urgently performed to rule out the possibility of infection. Any historic, physical, or surgical suspicion of infection necessitates staging the reconstruction secondary to its massive prolonged nature.

Debridement of the acetabular pseudocapsule proceeds until complete acetabular rim exposure is evident. All acetabular membranes are removed. Posterior dissection must be subperiosteal to protect the sciatic nerve. Any remaining posterior capsule is maintained to act as a retraction point for a self-retaining retractor placed in an anteroposterior manner. The tissue protects the sciatic nerve from any direct trauma. With large defects, anterior dissection must also proceed judiciously as the femoral neurovascular bundles or branches of the bundles can be encountered. The femoral extended trochanteric osteotomy allows for easier exposure in this direction if difficulty is encountered. Removal of components, cement, debris, and tissue is performed

routinely. It is essential to comprehend the inherent difficulties in removal of components and to have any removal devices appropriate to the product being removed.

With all acetabular components removed, debridement of the acetabulum must be completed. Acetabular defects are not always self-evident and some minimal reaming is undertaken to size the defect and create a spherical shape for acceptance of trial inserts. With the trial inserted, the amount of bone coverage can be estimated and correlated to the preoperative templating. When the most optimal trial is inserted and at least 50% of the cup uncovered, then an acetabular transplant is needed because press-fit will not be obtainable.

With allograft reconstruction, further dissection superiorly, posteriorly, and inferiorly is required for placement of the graft. Dissection is always subperiosteal to prevent neurovascular compromise. Posterior and anterior dissection was previously described. Rim exposure must be complete. Fixation of the graft is required along the remaining intact iliac wing. A periosteal elevator and a sponge are used to remove the abductor musculature. By maintaining subperiosteal dissection, the superior gluteal vessels and nerve can be preserved. Dissection should not extend into the greater sciatic foramen because disruption of the vessels can cause uncontrolled bleeding. Inferior exposure is required along the lateral wall of the ischium that will later act as a contact point for the reconstruction.

Acetabular exposure is not only a prelude for allograft acceptance, but is a prerequisite to exclude possible pelvic discontinuity. By removing the reactive granulomatous tissue and exposing the entire acetabular rim, the discontinuity is made evident. A pelvic reconstruction plate is used to bridge the defect between the ilium and ischium. It is fashioned along the posterior column and screwed into place to provide stability. Once the plate is in place, the preparation of the transplant can proceed. The antiprotrusio cages can be used as an alternative to the plate if screw fixation can be achieved both above and below the discontinuity.

By initially reaming the acetabular defect, the surgeon creates a hemispherical shape to the remaining bone for acceptance of the transplant (Fig. 3). This reaming also sizes the rim diameter. The aim in preparing the host and graft is to create a tongue and groove mortise that ensures intimate contact and stability of the construct. Transfer of load from the graft to the host can then occur along the posterior aspect of the graft and may promote biologic union of the graft. Also, the mortise prevents excess stresses at the screw fixation points allowing for improved stability until the graft unites to the host.

The acetabular transplant is shaped to buttress against the host bone. The graft's superior pubic and ischial ramii are cut at a point distal to the acetabular confluence with a length remaining to fill the defects present in the host pelvis. These graft extensions will buttress against the remaining host pubis and ischium, providing additional support. The transplant's iliac crest is cut in a curvilinear manner from the greater sciatic notch to the anterior inferior iliac spine (Fig. 4). This allows ample room for the graft to accept fixation without the bulk of excess bone and without the concern of fixation entering the acetabular cavity. The iliac crest flange is fashioned to allow best positioning of screws for purchase into the remaining host bone. Repeated trialing and trimming of

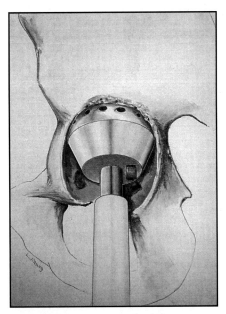

Fig. 3 The type IIIB acetabular defect is reamed spherically to create a tongue of bone superiorly to accept the allograft and to size the defect.

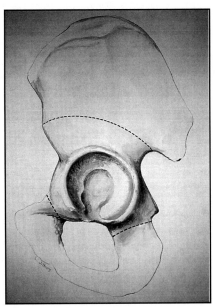

Fig. 4 The acetabular transplant is cut (as marked) to allow for acceptance into the host. Positioning of the cuts is determined by the amount of remaining host bone.

the graft are performed so that the appropriate amount and placement of bone resection are ensured. Resection should be conservative initially to maintain as much structural bone as possible and avoid the possibility of undersizing the graft. This can lead to poorer fixation, poor stability, early resorption, and ultimate failure.

The tongue of the mortise is created by the remaining host acetabular rim. The groove is created on the medial aspect of the graft where contact is being made with the host's acetabular rim (Fig. 5). A high-speed cylindrical burr and/or female reamer, sized 2 mm larger than the last male reamer used in the host acetabular defect, is used to score the medial side of the transplant. This creates a hemispherical defect, 1 to 1.5 cm in depth on the inner table of the graft, which will accept the remaining rim of host acetabulum. The position of the groove in the graft is templated to

the host bone and typically extends from the anterior inferior iliac spine to the ischium. The cylindrical burr is used to sculpt the groove to accept the irregularities in the host rim and to ensure that there is a tight tongue and groove fit. The medial portion of the graft should not be thinned to allow compromise of the articular surface or outer table because this will lead to loss of structural integrity and the possibility of transplant fracture. The transplant is seated in position and manipulated to ensure it is in its most stable position.

Once the graft has been trimmed, it is then impacted in place using an acetabular reamer or impactor. The transplant should be digitally manipulated to ensure that there is no toggling. The transplant should be positioned so that stability of the construct is obtained. The position of the transplant acetabulum is secondary, as the component insert can be repositioned to ensure joint stability. Commonly,

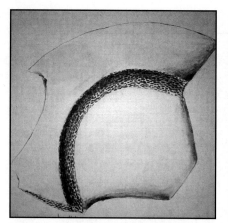

Fig. 5 The medial aspect of the graft is sculpted with a reamer or a burr to create a mortise that will contact with the tongue of bone as created in Figure 3.

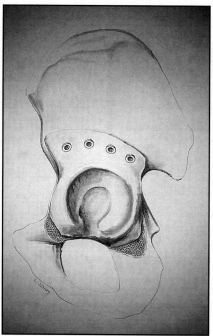

Fig. 6 The graft is impacted into position and then 6.5-mm cancellous screws are placed in a superior-medial direction to maintain position.

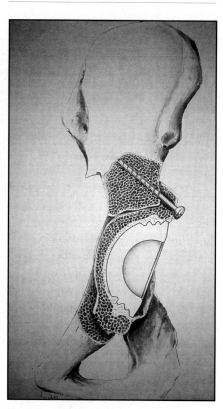

Fig. 7 Coronal view of transplant with screw fixation. Cup is cemented into allograft.

the transplant is positioned more vertical than the normal acetabulum. The construct is temporarily stabilized with 1 or 2 Steinman pins. Pin and screw placement are directed in the superior rim of the graft in the iliac wing. The aim is to direct screws in a proximal medial direction, along the joint force vectors (Fig. 6). This allows for compression at the host-transplant junction, optimizing contact, improving stability, and promoting union. Screw placement must be placed in the most structural bone possible without interfering with component insertion. The confluence of the host's acetabular columns has the best structural integrity, even in the failed acetabulum, as it continues to accept load from the component's vertical migration. Screw placement superior to this point will obtain weaker fixation as the iliac wing thins. It is optimal to obtain 3 to 4 screws with bicortical purchase into the host ilium. Once fixation is complete, manipulation should not produce motion in the construct. Large fragment, partially threaded cancellous screws are used to lag the transplant to the host. Washers are used to prevent the graft

from being crushed and to ensure adequate compressive force.

Acetabular preparation of the transplant proceeds in a routine fashion to remove cartilage and the subchondral bone. It is important to avoid overreaming because this will weaken the bone and possibly cause a fracture. Because the graft is avascular, cementing the acetabular component is the best option (Fig. 7). Cement anchor holes should be avoided because they too will cause fractures by creating a stress riser. The anchor holes also promote possible intrusion of cement at the host-transplant interface if the medial wall of the transplant is broached. This situation can prevent bone union and lead to possible early failure.

If a reconstruction cage is considered, preparation of the host acetabular shell continues as previously described. The transplant is then split in a vertical fashion so that any

remaining host bone will be loaded and in contact with the cage. The transplant is fixed to the host with screws or pins. The transplant is then reamed to a predetermined size to create a complete acetabular shell. With the disparity in bone quality between the host and the transplant, the reamer can easily ream eccentrically, producing an additional host columnar defect. Once the spherical defect is created, morcellized allograft is then impacted into the remaining defects and into the junction between the host and the transplant. A finishing reamer or a basket reamer on a T-handle can be used to manually impact and direct the graft into the defects. Excess allograft should not be used because it will excessively lateralize the acetabulum and prevent solid fixation of the cage to remaining structural bone. The last reamer size used will determine the size of the cage to be used.

The cage is then manipulated into position, an arduous task because the cage's proximal and distal extensions will impinge on bone and soft tissues. It is suggested that a malleable cage be used to allow for contouring to the transplant and host bone. A sharp retractor placed in the iliac wing retracts the abductor musculature and protects the superior gluteal structures when the proximal extent of the cage is placed. Inferiorly, the cage's extension can be either placed on the outer aspect of the ischial tuberosity and secured with screws or impaled into the substance of the ischium from the acetabular aspect. As with whole acetabular transplants, the reconstruction cage should be placed for optimal fit. Actual polyethylene component positioning can be altered for joint stability. Positioning and molding of the cage usually takes several attempts.

Reconstruction with the cage obtains stability by the cage press-fitting against the acetabular transplant and the remaining host acetabular rim, iliac wing, ischium, and/or pubis. The cage initially is fixed through its dome holes to ensure close approximation to the host bone and transplant. Initial screws would be placed superiorly and then posteriorly and anteriorly. More screws are then secured in the ischium and iliac wing. Once stabilized with screws, the construct will obtain further stability by pressurizing cement through the cage's remaining screw holes.

Prior to cementing the acetabulum into the transplant or the cage, trial reductions are performed with the femoral component. Because of the massive nature of the acetabular defect, proper orientation of the components can be deceiving. Trial reductions will optimize positioning

and are then matched with actual component insertion. These trials also determine if there are any impingement points with the reconstruction that would warrant trimming, to again alleviate the possibility of joint instability via a levering mechanism. Where there is significant soft-tissue loss, a constrained polyethylene liner may be considered (Fig. 8). Estimation of leg lengths and femoral component insertion depth are also assessed at this time. As discussed earlier, the transplant position is usually more vertical and retroverted than the normal acetabulum. The cup is placed in a more horizontal and anteverted position, leaving the posterior superior quadrant of the cup uncovered. This is not a cause for concern, and this area can be supported with a buttress of cement placed in this position.

Postoperative Care

Rehabilitation for acetabular transplants must be more guarded than that for routine acetabular revision arthroplasties. This is not only to protect the bony reconstruction but to also give time for the soft tissues to heal and strengthen. If the soft tissues were not already compromised from the multiple previous surgical procedures and lack of use, the extensive exposure will in itself cause some compromise. To prevent the possibility of postoperative dislocation, a hip abduction orthosis is worn for 3 months. Where there is obvious lack of muscle control as determined intraoperatively or postoperatively, a knee-ankle-foot extension is ordered. All patients are routinely braced because of the above-noted concerns. Toe touch weightbearing is continued for the first 3 months with progressive weightbearing continuing for an additional 3 months. Radiographic and clinical results are followed

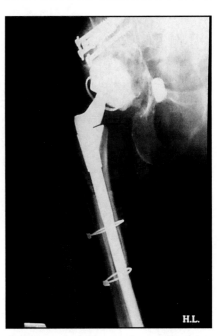

Fig. 8 Two-year follow-up of acetabular transplant. With the lack of abductor musculature, a constrained polyethylene cup was inserted to prevent dislocations.

monthly for the first 3 months, then at 6 months, biannually to 2 years, and then annually.

Antibiotic prophylaxis is continued for 5 days following surgery. This coverage will be continued until all wound drainage has stopped. Rehabilitation proceeds routinely as for any other hip arthroplasty procedure.

Results

We have reported on 20 whole acetabular transplant allografts that were performed on type IIIB defects.[23,24] Patients were initially diagnosed with osteoarthritis in 11 cases, trauma in 6, and with rheumatoid arthritis, developmental dysplasia, and radiation necrosis in the remaining 3. At the most recent follow-up of 31 months, 17 patients were available for assessment. All patients were reconstructed with a whole acetabular transplant allograft and a cemented acetabular compo-

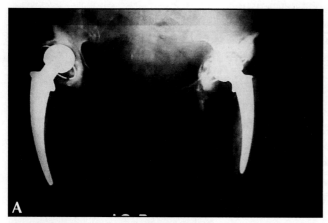 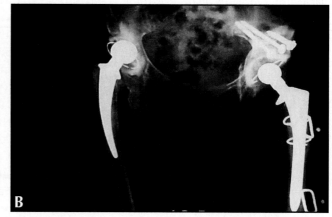

Fig. 9 A, Preoperative radiograph of a failed cemented acetabulum. With disruption of Kohler's line, loss of the teardrop, cement and lysis extending down the ischium over 15 mm and superiorly over 3 cm above the transverse obturator line, a type IIIB defect is present. **B**, Four-year follow-up of acetabular transplant with maintenance of cup and allograft position.

nent with the technique previously described. Follow-up was a minimum of 2 years (Fig. 9).

At 2 years, all grafts had radiographic evidence of union, with 1 graft union being confirmed by biopsy. Early migration of the graft was evident in most cases. Migration averaged 1.5 cm. One graft migrated 4 mm over 36 months and then ultimately failed. Three failures occurred, with 2 secondary to sepsis and 1 secondary to the abovementioned graft resorption and migration. Most grafts showed some continual minor lateral resorption. According to the modified D'Aubigne and Postel pain and walking score, patients improved from 3.7 preoperatively to 8.9 at final follow-up.[33]

The most common complication was instability, with 6 patients experiencing a dislocation event. Five patients were treated successfully with a brace and 1 required revision to a constrained cup. Two dislocations occurred anteriorly from excessive anteversion of the polyethylene cup, 1 secondary to patient noncompliance, and 3 others from poor musculature, multiple previous surgical procedures, and a history of recurrent dislocation. Consideration to the

abovementioned constrained acetabular liners is given if abductor musculature is absent or stability not within a safe range.

Infection occurred in 4 patients; 2 were treated with local debridement and antibiotics. One patient who has had a recurrence of the previously noted gram-negative infection is being treated with suppressive antibiotics and is asymptomatic despite radiographic evidence of failure. The last infection required resection arthroplasty as a curative treatment. The concern about possible recurrence of infection with these massive reconstructions has been raised but disputed by some authors.[34]

Stiehl[31] has also reported on 12 patients in whom reconstruction was with a pelvic allograft and a triradiate approach. Reconstruction included plating and stabilization of the anterior column. After a follow-up period between 14 and 84 months, 2 of these reconstructions have failed from loosening of the acetabular components that were press-fit in place, and 2 others developed sepsis, requiring removal of the entire graft and component construct. Six patients had good to excellent results, with improvement

in their hip scores of 40 points. After 8 months, all grafts showed evidence of remodeling radiographically, which was defined as probable incorporation. Complications were similar to the previous series reported with a 50% dislocation rate and the 18% infection rate.

Discussion

There has been a multitude of reports on the success or failure of revision arthroplasty and specifically revision arthroplasty with the use of allograft reconstruction.[35–38] There is, however, a multitude of surgical techniques that cannot be applied universally to all acetabular defects. The surgeon must be able to match the reconstruction method to the type of acetabular defect. Unfortunately, this inability of some surgeons to match acetabular defects to specific reconstruction methods has lead to miscommunication and confusion. Acceptance of an acetabular defect classification system is essential in order to develop a treatment protocol that can be applied appropriately to the patient population.

Presently, the short- and midterm results of porous ingrowth acetabular cups in the revision setting have been exceptional, and this method now can be accepted as the standard of care.[1-3] These exceptional results are, however, for less severe acetabular defects. For the more severe acetabular defects, different strategies of treatment must be instituted and a single alternate treatment strategy is not enough. The use of the same structural allografts and porous ingrowth cups has had mixed results when used unknowingly for different acetabular defects. For type IIIA acetabular defects, this reconstruction can provide the surgeon with success rates of 93% at an average 10.1-year follow-up, but when the same reconstruction is used for a type IIIB defect, success at 10-year follow-up may only be 40%.

Because of this discrepancy another reconstructive procedure is needed that includes the use of an acetabular transplant. The use of an acetabular transplant in reconstructing the deficient acetabulum has been successful but cannot be compared to the outstanding results obtained with porous ingrowth cups and lesser acetabular defects. The type IIIB acetabular defect has previously been treated as a unreconstructable acetabulum with a salvage operation considered to be the best procedure. Today reconstruction with an acetabular transplant is a more successful undertaking and should not be considered as a salvage procedure.

Other reconstructive procedures have been proposed, such as the use of acetabular reconstruction rings or impaction grafting. It is important to realize that these reconstructive measures should not be considered as an alternative but as an adjunct to these severe acetabular defects. When acetabular defects (such as type IIIB) are of such severity to warrant reconstruction, there is not enough bone to contain the cage or morcellized

graft. As mentioned in the discussion on surgical technique, an option is to create a contained defect with the use of a partial acetabular transplant and then to augment the remaining bone loss with reconstruction cage and/or graft. The results of this method are promising, but are anecdotal at this time.

As a caregiver, the surgeon should not only be able to recognize when to consider appropriate reconstruction, but also when to avoid it. The patient requires the support of the surgeon and the appropriate institution to handle the difficult postoperative rehabilitation and any possible complications that may ensue. Type IIIB reconstructions are therefore recommended in facilities that perform greater numbers of arthroplasties, thus having the resources to support the patient. The diligence required for a successful outcome with these procedures cannot be overemphasized, with the main goal being significant patient satisfaction by relieving pain and improving mobility.

A version of this chapter was published in the *Journal of Bone and Joint Surgery.*

References

1. Silverton CD, Rosenberg AG, Sheinkop MB, Kull LR, Galante JO: Revision total hip arthroplasty using a cementless acetabular component: Technique and results. *Clin Orthop* 1995;319:201–208.

2. Dorr LD, Wan Z: Ten years of experience with porous acetabular components for revision surgery. *Clin Orthop* 1995;319:191–200.

3. Petrera P, Rubash HE: Revision total hip arthroplasty: The acetabular component. *J Am Acad Orthop Surg* 1995;3:15–21.

4. More RC, Amstutz HC, Kabo JM, Dorey FJ, Moreland JR: Acetabular reconstruction with a threaded prosthesis for failed total hip arthroplasty. *Clin Orthop* 1992;282:114–122.

5. Namba RS, Clarke A, Scott RD: Bipolar revisions with bone-grafting for cavitary and segmental acetabular defects: A minimum 5-year follow-up study. *J Arthroplasty* 1994;9:263–268.

6. Sutherland CJ: Treatment of type III acetabular deficiencies in revision total hip arthroplasty

without structural bone-graft. *J Arthroplasty* 1996;11:91–98.

7. Cameron HU, Jung YB: Acetabular revision with a bipolar prosthesis. *Clin Orthop* 1990; 251:100–103.

8. Mallory TH, Vaughn BK, Lombardi AV Jr, Reynolds HM Jr, Koenig JA: Threaded acetabular components: Design rationale and preliminary clinical experience. *Orthop Rev* 1988;17: 305–314.

9. Murray WR: Acetabular salvage in revision total hip arthroplasty using the bipolar prosthesis. *Clin Orthop* 1990;251:92–99.

10. Scott RD: Use of a bipolar prosthesis with bone grafting in revision surgery. *Tech Orthop* 1987;2:84–86.

11. Slooff TJ, Buma P, Schreurs BW, Schimmel JW, Huiskes R, Gardeniers J: Acetabular and femoral reconstruction with impacted graft and cement. *Clin Orthop* 1996;324:108–115.

12. Wilson MG, Nikpoor N, Aliabadi P, Poss R, Weissman BN: The fate of acetabular allografts after bipolar revision arthroplasty of the hip: A radiographic review. *J Bone Joint Surg* 1989;71A: 1469–1479.

13. Czitrom AA, Gross AE, Langer F, Sim FH: Bone banks and allografts in community practice, in Bassett FH III (ed): *Instructional Course Lectures XXXVII*. Park Ridge, IL, American Academy of Orthopaedic Surgeons, 1988, pp 13–24.

14. Heekin RD, Engh CA, Vinh T: Morselized allograft in acetabular reconstruction: A postmortem retrieval analysis. *Clin Orthop* 1995; 319:184–190.

15. Gross AE, Allan DG, Catre M, Garbuz DS, Stockley I: Bone grafts in hip replacement surgery: The pelvic side. *Orthop Clin North Am* 1993;24:679–695.

16. D'Antonio JA, Capello WN, Borden LS, et al: Classification and management of acetabular abnormalities in total hip arthroplasty. *Clin Orthop* 1989;243:126–137.

17. Bradford MS, Paprosky WG: Acetabular defect classification: A detailed radiographic approach. *Semin Arthroplasty* 1995;6:76–85.

18. Padgett DE, Kull L, Rosenberg A, Sumner DR, Galante JO: Revision of the acetabular component without cement after total hip arthroplasty: Three to six-year follow-up. *J Bone Joint Surg* 1993;75A:663–673.

19. Weber KL, Callaghan JJ, Goetz DD, Johnston RC: Revision of a failed cemented total hip prosthesis with insertion of an acetabular component without cement and a femoral component with cement: A five to eight-year follow-up study. *J Bone Joint Surg* 1996;78A:982–994.

20. Sekundiak TD, Paprosky WG, Stewart RL: Long-term follow-up of distal femoral allografts with porous ingrowth acetabular cups: The fate of the allograft. Proceedings of the American Academy of Orthopaedic Surgeons 65th Annual Meeting, New Orleans, LA. Rosemont, IL, American Academy of Orthopaedic Surgeons, 1998, p 251.

21. Paprosky WG, Perona PG, Lawrence JM: Acetabular defect classification and surgical reconstruction in revision arthroplasty: A 6-year follow-up evaluation. *J Arthroplasty* 1994;9:33–44.

22. Garbuz D, Morsi E, Gross AE: Revision of the acetabular component of a total hip arthroplasty with a massive structural allograft: Study with a minimum five-year follow-up. *J Bone Joint Surg* 1996;78A:693–697.

23. Bradford MS, Paprosky WG: Total acetabular transplant allograft reconstruction of the severely deficient acetabulum. *Semin Arthroplasty* 1995;6:86–95.

24. Macdonald SJM, Krishnamurthy AB, Paprosky WG, Bradford MS: Acetabular transplants in revision total hip arthroplasty: When there are no alternatives. Proceedings of the American Academy of Orthopaedic Surgeons 63rd Annual Meeting, Atlanta, GA. Rosemont, IL, American Academy of Orthopaedic Surgeons, 1996, p 225.

25. Müller ME: Acetabular revision, in Salvati EA (ed): *The Hip: Proceedings of the Ninth Open Scientific Meeting of the Hip Society, 1981.* St. Louis, MO, CV Mosby, 1981, pp 46–56.

26. Berry DJ, Muller ME: Revision arthroplasty using an anti-protrusio cage for massive acetabular bone deficiency. *J Bone Joint Surg* 1992; 74B:711–715.

27. Peters CL, Curtain M, Samuelson KM: Acetabular revision with the Burch-Schnieder antiprotrusio cage and cancellous allograft bone. *J Arthroplasty* 1995;10:307–312.

28. Rosson J, Schatzker J: The use of reinforcement rings to reconstruct deficient acetabula. *J Bone Joint Surg* 1992;74B:716–720.

29. Zehntner MK, Ganz R: Midterm results (5.5-10 years) of acetabular allograft reconstruction with the acetabular reinforcement ring during total hip revision. *J Arthroplasty* 1994;9:469–479.

30. Mowe JC (ed): *Standards for Tissue Banking.* Arlington, VA, American Association of Tissue Banks, 1987.

31. Stiehl JB: Extensile anterior column acetabular reconstruction in revision total hip arthroplasty. *Semin Arthroplasty* 1995;6:60–67.

32. Younger TI, Bradford MS, Magnus RE, Paprosky WG: Extended proximal femoral osteotomy: A new technique for femoral revision arthroplasty. *J Arthroplasty* 1995;10: 329–338.

33. D'Aubigne RM, Postel M: Functional results of hip arthroplasty with acrylic prosthesis. *J Bone Joint Surg* 1954;36A:451.

34. Berry DJ, Chandler HP, Reilly DT: The use of bone allografts in two-stage reconstruction after failure of hip replacements due to infection. *J Bone Joint Surg* 1991;73A:1460–1468.

35. Hooten JP Jr, Engh CA Jr, Engh CA: Failure of structural acetabular allografts in cementless revision hip arthroplasty. *J Bone Joint Surg* 1994;76B:419–422.

36. Jasty M, Harris WH: Salvage total hip reconstruction in patients with major acetabular bone deficiency using structural femoral head allografts. *J Bone Joint Surg* 1990;72B:63–67.

37. Kwong LM, Jasty M, Harris WH: High failure rate of bulk femoral head allografts in total hip acetabular reconstructions at 10 years. *J Arthroplasty* 1993;8:341–346.

38. Pollock FH, Whiteside LA: The fate of massive allografts in total hip acetabular revision surgery. *J Arthroplasty* 1992;7:271–276.

Transfemoral Approach to the Deficient Proximal Femur

Allan E. Gross, MD, FRCSC

Introduction

The transfemoral approach is used when the host proximal femur is too deficient to provide proximal support for a new femoral implant. Under these circumstances, a proximal femoral allograft may be used to support a new implant. Alternative solutions would be a tumor prosthesis,[1] or a prosthesis using distal fixation.[2,3]

Indications

This approach is indicated when there is full circumferential loss of proximal femur measuring greater than 5 cm in length. Shorter defects can be managed by calcar-replacing implants and noncircumferential defects of any length can be managed by cortical strut allografts. This approach may also be used for removal of ingrown fully porous-coated prostheses with or without attempted salvage of host proximal femur. In addition, it greatly expedites removal of cement or ingrown porous-coated prostheses, and if enough proximal host femur can be salvaged and wired back, a distal press fit or fully porous coated prosthesis can be used.

Surgical Technique

A straight lateral incision is made that extends from just distal to the iliac crest to 5 or 6 cm beyond the junction of deficient and healthy host femur. Previous scars will probably

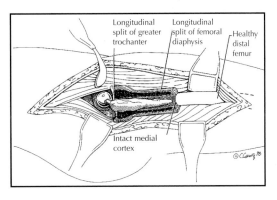

Fig. 1 Longitudinal split of deficient femur and greater trochanter. (Copyright © C. Chang)

have to be incorporated into the new incision. A Steinmann pin is inserted into the iliac crest through a separate stab incision to be used as a reference point for leg lengths.

The fascia lata is incised and the vastus lateralis and the anterior and posterior borders of the gluteus medius identified. The posterior fibers of the vastus lateralis are reflected off the posterior septum so that the bulk of the muscle is reflected anteriorly, exposing the lateral aspect of the femur. Only the deficient femur plus a few centimeters of healthy femur have to be exposed. Reflecting the vastus off the septum must be done carefully, dissecting out and cauterizing the perforating vessels as they are encountered. The vessels should be divided well anterior to the septum to avoid allowing a resected end to retract behind the septum, where hemostasis would be difficult to achieve.

The anterior, medial, and posterior aspects of the exposed femur should retain their soft-tissue attachments and blood supply.

The greater trochanter can be handled one of 3 ways. One choice is to split it longitudinally, as in the Wagner approach[3] (Fig. 1). Under these circumstances, the posterior half of the rough line is cleared of the origin of the vastus lateralis prior to splitting the trochanter longitudinally. In the second alternative, a trochanteric slide, the trochanter is osteotomized distal to the rough line in a posterior-anterior direction keeping all of the vastus still attached to the rough line so that the trochanter retains its proximal (gluteal) and distal (vastus) attachments[4] (Fig. 2). This method allows a more stable trochanteric reattachment and decreases the risk of trochanteric escape. The trochanter is retracted anteriorly after its posterior

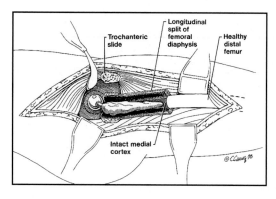

Fig. 2 Trochanteric slide and longitudinal split of femur. (Copyright © C. Chang)

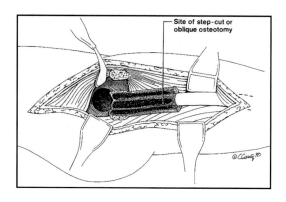

Fig. 3 Implant and cement has been removed showing intact medial cortex. (Copyright © C. Chang)

levering osteotomies against the femoral implant or cement in the canal. The deficient femur cracks anteriorly and posteriorly, and falls open distally to the transverse osteotomy. When this happens a spike of femur, usually on the medial side, will remain attached to the healthy distal femur, and this spike may be used to fashion a step-cut or an oblique osteotomy to help stabilize the graft-host junction (Fig. 3).

If a proximal femoral allograft is used, the graft-host junction is stabilized by cerclage wires around an oblique or step-cut osteotomy. Residual host femur with its soft-tissue attachments is wrapped around the allograft with cerclage wires. If it bridges the graft-host junction it will provide further stabilization, and it also serves as a vascularized autograft. The trochanter is reattached with cerclage wires, if it was split longitudinally, or by a trochanteric slide. If a transverse trochanteric osteotomy was performed, the trochanter is attached to the allograft, using horizontal and vertical wires that are passed through holes previously drilled in the lesser trochanter and lateral cortex of the allograft.

References

1. Malkani AL, Sim FH, Chao EY: Custom-made segmental femoral replacement prosthesis in revision total hip arthroplasty. *Orthop Clin North Am* 1993;24:727–733.

2. Engh CA, Glassman AH: Cementless revision of failed total hip replacement: An update, in Tullos HD (ed): *Instructional Course Lectures XL*. Park Ridge, IL, American Academy of Orthopaedic Surgeons, 1991, pp 189–197.

3. Wagner H, Wagner M: Conical stem fixation for cementless hip prostheses for primary implantation and revisions, in Morscher E (ed): *Endoprosthetics*. Berlin, Germany, Springer-Verlag, 1995, pp 258–270.

4. Glassman AH, Engh CA, Bobyn JD: A technique of extensile exposure for total hip arthroplasty. *J Arthroplasty* 1987;2:11–21.

attachments have been dissected off. In the third alternative, a transverse trochanteric osteotomy, the vastus must be dissected completely off the rough line so that the trochanter can be reflected proximally.

If the leg is not going to be lengthened more than 2 cm and extensive pelvic exposure is not required, a longitudinal split of the trochanter is fastest and easiest. If lengthening of more than 2 cm is required or more extensive exposure of the pelvis is indicated, a trochanteric slide is used. A trochanteric slide can easily be converted to a transverse trochanteric osteotomy if additional pelvic exposure is required.

In preparation for the femoral split, a transverse cut is made in the femur at the level to which the split will extend distally at the junction of deficient and healthy femur. This transverse osteotomy, which just extends through the lateral half of the femur, must be done carefully with an oscillating saw, leaving the medial femur intact. The medial femur, or at least a part of it, will remain attached to the distal femur when the femur is split, and it can be shaped into a step cut or an oblique osteotomy to help stabilize the graft-host junction later. The deficient femur is split in the midline laterally down to healthy host femur at the site of the transverse osteotomy. If the trochanter is being split longitudinally, the femoral split is continued proximally through the greater trochanter. If the trochanteric approach is via a trochanteric slide or a transverse osteotomy, the trochanter must be dealt with before the longitudinal split of the femur. The femoral split is done with an oscillating saw. The split is spread by

Impaction Morcellized Allografting and Cement

Tom J. J. H. Slooff, MD, PhD
B. Willem Schreurs, MD, PhD
Pieter Buma, PhD
Jean W. M. Gardeniers, MD, PhD

Introduction

Most total hip arthroplasties, cemented and cementless, fail because of aseptic loosening, a slow but progressive process that often results in loss of bone stock. The stability of the implant becomes compromised and the components may migrate. The key problems in revision surgery are how to manage the periprosthetic bone loss, how to achieve long-lasting stability, and how to restore hip mechanics. Although controversy still exists about the treatment of choice for the reconstruction of the failed total hip arthroplasty acetabular component, we prefer a biologic method, using impaction allografting with cement.

This chapter describes the essential general issues of bone grafting, particularly the use of morcellized grafts with cement and the rationale of the reconstruction method in acetabular revision arthroplasty. Subsequently, it describes the surgical technique, the supportive scientific studies, and the clinical and radiographic results of the reconstruction. Finally, current recommendations are presented and discussed.

General Issues

History

Bone grafting has a long history in medical science. According to folklore, it goes back to ancient times. The miracle of the saints, the twins Cosmas and Damianus, represents the first alleged bone and tissue transplant. The legend tells the history of a pious sexton, who was lying in the Roman Forum, exhausted from the pain of bone cancer in his leg. In a dream, the twin brothers came to help him, removed his diseased leg and transplanted the leg of a Moor who had just died. Because the Moor had darker skin than the sexton did, this miraculous event has been recorded as "The miracle of the black leg." Owing to the success of the operation, the twin brothers were canonized, inspiring artists over the years to create masterpieces portraying the event on canvas.

Back to reality! The early literature records that the Dutchmen Anthonie van Leeuwenhoek[1] and Job van Meekeren[2] performed excellent scientific work in the field of bone grafting and bone physiology. Anthonie van Leeuwenhoek, a contemporary of Jan van Swammerdam and Reinier de Graaf, gained international recognition through his research into microscopy and his production of the first thorough description of the histologic structure of bone. In a well-documented study published in 1668, van Meekeren, a surgeon from Amsterdam, described the first bone graft. The graft, taken from the skull of a dog, was used successfully to restore a traumatic defect in a soldier's skull. In this case, the graft material is known as a xenograft, which indicates bone donation from one species to another. An autograft refers to bone that is transplanted from one location to another within the same individual. In the tale of the Moor, the bone graft received by the sexton represents an allograft, because another member of the same species donated the bone.

Through the centuries, the use of autografts and allografts in surgical practice has varied widely. In the 18th and 19th centuries, bone grafting was not an accepted surgical procedure; it was considered to be experimental, with an unpredictable outcome. However, the technique was developed out

Reproduced from *Instructional Course Lectures 47*. Rosemont, IL, American Academy of Orthopaedic Surgeons, 1997.

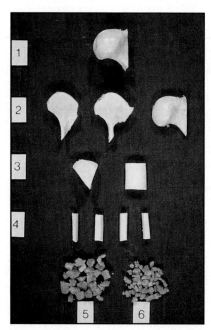

Fig. 1 Overview of the various types of bone graft: 1 to 3, solid, structural corticocancellous structural grafts; 4 to 6, cancellous morcellized grafts, from strips (4) to chips (5,6).

of sheer necessity in clinical practice, and even today clinical expertise runs ahead of science. At the end of the 19th century and the beginning of the 20th, famous surgeons such as Ollier[3] from France, Macewen[4] from Scotland, Curtis[5] from the United States, and Barth[6], Lexer[7], and Axhausen[8] from Germany stimulated the use of bone grafting. On the basis of animal experiments and clinical observations, they observed that the graft, whether it was an autograft or an allograft, largely lost its vitality and then became revitalized from the host bone. Major components in this process were considered to be the periosteum transplanted with the graft and the vascular network of the host.

The Present

Current knowledge about the histologic fate of a bone graft differs very little from the original ideas ex-

pressed in the past. It is generally accepted that to be incorporated, a graft, whether it is an autograft or an allograft, goes through a series of processes in which the donor bone and host become closely interconnected. The host supplies the blood vessels and viable bone cells, elements that are of vital importance to the incorporation and remodeling of the dead graft material. The graft stimulates the host's cellular activity, ultimately leading to new bone formation in and around the graft, which acts as a frame-like structure for bone apposition. Important factors that influence the success of incorporation are firm fixation of the bone graft to the bone bed of the host, extent of the surface area between the graft and host bone, the vascularity of the surrounding host tissue, and the load pattern in the graft. From our clinical experience it was established that the size and architecture of the bone graft also influence the incorporation process. The distinction between structural and morcellized allografts is based on this experience (Fig. 1).

Compact structural bone grafts are very dense, which strongly compromises the ingrowth of the blood vessels essential for revitalization of the graft. In the early stages of the incorporation process, only the contact surface of the graft undergoes partial and superficial breakdown to create space for revascularization. Consequently, there is only superficial union of the graft with the host bone. Subsequently the inner part of the graft remains dead bone. It weakens due to fatigue fractures and graft resorption. We have also observed that during this incomplete and slow incorporation process it is not always possible to maintain sufficient stability of a structural bone graft after surgical fixation

in a weightbearing part of the hip that is subject to considerable stress. This can also lead to movement and, thus, resorption of the graft. In contrast, impacted morcellized allografts are incorporated more uniformly and completely. Blood vessels can easily penetrate the open structure, which means rapid new bone apposition of the dead trabeculae without any loss of mechanical strength. It is well known that an individual's own bone, an autograft, incorporates better as compared to allograft due to the high osteogenic capacity and the absence of immunogenic reactions. However, it is not always possible to harvest sufficient quantities of an individual's own bone, and in elderly patients it is often of poor quality. Furthermore, the extra incision necessary to harvest the bone causes additional morbidity. For these reasons, in most cases it is necessary to use donor bone from a bone bank.

Impacted Morcellized Grafts and the Rationale for the Nijmegen Technique

The types of bone grafts used by different surgeons for acetabular reconstruction vary widely. Currently some surgeons[9,10] use morcellized allografts as routine. Others[11–13] advocate the use of structural cancellous or corticocancellous grafts, with or without cement. This chapter deals only with morcellized allografts used with polymethylmethacrylate (PMMA) bone cement.

In the past, various surgical revision techniques have been developed to compensate for bone loss and to restore the stability of the implant. Sotelo-Garza and Charnley[14] used large quantities of bone cement to close the defect and fill the acetabular cavity. However, it is evident that in revisions where only cement is used, the bone defects still remain. Also the thin, sclerotic and smooth acetabular bone bed provides an inadequate surface for successful mechanical bone-cement interlock. The literature reports poor clinical track records. Berry and Müller[15] recommended the use of rigid metal supporting rings to bridge acetabular defects. In our opinion, the addition of these rigid metal reinforcements to bone grafting will fail because of the mismatch between the more elastic pelvic bone and the rigid metal implants and the stress shielding of the graft. Other surgeons[16] used large diameter cementless acetabular implants that were supported only by the remaining host bone. They expected spontaneous new bone formation in and around the defect.

In the 1970s, a new application for bone grafting was introduced for the reconstruction of acetabular defects in primary and revision total hip arthroplasty. In primary total hip replacement, an acetabular defect was often a congenital peripheral, segmental acetabular rim defect (Fig. 2, *A*). A primary cavitary defect was seen fairly commonly in the advanced stages of rheumatoid arthritis. This defect has also been described as "protrusio acetabuli" (Fig. 2, *B*). In revision total hip replacement, the defects originated mostly from the damage to the bone by the loosening process and caused cavitary, segmental, or combined defects of the acetabulum (Fig. 2, *C* and *D*).

In 1975, Hastings and Parker[17] described the use of a combination of cemented total hip replacement and autogenous morcellized cancellous grafting in intrapelvic protrusio acetabuli. The graft was not impacted and was subsequently totally covered with a coarse mesh cup with a small rim.

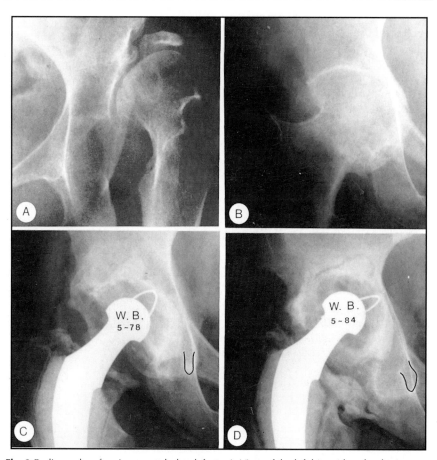

Fig. 2 Radiographs of various acetabular defects. **A,** View of the left hip with a dysplastic acetabulum, so-called dysplasia, which gave rise to secondary arthrosis. The femoral head has migrated in a cranial direction because of insufficient coverage. This is a case of a primary peripheral segmental rim defect. **B,** Preoperative radiograph of a woman with protrusio of the right acetabulum. The femoral head has migrated inwards and threatens to break through the medial wall of the acetabulum. The consequential bone loss is referred as a cavitary defect. **C,** Status after primary total hip arthroplasty that was performed in 1974. After some time both prosthetic components developed mechanical loosening. **D,** Clear signs of changes in position of the component and migration of the cup in a cranial and medial direction that resulted in bone loss and peripheral segmental rim defect. This is an example of a combined peripheral segmental and cavitary defect.

In 1978, McCollum and Nunley[18] reported their first experience with autogenous wafers of corticocancellous bone used to augment acetabular bone stock in 25 patients with protrusio acetabuli after failed total hip arthroplasty. A fine metal mesh was subsequently tucked into acetabular anchoring holes to distribute the forces across the acetabulum. To prevent the cement from penetrating into the graft, gelfoam was used to avoid direct contact between the cement and the graft. A cemented cup was combined with a ring when the medial wall was absent.

In 1983, Marti and Besselaar[19] introduced a technique for treating protruded and dysplastic acetabuli. Medial segmental defects were closed with a corticocancellous graft supplemented with autogenous chips. Intact acetabular host bone was compressed

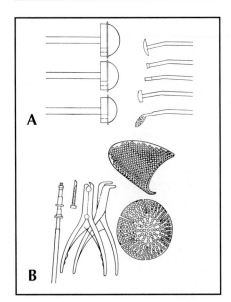

Fig. 3 A, The instrumentation used for acetabular impaction; **B,** Examples of the preformed metal reconstruction mesh and the special tools used to trim, cut, and fix the mesh.

to anchor the cement. Additionally, an Eichler ring was used. Peripheral segmental defects were repaired with segmental plugs taken from the pelvic crista and fixed with screws to the iliac wall.

In 1983, Roffman and associates,[20] in an animal model with intrapelvic protrusio, investigated the fate of autogenous chips under a layer of polymethylmethacrylate bone cement. Their model comprised a medial segmental defect. Histologic evaluation revealed the formation of bone from the acetabular wall toward the graft. The graft appeared viable, and new bone formation was induced along the surface adjoining the bone cement. Based on these experimental results in dogs, Mendes and associates[21] published the results of a clinical study on primary cemented arthroplasties combined with autogenous bone chips supported with a metal mesh for intrapelvic protrusio. Follow-up studies, the longest of

which were 6 years, showed clinical success in all patients.

In 1984, Slooff and associates[22] published their experience with a modified method using impacted morcellized allografts. Acetabular segmental defects were closed with corticocancellous slices or with flexible metal wire meshes. The contained acetabulum was tightly packed with allograft chips (sized 1 cm³). The cup was inserted after pressurizing the cement directly onto the graft. To correct structural acetabular integrity loss and impairment of implant mechanical support and hip joint mechanics, our treatment strategy sought to do the following: (1) repair hip mechanics by positioning the cup at the level of the anatomic acetabulum (teardrop); (2) close segmental defects with metal wire mesh to achieve containment (a cavitary defect remains); (3) replace the periprosthetic bone loss by augmenting the cavitary defect with morcellized allograft; and (4) restore stability by impacting the chips and using bone cement.

The X-Change Acetabular Revision Instrumentation System, developed in cooperation with Howmedica International, Staines, UK, was designed to achieve these goals (Fig. 3). In use since 1978, this surgical technique has been standardized and basically has not been changed.

Surgical Technique

The posterolateral approach was used in all cases. This enabled extensive exposure of all aspects of the acetabulum and proximal femur. Trochanteric osteotomy was seldom necessary. Identification of major landmarks was helpful for orientation if scarring and distortion disturbed the anatomy. These landmarks were the tip of the greater trochanter, the tendinous part of the gluteus max-

imus, the lower border of the gluteus medius and minimus, and the sciatic nerve. Aspiration of the hip was performed at this stage to obtain fluid for Gram staining and frozen sectioning to examine for possible infection.

The proximal part of the femur was exposed extensively and mobilized before the hip was dislocated. Exposure of the entire socket was achieved by removing all scar tissue, by performing circumferential capsulotomy, and by dividing the iliopsoas tendon. After removing the components and all the cement, the fibrous interface was freed completely from the irregular acetabular wall using sharp spoons and curettes. Special care was taken to locate the transverse ligament at the inferior side of the acetabulum. The socket was reconstructed from this level upwards. At least three specimens were taken from the interfacial fibrous membrane for frozen sectioning and bacterial culture. After taking these samples, systemic antibiotic therapy was started.

The acetabular floor and walls were examined meticulously for any hidden medial and/or peripheral segmental defects (Fig. 4, A). Using a pair of scissors, a flexible stainless steel mesh was trimmed and adapted to fit any of the defects and was rigidly fixed to the iliac wall with at least 3 screws. Any medial segmental defect was closed in a similar manner with a metal mesh. In this way, the acetabulum was contained and had become a cavitary defect (Fig. 4, B). Many small drill holes (2 mm) were made in the sclerotic acetabular wall to enhance surface contact and promote vascular invasion into the graft.

Deep frozen femoral heads from the hospital bone bank were divided into four equal parts. Substantial chips were cut with a rongeur or scissors. After cleaning the acetabulum,

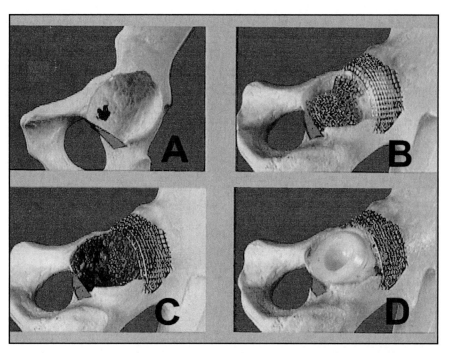

Fig. 4 The reconstruction technique. **A,** A combined segmental and cavitary defect. The medial wall defect is combined with a large rim defect and bone loss in the cranial part of the acetabulum. **B,** A preformed metal wire mesh closes the medial wall defect and a second wire mesh is used to reconstruct the acetabular rim. A confined cavitary defect remains. **C,** Solidly impacted morcellized allograft is molded in the defect and the new acetabulum is reconstructed at the level of the transverse ligament. **D,** Finally the new acetabular component is cemented directly on the impacted allograft, again at the level of the transverse ligament.

any existing small cavities were packed tightly with chips; then the entire socket was filled layer by layer. Impactors hammered the chips in situ, starting with the largest possible size impactor and ending with the most suitable size cup. Care was taken to reconstruct the anatomy of the hip with the new socket at the level of the transverse ligament. The acetabulum was reconstructed with a substantial layer of graft around the new cup, because the thickness of this graft layer must at least be 5 mm. After impaction, the whole acetabular hemisphere was covered with a layer of impacted allograft chips. However, it was evident that this layer was not of a uniform thickness, because the thickness depended locally on the depth of the acetabular defect. After impaction, the preexistent enlarged acetabular diameter had been reduced to a normal size (Fig. 4, *C*).

While the antibiotic-loaded cement was being prepared, pressure on the graft was maintained using a trial socket. After inserting and pressurizing the cement, the cup was placed and held in position with the pusher until the cement had polymerized (Fig. 4, *D*). Postoperative management included anticoagulation therapy for 3 months and systemic antibiotics for 24 hours. Indomethacin was administered for 7 days to prevent the development of heterotopic ossification. Mobilization of the patient was individualized according to the different circumstances of the revision arthroplasty. A period of 3 to 6 weeks of bed rest was

required after major acetabular reconstruction.

Scientific Studies

The scientific bases for bone impaction grafting and cement are the results of the animal experiments and laboratory examinations.

Animal Experiments

To obtain more insight into the mechanical stability of reconstructions using impacted morcellized allografts with cement, and to study the incorporation process of the graft, we performed 2 separate animal experiments using Dutch milk goats. For the femur, follow-up was relatively brief, so this study will concentrate primarily on the mechanical stability.[23] The longer follow-up periods available for the acetabulum made this study very useful as a detailed description of the histologic incorporation process.[24] Surgical techniques used to reconstruct acetabular and femoral deficiencies were similar to those used in humans.

Mechanical Study

The medullary cavity of the femur was prepared with hand-reamers. A concentric intramedullary graft could be impacted in a retrograde fashion, using a specially developed set of instruments.[25] Cement was inserted into this construction, followed by the insertion of the femoral stem. Tantalum pellets were fixed to the implant and the bone prior to insertion in order to allow Röntgen-Stereophotogrammatic Analysis (RSA).[26] The initial stability was analyzed in 4 specimens; the postoperative changes were evaluated in 8 goats sacrificed after 6 and 12 weeks. The prosthesis-bone construct was then loaded physiologically with a maximal load of 144% of body weight (Fig. 5). The loading

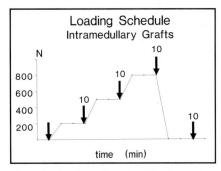

Fig. 5 The loading schedule of the femoral intramedullary grafts. Stereoradiographs were made 10 minutes after each step in load (arrows). (Reproduced with permission from Sloof TJ: Impaction grafting and cemented acetabular revision, in Villar (ed): *Revision Hip Arthroplasty*. Oxford, England, Butterworth Heinemann, 1997, pp 116–130.)

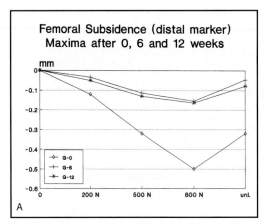

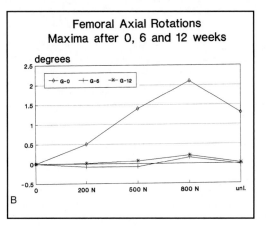

Fig. 6 A, Maximal femoral subsidence after 0, 6, and 12 weeks. Note increasing stability after incorporation of the graft. **B,** Maximal rotations of the graft after 0, 6, and 12 weeks show the same trend. (Reproduced with permission from Sloof TJ: Impaction grafting and cemented acetabular revision, in Villar (ed): *Revision Hip Arthroplasty*. Oxford, England, Butterworth Heinemann, 1997, pp 116–130.)

mode applied resulted in bending and rotational forces, which are important for testing the stability of hip prostheses.[25] Load was applied stepwise from 0 to 200, 500, and 800 N and again unloaded. Each loading period lasted 10 minutes. Stereoradiographs were taken before loading, after each loading step, and 10 minutes after the final unloading. Relative rotations and translations around and along the coordinate axes were calculated.

Six and 12 weeks after implantation the stability had clearly increased when compared to the initial stability of the stems immediately after insertion (Fig. 6). In the 6- and 12-week specimens, most of the motion was axial rotation and subsidence, both of which increased with increasing load. The maximum rotation was 0.24° under 800 N, but after unloading there was significant elastic recovery, which resulted in a maximum permanent rotation of 0.14°. There were no differences between the 6- and 12-week groups. Maximum subsidence under a load of 800 N was 0.164 mm and after unloading the maximum permanent subsidence was 0.078 mm.

Although there were no significant differences between the results of the 6- and 12-week specimens, there was a trend towards greater permanent displacement in the 12-week group. The standard deviations for translations and rotations observed during biomechanical testing were estimated to be 0.036 mm and 0.07°, respectively. The results of the mechanical testing showed an increased stability postoperatively as the graft became integrated into a new bony structure. This process could indeed be confirmed by histologic analysis.

Histologic Analysis

In another animal experiment, hand reamers were used to make a cavitary defect in the anterior-superior segment of the acetabulum. Impaction grafting of the resulting defect was performed in the same way as during clinical application to patients. The acetabular component was cemented.

In each time period, 3 goats were sacrificed, at intervals of 6, 12, 24, and 48 weeks. Different histologic techniques were applied, including fluorochrome labeling of new bone. Directly after the operation, the impacted graft consisted of fairly large pieces of trabecular bone, which displayed small microfractures at all levels (Fig. 7). The medullary fat had been squeezed out during impaction and had been replaced by a fibrin clot. After 6 weeks, a front of vascular sprouts accompanied by loose connective tissue, with many leukocytes, penetrated into the graft at a speed of about 70 mm per day. A very high dynamic bone turnover was observed in the graft in association with this

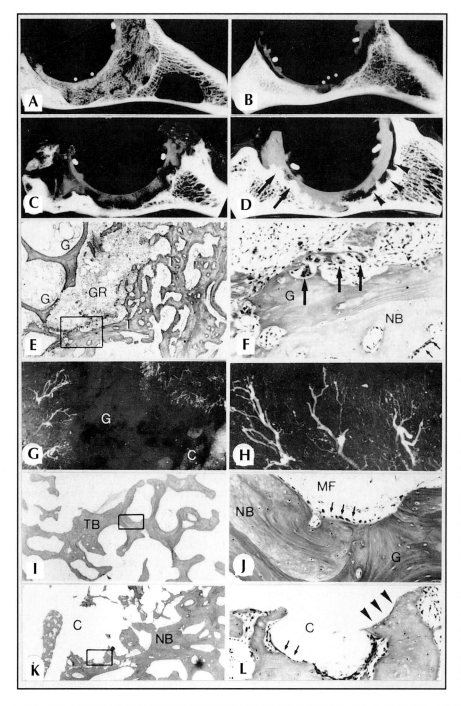

Fig. 7 A-D, Radiographs of thick sections through the acetabulum of the goat taken at 0 (**A**), 12 (**B**), 24 (**C**), and 48 weeks (**D**) after surgery. **A,** Note large pieces of graft and the clear transition zone to the host bone-bed. **B,** Complete consolidation of the graft with the host bone. The incorporation of the graft is almost completed. **C,** A radiolucent zone is present between the cement layer and the bone, indicating that a soft-tissue interface has been formed. **D,** Note local contact areas between bone and cement (arrows) and a radiolucent zone (arrow heads). Note also the dense bone adjacent the cement layer. **E,** Granulation tissue (GR) in the transition zone between a vital graft (G) and newly formed trabecular bone (T) 3 weeks after surgery. **F,** Enlargement of rectangular area outlined in **E**. Many osteoclastic bone cells (large arrows) resorb the graft (G) and osteoblasts (small arrows) synthesize new bone (NB). **G,** A vascularization front penetrates into the graft (G) 12 weeks after the surgery. Cement (C) had penetrated into the graft. **H,** Enlargement of left part of **G**. **I,** Structure of new trabecular bone after 12 weeks. **J,** Enlargement of rectangular area outlined in **I** showing active osteoblasts (arrows) and new bone (NB). Remnants of the graft (G) can be recognized by the empty osteocyte lacunae. **K,** Interface between new bone (NB) and the cement 48 weeks after surgery. Cement (C) that was removed during processing of the tissues, had penetrated deeply into the graft. **L,** Locally at higher magnification a very thin layer, 1 cell thick (arrows), of soft-tissue interface is present, while at other locations the new bone is in direct contact with the cement layer (arrowheads). **E, G, I, K** × 12.5; **F, H, J, L** × 125. (Reproduced with permission from Slooff TJ, Schimmel JW, Buma P: Cemented fixation with bone grafts. *Orthop Clin North Am* 1993;24:667–677.)

fibrovascular tissue, comprising bone graft resorption by osteoclasts and bone apposition by osteoblasts. After 6 weeks, this process resulted in a new trabecular structure in the revascularized areas. This structure consisted primarily of newly formed mainly woven bone with remnants of the graft. After 12 weeks, the percentage of graft in the new trabecular structure decreased further by bone remodeling, which produced lamellar bone. Radiographic and histologic evaluation demonstrated that the orientation of the newly formed trabecular bone was such that load transfer was possible from the cement layer to the host bone bed. At the graft-cement interface, a mixture was found of local areas where vital bone was in intimate contact with the cement layer, and other areas where fibrous tissue predominated. Between 24 and 48 weeks after surgery, the graft in the defect of the

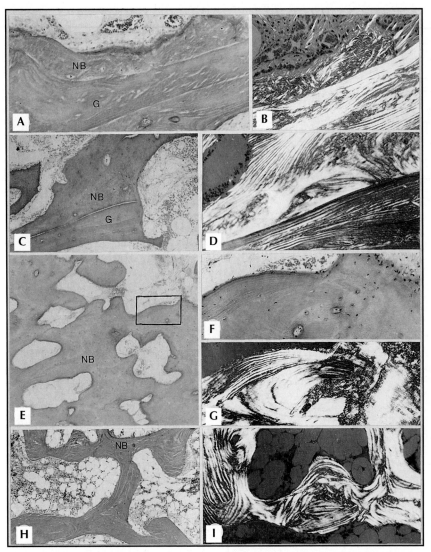

Fig. 8. A and **B,** Human core biopsy 4 months after impaction grafting in the acetabulum. Note new bone formation (NB) on remnant of graft (G). **B,** Same as **A** but with polarized light. Note woven bone formation (× 140). **C** and **D,** Eight months after impaction grafting. Graft (G) has been partially resorbed. New bone formation in the form of lamellar bone (× 60 and × 140, respectively). **E-G,** Fifteen months after impaction grafting. Graft remnants are extremely scarce. Detail of boxed area shows vital (**F**) lamellar (**G**) bone (× 35 and × 140, respectively). **H** and **I,** Normal lamellar (**I**) bony structure with vital cell rich hemopoetic tissue (**H**) in specimen 28 months after impaction grafting (× 60). (Figures A and B reproduced with permission from Buma P, Lamerigts N, Schreurs BW, et al: Impacted graft incorporation after cemented acetabular revision: Histological evaluation in 8 patients. *Acta Orthop Scand* 1996;67:536–540.)

acetabulum had been completely remodeled into lamellar bone.

From our histologic and mechanical results we conclude that the reconstruction technique provides sufficient initial stability to allow incorporation of the impacted acetabular and femoral grafts.

Human Data

Histologic analysis evaluation of graft incorporation is an alternative for radiographic techniques to assess the extent of incorporation into a new trabecular structure. We were able to collect 9 biopsies taken from 8 grafted acetabuli, 1 to 72 months after revision.[27] Revision in all these patients was done using the technique described by Slooff and associates.[22] In 1 patient, who developed persistent sciatic nerve problems after a huge reconstruction in which the center of rotation was created about 5 cm more distally, the whole reconstruction had to be removed after 28 months. Histologic inspection of almost the whole previous graft, including the graft-cement interface, was then possible.

At 1 month postrevision, no signs of graft incorporation were found. In 2 out of the 3 biopsies taken at 4 months, a front of new bone was now penetrating the avascular graft. At the revascularization front, which could be recognized on the basis of vital soft tissue, osteoid and woven bone formed on the original graft trabeculae and in the interstitial space (Fig. 8). Also, local osteoclastic resorption of the graft was found.

All of the specimens taken 8 to 28 months after revision showed different stages of graft incorporation. At 8 and 9 months, various amounts of graft remnants were embedded in a new trabecular structure. Initially, the newly formed bone was woven bone, and this was later remodeled into lamellar bone in the specimens with a longer follow-up period. The interface with the cement layer was histologically similar to that seen in earlier animal studies. Locally vital bone was in direct contact with the cement, but most locations showed a thin soft-tissue layer interfaced with the cement. The bone in the specimens with a follow-up of 15 months or longer closely resembled normal trabecular bone, with only a very few remnants of graft. Similar clinical results were reported after impaction grafting in the proximal femur.[28,29] The sequence of events was comparable to that which had previously been observed in animal experiments.[24,30–34]

From these scientific data, we conclude that impacted morcellized allograft with cement completely incorporates into a new trabecular structure and that the histologic pattern of graft incorporation is consistent in both the animal model and human biopsies.

Clinical Results

In 1984 we first reported the short-term results of bone impaction grafting in total hip replacement for acetabular protrusion.[22] In 40 patients, 43 acetabular reconstructions were performed. Of these, 21 arthroplasties were primary procedures in cases with protrusion and 22 were revisions after failed total hip arthroplasties with acetabular bone stock loss. Diagnosis of the cases was osteoarthritis (15), rheumatoid arthritis (15), or trauma. The defects were mainly contained. Autografts were used in all primary total hip arthroplasties, but allografts were used in all revisions. After a short-term follow-up of 2 years (range, 0.5 to 5.5 years) there were no revisions, but radiolucent lines were seen in 5 cases.

Our midterm results were presented in 1993 in a study of 88 acetabular hip revisions in 80 patients.[31] All hips were reconstructed with impacted morcellized bone grafts, and the average follow-up was 5.7 years (range, 2 to 11 years). The group consisted of 58 women and 22 men. The patients required surgery because of primary osteoarthritis (49), secondary osteoarthritis (22), or rheumatoid arthritis (9). Defects were classified according to the American

Academy of Orthopaedic Surgeons' classification system as cavitary (42 cases) or combined segmental-cavitary (38 cases). At this midterm 5.7-year follow-up, 4 acetabular re-revisions had been performed, 2 for septic loosening and 2 for aseptic loosening. The postoperative Harris Hip Scores (HHS) averaged 87; the preoperative HHS was estimated at 44. Six cases were defined as radiologic failures, 1 case because of progressive radiologic loosening in all 3 zones, according to DeLee and Charnley.[35] Using a computer-digitizing program, in the other 5 cases radiologic loosening was suspected because of progressive migration.

However, only long-term follow-up can prove the true clinical value of a surgical technique. The most reliable criterion in long-term follow-up of primary hip arthroplasties and revision hip arthroplasties is the survival rate of the prosthesis using the moment of re-revision as the end point.[36] All patients who underwent acetabular reconstruction and revision surgery with impacted morcellized bone grafts at our department with a follow-up of at least 10 years were enrolled in our study (to be published).

In this long-term study, 62 acetabular revisions were performed with impacted morcellized bone grafts and a cemented cup for failed acetabular components in 58 patients.[37] Two cases (2 hips) were lost to follow-up. Ten patients (10 hips) died within 10 years after the operation. None had a re-revision. Forty-six patients (50 hips) had a follow-up of 10 years or more (range, 10 to 15 years; average, 11.8 years). The defects were classified as cavitary in 37 and combined in 23 cases. There were no solitary segmental defects in this group of patients. Five acetabular re-revisions

had been performed. These were due to septic loosening in 2 cases (3 and 6 years postoperative) and aseptic loosening in 3 cases (6, 9, and 12 years postoperative).

The overall survival rate was 90% when all loosenings were taken into account. But excluding the 2 infections, the survival rate for aseptic loosening only was 94% at an average of 11.8 years follow-up. Using the same criteria as mentioned above, there were 4 radiographic failures without clinical symptons of loosening.

Current Recommendations

Before attempting acetabular reconstruction with bone impaction grafting and cement, a surgeon should be informed as thoroughly as possible about the clinical, scientific, and technical details of this reconstruction method, developed at the hospitals in Nijmegen and Exeter. Experimental studies and clinical observations have clearly shown that impacted morcellized allografts lead to a predictable result: complete and rapid incorporation without impairing the strength of the graft during the process (Fig. 9). This is in contrast with the use of structural bone grafts, which incorporate incompletely, with unpredictable results.[38,39] The structural grafts that are generally used are parts of degenerative femoral heads, and this may be the cause of the incomplete incorporation. Furthermore, because of the existing mismatch of the contact surfaces, it is very difficult to achieve permanent fixation of structural cancellous grafts to host bone. This lack of fixation can lead to instability of the graft and eventual resorption.

If segmental acetabular defects are present, it is mandatory to close them in order to achieve adequate impaction. We advocate the use of

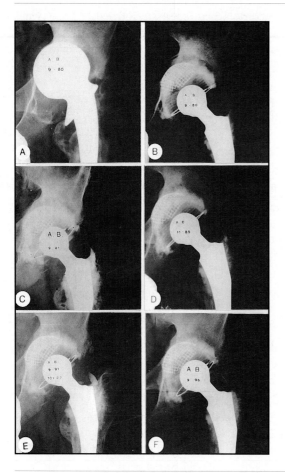

Fig. 9 A, Radiograph of a 36-year-old patient with a hemiprosthesis of the right hip that had been implanted 6 years following failed osteosynthesis of a femoral neck fracture. The metal head of the prosthesis is protruding through the acetabulum, causing central segmental defect of the acetabulum. **B-F,** Serial radiographs directly after (**B**), 1 year after (**C**), 5 years after (**D**), 10 years after (**E**), and 16 years (**F**), after reconstruction with impacted allograft bone chips. No migration, no signs of loosening, and a homogeneous structure of the graft are visible.

hip surgery, in general, make this procedure very unpopular for hospital administration and orthopaedic surgeons. The resource issues of these reconstruction techniques of the hip are significant and are mainly defined by the type of implant, the fixation method (with or without cement), and the use of banked bone. However, the cost aspects of special and custom-made prostheses must not be underestimated.

References

1. van Leeuwenhoek A: Microscopical observations about blood, milk bones, the brain, spittle, cuticula, sweat, fat and tears. *Philos Trans R Soc Lond* 1674;9:121–131.

2. van Meekeren J: *Heel-en Geneeskundige Aanmerkingen*. Amsterdam, The Netherlands, L Commelijn, 1668.

3. Ollier L: *Traité Experimental et Clinique de la Regeneration des os et de la Production Artificielle du Tissu Osseux*. Paris, France, Victor Masson, 1867.

4. Macewen W: Observations concerning transplantation of bones. *Proc Roy Soc Lond* 1881;32:232–247.

5. Curtis BF: Cases of bone implantation and transplantation for cyst of tibia, osteomyelitic cavities, and ununited fractures. *Am J Med Sci* 1893;106:30–37.

6. Barth A: Ueber histologische Befunde nach Knochenimplantationen. *Arch Klin Chir* 1893;46:409–417.

7. Lexer E: Die Verwendung der freien Knochenplastik nebst Versuchen über Gelenkversteifung und Gelenktransplantation. *Arch Klin Chir* 1908;86:939–954.

8. Axhausen G: Arbeiten aus dem Gebiet de Knochenpathologie und Knochenchirurgie 1: kritische bemerkungen und neue Beiträge zur freien Knochentransplantation. *Arch Klin Chir* 1911;94:241–281.

9. Hirst P, Esser M, Murphy JC, et al: Bone grafting for protrusio acetabuli during total hip replacement: A review of the Wrightington method in 61 hips. *J Bone Joint Surg* 1987;69B:229–233.

10. Olivier H, Sanouiller JL: Acetabular reconstruction using spongious grafts in reoperation of hip arthroplasties. *Rev Chir Orthop Repar Appar Mot* 1991;77:232–240.

11. Gross AE, Lavoie MV, McDermott P, et al: The use of allograft bone in revision of total hip arthroplasty. *Clin Orthop* 1985;197:115–122.

12. Harris WH, Crothers O, Oh I: Total hip replacement and femoral-head bone-grafting for severe acetabular deficiency in adults. *J Bone Joint Surg* 1977;59A:752–759.

flexible wire meshes, which are adapted and fixed to the pelvis by screw fixation. Impaction of the morcellized grafts results in a stable and rough surface that improves the mechanical cement-bone interlock and the adaptation of the chip closely to the irregular surface of the host bone bed. Rigid impaction reduces gap formation between the host and graft, promoting the union process. The stability of the reconstruction is further improved by pressurizing the cement onto the graft.

As previously mentioned, the use of substantially sized morcellized allografts approximately 1 cm in each dimension is recommended for the acetabulum. Reduction of the chip size can cause early migration of the acetabular cup during the incorpora-

tion process because of the lack of initial stability.

In 1988, Hungerford and Jones[40] expressed their concern about allowing cement to be in direct contact with a morcellized allograft. Positive results with this combination have been reported by Roffman and associates,[20] and have been confirmed by the results of histologic studies performed by Schimmel[24] and Schreurs[34] in animal models.

As reported by other investigators, no difference was observed between the radiologic evaluation of autogenous grafts and that of allografts. However, in our view radiographic evaluation of bone incorporation is difficult. Because allograft bone can be available in sufficient quantities, there is no limit to the quantity of graft used. The economics of revision

13. Harris WH: Allografting in total hip arthroplasty: In adults with severe acetabular deficiency including a surgical technique for bolting the graft to the ilium. *Clin Orthop* 1982;162:150–164.

14. Sotelo-Garza A, Charnley J: The results of Charnley arthroplasty of the hip performed for protrusio acetabuli. *Clin Orthop* 1978;132:12–18.

15. Berry DJ, Müller ME: Revision arthroplasty using an anti-protrusio cage for massive acetabular bone deficiency. *J Bone Joint Surg* 1992;74B:711–715.

16. Harris WH: Management of the deficient acetabulum using cementless fixation without bone grafting. *Orthop Clin North Am* 1993;24:663–665.

17. Hastings DE, Parker SM: Protrusio acetabuli in rheumatoid arthritis. *Clin Orthop* 1975;108:76–83.

18. McCollum DE, Nunley JA: Bone grafting in acetabular protrusio: A biologic buttress, in Nelson CL (ed): *The Hip: Proceedings of the Sixth Open Scientific Meeting of the Hip Society, 1978.* St. Louis, MO, CV Mosby, 1978, pp 124–146.

19. Marti RK, Besselaar PP: Bone grafts in primary and secondary total hip replacement, in Marti RK (ed): *Progress in Cemented Total Hip Surgery and Revision.* Amsterdam, The Netherlands, Excerpta Medica, 1983, pp 107–129.

20. Roffman M, Silbermann M, Mendes DG: Incorporation of bone graft covered with methylmethacrylate onto the acetabular wall: An experimental study. *Acta Orthop Scand* 1983;54:580–583.

21. Mendes DG, Roffman M, Silbermann M: Reconstruction of the acetabular wall with bone graft in arthroplasty of the hip. *Clin Orthop* 1984;186:29–37.

22. Slooff TJ, Huiskes R, van Horn J, et al: Bone grafting in total hip replacement for acetabular protrusion. *Acta Orthop Scand* 1984; 55:593–596.

23. Schreurs BW, Huiskes R, Slooff TJJH: The initial stability of hip prosthesis in combination with femoral intramedullary bonegraft, in Odgaard A, Kjaersgaard-Andersen P, Sojbjerg JO (eds): *European Biomechanics: Proceedings of the 7th Meeting of the European Society of Biomechanics.* Aarhus, Denmark, European Society of Biomechanics, 1990, p A14.

24. Schimmel JW, Buma P, Versleyen D, Huiskes R, Slooff TJ: Acetabular reconstruction with impacted morcellized cancellous allografts in cemented hip arthroplasty: A histologic and biomechanical study on the goat. *J Arthroplasty* 1998;13:438–448.

25. Schreurs BW, Buma P, Huiskes R, et al: Morsellized allografts for fixation of the hip prosthesis femoral component: A mechanical and histological study in the goat. *Acta Orthop Scand* 1994;65:267–275.

26. Selvik G: *A Roentgen Stereophotogrammetric Method for the Study of the Kinematics of the Skeletal System.* Lund, Sweden, University of Lund, 1974. Thesis.

27. Buma P, Lamerigts N, Schreurs BW, et al: Impacted graft incorporation after cemented acetabular revision: Histological evaluation in 8 patients. *Acta Orthop Scand* 1996;67:536–540.

28. Ling RS, Timperley AJ, Linder L: Histology of cancellous impaction grafting in the femur: A case report. *J Bone Joint Surg* 1993;75B:693–696.

29. Nelissen RG, Bauer TW, Weidenhielm LR, et al: Revision hip arthroplasty with the use of cement and impaction grafting: Histological analysis of four cases. *J Bone Joint Surg* 1995;77A:412–422.

30. Buma P, Schreurs BW, Versleyen D, et al: Histological evaluation of allograft incorporation after cemented and non-cemented hip arthroplasty in the goat, in Older J (ed): *Bone Implant Grafting.* London, England, Springer Verlag, 1992, pp 13–17.

31. Slooff TJ, Schimmel JW, Buma P: Cemented fixation with bone grafts. *Orthop Clin North Am* 1993;24:667–677.

32. Slooff TJ , Buma P, Schreurs BW, et al: Acetabular and femoral reconstruction with impacted grafts and cement. *Clin Orthop* 1996;324:108–115.

33. Slooff TJ, Buma P, Schimmel JW, et al: Impaction grafting and cement in acetabular revision arthroplasty, in Czitrom AA, Winkler H (eds): *Orthopaedic Allograft Surgery.* Wien, Germany, Springer-Verlag, 1996, pp 125–134.

34. Schreurs BW: *Reconstructive Options in Revision Surgery of Failed Total Hip Arthroplasties.* Nijmegen, The Netherlands, University of Ku Nijmegen, 1994. Thesis.

35. DeLee JG, Charnley J: Radiological demarcation of cemented sockets in total hip replacement. *Clin Orthop* 1976;121:20–32.

36. Malchau H, Herberts P: Surgical and cemented technique in total hip replacement: A revision-risk study of 136,000 primary operations. Proceedings of the American Academy of Orthopaedic Surgeons 63rd Annual Meeting, Atlanta, GA. Rosemont, IL, American Academy of Orthopaedic Surgeons, 1996.

37. Schreurs BW, Buma P, Gardeniers JW, et al: Acetabular reconstruction with impacted morcellized cancellous bone grafts in cemented revision hip arthroplasty: A ten- to 15-year follow-up study. Proceedings of the American Academy of Orthopaedic Surgeons 65th Annual Meeting, New Orleans, LA. Rosemont, IL, American Academy of Orthopaedic Surgeons, 1998.

38. Enneking WF, Mindell ER: Observations on massive retrieved human allografts. *J Bone Joint Surg* 1991;73A:1123–1142.

39. Stevenson S, Xiao Qing Li, Martin B: The fate of cancellous and cortical bone after transplantation of fresh and frozen tissue-antigen-matched and mismatched osteochondral allografts in dogs. *J Bone Joint Surg* 1991; 73A:1143–1156.

40. Hungerford DS, Jones LC: The rationale of cementless revision of cemented arthroplasty failures. *Clin Orthop* 1988;235:12–24.

Hip and Knee: Reconstruction

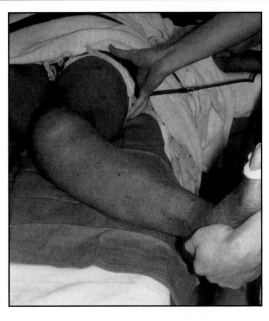

Surgical Management of Inflammatory Arthritis of the Adult Hip and Knee

Steven A. Stuchin, MD
Norman A. Johanson, MD
Paul F. Lachiewicz, MD
Michael A. Mont, MD

Introduction

Patients with inflammatory arthritis often present a complicated medical and surgical challenge. Multijoint and multiorgan involvement is compounded with immunosuppressive chemotherapeutic drugs. Compromised bone stock and poor soft-tissue quality increase the surgical risks. Successful surgical management depends on anticipation of the common pitfalls and patterns of disease and the ability to delineate and implement a campaign for long-term care that may require a number of procedures staged over months to years. The impact of each intervention must be understood and integrated into a plan designed to maximize a patient's ability to ambulate and transfer, while exposing the patient to a minimum of risk.

The decisions surrounding the surgical treatment of polyarticular inflammatory arthritis are in many respects as much an art as they are science. Many important considerations that pertain to the patient's global status, the particular regions of involvement, and the tempo of the disease need to be enumerated, prioritized, and integrated into the final surgical

plan. However, rather than employing a "paint-by-numbers" approach to surgical treatment, a series of hierarchical principles should be used initially to plan out the type and order of procedures before actually deciding on a rational approach to surgical staging that is based on relevant time-tested principles.

Indications for Surgery

Pain

Joint pain that cannot be relieved by nonsurgical means is the primary indication for surgery. Because of multiple joint involvement, ambulation is often a tenuous compromise made among marginally functional hips, knees, feet, and ankles. Increased pain may disrupt this compromise, putting the patient in a wheelchair. Even if the painful joint is not the most clinically deformed or radiographically involved, it should have surgical priority.

Function

Pain usually is linked to functional disturbance, which often is the patient's primary concern.[1] Questions that approach the functional compromises that are directly related to pain,

such as walking distance, stair-climbing, occupational duties, and housework, are useful as proxy measures for pain. However, there may be other causes of functional loss, such as generalized fatigue and weakness, that would not necessarily be helped by surgery. An accurate history is essential to establish a causal relationship between a specific articular or periarticular pain pattern and the patient's functional status. Once this has been established, the analysis of the patient's functional decline can become a useful adjunct to evaluating the severity and global impact of pain.

Deformity

Patients with inflammatory arthritis often develop severe deformities, particularly in the hands, wrists, feet, ankles, and knees. The disfiguring peripheral deformities are often striking, but it is surprising how well tolerated they may be in some patients who are treated nonsurgically, using assistive devices. However, because of the exquisite interrelationship of the lower extremity joints, factors that affect 1 joint may have profound implications for the entire locomotor system. A severe varus, valgus, rotational, or flexion deformity of the knee may have significant impact on the efficiency of rehabilitation and the ultimate outcome of surgery in the hip, ankle, or foot. In such cases, correction of the deformity may be required prior to performing surgery on more painful joints.[2] The relationship between valgus knee arthritis and planovalgus foot deformities should be taken into account when planning lower extremity surgery.[3] If a hindfoot valgus or rotational deformity is overcorrected prior to the correction of valgus knee alignment, overloading of the lateral side of the foot may result. If the foot or ankle deformities are severe enough to jeopardize knee rehabilitation, they should be corrected first. Otherwise the knee should be treated first and foot and ankle symptoms monitored during the following months. Deformities of the hindfoot should be treated before forefoot deformities because of the tendency to alter load-bearing patterns of the forefoot with hindfoot surgery and the reported tendency for the results of forefoot surgery to be compromised by severe ankle valgus deformity.[3] This is particularly true when the midfoot is rigid, which transfers excessive loads distally to the metatarsal heads.

Regional Priorities
Cervical Spine
Inflammatory involvement at the atlanto-occipital, atlantoaxial, or sub-axial joints makes instability of the cervical spine a potentially devastating orthopaedic problem. A continuous surveillance of the onset and progression of symptoms and radiographic signs should be conducted. Symptoms of neck pain, occipital pain, weakness, spasticity, or vertebral artery compromise, in combination with significant radiographic findings of cervical instability, should be given

the highest priority for surgical treatment.[4] Early diagnosis through screening of patients may help prevent progression to intractable neurologic symptoms and technically difficult surgical procedures that have high complication rates and compromised outcomes. The actual threshold for cervical spine surgery in inflammatory arthritis has not been precisely defined, but certain radiographic parameters have been identified as indicators for surgery: (1) atlantoaxial subluxation of greater than 9 mm, (2) superior migration of the odontoid into the foramen magnum, (3) magnetic resonance imaging (MRI) evidence of spinal cord or brainstem compression, and (4) sub-axial instability of greater than 4 mm.[4]

Upper Extremities
Panning for lower extremity surgery must include an evaluation of the upper extremities. For patients using ambulatory aids, walkers, crutches, and canes, the upper extremities are part of the locomotor system (Fig. 1). Furthermore, because patients who undergo hip or knee surgery invariably require assistive devices in the postoperative period, appropriate considerations are paramount. In polyarticular inflammatory arthritis involving both upper and lower extremities, it is useful to obtain an occupational therapy evaluation for assessment of the various joints' relative functional disturbances. This process provides helpful information for the prioritization of surgical procedures. The functional impact of stiff and painful upper extremity joints can be better assessed when the patient is observed performing a series of standardized tasks, such as dressing, opening containers, eating, and using walking supports. Assistive devices, including rolling and platform walkers and modified crutches

and canes, may be ordered in advance to allow patients to best use compromised upper extremities to enhance ambulation. A patient's own reaction to the current situation and attitude toward his or her disease is usually revealed through the assessment process, thus giving clues regarding the optimal prioritization of surgery.

Hip and Knee
Hip and knee reconstructive procedures take high priority because they often make the difference between an ambulatory and independent patient and one who must depend on a wheelchair and the help of others for activities of daily living. In the absence of severe disabling knee pain or deformity the hip should be surgically treated first[5] (Fig. 2). The recovery from hip replacement is faster than for total knee replacement, and the rehabilitation of a total hip depends less on a mobile knee than rehabilitation of a knee replacement depends on a mobile hip for an optimal result. A caveat in the prioritization of hip and knee surgery is that a severe valgus knee deformity can contribute to dislocation of a total hip replacement because of the resulting excessive hip adduction and internal rotation. Therefore, even if hip and knee symptoms are similar, in this case it may be safer to proceed with knee replacement first.[2] Additionally, patients with advanced bilateral knee contractures may also be considered for initial knee replacement in order to allow them to assume a vertical position.

Foot and Ankle
Severe ankle and hindfoot arthritis should be treated surgically prior to undertaking forefoot reconstruction. The typical ankle and foot alignment in inflammatory arthritis is a valgus hindfoot deformity and a severely

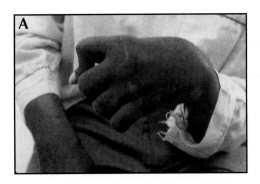
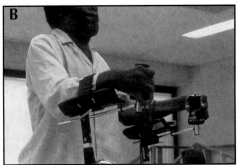
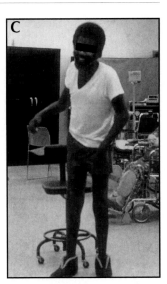

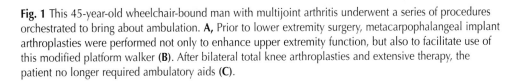

Fig. 1 This 45-year-old wheelchair-bound man with multijoint arthritis underwent a series of procedures orchestrated to bring about ambulation. **A,** Prior to lower extremity surgery, metacarpophalangeal implant arthroplasties were performed not only to enhance upper extremity function, but also to facilitate use of this modified platform walker **(B)**. After bilateral total knee arthroplasties and extensive therapy, the patient no longer required ambulatory aids **(C)**.

pronated forefoot, often with hallux valgus, clawing of the lesser toes, and callus formation (bunion) over the metatarsal heads. In extreme cases, a callus forms under the navicular. An ankle or subtalar arthrodesis may correct the hindfoot deformity and can have significant impact on the loading of the forefoot, sometimes for the better if the load is distributed more favorably. The forefoot should be reevaluated following hindfoot or ankle surgery to assess the patient's symptoms and function prior to considering a forefoot reconstruction. Open lesions of the dorsal or plantar aspects of the feet should be addressed prior to any implant surgery because of the risk of metastatic infection. After total hip or knee replacement, the patient's functional status is often improved to the point where a previously quiescent foot or ankle problem may interfere with further progress in rehabilitation. In rare cases, a foot or ankle problem, usually a deformity, is so severe that foot or ankle surgery is needed prior to undertaking hip or knee surgery.[3] For this to be indicated, it must be demonstrated that without surgery on the foot or ankle, the rehabilitation

from hip or knee surgery would be extremely difficult.

Bilateral Surgery

The patient with polyarticular inflammatory arthritis may become overwhelmed with multiple joint problems that must be surgically treated within a relatively short period of time to avoid the downward spiral toward functional dependency. Bilateral surgery in the hips, knees, and forefeet should be performed whenever the surgical indications exist and the patient is medically and psychologically able to undergo the procedures.[6] The extent of flexion contracture that may develop in patients is so great that without bilateral surgery, standing unassisted, let alone ambulation, may not be possible. Bilateral total hip replacement followed in 10 days to 2 weeks by bilateral total knee replacement has been found to be effective in selected, highly motivated patients. Ankle arthrodesis or triple arthrodesis for bilateral problems should be performed 1 side at a time because prolonged nonweightbearing would have a significant impact on the patient's functional status. In addition, in a nonweightbearing patient, the proba-

bility of enhanced disuse osteopenia would be significantly increased, especially in conjunction with steroid use.

Preoperative Evaluation and Planning

The multisystem nature of the inflammatory arthritides make for some complicated but well-recognized pitfalls in the preoperative evaluation and planning for surgery. The organ systems generally at risk include the following.

The Skin

Psoriasis Patients with psoriatic arthritis are at increased risk for infection. Skin lesions may harbor bacteria. Dermatologic care, especially at planned incision sites, may be helpful. Risks for infection after hip replacement have been found to be as high as 9.1% for superficial and 5.5% for deep infection.[7] Interestingly, knee replacement risks have been reported as no greater than osteoarthritis in some studies[8] and at greater risks in others.[9]

Ulceration Rheumatoid vasculitis may cause skin ulceration. Pressure sores over foot deformities and over the sacrococcygeal region in wheel-

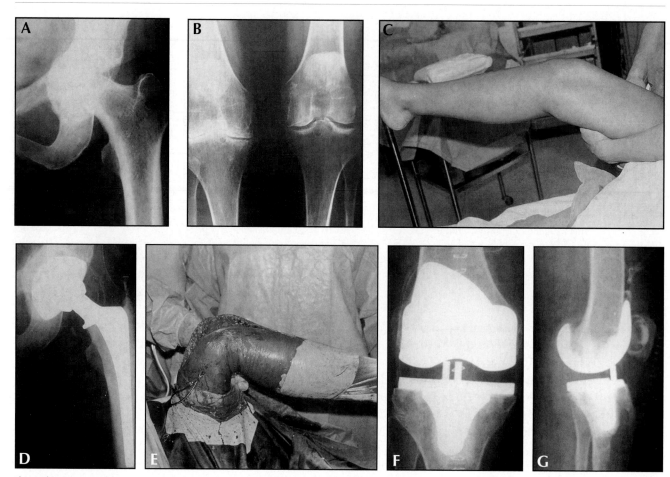

Fig. 2 This 57-year-old woman presented with a painful left hip with protrusio deformity (**A**), and an equally painful right knee with severe limitation of motion (**B** and **C**). She underwent hybrid hip arthroplasty. The hip center of motion was restored using this cementless socket pressfit at the rim and morcellized autogenous femoral head graft (**D**). Knee motion was enhanced by employing a quadriceps V-Y resection (**E**). Because there was underlying ligamentous integrity, a minimally constrained implant was used (**F** and **G**).

chair- and bed-bound patients may also cause skin breakdown, resulting in local infection that may seed distal surgical sites. Careful inspection and appropriate local care should be undertaken prior to planned surgery.

The Spine

Cervical Spine Rheumatoid arthritis may cause instability, especially at C1-C2. The hyperextension of the neck necessary for intubation and anesthesia may cause severe neurologic compromise in the presence of instability. Radiographs of the cervical spine, including flexion-extension instability studies, should be obtained. In a study

by Collins and associates,[10] 61% of 113 patients with rheumatoid arthritis who had total hip or total knee replacement had radiographic cervical spine instability. However, 50% of these patients were asymptomatic and had no physical findings.[10] Surgical stabilization of the cervical spine is not required prior to total joint replacement, but care should be taken during intubation and patient positioning. To avoid problems with the cervical spine, and because it can be difficult to intubate patients who have juvenile rheumatoid arthritis (due to temporomandibular joint problems and micrognathia), regional anesthesia may

be indicated. In patients with ankylosing spondylitis, fiberoptic nasotracheal intubation and general anesthesia are often employed.

Thoracolumbar Spine Ankylosing spondylitis may fuse spinal elements, creating a bone block to spinal or epidural anesthesia techniques (Fig. 3). Limited chest-wall expansion obligates diaphragmatic respiration. Pulmonary function studies should be performed in this patient population. Patients undergoing total hip replacement in the lateral position may experience marked respiratory compromise if a positioning device is used to stabilize the pelvis. These devices, which frequently compress the lower abdomen as well as the pelvis, can prevent excursion of the diaphragm, especially in patients with large abdominal girth. Careful positioning at surgery, alteration of surgical approach to use the supine position, use of less restrictive positioning devices, and close communication with the anesthesiologist should be borne in mind.

Head and Neck
Rheumatoid arthritis may affect the temporomandibular joints, making intubation difficult. It also may affect the cricoarytenoid cartilage, interfering with intubation.

The Lungs
Rheumatoid Arthritis Rheumatoid involvement of the lung may compromise function. Pulmonary evaluation may be important.

Ankylosing Spondylitis Limited chest wall expansion may have serious consequences, as noted previously.

The Intestines
Ileitis and colitis are associated with arthritis. Hematogenous seeding of an implant from bowel infection is a risk of surgery. Hip wounds should be protected from potential outflow of colostomy sites.

The Hematopoietic System
Patients may be chronically anemic. Strategies for blood conservation, replacement, and donation are paramount, because the normal reticulocyte response may not occur. Multiply operated-on patients may have undergone previous transfusions, which, coupled with autoimmune problems, can severely limit blood replacement options.

The Immune System
Immune system suppression is caused by these diseases and is further com-

promised by the drugs used to treat them. Methylmethacrylate has been shown to inhibit white cell function as well.[11] Furthermore, patients who are taking steroids may not present with classic signs of infection. Blood tests are often equivocal. Steroids raise the white blood cell count. An elevated erythrocyte sedimentation rate is common in arthritis. A high index of suspicion is important. Meticulous attention must be paid to surgical technique and postoperative wound care. Hematomas and draining wounds should be treated appropriately.

The Bone
Bone quality and density vary. Steroid-dependent rheumatoid arthritis may make for large intramedullary canals and weak bone. Juvenile arthritis may leave joints very small, with exceedingly tight canals. Appropriate preoperative planning is necessary to insure appropriately sized components for arthroplasty. The surgeon should be familiar with a variety of cemented and cementless fixation techniques.

The Soft Tissues
Contractures of muscle, capsule, and ligament frequently require release. Hip flexion and adduction contractures may require iliopsoas and adductor releases. Stiff knees may require a quadriceps-lengthening procedure (Fig. 2, *E* and *F*).

Ankylosing spondylitis may be complicated by heterotopic ossification after total hip arthroplasty (Fig. 4). Prophylactic treatment with radiation therapy or pharmacologic agents should be planned. In spite of treatment, the fibroblastic response after surgery may limit hip motion even without heterotopic ossification.[12]

The Other Joints
Upper Extremities Upper extremity function may be an important con-

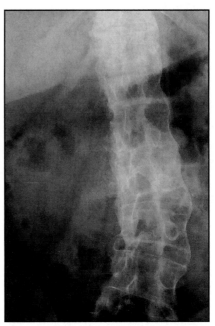

Fig. 3 Ankylosing spondylitis has resulted in fusion across extensive areas of the spine.

sideration in patients who require ambulatory aids for walking and transfers. The weight transfers and stresses that will be applied to the arms and shoulders in the postoperative period must be considered. Modified walkers and crutches that transfer forces away from weakened or disabled joints should be available. These may include platform attachments to walkers and crutches and rolling walkers. If the expected protocol for a given implant or surgical technique requires a period of limited weightbearing, this surgical approach may need to be reconsidered for certain patients.

Lower Extremities Foot and ankle problems must be addressed to allow for proper ambulation. Patients who have multijoint problems will require a well-thought-out plan in order to accommodate what may be multiple surgical procedures staged over time and accompanied by appropriate therapy to maximize their gains.

Nutrition

Rheumatoid arthritis is traditionally considered a catabolic, wasting disease. While many patients are underweight, a significant number are overweight but, paradoxically, are still malnourished. Nutritional assessment and care may limit wound healing and infection problems.[13]

Medications

Attaining medical control of these diseases can be difficult. Stopping all medications prior to surgery may exacerbate disease and cause undue suffering.

Nonsteroidal Anti-Inflammatory Drugs (NSAIDs) The half life for antiplatelet activity of these drugs is different for each medication. Aspirin may be effective for much longer than ibuprofen. In appropriate circumstances, it may not be necessary to stop all drugs of this class 1 week before surgery, as has been traditional in some centers. Consultation with rheumatology and judicious drug substitution may make it possible to continue these medications to the day before surgery and still avoid the theoretical bleeding problems that platelet inhibition can cause.[14]

Steroids Steroid-dependent patients may require stress doses at the time of surgery, and they should be monitored for steroid insufficiency should complications of surgery bring about undue stresses. However, in a study by Friedman and associates[15] of 28 patients who had 35 major orthopaedic procedures without stress-dose steroids, no patient, including 17 with rheumatoid arthritis, had any evidence of adrenocorticoid deficiency. These investigators concluded that supplemental exogenous stress glucocorticoids are not needed to meet the demands of surgical stress in these patients.

Chemotherapeutic Agents Antineoplastic and antimetabolic agents, including methotrexate and penicillamine, may delay wound healing and contribute to immunosuppression.[16,17] Methotrexate, a second-line or disease-modifying antirheumatic drug, inhibits the division of immune cells active in inflammatory pathways, with an increased risk of infection as a potential consequence. The effect of methotrexate on the risk of infection and delayed wound healing is controversial and unsettled. In a 10-year retrospective study, Perhala and associates[16] concluded that weekly low-dose methotrexate does not increase the risk of postoperative infection or affect wound healing in rheumatoid arthritis patients who undergo total joint replacement. However, in another study, of 38 patients who underwent elective surgery, there were 4 infections or dehiscences in 19 procedures on patients who continued methotrexate perioperatively, compared to no complications in 34 procedures on patients who discontinued methotrexate 4 weeks before surgery.[17]

While only too often these diseases culminate in the surgical ablation of a joint by replacement or fusion, the young age and at times active lifestyle of many patients mandates that every effort be made to preserve or protect biologic articular surfaces when possible. Several diseases and disease states may lend themselves to this kind of thinking.

Osteonecrosis

Osteonecrosis affecting the hips of patients with systemic lupus erythematosus involves the femoral head before any joint cartilage destructive changes have occurred. In these patients, joint-preserving procedures, such as core decompression, bone grafting, and osteotomies, can be at-tempted with some success. The osteonecrosis that arises in the femoral heads of patients with rheumatoid arthritis and ankylosing spondylitis occurs synchronously with the joint destruction by the inflammatory disease, which attacks both the femoral and acetabular cartilage. This makes it impossible to save the osteonecrotic femoral heads in these patients. As a result, rheumatoid arthritis patients with osteonecrosis are treated symptomatically or based on their joint inflammatory disease. This section will detail hip-preserving surgical approaches for patients with systemic lupus erythematosus and those with rheumatoid arthritides.

Systemic Lupus Erythematosus

Unlike patients with the other inflammatory arthritides, patients with systemic lupus erythematosus (SLE) most commonly do not have significant deformity or radiographic evidence of erosive disease in their hip joint. Arthralgias and/or myalgias, in the absence of overt arthritis, are the rule. However, osteonecrosis of the femoral head is common in patients with SLE, ranging in large series from 2.8% to 40%.[18–34] In addition, approximately 20% of these patients develop osteonecrosis in other joints,[35] making the effects of this disease even more devastating.

The importance of buying time for the femoral head in this young, often bilaterally affected group (80% in most studies) of patients must not be underestimated. The results of total joint arthroplasty performed for osteonecrosis have been extensively reported to fall short of the successes that are seen with other patients undergoing total hip replacement. In 27 separate reports,[36] only 1 showed favorable results in patients with osteonecrosis compared to matched groups with other diagnoses. Examples of studies with high failure rates in osteonecrosis patients include Cornell and associates,[37] who reported on 11 failures of 28 hips (39%). In addition, these patients are generally under treatment with large doses of corticosteroids, which makes them susceptible to infections. Even with the present and future improvements in total hip replacement, it is extremely desirable to delay or avoid the need for arthroplasty in these patients. The surgeon should appreciate that these SLE patients have a near-normal life expectancy, which may be greater than 50 years. Thus, it is important to prolong the time before total hip arthroplasty in patients with SLE.

The multitude of treatments for osteonecrosis of the femoral head reflects both the magnitude of the problem and the lack of a clearly superior method. For small lesions in young patients who have early disease without involvement of the acetabulum, options such as core decompression, corrective osteotomy, and vascularized and nonvascularized bone grafting have been used.[36] The treatment should be viewed as a continuum. Core decompression is indicated for early cases and limited femoral resurfacing or total hip arthroplasty for the most advanced, with osteotomy and bone grafting reserved for the patient with intermediate disease involvement.

Most authors have not found a difference in outcome when SLE patients with osteonecrosis treated by various methods are compared to non-SLE patients[16,25,28,38,39,40] The fate of the femoral head in these patients has been found in multiple studies to depend mostly on the size and stage of the lesion.[41,42] Although there are multiple staging systems, a simple way to conceptualize treatment is to separate hips into pre- and postcollapse groups. Precollapse hips that

have small or medium-sized lesions can be treated with core decompression, osteotomies, and/or nonvascularized and vascularized bone-grafting. With postcollapse hips, there are fewer choices. Occasionally, bone grafting and limited femoral resurfacing can be done, but often the only option is total hip arthroplasty. Most studies have shown that nonsurgical management yields poor results with greater than 85% of hips treated with various methods of restricted weightbearing going on to total hip arthroplasties within 3 years.[36,40] The rest of this section will deal with various methods of surgical treatment. Because most studies lump all osteonecrosis patients together, the following sections will focus on the treatments in general, referring to patients with SLE when possible.

Surgical Treatment for Precollapse Disease Four types of surgical treatment are used to treat precollapse disease. The 4 are core decompression, osteotomy, nonvascularized bone grafting, and vascularized bone grafting.

The rationale for the first of these, core decompression, is based on the reduction of bone marrow pressure and improvement in bone blood flow, which may enhance the process of creeping substitution by stimulating neovascularization in the drilled channel(s).[36,43] Satisfactory clinical results were reported for this procedure in 63.5% of 1,206 hips in 24 studies of core decompression in a recent literature review.[40] This study looked at all osteonecrosis patients but did not stratify into a group those patients with SLE.

In a recent cross-sectional study of 50 patients (79 hips) with corticosteroid-associated osteonecrosis of the femoral head there were 31 hips in 18 patients with SLE.[28] In the SLE patients, 21 (67%) were converted to a

total hip arthroplasty at an average of 51 months (range, 5 to 180 months). The major risk factors for disease progression were late stage of the disease at presentation (postcollapse) and the extent of the lesion (necrotic angle greater than 200°). Five of 15 (33%) precollapse hips progressed as did all 16 (100%) postcollapse hips. Necrotic angles > 200° at presentation all progressed to hip replacement (9 hips). Conversely, if the necrotic angle was < 200°, 50% progressed to hip replacement. There were no statistical etiology-related differences in outcome ($p = 0.4$) for directly matched groups of SLE and non-SLE patients undergoing core decompression. Thus, the majority of osteonecrotic hips in SLE patients had reached postcollapse disease (52% versus 31% in non-SLE patients), which portended a poor outcome. In summary, it appears that core decompression should be reserved for small, early stage lesions, which makes a high suspicion for osteonecrosis in SLE patients all the more important so that the diagnosis is made as early as possible.

The aim of an osteotomy, second of the 4 treatment types, is to remove the osteonecrotic area, which usually involves the posterolateral part of the femoral head, and to replace it by relatively unaffected sound bone.[44,45] Some researchers believe that the beneficial effects of osteotomies may result from a reduction of venous hypertension and intramedullary pressure.[46]

Multiple reports have detailed the use of various types of osteotomies for the salvage of precollapse and early collapsed femoral heads. A recent review of corrective osteotomies for osteonecrosis of the femoral head, at a mean follow-up of 11.5 years (range, 5 to 18 years),[45] revealed 28 hips (76%) with excellent and good Harris Hip Scores. Six of the 9 failures were in the group of 16 hips that had a corticosteroid association. Conversely, in the 20 hips without a corticosteroid association, 17 (85%) had good or excellent Harris Hip Scores at final follow-up. Seven patients (8 hips) had SLE, with 4 successful results. The 3 failures were in hips with large lesions. Other reports have not stratified the results of these operations by diagnosis of SLE. The results in patients with SLE are probably also based on the size of the lesion rather than the diagnosis.

The third form of treatment for osteonecrosis, nonvascularized bone grafting, includes 3 general categories; (1) cortical bone grafting through a core decompression tract;[47](2) bone grafting through a window made in the femoral neck;[48] and (3) bone grafting through a trapdoor in the articular cartilage.[49,50] Cortical strut grafting employs graft, harvested from the ilium, fibula, or tibia, and placed into a core tract in the femoral head. Historical reports have had unfavorable long-term results.[36] Recently there have been better success rates reported by Bridges and associates,[17] Rosenwasser and associates,[48] and Mont and associates.[51] In the latter study, bone grafting through a so-called trapdoor was made through the articular cartilage and subchondral bone in a manner similar to that used by several surgeons for late-stage osteonecrosis of the femoral head.[23,27,40,48] In this report of 30 cases, 6 patients (9 hips) had SLE. Overall, 22 (73%) of the 30 hips had good (4 hips) or excellent (16 hips) results, and 6 of the 9 patients with SLE were in this group.

The fourth option for patients with osteonecrosis is vascularized fibular grafting. There have been variable outcomes from different centers, ranging from 60% to 90% success at short-term follow-up (under 3 years).[36,52–54] Urbaniak and associates[52] recently reported an 87% success rate in patients with pre- and postcollapse disease. This is certainly an excellent option, but it requires much technical expertise and lengthy operating time. Patient morbidity is probably similar to or greater than that of osteotomies with the need to sacrifice part of the fibula and the prolonged weightbearing restriction (6 months). We believe that a rational approach would be the use of osteotomies or nonvascularized bone grafting procedures in patients with small lesions (less than 200° combined necrotic angles) and the use of vascularized fibular grafting in larger lesions.

Postcollapse Disease The use of a limited femoral endoprosthesis for osteonecrosis of the femoral head has not gained widespread acceptance, perhaps because of the poor results of total articulating resurfacing arthroplasties. However, resurfacing only the femoral head avoids the reasons for failure associated with the thin polyethylene used when both sides of the joint are resurfaced. Resurfacing of only the femoral side using this prosthesis has been favorably reported upon in short-term clinical and radiographic follow-up.[4,55–58] Scott and associates[58] reported good or excellent results in 22 of 25 hips (88%) at a mean follow-up of 37 months (range, 25 to 60 months), and Bridges and associates[17] found 18 of 21 hips (86%) with good and excellent results at a mean follow-up of 4 years (range, 3 to 7 years). Amstutz and associates[59] have recently reported on the use of a stemless titanium surface hemiarthroplasty in 10 hips with osteonecrosis. At an average follow-up of 11 years (range, 10 to 12 years), 5 hips were functioning satisfactorily. The other 5 hips were revised at an average of 7.8 years (range, 3.3 to 10.3 years) postoperatively. We have recently reviewed the long-term results of 33 femoral resurfacing procedures (25 patients) that had been performed for postcollapse disease.[56] At a mean of 10.5 years (range, 2 to 14 years) postoperatively, 20 hips (61%) had good and excellent results according to the Harris hip-scoring system. Seven patients (9 hips) in this study had SLE with 6 good clinical outcomes. The results of these studies suggest that femoral head resurfacing with an endoprosthesis can be a successful intermediate treatment for patients with postcollapse disease and large lesions, which would not be amenable to other treatment options except for total hip arthroplasty. Furthermore, improvements in design and size availability will likely improve on current reported results.

Rheumatoid Arthritis

Salvage Procedures Osteotomy of the hip has not been found to be successful in patients with rheumatoid arthritis and should not be considered. Likewise, arthrodesis is not a viable option, because these patients have multiple joint involvement and a unilateral fusion cannot be expected to enable the patient to have significant functional gains. However, in the rare young patient with unilateral disease it could be considered. Synovectomy has been used in only a few reports, more commonly for juvenile rheumatoid arthritis.[60–63] Gains in pain scores have been realized when there is minimal joint destruction. A technique that uses arthroscopy of the hip in juvenile chronic arthritis is used more for diagnosis than for treatment. There are few studies about the use of this technique in adults. The few sporadic reports of this procedure have not detailed the greater than short-term outcome of this procedure. In the knee, as in the hip, osteonecrosis occurring in rheumatoid arthritis has a markedly different treatment and prognosis when compared to osteonecrosis patients with SLE.

The knee is the second most common location for osteonecrosis, although it occurs much less often than in the hip. In 1 report, there were 620 patients presenting with osteonecrosis of the hip. At the same time, only 61 patients (9% of hip patients) presented with findings in the knee.[35,64] Treatment options for the knee have included nonsurgical therapy, such as restricted weightbearing, analgesics, and observation.[35,64,65] Unfortunately, these treatment methods have led to a clinical failure rate greater than 80% in 1 report (26 of 32 knees) at an average follow-up of 11 years.[64] There have been few reports focusing specifically on the surgical treatment of this problem, which will be discussed in the rest of this section.

Core Decompression In a study of 47 knees treated by core decompression of the distal femur, good or excellent results were obtained in 73% of the knees at an average follow-up of 11 years (range, 4 to 16 years).[64] Of the 13 failures of core decompression, 7 avoided a knee replacement for greater than 5 years. This long-term follow-up suggests that core decompression may slow the rate of symptomatic progression of osteonecrosis of the knee. In addition, core decompression may extend the symptom-free interval in certain patients and may delay the need for more extensive procedures, such as total knee arthroplasty.

Joint-preserving surgical treatment modalities, including arthroscopic debridement,[66] vascularized bone grafting, and resurfacing with osteoarticular allografts,[67,68] have

been reported only in anecdotal case report studies.

Total Knee Replacement Patients who have secondary arthrosis from severe disease have few options other than either unicompartmental[41] or total knee arthroplasty[69,70] despite their young age. There has been only 1 study of total knee arthroplasty in this specific patient population.[70] In that study, 31 porous-coated anatomic (Howmedica, Rutherford, NJ) total knee replacements were performed in 21 patients under 50 years of age who had osteonecrosis of the femoral and tibial condyles. Seventeen of the 21 patients had SLE. At a mean follow-up of 8.2 years (range, 2 to 16 years), there were 17 good and excellent results at final follow-up (55%). There were 11 knees revised for aseptic loosening, and 3 additional knees were ultimately revised for deep sepsis. Only 11 of the 25 successful outcomes (44%) were in the SLE population. The results of total knee arthroplasty in this group of patients were inferior to results in groups of young patients with other diagnoses. In the future, refinements in prosthetic design may improve on these results.

Synovectomy and Osteotomy The results of joint synovectomy were reviewed by Granberry and Brewer.[61,71] They concluded that the most consistent benefit from this procedure is relief of pain. The procedure is best done early in the disease. It is also best done in patients with monarticular or pauciarticular arthritis. The prognosis following synovectomy is poor when the sedimentation rate is elevated, when the disease has onset in small joints, and when films reveal periostitis or erosions. Early stage of involvement is defined as persistent synovitis for greater than 6 months, despite appropriate conventional medical therapy, and no loss of articular cartilage or stability of the knee.

Inflammatory disease is a contraindication for the performance of a high tibial osteotomy. This is probably because the rheumatoid process is perpetuated in a given joint by the retention of articular cartilage.

Total Hip Replacement

The disorders of the hip in adult-onset rheumatoid arthritis, juvenile rheumatoid arthritis, and ankylosing spondylitis require specific considerations for total hip arthroplasty.

Adult-Onset Rheumatoid Arthritis

Rheumatoid synovitis and early arthritis of the hip joint are frequently subclinical and are often overlooked in patients with polyarticular arthritis. In 1 Scandinavian study of 64 patients with rheumatoid arthritis, 15% of hip joints showed impaired function after 1 year of disease.[72] This progressed to 28% involvement after 5 years. Synovitis of the hip is difficult to determine by clinical examination. Using ultrasonography, hip synovitis (defined by the presence of fluid, synovial thickening, or a bulging capsule) was found in 13 of 76 patients (17%) in the early phase of their disease (median duration, 3 years).[72] Seven of these 13 patients were asymptomatic. In the same study by Eberhardt and associates,[72] the prevalence of progressive hip joint involvement requiring joint arthroplasty was 15% after 6 years of disease. Progression of arthritis occurred despite medical treatment.

In adult-onset rheumatoid arthritis, hip involvement is usually characterized radiographically by concentric joint space narrowing, caused by the generalized loss of articular cartilage. Cysts and erosions are frequently seen. With progression of the disease, medial and/or axial migration of the femoral head with protrusio acetabulae occurs. Using an anteroposterior pelvic radiograph, protrusio acetabulae can be quantified using the method of Ranawat and associates.[73] This method also permits localization of the original position of the acetabulum. Protrusio acetabulae is usually progressive, and careful radiographic follow-up of patients is recommended. In a study of 9 hips (in 7 patients), axial (medial) migration occurred first and progressed at an average rate of 2.65 mm per year.[73] However, superior migration progressed more rapidly (mean, 4.0 mm per year).

Rheumatoid arthritis of the hip is also characterized by periarticular osteopenia, as well as generalized osteoporosis. Periarticular osteopenia of the hip in rheumatoid arthritis has been evaluated and compared to the osteoarthritic hip by histomorphometry in 35 patients undergoing total hip arthroplasty.[74] Bone turnover, as measured by osteoid volume and surface, resorptive surface, and appositional rate were increased in the acetabular biopsies from 42 rheumatoid hips compared to 61 osteoarthritic hips. Only osteoid surface was increased in the proximal femoral biopsies from the rheumatoid hips. These histomorphometric findings of increased osteoid and resorptive activity in the acetabulum may partially explain the high rate of acetabular component loosening and migration reported after cemented total hip replacement in rheumatoid patients.

Juvenile Rheumatoid Arthritis

Juvenile rheumatoid arthritis (JRA) affects approximately 100,000 children per year in the United States. The knee and ankle are the most commonly involved joints in the lower extremity. The hip joint may be involved in 10% to 60% of patients, but total hip arthroplasty will be required for only a small percentage of these patients. Hip involvement in these patients has 5 common radiographic patterns: typical concentric joint space narrowing, as seen in adult-onset rheumatoid arthritis; axial or superior (or both) protrusio acetabulae; subluxation; acetabular or femoral dysplasia; and ankylosis.[75,76] As with adult-onset disease, JRA is a systemic disease and there may be multisystem involvement. In 1 study of 39 patients with JRA who were younger than 30 years old at the time of total hip arthroplasty, the overall mortality was 18% (7 of 39 patients died) at an average age of 27.6 years.[77] However, only 1 patient died perioperatively, from gastrointestinal bleeding and respiratory arrest.

Ankylosing Spondylitis

Although both sexes are affected by this seronegative spondyloarthropathy, males generally have more severe disease. The disorder is an enthesopathy, with inflammation at the site of ligament insertion into bone. The disease develops in the second or third decades. Sacroiliac joint involvement is required for diagnosis. Approximately 90% of white patients are HLA-B27 positive. Asymmetric, usually lower joint involvement occurs in 20% of patients at presentation and in 33% at some stage of the disease. The hip is involved by a typical erosive destructive arthropathy. Spinal stiffness and deformity will exacerbate the limited range of motion of the hip. Ankylosis of the hip joints may be seen in up to 21% of patients, and the range of motion is severely restricted in most patients. In 1 study of 73 hips undergoing arthroplasty, the mean arc of flexion preoperatively was 47° (33° flexion contracture), the mean lateral motion was 10° and mean rotation was only 11°.[12]

Hip Fractures in Rheumatoid Patients

Patients with rheumatoid arthritis have an increased risk of fracture of the proximal femur-femoral neck and intertrochanteric fractures. This is likely related to the generalized osteoporosis and periarticular osteopenia that occurs with the disease and concomitant treatment with corticosteroids. At least, in part, due to bone quality, a high rate of failure of fixation devices for these fractures has been reported. In 1 study of 52 femoral neck fractures in 50 rheumatoid patients, 12 of 20 fractures treated by internal fixation had a serious complication, and 7 of 11 displaced fractures had revision surgery.[78] Therefore, displaced fractures of the femoral neck in older rheumatoid patients, or those with hip joint involvement, should be treated by total hip arthroplasty.[78,79] Nondisplaced femoral neck fractures should have internal fixation if the hip joint is not involved. In a study of 33 intertrochanteric femur fractures in patients with rheumatoid arthritis, prefracture involvement of the hip joint was seen in only 3 patients (9%).[80] Of 30 patients treated with a sliding hip-screw-plate device, 11 had a complication, including osteonecrosis in 3 (10%), nonunion in 2 (6.5%), and loss of fixation (fracture collapse) in 8 (24%). Total hip arthroplasty may be indicated for primary treatment of intertrochanteric hip fractures when there is rheumatoid hip joint involvement or as a salvage procedure for failure of the fixation device. However, intertrochanteric fractures in these patients should usually be treated initially with internal fixation and protected weightbearing.

Clinical Manifestations

When rheumatoid arthritis involves the hip joint, the disease may be particularly devastating because the patients are young (mean, 41 years in 1 study),[81] the involvement is frequently bilateral, and the patients are severely disabled by pain and inability to ambulate or transfer. Some patients with severe multiple lower extremity involvement may be confined to a wheelchair. Pain in the groin, buttock, or thigh is the usual presenting complaint, but occasionally patients with hip arthritis will present with only knee pain. On examination, range of motion of the hip will usually be painful and restricted. Hip flexion and adduction contractures of variable amounts may be present. It is also important to evaluate the upper extremities to determine triceps strength and the patient's ability to use assistive devices for ambulation. The knees, ankles, and feet should be evaluated for arthritic involvement, because axial deformity or flexion contractures of the knees and open skin lesions of the ankles or feet influence the orthopaedic treatment plan.

Treatment

The systemic disease manifestations and polyarthritis of rheumatoid arthritis are usually treated with a wide variety and combinations of medications by rheumatologists or internists. Total hip arthroplasty is the well-accepted surgical procedure for relief of pain and disability in patients with adult-onset rheumatoid arthritis. It is also indicated in patients severely disabled by JRA, provided that the patient is psychologically mature, motivated, and able to participate in postoperative rehabilitation. The beneficial effects of total hip arthroplasty for relief of pain and improvement in function and quality of life are well established.[82] There is no role for osteotomy or arthrodesis of the hip in this patient population. There is often severe

involvement of both hip and knee joints in these patients.[83] In general, unilateral or bilateral total hip arthroplasty is recommended initially, because rehabilitation of total knee arthroplasties would be inhibited by a stiff, painful, or deformed hip. However, we recommend total knee arthroplasty initially if the knee has a fixed flexion contracture of 45° or greater.

Total hip arthroplasty in rheumatoid patients may be performed through an anterior, direct lateral, transtrochanteric, or posterior approach. Because of the high reported incidence of nonunion in rheumatoid patients,[73] the transtrochanteric approach should be avoided, except in hips with severe protrusio acetabulae, in which the hip cannot be dislocated or additional exposure is required for acetabular reconstruction. In these situations, we, using a posterior approach, remove a section of bone from the femoral neck and then remove or ream the remaining femoral head from the acetabulum. There is a risk of fracture of the femur during exposure because of generalized osteoporosis. Protrusio acetabulae should be grafted (with a bulk autograft or packed reamings from the femoral head) in order to place the acetabular component within 5 mm of the original anatomic position (Fig. 2, A and D). Increased loosening of cemented acetabular components has been correlated with positioning of the component outside this location.[76]

Cemented Total Hip Arthroplasty Cemented total hip arthroplasty has been considered to be the "gold standard" for the treatment of end-stage hip joint disease associated with rheumatoid arthritis. Poss and associates[84] showed that these patients generally maintain good function and relief of pain at 6 to 11 years after surgery. However, patients with

rheumatoid arthritis had a 2.6 times greater incidence of deep infection than patients with osteoarthritis. Unger and associates[85] reported 83 cemented total hip arthroplasties in 51 rheumatoid patients (mean age, 40 years) at a mean of 12 years after surgery. The overall rate of revision was 13%, but an additional 11 acetabular and 2 femoral components were radiographically loose. Cemented component loosening was accelerated in patients with JRA, although the clinical results were generally satisfactory. Lachiewicz and associates[76] reported radiographic loosening in 26% of acetabular components and 8% of femoral components in 62 hips followed for a mean of 6 years. Chmell and associates[77] reported 55 cemented hips in 33 patients (who were younger than 30 years old) followed for 11 years. Although 76% of hips were not painful, the overall rate of reoperation was 45%. Revision was performed in 12 of 66 femoral components (18%) and 23 of 66 acetabular components (35%). Survivorship analysis at 15 years was 85% for the femoral component and 61% for the acetabular component. However, in all series, so-called first-generation cement techniques and prostheses were used. Long-term results with the cemented Charnley prosthesis have confirmed that acetabular loosening and migration is a major problem.[86] To our knowledge, there are no published reports of the results of hips implanted in rheumatoid patients using so-called second and third generation cementing techniques.

A bipolar hemiarthroplasty has been recommended as a conservative approach for patients with JRA when combined with a porous-coated or press-fit femoral component.[87] However, in a study of 25 bipolar arthroplasties at a mean follow-up of only 32 months, 24% of the hips had progressive central migration of the bipolar shell, at a rate of 1 to 2 mm per year. Although no patient had groin pain, this approach is generally not now recommended.

Uncemented Total Hip Arthroplasty There is considerable concern about the early and long-term stability of uncemented total hip arthroplasty components in rheumatoid patients. Osteopenic bone, increased osteoid and bone turnover as seen on histomorphometry, protrusio acetabulae, and deformities of the proximal femur may affect fixation of these components. In addition, the effect of commonly used antirheumatic medications on bone ingrowth and remodeling in vivo are not known.

There are few reports of the results of uncemented, porous-coated total hip arthroplasty in patients with rheumatoid arthritis or JRA. Cracchiolo and associates[88] reported good results in 37 hips in patients with adult- or juvenile-onset rheumatoid arthritis at a mean follow-up of 3.7 years. However, there was an 8% incidence of intraoperative fracture of the femur in this series.

Lachiewicz[81] has followed up 35 so-called first-generation uncemented total hip arthroplasties (Harris-Galante) in 25 patients with adult-onset rheumatoid arthritis or JRA for a mean of 4.5 years. Eighty-six percent had a good or excellent clinical result. There was no migration of the acetabular component, but nonprogressive subsidence of 3 femoral components was seen. However, longer follow-up is necessary to determine the prevalence of osteolysis and loosening that require revision. There are few studies directly comparing the results of cemented and uncemented components in rheumatoid patients.[89] Hybrid total hip arthroplasty (uncemented acetabular component and cemented

femoral component) has been recommended for a wide variety of arthritic disorders, but there are no published reports of the results of this type of reconstruction in rheumatoid patients.

Because of the high prevalence of late cemented acetabular component loosening, the use of uncemented acetabular components is recommended for all patients with rheumatoid arthritis. Bone grafting is recommended for protrusio acetabulae, so that the uncemented component is located at or near the anatomic position. Uncemented, circumferential proximally porous-coated titanium femoral components are generally used in patients younger than 60 years of age. Cemented components, using so-called third-generation techniques, are implanted in older patients.

Total Hip Arthroplasty in Ankylosing Spondylitis In patients with ankylosing spondylitis, cemented total hip arthroplasty has been reported to provide excellent relief of pain and improvement in range of motion. In 1 study, the mean postoperative flexion arc improved 46° (total 93°), lateral motion improved 30° (total 40°), and mean rotation improved 43°.[82] However, in another study, there was only 75° mean improvement in motion.[90] It has been reported that these patients are at particular risk for the development of heterotopic ossification. Bisla and associates[91] reported an overall incidence of 61.7% (21 of 34 hips), with Brooker Class III or IV ossification in 26% of hips. A literature review of 302 hips in patients with this disorder revealed that some heterotopic bone was observed in 54% of these hips, but a clinically important amount was seen in only 9% of hips (Fig. 4).[12] Patients who are at an increased risk of severe heterotopic ossification are those with complete ankylosis preop-

eratively, those having a reoperation, or those with an acute postoperative infection.

Prophylaxis for heterotopic ossification should be strongly considered in this patient population and especially in high-risk patients. Indomethacin and irradiation are effective means of prophylaxis. Both a single 8 Gy dose and divided 10 Gy doses of limited field irradiation have been reported to be effective in patients who were considered high risk for heterotopic ossification.

The longest follow-up of total hip replacements in ankylosing spondylitis was a series of 53 hips in 31 patients followed for a mean of 6.3 years.[12] However, 10 surface replacements, 5 uncemented arthroplasties, and 8 revisions were included in this study. Only 1 primary cemented hip was revised for aseptic loosening. However, there was a high incidence of radiolucent lines at the bone cement interface of the acetabular component. Although there are no reports of uncemented components in patients with ankylosing spondylitis, use of an uncemented acetabular component is recommended in all patients with this disorder and uncemented femoral components are recommended in patients younger than age 50.

Revision Surgery

There are few reports of the results of revision total hip surgery in patients with rheumatoid arthritis. Raut and associates[92] reported 37% radiographic failure of 41 cemented Charnley acetabular revisions and 2 of 15 cemented Charnley femoral revisions at a mean follow-up of 7 years.[92] Bone grafting of defects and uncemented porous-coated components with screw fixation are probably a better choice for acetabular revisions in these patients. The optimal method of

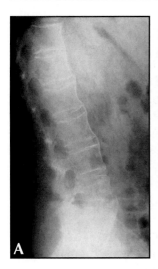
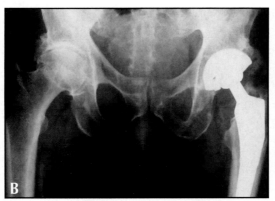
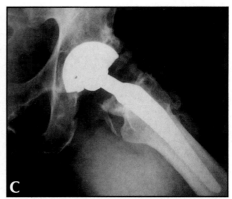

Fig. 4 This 62-year-old man presented with limitation of motion after total hip arthroplasty. **A,** His spine indicates bony bridging developing over several vertebral levels. **B** and **C,** hip radiographs show heterotopic ossification.

femoral component fixation for revisions in rheumatoid patients is unknown and should be individualized, based on the mode of failure, patient age, and the anatomy and bone deficiencies of the proximal femur.

Postoperative Care Although controversial, prophylactic antibiotics are recommended for patients with rheumatoid arthritis before dental work, colonoscopy, and other procedures associated with significant bacteremia. As mentioned previously, these patients, who are considered to be immunocompromised hosts, are at high risk, compared to osteoarthritic patients, for late infection of total hip arthroplasty. We recommend cephalexin, with 1 dose given prior to and 1 dose after dental work or other invasive procedure. For patients who are allergic to penicillin, erythromycin or clindamycin is recommended. Open ulcerations or cellulitis of the lower extremity should be treated aggressively with systemic antibiotics and local wound care to prevent metastatic infections.

Total Knee Replacement

In rheumatoid arthritis, 1 or both knees may be affected in almost 90% of patients.[93] This makes for a large

population of patients often younger than other diagnostic groups. Improved medical understanding of chemotherapeutic disease control coupled with young age and expectations for high activity level create significant risks for survivorship of total knee replacements in this population. Furthermore, not only does the disease itself compromise bone stock, the medications used to treat it will further inhibit bone metabolism. Steroids, nonsteroidal drugs, and even anticoagulants have all been implicated in issues of metabolism and fixation.[94–98] Inflammatory arthritis may also bring about marked ligament imbalance, causing unequal loading, with bone stock and joint balancing problems.[93,99,100]

Successful knee arthroplasty in inflammatory arthritis has been attributed to low demand and limited rehabilitation goals. However, long-term survivorship and durable fixation may be associated with factors other than limited stress, because activity level may significantly increase after successful surgery. Reports of durable results in patients with osteoarthritis suggest that this may be the case.[101–104]

Additionally, while rheumatoid bone may be more prone to osteope-

nia, the actual incidence of mechanically insufficient bone may be limited. Hvid[105] demonstrated that tibial bone strength in biopsy is lower in rheumatoid than osteoarthritis specimens, but the difference is not great and is not related to steroids. Also, markedly low bone strength is uncommon.

With acceptable bone quality, results of cementless total knees are comparable to those of cemented devices in inflammatory arthritis.[106] Accordingly, the choice of fixation methods is dependent on the clinical situation, and the surgeon's judgment and expertise.

After considerations of bone quality, and fixation, issues of joint alignment and stability are paramount. Patients with inflammatory arthritis may be subject to all manner and degree of multiplanar joint deformity and ligament contracture. Techniques for ligament balancing have been reported extensively. Saving or substituting for the posterior cruciate ligament has become a common controversy, with no clear winner apparent. For patients with significant soft-tissue imbalance, the more important and less described issue becomes what level of constraint to employ and when.

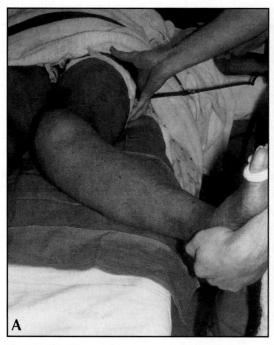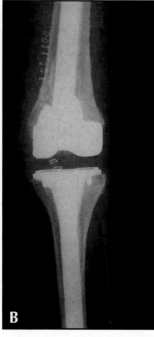

Fig. 5 A, This 72-year-old woman presented with severe valgus deformity and medial collateral ligament insufficiency, which necessitated the use of an implant with both posterior and medial-lateral constraint. **B,** Long pressfit stems were used to offload the forces this increased level of constraint can cause at the cement-bone interface.

Reports of the original total condylar knee showed 91% good to excellent results in deformities ranging from 37° varus to 33° valgus and up to 45° of flexion contracture. Because this device sacrificed the posterior cruciate ligament (PCL) without substituting for it, it is clear that satisfactory results are not dependent on the PCL. However, 3% of cases showed posterior instability, leading the investigators to state that "We believe that there is virtually no degree of deformity and instability...that cannot be corrected. There are occasional bizarre knees [that] require a more constrained prosthesis; they constitute about 0.5% of our cases."[107]

The posterior stabilized prosthesis was developed in part to compensate for posterior laxity. "Errors in surgical technique can lead to laxity of the prosthesis in flexion which may allow posterior subluxation; the cor-rect tightness in flexion is also difficult to obtain after an extensive ligament release."[108]

Interestingly, reports of posterior stabilized knees show 87% good to excellent results. This readily compares to the 91% good to excellent results found in the original total condylar.[109] Clearly then, when it is a matter of choice, the surgeon may preserve, substitute, or even sacrifice the PCL and still obtain good results.

Extensive ligament release in both primary and revision knees may make for an overlarge gap in flexion where the collateral ligaments are most slack. In extension, collateral ligaments tighten and stability is more readily achieved. Inserting a polyethylene spacer of appropriate thickness when the knee is in flexion may excessively raise the joint line or not allow sufficient extension. Here,

the situation mandates the surgeon's choice to be posterior stabilization.

Patients with severe ligament unbalance or medial collateral ligament insufficiency require constraint in the medial-lateral plane. The total condylar III knee is the classic device designed for this purpose and the one with the best long-term follow-up. In primary knees, 90% good to excellent results can still be obtained. In revision surgery, good to excellent results drop to 50%[110–113] (Fig. 5). Hinged devices have shown disappointing long-term results, but they may still have a place in complex cases in elderly low-demand patients.[111]

Conclusion

The surgical management of inflammatory arthritis can bring about dramatic and gratifying results for the patient and surgeon. Advances in medical management have made for healthier patients. Societal demands and expectations are such that patients accept limitations but look forward to increasingly active lives. The nature of the diseases and the limitations of our technology are such that few surgical procedures can be considered definitive in younger, increasingly active patients who have inflammatory arthritis. Nonetheless, with careful planning and an understanding of the sequence and interplay of the various joint procedures, complications can be minimized, and predictable durable results can be achieved.

References

1. Johanson NA, Charlson ME, Szatrowski TP, Ranawat CS: A self-administered hip-rating questionnaire for the assessment of outcome after total hip replacement. *J Bone Joint Surg* 1992;74A:587–597.

2. Sculco TP: The knee, in Sculco TP (ed): *Surgical Treatment of Rheumatoid Arthritis.* St. Louis, MO, Mosby-Year Book, 1992, pp 237–264.

3. Figgie MP, Sobel M, Geppert MJ: The hind-foot, in Sculco TP (ed): *Surgical Treatment of*

Rheumatoid Arthritis. St. Louis, MO, Mosby-Year Book, 1992, pp 273–313.

4. Sculco TP, Alexiades M: The cervical spine, in Sculco TP (ed): *Surgical Treatment of Rheumatoid Arthritis*. St. Louis, MO, Mosby-Year Book, 1992, pp 103–125.

5. Maynard MJ, Ranawat CS, Flynn WF Jr: The hip, in Sculco TP (ed): *Surgical Treatment of Rheumatoid Arthritis*. St. Louis, MO, Mosby-Year Book, 1992, pp 211–236.

6. Sculco TP: Bilateral hip and knee replacement, in Sculco TP (ed): *Surgical Treatment of Rheumatoid Arthritis*. St. Louis, MO, Mosby-Year Book, 1992, pp 265–271.

7. Menon TJ, Wroblewski BM: Charnley low-friction arthroplasty in patients with psoriasis. *Clin Orthop* 1983;176:127–128.

8. Beyer CA, Hanssen AD, Lewallen DG, Pittelkow MR: Primary total knee arthroplasty in patients with psoriasis. *J Bone Joint Surg* 1991;73B:258–259.

9. Stern SH, Insall JN, Windsor RE, Inglis AE, Dines DM: Total knee arthroplasty in patients with psoriasis. *Clin Orthop* 1989;248:108–110.

10. Collins DN, Barnes CL, FitzRandolph RL: Cervical spine instability in rheumatoid patients having total hip or knee arthroplasty. *Clin Orthop* 1991;272:127–135.

11. Petty W, Spanier S, Shuster JJ, Silverthorne C: The influence of skeletal implants on incidence of infection: Experiments in a canine model. *J Bone Joint Surg* 1985;67A:1236–1244.

12. Kilgus DJ, Namba RS, Gorek JE, Cracchiolo A III, Amstutz HC: Total hip replacement for patients who have ankylosing spondylitis: The importance of the formation of heterotopic bone and of the durability of fixation of cemented components. *J Bone Joint Surg* 1990;72A:834–839.

13. Gherini S, Vaughn BK, Lombardi AV Jr, Mallory TH: Delayed wound healing and nutritional deficiencies after total hip arthroplasty. *Clin Orthop* 1993;293:188–195.

14. Schafer AI: Effects of nonsteroidal antiinflammatory drugs on platelet function and systemic homeostasis. *J Clin Pharmacol* 1995;35:209–219.

15. Friedman RJ, Schiff CF, Bromberg JS: Use of supplemental steroids in patients having orthopaedic operations. *J Bone Joint Surg* 1995;77A:1801–1806.

16. Perhala RS, Wilke WS, Clough JD, Segal AM: Local infectious complications following large joint replacement in rheumatoid arthritis patients treated with methotrexate versus those not treated with methotrexate. *Arthritis Rheum* 1991;34:146–152.

17. Bridges SL Jr, Lopez-Mendez A, Han KH, Tracy IC, Alarcon GS: Should methotrexate be discontinued before elective orthopedic surgery in patients with rheumatoid arthritis? *J Rheumatol* 1991;18:984–988.

18. Abeles M, Urman JD, Rothfield NF: Aseptic necrosis of bone in systemic lupus erythematosus: Relationship to corticosteroid therapy. *Arch Intern Med* 1978;138:750–754.

19. Asherson RA, Liote F, Page B, et al: Avascular necrosis of bone and antiphospholipid antibodies in systemic lupus erythematosus. *J Rheumatol* 1993;20:284–288.

20. Bergstein JM, Wiens C, Fish AJ, Vernier RL, Michael A: Avascular necrosis of bone in systemic lupus erythematosus. *J Pediatr* 1974;85:31–35.

21. Cruess RL: Cortisone-induced avascular necrosis of the femoral head. *J Bone Joint Surg* 1977;59B:308–317.

22. Cruess RL: Steroid-induced osteonecrosis: A review. *Can J Surg* 1981;24:567–571.

23. Dubois EL, Cozen L: Avascular (aseptic) bone necrosis associated with systemic lupus erythematosus. *JAMA* 1960;174:966–971.

24. Glick JM: Hip arthroscopy using the lateral approach, in Bassett FH III (ed): *Instructional Course Lectures XXXVII*. Park Ridge, IL, American Academy of Orthopaedic Surgeons, 1988, pp 223–231.

25. Hungerford DS, Zizic TM: II: Treatment of ischemic necrosis of bone in systemic lupus erythematosus. *Medicine* 1980;59:143–148.

26. Kalla AA, Learmonth ID, Klemp P: Early treatment of avascular necrosis in systemic lupus erythematosus. *Ann Rheum Dis* 1986;45:649–652.

27. Leventhal GH, Dorfman HD: Aseptic necrosis of bone in systemic lupus erythematosus. *Semin Arthritis Rheum* 1974;40:73–93.

28. Mont MA, Fairbank AC, Petri M, Hungerford DS: Core decompression for osteonecrosis of the femoral head in systemic lupus erythematosus. *Clin Orthop* 1997;334:91–97.

29. Ono K, Tohjima T, Komazawa T: Risk factors of avascular necrosis of the femoral head in patients with systemic lupus erythematosus under high-dose corticosteroid therapy. *Clin Orthop* 1992;277:89–97.

30. Petri M: Musculoskeletal complications of systemic lupus erythematosus in the Hopkins Lupus Cohort: An update. *Arthritis Care Res* 1995;8:137–145.

31. Petri M, Baker J, Goldman D: Risk factors for osteonecrosis in lupus. *Am Coll Rheumatol Proc* 1992;31:119.

32. Prupas HM, Patzakis M, Quismorio FP Jr: Total hip arthroplasty for avascular necrosis of the femur in systemic lupus erythematosus. *Clin Orthop* 1981;161:186–190.

33. Zelicof SB, Aranow C, Weinstein A, Leslie D, Solomon C: The prevalence and natural history of clinically occult avascular necrosis of the hip in SLE. *Orthop Trans* 1995;18:1044,1994–1995.

34. Zizic TM, Hungerford DS, Stevens MB: Ischemic bone necrosis in systemic lupus erythematosus: I. The early diagnosis of ischemic necrosis of bone. *Medicine* 1980;59:134–142.

35. Mont MA, Hungerford DS: Osteonecrosis of the shoulder, knee, and ankle, in Urbaniak JR, Jones JP Jr (eds): *Osteonecrosis: Etiology, Diagnosis, and Treatment*. Rosemont, IL, American Academy of Orthopaedic Surgeons, 1997, pp 429–436.

36. Mont MA, Hungerford DS: Non-traumatic avascular necrosis of the femoral head. *J Bone Joint Surg* 1995;77A:459–474.

37. Cornell CN, Salvati EA, Pellici PM: Long-term follow-up of total hip replacement in patients with osteonecrosis. *Orthop Clin North Am* 1985;16:757–769.

38. Camp JF, Colwell CW Jr: Core decompression of the femoral head for osteonecrosis. *J Bone Joint Surg* 1986;68A:1313–1319.

39. Fairbank AC, Bhatia D, Jinnah RH, Hungerford DS: Long-term results of core decompression for ischaemic necrosis of the femoral head. *J Bone Joint Surg* 1995;77B:42–49.

40. Mont MA, Carbone JJ, Fairbank AC: Core decompression versus nonoperative management for osteonecrosis of the hip. *Clin Orthop* 1996;324:169–178.

41. Kerboul M, Thomine J, Postel M, Merle d'Aubigné R: The conservative surgical treatment of idiopathic aseptic necrosis of the femoral head. *J Bone Joint Surg* 1974;56B:291–296.

42. Steinberg ME, Bands RE, Parry S, Hoffman E, Chan T, Hartman KM: Does lesion size affect outcome in avascular necrosis? *Orthop Trans* 1992;16:706–707.

43. Stulberg BN, Davis AW, Bauer TW, Levine M, Easley K: Osteonecrosis of the femoral head: A prospective randomized treatment protocol. *Clin Orthop* 1991;268:140–151.

44. Dean MT, Cabanela ME: Transtrochanteric anterior rotational osteotomy for avascular necrosis of the femoral head: Long-term results. *J Bone Joint Surg* 1993;75B:597–601.

45. Mont MA, Fairbank AC, Krackow KA, Hungerford DS: Corrective osteotomy for osteonecrosis of the femoral head: The results of a long-term study. *J Bone Joint Surg* 1996;78A:1032–1038.

46. Arnoldi CC: Vascular aspects of degenerative joint disorders: A synthesis. *Acta Orthop Scand* 1994; 261(suppl):1–82.

47. Buckley PD, Gearen PF, Petty RW: Structural bone-grafting for early atraumatic avascular necrosis of the femoral head. *J Bone Joint Surg* 1991;73A:1357–1364.

48. Rosenwasser MP, Garino JP, Kiernan HA, Michelsen CB: Long term followup of thorough debridement and cancellous bone grafting of the femoral head for avascular necrosis. *Clin Orthop* 1994;306:17–27.

49. Meyers MH: The treatment of osteonecrosis of the hip with fresh osteochondral allografts and with the muscle pedicle graft technique. *Clin Orthop* 1978;130:202–209.

50. Meyers MH, Convery FR: Grafting procedures in osteonecrosis of the hip. *Semin Arthroplasty* 1991;2:189–197.

51. Mont MA, Einhorn TA, Sponseller PD, Hungerford DS: The Trapdoor procedure using autogenous cortical and cancellous bone grafts for osteonecrosis of the femoral head. *J Bone Joint Surg* 1998;80B:56–62.

52. Urbaniak JR, Coogan PG, Gunneson EB, Nunley JA: Treatment of osteonecrosis of the

femoral head with free vascularized fibular grafting: A long-term follow-up study of one hundred and three hips. *J Bone Joint Surg* 1995;77A:681–694.

53. Vail TP, Urbaniak JR: Donor-site morbidity with use of vascularized autogenous fibular grafts. *J Bone Joint Surg* 1996;78A:204–211.

54. Yoo MC, Chung DW, Hahn CS: Free vascularized fibula grafting for the treatment of osteonecrosis of the femoral head. *Clin Orthop* 1992;277:128–138.

55. Hungerford DS, Lennox DW: Diagnosis and treatment of ischemic necrosis of the femoral head, in Evarts CM (ed): *Surgery of the Musculoskeletal System*, ed 2. New York, NY, Churchill Livingstone, 1990, vol 3, pp 127.

56. Krackow KA, Mont MA, Maar DC: Limited femoral endoprosthesis for avascular necrosis of the femoral head. *Orthop Rev* 1993;22: 457–463.

57. Nelson CL, Walz BH, Gruenwald JM: Resurfacing of only the femoral head for osteonecrosis: Long-term follow-up study. *J Arthroplasty* 1997;12:736–740.

58. Scott RD, Urse JS, Schmidt R, Bierbaum BE: Use of TARA herniarthroplasty in advanced osteonecrosis. *J Arthroplasty* 1987;2:225–232.

59. Amstutz HC, Grigoris P, Safran MR, Grecula MI, Campbell PA, Schmalzried TP: Precision-fit surface hemiarthroplasty for femoral head osteonecrosis: Long-term results. *J Bone Joint Surg* 1994;76B:423–427.

60. Albright JA, Albright JP, Ogden JA: Synovectomy of the hip in juvenile rheumatoid arthritis. *Clin Orthop* 1975;106:48–55.

61. Granberry WM, Brewer EJ Jr: Early surgery in juvenile rheumatoid arthritis, in Calandruccio RA (ed): American Academy of Orthopaedic Surgeons *Instructional Course Lectures XXIII*. St. Louis, MO, CV Mosby, 1974, pp 32–37.

62. Kelly IG: Surgical treatment of the rheumatoid hip. *Ann Rheum Dis* 1990;2(suppl):858–862.

63. Mogensen B, Brattstrom H, Ekelund L, Svantesson H, Lidgren L: Synovectomy of the hip in juvenile chronic arthritis. *J Bone Joint Surg* 1982;64B:295–299.

64. Mont MA, Tomek IM, Hungerford DS: Core decompression for avascular necrosis of the distal femur: Long term followup. *Clin Orthop* 1997;334:124–130.

65. Ecker ML, Lotke PA: Spontaneous osteonecrosis of the knee. *J Am Acad Orthop Surg* 1994;2:173–178.

66. Miller GK, Maylahn DJ, Drennan DB: The treatment of idiopathic osteonecrosis of the medial femoral condyle with arthroscopic debridement. *Arthroscopy* 1986;2:21–29.

67. Flynn JM, Springfield DS, Mankin HJ: Osteoarticular allografts to treat distal femoral osteonecrosis. *Clin Orthop* 1994;303:38–43.

68. Meyers MH, Akeson W, Convery FR: Resurfacing the knee with fresh osteochondral allograft. *J Bone Joint Surg* 1989;71A:704–713.

69. Bergman NR, Rand JA: Total knee arthroplasty in osteonecrosis. *Clin Orthop* 1991;273:77–82.

70. Mont MA, Myers TH, Krackow KA, Hungerford DS: Total knee arthroplasty for corticosteroid associated avascular necrosis of the knee. *Clin Orthop* 1997;338:124–130.

71. Brewer EJ (ed): *Juvenile Rheumatoid Arthritis*. Philadelphia, PA, WB Saunders, 1970.

72. Eberhardt K, Fex E, Johnsson K, Geborek P: Hip involvement in early rheumatoid arthritis. *Ann Rheum Dis* 1995;54:45–48.

73. Ranawat CS, Doff LD, Inglis AE: Total hip arthroplasty in protrusio acetabuli of rheumatoid arthritis. *J Bone Joint Surg* 1980;62A:1059–1065.

74. Akesson K, Onsten L, Obrant KJ: Periarticular bone in rheumatoid arthritis versus arthrosis: Histomorphometry in 103 hip biopsies. *Acta Orthop Scand* 1994;65:135–138.

75. Isdale IC: Hip disease in juvenile rheumatoid arthritis. *Ann Rheum Dis* 1970;29:603–608.

76. Lachiewicz PF, McCaskill B, Inglis A, Ranawat CS, Rosenstein BD: Total hip arthroplasty in juvenile rheumatoid arthritis: Two to eleven-year results. *J Bone Joint Surg* 1986;68A: 502–508.

77. Chmell MJ, Scott RD, Thomas WH, Sledge CB: Total hip arthroplasty with cement for juvenile rheumatoid arthritis: Results at a minimum of ten years in patients less than thirty years old. *J Bone Joint Surg* 1997;79A:44–52.

78. Bogoch E, Ouellette G, Hastings D: Failure of internal fixation of displaced femoral neck fractures in rheumatoid patients. *J Bone Joint Surg* 1991;73B:7–10.

79. Asai T, Nagaya L, Miyake N, Kondo K, Tsukamoto M: The treatment of intrascapular hip fractures with total hip arthroplasty in rheumatoid arthritis. *Bull Hosp Jt Dis* 1993;53:29–33.

80. Bogoch ER, Ouellette G, Hastings DE: Intertrochanteric fractures of the femur in rheumatoid arthritis patients. *Clin Orthop* 1993;294:181–186.

81. Lachiewicz PF: Porous-coated total hip arthroplasty in rheumatoid arthritis. *J Arthroplasty* 1994;9:9–15.

82. Kirwan JR, Currey HL, Freeman MA, Snow S, Young PJ: Overall long-term impact of total hip and knee joint replacement surgery on patients with osteoarthritis and rheumatoid arthritis. *Br J Rheumatol* 1994;33:357–360.

83. McDonagh JE, Ledingharn J, Deighton CK, Griffiths ID, Pinder IM, Walker DJ: Six-year follow-up of multiple joint replacement surgery to the lower limbs. *Br J Rheumatol* 1994;33:85–89.

84. Poss R, Maloney JP, Ewald FC, et al: Six- to 11-year results of total hip arthroplasty in rheumatoid arthritis. *Clin Orthop* 1984; 182:109–116.

85. Unger AS, Inglis AE, Ranawat CS, Johanson NA: Total hip arthroplasty in rheumatoid arthritis: A long-term follow-up study. *J Arthroplasty* 1987;2:191–197.

86. Onsten I, Bengner U, Besjakov J: Socket migration after Charnley arthroplasty in rheumatoid arthritis and osteoarthritis: A

roentgen stereophotogrammetric study. *J Bone Joint Surg* 1993;75B:677–680.

87. Wilson MG, Scott RD: The bipolar socket in juvenile rheumatoid arthritis: A two-to five year follow-up study. *J Orthop Rheumatol* 1989;2:133–143.

88. Cracchiolo A III, Severt R, Moreland J: Uncemented total hip arthroplasty in rheumatoid arthritis diseases: A two-to six-year follow-up study. *Clin Orthop* 1992;277:166–174.

89. Kirk PG, Rorabeck CK, Boume RB, Burkart B: Total hip arthroplasty in rheumatoid arthritis: Comparison of cemented and uncemented implants. *Can J Surg* 1993;36:229–232.

90. Walker LG, Sledge CB: Total hip arthroplasty in ankylosing spondylitis. *Clin Orthop* 1991;262:198–204.

91. Bisla RS, Ranawat CS, Inglis AE: Total hip replacement in patients with ankylosing spondylitis with involvement of the hip. *J Bone Joint Surg* 1976;8A:233–238.

92. Raut VV, Siney PD, Wroblewski BM: Cemented revision Charnley low-friction arthroplasty in patients with rheumatoid arthritis. *J Bone Joint Surg* 1994;6B:909–911.

93. Sledge CB, Walker PS: Total knee arthroplasty in rheumatoid arthritis. *Clin Orthop* 1984; 182:127–136.

94. Trancik TM, Mills W: The effects of several non-steroidal anti-inflammatory medications on bone ingrowth into a porous coated implant. *Trans Orthop Res Soc* 1989;14:338.

95. Keller JC, Tranck TM, St. Mary T, Hautanierni JA, Friedman RJ: Untitled. *Trans Orthop Res Soc* 1987;12:437.

96. Longo JA, Magee FP, Hedley AK, Weinstein AM: The effect of chronic indomethacin on fixation of porous implants to bone. *Trans Orthop Res Soc* 1989;14:337.

97. Magee FP, Longo JA, Emmanual JE, Van De Wyngaerde DG, Hedley AK: The effect of naprosyn on bone ingrowth. *Trans Orthop Res Soc* 1990;15:166.

98. Lavernia CJ, Yoshida G, Reindel E, Cook S, Woo SL-Y, Convery FR: Effects of warfarin on the ingrowth kinetics of porous coated devices. *Trans Orthop Res Soc* 1988;13:312.

99. Hungerford DS, Krackow KA, Kenna RV: Two-to five-year experience with a cementless porous-coated total knee prosthesis, in Rand JA, Dorr LD (eds): *Total Arthroplasty of the Knee: Proceedings of the Knee Society 1985–1986*. Rockville, MD, Aspen Publishers, 1987, pp 215–235.

100. Hvid I, Kjaersgaard-Andersen P, Wethelund JO, Sneppen O: Knee arthroplasty in rheumatoid arthritis: Four- to six-year follow-up study. *J Arthroplasty* 1987;2:233–239.

101. Sarokhan AJ, Scott RD, Thomas WH, Sledge CB, Ewald FC, Cloos DW: Total knee arthroplasty in juvenile rheumatoid arthritis. *J Bone Joint Surg* 1983;65A:1071–1080.

102. Sledge CB, Walker PS: Total knee replacement in rheumatoid arthritis, in Insall JN (ed): *Surgery of the Knee*. New York, NY, Churchill Livingstone, 1984, p 697.

103. Ranawat CS, Padgett DE, Ohashi Y: Total knee arthroplasty for patients younger than 55 years. *Clin Orthop* 1989;248:27–33.

104. Stern SH, Bowen MK, Insall JN, Scuderi GR: Cemented total knee arthroplasty for gonarthrosis in patients 55 years old or younger. *Clin Orthop* 1990;260:124–129.

105. Hvid I: Trabecular bone strength at the knee. *Clin Orthop* 1988;227:210–221.

106. Stuchin SA, Ruoff M, Matarese W: Cementless total knee arthroplasty in patients with inflammatory arthritis and compromised bone. *Clin Orthop* 1991;273:42–51.

107. Insall JN, Hood RW, Flawn LB, Sullivan DJ: The total condylar knee prosthesis in gonarthrosis: A five- to nine-year follow-up of the first one hundred consecutive replacements. *J Bone Joint Surg* 1983;65A:619–628.

108. Insall JN, Lachiewicz PF, Burstein AH: The posterior stabilized condylar prosthesis: A modification of the total condylar design: Two to four-year clinical experience. *J Bone Joint Surg* 1982;64A:1317–1323.

109. Stern SH, Insall JN: Posterior stabilized prosthesis: Results after follow-up of nine to twelve years. *J Bone Joint Surg* 1992;74A:980–986.

110. Donaldson WF III, Sculco TP, Insall JN, Ranawat CS: Total condylar III knee prosthesis: Long-term follow-up study. *Clin Orthop* 1988;226:21–28.

111. Hohl WM, Crawfurd E, Zelicof SB, Ewald FC: The total condylar III prosthesis in complex knee reconstruction. *Clin Orthop* 1991;273:91–97.

112. Rosenberg AG, Verner JJ, Galante JO: Clinical results of total knee revision using the total condylar III prosthesis. *Clin Orthop* 1991;273:83–90.

113. Karpinski MR, Grimer RJ: Hinged knee replacement in revision arthroplasty. *Clin Orthop* 1987;220:185–191.

13

Evaluation and Treatment of Infection at the Site of a Total Hip or Knee Arthroplasty

Arlen D. Hanssen, MD
James A. Rand, MD

Infection following total joint replacement remains a major problem that has not been solved during the last 30 years. The prevalence of infection at the Mayo Clinic between 1969 and 1996 was 1.7% of 30,680 total hip arthroplasties and 2.5% of 18,749 total knee arthroplasties. After primary operations, the rate of infection was 1.3% of 23,519 hips and 2.0% of 16,035 knees. After revision operations, the rate was 3.2% of 7,161 hips and 5.6% of 2,714 knees (Table 1). The rate of infection has been remarkably constant despite the use of different regimens of antibiotic prophylaxis, operating-room configurations, surgical techniques, and modes of fixation of the implant. Factors leading to deep infection must be considered with respect to the host, wound, surgical technique, operating-room environment, and microbiologic characteristics of the infecting organisms. A prompt diagnosis of infection will facilitate treatment and minimize morbidity.

Etiology

As stated, in discussing the etiology of infection, the host, wound, operating-room environment, surgical technique, and microbiologic characteristics of infecting organisms must be considered. The patient as host is an important risk factor for infection. The surgical wound is contaminated to some extent in all procedures, but the immune-defense mechanisms of the host prevent infection in most instances. Immunocompromised patients are clearly at increased risk for deep infection, as are patients who have rheumatoid arthritis.[1,2] In a series of 4,171 total knee replacements, an infection developed after 16 (0.9%) of 1,854 replacements in patients who had osteoarthrosis compared with 45 (2.2%) of 2,076 replacements in those who had rheumatoid arthritis.[2] In a series of 4,240 total hip, knee, and elbow arthroplasties, the rate of infection was 2.6 times greater in patients who had rheumatoid arthritis than it was in those who had osteoarthrosis.[1] In one study, 17 (4%) of 425 male patients with polyarticular rheumatoid arthritis had an infection following total knee replacement.[2] In another study, male patients who had polyarticular rheumatoid arthritis were found to be at risk for more than 1 infection: of 145 patients who had an infection following total joint replacement, 27 (19%) had a subsequent infection and 19 of those 27 patients had a diagnosis of rheumatoid arthritis.[3]

Patients who have diabetes mellitus also are at increased risk for deep infection. In a series of 66 knees in 46 diabetic patients (6 of whom were lost to follow-up, leaving 59 knees in 40 patients), 4 knees (7%) became infected after total knee arthroplasty.[4] The increased rate of infection was associated with complications related to wound-healing in 8 (12%) of the original 66 knees. In another study, of 68 knees in 51 patients with diabetes mellitus who were followed for 8 years after a total knee arthroplasty, there were 21 complications (31%); in a matched-case group consisting of 68 knees, 2 (3%) became infected.[5] In a third study, the rate of infection following total hip arthroplasty in 44 patients (62 hips) who had diabetes mellitus was 6%, which was significantly higher than the rate in non-diabetic osteoarthrotic patients ($p < 0.001$) and non-diabetic rheumatoid patients ($p < 0.01$).[6] However, in a fourth study, of 93 total hip arthroplasties in patients with diabetes mellitus who were followed for 4 years, there were no infections.[7]

Poor nutrition is another factor influencing deep infection. It was reported that wound complications occurred more frequently in patients with malnutrition as indicated by a total lymphocyte count of less than 1,500/mm³ (1.5×10^9/l) or a serum albumin level of less than 3.5 g/dl (35

Table 1
Prevalence of infection after total joint arthroplasty for the years 1969 through 1996

	Knee Arthroplasties	Hip Arthroplasties
Primary procedures		
Total number performed	16,035	23,519
Percentage followed by infection	2.0	1.3
Revision procedures		
Total number performed	2,714	7,161
Percentage followed by infection	5.6	3.2
Overall		
Total number performed	18,749	30,680
Percentage followed by infection	2.5	1.7

g/l).[8–10] In a study of 103 total hip arthroplasties, a serum transferrin level of less than 226 mg/dl (2.26 g/l) was the only variable indicating malnutrition that was significantly associated with delayed wound-healing ($p < 0.002$).[11]

Other risk factors for deep infection include obesity, urinary-tract infection, and oral use of steroids.[2] In a series of 182 total knee arthroplasties in obese patients, there were no infections.[12] Deep infection developed after total knee arthroplasty in 4 (17%) of 24 knees in patients who had psoriasis.[13]

Previous surgery on the affected joint increases the rate of deep infection as much as 2-fold after total knee arthroplasty and as much as 3-fold after total hip arthroplasty.[14,15] Wilson and associates[2] noted that the rate of infection in patients who had osteoarthrosis was 1.4% when the affected knee had been operated on previously, compared with 0.3% when it had not. Poss and associates[1] reported an 8-fold increase in the risk of infection in patients who had had a revision compared with those who had had a primary total hip arthroplasty. In a study of 3,215 total hip arthroplasties, infection was found to be related to previous surgery, prolonged operative time, positive intraoperative cultures, or an unrecognized preoperative infection.[16] In a study of 65 knee

replacements in patients who had had a previous knee infection, the overall risk of infection was 8% (5 knees), with 2 (4%) of 45 knees that had had septic arthritis and 3 (15%) of 20 that had had osteomyelitis becoming infected.[17] A study of 3,051 total hip arthroplasties revealed a significantly ($p < 0.001$) increased risk of infection in patients who had had a revision of a previous arthrodesis or had a history of infection.[18]

Particles of debris, advanced age, and prolonged preoperative hospitalization also are potential risk factors for infection. In a series of 23,649 general surgical patients, the rate of infection was 1.1% for patients who had been admitted to the hospital on the day of surgery, compared with 4.3% for those who had been hospitalized for 2 weeks before surgery (no numbers were given).[19]

Any active site of concurrent infection may allow hematogenous seeding of the surgical site. In a consecutive series of 803 total hip arthroplasties, the rate of infection was threefold greater in patients who had a concurrent remote infection than in those who did not.[15]

The type of reconstruction also influences the risk of deep infection. Large, hinged total knee implants have been associated with rates of infection ranging from 17 (11%) of 156 to 8 (16%) of 50.[1,20] In a study of 659 hips

that had a total hip arthroplasty, 4 (3%) of 125 that had had the procedure with use of structural bone graft had an infection compared with 1 (0.2%) of 534 that had not.[21] All procedures were performed with use of prophylactic antibiotics, vertical laminar airflow, and helmet aspirator suits.

The operating-room environment is an important factor that influences contamination of the surgical wound. Variables affecting the operating room include the number of personnel, the amount of traffic, preparation of the surgical site, the use of airflow, and the dress of the surgical team. The major source of bacteria within the operating room is people. In 1 study, the number of colony-forming units was 34-fold greater when the room was occupied than when it was empty.[22] Some individuals shed a large number of bacteria.[23] Exclusion of such individuals and minimization of the number of people in the room decrease the potential for contamination of the wound. The use of a helmet aspirator suit can decrease bacterial environmental air settle-plate counts in the operating room compared with those associated with use of a standard gown and hood ($p < 0.005$).[23] A helmet aspirator suit should be worn by individuals in the operating room who shed an increased number of bacteria. Such a suit also is useful in preventing contamination of the surgical team by blood from the surgical site, as such blood may contain human immunodeficiency virus, hepatitis virus, or infectious bacteria.[24] The suit also can prevent contamination of the surgical wound by fragments of cement that strike the surgeon during removal and fall into the wound during a revision.

The use of standard operating-room clothing and gowns is less effective in preventing contamination than the use of a polypropylene coverall.[25,26] Even in an ultraclean-air operating room, bacterial counts were 4.4 times higher during preparation and draping of the wound by an unscrubbed, ungowned assistant and 2.4 times higher during preparation and draping by a gowned assistant than they were intraoperatively.[27] Shaving and preparation of the surgical site should be performed immediately before surgery, as areas of skin damage may harbor bacteria. A wide variety of skin-cleaning agents are effective for preparation of the surgical site.[23] In one study, use of an iodophor-incorporated drape during 649 total knee arthroplasties was associated with a rate of infection of only 0.5% (3 infections).[28] In another study, use of an iodophor-incorporated drape was significantly ($p = 0.05$) better than other methods of skin-site preparation in preventing recolonization of the skin by bacteria.[29] Other variables that increase the potential for contamination of the surgical wound include use of a splash basin to wash or store instruments, prolonged use of a suction tip, and perforations in gloves.[30–32]

The role of laminar airflow in controlling infection has remained controversial. Lidwell and associates,[33] in a multicenter study, reported that infection developed after 63 of 4,133 hip and knee arthroplasties performed in a conventional operating room compared with 23 of 3,923 such procedures performed in a room with laminar airflow. Infection developed in 34 of 5,831 hips in patients who had antibiotic prophylaxis compared with 52 of 2,221 hips in patients who did not. However, the prophylactic use of antibiotics was not strictly controlled. The data reported by Lidwell and associates[33,34] suggest a combined beneficial effect of laminar airflow and prophylactic antibiotics. Charnley[35] found that the rate of infection after total hip arthro-

plasty decreased from 3.1% of 1,080 when laminar airflow was not used to 1.4% of 909 when it was. Other investigators have also reported that laminar airflow decreases the prevalence of infection.[36–39] Ritter and associates[26] attributed this decrease to a 92% reduction in bacteria within the clean-air area. Laminar airflow appears to diminish the prevalence of contamination of the surgical instruments while they are exposed on the instrument table.[22]

The effect of laminar airflow during hip arthroplasty may be different from that during knee arthroplasty. In one study, the rate of infection after hip arthroplasty decreased, from 11 (1.4%) of 761 hips to 13 (0.9%) of 1,518 hips, when laminar airflow had been used; however, the rate of infection after knee arthroplasty increased, from 8 (1.4%) of 573 knees to 12 (3.9%) of 310 knees, when laminar airflow had been used.[40] This difference was thought to be related to the positioning of the operating-room personnel between the airflow and the surgical wound during the knee arthroplasties.

Another approach that has been used to control the operating-room environment is the use of ultraviolet light. Lowell and associates[41] reported that the rate of infection was 0.5% of 1,712 hips when arthroplasty was performed in an operating room equipped with ultraviolet light compared with 3% of 621 hips when the procedure was performed in a conventional operating room. As demonstrated by continuous air-sampling adjacent to a total hip-arthroplasty incision, use of a combination of ultraviolet light and occlusive clothing decreased the number of colony-forming units per cubic meter to 0.5 compared with 7.7 with use of laminar airflow.[42]

The surgical technique is an important variable that influences the potential for deep infection. Meticulous handling of tissue is necessary to minimize devitalization and hematoma. Increased surgical time has been reported to be associated with an increased risk of infection.[35] The time should be minimized to decrease the time for potential contamination of the wound. Previous incisions should be used to prevent areas of skin necrosis between an old and a new incision. Whenever there is a need to reoperate because of persistent drainage, a hematoma, or an area of wound necrosis, there is an increased risk of deep infection. Brown and associates[27] found that hips with a history of drainage after an operation had a 3.2 times higher risk of infection than those that had healed normally. Therefore, meticulous hemostasis and wound closure are essential.

The microbiology of deep infection as well as the interactions among biomaterials, the patient, and contaminating microorganisms must be considered. Microorganisms that may be responsible for infection at the site of a total joint arthroplasty include aerobic and anaerobic organisms, fungi, mycobacteria, and Brucella.[43,44] An inability to identify the organism causing some clinical infections may be due to failure to culture for fastidious organisms or it may be due to the fact that the organism was suppressed by previous treatment with antibiotics. The most frequent pathogenic organisms are *Staphylococcus aureus* and *Staphylococcus epidermidis*. However, each hospital must constantly review the types of organisms causing infection, as these may change over time. Antibiotic prophylaxis must be directed at the most common pathogens in each hospital setting. The increasing frequency of infections caused by organisms such as methicillin-resistant *Staphylococcus aureus* and vancomycin-resistant Enterococcus species, which are generally resistant to more than one antibiotic, provides a dilemma with regard to prophylaxis and treatment.

There have been numerous experimental studies evaluating the susceptibility of the patient to infection adjacent to implant materials. Polymethylmethacrylate, stainless steel, cobalt-chromium alloy, and polyethylene all have been found to increase susceptibility to infection.[45–49] Polymethylmethacrylate, especially when polymerized in vivo, impairs the chemotaxis, phagocytosis, and killing ability of polymorphonuclear leukocytes.[46] The prosthesis, which acts as a large foreign body, provides a biomaterial that can be colonized by a contaminating microorganism. Biomaterials are surrounded by an immunoincompetent zone that predisposes to infection.[50] Bacteria have the ability to bind to biomaterials with use of physical forces, chemical binding, and specific receptors to surface proteins.[50] *Staphylococcus epidermidis* has a high rate of adhesion to polyethylene.[50] Bacterial resistance to antibiotics is related to the production of a glycocalyx slime that impairs antibiotic access and killing by host-defense mechanisms.[50–54] Recently, bacteria were found to persist in vitro on the surface of antibiotic-impregnated cement.[55] The presence of a glycocalyx can result in unreliable in vitro testing for the minimum inhibitory concentration of antibiotic that is needed to treat an infection. The more virulent organisms causing infection include methicillin-resistant staphylococci, gram-negative bacilli, group-D streptococci, enterococci, and organisms that elaborate a glycocalyx.[56] Less virulent organisms include methicillin-sensitive staphylococci, anaerobic cocci, and streptococci other than group D.[57]

The diagnosis of infection must begin with the careful recording of the history, which should include a search for host factors predisposing to infection or problems with wound-healing, and a physical examination, which should include an assessment of effusion, warmth, tenderness, and drainage. The only finding that is consistently associated with infection is pain.[58] Radiographs should be evaluated carefully for loosening of the implant, periosteal new-bone formation, periprosthetic bone resorption, and ectopic bone. The most consistent radiographic finding is progressive prosthetic loosening.

Hematologic testing may include the white blood-cell count (WBC), the erythrocyte sedimentation rate (ESR), and the C-reactive protein (CRP) level. However, neither the WBC nor the ESR is consistently elevated in the presence of deep infection.[58,59] In a series of 72 infections at the sites of total joint arthroplasties, the ESR had a sensitivity of 60% and a specificity of 65%.[56] The CRP level is generally elevated initially after an uncomplicated total hip arthroplasty, returning to normal within 3 weeks.[60,61] The CRP level is normal in patients who have mechanical loosening but remains elevated in those who have septic loosening.[61]

Bone scans may be of the technetium-99, indium-111 white blood-cell, monoclonal antibody, or polyclonal antibody type. The technetium-99 scan has been used widely but is very nonspecific. Levitsky and associates,[56] in a series of 72 total joint arthroplasties, reported a sensitivity of 33%, a specificity of 86%, a positive predictive value of 30%, and a negative predictive value of 88%. In a series of 38 knees that had been painful following a total knee arthroplasty and had been evaluated with use of indium-111 white blood-cell scans before a reoperation, the accuracy of the scans was 84%, the sensitivity was 83%, and the specificity was 85%.[62] In a series of 92 total hip arthroplasties that had been performed with cement, use of a technetium-99m-sulfur colloid scan in addition to an indium-111 leukocyte scan improved sensitivity to 100%, specificity to 97%, and accuracy to 98%.[63] Indium-111 polyclonal antibody scans provided a sensitivity, specificity, and accuracy of 100% in a series of 25 patients,[64] and they provided a sensitivity of 98% and a specificity of 94% for 25 patients in another series;[65] however, the use of these scans was not specifically studied with respect to total joint arthroplasty.[64,65] Monoclonal antibody scans used for imaging of bones and joints had a sensitivity of 90%, a specificity of 85%, and an accuracy of 88% in a series of 53 patients,[66] and they had a sensitivity of 93%, a specificity of 89%, and an accuracy of 90% in 62 patients in another series.[67]

Aspiration of the joint has been controversial. Studies of the aspirate should include culture, determination of the glucose level in synovial fluid, and a cell count. In a series of 72 infections at the sites of joint arthroplasties, aspiration had a positive predictive value of 75% and a negative predictive value of 94%.[56] Barrack and Harris[68] found that cultures of material aspirated from the hip were positive for 6 of 10 infected hips and 34 of 291 noninfected hips. Lachiewicz and associates,[69] in a study of aspiration performed before 193 revision total hip arthroplasties, found an accuracy of 96%, a specificity of 97%, and a sensitivity of 92%. Those authors recommended aspiration if the prosthesis had been in place for less than 5 years and the erythrocyte sedimentation rate was abnormal. In another study, aspiration of 64 knees before revision had a sensitivity and specificity of 100%.[70] Polymerase chain-reaction testing may provide increased sensitivity for the diagnosis of infection, but it also may increase the number of false-positive results.[71]

Pathologic evaluation of tissue at the time of surgery may be necessary to confirm infection in difficult cases. Tissue should be obtained from the bone-cement or prosthesis-bone interface as well as from abnormal-appearing areas of synovial tissue. Five polymorphonuclear leukocytes per high-power field has been recommended as the criterion for the diagnosis of infection.[72] In a study of knee arthroplasty, there was pathologic evidence of acute inflammation in 14 of 15 knees that were infected and in 1 of 40 knees that were not infected.[70] In a series of 33 total hip and knee revisions, the sensitivity of analysis of frozen sections was 100% and the specificity was 96%.[73]

Therefore, a high index of suspicion is necessary for the diagnosis of infection following total joint arthroplasty. It is essential that a careful history be obtained to assess host risk factors and wound-healing. Physical examination of the affected joint, with assessment of the skin, effusion, and tenderness, should be performed. High-quality radiographs must be examined for areas of loosening and bone resorption. Ancillary evaluation with hematologic tests, bone scans, and aspiration of the joint can provide additional information about selected patients. A final decision at the time of the revision may need to be made on the basis of the findings of pathologic evaluation of tissue. There is no single test that

can reliably predict a diagnosis of infection in all patients. The use of combined studies often can provide a reasonable indication of the probability of infection.

Infection at the Site of a Total Hip Arthroplasty

Options for the treatment of infection at the site of a total hip arthroplasty include long-term antibiotic suppression, debridement with retention of the prosthesis, definitive resection arthroplasty, arthrodesis, and reinsertion of another prosthesis (reimplantation).[74] When feasible, reimplantation is generally the most desirable method of treatment for most patients, as it has been associated with improved functional outcome and greater patient satisfaction. Contraindications to reimplantation include persistent infection; medical conditions preventing multiple surgical procedures; severe soft-tissue damage, such as absent function of the abductor muscles or limited skin or muscle over the hip; and systemic conditions that highly predispose toward reinfection.

The central controversies with regard to reimplantation involve aspects of antibiotic therapy, such as use of local antibiotic-delivery systems; the proper time interval between removal of the prosthesis and reimplantation; use of antibiotic-impregnated bone cement for fixation of the prosthesis; use of a prosthesis inserted without cement; and use of bone graft, specifically structural allograft, for reconstruction. The small numbers of patients in most reports have hindered accurate analysis of these controversial treatment variables. Furthermore, differences in outcome between older and more contemporary series may reflect differences in ancillary treatment modalities. Finally, analyses of

the outcomes of treatment of infection following total hip arthroplasty should not include patients who have an endoprosthesis or an internal fixation device.[58,75–82] Cherney and Amstutz[76] noted that "there was a higher infection rate in the patients who had had an infection following a prior total hip-joint replacement. . . . Infections following internal fixation of fractures or from hematogenous spread may be more readily curable." In the analyses that follow, only patients who had an infection at the site of a hip prosthesis are included when multiple series are combined to assess the effect of different treatment variables.

Antibiotic Therapy

The primary controversies with respect to antibiotic therapy include the duration and route of administration and the efficacy of local delivery systems.

The optimum duration of antibiotic therapy has not been definitively established, and the use of antibiotic-impregnated cement has altered current recommendations. Although there are some general guidelines for the use of intravenous antibiotic therapy, there is no consensus on the proper use of oral antibiotic therapy for patients who have an infection at the site of a total hip arthroplasty. Recommendations have generally been for 4 to 6 weeks of intravenous administration; however, the reported durations have been extremely variable, ranging from 0 to 9 weeks of intravenous therapy and no oral therapy to more than 2 years of oral therapy.[83–90]

The most consistent results have been achieved with the duration of antibiotic therapy that is included in a 2-stage reimplantation protocol consisting of resection arthroplasty, 6 weeks of intravenous administration of antibiotics in doses that achieve a serum bactericidal titer of at least 1:8, and subsequent reinsertion of a new prosthesis.[80,88,91] By definition, the use of this strict protocol prevents comparison of different durations of antibiotic therapy, but its rate of success is persuasive, with reinfection developing in only 3 (9%) of 32 hips.[80] Of 4 patients who had a bactericidal titer of less than 1:8, 2 had a reinfection; this rate of reinfection was significantly higher than the rate for the other 28 patients ($p = 0.035$).[80] Those authors stated that reimplantation is contraindicated if a bactericidal titer of at least 1:8 cannot be achieved. The importance of the serum bactericidal titer in that report may have been overstated, as both patients who had an inadequate titer and a reinfection had a number of other confounding variables. Both had had a polymicrobial infection; one was elderly, with multiple medical problems; and the other had needed multiple debridements and transposition of the vastus lateralis muscle for wound-healing. Additionally, the use of gentamicin-impregnated beads in 4 patients and of antibiotic-impregnated bone cement for fixation of the prosthesis in 17 patients potentially affected the authors' conclusion regarding the efficacy and necessity of serum bactericidal-titer testing.[80] Finally, the method for this type of testing is difficult to duplicate consistently within and between laboratories, and the minimum inhibitory concentration achieved with use of agar or broth dilution appears to be the best guide for antibiotic therapy.[92]

In another retrospective study, 35 patients received antibiotics intravenously for less than 4 weeks and 44, for 4 weeks or more.[81] The strength of this study is that the confounding variables of antibiotic-

impregnated beads or spacers and antibiotic-impregnated cement for fixation of the prosthesis were not present. Although reinfection occurred in 7 (20%) of the 35 patients who had therapy for less than 4 weeks compared with 4 (9%) of the 44 who had therapy for 4 weeks or more, this difference was not found to be significant with the number of patients available for study ($p = 0.19$).[81] Multivariate analysis of a subgroup of the patients who were infected with an organism that was determined to be more virulent revealed that 3 of 7 who were managed for less than 4 weeks had a reinfection compared with only 1 of 13 who were managed for 4 weeks or more. Again, with the numbers available, this difference was not found to be significant ($p = 0.055$), but these findings strongly suggest that at least 4 weeks of intravenous therapy is probably advisable.

Although many investigators have thought that gram-negative infections are more difficult to treat,[76,79,93,94] others have found no difference in the prevalence of reinfection with gram-negative organisms.[78,80–82] Some bacteria form an exopolysaccharide-glycocalyx slime that shields microbial growth from antibodies and antibiotics.[52] It has been suggested that, when colonization takes place on a surface, resistance to antibiotics is related to bacterial metabolic changes that are specific to the organism and the type of biomaterial substrate.[54] Comparisons of susceptibility to antibiotics between suspended bacteria and surface-adherent bacteria have revealed consistently higher minimum inhibitory concentrations for adherent bacteria, and this effect was greater when bacteria had adhered to bone cement than when they had adhered to polyethylene.[54] This varying susceptibility to antibiotics, based

on the specific organism as well as the specific biomaterial, has extraordinary relevance to many treatment concepts. For example, the increased resistance of the infecting organism to antibiotics that is induced by surface adherence to a retained piece of bone cement is not accounted for by serum bactericidal-titer and minimum inhibitory-concentration testing as currently performed.

Although it has been traditionally accepted that intravenous administration of antibiotics is more effective than oral administration, there are several factors that may call this tenet into question. Many new antibiotics that are given orally are absorbed more effectively than older antibiotics, and several of these new agents are effective against organisms that previously could be treated only intravenously. Given good patient compliance and serum-testing to evaluate the efficacy of absorption, many investigators currently are interested in whether oral administration can replace portions of the therapy formerly reserved for intravenous administration. If this approach proves equally effective, the potential benefits will include a marked reduction in overall healthcare costs. Efficacy studies currently are being performed to evaluate different combinations of orally administered antibiotics for the treatment of infections at the sites of orthopaedic implants.[95] Oral administration also can be used to supplement a course of intravenous administration, either for a defined period or for chronic longterm suppression.

Because there are not yet any established guidelines for the duration of oral antibiotic therapy, treatment must be individualized for each patient.[83–90] Many current drug trials are being performed to address the issue of the duration of oral administration. In general, the oral use of antibiotics for chronic suppression is reserved for elderly patients or for those in whom removal of the prosthesis would be prohibitively difficult. Also, the antibiotic must be relatively nontoxic and tolerated by the patient. If the patient is expected to live for a long duration, it is probably best to avoid prolonged oral therapy in order to prevent the emergence of multiresistant organisms, the formation of excessive scar tissue, and the progressive loss of bone stock.

Local Delivery of Antibiotics

The use of local antibiotic-delivery systems in the form of antibiotic-impregnated beads or spacers also has changed traditional regimens of intravenous antibiotic therapy. These delivery systems result in local levels of antibiotics that far exceed those attained with systemic antibiotic therapy. Despite remarkably high levels of antibiotics in adjacent cortical bone, the efficacy of antibiotic-impregnated cement in the treatment of infection at the site of a total hip arthroplasty has not been established with use of comparative clinical studies, to our knowledge; however, the clinical experience with antibiotic-impregnated cement has been widespread.[78,80,85,87,88,90,91,96–113] Several different factors, such as variability in the type and amount of antibiotic added to bone cement, probably account for the inability to demonstrate the efficacy of local delivery. Most of the commonly used antibiotics leach from a variety of different acrylic bone cements.[114–123] The antibiotics that are most frequently added to bone cement in the United States include tobramycin, gentamicin, and vancomycin.[99] It is important to note that some antibiotics should not be mixed with bone cement. Lincomycin and tetracycline

are deactivated by the bone-cement polymerization process, and rifampin produces a black, tacky composite that does not harden for several days.[115,122]

There are many variables affecting elution of antibiotics from bone cement. Antibiotics elute in greater amounts and over more sustained time-intervals from Palacos bone cement than from Simplex-P, CMW, or Sulfix acrylic bone cement.[115,119] Most investigators have determined that vancomycin elutes effectively and maintains bioactivity after elution from bone cement.[115,120,121,124] The total elution of an antibiotic is highly dependent on the porosity and surface characteristics of the bone cement as well as on the type of antibiotic being used.[116,124–126] A combination of 2 antibiotics improves the elution of both agents.[124] Large amounts (as much as 8 or 9 g) of antibiotic powder may be added to cement beads or spacers. However, only 1 to 2 g of antibiotic powder per 40 g of cement is recommended for fixation of the prosthesis so as to avoid major mechanical weakening of the bone cement.

A distinct disadvantage of the use of cement beads about the hip joint is the extreme difficulty in removing these beads after approximately 6 weeks of implantation. Biodegradable antibiotic delivery systems that are currently under investigation should eliminate this problem. An alternative method is the use of antibiotic-impregnated spacers, which allows local delivery of antibiotics, minimizes limb shortening, limits scar formation, and facilitates reimplantation.[100,107,113,116] (This method will be discussed later, in the section on delayed reconstruction.) However, the efficacy of this antibiotic-depot method has not yet been proved in a clinical trial. Additional investigation

is necessary to elucidate the numerous issues related to antibiotic therapy.

Timing of the Reconstruction and Use of Antibiotic-Impregnated Bone Cement

The choice of surgical technique (direct exchange or delayed reconstruction) is one of the principal decisions with regard to the treatment of infection at the site of a total hip arthroplasty. Potential advantages of direct exchange include less morbidity (because the need for resection arthroplasty is avoided), reductions in cost (because a second hospitalization and surgical procedure are not needed), and avoidance of technical difficulties associated with delayed implantation. A distinct disadvantage of direct exchange is the inability to use bone cement mixed with specific antibiotics selected on the basis of cultures of tissue samples obtained intraoperatively. Some reports have detailed success of direct exchange as the final outcome of repeated exchanges;[93] however, the final outcome and total cost of initial treatment with direct exchange have not been fully elucidated. In contrast to direct exchange, delayed reconstruction allows observation of the patient's response to therapy. Disadvantages include the hardships associated with resection arthroplasty, technical difficulties, and the cost of a second procedure.

In a comparative study of direct exchange, reimplantation within 4 weeks (average, 2.1 weeks), and reimplantation delayed for more than 4 weeks (average, 12.7 weeks), the group that had 2-stage early reimplantation had the best functional results, the lowest rate of mortality, and the best rate of resolution of the infection.[101] The primary interests of proponents of delayed reconstruction include determining the shortest acceptable delay between resection arthroplasty and reimplantation in order to minimize hardship to the patient, improving the functional results, and decreasing the difficulty of revision procedures while maintaining the lowest possible rate of reinfection.

Direct Exchange

To our knowledge, the largest reported experience with direct-exchange procedures involved 577 hips that were infected after a total hip arthroplasty.[93] The findings suggested that overall results can be improved by careful selection of patients, as gram-positive infections were associated with a better prognosis than were gram-negative infections. General contraindications to the direct-exchange technique included the presence of a gram-negative organism, an actively discharging sinus, or overt purulence at the time of revision.[93] In a study in which these strict selection criteria had been used and in which antibiotic-impregnated cement had been employed for fixation of the prosthesis, all 30 patients had had resolution of the infection at the time of follow-up, at 2 to 8 years.[105] When these generally accepted criteria had not been used, in a study of direct exchange in 57 hips that had an infection with a draining sinus at the site of a total arthroplasty, the rate of resolution of the infection was 86% (49 hips) at an average of 7 years.[108]

The use of antibiotic-impregnated bone cement for fixation of the prosthesis seems to be quite important when the direct-exchange method is employed. A review of multiple series revealed that direct exchange with use of plain bone cement was successful in 40 (60%) of 67 hips that had an infection after total hip arthroplasty.[76,79,127–129] These results are in marked contrast to the reported success rate of 1,352 (83%) of 1,630 hips after use of antibiotic-impregnated cement.[78,84–87,89,90,93,96,98,101,102,105,108,111,127,128,130–132] Although the direct-exchange technique has been used far more commonly in Europe than in North America, if it is thought appropriate for an individual patient, use of strict preoperative selection criteria as well as antibiotic-impregnated cement for fixation of the prosthesis is strongly recommended. The ratio of antibiotics in bone cement that is needed for fixation of the prosthesis is not universally accepted. In a 12-year survival analysis of 239 hip prostheses, there was no demonstrable difference with regard to mechanical loosening between hips in which a ratio of less than 2.5 g of antibiotic per 40 g batch of bone cement had been used and those in which a ratio of 2.5 to 4.5 g/40 g of cement had been used.[117] The current recommendation in North America is for 0.6 to 1.2 g of tobramycin combined with 0.5 to 1.0 g of vancomycin per 40 g batch of bone cement.[116]

Delayed Reconstruction

The success that has been achieved with use of delayed-reconstruction techniques in the absence of antibiotic-impregnated bone cement strongly supports the concept that delayed reconstruction is an important variable. A review of multiple series of hips treated with delayed reconstruction and bone cement without antibiotics revealed that 130 (82%) of 159 hips had a successful result at the time of the latest follow-up.[76,80,81,97,128,129,133–135] It is important to note that none of the patients in these series were managed with antibiotic-impregnated beads or spacers between the time of the resection arthroplasty and the reimplantation. A review of multiple series of patients managed with delayed reimplantation and use of antibiotic-impregnated cement for fixation of the prosthesis revealed that 354 (90%) of 392 had a successful outcome.[78,80,84,85,87,89,96,100,110,113,117,136] A separate analysis of hips treated with antibiotic-impregnated beads or spacers for local delivery of antibiotics showed that a successful outcome was achieved in 174 (92%) of 189 hips.[78,85,89,100,113,136] It is difficult to determine, from these data, whether local delivery of antibiotics has an independent beneficial effect. If reimplantation is being performed because of reinfection after a previous attempt at reimplantation for the treatment of infection, then delayed reconstruction with use of antibiotic-impregnated cement provides the best chance for a successful outcome.[137]

The prosthesis of antibiotic-loaded acrylic cement (PROSTALAC) was developed in an effort to reduce morbidity and decrease the technical difficulties associated with delayed reconstruction.[113,116,138] This concept is, in reality, a hybrid of direct exchange and delayed reconstruction. The prosthesis consists of a thin polyethylene acetabular component and a modular stainless-steel femoral endoskeleton coated with antibiotic-loaded cement, which acts as a local antibiotic-delivery system to maintain limb length and anatomic relationships and to facilitate mobility while the patient awaits definitive reconstruction. The rate of success with use of these implants has been encouraging; in 1 series, only 3 (6%) of 48 hips had a reinfection.[113] The PROSTALAC implant merits further evaluation to explore the possibility of lower health-care costs as a result of the patient being more independent and having a higher level of function and to assess the effect of local delivery of antibiotics.

The timing of the reconstruction and the use of antibiotic-impregnat-

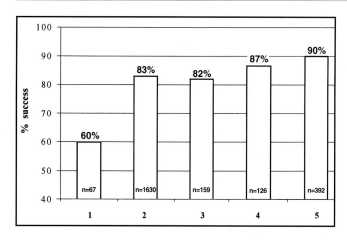

Fig. 1 Bar graph showing effects of the timing of the reconstruction and the use of antibiotic-impregnated bone cement. Combination of the results from multiple series reveals that delayed reconstruction and antibiotic-impregnated bone cement exert independent, beneficial effects on the outcome of reimplantation performed because of infection at the site of a total hip arthroplasty. 1 = direct exchange with bone cement without antibiotics;[76,79,127–129] 2 = direct exchange with antibiotic-impregnated cement;[78,84–87,89,90,93,96,98,101,102,105,108,111,128,130–132] 3 = delayed reconstruction with bone cement without antibiotics;[76,80,81,97,127,128,133–135] 4 = delayed reconstruction with insertion of the prosthesis without cement;[82,97,112,135,139,140] and 5 = delayed reconstruction with antibiotic-impregnated cement.[78,80,84,85,87,89,96,100,110,113,117,136]

ed cement are 2 closely linked variables that exert an independent influence on the outcome of treatment of infection at the site of a total hip arthroplasty. The apparent effect of these 2 variables is demonstrated by a review of the results of multiple series (Fig. 1). In the absence of antibiotic-impregnated bone cement, the results of direct-exchange techniques are vastly inferior. However, when the reconstruction is performed after a delay following removal of the implant, the results obtained without use of antibiotic-impregnated cement are similar to those achieved with direct exchange with use of antibiotic-impregnated cement. Finally, although analyses based on combined series have major shortcomings, delayed reconstruction combined with use of antibiotic-impregnated bone cement appears to provide the highest rate of success of treatment of infection at the site of a total hip arthroplasty.

Insertion of the Prosthesis Without Cement

Studies have demonstrated deleterious effects of bone cement on chemotaxis, phagocytosis, and opsonization of leukocytes in humans and higher rates of infection with use of polymethylmethacrylate than with use of other biomaterials in canine models.[17,29,131] Accordingly, the results of reimplantation of prostheses without cement have been investigated. When several series in which this approach was used are combined, the rate of successful eradication of infection is found to be 109 (87%) of 126 patients.[82,97,112,135,139,140] The use of antibiotic-impregnated beads in the interval between resection arthroplasty and reimplantation yielded a successful result in 51 (88%) of 58 patients.[139,140] Again, it is difficult to determine, on the basis of this analysis, whether or not local delivery of antibiotics from the cement beads in these studies provided any substantial benefit. It is important to note that rather worrisome rates of loosening and inferior functional results have been reported after the insertion of femoral prostheses without cement for the treatment of infection at the site of a hip arthroplasty.[82,112] Insertion of the femoral component with cement combined with insertion of the acetabular component without cement has provided better functional results than have femoral and acetabular reconstructions done without cement.[112] Currently, most of the delayed reimplantations that we perform involve insertion of the acetabular component without ce-

ment and fixation of the femoral component with antibiotic-impregnated cement.

Bone-Grafting

The use of structural bone graft for reimplantation of a prosthesis in a patient who had had an infection at the site of a total hip arthroplasty was not associated with an increased risk of reinfection in several studies;[80,82,97,104,112,139] however, none of these studies involved the use of massive structural bone graft. Two reports on the use of massive structural allograft for reconstruction of large acetabular or femoral defects in a total of 57 patients, with all components fixed with antibiotic-impregnated bone cement, did not reveal an increased risk of reinfection.[102,141]

An alternative method for the treatment of patients who have massive bone defects is a 3-stage reconstruction.[82] The first stage consists of resection arthroplasty and subsequent therapy with antibiotics; the second stage, performed 3 to 6 months later, consists of bone-grafting with use of a 50-50 particulate mixture of cancellous autogenous graft and allograft; and the third stage, performed 9 to 12 months after the bone-grafting, consists of insertion of a new prosthesis without cement. All of the patients in this small subset had a successful outcome.[82] This technique warrants consideration, particularly for the acetabulum, for patients who have extensive bone loss, as bone graft appears to incorporate more readily in this region than in the femur. The use of massive structural allografts for delayed reconstruction in patients who have an infection at the site of a total hip arthroplasty appears to be increasing.

References

1. Poss R, Thornhill TS, Ewald FC, Thomas WH, Batte NJ, Sledge CB: Factors influencing the incidence and outcome of infection following total joint arthroplasty. *Clin Orthop* 1984;182:117–126.

2. Wilson MG, Kelley K, Thornhill TS: Infection as a complication of total knee-replacement arthroplasty: Risk factors and treatment in sixty-seven cases. *J Bone Joint Surg* 1990;72A:878–883.

3. Luessenhop CP, Higgins LD, Brause BD, Ranawat CS: Multiple prosthetic infections after total joint arthroplasty: Risk factor analysis. *J Arthroplasty* 1996;11:862–868.

4. England SP, Stern SH, Insall JN, Windsor RE: Total knee arthroplasty in diabetes mellitus. *Clin Orthop* 1990;260:130–134.

5. Papagelopoulos PJ, Idusuyi OB, Wallrichs SL, Morrey BF: Long term outcome and survivorship analysis of primary total knee arthroplasty in patients with diabetes mellitus. *Clin Orthop* 1996;330:124–132.

6. Menon TJ, Thjellesen D, Wroblewski BM: Charnley low-friction arthroplasty in diabetic patients. *J Bone Joint Surg* 1983;65B:580–581.

7. Moeckel B, Huo MH, Salvati EA, Pellicci PM: Total hip arthroplasty in patients with diabetes mellitus. *J Arthroplasty* 1993;8:279–284.

8. Greene KA, Wilde AN, Stulberg BN: Preoperative nutritional status of total joint patients: Relationship to postoperative wound complications. *J Arthroplasty* 1991;6:321–325.

9. Jensen JE, Jensen TG, Smith TK, Johnston DA, Dudrick SJ: Nutrition in orthopaedic surgery. *J Bone Joint Surg* 1982;64A:1263–1272.

10. Smith TK: Nutrition: Its relationship to orthopedic infections. *Orthop Clin North Am* 1991;22:373–377.

11. Gherini S, Vaughn BK, Lombardi AV Jr, Mallory TH: Delayed wound healing and nutritional deficiencies after total hip arthroplasty. *Clin Orthop* 1993;293:188–195.

12. Stern SH, Insall JN: Total knee arthroplasty in obese patients. *J Bone Joint Surg* 1990;72A:1400–1404.

13. Stern SH, Insall JN, Windsor RH, Inglis AE, Dines DM: Total knee arthroplasty in patients with psoriasis. *Clin Orthop* 1989;248:108–110.

14. Rand JA, Fitzgerald RH Jr: Diagnosis and management of the infected total knee arthroplasty. *Orthop Clin North Am* 1989;20:201–210.

15. Surin VV, Sundholm K, Bäckman L: Infection after total hip replacement: With special reference to a discharge from the wound. *J Bone Joint Surg* 1983;65B:412–418.

16. Fitzgerald RH Jr, Nolan DR, Ilstrup DM, Van Scoy RE, Washington JA II, Coventry MB: Deep wound sepsis following total hip arthroplasty. *J Bone Joint Surg* 1977;59A:847–855.

17. Jerry GJ Jr, Rand JA, Ilstrup D: Old sepsis prior to total knee arthroplasty. *Clin Orthop* 1988;236:135–140.

18. Schmalzried TP, Amstutz HC, Au MK, Dorey FJ: Etiology of deep sepsis in total hip arthroplasty: The significance of hematogenous and recurrent infections. *Clin Orthop* 1992;280:200–207.

19. Cruse PJ, Foord R: A five-year prospective study of 23,649 surgical wounds. *Arch Surg* 1973;107:206–210.

20. Rand JA, Chao EY, Stauffer RN: Kinematic rotating-hinge total knee arthroplasty. *J Bone Joint Surg* 1987;69A:489–497.

21. Schutzer SF, Harris WH: Deep-wound infection after total hip replacement under contemporary aseptic conditions. *J Bone Joint Surg* 1988;70A:724–727.

22. Ritter MA, Eitzen HE, French ML, Hart JB: The effect that time, touch and environment have upon bacterial contamination of instruments during surgery. *Ann Surg* 1976;184:642–644.

23. Ritter MA, Eitzen HH, Hart JB, French ML: The surgeon's garb. *Clin Orthop* 1980;153:204–209.

24. Smith RC, Mooar PA, Cooke T, Sherk HH: Contamination of operating room personnel during total arthroplasty. *Clin Orthop* 1991;271:9–11.

25. Blomgren G, Hoborn J, Nyström B: Reduction of contamination at total hip replacement by special working clothes. *J Bone Joint Surg* 1990;72B:985–987.

26. Ritter MA, French ML, Hart JB: Microbiological studies in a horizontal wall-less laminar air-flow operating room during actual surgery. *Clin Orthop* 1973;97:16–18.

27. Brown AR, Taylor GJ, Gregg PJ: Air contamination during skin preparation and draping in joint replacement surgery. *J Bone Joint Surg* 1996;78B:92–94.

28. Ritter MA, Campbell ED: Retrospective evaluation of an iodophor-incorporated antimicrobial plastic adhesive wound drape. *Clin Orthop* 1988;228:307–308.

29. Johnston DH, Fairclough JA, Brown EM, Morris R: Rate of bacterial recolonization of the skin after preparation: Four methods compared. *Br J Surg* 1987;74:64.

30. Baird RA, Nickel FR, Thrupp LD, Rucker S, Hawkins B: Splash basin contamination in orthopaedic surgery. *Clin Orthop* 1984;187:129–133.

31. Greenough CG: An investigation into contamination of operative suction. *J Bone Joint Surg* 1986;68B:151–153.

32. Sanders R, Fortin P, Ross E, Helfet D: Outer gloves in orthopaedic procedures: Cloth compared with latex. *J Bone Joint Surg* 1990;72A:914–917.

33. Lidwell OM, Lowbury EJ, Whyte W, Blowers R, Stanley SJ, Lowe D: Effect of ultraclean air in operating rooms on deep sepsis in the joint after total hip or knee replacement: A randomised study. *Br Med J (Clin Res Ed)* 1982;285:10–14.

34. Lidwell OM: Clean air at operation and subsequent sepsis in the joint. *Clin Orthop* 1986;211:91–102.

35. Charnley J: Postoperative infection after total hip replacement with special reference to air contamination in the operating room. *Clin Orthop* 1972;87:167–187.

36. Brady LP, Enneking WF, Franco JA: The effect of operating-room environment on the infection rate after Charnley low-friction total hip replacement. *J Bone Joint Surg* 1975;57A:80–83.

37. Glynn MK, Sheehan JM: An analysis of the causes of deep infection after hip and knee arthroplasties. *Clin Orthop* 1983;178:202–206.

38. Marotte JH, Lord GA, Blanchard JP, et al: Infection rate in total hip arthroplasty as a function of air cleanliness and antibiotic prophylaxis: 10-year experience with 2,384 cementless Lord Madreporic prostheses. *J Arthroplasty* 1987;2:77–82.

39. Nelson JP, Glassburn AR Jr, Talbott RD, McElhinney JP: The effect of previous surgery, operating room environment, and preventive antibiotics on postoperative infection following total hip arthroplasty. *Clin Orthop* 1980;147:167–169.

40. Salvati EA, Robinson RP, Zeno SM, Koslin BL, Brause BD, Wilson PD Jr: Infection rates after 3175 total hip and total knee replacements performed with and without a horizontal unidirectional filtered air-flow system. *J Bone Joint Surg* 1982;64A:525–535.

41. Lowell JD, Kundsin RB, Schwartz CM, Pozin D: Ultraviolet radiation and reduction of deep wound infection following hip and knee arthroplasty. *Ann NY Acad Sci* 1980;353:285–293.

42. Berg M, Bergman BR, Hoborn J: Ultraviolet radiation compared to an ultra-clean air enclosure: Comparison of air bacteria counts in operating rooms. *J Bone Joint Surg* 1991;73B:811–815.

43. Agarwal S, Kadhi SK, Rooney RJ: Brucellosis complicating bilateral total knee arthroplasty. *Clin Orthop* 1991;267:179–181.

44. Hanssen AD, Osmon DR, Nelson CL: Prevention of deep periprosthetic joint infection. *J Bone Joint Surg* 1996;78A:458–471.

45. Petty W: The effect of methylmethacrylate on chemotaxis of polymorphonuclear leukocytes. *J Bone Joint Surg* 1978;60A:492–498.

46. Petty W: The effect of methylmethacrylate on bacterial phagocytosis and killing by human polymorphonuclear leukocytes. *J Bone Joint Surg* 1978;60A:752–757.

47. Petty W, Spanier S, Shuster JJ: Prevention of infection after total joint replacement: Experiments with a canine model. *J Bone Joint Surg* 1988;70A:536–539.

48. Petty W, Spanier S, Shuster JJ, Silverthorne C: The influence of skeletal implants on incidence of infection: Experiments in a canine model. *J Bone Joint Surg* 1985;67A:1236–1244.

49. Schurman DJ, Johnson BL Jr, Amstutz HC: Knee joint infections with Staphylococcus aureus and Micrococcus species: Influence of antibiotics, metal debris, bacteremia, blood, and steroids in a rabbit model. *J Bone Joint Surg* 1975;57A:40–49.

50. Gristina AG: Implant failure and the immuno-incompetent fibro-inflammatory zone. *Clin Orthop* 1994;298:106–118.

51. Gristina AG: Biomaterial-centered infection: Microbial adhesion versus tissue integration. *Science* 1987;237:1588–1595.

52. Gristina AG, Costerton JW: Bacterial adherence to biomaterials and tissue: The significance of its role in clinical sepsis. *J Bone Joint Surg* 1985;67A:264–273.

53. Gristina AG, Kolkin J: Total joint replacement and sepsis. *J Bone Joint Surg* 1983;65A:128–134.

54. Naylor PT, Myrvik QN, Gristina A: Antibiotic resistance of biomaterial-adherent coagulase-negative and coagulase-positive staphylococci. *Clin Orthop* 1990;261:126–133.

55. Kendall RW, Duncan CP, Smith JA, Ngui-Yen JH: Persistence of bacteria on antibiotic loaded acrylic depots: A reason for caution. *Clin Orthop* 1996;329:273–280.

56. Levitsky KA, Hozack WJ, Balderston RA, et al: Evaluation of the painful prosthetic joint: Relative value of bone scan, sedimentation rate, and joint aspiration. *J Arthroplasty* 1991;6:237–244.

57. Fitzgerald RH Jr: Total hip arthroplasty sepsis: Prevention and diagnosis. *Orthop Clin North Am* 1992;23:259–264.

58. Fitzgerald RH Jr, Jones DR: Hip implant infection: Treatment with resection arthroplasty and late total hip arthroplasty. *Am J Med* 1985;78:225–228.

59. Hanssen AD, Rand JA, Osmon DR: Treatment of the infected total knee arthroplasty with insertion of another prosthesis: The effect of antibiotic-impregnated bone cement. *Clin Orthop* 1994;309:44–55.

60. Niskanen RO, Korkala O, Pammo H: Serum C-reactive protein levels after total hip and knee arthroplasty. *J Bone Joint Surg* 1996;78B:431–433.

61. Shih LY, Wu JJ, Yang DJ: Erythrocyte sedimentation rate and C-reactive protein values in patients with total hip arthroplasty. *Clin Orthop* 1987;225:238–246.

62. Palestro CJ, Kim CK, Swyer AJ, Capozzi JD, Solomon RW, Goldsmith SJ: Total hip arthroplasty: Periprosthetic indium-111-labeled leukocyte activity and complementary technetium-99m-sulfur colloid imaging in suspected infection. *J Nucl Med* 1990;31:1950–1955.

63. Rand JA, Brown ML: The value of indium 111 leukocyte scanning in the evaluation of painful or infected total knee arthroplasties. *Clin Orthop* 1990;259:179–182.

64. Oyen WJ, Claessens RA, van Horn JR, van der Meer JW, Corstens FH: Scintigraphic detection of bone and joint infections with indium-111-labeled nonspecific polyclonal human immunoglobulin G. *J Nucl Med* 1990;31:403–412.

65. Datz FL, Anderson CH, Ahluwalia R, et al: The efficacy of indium-111-polyclonal IgG for the detection of infection and inflammation. *J Nucl Med* 1994;35:74–83.

66. Becker W, Palestro CJ, Winship J, et al: Rapid imaging of infections with a monoclonal antibody fragment (LeukoScan). *Clin Orthop* 1996;329:263–272.

67. Hakki S, Harwood SJ, Morrissey MA, Camblin JG, Laven DL, Webster WB Jr: Comparative study of monoclonal antibody scan in diagnosing orthopaedic infection. *Clin Orthop* 1997;335:275–285.

68. Barrack RL, Harris WH: The value of aspiration of the hip joint before revision total hip arthroplasty. *J Bone Joint Surg* 1993;75A:66–76.

69. Lachiewicz PF, Rogers GD, Thomason HC: Aspiration of the hip joint before revision total hip arthroplasty: Clinical and laboratory factors influencing attainment of a positive culture. *J Bone Joint Surg* 1996;78A:749–754.

70. Duff GP, Lachiewicz PF, Kelley SS: Aspiration of the knee joint before revision arthroplasty. *Clin Orthop* 1996;331:132–139.

71. Mariani BD, Martin DS, Levine MJ, Booth RE Jr, Tuan RS: Polymerase chain reaction detection of bacterial infection in total knee arthroplasty. *Clin Orthop* 1996;331:11–22.

72. Mirra JM, Marder RA, Amstutz HC: The pathology of failed total joint arthroplasty. *Clin Orthop* 1982;170:175–183.

73. Feldman DS, Lonner JH, Desai P, Zuckerman JD: The role of intraoperative frozen sections in revision total joint arthroplasty. *J Bone Joint Surg* 1995;77A:1807–1813.

74. Garvin KL, Hanssen AD: Infection after total hip arthroplasty: Past, present, and future. *J Bone Joint Surg* 1995;77A:1576–1588.

75. Balderston RA, Hiller WD, Iannotti JP, et al: Treatment of the septic hip with total hip arthroplasty. *Clin Orthop* 1987;221:231–237.

76. Cherney DL, Amstutz HC: Total hip replacement in the previously septic hip. *J Bone Joint Surg* 1983;65A:1256–1265.

77. Colyer RA, Capello WN: Surgical treatment of the infected hip implant: Two-stage reimplantation with a one-month interval. *Clin Orthop* 1994;298:75–79.

78. Garvin KL, Evans BG, Salvati EA, Brause BD: Palacos gentamicin for the treatment of deep periprosthetic hip infections. *Clin Orthop* 1994;298:97–105.

79. Jupiter JB, Karchmer AW, Lowell JD, Harris WH: Total hip arthroplasty in the treatment of adult hips with current or quiescent sepsis. *J Bone Joint Surg* 1981;63A:194–200.

80. Lieberman JR, Callaway GH, Salvati EA, Pellicci PM, Brause BD: Treatment of the infected total hip arthroplasty with a two-stage reimplantation protocol. *Clin Orthop* 1994;301:205–212.

81. McDonald DJ, Fitzgerald RH Jr, Ilstrup DM: Two-stage reconstruction of a total hip arthroplasty because of infection. *J Bone Joint Surg* 1989;71A:828–834.

82. Nestor BJ, Hanssen AD, Ferrer-Gonzalez R, Fitzgerald RH Jr: The use of porous prostheses in delayed reconstruction of total hip replacements that have failed because of infection. *J Bone Joint Surg* 1994;76A:349–359.

83. Canner GC, Steinberg ME, Heppenstall RB, Balderston R: The infected hip after total hip arthroplasty. *J Bone Joint Surg* 1984;66A:1393–1399.

84. Carlsson AS, Josefsson G, Lindberg L: Revision with gentamicin-impregnated cement for deep infections in total hip arthroplasties. *J Bone Joint Surg* 1978;60A:1059–1064.

85. Hope PG, Kristinsson KG, Norman P, Elson RA: Deep infection of cemented total hip arthroplasties caused by coagulase-negative staphylococci. *J Bone Joint Surg* 1989;71B:851–855.

86. Miley GB, Scheller AD Jr, Turner RH: Medical and surgical treatment of the septic hip with one-stage revision arthroplasty. *Clin Orthop* 1982;170:76–82.

87. Murray WR: Use of antibiotic-containing bone cement. *Clin Orthop* 1984;190:89–95.

88. Salvati EA, Chekofsky KM, Brause BD, Wilson PD Jr: Reimplantation in infection: A 12-year experience. *Clin Orthop* 1982;170:62–75.

89. Sanzén L, Carlsson AS, Josefsson G, Lindberg LT: Revision operations on infected total hip arthroplasties: Two- to nine-year follow-up study. *Clin Orthop* 1988;229:165–172.

90. Wroblewski BM: One-stage revision of infected cemented total hip arthroplasty. *Clin Orthop* 1986;211:103–107.

91. Salvati EA, Callaghan JJ, Brause BD, Klein RF, Small RD: Reimplantation in infection: Elution of gentamicin from cement and beads. *Clin Orthop* 1986;207:83–93.

92. Rosenblatt JE: Laboratory tests used to guide antimicrobial therapy. *Mayo Clin Proc* 1991;66:942–948.

93. Buchholz HW, Elson RA, Engelbrecht E, Lodenkämper H, Röttger J, Siegel A: Management of deep infection of total hip replacement. *J Bone Joint Surg* 1981;63B:342–353.

94. Coventry MB: Treatment of infections occurring in total hip surgery. *Orthop Clin North Am* 1975;6:991–1003.

95. Drancourt M, Stein A, Argenson JN, Roiron R, Groulier P, Raoult D: Oral treatment of Staphylococcus spp. infected orthopaedic

implants with fusidic acid or ofloxacin in combination with rifampicin. *J Antimicrob Chemother* 1997;39:235–240.

96. Antti-Poika I, Santavirta S, Konttinen YT, Honkanen V: Outcome of the infected hip arthroplasty: A retrospective study of 36 patients. *Acta Orthop Scand* 1989;60:670–675.

97. Berry DJ, Chandler HP, Reilly DT: The use of bone allografts in two-stage reconstruction after failure of hip replacements due to infection. *J Bone Joint Surg* 1991;73A:1460–1468.

98. Elson RA, Jephcott AE, McGechie DB, Verettas D: Antibiotic-loaded acrylic cement. *J Bone Joint Surg* 1977;59B:200–205.

99. Heck D, Rosenberg A, Schink-Ascani M, Garbus S, Kiewitt T: Use of antibiotic-impregnated cement during hip and knee arthroplasty in the United States. *J Arthroplasty* 1995;10:470–475.

100. Hovelius L, Josefsson G: An alternative method for exchange operation of infected arthroplasty. *Acta Orthop Scand* 1979;50:93–96.

101. Ketterl R, Henley MB, Stübinger B, Beckurts T, Claudi B: Analysis of three operative techniques for infected total hip replacements. *Orthop Trans* 1988;12:715.

102. Loty B, Postel M, Evrard J, et al: One stage revision of infected total hip replacements with replacement of bone loss by allografts: Study of 90 cases of which 46 used bone allografts. *Int Orthop* 1992;16:330–338.

103. Lynch M, Esser MP, Shelley P, Wroblewski BM: Deep infection in Charnley low-friction arthroplasty: Comparison of plain and gentamicin-loaded cement. *J Bone Joint Surg* 1987;69B:355–360.

104. Morscher E, Babst R, Jenny H: Treatment of infected joint arthroplasty. *Int Orthop* 1990;14:161–165.

105. Nasser S, Lee YF, Amstutz HC: Direct exchange arthroplasty in 30 septic total hip replacements without recurrent infection. *Orthop Trans* 1989;13:519.

106. Nelson CL, Evans RP, Blaha JD, Calhoun J, Henry SL, Patzakis MJ: A comparison of gentamicin-impregnated polymethylmethacrylate bead implantation to conventional parenteral antibiotic therapy in infected total hip and knee arthroplasty. *Clin Orthop* 1993;295:96–101.

107. Oxborrow NJ, Stamer J, Andrews M, Stone MH: New uses for gentamicin-impregnated polymethyl methacrylate spacers in two-stage revision hip arthroplasty. *J Arthroplasty* 1997;12:709–710.

108. Raut VV, Siney PD, Wroblewski BM: One-stage revision of infected total hip replacements with discharging sinuses. *J Bone Joint Surg* 1994;76B:721–724.

109. Raut VV, Orth MS, Orth MC, Siney PD, Wroblewski BM: One stage revision arthroplasty of the hip for deep gram negative infection. *Int Orthop* 1996;20:12–14.

110. Tsukayama DT, Estrada R, Gustilo RB: Infection after total hip arthroplasty: A study of

the treatment of one hundred and six infections. *J Bone Joint Surg* 1996;78A:512–523.

111. Wagner H, Wagner M: Infected hip joint prosthesis: Viewpoints for 1-stage and 2-stage prosthesis exchange. Orthopäde 1995;24:314–318.

112. Wang JW, Chen CE: Reimplantation of infected hip arthroplasties using bone allografts. *Clin Orthop* 1997;335:202–210.

113. Younger AS, Duncan CP, Masri BA, McGraw RW: The outcome of two-stage arthroplasty using a custom-made interval spacer to treat the infected hip. *J Arthroplasty* 1997;12:615–623.

114. Baker AS, Greenham LW: Release of gentamicin from acrylic bone cement: Elution and diffusion studies. *J Bone Joint Surg* 1988;70A:1551–1557.

115. Beeching NJ, Thomas MG, Roberts S, Lang SD: Comparative in-vitro activity of antibiotics incorporated in acrylic bone cement. *J Antimicrob Chemother* 1986;17:173–184.

116. Duncan CP, Masri BA: The role of antibiotic-loaded cement in the treatment of an infection after a hip replacement, in Jackson DW (ed): *Instructional Course Lectures 44*. Rosemont, IL, American Academy of Orthopaedic Surgeons. 1995, pp 305–313.

117. Elson R: One-stage exchange in the treatment of the infected total hip arthroplasty. *Semin Arthroplasty* 1994;5:137–141.

118. Hill J, Klenerman L, Trustey S, Blowers R: Diffusion of antibiotics from acrylic bone-cement in vitro. *J Bone Joint Surg* 1977;59B:197–199.

119. Hoff SF, Fitzgerald RH Jr, Kelly PJ: The depot administration of penicillin G and gentamicin in acrylic bone cement. *J Bone Joint Surg* 1981;63A:798–804.

120. Kuechle DK, Landon GC, Musher DM, Noble PC: Elution of vancomycin, daptomycin, and amikacin from acrylic bone cement. *Clin Orthop* 1991;264:302–308.

121. Lawson KJ, Marks KE, Brems J, Rehm S: Vancomycin vs tobramycin elution from polymethylmethacrylate: An in vitro study. *Orthopedics* 1990;13:521–524.

122. Levin PD: The effectiveness of various antibiotics in methyl methacrylate. *J Bone Joint Surg* 1975;57B:234–237.

123. Marks KE, Nelson CL, Lautenschlager EP: Antibiotic-impregnated acrylic bone cement. *J Bone Joint Surg* 1976;58A:358–364.

124. Penner MJ, Masri BA, Duncan CP: Elution characteristics of vancomycin and tobramycin combined in acrylic bone-cement. *J Arthroplasty* 1996;11:939–944.

125. Brien WW, Salvati EA, Klein R, Brause B, Stern S: Antibiotic impregnated bone cement in total hip arthroplasty: An in vivo comparison of the elution properties of tobramycin and vancomycin. *Clin Orthop* 1993;296:242–248.

126. Masri BA, Duncan CP, Beauchamp CP, Paris NJ, Arntorp J: Effect of varying surface patterns on antibiotic elution from antibiotic-loaded bone cement. *J Arthroplasty* 1995;10:453–459.

127. Hughes PW, Salvati EA, Wilson PD Jr, Blumenfeld EL: Treatment of subacute sepsis of the hip by antibiotics and joint replacement: Criteria for diagnosis with evaluation of twenty-six cases. *Clin Orthop* 1979;141:143–157.

128. Hunter GA: The results of reinsertion of a total hip prosthesis after sepsis. *J Bone Joint Surg* 1979;61B:422–423.

129. Lai KA, Shen WJ, Yang CY, Lin RM, Lin CJ, Jou IM: Two-stage cementless revision THR after infection: 5 recurrences in 40 cases followed 2.5-7 years. *Acta Orthop Scand* 1996;67:325–328.

130. Herzog R, Morscher E: Treatment of infected total prosthesis arthroplasty of the hip joint. *Orthopäde* 1995;24:326–334.

131. Johnston RC, Katz RP, Sullivan PM, Kratz PK: A minimum ten year follow-up study of one stage reimplantation of the infected total hip. Proceedings of the 61st Annual Meeting of the American Academy of Orthopaedic Surgeons, New Orleans, LA. Rosemont, IL, American Academy of Orthopaedic Surgeons, 1994, p 30.

132. Mulcahy DM, O'Byrne JM, Fenelon GE: One stage surgical management of deep infection of total hip arthroplasty. *Ir J Med Sci* 1996;165:17–19.

133. Goodman SB, Schurman DJ: Outcome of infected total hip arthroplasty: An inclusive, consecutive series. *J Arthroplasty* 1988;3:97–102.

134. Talbott RD, Glassburn AR Jr, Nelson JP, McElhinney JP, Greenberg RL: Implantation of total hip arthroplasty after known deep infection. *Orthop Trans* 1980;4:97.

135. Wilson MG, Dorr LD: Reimplantation of infected total hip arthroplasties in the absence of antibiotic cement. *J Arthroplasty* 1989;4:263–269.

136. Harle A: Infection management in total hip replacement. *Arch Orthop Trauma Surg* 1989;108:63–71.

137. Pagnano MW, Trousdale RT, Hanssen AD: Outcome after reinfection following reimplantation hip arthroplasty. *Clin Orthop* 1997;338:192–204.

138. Kendall RW, Duncan CP, Beauchamp CP: Bacterial growth on antibiotic-loaded acrylic cement: A prospective in vivo retrieval study. *J Arthroplasty* 1995;10:817–822.

139. Gustilo RB, Tsukayama D: Treatment of infected cemented total hip arthroplasty with tobramycin beads and delayed revision with a cementless prosthesis and bone grafting. *Orthop Trans* 1988;12:739.

140. Lai KA, Yang CY, Lin RM, Jou IM, Lin CJ: Cementless reimplantation of hydroxyapatite-coated total hips after periprosthetic infections. *J Formos Med Assoc* 1996;95:452–457.

141. Alexeeff M, Mahomed N, Morsi H, Garbuz D, Gross A: Structural allograft in two-stage revisions for failed septic hip arthroplasty. *J Bone Joint Surg* 1996;78B:213–216.

Knee: Adult Reconstruction

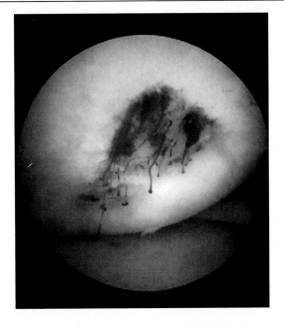

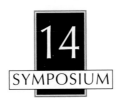

Distal Femoral Varus Osteotomy: Indications and Surgical Technique

Matthew J. Phillips, MD
Kenneth A. Krackow, MD

Introduction

Valgus deformity around the knee is much less frequent than varus deformity. Conditions more commonly associated with valgus deformity include rheumatoid arthritis, renal osteodystrophy, rickets, overcorrected proximal tibial valgus osteotomy, and infantile polio. Primary osteoarthritis and posttraumatic arthritis can also present with significant valgus deformity.[1] The primary pathologic features of the valgus knee are tight lateral soft-tissue structures, varying degrees of medial laxity, and lateral femoral condyle hypoplasia.[1] Treatment options available for the valgus, arthritic knee include nonsurgical measures, arthroscopic debridement, osteotomy, unicompartmental arthroplasty, and total knee arthroplasty (TKA). The purpose of this chapter is not to argue the merits of the various treatment options but rather to make a case for distal femoral varus osteotomy and to provide the reader with a detailed technique for the procedure.

Indications

The basic indications for any knee osteotomy generally have an inverse relationship to those for total knee or even unicompartmental knee arthroplasty. TKA is more predictable in terms of initial pain relief and later durability than knee osteotomy. However, it is always necessary to question the suitability of artificial joints, ie, metal and plastic arthroplasty, in younger and more active patients for fear of problems of loosening, osteolysis, and the need for multiple revisions over the years.

It is not unreasonable to expect today that a good proportion of patients aged 30 to 55 years or even 60 will live to be 90 or even 95 years of age. If they enter into the realm of TKA, they will be requiring arthroplasty function for a total of 30 to 65 years. It is simply not possible to extrapolate 10-, 15-, and even 20-year survivorship studies, done largely on older patients, to the requisite 30- to 65-year periods. The prospects for satisfactory multiple revisions in these patients over these periods of time are another concern. For these reasons, there must often be a search for some alternative management of arthrosis in the younger, more active patient.

More specifically, with regard to indications, we can say that the basic indications for distal femoral osteotomy are principally lateral compartment tibiofemoral arthrosis, in com-

bination with a valgus deformity, present in a patient too young or too active for the comfortable selection of TKA. In addition, there are such well-recognized factors as synovitis states, for example, rheumatoid arthritis and crystalline arthropathies, which portend a lesser likelihood of satisfactory outcomes with osteotomy treatment. Also, there may be concern for problems such as decreased range of motion, flexion contracture, and ligamentous instability in certain cases. However, some of these are only relative contraindications or negative factors, and the appropriate decision may depend very much on the complementary undesirability of TKA because of unquestionably young age or strenuous work practices, etc.

A commonly asked question is whether the indication for osteotomy is based on deformity alone. For cases of distal femoral osteotomy and valgus deformity, this consideration may initially be a cosmetic one. If the physician and patient can come to a satisfactory conclusion based on cosmetic considerations alone, then we see no reason not to proceed with such surgery. If the question is really one of attempting to prevent arthrosis, the situation may be different. We

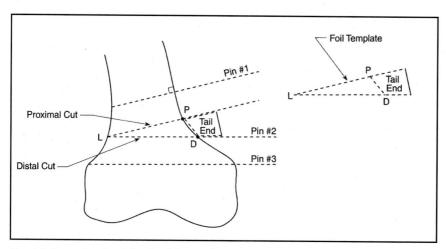

Fig. 1 Schematic of a right distal femur showing pin placements, proximal and distal cuts, and creation of a foil template.

are not aware of any good literature citations that establish guidelines for recommendations on this point. Our own recommendations in this situation are to wait for some sign of degeneration or progression of the deformity. Long, standing lower extremity radiographs are our recommended means of following lower extremity deformity. Films several years apart can be obtained, and at the first sign of progression of wear or increase in deformity surgery can be offered. The assumption here is that the patient is quite young.

The published results of distal femoral osteotomy have been generally good. McDermott and associates[2] reported a 92% success rate at 4 years after surgery. Healy and associates[3] had 93% good or excellent results after 4 years. Overcorrection and undercorrection are both associated with poorer results. We typically aim for 4° of mechanical axis varus. Others have recommended a 0° tibiofemoral angle (6° of mechanical axis varus)[2] or a mechanical axis that is just medial to the midportion of the tibial plateau.[4] For us, 4° of varus has been both clinically and cosmetically acceptable.

Cosmesis can be an important issue in osteotomy.[5] It has been our experience that a valgus producing osteotomy creates a relatively obvious clinical valgus deformity, which may be cosmetically unappealing to the patient. On the other hand, varus osteotomy of a valgus deformity generally leads to a significant cosmetic improvement, as if the eye is more esthetically accepting of mild varus and more sensitive to mild valgus deformity.

Surgical Technique
The patient is positioned supine on the operating table, with folded sheets rolled under the buttock of the operative side. An image intensification fluoroscope is brought in and tested so that one is confident that the hip and also the knee can be seen without any interference from the table. We will be using fluoroscopic assessment of the Bovie cord passing from the center of the femoral head to the center of the ankle and checking where that crosses the knee to assure alignment. A tourniquet is used, but it is used as a sterile tourniquet. The draping basically goes from the groin on down so that as

much of the extremity as possible is visually apparent and the general appearance of alignment can be assessed.

The foil template, used as described below, can be made ahead of time and sterilized or made on the table. The template is made from one side of the foil envelope in which most surgical knife blades are packaged. A steel Zimmer goniometer can be set to the osteotomy angle and the foil bent along the edges of that goniometer so that the surgeon can cut out and angle a template equal to the angle of the correction (Fig. 1).

The surgeon stands to the patient's opposite side, that is the left side for a right distal femoral osteotomy. After routine preparation and draping and placement and inflation of the tourniquet, a nearly midline, relatively long incision is made. It is basically a total knee replacement incision extending at least distally to the level of the tibial tubercle. This length is not absolutely necessary, but it does facilitate easier retraction and better appreciation of bony landmarks. The precapsular plane is developed over the knee itself in the medial aspect. This development allows the surgeon to know exactly where he/she is with regard to placement of the blade and provides good confidence that the blade will be in the appropriate bone and not exiting anywhere inappropriately. The knee joint specifically is not opened.

The deep fascia proximal to the patella is incised over the quadriceps tendon and retracted peripherally, medially, and posteriorly as the vastus medialis is separated from this fascia and retracted anteriorly and laterally. This is basically a sub-vastus exposure. When as much of the vastus medialis as possible has been "shelled-out" of this fascial envelope, a Bovie is used to divide the muscle at the inferior proximal aspect, leaving approximately 1 cm of muscle cuff on the fascia, close to the femur. This technique minimizes the risk of injury to the femoral vessels.

The vastus medialis is initially retracted with sharp, relatively shallow, rake retractors or small Myerdings. After enough of the medial femoral metaphysis and diaphysis have been exposed, a longitudinal medial incision into the periosteum is made and, with very careful subperiosteal dissection anteriorly and posteriorly at the level of the osteotomy, the surgeon is then able to place subperiosteal retractors. We typically use malleable retractors 1 cm in width, especially anteriorly, and perhaps a narrow dull-tipped Hohman retractor posteriorly.

The posterior subperiosteal dissection is carried just cephalad to the proximal margin of the femoral condyles and above the origins of the gastrocnemius. This dissection, plus the palpation of the end of the femur deep to the capsule with the knee bent, are the key elements that assure the surgeon of the appropriate level for osteotomy and blade plate placement. Next, the entry point is estimated for the blade plate. This entry is just anterior to the origin of the medial collateral ligament and basically central in a proximal-distal direction with regard to the medial femoral condyle. In the anterior-posterior dimension, the entry point is relatively anterior, so that the blade will lie along the shaft. After marking the entry point with a cautery, the surgeon can measure back to the osteotomy level, ie, the distance to the distal cut. The step-off on an AO blade plate is about 2 cm. The cut can actually be 2.5 cm to 2.75 cm from the entry point of the blade. The goal is to maximize the amount of bone

between the under surface of the blade and the osteotomy.

Having marked the entry point for the seating chisel and the level for the distal osteotomy, it is now possible to estimate the location of the proximal osteotomy and then to place the first alignment pin, referred to as pin #1. This 1/8-in Steinmann pin is placed perpendicular to the shaft of the femur, approximately 1½- to 2-cm proximal to the anticipated level of the proximal osteotomy. This pin will be used to guide the osteotomy, that is, the proximal osteotomy, ensuring that the osteotomy is perpendicular to the shaft of the femur. The pin will also be compared with what is described below as pin #3, assuring that when pin #1 and pin #3 are parallel, the angular correction has been obtained. Note: When placing all pins, go completely through the lateral cortex.

Pin #2 is placed at the indicated level of the distal osteotomy. The angle between pin #2 and pin #1 is the one chosen for the osteotomy. This angular relationship is established by using the metal goniometer, which has been locked in the position of the desired correction. The goniometer is held by an assistant so that it is parallel to pin #1, and with eyeball alignment pin #2 is placed parallel to the other limb of the goniometer. We find this freehand technique more reliable than using drill guides. Drill guides capture the tail end of a Steinmann pin but don't secure the point that enters the bone. Typical wandering of the pin points as they attempt to enter the bone can lead to errors of placement of the pins when the drill guide is removed.

A third pin is placed about 1-cm proximal and anterior to pin #2. This position is chosen so as to be out of the way of the seating chisel

entry points and the ultimate predicted blade plate position. Pin #3 is parallel to pin #2.

Pins #1 and #3 will be used as guides for the saw blade. Again, when the osteotomy is closed, they should be parallel. This position assures maintenance of rotation, assuming that the pins were put in neutral rotation to the bone and to one another. Also, their parallelism assures that the angular correction was as planned.

Pin #1 is removed. It should be emphasized that each of these Steinmann pins—#1, #2, and #3— is drilled from medial to lateral and indeed are drilled all the way through the lateral cortex. This point, which will become important later, is also important now, as hole #2 is used to measure the thickness of the bone at the level of the distal cut using a standard large AO depth gauge. We relocate the plate and seating chisel entry point and place the seating chisel at the entry point, parallel to pin #3 as seen from anterior to posterior. The seating chisel is impacted 2 to 3 cm and is then removed.

An important feature of this particular technique is that the seating chisel is not used to select the final, definitive position of the blade plate but mainly, or only, the entry point. The blade plate will be placed later almost as one would place a staple. This feature of the technique makes it much easier to align the blade plate accurately to the more proximal shaft. An adequately sized piece of distal bone ensures that this technique can be used without questioning the safety of the blade. In other words, it differs from a hip osteotomy in that there is a big distal target.

After the seating chisel is removed, the previously marked distal osteotomy level, ie, the location occupied by pin #2, is identified. This location can be adjusted before starting the distal cut if the seating chisel has changed the expected position. Before starting the distal osteotomy, its location should be clearly drawn on the bone with a skin marking pen or with a cautery. It is usually made in a straight anterior-posterior line, ie, a line that appears perpendicular to the shaft of the femur. After drawing a distal osteotomy line and having measured the thickness of the bone with a standard depth gauge used through the holes for pin #2, the foil template is cut corresponding to the thickness of the bone (Fig. 1).

What we refer to as the "tail end" of the template is used to mark the starting point for the level of the proximal cut, which is parallel to pin #1. The piece of foil cut away should be a triangle congruent to the wedge of bone to be resected. When looking from anterior to posterior at the resected bone wedge, it should represent a triangle congruent to the resected apex angle of the foil (Fig. 1).

Before starting the distal osteotomy, pin #3 is in place and pins #1 and #2 are removed. When starting the distal osteotomy, and, later, when starting the proximal cut as well, the saw is used to cut into the peripheral cortex along the line drawn, taking care to etch that line, but with less attention to having the saw blade parallel to the guide pin, pin #3. After the saw has etched the drawn cut line, the blade is adjusted to be parallel to guide pin #3 and the saw cut is undertaken. Protecting retractors should be in place, and we usually place a sponge between the posterior retractor and the soft tissues. In addition to trying to effect adequate protection of the soft tissues, care is also taken to attempt not to strip more periosteum than is necessary, ideally nothing more than the periosteum covering the resection wedge. The

distal cut is made approximately 2/3 to 3/4 of the way across the femur.

In the case of a large extremity, during wedge resection, especially when making the second cut, thought must be given to preventing the weight of the leg from inadvertently cracking through residual thin lateral cortex. This problem can be avoided by having an assistant support the knee. Although the overall position is one of knee flexion with hip external rotation, it is still possible to support the lateral knee to keep gravity from completing the osteotomy in a way that typically leads to a proximally directed spike on the distal fragment.

After the distal osteotomy has been completed to the desired distance, pin #3 is removed. A 7/64-in pin is then placed into the holes made for pin #1. This selection provides accurate alignment of the pin and instant ease of placement through both bone holes. When starting the proximal cut, care is taken again simply to etch the osteotomy without making certain that the saw blade is parallel to the pin. After the osteotomy has been etched, the saw blade is made parallel to pin #1.

After beginning to etch the proximal cut, the tail end of the foil template is brought up to the bone to ascertain that the distance between the distal cut and the proximal cut is as planned (Fig. 1). In using the tail end of the foil template to check the width of the base of the wedge, it is important, as shown in the diagram, to keep the proximal and distal edges of this part of the template parallel to the respective pins.

After most of the proximal cut has been made, the surgeon returns alternatively to the distal and back to the proximal osteotomy to complete the wedge resection. It is important

to realize that if a saw blade is taken all of the way across the bone and through the lateral cortex, the width of the saw blade itself, the kerf, will create a small lateral defect and laxity of the soft tissues. Therefore, the saw blade is not advanced quite all the way across; rather, the osteotomy is completed with a sharp osteotome. The osteotomy is then opened a bit and the saw blade is passed along to smooth off the residual bone without creating a lateral kerf.

Great care must be taken to create flat surfaces that reduce nicely. During trial closure or osteotomy reduction, pins #1 and #3 are in place. Care is taken to trim the bone and adjust the fit so that the surfaces will be parallel when the osteotomy is well closed. Once the surgeon is confident of this position, an oblique 1/8-in Steinmann pin is passed from posteriorly in the distal fragment in a proximal lateral direction to temporarily stabilize the osteotomy. The knee can be extended, the hip internally rotated somewhat, and the extremity basically put back into a neutral position. The fluoroscope is brought in and the overall alignment is checked with the image and Bovie cord. The Bovie cord is pulled taut in position over the center of the femoral head and is visually positioned over the center of the ankle. Then the fluoroscope is brought over the knee, taking care that the rotation of the C-arm is neutral to the anteroposterior axis of the knee. The point of traverse of the Bovie cord is visualized. The goal is to have it traverse approximately 30% to 40% of the way between the midpoint of the distal femur and the medial edge of the radial femoral condyle. This traverse point approximates the junction between the medial or most lateral third of the medial compartment and the central third of the medial compartment.

When reduction and alignment have been assured, the offset at the osteotomy is inspected. Judging from the measured thickness of the bone taken with the depth gauge through hole #2, as well the radiograph, the length of the blade can be selected. Thus, both parameters for the blade plate, namely blade length and offset, are provided.

The blade plate, grasped with the specific plate-holding instrument, is placed into the previously made seating chisel spot and is adjusted so that the side plate is directed to its proper position along the shaft of the femur. In general, the blade should be directed from somewhat anteromedial to somewhat posterolateral, allowing it to sit better on the medial femoral condyle. If the side plate position is not correct, extract the plate and redirect it slightly. Because the medial bone is relatively soft, this is not difficult to do. This is the point at which we have made blade plating more analogous to staple placement and have eliminated a lot of the problems associated with use of a fully impacted seating chisel. It is general-ly not necessary to use a plate clamp such as a Verbrug.

Some decision must be made about the amount of compression to be applied. It is important to note two things: (1) overcompression can lead to a change in the angulation, and (2) overcompression of a step-off arrangement can actually lead to the blade plate's breaking the bone, ie, pulling through proximally. Note that it is permissible to medialize the shaft slightly, if that is necessary for fitting the best selected blade plate.

Care should be taken before definitive blade plate placement to palpate posteriorly and anteriorly in order to ensure that rotation has been maintained and that no troublesome step-offs exist. Imaging and the fluoroscope can be used to follow any particular step, but this is rarely necessary once the surgeon has become confident about the location of the blade and is able to feel and see the direction of the osteotomy itself. The wound is closed routinely with suction drainage.

Postoperatively, we immobilize patients in a bulky Jones' dressing and a knee immobilizer. We allow them touch-down weightbearing with crutches. They are followed every 2 weeks in the clinic with radiographs. After the first 2 weeks we generally allow patients to remove the immobilizer 3 times a day for gentle range of motion. At the first sign of radiographic healing, typically 6 weeks, we discontinue the immobilizer and begin a gradual increase in weightbearing. Formal physical therapy is usually not necessary.

References

1. Murray PB, Rand JA: Symptomatic valgus knee: The surgical options. *J Am Acad Orthop Surg* 1993;1:1–9.

2. McDermott AG, Finklestein JA, Farine I, Boynton EL, MacIntosh DL, Gross A: Distal femoral varus osteotomy for valgus deformity of the knee. *J Bone Joint Surg* 1988;70A:110–116.

3. Healy WL, Anglen JO, Wasilewski SA, Krackow KA: Distal femoral varus osteotomy. *J Bone Joint Surg* 1988;70A:102–109.

4. Morrey BF, Edgerton BC: Distal femoral osteotomy for lateral gonarthrosis, in Eilert RE (ed): *Instructional Course Lectures XLI*. Park Ridge, IL, American Academy of Orthopaedic Surgeons, 1992, pp 77–85.

5. Phillips MJ, Krackow KA: High tibial osteotomy and distal femoral osteotomy for valgus or varus deformity around the knee, in Cannon WD Jr (ed): *Instructional Course Lectures 47*. Rosemont, IL, American Academy of Orthopaedic Surgeons, 1998, pp 429–436.

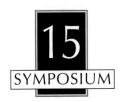

Proximal Valgus Tibial Osteotomy for Osteoarthritis of the Knee

Carol R. Hutchison, BSC, MD, MEd, FRCSC
Brian Cho, MD
Natalie Wong, MD
Zoe Agnidis, MSc, PT
Allan E. Gross, MD, FRCSC

Introduction

Although the incidence of proximal valgus osteotomy for osteoarthritis has decreased because of advances in total knee arthroplasty,[1] there is still a need for this operation in the young, high-demand patient with medial compartment osteoarthritis. In a study of unselected knees, Insall and associates[2] reported a success rate of 61% at 10 years. A more recent publication, based on a separate cohort of younger patients, reported a success rate of 82% and recommended this operation for patients younger than 60 years of age who wished to participate in vigorous sports or work activities (running, jumping, heavy lifting, etc).[3] Other reports in the literature have success rates ranging from 60% to 70% at 10 years.[4–7]

Proximal tibial osteotomy is a technically demanding procedure with the potential for intraoperative and postoperative complications.[8] Tibial osteotomy also makes total knee replacement technically more difficult although still yielding results comparable to those in patients who have not had a previous osteotomy.[9–11]

The prerequisites for osteotomy to realign the knee may be consid-

ered under the headings patient characteristics, disease characteristics, and joint characteristics. The patient characteristics are males younger than 60, females premenopausal with a high-demand lifestyle, and occupation. The disease characteristics are noninflammatory and unicompartmental. The joint characteristics are stable, no subluxation, flexion of at least 90°, and flexion deformity of less than 15°.

There have been many surgical techniques described to realign the proximal tibia into valgus: closing wedge osteotomy proximal to or distal to or at the insertion of the patellar tendon,[6,12,13] dome osteotomy,[14] and, for severe deformities of over 15°, double osteotomy (both femur and tibia). For multiplanar deformity, or where lengthening as well as angular correction is required, Ilizarov techniques may be required.[15–17] Various methods of fixation have been used, including staples, plates, external fixators, and plaster.[8]

We have used a surgical technique for proximal tibial osteotomy that addresses the potential complications of this operation and some of the difficulty of later total knee replacement.

This technique has been previously reported as a combined osteotomy of the tibial tubercle and the proximal tibia in order to address both patellofemoral and medial compartmental osteoarthritis.[18–21] We have used a similar technique, not to address bicompartmental disease, but to gain better and safer exposure to the proximal tibia, better bone for fixation, and loss of bone stock that is distal rather than proximal to the tubercle so that it interfers less with later total knee replacement. Osteotomy of the tubercle allows it to be elevated anteriorly, giving access to the proximal tibia at and just distal to the patellar tendon insertion. This procedure allows the closing wedge valgus osteotomy of the proximal tibia to be slightly more distal, which decreases the possibility of the staples or the osteotomy infringing on the articular surface. In addition, the bone is stronger, providing better fixation. Also, posterior exposure of the proximal tibia is facilitated because the joint capsule is well proximal to the site of osteotomy, and by excising only the superomedial part of the fibula, leaving the lateral cortex, the lateral ligament and the peroneal nerve are protected. We do not advocate debridement at the time of osteotomy because of the potential for joint stiffness and also because most of these patients have already undergone prior arthroscopic surgery.

Surgical Technique

A straight midline incision is made from the upper pole of the patella to 4 to 6 cm distal to the tibial tuberosity. Horizontal incisions are not used because of the possibility of future total knee arthroplasty. The dorsiflexor muscle mass is dissected off the proximal tibia for a distance of 2 to 4 cm, staying well proximal to the bifurcation of the artery. The head of the fibula is identified, and its proximal medial portion, which is the articular surface, is excised. The proximal lateral cortex is left intact to protect the lateral ligament and the peroneal nerve.

The patellar tendon insertion is identified. The tuberosity is then osteotomized and elevated anteriorly, just enough to protect the patellar tendon insertion, at which level the osteotomy is performed (Fig. 1). The proximal limb of the osteotomy is made parallel to the joint at the level of the insertion of the patellar tendon, which has been elevated anteriorly. The distal limb of the osteotomy starts at the predetermined distance according to the size of the wedge required to achieve 3° of overcorrection of the biomechanical axis. The size of the wedge is determined by measuring the biomechanical axis on a 3-foot standing radiograph. The number of degrees required to obtain 3° of overcorrection is calculated and, using a goniometer, the size of wedge to be removed is measured on the radiograph at the level of the osteotomy.

The osteotomy is done with an oscillating saw. The posterior cortex is osteotomized under direct vision after the rest of the wedge has been

removed. The medial cortex, which has been left intact, is perforated in multiple sites from anterior to posterior by a narrow osteotome or a drill bit. The osteotomy is then gently closed and held with 2 stepped staples. The excised wedge is morcellized and used as bone graft around the staples. Anteroposterior and lateral radiographs are taken to confirm staple position and adequate correction.

The tuberosity is left in its original bed and actually bridges the osteotomy. Bone graft is placed along the tuberosity. Internal fixation is not required. Anterolateral fasciotomy is carried out, a drain is left in the anterior compartment, and closure is done. Well-padded plaster slabs are applied and molded into valgus. A molded cast is applied a few days later. The patient is kept nonweightbearing for 2 or 3 weeks. Knee mobilization is started at 2 to 3 weeks. The patient resumes full activities after 3 months (Fig. 1).

Clinical Study

This surgical technique was used by the senior author on 321 knees in 279 patients. Twenty-six patients were lost to follow-up, leaving 292 knees in 253 patients. Determination of duration of time of tibial osteotomy to total knee arthroplasty was obtained through chart review and telephone interview. A Kaplan Meier survival analysis with a minimum 2-year follow-up was carried out.[22]

Sixty-two knees had gone on to total knee arthroplasty. Eight of 89 that were followed up less than 5 years, 28 of 72 knees from 5 to 10 years, and 26 of 131 that were followed up for more than 10 years were converted to total knee arthroplasty. The Kaplan Meier minimum 2-year survival analysis included 241 knees. At 5 years, 98% of patients had not undergone total knee arthroplasty. At

10 years 83% had not gone on to total knee arthroplasty.

Discussion

Proximal tibial valgus osteotomy has proven to be an effective operation for medial compartment osteoarthritis in the patient who is of too high demand by reason of age, size, occupation, or lifestyle for unicompartmental or total knee arthroplasty. The literature reports success rates of 80% to 90% at 5 years[4,6] and 60% to 70% at 10 years.[4-7] Our survivorship at 10 years is 83%. High-demand patients do better than low-demand patients, and males do better than females.[3]

This procedure has declined in popularity because of the improved technology and results of total knee arthroplasty and also because it makes subsequent total knee replacement technically more difficult to perform. The problems of total knee replacement after proximal tibial osteotomy include contracture of the patellar tendon, making eversion of the patella and exposure more difficult; loss of lateral tibial plateau bone stock, if a closing wedge technique was used; and valgus alignment, which may be excessive.[9-11] Despite these problems, the results are comparable to total knee replacement without prior osteotomy.[9-11] Proximal tibial osteotomy does not, therefore, preclude later total knee arthroplasty and should be part of the surgical spectrum for the osteoarthritic knee if the right prerequisites and indications exist. The technical difficulty of proximal tibial osteotomy is also a deterrent, and so are the potential complications, which include intra-articular fracture, peroneal nerve injury, exposure of the posterior cortex, and difficulty of fixation.

The surgical technique described in this paper obviates many of the complications associated with proxi-

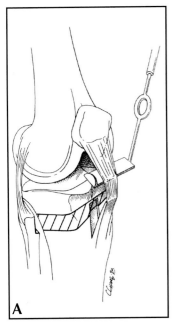 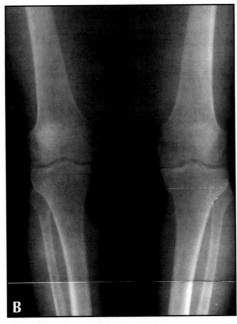 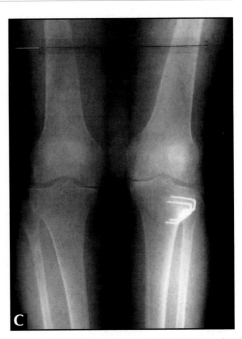

Fig. 1 A, This drawing illustrates the partial excision of the fibular head, elevation of the tibial tubercle and patellar tendon, and the closing wedge osteotomy. (Copyright © C. Chang) **B,** The standing anteroposterior radiograph shows a 58-year-old male with varus deformities of both knees and symptomatic osteoarthritis of the medial compartment of the left knee. **C,** Eight years after valgus osteotomy of the left knee.

mal tibial osteotomy and the potential difficulty of later total knee replacement. By elevating the tibial tubercle, the patellar tendon is protected and retracted anteriorly, allowing access to a part of the proximal tibia that is not normally accessible. In this way, the osteotomy can be performed more distally in stronger bone that is still metaphyseal, not diaphyseal, so that union is not delayed. Fixation, therefore, is stronger and is also well away from the joint surface. The more distal site of the osteotomy avoids intra-articular extension and also allows better exposure of the posterior tibial cortex because it is distal to the capsule. Excising of the superomedial proximal fibula and sparing the lateral cortex protects the lateral ligament and the peroneal nerve. The bone that is excised as part of the closing wedge is distal to the patellar tendon insertion and interferes less with total knee replacement.

If the deformity is so severe as to require removal of a wedge of more than 1.5 cm, an alternative technique should be used. A dome osteotomy with internal or external fixation can be used for severe deformity.[14] Ilizarov technology can be used for severe or complex multiplanar deformity.[15–17] Both the distal femur and proximal tibia can be osteotomized to correct a severe deformity so that less of a wedge has to be removed from the tibia.

Unicompartmental replacement may be used for unicompartmental disease,[23,24] but the same criteria should be applied as for total knee replacement. This procedure is not appropriate for the young, high-demand patient and provides problems with bone stock for later total knee replacement.[10]

In summary, therefore, valgus osteotomy of the proximal tibia still plays a role in the treatment of osteoarthritis of the medial compartment of the knee. The surgical tech-

nique used should allow adequate overcorrection of 2° to 3°, good fixation, and should avoid intraoperative complications and not make later total knee replacement too difficult. Successful surgery will allow the patient to return to full unrestricted activities for at least 10 years.

References

1. Wright J, Heck D, Hawker G, et al: Rates of tibial osteotomies in Canada and the United States. *Clin Orthop* 1995;319:266–275.

2. Insall JN, Joseph DM, Msika C: High tibial osteotomy for varus gonarthrosis: A long-term follow-up study. *J Bone Joint Surg* 1984;66A:1040–1048.

3. Nagel A, Insall JN, Scuderi GR: Proximal tibial osteotomy: A subjective outcome study. *J Bone Joint Surg* 1996;78A:1353–1358.

4. Rudan JF, Simurda MA: Valgus high tibial osteotomy: A long-term follow-up study. *Clin Orthop* 1991;268:157–160.

5. Ivarsson I, Myrnerts R, Gillquist J: High tibial osteotomy for medial osteoarthritis of the knee: A 5 to 7 and 11 year follow-up. *J Bone Joint Surg* 1990;72B:238–244.

6. Coventry MB, Ilstrup DM, Wallrichs SL: Proximal tibial osteotomy: A critical long-term study of eighty-seven cases. *J Bone Joint Surg* 1993;75A:196–201.

7. Yasuda K, Majima T, Tsuchida T, Kaneda K: A ten- to 15-year follow-up observation of high tibial osteotomy in medial compartment osteoarthritis. *Clin Orthop* 1992;282:186–195.

8. Waugh W: Tibial osteotomy in the management of osteoarthritis of the knee. *Clin Orthop* 1986;210:55–61.

9. Bergenudd H, Sahlström A, Sanzén L: Total knee arthroplasty after failed proximal tibial valgus osteotomy. *J Arthroplasty* 1997;12:635–638.

10. Gill T, Schemitsch EH, Brick GW, Thornhill TS: Revision total knee arthroplasty after failed unicompartmental knee arthroplasty or high tibial osteotomy. *Clin Orthop* 1995;321:10–18.

11. Mont MA, Alexander N, Krackow KA, Hungerford DS: Total knee arthroplasty after failed high tibial osteotomy. *Orthop Clin North Am* 1994;25:515–525.

12. MacIntosh DL, Welsh RP: Joint debridement: A complement to high tibial osteotomy in the treatment of degenerative arthritis of the knee. *J Bone Joint Surg* 1977;59A:1094–1097.

13. Jackson JP, Waugh W: Tibial osteotomy for osteoarthritis of the knee. *J Bone Joint Surg* 1961;43B:746–751.

14. Maquet P: The biomechanics of the knee and surgical possibilities of healing osteoarthritic knee joints. *Clin Orthop* 1980;146:102–110.

15. Catagni MA, Guerreschi F, Ahmad TS, Cattaneo R: Treatment of genu varum in medial compartment osteoarthritis of the knee using the Ilizarov method. *Orthop Clin North Am* 1994;25:509–514.

16. Paley D, Maar DC, Herzenberg JE: New concepts in high tibial osteotomy for medial compartment osteoarthritis. *Orthop Clin North Am* 1994;25:483–498.

17. Paley D, Tetsworth K: Mechanical axis deviation of the lower limbs: Preoperative planning of uniapical angular deformities of the tibia or femur. *Clin Orthop* 1992;280:48–64.

18. Bourguignon RL: Combined Coventry-Maquet tibial osteotomy: Preliminary report of two cases. *Clin Orthop* 1981;160:144–148.

19. Hofmann AA, Wyatt RW, Jones RE: Combined Coventry-Maquet procedure for two-compartment degenerative arthritis. *Clin Orthop* 1984;190:186–191.

20. Nguyen C, Rudan J, Simurda MA, Cooke TD: High tibial osteotomy compared with high tibial and Maquet procedures in medial and patellofemoral compartment osteoarthritis. *Clin Orthop* 1989;245:179–187.

21. Sasaki T, Yagi T, Monji J, Yasuda K, Tsuge H: High tibial osteotomy combined with anterior displacement of the tibial tubercle for osteoarthritis of the knee. *Int Orthop* 1986;10:31–40.

22. Kaplan EL, Meier P: Nonparametric estimation from incomplete observations. *J Am Stat Assoc* 1958;53:457–481.

23. Marmor L: Unicompartmental knee arthroplasty: Ten- to 13-year follow-up study. *Clin Orthop* 1988;226:14–20.

24. Kozinn SC, Scott RD: Surgical treatment of unicompartmental degenerative arthritis of the knee. *Rheum Dis Clin North Am* 1988;14:545–564.

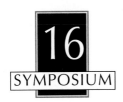

Arthroscopic Management for Degenerative Arthritis of the Knee

Michael J. Stuart, MD

Treatment of degenerative arthritis of the knee in the young patient remains a formidable challenge because no reliable method to date can reconstitute hyaline cartilage. Restoration of articular cartilage defects is currently under investigation and involves 3 principal methods: repair, regeneration, or replacement. The ability for the body to repair hyaline cartilage is very limited, but the future may allow local recruitment of cells by growth factor stimulation. Other biologic solutions for isolated defects include cartilage regeneration by periosteal or perichondrial autografting, with or without addition of chondrocytes or undifferentiated cells suspended in a matrix. Replacement of articular defects is performed by inserting autogeneic osteochondral plugs (mosaicplasty) or fresh osteochondral allografts. These intriguing experimental protocols are not indicated for the knee with global degenerative changes. Osteoarthritis of the knee is treated initially with a nonsurgical program of activity modification, physical therapy for strengthening and low-impact aerobic conditioning, non-steroidal anti-inflammatory medication, weight loss, energy-absorbing insoles, ambulatory aids, bracing, and intra-articular steroid or hyaluronan injections. Symptoms that are refrac-

tory to this treatment may require surgical management, which has traditionally included open or arthroscopic debridement, osteotomy, or prosthetic arthroplasty. Proximal tibial and distal femoral osteotomy remain viable options for unicompartmental osteoarthritis and associated malalignment in selected patients. Prosthetic arthroplasty is a reproducible, end-stage reconstructive procedure that cannot be applied to a young, athletic population with degenerative disease.

Although the arthroscope is a valuable tool for the treatment of many knee disorders, limited goals are expected when this technology is applied to the arthritic knee.

According to Burks,[1] the general objectives of arthroscopy for the painful osteoarthritic knee are: (1) to define pathology and plan treatment, (2) to treat a specific, concurrent problem (example: degenerative meniscal tear), and (3) to prolong the use of the knee. Routine arthroscopy has not been helpful in predicting the outcome of proximal tibial osteotomy, patellectomy, or prosthetic arthroplasty.[2] Arthroscopic lavage and debridement has resulted in short-term symptomatic relief in the majority of patients; however, the true natural history of the disease process is probably not altered. The available

literature is confusing because of nebulous inclusion criteria, inadequate study designs, and limited outcome-based analyses. The controversy surrounding arthroscopic debridement of the osteoarthritic knee was clearly stated by the Editor-in-Chief of *Arthroscopy: The Journal of Arthroscopy and Related Surgery*: "There is no evidence thus far that irrigation, debridement, and/or abrasion arthroplasty produce relief for more than a few months or, at most, several years." "Can we justify the cost and effectiveness of such a procedure?"[3] Orthopaedists are often faced with a difficult decision, because while we do not want to deny our patients an opportunity for reduced pain and improved quality of life, we do not want to indiscriminately perform an unpredictable procedure. Three fundamental questions raised by Sharkey[4] remain unanswered: (1) Does arthroscopy for osteoarthritis change the natural history of the disease? (2) Is the outcome of arthroscopic debridement related to a placebo effect? (3) How can any improvement from arthroscopic debridement be explained on a cellular or biochemical level? Additional basic science and clinical research are needed to clarify the role of arthroscopic techniques in the context of the size and stage of the lesion. No prospective, randomized, blinded clinical trials have accurately evaluated arthroscopic treatment for the degenerative knee.

Arthroscopic Debridement

Surgical debridement of the degenerative knee is a variable procedure that may involve lavage, partial meniscectomy, limited synovectomy, excision of osteophytes, loose body removal, and cartilage shaving. Removal of the mechanical, irritating products of joint degeneration has been postulated to relieve symptoms and arrest disease progression.[5] The theoretical explanations for the perceived improvement include the anesthetic effect of saline, the removal of particulate debris and degradative enzymes, and the interruption of pain impulses by chloride ions.

Debridement of the knee using the arthroscope eliminated the long surgical incision and extensor mechanism disruption associated with an open procedure.[6,7] The published results of arthroscopic debridement are variable, and the recommendations are inconsistent. Sprague[8] endorsed the procedure because of the small risk and improvement in 74% of his patients after 1 year. A retrospective review of 109 patients by Timoney and associates[9] revealed an early failure rate of 27% at 6 months and only 45% good results at 4 years following arthroscopy, but these researchers concluded that the surgery was useful in selected patients. Arthroscopic removal of an unstable meniscal fragment combined with joint lavage was shown by Rand[10] to be beneficial; however, advanced degenerative changes adversely affected the results. The procedure was felt to be indicated for individuals with symptoms typical of a degenerative meniscal tear, but without malalignment or radiographic evidence of advanced arthritis. Other authors have

suggested that a meniscus tear may be an incidental finding in the arthritic knee, because there was no difference in the results of surgery in patients with and without meniscus tears.[9] Preoperative radiographic assessment was also found to correlate with outcome in a retrospective review of arthroscopy in patients over the age of 50.[11] Good to excellent results were obtained in 68% of the knees with a joint space greater than 1 mm and in only 29% of the knees with a joint space less than 1 mm on nonweight-bearing radiographs.

Salisbury and associates[12] recommended that patients with genu varum be excluded from consideration for arthroscopic debridement, because relief of pain and good results were obtained in 94% of normally aligned knees and only 32% of varus knees. Sixty percent of the 441 patients retrospectively studied by Ogilvie-Harris and Fitsialos[13] had at least 2 years of symptomatic relief following arthroscopic treatment of degenerative arthritis. The best results were obtained in patients with mild disease, normal alignment, and an unstable meniscus tear. Bicondylar disease, malalignment, and chondrocalcinosis were associated with a much lower success rate. The authors recommended arthroscopy in the presence of degenerative changes in patients with mechanical symptoms like locking and giving way. Baumgaertner and associates[14] reported on the arthroscopic debridement of 49 knees, two thirds of which had radiographic evidence of severe arthritis. Shorter duration of symptoms, mechanical symptoms, mild to moderate radiographic changes, and crystal deposition correlated with improved results. Forty-seven percent of the procedures were deemed failures by 33 months following surgery.

McLaren and associates[15] were unable to identify any factors that correlated with outcome. Their retrospective review of 171 patients led to the conclusion that marked, but unpredictable, improvement in symptoms after arthroscopic debridement is seen in 1 patient out of 3. A prospective review of 254 patients with degenerative arthritis and moderate to severe knee pain involved reexamination at nearly 4 years following arthroscopic debridement.[16] Minimal discomfort and improved function were reported by 75% of patients, and 85% were satisfied with the treatment. The best results were noted when meniscal debridement alone was performed in knees with less severe degenerative changes. The authors concluded that the procedure offers worthwhile relief of symptoms, but no control group was included in the prospective analysis.

The discrepancies in the literature are explained by the varied entrance criteria, procedures, and outcome measures. The degenerative process in osteoarthritis is unrelated to crystalline, infectious, or inflammatory arthropathy, which may be improved with arthroscopic lavage, debridement, or synovectomy.[4] The inherent selection bias and intervention bias make it difficult to establish the role of arthroscopic debridement in the arthritic knee. A prospective pilot study of 20 patients with moderate unilateral osteoarthritis randomly assigned the involved knee to arthroscopic lavage only or arthroscopic debridement with removal of all osteophytes.[17] Objective measurements of quadriceps isokinetic torque at 6 and 12 weeks showed some improvement after joint lavage but not after debridement. Neither procedure significantly improved the patients' symptoms.

Merchan and Galindo[18] randomized 80 patients into surgical and nonsurgical groups using strict entrance criteria. Patients were selected if they had no patellofemoral involvement, limited radiographic degenerative changes, a normal mechanical axis, pain of sudden onset or pain present for less than 6 months, and no history of previous surgery. Although a surgical control group was not included, arthroscopic surgery proved to be a useful technique according to the Hospital for Special Surgery (HSS) Rating Score at a mean follow-up of 2 years. These authors and others point out that the main benefit of arthroscopy is the treatment of other problems that coexist with osteoarthritis.

Arthroscopic surgery for degenerative arthritis may provide transient pain relief by a placebo effect. A prospective, randomized, placebo-controlled pilot study was carried out by Moseley and associates[19] on 10 patients with symptomatic osteoarthritis of the knee. All patients and the physicians who performed the postoperative assessment were blinded as to treatment. Five subjects were randomly assigned to a "placebo" arthroscopy with only skin puncture wounds, 3 patients underwent arthroscopic lavage, and 2 patients had a "standard" arthroscopic debridement. All 5 patients who received the puncture wounds reported improvement in their knee pain at 6 months following surgery. Four of the 5 judged the procedure to be worthwhile and recommended the operation to family and friends. Activity level and physical examination parameters were unchanged when compared to preoperative measures. The patients who had the arthroscopic lavage and the arthroscopic debridement reported similar results. This pilot study introduces some skepticism on the mechanism of pain relief following arthroscopic treatment of osteoarthritis. A larger study with a similar design is required to make a more definitive statement on the placebo effect of arthroscopy and the true efficacy of debridement of the arthritic knee. Randomized, controlled, clinical trials, with entrance criteria, sufficient patient numbers, blinding, and reproducible outcome measures, will yield much more reliable information than retrospective or uncontrolled prospective studies.[20]

Arthroscopy cannot be expected to have any appreciable effect on the natural history of the disease process. Joint debridement provides somewhat unpredictable short-term symptomatic improvement in some patients, but it does not address the underlying problem of articular surface chondral damage. Irrigation and debridement may in theory slow down the degradative pathway by transiently diluting the concentration of inflammatory mediators and catabolic enzymes. Carefully selected patients with acute or short-term symptoms (less than 6 months), normal limb alignment, and mild or moderate unicompartmental degenerative disease can be considered for arthroscopic treatment if a nonsurgical program is unsuccessful. Indications for arthroscopic debridement, partial meniscectomy, and/or loose body removal include a discrete chief complaint, such as the acute onset of well-localized joint line pain, persistent effusion, catching or locking, and mild to moderate radiographic degenerative changes (Fig. 1). The success of the arthroscopic procedure may be because the symptoms, which are due to an acute injury or an associated internal mechanical problem, are not exclusive to the osteoarthritic knee. Patients should be counseled about the underlying disease process, the limited goals of the arthroscopic procedure, and the possible need for reconstructive surgery in the future.

Subchondral Drilling/Microfracture

Arthroscopic drilling or picking (microfracture) of the subchondral bone has been performed along with debridement to treat localized areas of articular loss in the degenerative knee (Fig. 2). The resultant hematoma may transform into reparative fibrocartilage with partial restoration of joint surface contour, improved symptoms, and delayed need for reconstructive surgery. Richards and Lonergan[21] reported on 22 patients treated with arthroscopic debridement and drilling. Symptomatic improvement was reported in 80% at 25-month follow-up by retrospective analysis. Full-thickness chondral defects have also been treated arthroscopically with a debridement and microfracture technique.[22] The patients were not classified as having osteoarthritis, but the overwhelming majority were categorized with "chronic full-thickness cartilage loss with exposure of subchondral bone and deep fissures or cobblestone edges." An awl is used to make multiple holes or "microfractures" in the exposed subchondral bone of the defect. The awl is assumed to generate less heat and thermal damage than a drill. The perforations promote adhesion of the blood clot to the subchondral bone, which may enhance fibrocartilage formation. A continuous passive motion (CPM) machine is recommended for 6 to 8 hours per day and touch weight-bearing is recommended for 8 weeks following surgery. Limited information is available on the results of this arthroscopic technique.

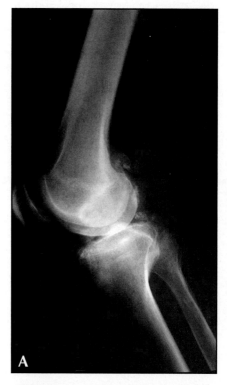

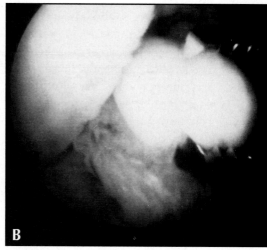

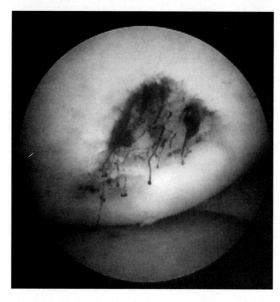

Fig. 1 A, Lateral radiograph of an arthritic knee with multiple intra-articular osseous loose bodies. **B,** Arthroscopic photograph of loose body removal.

Fig. 2 Arthroscopic photograph of a full-thickness chondral defect on the femoral articular surface after picking (microfractures) of the base.

stressed that no extrapolation of the analysis to functional outcome status of the patients is possible. Their patients showed significant improvement in postoperative function scores for pain, activities of daily living, strenuous sports, strenuous work, and sedentary work. These gains appeared slowly over a 3-year period and were maintained for at least 5 years.

Arthroscopic debridement and drilling or microfracture of the exposed subchondral bone is a technique that promotes fibrocartilage ingrowth at the site of full-thickness articular surface defects of the knee. No firm conclusions can be made at the present time as to the indications, limitations, and efficacy of this procedure. The appearance of the articular surface and short-term subjective symptoms are improved with fibrocartilaginous ingrowth, but the durability of this reparative tissue remain in question. Drilling or microfracture can be considered for isolated

Steadman and colleagues have performed debridement and microfracture on 298 patients since 1985. A subset of this group, 77 patients who underwent second look arthroscopy, was reviewed by Rodrigo and associates.[22] Continuous passive motion for 6 hours daily for 8 weeks appeared to result in better gross healing of the lesion when evaluated by arthroscopic visualization compared with the same treatment without CPM. Pain improvement was maintained in 63% of the CPM group and 55% of the non-CPM group at 6 years following chondroplasty. The authors

full-thickness chondral defects in the femoral articular surface in patients with normal limb alignment and little or no degenerative changes.

Abrasion Arthroplasty

Arthroscopic abrasion arthroplasty has also been promoted as a technique that stimulates cartilage regeneration. Removal of superficial necrotic bone exposes the vascular network, which results in blood clot attachment to the surface. Fibrous tissue is formed and undergoes metaplasia to reparative fibrocartilage composed predominantly of type I and type III collagen. The function and longevity of this tissue remain unknown, although arthroscopic biopsy and radiographs confirm its integrity at up to 4 years postoperatively.[23]

The surgical technique and the clinical experience of arthroscopic abrasion arthroplasty are the result of the pioneering work of Dr. Lanny Johnson.[23] Contrary to previous experimental evidence, Johnson observed that intracortical defects created in a sclerotic lesion without penetration of the subchondral bone uncovered small blood vessels. Second look arthroscopy revealed islands of repair tissue at the sites of the superficial debridement. The abraded sclerotic lesions remained vascular for 8 weeks, and protection from weightbearing during this period was essential for fibrocartilage transformation to occur. Johnson recommends performing the abrasion with a motorized cutting device to a depth of 1 to 2 mm. Biologic adherence to solid tissue is promoted by extending the abrasion for 1 or 2 mm into the adjacent degenerative cartilage. Partial-thickness degenerative hyaline cartilage should never be removed in favor of reparative fibro-

cartilage. Nonweightbearing ambulation is recommended for 8 weeks following surgery.

Arthroscopic abrasion arthroplasty was performed on 104 patients with rest or night pain and radiographic evidence of degenerative arthritis.[23] Ninety-five patients (99 knees) responded by questionnaire or returned for examination at a minimum of 2 years following surgery. Subjective assessment included 78% better, 15% unchanged, and 7% worse. No complications occurred, and 7 reoperations were performed, including 1 arthrotomy, 3 osteotomies, and 3 total knee arthroplasties. Comparative pre- and postoperative standing radiographs were available for 64 knees. Thirty-one had a wider joint space due to presumed regeneration of fibrocartilage. Follow-up biopsy at 4 years postoperatively showed typical fibrocartilage repair with positive staining for mucopolysaccharides and reformation of the tidemark. Friedman and associates[24] performed abrasion arthroplasty and mechanical debridement in 73 patients with improvement of symptoms in 60%. Pain was still present to some degree in 83% of patients after an average follow-up of only 12 months. The best results were obtained in patients younger than 40 years.

The arthroscopic treatment of unicompartmental gonarthrosis was studied retrospectively by Bert and Maschka[25] by a review of 67 patients with debridement alone and 59 patients with abrasion arthroplasty and debridement. The patients who refused to remain nonweightbearing for 6 weeks following surgery were offered arthroscopic debridement alone. The HSS score was used to grade the results at 5 years following surgery. The abrasion arthroplasty group included 51% good or excellent

results, 16% fair results, and 33% poor results. Interestingly, one third of the 30 knees with radiographic evidence of joint space widening had no improvement or actually became worse. The group treated by debridement alone included 66% good or excellent results, 13% fair results, and 21% poor results. Twelve of the knees with a poor result actually became worse, and 10 of these required a total knee arthroplasty. The results were not influenced by patient age, weight, previous surgery, extent of unicompartmental disease, and limb malalignment. Akizuki and associates[26] prospectively evaluated patients undergoing a proximal tibial osteotomy to determine if abrasion of eburnated bone would promote cartilage regeneration. Second look arthroscopy at 12 months showed a smoother articular surface in the abrasion group. Fibrocartilage comprised 64% of the regenerated tissue. There was no difference in the clinical outcome between the 2 cohorts at 2- to 9-year follow-up.

Meticulous surgical technique can apparently stimulate the formation of reparative fibrocartilage. Abrasion arthroplasty is contraindicated in patients with inflammatory arthritis or in the presence of significant knee stiffness, deformity, or instability. This procedure should also be avoided in patients who are unwilling or unable to comply with the postoperative regimen of nonweightbearing for 2 months. The durability of this repair tissue remains a concern, and the long-term results of this procedure require further study. Arthroscopic abrasion arthroplasty for localized degenerative arthritis even in a compliant patient with rest pain and no associated malalignment or instability is unpredictable.

Complications

Complications in arthroscopy are infrequent and usually minor, but the risk increases as procedures become more technically demanding.[27,28] Arthroscopic treatment of degenerative arthritis is associated with low morbidity, and serious complications are very infrequent. The overwhelming majority of the retrospective series in the literature fail to report complications even though they undoubtedly must occur. Complication rates that have been reported range from 7% to 31%.[8–10] The documented complications of knee arthroscopy are shown in Outline 1.

Careful preoperative screening and meticulous attention to surgical detail will minimize these complications. Arthroscopic treatment of the degenerative knee should not be taken lightly, because there are inherent risks involved with any surgical procedure.

Conclusion

Hyaline articular cartilage is and must be remarkably durable in order to tolerate the repetitive impact and shearing loads that are constantly applied. This complex material is critical to joint function, but it has very limited potential for repair. The etiology of osteoarthritis remains obscure. The etiology of posttraumatic degenerative arthritis is multifactorial. Chondral and osteochondral fractures, loss of the menisci, recurrent instability, and axial malalignment appear to contribute to the deterioration of the knee joint surfaces.[29] Prevention of this deterioration is critical, because there are no reliable methods available at the present time to restore the articular cartilage of the knee. Correction of the mechanical axis and elimination of pathologic laxity are fundamental issues that must be recognized and addressed.

Despite the success of prosthetic arthroplasty, degenerative arthritis remains an unsolved problem in the younger, more active patient. The arthroscope remains an appealing tool, which may be able to help "buy some time" before the definitive reconstructive procedure is required. Treatment of osteoarthritis and chronic chondral injuries with arthroscopic debridement, partial meniscectomy, and chondroplasty provide unpredictable, incomplete, and transient symptomatic relief. The durability of any repair tissue that forms remains a concern and the long-term results of this procedure require further study. Arthroscopic surgery can relieve some symptoms, but additional basic science research and well-designed clinical protocols are necessary to determine if further joint surface deterioration is prevented or only delayed. Randomized, controlled trials with de-fined entrance criteria, sufficient patient numbers, and valid, reproducible outcome measures will provide the most unbiased assessment of the risks and benefits of arthroscopic procedures for degenerative arthritis of the knee.

Carefully selected patients with normal limb alignment and mild or moderate degenerative disease can be considered for arthroscopic treatment if a nonsurgical program is unsuccessful. Indications for arthroscopic debridement, partial meniscectomy, and/or loose body removal include a discrete chief complaint, the acute onset of well-localized joint line pain, a persistent effusion, and mechanical symptoms, such as catching or locking. The single most important factor when considering arthroscopic intervention is axial alignment of the leg. If the mechanical axis passes through the lesion, any arthroscopic procedure is likely to be unsuccessful. Arthroscopic surgical technique involves excision of only the unstable meniscal fragments, with restoration of a smooth, balanced, contoured rim. Osteophytes are removed with a small osteotome or a burr only if they appear to cause painful impingement or block knee motion. Subchondral bone drilling or microfracture are performed in cases of isolated, focal full-thickness articular cartilage defects on the medial or lateral femoral condyle. The remainder of the knee must not be significantly involved and the patient must be willing to comply with the postoperative program of continuous passive motion and touch-weightbearing ambulation. Patients must be counseled about the underlying disease process, the limited goals of the arthroscopic procedure, the potential complications, and the possible need for reconstructive surgery in the future.

References

1. Burks RT: Arthroscopy and degenerative arthritis of the knee: A review of the literature. *Arthroscopy* 1990;6:43–47.

2. Keene JS, Monson DK, Roberts JM, Dyreby JR Jr: Evaluation of patients for high tibial osteotomy. *Clin Orthop* 1989;243:157–165.

3. Casscells SW: What, if any, are the indications for arthroscopic debridement of the osteoarthritic knee? *Arthroscopy* 1990;6:169–170.

4. Sharkey PF: The case against arthroscopic debridement. *J Arthroplasty* 1997;12:467–469.

5. Magnuson PB: Joint debridement: Surgical treatment of degenerative arthritis. *Surg Gynecol Obstet* 1941;73:1–9.

6. Insall JN: Intra-articular surgery for degenerative arthritis of the knee: A report of the work of the late K.H. Pridie. *J Bone Joint Surg* 1967;49B:211–228.

7. Insall J: The Pridie debridement operation for osteoarthritis of the knee. *Clin Orthop* 1974;101:61–67.

8. Sprague NF III: Arthroscopic debridement for degenerative knee joint disease. *Clin Orthop* 1981;160:118–123.

9. Timoney JM, Kneisl JS, Barrack RL, Alexander AH: Arthroscopy update #6: Arthroscopy in the osteoarthritic knee. Long-term follow-up. *Orthop Rev* 1990;19:371–373.

10. Rand JA: Role of arthroscopy in osteoarthritis of the knee. *Arthroscopy* 1991;7:358–363.

11. Anderson JK, Goldstein WM: Arthroscopy in patients over the age of 50 years. *Am J Arthroscopy* 1991;1:15–18.

12. Salisbury RB, Nottage WM, Gardner V: The effect of alignment on results in arthroscopic debridement of the degenerative knee. *Clin Orthop* 1985;198:268–272.

13. Ogilvie-Harris DJ, Fitsialos DP: Arthroscopic management of the degenerative knee. *Arthroscopy* 1991;7:151–157.

14. Baumgaertner MR, Cannon WD Jr, Vittori JM, Schmidt ES, Maurer RC: Arthroscopic debridement of the arthritic knee. *Clin Orthop* 1990;253:197–202.

15. McLaren AC, Blokker CP, Fowler PJ, Roth JN, Rock MG: Arthroscopic debridement of the knee for osteoarthrosis. *Can J Surg* 1991;34:595–598.

16. Aichroth PM, Patel DV, Moyes ST: A prospective review of arthroscopic debridement for degenerative joint disease of the knee. *Int Orthop* 1991;15:351–355.

17. Gibson JN, White MD, Chapman VM, Strachan RK: Arthroscopic lavage and debridement for osteoarthritis of the knee. *J Bone Joint Surg* 1992;74B:534–537.

18. Merchan EC, Galindo E: Arthroscope-guided surgery versus nonoperative treatment for limited degenerative osteoarthritis of the femorotibial joint in patients over 50 years of age: A prospective comparative study. *Arthroscopy* 1993;9:663–667.

19. Moseley JB Jr, Wray NP, Kuykendall D, Willis K, Landon G: Arthroscopic treatment of osteoarthritis of the knee: A prospective, randomized, placebo-controlled trial. Results of a pilot study. *Am J Sports Med* 1996;24:28–34.

20. Laupacis A, Rorabeck CH, Bourne RB, Feeny D, Tugwell P, Sim DA: Randomized trials in orthopaedics: Why, how, and when? *J Bone Joint Surg* 1989;71A:535–543.

21. Richards RN Jr, Lonergan RP: Arthroscopic surgery for the relief of pain in the osteoarthritic knee. *Orthopedics* 1984;7:1705–1707.

22. Rodrigo JJ, Steadman JR, Silliman JF, Fulstone HA: Improvement of full-thickness chondral defect healing in the human knee after debridement and microfracture using continuous passive motion. *Am J Knee Surg* 1994;7:109–116.

23. Johnson LL: Arthroscopic abrasion arthroplasty historical and pathologic perspective: Present status. *Arthroscopy* 1986;2:54–69.

24. Friedman MJ, Berasi CC, Fox JM, Del Pizzo W, Snyder SJ, Ferkel RD: Preliminary results with abrasion arthroplasty in the osteoarthritic knee. *Clin Orthop* 1984;182:200–205.

25. Bert JM, Maschka K: The arthroscopic treatment of unicompartmental gonarthrosis: A five-year follow-up study of abrasion arthroplasty plus arthroscopic debridement and arthroscopic debridement alone. *Arthroscopy* 1989;5:25–32.

26. Akizuki S, Yasukawa Y, Takizawa T: Does arthroscopic abrasion arthroplasty promote cartilage regeneration in osteoarthritic knees with eburnation? A prospective study of high tibial osteotomy with abrasion arthroplasty versus high tibial osteotomy alone. *Arthroscopy* 1997;13:9–17.

27. Rodeo SA, Forster RA, Weiland AJ: Neurological complications due to arthroscopy. *J Bone Joint Surg* 1993;75A:917–926.

28. Committee on Complications of the Arthroscopy Association of North America: Complications in arthroscopy: The knee and other joints. *Arthroscopy* 1986;2:253–258.

29. Stuart MJ: Treatment of chronic chondral Injuries. *Sports Med Arthroscopy Rev* 1994;2:50–58.

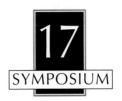

Unicondylar Arthroplasty: An Option for High-Demand Patients With Gonarthrosis

Gerard A. Engh, MD
James P. McAuley, MD

Unicondylar knee arthroplasty (UKA) is rarely considered a surgical option for an osteoarthritic patient younger than 60 years of age primarily because of the widespread opinion that an implant of any type is contraindicated in younger, active individuals. When no acceptable nonarthroplasty treatments are available, most orthopaedists perform a total knee arthroplasty (TKA). Controversy exists regarding the durability of a UKA when compared to the durability of a TKA. However, unicompartmental arthroplasty is an acceptable alternative for the young, active patient with osteoarthritis if the clinical results are predictable and better than other arthroplasty and nonarthroplasty surgical options (ie, osteotomy), and if the revision of the unicondylar implant, if and when it fails, does not compromise the durability of a subsequent TKA.

To address the effectiveness of UKA, we have examined 4 basic questions: (1) What are the clinical results and the durability of UKA in relatively young, active individuals? (2) How do the morbidity and complications of UKA compare to those of other surgical procedures? (3) How difficult is the revision of a UKA or the conversion to a TKA? (4)

What is the durability of a TKA following revision of a failed UKA?

Results of Unicondylar Arthroplasty

No clinical results have been reported that specifically address unicondylar arthroplasty and its durability in active, osteoarthritic individuals younger than 60 years of age. We can extract useful information from relatively long-term outcome studies of unicondylar arthroplasties in a general patient population[1-5] (Table 1). However, these studies do not stratify patients by either age or activity level. Unicondylar revision rates are reported, but there is no correlation of the demographic data in the revised versus the nonrevised groups.

In our analysis, we stratified unicondylar replacements in 5 relatively long-term studies[1-5] (Table 1). All-

polyethylene, nonmodular implants, used in arthroplasties performed primarily during the 1970s and early 1980s, provide long-term results for evaluation. Each of the 5 studies included between 40 and 80 cases for clinical review. In these studies, a total of 290 knees was followed for an average of 10 years. The average patient age in each group was relatively similar (Table 1).

Fifty-one of the 290 knees required revision, for an overall revision rate of 18% at 10 years. When examining the cases that required revision, we found that the most common failure modes of these nonmodular components were aseptic loosening (N = 22) and progressive arthritis (N = 17). Analysis of the cases led to the conclusion that aseptic loosening was often secondary to the use of thin, tibial polyethylene

Table 1
Unicondylar outcome studies

Study	Follow-up Interval (years)	No. of Knees	Mean Age (years)	Gender	Revision Rates No. (%)
Marmor[1]	11	60	63	% F > M	21 (35%)
Capra and Fehring[2]	8.3	45	63	Unknown	6 (6.25%)
Cartier and Sanouiller[3]	12	60	65	% M > F	7 (12%)
Stockelman and Pohl[4]	7.5	48	65	% M > F	4 (8%)
Scott et al[5]	10	77	71	% F > M	13 (18%)

components; whereas progressive arthritis was commonly caused by overcorrection of the patient's varus deformity into a valgus position.

There are two European studies with results similar to those of the five studies previously discussed. The survivorship of over 2,000 single-compartment replacements from a prospective, nationwide multicenter investigation in Sweden was 90% at 6 years.[6] In another prospective clinical study at the Bristol Royal Infirmary in England, the cumulative success rate (not the revision rate) was 76.4% at 9 years with the St. Georg Sledge implant.[7] Failed cases in this study included revision cases as well as cases in which patients had pain or dissatisfaction. Only 6% (7/115) of the knees in this study were revised.

It is reasonable to assume that failure rates from the aforementioned studies would have been greater in younger, more active patients. However, the overall failure rates would be lower with the elimination of tibial components with thin polyethylene, a design flaw in early unicondylar components.[1] The authors believe that when an implant of adequate polyethylene thickness is used, an 18% revision rate or an 82% success rate at 10-year follow-up represents a more realistic outlook for the durability of a UKA in a high-demand patient population.

Currently 239 unicondylar arthroplasties are being followed at the Anderson Clinic (Alexandria, VA) where we recently evaluated a subset of the 49 UKAs performed in patients 40 to 60 years of age. The arthroplasty was performed on the medial compartment in all but 1 of these cases. The average patient weight was 191 pounds. The average length of follow-up was 7.1 years. Three patients were lost to follow-up. At the 7-year interval, the revision rate was 28%

(13/46). Failure secondary to polyethylene wear accounted for 10 of the 13 revisions. Eight of 9 unicondylar implants that failed secondary to polyethylene wear were Robert Brigham (Johnson & Johnson, Raynham, MA) 6-mm metal-backed tibial components (actual polyethylene thickness of 4 mm). This particular component, subsequently discontinued by the manufacturer, was used in 9 of the 46 cases in this series. Only 5 failures occurred in the other 37 cases, thereby providing a much more acceptable success rate of 86% at 7.1 years. We estimate that the success rate of UKA in younger, active patients would most likely be about 80% at 10 years, as long as an implant of adequate polyethylene thickness and proven design is selected.

Perioperative Morbidity and Patient Satisfaction

After UKA, there is greater patient satisfaction and less perioperative morbidity than with other surgical options. Broughton and associates[8] reported fewer systemic complications and wound problems, as well as better function and movement with 42 unicondylar arthroplasties compared to 49 high tibial osteotomies. When patients were examined 5 to 10 years postoperatively, 76% of the UKAs rated "good" on a modified Hospital for Special Surgery knee rating score (Baily score) as compared to 43% following osteotomy. Similarly, in a comparative study with 12- to 17-year follow-up, Weale and Newman[9] found that in 80% of the surviving UKAs, patients reported either no pain or mild pain, whereas patients reported no pain or mild pain in only 43% of the surviving osteotomy cases.

When compared to TKA, unicondylar arthroplasty has a lower rate of perioperative problems. Because

blood loss is minimal, a transfusion is rarely needed with UKA, whereas 50% of patients require a transfusion for TKA.[10] Manipulation, reoperation for lysis of adhesions, and the extensor mechanism problems that can occur with TKA are extremely unlikely with unicondylar replacement.[10] Rougraff and associates[10] reported a need for reoperation in 20% of TKAs as compared to 4% of UKAs. In osteoarthritic patients, the infection rate as reported from the Swedish nationwide study of 8,000 knee replacements was significantly less with UKA.[6] The 6-year rate of revision for infection in a single-compartment replacement was 0.8% compared to 2% for 2- or 3-compartment replacements.[6]

In comparison to other surgical options, patient satisfaction and function are optimal after UKA. Our experience with UKA at the Anderson Clinic, and other studies, confirm that the range of motion, averaging between 120° and 130° of flexion, is excellent with unicondylar arthroplasty.[3,4,11] This range of motion enhances a patient's functional potential, such as stair climbing and getting in and out of cars. With a single-compartment arthroplasty, the preserved anterior cruciate ligament and unresurfaced patella help maintain proprioception of the knee. In addition, the need for postoperative ambulatory aids is less likely with a UKA than with a TKA.[10]

Revision of a Unicondylar Implant

The degree of difficulty the surgeon encounters when revising a unicondylar arthroplasty to a TKA depends on the amount of bone removed at the time of the UKA, the bone damage that occurred with implant failure, and the bone loss that accompanies component removal. In the 1970s and early 1980s, the most common failure mechanism was aseptic loosening. Thin, all-polyethylene tibial components that buckled,[12] components with no tibial lugs,[13] and poor bone coverage resulting in inadequate initial fixation were major contributing factors to these failures. Additional tibial bone loss was caused by component migration, cement fragmentation, and small areas of secondary osteolysis. Femoral bone was often severely damaged from both aseptic loosening and difficult component removal (Fig. 1). Some of the early unicondylar implant designs featured narrow femoral components that did not adequately cover the femoral condyle and large fixation lugs or spikes that sacrificed bone with implant removal.[13–15]

Because of severe bone damage, the revision of these early unicondylar designs was difficult and less predictable than anticipated by advocates of UKA. Two early reports of unicondylar conversion to TKA revealed that 76% of the cases in the Padgett and associates[14] study, and almost 50% of the cases in the Barrett and Scott study[15] required bone grafting, long-stemmed components, and, on occasion, a custom-designed implant to manage the bone defects.

Bone loss was the only difficulty reported in these studies of unicondylar revisions. Primary components were used as the revision implant in almost all cases. In the study by Barrett and Scott,[15] 93% of knees were revised with cruciate-sparing components. In a study by Padgett and associates,[14] almost all of the cases were revised with total condylar (manufacturer unspecified) or posterior-stabilized implants. In most cases, bone defects were filled with cement or autogenous bone graft (3 cases in each study mentioned). In a few cases, the cement was reinforced with screws or mesh.

With more recent designs, the revision of a failed UKA has been more successful because of diminished bone loss and the availability of modular, stemmed components. Whereas aseptic loosening accounted for most of the failures with the early, all-polyethylene unicondylar designs, polyethylene wear has been the most common failure mode of metal-backed tibial implants. The clinical results of 31 revisions of failed metal-backed Robert Brigham (Johnson & Johnson, Raynham, MA) unicondylar implants were comparable to those of primary TKA.[13] After revision, patients averaged 115° of flexion and 91 points on the Knee Society score. Cruciate-retaining total knee components were satisfactory as the revision prosthesis in 30 out of 31 cases. In the revision procedures, 2 femoral wedges, 4 tibial wedges, and 7 cancellous bone grafts were used to repair the bone loss.

At the Anderson Clinic, 13 revisions were performed in patients between the ages of 40 and 60 at the time of their UKA. The time interval between the UKA and the conversion to a TKA averaged 77.7 months (range, 14 to 110 months). All of the revised cases included metal-backed tibial components. Polyethylene wear was the major cause of failure in 12 of the 13 revisions. Because metal debris was present in all of these cases, a complete synovectomy was performed as part of the revision procedure. In every case, a primary implant system was used in the revision procedure; 11 of these 13 implants were cruciate-retaining devices (Fig. 2). In 9 of the 13 revisions, satisfactory tibial metaphyseal bone was present to support a primary tibial component without bone grafts or wedges. A modular stem was used in 3 revision cases: 2 in association with a metal wedge, and 1

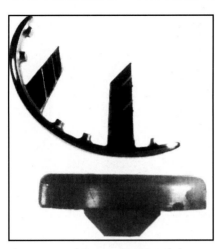

Fig. 1 Large spikes on a St. Georg Sledge femoral component can result in bone loss with component removal. (Reproduced with permission from Mackinnon J, Young S, Baily RA: The St Georg sledge for unicompartmental replacement of the knee: A prospective study of 115 cases. *J Bone Joint Surg* 1988; 70B:217–223.)

in conjunction with an autograft. In 1 revision a 5-mm wedge was used without a stemmed component.

The difficulty of a subsequent revision to a TKA must be considered when determining whether to perform a UKA or a high tibial osteotomy (HTO) in a young, active individual. After osteotomy, a TKA is more difficult but for different reasons. The difficulty of the revision when a UKA fails comes with managing bone loss. However, in revision after HTO, adequate surgical exposure can be difficult to obtain because of the reduced distance from the tibial plateau to the tibial tubercle. A second difficulty after HTO occurs with achieving ligament balance (Fig. 3). A valgus extra-articular deformity of the proximal tibia is created following an osteotomy. When tibial resection at 90° to the tibial mechanical axis is performed, more bone is removed from the medial tibial plateau, a situation opposite to the usual tibial resection made for TKA.

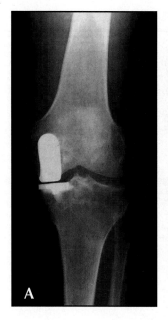
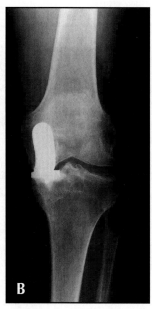
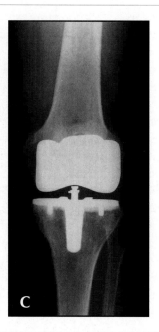

Fig. 2 A, The early postoperative radiograph of a Robert Brigham (Johnson & Johnson, Raynham, MA) metal-backed unicondylar tibial component with excellent component-to-component alignment. A minimal amount of bone has been removed from the tibia. The polyethylene is only 4 mm thick. **B,** Failure secondary to polyethylene wear occurred at 4 years after UKA. No additional bone loss is apparent on radiographic evaluation. Bone loss should not be a problem at the time of revision surgery. **C,** The revision component is a primary, cruciate-retaining implant. Bone loss was not a problem in this revision.

Because extra bone that is removed from the medial plateau creates medial instability of the knee, it may be necessary to imbricate the medial ligaments to avoid postoperative instability.[16] In more severe cases, the deformity created with the osteotomy may need to be corrected before, or as part of, the conversion to a TKA (Fig. 4).

The potential complications of TKA following UKA, therefore, differ from those after HTO. Studies comparing the outcomes of TKA after HTO emphasize the increased risk of wound healing, difficulty with surgical exposure, and possibility of infection following osteotomy.[17] Conversely, aseptic loosening because of implant instability with bone loss may be an increased risk factor.[18]

Durability of the Revision TKA

The durability of TKA following revision of a failed unicondylar replacement should relate to the age and activity level of the patient, the extent of bone loss at the time of revision, and the mechanism for managing the bone defects. As previ-

ously discussed, there are no studies that specifically address unicondylar revision in the younger, active patient; therefore we must rely on the published literature for information on the general patient population.

Padgett and associates[14] reported radiolucent lines around 9 tibial bone defects that were filled with bone cement alone and not reinforced with screws or mesh. Eight developed radiolucent lines at least 1 mm thick. Two of these cases required subsequent revision of the tibial component for loosening. These were the only failures resulting in revision from the 21 cases with 2- to 10-year follow-up. Barrett and Scott[15] reported inferior results with unicondylar revision after an average follow-up of 4.6 years. Four of 29 unicondylar revisions required re-revision; 3 for tibial loosening. No failures occurred in the 12 cases that were managed with a stemmed component or in which the bone defect was repaired with bone graft, wedges, or screw-cement augmentation.

More recently, Levine and associates[13] reviewed the outcome of 31

unicondylar revisions and found that the results were similar to those of primary TKA. In the unicondylar revision series, Knee Society scores averaged 91 (knee score) and 81 (function), with an average follow-up interval of 45 months. The one re-revision was performed for infection. No significant tibial or femoral radiolucent lines suggestive of component loosening were identified in any of the cases.

We are unable to draw valid conclusions from the small number of young patients (N = 13) who have undergone revision of a UKA to TKA. However, the results are similar to our overall series (N = 35) of revision of UKA to TKA.

In our overall series, the average age of the patients at unicondylar arthroplasty was 60 years and the average weight was 188 pounds. The average interval to revision was 61 months. The reason for revision was polyethylene wear in 26 cases at an average of 75 months and aseptic loosening in 9 cases at an average of 20 months. Three patients were successfully revised to another unicompartmental arthroplasty. Twenty-six of the remaining 32 cases were revised to a cruciate-sparing TKA. Stemmed tibial components were used in 14 patients, and wedges in 9 patients. There was no need for allograft in any of the revision procedures. The unresected surfaces of the knee provided an abundant source of autogenous bone graft that was used to repair bone defects. Autograft bone, from local bone resection, was used in 8 patients. At an average 38-month follow-up after revision, the Knee Society knee scores of these patients averaged 86 and the function scores averaged 76. The average range of motion in these patients was 114°.

There were few complications in this series. One patient had a tibial fracture that occurred at the tip of the component stem. Two patients developed an asymptomatic deep venous thrombosis detected by routine Doppler screening at 6 weeks. No treatment was needed in either patient. Two medical complications included 1 case of a gastrointestinal bleed and 1 small cerebrovascular accident. Two patients underwent manipulation for stiffness in the knee.

There were 5 reoperations (2 revisions) in this series of 35 patients. Three were arthroscopic procedures: 2 for a patellar clunk, both at 18 months postrevision, and 1 for pain, which continues to be of unknown etiology. One patient had a re-revision of the tibial insert for polyethylene wear 78 months after the conversion arthroplasty. Two years later, this patient had an excellent result, with scores of 100 and 90 and range of motion of 0 to 125°. This patient's radiographs show no radiolucencies or osteolysis. The second re-revision patient underwent a polyethylene exchange and patellar component revision at 102 months after uni-

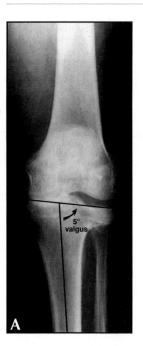
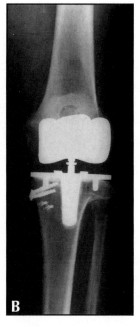

Fig. 3 A, A valgus deformity of the tibia has been created with this high tibial osteotomy. A 90° tibial resection will create medial instability by removing more bone from the medial tibial plateau. **B,** Medial ligament advancement was required. Mitek anchors (Mitek, Westwood, MA) and a staple were used to achieve ligament balance.

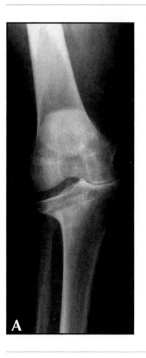
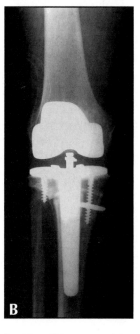

Fig. 4 A, A severe valgus deformity of the tibia was created with a high tibial osteotomy. **B,** The tibial deformity was corrected with an osteotomy, as part of the conversion to a knee arthroplasty. A long-stemmed component was required to stabilize the osteotomy and ligament advancement was needed to provide knee stability.

condylar revision. Therefore, in the Anderson Clinic series of 35 patients, 33 (94%) have undergone successful conversions of a UKA. These results are more encouraging than those of revision of a TKA and similar to the outcomes of a primary TKA.

In conclusion, a UKA can provide a young, active patient pain relief and

excellent function for a number of years. The durability of the UKA is approximately 80% at 10 years. The morbidity and complication rate is less than that with HTO or TKA. When the conversion arthroplasty is necessary, the patient will then be at a more appropriate age to undergo TKA. Although the revision of a failed unicondylar implant rarely requires a revision component, it may require an augment or bone graft. Fortunately, abundant autograft bone is available with a unicondylar revision; an option that is not available with total knee revision. The clinical results of the TKA following UKA are encouraging and appear to be similar to those of primary TKA, but the durability compared to primary TKA is unknown. Recognizing the importance of adequate tibial component polyethylene thickness and conservation of bone in a unicondylar arthroplasty, the authors conclude that an all-polyethylene tibial component for unicondylar implants may be the best option.

References

1. Marmor L: Unicompartmental arthroplasty of the knee with a minimum ten-year follow-up period. *Clin Orthop* 1988;228:171–177.

2. Capra SW Jr, Fehring TK: Unicondylar arthroplasty: A survivorship analysis. *J Arthroplasty* 1992;7:247–251.

3. Cartier P, Sanouiller J-L, Grelsamer RP: Unicompartmental knee arthroplasty surgery: 10-year minimum follow-up period. *J Arthroplasty* 1996;11:782–788.

4. Stockelman RE, Pohl KP: The long-term efficacy of unicompartmental arthroplasty of the knee. *Clin Orthop* 1991;271:88–95.

5. Scott RD, Cobb AG, McQueary FG, Thornhill TS: Unicompartmental knee arthroplasty: Eight- to 12-year follow-up evaluation with survivorship analysis. *Clin Orthop* 1991;271: 96–100.

6. Knutson K, Lindstrand A, Lidgren L: Survival of knee arthroplasties: A nation-wide multicentre investigation of 8000 cases. *J Bone Joint Surg* 1986;68B:795–803.

7. Mackinnon J, Young S, Baily RA: The St Georg sledge for unicompartmental replacement of the knee: A prospective study of 115 cases. *J Bone Joint Surg* 1988;70B:217–223.

8. Broughton NS, Newman JH, Baily RA: Unicompartmental replacement and high tibial osteotomy for osteoarthritis of the knee: A comparative study after 5-10 years' follow-up. *J Bone Joint Surg* 1986;68B:447–452.

9. Weale AE, Newman JH: Unicompartmental arthroplasty and high tibial osteotomy for osteoarthrosis of the knee: A comparative study with a 12- to 17-year follow-up period. *Clin Orthop* 1994;302:134–137.

10. Rougraff BT, Heck DA, Gibson AE: A comparison of tricompartmental and unicompartmental arthroplasty for the treatment of gonarthrosis. *Clin Orthop* 1991;273:157–164.

11. Laurencin CT, Zelicof SB, Scott RD, Ewald FC: Unicompartmental versus total knee arthroplasty in the same patient: A comparative study. *Clin Orthop* 1991;273:151–156.

12. Marmor L: Unicompartmental knee arthroplasty: Ten- to 13-year follow-up study. *Clin Orthop* 1988;226:14–20.

13. Levine WN, Ozuna RM, Scott RD, Thornhill TS: Conversion of failed modern unicompartmental arthroplasty to total knee arthroplasty. *J Arthroplasty* 1996;11:797–801.

14. Padgett DE, Stern SH, Insall JN: Revision total knee arthroplasty for failed unicompartmental replacement. *J Bone Joint Surg* 1991;73A: 186–190.

15. Barrett WP, Scott RD: Revision of failed unicondylar unicompartmental knee arthroplasty. *J Bone Joint Surg* 1987;69A:1328–1335.

16. Krackow KA, Holtgrewe JL: Experience with a new technique for managing severely overcorrected valgus high tibial osteotomy at total knee arthroplasty. *Clin Orthop* 1990;258:213–224.

17. Jackson M, Sarangi PP, Newman JH: Revision total knee arthroplasty: Comparison of outcome following primary proximal tibial osteotomy or unicompartmental arthroplasty. *J Arthroplasty* 1994;9:539–542.

18. Gill T, Schemitsch EH, Brick GW, Thornhill TS: Revision total knee arthroplasty after failed unicompartmental knee arthroplasty or high tibial osteotomy. *Clin Orthop* 1995;321:10–18.

Specialized Surgical Exposure for Revision Total Knee: Quadriceps Snip and Patellar Turndown

Robert L. Barrack, MD

Adequate exposure is the first step in successfully performing a revision total knee arthroplasty. In order to safely and expeditiously remove the implants that are in place and insert trials and components, flexion well beyond 90°, to about 110°, is required.[1] In addition, it is preferable to be able to evert the patella and dislocate the tibia anteriorly. If a patient has less than 80° to 90° of passive flexion under anesthesia, the standard medial parapatellar approach may not provide adequate exposure. Initially, it is useful to start the midline incision more proximally in order to establish normal tissue planes above the extensor mechanism. It is also useful to take additional time to define the borders of the rectus tendon and the vastus lateralis and medialis insertions into the patella. The medial parapatellar capsular incision begins at the proximal extent of the rectus tendon and ends distally, 1 cm medial to the tibial tubercle. **(CD–18.1)**

After medial arthrotomy, any adhesions in the suprapatellar pouch and medial and lateral gutters should be released. Access to the lateral gutter is more difficult following standard medial arthrotomy. A medial capsular release is typically carried past the midcoronal plane, usually to the posteromedial corner of the knee just in front of the semimembranosus insertion. External rotation of the tibia following medial release and clearing the gutters and suprapatellar pouch usually increases knee flexion to some degree. The next maneuver that improves exposure is to place traction on the patella as the knee is flexed and an attempt is made to evert the patella. This traction places the fibers of the patellofemoral ligament, which extends from the lateral epicondyle to the lateral border of the patella, under tension. Routine release of these fibers assists in patellar eversion, mobilization, and tracking.[2,3] After all of these maneuvers, passive knee flexion and patellar eversion are assessed. If flexion well beyond 90° cannot be accomplished without excessive tension on the patellar tendon, and patellar eversion cannot be accomplished, additional steps must be taken in order to accomplish these goals.

The two basic approaches to achieving more flexion are either proximally, through the extensor mechanism, or distally, through the tibial tubercle. If a proximal approach is elected, the options include dividing the quadriceps tendon, lateral retinaculum, vastus lateralis tendon, or some combination of the three. Isolated division of the rectus tendon to improve exposure during knee arthroplasty has been called the quadriceps snip and is attributed to Insall.[4] Early on, it was described as a transverse cut across the proximal portion of the rectus tendon[2] (Fig. 1). Later, it was modified to be a 45° oblique incision placed from distal to proximal (Fig. 2). The oblique incision has a number of potential advantages in that it is directed in line with the vastus lateralis muscle and away from the superior geniculate artery and the vastus lateralis tendon. It also allows more leeway in closing the defect. If adequate exposure is not obtained with the rectus snip, it can be combined with a lateral retinacular release placed longitudinally approximately 1 cm lateral to the lateral border of the patella (Fig. 3). A more recent modification of the rectus snip angles the 45° oblique incision distally, rather than proximally[2] (Fig. 4). This incision has the advantage of being more extensile, because it can more easily be converted into a complete patellar turndown. **(CD–18.2)**

The advantages of the quadriceps snip are that it is technically easy, it spares the major vascular supply to the patella (the superior lateral geniculate artery), the postoperative rehabilitation does not have to be modified, and it has not been associated with such

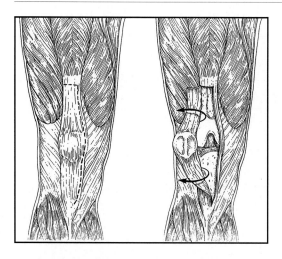

Fig. 1 Early description of quadriceps snip involved transverse sectioning of the rectus tendon.

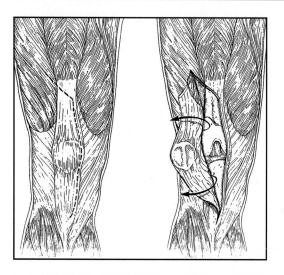

Fig. 2 Modification of quadriceps snip extends obliquely from distal to proximal.

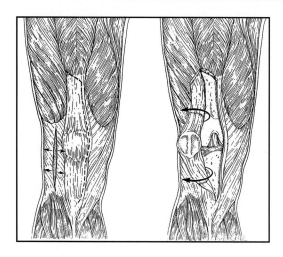

Fig. 3 Combination of the quadriceps snip and lateral release provides adequate exposure for most revision total knees.

knee performed through a standard approach.[5] Another review of 31 revision total knees performed with a quadriceps snip reported the results to be equivalent to 63 revision knees done with a standard medial parapatellar approach based on The Knee Society clinical, functional, and total scores, range of motion, extension lag, patellofemoral pain, and patient satisfaction.[6] The rectus snip has been reported to be applicable to most, if not all, stiff or ankylosed knees.[5] Other reports have stated that this technique is only effective with mild to moderate stiffness, and more extensive procedures are necessary for very stiff knees.[1,2] In this scenario, the rectus snip can be combined with a tibial tubercle osteotomy or converted to a patellar turndown.

The patellar turndown was described by Insall in 1983 as a modification of the Coonse and Adams approach.[5,7] It consists of a standard medial parapatellar capsular incision combined with an oblique distal cut from the proximal extent of the arthrotomy across the rectus tendon, vastus lateralis tendon, and lateral retinaculum (Fig. 5). It provides rapid, wide exposure to the stiff or ankylosed knee and gives easy access to the lateral gutter through the oblique arm of the incision, which allows lysis of dense adhesions and rapid mobilization of the extensor mechanism. It releases all tension on the patellar tendon insertion and all but eliminates the risk of patellar tendon avulsion. It also allows easy access to the central anterior portion of the proximal tibia, which is particularly helpful during trial reductions because the majority of revision tibial components are modular. Most of these components require direct front loading of the inserts, which can place very high tension on the patellar tendon in the stiff knee as retractors are levered laterally to allow insert placement. The patellar

postoperative complications as extension lag. Objective assessment consisting of isokinetic testing of total knee patients who had undergone a quadriceps snip revealed that their operated knee was not as strong as the contralateral normal knee, but it did not differ significantly from a total

turndown makes this potentially dangerous portion of the case safe and easy. **(CD–18.3)**

Repair of the patellar turndown should be performed with heavy nonabsorbable suture. The VY incision allows advancement of a centimeter or more, if necessary. The rectus and vastus lateralis tendons are repaired, but some or all of the lateral retinaculum is typically left open to improve flexion and patellar tracking. This approach is not without difficulties, however. Reattachment at the appropriate level of tension can be difficult. If the knee flexes easily beyond 90° after a few trial sutures are placed, the repair should be redone with more proximal reattachment of the patellar turndown. If the quadriceps is overlengthened, an extension lag can result, which can be functionally significant. The incidence of extension lag of 10° or greater has been reported at 10% to 15%.[6,8] Trousdale and associates[8] reported significant extension weakness following VY quadricepsplasty compared to a contralateral normal knee, but not compared to a total knee, just as Garvin and associates[5] reported with the rectus snip. **(CD–18.4)**

The patellar turndown approach requires modification of postoperative rehabilitation to protect the repair. Originally 2 weeks of immobilization was recommended following patellar turndown.[4,9] More recently, immediate continuous passive motion, starting at 0° to 30° has been recommended.[10] The point at which the original repair comes under tension should be noted and passive motion can be increased 10° per day until that degree of flexion is obtained.[8] Active flexion and passive extension can be started immediately, but it is probably prudent to delay straight leg raises and other active extension exercises

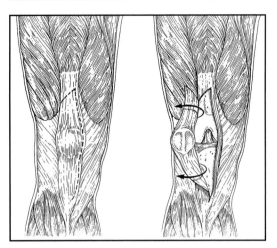

Fig. 4 Oblique incision oriented distally can easily be extended into patellar turndown.

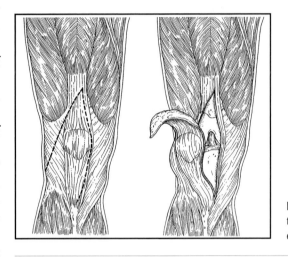

Fig. 5 Patellar turndown transects the rectus, vastus lateralis, and lateral retinaculum.

until there has been adequate time for early tendon healing to occur.

Other potential difficulties with the patellar turndown have been noted, including difficulty in using it more than once.[11] If a knee is infected and multiple surgical exposures may be needed, difficulty may be encountered in performing and repairing a patellar turndown repeatedly. The final potential problem that has been noted is the risk of devascularizing the patella and extensor mechanism by carrying an oblique incision through the lateral retinaculum,[10] which invariably transects the lateral superior genicular artery. The patellar turndown approach is thought by

some to spare the inferolateral genicular blood supply to the extensor mechanism.[12] Other authors, however, have noted that this vessel is normally interrupted during lateral meniscectomy.[1] Scott and Siliski[10] modified the patellar turndown to avoid interruption of the vascular supply of the patella. The distal extent of the incision they described carried the apex distally for 3 cm along the insertion of the vastus lateralis muscle (Fig. 6). It therefore stops proximal to the superior geniculate artery and does not actually include a lateral retinacular release. This approach was termed the modified VY quadricepsplasty.[10] While preserving the blood

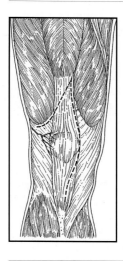

Fig. 6 Modified VY quadriceps-plasty curves along the edge of the vastus lateralis tendon avoiding the lateral superior genicular artery.

supply to the patella, it does not provide as extensive exposure or relief of tension on the patellar tendon. Maintenance of the blood supply may be more of a theoretical advantage, as Ritter and associates[13] found no difference in the rate of patellar complications including radiolucency, loosening, or fracture, with preservation of the superior geniculate artery. They concluded that saving the superior lateral geniculate artery was not necessary.

The combination of quadriceps snip and lateral release is adequate for exposing the majority of revision to-tal knees.[6] For knees with moderate or severe degrees of ankylosis, conversion to a patellar turndown may be necessary. This approach greatly expedites performing revision knee replacement in the setting of ankylosis and minimizes the risk of patellar tendon avulsion, which is among the most devastating complications of knee arthroplasty. The reconstruction is proximally in the thigh where the vasculature and soft-tissue coverage are excellent so that wound healing problems do not occur. The only complication of significance is extension weakness and lag, which is transient more than 90% of the time and is rarely functionally debilitating in the few cases in which it does persist.

References

1. Younger ASE, Duncan CP, Masri BA: Surgical exposures in revision total knee arthroplasty. *J Am Acad Orthop Surg* 1998;6:55–64.

2. Rosenberg AG: Surgical technique of posterior cruciate sacrificing, and preserving total knee arthroplasty, in Rand JA (ed): *Total Knee Arthroplasty*. New York, NY, Raven Press, 1993, pp 115–153.

3. Krackow KA: Surgical procedure, in Krackow KA (ed): *The Technique of Total Knee Arthroplasty*. St. Louis, MO, CV Mosby, 1990, pp 168–237.

4. Insall JN: Surgical approaches, in Insall JN, Windsor RE, Scott WN, Kelly MA, Aglietti P (eds): *Surgery of the Knee*, ed 2. New York, NY, Churchill Livingstone, 1993, pp 135–148.

5. Garvin KL, Scuderi G, Insall JN: Evolution of the quadriceps snip. *Clin Orthop* 1995;321: 131–137.

6. Barrack RL, Smith P, Munn B, Engh GA, Rorabeck C: Comparison of tibial tubercle osteotomy and quadriceps turndown in revision TKA. *Clin Orthop*, in press.

7. Coonse K, Adams JD: A new operative approach to the knee joint. *Surg Gynecol Obstet* 1943;77:344–347.

8. Trousdale RT, Hanssen AD, Rand JA, Cahalan TD: V-Y quadricepsplasty in total knee arthroplasty. *Clin Orthop* 1993;286:48–55.

9. Aglietti P, Windsor RE, Buzzi R, Insall JN: Arthroplasty for the stiff or ankylosed knee. *J Arthroplasty* 1989;4:1–5.

10. Scott RD, Siliski JM: The use of a modified V-Y quadricepsplasty during total knee replacement to gain exposure and improve flexion in the ankylosed knee. *Orthopedics* 1985;8:45–48.

11. Stiehl JB, Anouchi Y, Dennis DA, et al: Symposium: Revision total knee replacement. *Contemp Orthop* 1995;30:249–276.

12. Peters PC Jr: Surgical exposure for revision total knee arthroplasty, in Engh GA, Rorabeck CH (eds): *Revision Total Knee Arthroplasty*. Baltimore, MD, Williams & Wilkins, 1997, pp 195–204.

13. Ritter MA, Herbst SA, Keating EM, Faris PM, Meding JB: Patellofemoral complications following total knee arthroplasty: Effect of a lateral release and sacrifice of the superior lateral geniculate artery. *J Arthroplasty* 1996;11: 368–372.

Reference to Video

Barrack R: *Specialized Surgical Exposures for Revision Total Knee: Quadriceps Snip and Patellar Turndown*. Rosemont, IL, American Academy of Orthopaedic Surgeons, Annual Meeting, 1998.

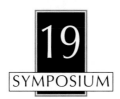

Medial Epicondylar Osteotomy: A Technique Used With Primary and Revision Total Knee Arthroplasty to Improve Surgical Exposure and Correct Varus Deformity

Gerard A. Engh, MD

Indications

A medial epicondylar osteotomy (Fig. 1) is a surgical technique for correcting the soft-tissue contractures associated with varus deformity and fixed-flexion deformity in difficult primary and revision knee replacement procedures.[1] Historically, the correction of varus deformity has required extensive stripping of the capsule and ligaments from the medial side of the tibia. An epicondylar osteotomy provides a method for achieving ligament balance by correcting the soft-tissue contractures on the femoral side of the knee. The osteotomy enhances the exposure of the posterior capsule, where additional releases are often necessary to fully correct the varus deformity and large flexion contractures (> 20°) often associated with advanced degenerative arthritis.

When an epicondylar osteotomy is performed, it is possible to correct contractures without cutting or stripping ligaments. The osteotomy releases the medial collateral ligaments with a wafer of bone from the femur, thereby permitting the tibia to displace forward with external tibial rotation. In flexion, the knee is angulated to a valgus position and the tibia

is externally rotated to enhance lateral subluxation of the patella. The medial side of the knee is destabilized in flexion. Stability is reestablished when the osteotomized fragment of bone is reattached to the condyle and the medial parapatellar arthrotomy is repaired. Conventional releases that essentially create a grade 3 ligament tear by stripping from bone or sectioning ligaments are avoided. With an epicondylar osteotomy, however, the undamaged ligaments remain attached to the epicondyle and are intact when the osteotomy is repaired.

Optimal knee stability in both flexion and extension is possible through the repair of an epicondylar osteotomy. Even if the epicondyle is not reattached and heals by fibrous union, the repair of the medial retinaculum and capsule restores stability to the medial side of the knee. Specifically, stability in flexion is provided when the joint capsule is repaired along the medial edge of the patella. The repair of the medial capsular arthrotomy functionally restores the medial patellofemoral ligament and prevents the epicondyle from migrating posteriorly. Stability in extension is provided by proximal tension from the adductor magnus

tendon to the osteotomized epicondyle. The posteromedial capsule provides additional stability to the medial side of the knee.

Special situations in which medial epicondylar osteotomy may be indicated are in cases of severe capsular fibrosis that make exposure difficult, revision cases with distal femoral bone deficiencies to be reconstructed with an allograft-composite, dislocated knees (with intact cruciate ligaments) that cannot be reduced, and the conversion of a knee fusion to a total knee arthroplasty. In these situations, surgical exposure is enhanced by the osteotomy and stability is reestablished when the wafer of bone with the intact collateral ligaments is attached to the medial femoral condyle.

Surgical Technique

The surgery begins with a standard medial parapatellar, midline, or vastus-splitting approach. The capsule is incised and reflected from the medial metaphyseal flare of the tibia to the midcoronal plane of the tibia. If the patient has less than 90° of preoperative knee flexion, a quadriceps snip or tibial tubercle osteotomy may be needed to relax the extensor mecha-

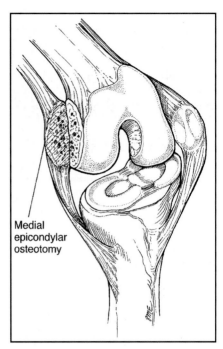

Fig. 1 The osteotomized epicondyle with intact adductor magnus tendon and collateral ligaments is displaced posterior to the medial femoral condyle. Exposure is enhanced by external rotation and varus angulation of the knee in a flexed position.

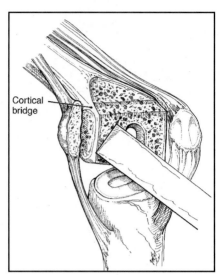

Fig. 2 A cortical bridge is established between the anterior femoral bone resection and the osteotomized medial femoral epicondyle. Sutures are passed beneath this bridge of cortical bone to anchor the repair of the epicondyle.

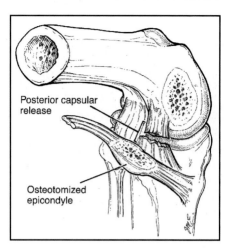

Fig. 3 The posteromedial capsule, including fibers of the posterior oblique ligament, is released with a cautery to fully correct varus deformity and flexion contracture of the knee.

nism and permit lateral displacement and eversion of the patella.

An epicondylar osteotomy is performed with the knee in 90° of flexion or at the maximum knee flexion possible if the 90° position is unobtainable. Osteophytes are removed from the rim of the medial femoral condyle so that the medial epicondyle is clearly visible. The adductor tubercle and the insertion of the adductor magnus tendon are identified by palpating the proximal end of the medial femoral condyle. To demarcate the osteotomy, the surgeon uses a cautery to incise the synovium.

The osteotomy is begun just proximal to the rim of previously excised osteophytes. A 1-¼-in osteotome is oriented parallel to the long axis of the femur (Fig. 2) and advanced to release a segment of bone

1 cm thick and 4 cm in diameter. The attachments of the medial collateral ligaments and the adductor magnus tendon insertion to the epicondyle remain attached to this wafer of bone. The osteotomy is completed and the segment of bone hinged open when the osteotomized epicondylar fragment is displaced posterior to the medial femoral condyle. Once the osteotomy is completed, the posterior compartment is easily accessed from the medial side, if additional release is indicated.

To fully correct a varus deformity, the surgeon releases the posteromedial capsule, including the posterior oblique ligament, particularly when a large flexion contracture is present. This ligament complex originates from the medial side of the femur posterior to the adductor tubercle and distal to the linea aspera. A cautery is used to release the capsule close to its femoral origin (Fig. 3). The release is continued until the

knee is correctly aligned in extension and balanced tension is achieved within the soft tissues on the medial and lateral sides of the knee.

Repair of the Epicondylar Osteotomy

When an epicondylar osteotomy is performed, knee stability in extension is maintained through the proximal to distal continuity of soft-tissue structures that attach to the epicondyle and adductor tubercle. An epicondylar osteotomy is analogous to a trochanteric slide used in total hip arthroplasty. A sleeve of soft tissue is maintained through the osteotomized segment of bone. Just as in revision hip arthroplasty when the trochanter is reattached in a more proximal position with leg lengthening, the osteotomized bone is positioned more distally on the medial femoral condyle with correction of severe varus deformity. Bone of the epicondyle that overhangs the femoral component at the joint line is trimmed to permit apposition of the epicondyle against the medial femoral condyle.

Knee stability in flexion is re-established when the epicondyle is reattached to the medial side of the femur. With the repair of the medial capsular arthrotomy, the epicondyle is repositioned near its condylar origin and reasonably good stability is restored to the medial side of the knee. However, the epicondyle is not rigidly stable with capsular closure alone. A nonunion may result, with heterotopic bone forming in the vicinity of the epicondyle. Therefore, optimal knee stability is achieved by reattaching the medial epicondyle to the femur with #2 (or heavier) non-absorbable sutures.

The osteotomy is repaired with the knee at 90° of flexion. The epicondyle is brought into position when the epicondyle is lifted with a clamp or towel clips as far anterior on the condyle as permitted by the medial collateral ligaments attached to the epicondyle. A cortical bridge between the anterior femoral resection and the medial epicondylar osteotomy is established when a primary or revision total knee arthroplasty is performed (Fig. 2). This bridge serves as an anchor for those sutures that are passed through the medial femoral condyle.

Sutures are placed under the anterior cortical bridge of the condyle and through the epicondylar fragment. With the osteotomized fragment held in position against the medial femoral condyle, 2 or 3 heavy sutures are secured. The surgeon tests the stability of the repaired osteotomy by flexing and extending the knee while inspecting the osteotomy site for motion. Cancellous screws with washers are rarely needed to repair the osteotomized bone fragment. If the epicondyle will not reposition to the condyle, it may be necessary to release some of the medial capsule from the posterior aspect of the epicondylar fragment.

Rehabilitation Following Epicondylar Osteotomy
Range of motion and strengthening exercises are encouraged following a total knee arthroplasty with an epicondylar osteotomy. At the surgeon's discretion, a continuous passive motion device can be used to enhance the early restoration of knee flexion.

A postoperative knee brace is not necessary after an epicondylar osteotomy. Repairing the osteotomized fragment should provide sufficient flexion stability on the medial side. However, if the fragment cannot be satisfactorily reattached to the medial femoral condyle, the patient should be placed in a knee immobilizer with limited flexion. The immobilizer prevents the osteotomized fragment of bone from moving during knee flexion. For adequate healing of the osteotomy and restoration of optimum stability in flexion, the knee should be kept in the immobilizer for 6 weeks.

If heterotopic bone does develop proximal to an epicondylar osteotomy, it has not inhibited excursion of the knee and has not compromised the range of motion achieved after knee arthroplasty. In my experience, this bone has not been associated with any clinical symptoms. Likewise, a fibrous union of the epicondyle has not been associated with either knee instability or pain.

Additional Indications for an Epicondylar Osteotomy
The Medial Epicondylar Osteotomy and Severe Capsular Fibrosis
Capsular fibrosis with a loss of soft-tissue compliance compromises the exposure of a failed total knee. Even with full release of the extensor mechanism, knee flexion may be blocked because of a loss of soft-tissue compliance and a hypertrophic

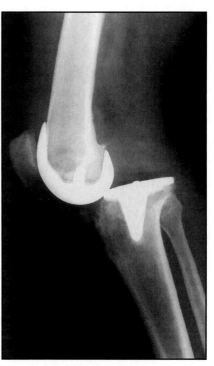

Fig. 4 A posterior tibial dislocation of a cruciate-retaining total knee component that required a medial epicondylar osteotomy for surgical exposure during revision total knee arthroplasty.

barrier of soft tissue within the posterior compartment of the knee. An osteotomy of the medial epicondyle permits adequate knee flexion for component removal. After the osteotomy and component removal have been completed, the thick capsular tissue in the back of the knee is accessible. Removing this tissue barrier to knee flexion also improves the patient's postoperative range of motion.

Epicondylar Osteotomy and Allograft Reconstruction
When a massive distal femoral allograft is needed in revision total knee arthroplasty, osteotomizing both epicondyles is beneficial. Maintaining a contiguous sleeve of soft tissue through the epicondyles makes it possible to destabilize the knee and

achieve adequate surgical exposure. Repositioning and attaching the epicondyles to the sides of a distal femoral allograft with heavy suture material will restore stability to the knee. With time, the epicondyle will heal to an allograft. A rigid repair of the host epicondyles to a distal femoral allograft eliminates the need for a varus-valgus or rotating hinge prosthesis.

Epicondylar Osteotomy and Knee Dislocation

It is rare to encounter a posterior tibial dislocation of a posterior-stabilized implant, and a dislocation is even less likely with a cruciate-retaining component (Fig. 4). With such a dislocation, it may be impossible to reduce the knee with intact collateral ligaments because the tibia cannot be brought forward from behind the femur. An osteotomy of the medial epicondyle destabilizes the knee in flexion, permitting the dislocation to be reduced. After the reduction, the osteotomized epicondyle can be reattached to restore the appropriate tension for adequate knee stability. In my own experience, this technique has been necessary in 2 cases of recalcitrant knee dislocations that could not be reduced prior to an epicondylar osteotomy.

Epicondylar Osteotomy and Take-Down of Knee Fusions

In unusual circumstances, a malunion of a knee fusion may need to be converted to a total knee arthroplasty. When the take-down of a fusion is indicated, the epicondylar osteotomy performed in conjunction with the knee arthroplasty enhances surgical exposure. It also provides an opportunity to restore optimal stability by directly reattaching the wafer of bone, with the collateral ligaments intact, to the femur. In this situation, it is essential that the osteotomized epicondylar fragments are properly positioned to achieve stability throughout an arc of motion.

Pitfalls of a Medial Epicondylar Osteotomy

A medial epicondylar osteotomy alone may not fully correct large fixed deformities on the medial side of the knee. In such cases, the posteromedial capsule is contracted and must be fully divided to correct fixed deformities and optimize ligament balance. Whenever the deformity is not fully corrected with an epicondylar osteotomy, a release of the posteromedial capsule is necessary (Fig. 3). This release should continue until the medial side will open slightly in extension with a valgus stress.

The wafer of bone released with a medial epicondylar osteotomy should be at least 1 cm thick. Thinner wafers of bone tend to fragment, making rigid reattachment to the femoral condyle more difficult. The best way to avoid releasing a wafer of bone that is too thin is to direct the osteotome to exit the condyle proximal to the adductor tubercle.

In knees with severe varus and large flexion contractures, this bone wafer may be difficult to reduce on the medial femoral condyle. In this situation, a cautery is used to release the soft tissues attached to the posterior rim of the epicondylar fragment until the epicondyle can be brought forward, reapproximated, and repaired in a more anterior location on the condyle.

The correction of a severe varus deformity with releases on the femoral side may displace the osteotomized epicondyle to a more distal position on the femur. The fragment should be reattached to the medial femoral condyle at this more distal location. When the epicondylar fragment cannot be anatomically relocated to the condyle, any joint line overhang of the epicondylar fragment is removed with a rongeur.

Summary

The epicondylar osteotomy is a valuable tool for use in both primary and revision knee arthroplasty. Without damaging the ligamentous structures, this technique provides the surgeon with a means of accessing the knee, correcting deformity, and restoring knee stability. I have not experienced any clinical problems associated with this procedure.

Reference

1. Engh GA, McAuley JP: Joint line restoration and flexion-extension balance with revision total knee arthroplasty, in Engh GA, Rorabeck CH (eds): *Revision Total Knee Arthroplasty*. Baltimore, MD, Williams & Wilkins, 1997, pp 242–245.

The Quadriceps Myocutaneous Composite Flap for the Exposure of the Distal Femur and Knee in Tumor Resection and Reconstruction

Robert M. Kerry, MB, FRCS (Orth)
Bassam A. Masri, MD, FRCSC
Christopher Beauchamp, MD, FRCSC
Clive P. Duncan, MD, FRCSC

Introduction

The wide resection of tumors of the distal femur requires extensive circumferential surgical exposure to allow resection of the biopsy track, whether it is located laterally or medially, as well as the meticulous dissection of the contents of the popliteal fossa, and protection of the vital structures that lie within it. The standard surgical approach is through a longitudinal incision that incorporates the biopsy track. The exposure of the popliteal vascular structures and of the tibial nerve is easier through a medial incision, yet the exposure of the common peroneal nerve is simpler through a lateral exposure. When one incision is used, the opposite side has to be exposed after wide flaps are elevated.

In this chapter, we describe an approach that offers the advantages of both medial and lateral incisions without compromising the integrity of the soft-tissue flaps. This approach uses a U-shaped proximally based myocutaneous flap, which affords excellent exposure of the whole distal femur and knee joint and allows a choice of treatment options for the extensor mecha-

nism. Its most common application is in musculoskeletal oncology, but the approach does have a potential application in complex reconstruction for other reasons and in the management of injuries of uncommon severity.

Anatomic Basis

Until the cutaneous vascular anatomy was fully understood, there were strict limits to the size of cutaneous flaps that could be raised and remain viable. Flap necrosis was an ever present risk. Flaps were largely based on geometric ratios rather than on particular feeding vessels and a strict anatomic understanding.

Much information of extreme value had been identified but was not widely appreciated. Seven years before the discovery of X-rays, Manchot[1] completed his treatise *Die Hautarterien des menschlichen Körpers–The Skin Arteries of the Body*. Recently this has been translated into English.[2] His mapping of vascular territories and cutaneous perforators was remarkably accurate, considering that radiography was not available to him. In the 1930s, with the benefit of radiography and injection techniques, Salmon[3] was

able to repeat the work of Manchot and also map the blood supply of every muscle of the body.[4] His work has also recently been translated into English.[5] Considerable further clarification of the vascular territories of the body has been provided in a number of studies by Taylor and Palmer,[6] including introduction of the concept of the angiosome–a composite unit of skin and underlying deep tissue based on a single source artery. They also pointed out that most muscles span at least 2 angiosomes and, due to the complex arrangement of choke vessels that connect neighboring vascular territories, if a flap is raised on the vessels of one angiosome the tissue of the adjacent angiosome can be captured with safety. Necrosis is only likely to occur in the next or subsequent angiosome. These studies provide a sound anatomic basis for flap design, and they demonstrate that in certain areas very large flaps can be raised without a major risk of necrosis. The fact that the entire lower limb can perfuse through the anastamosis around the hip joint in the case of chronic common femoral artery occlusion is indicative of the potential for raising

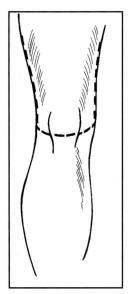

Fig. 1 Skin incision.

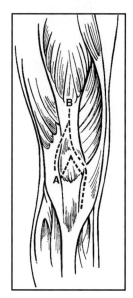

Fig. 2 Division of the extensor mechanism. Patellar osteotomy (**A**), quadriceps turndown (**B**).

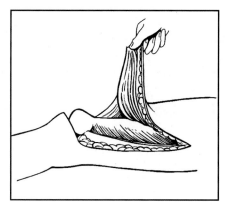

Fig. 3 Composite flap raised exposing distal femur.

large, well-vascularized flaps, distal to that anastamosis.

This increasing understanding has been mirrored by clinical advances. Large anterior thigh flaps with disarticulation of the femur have been described by several authors for closure of massive decubitus ulcers in the paraplegic patient.[7–10] Anterior thigh flaps have also been described for closure of hemipelvectomy defects, with greater reliability than the traditional posterior flap.[11,12] These flaps have been based on the quadriceps, tensor fascia lata, and proximal sartorius muscles and the overlying skin with a blood supply based on the femoral vessels, particularly the lateral femoral circumflex artery.

The approach we describe is based on the same anatomic features but, rather than being used for coverage of a defect following limb ablation, it allows excellent exposure for resection of tumors followed by complex reconstruction.[13]

Indications

The approach is of use whenever wide surgical exposure of the entire distal femur is required. The most common indications are the wide excision of malignant tumors of the distal femur, and the management of complex intra-articular pathologic fractures of the distal femur, particularly when associated with large benign, yet aggressive lesions.

Surgical Technique
The Exposure and Resection
The patient is positioned supine with the affected limb draped free. A U-shaped skin incision is created using medial and lateral incisions along the line of the femur which are joined distally by a transverse anterior incision at the level of the patella (Fig. 1). The extensor mechanism can be divided either by a patellar osteotomy or by a distally based V-shaped division of the quadriceps tendon (Fig. 2). The entire quadriceps muscle can then be raised from the anterior surface of the femur (Fig. 3). Laterally, the muscle is raised from the lateral intermuscular septum, ligating any perforating vessels from the posterior

compartment as they are identified. Medially, a subvastus approach is performed, taking care to identify branches of the descending geniculate vessels and to identify the main femoral neurovascular bundle in the vasto-adductor interval. The adductors are raised off the distal femur and adductor tubercle. If an extra-articular excision is required, the dissection can stay clear of the suprapatellar pouch, and a small portion of the deep surface of the tendon can be excised with the tumor. A coronal osteotomy of the patella can then be performed, and the articular surface can remain attached to the resection specimen. The anterior portion of the patella can then be reflected distally, taking great care to stay extrasynovial, and to separate the patellar tendon from the underlying fat pad. The proximal tibia can then be exposed. With the knee flexed, the popliteal fossa contents can be separated from the distal femur, and the geniculate vessels can be ligated to allow mobilization of the popliteal vessels. An osteotomy of the proximal tibia can then be performed. The entire knee joint can then be removed, along with the tumor, by performing an osteotomy of the femur. If an extra-articular resection is not required, a similar technique can be used, in which the knee joint is entered, and the distal femur is resected by disarticulating the knee joint and by performing a femoral osteotomy.

The Reconstruction

A number of surgical options are available for reconstruction. Despite a well recognized and significant risk of major complications, allograft replacement can provide a durable reconstruction with good function either alone, with a knee arthrodesis, or with a condylar total knee replacement. Another option is to replace the bony deficit with a modular or custom-made segmental replacement implant. After reimplantation, the extensor mechanism can be repaired through the site of its division, whether it be bone or soft tissue. Postoperatively, the knee should be protected in extension for 6 weeks to allow healing of the extensor mechanism. One of the advantages of a tenotomy of the quadriceps tendon is that when a substantial portion of the quadriceps muscle is resected with the tumor, the remaining extensor mechanism can be centralized into the patella to ensure proper patellar tracking postoperatively.

Complications

The major complications relate to the extensor mechanism. A mild extensor lag is the most common complication. This extensor lag, however, is early, and tends to resolve with time, provided that sufficient quadriceps muscle remains after tumor excision. Patellar nonunion after osteotomy may also occur despite stable fixation but usually responds to repeat internal fixation and bone grafting. Patellar internal fixation devices often require removal for symptomatic prominence. Persistent and significant functional impairment has not, however, occurred. In the 15 cases done to date, we have not seen any cases of flap necrosis, even in patients who had received preoperative radiotherapy. Allograft-related complications are relatively common, in keeping with the experience of others.[14-16] Host allograft nonunion, the most common of these, usually responds well to autogenous bone grafting. Infection and fracture are more serious, but even these complications do not usually represent an unsalvageable limb.

Conclusion

A sound understanding of the blood supply to the thigh makes possible the elevation of a very large myocutaneous flap, giving excellent exposure of the entire distal femur in oncologic surgery. This technique allows adequate tumor resection with a number of reconstructive possibilities. The complication rate has been acceptably low.

References

1. Manchot C (ed): *Die Hautarterien des Menschlichen Körpers*. Leipzig, Germany, Vogel, 1889.

2. Manchot C (ed): *The Cutaneous Arteries of the Human Body*. New York, NY, Springer-Verlag, 1983.

3. Salmon M (ed): *Artères de la Peau*. Paris, France, Masson et cie, 1936.

4. Salmon M (ed): *Les Artères des Muscles des Membres et du Tronc*. Paris, France, Masson et cie, 1933.

5. Salmon M, Taylor GI, Tempest MN (eds): *Arteries of the Skin*. London, England, Churchill Livingstone, 1988.

6. Taylor GI, Palmer JH: The vascular territories (angiosomes) of the body: Experimental study and clinical applications. *Br J Plast Surg* 1987;40:113–141.

7. Conway H, Stark RB, Weeter JC, Garcia FA, Kavanaugh JD: Complications of decubitus ulcers in patients with paraplegia. *Plast Reconstr Surg* 1951;7:117–130.

8. Georgiade N, Pickrell K, Maguire C: Total thigh flaps for extensive decubitus ulcers. *Plast Reconstr Surg* 1956;17:220–225.

9. Spira M, Hardy SB: Our experiences with high thigh amputations in paraplegics. *Plast Reconstr Surg* 1963;31:344–352.

10. Weeks PM, Brower TD: Island flap coverage of extensive decubitus ulcers. *Plast Reconstr Surg* 1968;42:433–436.

11. Frey C, Matthews LS, Benjamin H, Fidler WJ: A new technique for hemipelvectomy. *Surg Gynecol Obstet* 1976;143:753–756.

12. Mnaymneh W, Temple W: Modified hemipelvectomy utilizing a long vascular myocutaneous thigh flap: Case report. *J Bone Joint Surg* 1980;62A:1013–1015.

13. Beauchamp CP, Duncan CP: Resection of the distal femur via a trans-patellar/ligament myocutaneous flap, in Brown KLB (ed): *Complications of Limb Salvage: Prevention, Management and Outcome*. Montreal, Canada, International Symposium on Limb Salvage (ISOLS), 1991, pp 303–305.

14. Vander Griend RA: The effect of internal fixation on the healing of large allografts. *J Bone Joint Surg* 1994;76A:657–663.

15. Dick HM, Strauch RJ: Infection of massive bone allografts. *Clin Orthop* 1994;306:46–53.

16. Berrey BH Jr, Lord CF, Gebhardt MC, Mankin HJ: Fractures of allografts: Frequency, treatment, and end-results. *J Bone Joint Surg* 1990;72A:825–833.

Planning for Revision Total Knee Arthroplasty

James A. Rand, MD

In planning for revision of a failed total knee arthroplasty, it is important to understand the mechanism(s) of failure, determine the prior implant type, evaluate the patient for soft-tissue abnormalities as well as bone loss, and plan for management of these problems. More than 1 alternative should be available at the time of surgery, because an alternative technique may be necessary. The principles of total knee arthroplasty must be carefully adhered to, followed by an appropriate rehabilitation plan.

Mechanisms of Failure

It is essential to determine the etiology of failure of the prior prosthesis. Failure may arise from any of the following 3 basic areas: (1) patient selection; (2) implant design; (3) surgical technique.

Patient Selection

Appropriate patient selection is important in knee arthroplasty. The noncompliant patient who places increased stresses across the joint arthroplasty may predispose to mechanical failure from loosening, or due to polyethylene wear. This problem arises most frequently in knee arthroplasties performed for traumatic arthritis in the young patient. The patient who has a knee arthroplasty with an associated anatomic abnormality from bowing or malalignment of the femur or tibia

from prior fracture presents a technical challenge to achieve optimum alignment at the time of the initial arthroplasty. If optimum alignment is not achieved, the risk of subsequent loosening and failure will be increased.[1] Management of these complex deformities requires careful preoperative planning to determine whether an associated osteotomy will be required, either prior to or in conjunction with the arthroplasty, to obtain correct limb alignment. Deformities close to the joint have a greater effect on alignment and are more problematic than deformities distant from the knee. Deformity in the coronal plane is more problematic than sagittal plane deformity. Deformity in the supracondylar area of the femur is more difficult to manage than tibial deformity. A coronal plane malunion of 20° or greater in the supracondylar area usually necessitates an osteotomy, either prior to or in conjunction with total knee arthroplasty, in order to obtain correct alignment and not have ligament imbalance.[2]

Another abnormality that may occur following osteotomy or trauma is offset of the metaphysis referable to the diaphysis of the femur or tibia. An offset abnormality can result in difficulty in appropriate seating and implant size selection, which can lead to subsequent failure (Fig. 1). A custom implant with an offset or bowed

stem may be necessary for fixation. The presence of significant ipsilateral hip disease can also cause failure of a knee replacement. The patient with a prior Girdlestone arthroplasty of the hip who develops lateral compartmental knee arthritis and valgus deformity because of the abnormal mechanics of gait will continue to have these abnormal mechanical forces after the total knee arthroplasty. If the hip problem is not corrected, the same abnormal forces will be placed across the knee prosthesis, leading to mechanical failure. The patient with a chronic pain syndrome or reflex sympathetic dystrophy who undergoes knee arthroplasty will present with failure due to pain. These problems do not improve with additional surgery and must be carefully evaluated as failure mechanisms intrinsic to the patient. Katz and associates[3] have reported a prevalence of reflex sympathetic dystrophy after knee arthroplasty of 0.8%. These patients present with limited flexion, excessive pain, and cutaneous hypersensitivity.

Mont and associates[4] reported on the results of reoperation for a painful total knee arthroplasty in 27 knees followed up for 42 months. Only 41% achieved a satisfactory result. The other 59% had unsatisfactory results overall. The highest success rate was 60% in the group that presented with pain and limited

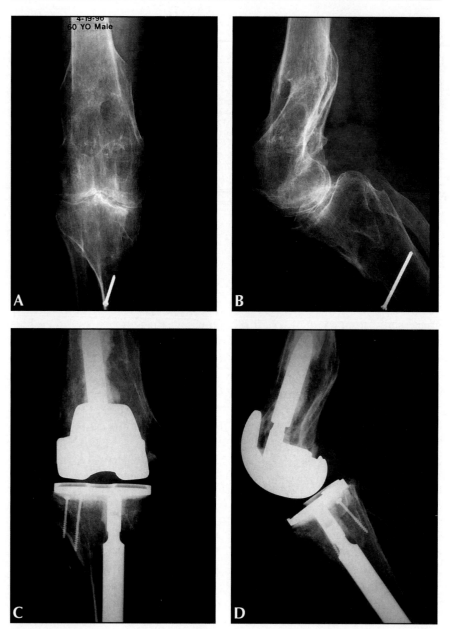

Fig. 1 A, Anteroposterior and **B,** lateral radiographs of posttraumatic arthritis with offset of tibial metaphysis. **C,** Anteroposterior and **D,** lateral radiographs after total knee arthroplasty with offset stem tibial component.

may have persistent pain and dysfunction after knee arthroplasty, and these symptoms are unrelated to the function of the prosthesis. Referred pain from ipsilateral hip arthritis or lumbar spine disease should be excluded.

Implant Design

Poor implant design was a recognized mode of failure with early implants, such as the polycentric or geometric resurfacing prostheses, or with the fixed hinge designs such as the Guepar. These implants had an unacceptable rate of loosening and were abandoned. More modern implant designs have been identified as having a high prevalence of polyethylene wear. The PCA (Howmedica Inc, Rutherford, NJ) design has been recognized as being prone to catastrophic failure from polyethylene wear, as have the Synatomic (DePuy Inc, Warsaw, IN) and Arizona (DePuy Inc, Warsaw, IN) designs.[5,6] The increased polyethylene wear has led to problems of osteolysis with bone resorption and implant loosening (Fig. 2). Other implant-related problems include those with designs such as the Miller-Galante I (Zimmer Inc, Warsaw, IN), which had a high prevalence of patellar maltracking and instability due to a shallow trochlear groove,[7] or the kinematic rotating hinge (Howmedica Inc, Rutherford, NJ), which had an unacceptable prevalence of implant breakage.[8] Metal-backed patellae are predisposed to problems of polyethylene wear.

Surgical Technique

The most frequent reasons for nonseptic failure relate to problems with surgical technique. These may be grouped into problems affecting the extensor mechanism and problems

motion, while the group operated on for pain alone had only a 17% success rate.[4] The patient who presents with significant soft-tissue deficiencies is at risk of an unsatisfactory result. The patient with marked weakness in the extensor mechanism from an old quadriceps rupture, or the patient who has marked scarring and soft-

tissue deformity may not achieve a satisfactory range of motion and may have persistent weakness or pain. Another source of persistent unsatisfactory results after knee arthroplasty is the patient with neurologic dysfunction and a central pain syndrome. Patients with demyelinating disorders or peripheral neuropathy

related to malalignment, implant malposition, incorrect implant size, soft-tissue imbalance, or poor implant fixation.

Extensor mechanism problems are some of the more frequent reasons for reoperation after current condylar knee designs. Patellofemoral problems include instability, patellar fracture, metal-backed patellar wear, patellar implant loosening, and a variety of peripatellar soft-tissue problems such as the patellar clunk syndrome.[9] In many of these instances, the abnormality can be traced to implant malpositioning, failure to balance the extensor mechanism at the time of surgery, or an abnormality in the technique of patellar resurfacing. Malalignment of the limb into excessive valgus or varus places increased loads across the prosthesis and predisposes to mechanical loosening as well as abnormal polyethylene wear. Implant malpositioning can have adverse effects on limb alignment and extensor mechanism tracking, and can affect soft-tissue balancing about the knee, leading to instability in the tibiofemoral articulation or limitation of motion. Selection of the incorrect implant size affects soft-tissue balance and may result in soft-tissue impingement if there is overhang of the implant, especially of the tibial component on the medial aspect of the knee, where it can impinge on the medial collateral ligament. Selection of the incorrect implant constraint, such as a posterior cruciate-sacrificing but nonstabilized knee in the patient with prior patellectomy, can result in abnormal joint laxity, posterior tibial subluxation, and extensor mechanism pain and weakness.[10] Failure to balance the soft tissues, both in the varus-valgus and the anterior-posterior planes, can result in a knee that is unstable in

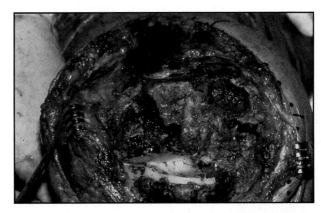

Fig. 2 Operative photograph of femoral osteolysis associated with polyethylene wear.

flexion or is excessively tight, with limitation of motion. Abnormal soft-tissue forces can place increased stresses on the interfaces, leading to accelerated loosening or accelerated polyethylene wear.

One of the most common reasons for failure of knee arthroplasty is that of deep infection, which may often be unrecognized (Table 1). A careful search of patient history factors that may predispose to infection, combined with a careful physical examination and appropriate use of radiographs, bone scans, aspiration, and hematologic testing, will help to eliminate this potential cause of failure.

Define Bone and Soft-Tissue Deficiency

Identification of problems that must be anticipated and corrected at the time of surgery must begin with an evaluation of what has been lost at the previous surgical procedure. The initial assessment must begin with a careful evaluation of the soft tissues. Evaluation should begin with the skin, because areas of prior scar, skin grafting, or soft-tissue defect may make revision surgery impractical unless these problems are addressed with a soft-tissue procedure by a plastic surgeon either prior to or at the time of arthroplasty[11] (Fig. 3). The integrity of the ligaments, both

Table 1

Infection rates in primary surgery 1969-1996

Joint	Number	Infection %
Ankle	219	3.7
Elbow	804	7.8
Hip	23,519	1.3
Knee	16,035	2.0
Shoulder	2,068	1.2

Infection rates in revision surgery 1969-1996

Joint	Number	Infection %
Ankle	7	0
Elbow	208	7.7
Hip	7,161	3.2
Knee	2,714	5.6
Shoulder	253	3.2

collaterals and cruciates, should be evaluated by a careful examination, review of the prior surgical notes, and the type of implant. The patient who has a deficient cruciate or collateral ligament will require the appropriate constrained prosthesis for revision. Failure to consider the soft-tissue needs may result in a selection of an implant design with inadequate intrinsic stability, which can lead to failure. The extensor mechanism must be carefully evaluated to be sure that it is correctly aligned, as well as intact and functioning. The patient with a patellar tendon rupture will not have adequate function unless the extensor mechanism can be reconstructed at the time of revision. This reconstruction may necessitate

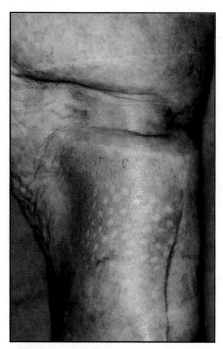

Fig. 3 Operative photograph of knee for reimplantation for infection with prior local rotational flaps and skin grafts.

having allografts available for reconstruction in longstanding ruptures,[12] or appropriate intrinsic soft tissues such as hamstring tendons available for acute or early ruptures. If the extensor mechanism is malaligned, plans will have to be undertaken to obtain correct alignment and tracking of the extensor mechanism.

Bone deficiency is commonly encountered at the time of revision knee arthroplasty. Bone loss affects the femur, tibia, and patella. In the femur, bone loss tends to be distal and posterior, and these are often combined. In the tibia, bone loss may be central or peripheral or combined. Patellar bone loss tends to be concave with a central deficiency. In any of these locations the bone loss may be symmetric or asymmetric. The patient with osteolysis often has substantially more bone loss at the time of surgery than is appreciated on review of the preoperative radiographs. These potential deficiencies must be anticipated to plan for appropriate modular augments or bone graft. The patient with associated extra-articular deformity from prior fracture or bowing must be carefully evaluated preoperatively to determine if associated osteotomy or other corrective procedures will be required or if custom implants with offset stems will be needed to fit the underlying bone abnormalities.

Reconstructive Needs

The prior evaluation of the soft tissues will determine the need for associated plastic surgical intervention, which may be in the form of preoperative soft-tissue expansion or in the form of muscle flaps at the time of revision or prior to revision. If an allograft is going to be required for reconstruction of an extensor mechanism, it must be carefully planned, to be sure the right type and quality is available for the revision procedure.

Careful templating of radiographs is essential in planning for revision.[13] True anteroposterior (AP) and lateral radiographs of the affected knee of known radiographic magnification are important to determine the implant size (Fig. 4). Fluoroscopically positioned radiographs can be helpful in identifying areas of osteolysis or subtle loosening.[14] A full-length standing radiograph of the lower extremity will help to define areas of extra-articular deformity, such as fracture or bowing, and will allow planning for long-stemmed implants. AP and lateral radiographs of the contralateral normal knee with known radiographic magnification can be helpful in planning for the appropriate size of implant. Once the implant size is selected from the intact knee, it can then be placed onto the operative knee to determine if there are substantial bone deficiencies distally and posteriorly that are likely to need to be corrected at the time of revision to achieve appropriate collateral ligament tensioning and kinematics.

Areas of bone deficiency can be dealt with by cement filling, by bone grafting, or by augmented or custom implants. Although cement filling may function well for localized central deficiencies with an intact peripheral rim, cement does not provide optimum load distribution in most instances. Modular bone augments are available from most manufacturers and can be used to deal with areas of condylar deficiency on either the tibia or femur. The modular augments are quite useful in assisting with restoration of the joint line on the femoral side and with flexion-extension balancing. In cases of more substantial bone loss or global metaphyseal deficiency, allografts of either the proximal tibia or distal femur will need to be selected. Only in rare instances, such as the revision of the failed unicompartmental arthroplasty, is autograft available. In most cases, allograft reconstruction will be required for revision surgery. In cases of contained defects, a morcellized graft may be used, but in the case of peripheral defects, structural grafting will usually be required. True AP and lateral high quality radiographs of the allograft need to be obtained with known magnification for templating to determine the appropriate size for the anticipated bone deficiency at the time of revision.

Planning for the revision implant is essential. With modular implant systems, the degree of constraint can often be varied within a single system, which facilitates a revision. The assessment of the integrity of the collateral and cruciate ligaments is important in implant selection, as is the need for intramedullary stems or augments. Usually a posterior stabilized prosthesis should be used for most revision procedures. A more constrained condylar implant should be selected in the case of difficult soft-tissue balancing. For a patient with a marked deficiency of a collateral ligament and severe deformity, there remains a role for a hinged prosthesis. In planning for the implant, it is important to template the radiograph of the failed arthroplasty to determine the alignment of the stem, the fit of the condylar portion of the prosthesis, the extent of bone deficiency, and whether or not the stem will be press-fit or cemented. In instances of marked metaphyseal bone loss or prior osteotomy, a customized implant or an implant with an offset stem may be necessary in order to obtain adequate alignment of the prosthesis into the remaining bone. These customized implants require careful templating and planning in order to have them available at the time of the revision.

Surgical Planning

A review of the prior surgical note can be extremely useful in planning for revision. Determining the size of the prosthesis, type of implant, and any difficulties encountered by the prior surgeon is useful in planning for revision. The type of prior exposure used in the patient, and the presence of any associated bone or soft-tissue abnormalities should be carefully reviewed.

Exposure of the knee in revision can be difficult. It is important to be aware of the location of prior incisions and to select the most lateral anterior incision that allows access to the knee, to prevent areas of skin necrosis between the old and new incision.

The standard anteromedial approach may be adequate in the knee

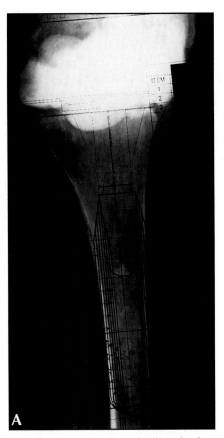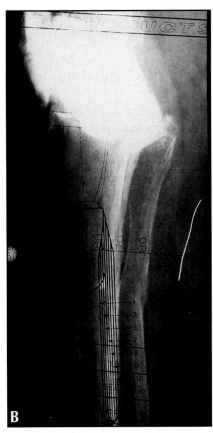

Fig. 4 A, Anteroposterior and **B,** lateral radiographs of a resection arthroplasty for an infected total knee with template for custom tibial component.

with a good range of motion and soft-tissue laxity. However, the patient with limited motion or stiffness may require an alternative exposure. The V-Y quadricepsplasty is an excellent technique to achieve exposure and addresses contracture in the extensor mechanism by allowing lengthening. It has the disadvantages of requiring protected rehabilitation after the quadricepsplasty, and it does slightly weaken the extensor mechanism.[15]

The rectus snip is another alternative exposure technique that consists of an oblique incision across the rectus tendon. This has the advantage of allowing side-to-side repair and no specialized rehabilitation. The quadriceps snip results in only mild weakening of the quadriceps, with 16 of 16 knees having a satisfactory result at

2.5 years.[16] Tibial tubercle osteotomy may be necessary to gain exposure in the severely contracted knee. Tibial tubercle osteotomy has the advantage of allowing repositioning of the tibial tuberosity in a more proximal location to address a patella infera. It has the potential disadvantages of fracture of the tibial tubercle or associated tibial fracture, which occurred in 2 instances each in 136 knees in 1 series.[17] Marked tibial bone loss is a relative contraindication for tibial tubercle osteotomy. An alternative exposure technique is a subperiosteal dissection of the entire distal femur, the so-called femoral peel. This exposure would be selected for the severely contracted knee, such as is experienced in a delayed reimplantation for infection. The femoral peel necessitates the use of a constrained condylar prosthesis for revision.

Implant removal may be relatively easy if the implants are loose. In the case of a securely fixed implant, special implant removal equipment may be required. High speed cutting burrs, such as the Midas Rex (Midas Rex, Forth Worth, TX) or Anspach (Zimmer Inc, Warsaw, IN) device, should be available to allow dissection at the implant cement interface in order to preserve bone. Multiple osteotomes, including flexible osteotomes, should be available in order to assist in freeing the interfaces and allowing implant removal. A variety of implant extractors are available for use in implant removal, but they must be used in a gentle fashion to prevent excessive bone loss. A Gigli saw is an excellent instrument for dissecting interfaces adjacent to secure implants to assist in implant removal with minimal loss of bone. Some implants, such as constrained hinges, have a specific assembly and disassembly sequence and may require specialized tools for their removal. It is therefore helpful to review the implant type with the manufacturer's representative if the surgeon is unfamiliar with the specific device.

A rehabilitation plan will need to be formulated based on the anticipated bone defect and soft-tissue management at revision. A carefully supervised rehabilitation program is helpful in avoiding potential complications, such as patellar ligament avulsion, during rehabilitation.

In conclusion, begin by defining the mechanism or mechanisms of failure and any specific problems and deficiencies in the soft tissues and bone. Plan reconstruction to restore the normal joint line and kinematics of the knee with management of bone deficiency and restoration of alignment. Always have more than 1 option available for management of a complex problem, including implants with increased constraint if soft-tissue balancing cannot be adequately achieved. A carefully planned and supervised rehabilitation will help to maximize the results of revision knee arthroplasty.

References

1. Rand JA, Franco MG: Revision considerations for fractures about the knee, in Goldberg VM (ed): *Controversies of Total Knee Arthroplasty*. New York, NY, Raven Press, 1991, pp 235–247.

2. Wolff AM, Hungerford DS, Pepe CL: The effect of extraarticular varus and valgus deformity on total knee arthroplasty. *Clin Orthop* 1991;271:35–51.

3. Katz MM, Hungerford DS, Krackow KA, Lennox DW: Reflex sympathetic dystrophy as a cause of poor results after total knee arthroplasty. *J Arthroplasty* 1986;1:117–124.

4. Mont MA, Serna FK, Krackow KA, Hungerford DS: Exploration of radiographically normal total knee replacements for unexplained pain. *Clin Orthop* 1996;331:216–220.

5. Kim YH, Oh JH, Oh SH: Osteolysis around cementless porous-coated anatomic knee prostheses. *J Bone Joint Surg* 1995;77B:236–241.

6. Peters PC Jr, Engh GA, Dwyer KA, Vinh TN: Osteolysis after total knee arthroplasty without cement. *J Bone Joint Surg* 1992;74A:864–876.

7. Rosenberg AG, Barden RM, Galante JO: Cemented and ingrowth fixation of the Miller-Galante prosthesis: Clinical and roentgenographic comparison after three- to six-year follow-up studies. *Clin Orthop* 1990;260:71–79.

8. Rand JA, Chao EY, Stauffer RN: Kinematic rotating-hinge total knee arthroplasty. *J Bone Joint Surg* 1987;69A:489–497.

9. Beight JL, Yao B, Hozack WJ, Hearn SL, Booth RE Jr: The patellar "clunk" syndrome after posterior stabilized total knee arthroplasty. *Clin Orthop* 1994;299:139–142.

10. Martin SD, Haas SB, Insall JN: Primary total knee arthroplasty after patellectomy. *J Bone Joint Surg* 1995;77A:1323–1330.

11. Markovich GD, Dorr LD, Klein NE, McPherson EJ, Vince KG: Muscle flaps in total knee arthroplasty. *Clin Orthop* 1995;321:122–130.

12. Emerson RH Jr, Head WC, Malinin TI: Extensor mechanism reconstruction with an allograft after total knee arthroplasty. *Clin Orthop* 1994; 303:79–85.

13. Rand JA: Preoperative planning and templating in Rand JA (ed): *Total Knee Arthroplasty*. New York, NY, Raven Press, 1993, pp 93–114.

14. Fehring TK, McAvoy G: Fluoroscopic evaluation of the painful total knee arthroplasty. *Clin Orthop* 1996;331:226–233.

15. Trousdale RT, Hanssen AD, Rand JA, Cahalan TD: V-Y quadricepsplasty in total knee arthroplasty. *Clin Orthop* 1993;286:48–55.

16. Garvin KL, Scuderi G, Insall JN: Evolution of the quadriceps snip. *Clin Orthop* 1995;321:131–137.

17. Whiteside LA: Exposure in difficult total knee arthroplasty using tibial tubercle osteotomy. *Clin Orthop* 1995;321:32–35.

Bone Loss With Revision Total Knee Arthroplasty: Defect Classification and Alternatives for Reconstruction

Gerard A. Engh, MD
Deborah J. Ammeen, BS

Introduction

Bone loss and the associated soft-tissue laxity make the revision of a failed knee arthroplasty more challenging and less predictable than primary total knee arthroplasty (TKA). Today, the three most common reasons for knee revision are: aseptic loosening, osteolysis from polyethylene wear, and infection. Each of these failure mechanisms results in bone loss. Iatrogenic damage also occurs when a failed implant and the adjacent cement mantle are removed. When revising a knee with bone loss, the surgeon must focus on preserving bone and stabilizing the implants on strong, structurally intact viable bone. Augments and/or bone grafts are used to re-create a relatively normal anatomic joint-line level, restore flexion-extension stability with the least-constrained implant available, and eliminate hyperextension of the knee by restoring appropriate leg length. Classifying bone defects to describe the extent and location of bone damage is helpful when planning a revision arthroplasty. The severity of bone loss influences the type of prosthesis required, the need for bone grafts, and any special equipment that will be necessary.

The Frequency of Bone Defects

In many knees that require revision arthroplasty, bone defects are minor and adequate cancellous bone is present for cement interdigitation. In this situation, a primary component or a revision component without a stem can be used. Knees that have larger bone defects are best repaired with a long-stemmed revision component and augments or bone grafts to avoid joint-line elevation.

Goals of Revision Total Knee Arthroplasty

The goal of revision surgery, a pain-free, stable knee with a functional range of motion, may be difficult to achieve. In revision surgery, knee kinematics are restored, as much as possible, when a solid base of support for the components is provided at or near a normal joint-line level. This is accomplished by preserving all strong and viable metaphyseal bone that remains after the implant is removed and repairing bone defects with cement, metal wedges, or bone grafts. The collateral ligaments provide knee stability when an implant similar in size and configuration to the patient's femur is used and leg length is restored after the bone loss is repaired.

Implant Selection

An implant with the least amount of constraint required for satisfactory knee stability should be used in the revision. Linked implants, including rotating hinges and salvage tumor prostheses, are rarely indicated and should be reserved for cases that cannot be managed by applying the principles of bone repair, joint-line restoration, and proper flexion-extension balance.

Bone damage compromises the fixation interface for the component, particularly when it involves the loss of cancellous bone necessary for cement interdigitation. For this reason, a stem should be added to the revision component to transfer loads to the diaphyseal segment of the bone. A stem is essential if a varus-valgus-constrained implant is used.

Stratifying Bone Defects to Select the Method of Management

In general, clinical outcome studies of revision TKA have focused on the type of prosthesis used or on the mechanism by which the arthroplasty failed. No attempt has been made to examine the results of revision surgery on the basis of the extent of bone loss or the degree of soft-tissue

Type 1 defect
(Intact metaphyseal bone)
    Good cancellous bone at or near a normal
    joint-line level
Type 2 defect
(Damaged metaphyseal bone)
    Loss of cancellous bone that requires
    cement fill, augments, or small bone grafts
    to restore a reasonable joint-line level
Type 3 defect
(Deficient metaphyseal bone)
    Deficient bone that compromises a major
    portion of either condyle or plateau; these
    defects usually require a large structural
    allograft, a rotating hinged component, or
    custom component

*Anderson Orthopaedic Research Institute

Table 1
AORI* bone defect classification guidelines

	Preoperative Radiographs	Surgical Management
Type 1 defect (Intact metaphyseal bone)	A full metaphyseal segment	
Femur	Metaphyseal bone intact distal to the epicondyles No component subsidence or osteolysis	No augments, structural bone grafts, or cement fill > 1 cm
Tibia	Metaphyseal bone intact above the tibial tubercle No component subsidence or osteolysis	
Type 2 defect (Damaged metaphyseal bone)	A shortened metaphyseal flare	
Femur	Component subsidence or joint-line elevation of the failed component Small osteolytic defects in bone distal to the epicondyles	Joint-line restoration with augments (> 4 mm), particulate or chunk bone graft, or > 1 cm cement fill; joint-line elevation with a primary component as the revision implant
Tibia	Component subsidence or position up to or below the tip of the fibular head; a shortened tibial metaphyseal flare	
Type 3 defect (Deficient metaphyseal bone)	A deficient metaphyseal segment	
Femur	Bone damage to or above the level of the epicondyles Component subsidence to the epicondyles	A reconstructed condyle or plateau with structural graft or cement, or a custom or hinged component
Tibia	Bone damage or component subsidence to the tibial tubercle	

*Anderson Orthopaedic Research Institute

laxity. Established guidelines are needed for selecting the best revision prosthesis and method of reconstruction according to bone damage. By applying a bone defect classification to all revision arthroplasty cases and subsequently analyzing the outcome data, the surgeon can formulate answers to important questions as: (1) When is a stem needed with a revision component? (2) Should the stem or just the component be cemented? (3) What works better, morselized or structural bone graft? and (4) When is a salvage prosthesis needed?

Anderson Orthopaedic Research Institute (AORI) Bone Defect Classification

The AORI bone defect classification[1] uses the same categories to describe femoral as well as tibial bone loss (Outline 1). Bone defects are initially classified when the preoperative radiographs are examined. Type 1 defects have essentially healthy cancellous bone. Type 2 defects have bone damage that requires the use of an augment, bone graft, or cement fill to repair the bone defect. Type 3 defects have bone loss that requires

repair of the bone segment with structural bone graft or replacement with a custom or hinged component. Criteria have been established and should be adhered to when one is classifying bone defects (Table 1).

When each component is removed (femoral and/or tibial), the underlying bone defect is classified. Preoperative radiographs that reveal femoral damage to the level of the epicondyles or tibial damage down to the tubercle usually indicate a type 3 bone defect. The classification may change on the basis of the intraoperative examination of the bone damage and the method of reconstruction. For example, if a major structural

allograft or a hinged or a custom component is required to reconstruct the knee, the bone defect is classified as a type 3.

Postrevision radiographs should be used to confirm the bone defect classification. The metaphyseal segment of the femur and tibia has a distinct profile on the anteroposterior (AP) radiograph (Fig. 1). The widened segment of bone that constitutes the metaphyseal flare of the tibia should be evident on the radiograph of a type 1 tibial defect. Radiographs of a type 1 femoral defect should demonstrate an intact segment of bone distal to the epicondyles. Radiographs that demonstrate either joint-line elevation of

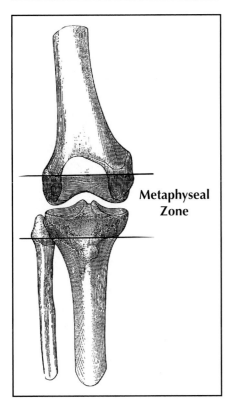

Fig. 1 The metaphyseal region of the knee. (Reproduced with permission from Engh GA: Bone defect classification, in Engh GA, Rorabeck CH (eds): *Revision Total Knee Arthroplasty*. Baltimore, MD, Williams & Wilkins, 1997, pp 63–120.)

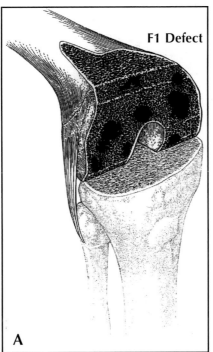

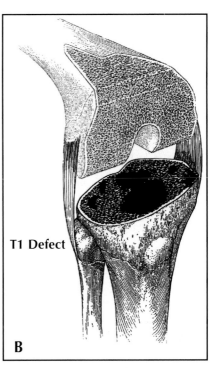

Fig. 2 A, Type 1 femoral defect (F1). **B,** Type 1 tibial defect (T1). (Reproduced with permission from Engh GA: Bone defect classification, in Engh GA, Rorabeck CH (eds): *Revision Total Knee Arthroplasty*. Baltimore, MD, Williams & Wilkins, 1997, pp 63–120.)

the component or a repaired segment filled with an augment or cement generally indicate a type 2 defect. When a type 3 bone defect has been repaired with an allograft, the host-allograft junction and the altered texture of the bone graft relative to the host bone are usually apparent on radiographic examination.

Alternatives for Management
Type 1 Bone Defects
It is appropriate to use contemporary primary total knee implants as the revision components when most type 1 bone defects are encountered (Fig. 2). With a type 1 defect, the most common mechanisms of failure are failed metal-backed patellae, failed uni-

condylar arthroplasties, and cases of polyethylene wear without osteolysis.

The failed primary implant is carefully removed with osteotomes to separate the implant from its cement mantle. Loose cement, debris, and any membranous tissue are then removed. Cement that is firmly attached can be retained as long as the possibility of infection has been ruled out. If the femoral component is being revised, it is important to maintain the dimensions of the posterior femoral condyles so that an implant with full AP condylar dimensions can be used to provide stability in flexion. Small cancellous defects may remain when the primary component and cement are removed. These defects can be filled with particulate bone graft or cement. If the posterior cruciate ligament is no longer functional, a posterior-stabilized implant should be used for the revision.

In some circumstances, a revision component is appropriate even when no measurable bone defect is present. This situation occurs when the bone is intact but structurally weak from osteoporosis and stress shielding from the primary components, or when instability of the knee requires that a more constrained implant design be used for the revision.

Type 2 Bone Defects
The most common cause of type 2 bone defects is aseptic loosening of a primary component (Fig. 3). Implant subsidence leads to progressive loss of bone beneath the component. The loose component often migrates to an angulated position with more extensive bone loss in one condyle or plateau. When only one condyle or plateau is involved, the bone on the uninvolved side is preserved at revision surgery to maintain a rela-

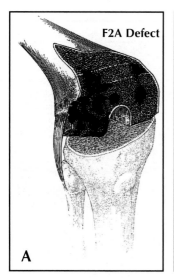
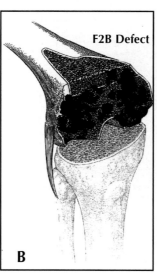
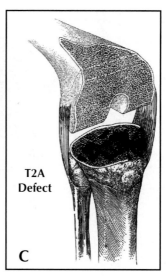
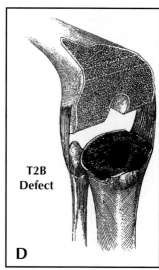

Fig. 3 A, Type 2A femoral defect (F2A). **B,** Type 2B femoral defect (F2B). **C,** Type 2A tibial defect (T2A). **D,** Type 2B tibial defect (T2B). (Reproduced with permission from Engh GA: Bone defect classification, in Engh GA, Rorabeck CH (eds): *Revision Total Knee Arthroplasty*. Baltimore, MD, Williams & Wilkins, 1997, pp 63–120.)

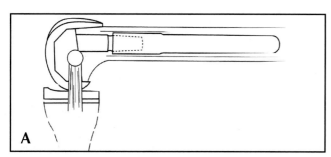
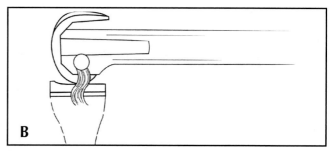

Fig. 4 A, The anterior stem location on the femoral component restores stability in flexion by positioning the femoral condyles posterior to the epicondylar axis. **B,** A stem position near the center of the femoral component leaves the implant prominent anteriorly. There is no tension on the collateral ligaments in flexion.

tively normal joint line. Modular augments permit repair of the damaged condyle or plateau without sacrificing the relatively healthy bone on the uninvolved side.

Contemporary modular revision implant systems are ideal for managing type 2 defects. These systems offer a variety of augment thicknesses and stems of different diameters and lengths. With a suitably large component, augments are used to restore an appropriate joint-line level and achieve knee stability in both flexion and extension. Stems are used to transfer loads from the damaged metaphyseal

region to the diaphyseal bone.

Type 2 defects may involve one condyle or plateau (type 2A) or both condyles or plateaus (type 2B). Preoperative radiographs of a type 2A defect often demonstrate the angular position of a loose component that has subsided. Intraoperatively, augments are added to the cutting guides (on the side with the bone defect) and the knee is reconstructed to the length of the relatively normal condyle or plateau. This procedure restores stability in extension. Stability in flexion is restored when a femoral component with an appropriately large AP

dimension is used to tense the flexion gap.

Type 2B defects are commonly encountered in patients who have undergone multiple revisions. A patient with a type 2B defect may present with a stiff knee and a large flexion contracture or with an unstable knee that becomes increasingly unstable as a loose implant subsides. To achieve full knee extension when a type 2B defect with a large flexion contracture is reconstructed, the surgeon must place the femoral component at a more proximal location. In this situation, the joint line is intentionally being raised; therefore, the distal femoral bone defects from component migration are not repaired. The postoperative radiographs confirm the joint-line elevation of the femoral component.

In an unstable knee with a type 2B defect, large augments are required to tense the ligaments and restore stability. A relatively large femoral component is necessary for flexion stability. Both distal and posterior augments are usually needed on the femoral component. The stem of the revision femoral component needs to attach anteriorly on the component (Fig. 4). The anterior stem location on the femoral component reestablishes the anatomic posterior offset of the posterior femoral condyles, thus restoring knee stability in flexion.

Type 3 Bone Defects

Prior to the introduction of modular revision total knee implants, type 3 bone defects (Fig. 5) were frequently managed with cement fill and a primary short-stemmed component or a custom implant. However, in such cases, failure often occurred, either by aseptic loosening or progressive knee instability. Contemporary modular revision components were designed to address these bone deficiencies through the use of modular augments, stems, and constrained inserts. However, modular revision components that work well for type 2 bone defects are not sufficient to manage the depth of a type 3 defect that involves extensive bone loss or ligament instability.

The deficient bone of a type 3 bone defect is best replaced with an allograft or an implant with large or custom augments. Occasionally, knee stability is compromised as a result of component migration and the loss of collateral ligament attachments to the epicondyles. In this case, a condylar

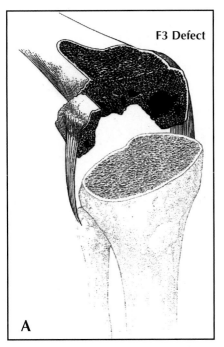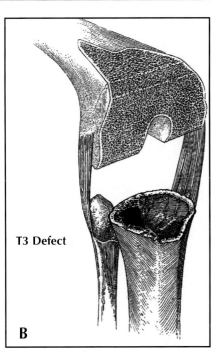

Fig. 5 A, Type 3 femoral defect (F3). **B,** Type 3 tibial defect (T3). (Adapted with permission from Engh GA: Bone defect classification, in Engh GA, Rorabeck CH (eds): *Revision Total Knee Arthroplasty*. Baltimore, MD, Williams & Wilkins, 1997, pp 63–120.)

replacement prosthesis (a rotating-hinge component) is an acceptable alternative. Fixed-hinge components are contraindicated due to the reported high incidence of both septic and aseptic loosening.[2,3]

The preoperative radiographs of a type 3 femoral bone defect reveal bone loss to the level of the femoral epicondyles. The AP and lateral radiographs may demonstrate bone loss from osteolysis with lytic changes proximal to the femoral component, or they may show component migration to the level of the epicondyle on one or both sides. Often the femoral component subsides within the confines of the epicondyles, thereby creating a large cavitary lesion. Particularly when only one condyle is involved, this type of bone defect can be successfully filled and/or reconstructed with a structural femoral head allograft. Alternatively, large chunks of allograft bone can be cut into ½-inch

cubes and impacted into the bone defect. When used with a long-stemmed component, these techniques work quite well to prevent graft collapse and control implant subsidence. Although cementless component fixation has been successful in conjunction with allograft repair,[4] the risk of component subsidence and an unsatisfactory clinical result with knee instability make cemented component fixation preferable.

There are 3 options for managing a type 3 bone defect that involves both femoral condyles: a femoral head allograft for each condyle, a composite distal femoral allograft, or a rotating-hinge prosthesis. If deep cavitary bone defects in both condyles or plateaus are contained within a peripheral shell of bone, two femoral heads fill the defect well (Fig. 6). The peripheral shell of bone provides stability for the femoral head allografts.

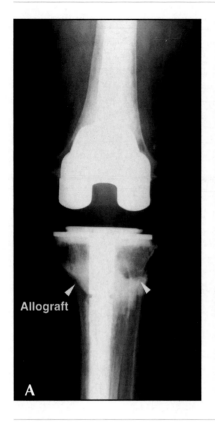

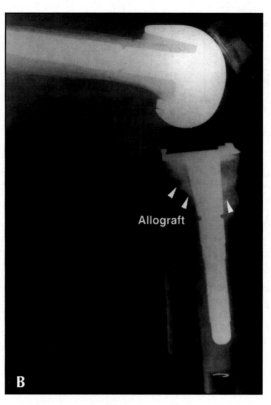

Fig. 6 A, A cemented long-stemmed tibial component and 2 large structural femoral head allografts have been used for type 3 tibial (T3) bone defect reconstruction. For bone defect repairs using an allograft, we prefer to use a cemented component, but a press-fit stem. **B,** The femur has been revised with augments and cement fill. A structural allograft has been used to repair the T3 tibial defect.

A female hemispherical reamer is used to remove the cartilage and subchondral bone from the femoral head allograft. Next, the condylar defect is reamed to a diameter 2 mm smaller than the graft diameter to remove dense sclerotic bone and create a hemispheric shape to the bone defect. The graft is then impacted into the prepared bone defect or attached with K-wires. Once the allografts are in place, the arthroplasty resection instruments are used to prepare the femur for the revision component. After the revision prosthesis is implanted, the K-wires that were inserted for temporary graft stability are removed.

A composite (distal femoral allograft and a long-stemmed revision prosthesis) is particularly applicable for severe type 3 femoral bone defects with peripheral bone loss that includes the attachments of the epicondyles. Allograft composites should

be considered for comminuted supracondylar fractures that cannot be stabilized, for failed hinged components, and for rerevisions with massive bone loss from recurrent aseptic loosening.

Preoperative planning for an allograft composite begins with quality radiographs of the patient's knees. Radiographs of the patient's unoperated knee are important because they provide a template for selecting an allograft of similar dimensions. The allograft should be of the same cadaveric bone segment and from the same side as the bone segment undergoing reconstruction (ie, right distal femur for a right distal femoral composite revision). The extent of bone damage above the failed total knee must be considered when the length of the allograft required for the revision is being determined. The stem of the revision prosthesis must be long enough to extend at least 5 cm beyond the damaged bone segment.

The first step in preparing the distal femur for an allograft composite is to osteotomize the femoral epicondyles of the host bone. The epicondyles will be attached to the allograft once the revision component is implanted. After the failed components are removed, the distal femur is step cut in the coronal plane. The longer portion of the step cut is on the less-damaged side of the host femur. The femoral canal is reamed by hand with progressively larger, rigid intramedullary reamers until a tight fit of the reamer is achieved.

Revision arthroplasty is then performed on the distal femoral allograft. The intramedullary canal of the allograft is opened to the same diameter as the largest reamer used to prepare the host femur. The length of the graft is adjusted by placement of the condyles of the revision femoral component against the prepared proximal tibia. The knee is distracted

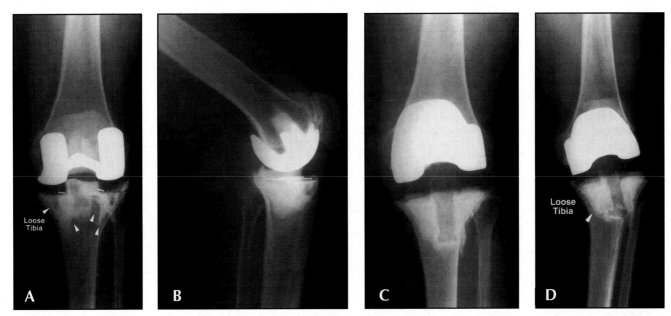

Fig. 7 A, This Geometric (Zimmer, Warsaw, IN) total knee arthroplasty has failed by aseptic loosening of the tibial component. The preoperative tibial bone defect classification is a T3 (type 3 tibial). **B,** This lateral radiograph confirms an F2/T3 (type 2 femoral/type 3 tibial) defect classification. The posterior condyles were removed with the index arthroplasty. Cement fill extends far distal to the fibular head. **C,** The F2/T3 bone defects were managed with primary components and cement fill on the tibial side. **D,** The femoral component has subsided into valgus and the tibial component into varus. Cement fill is unsatisfactory for managing large bone defects. The anticipated bone defect classification is an F3/T3 (type 3 femoral/type 3 tibial).

and the graft marked for length at the level of the proximal step cut on the femur. The stem of the trial femoral component, intercalated through the allograft, is then inserted into the patient's femoral canal and advanced until the graft contacts the longer side of the step cut femur. The allograft is marked and resected with a step cut to fit the distal femur when the step cuts are fully engaged. The final length of the allograft is adjusted by removal of additional bone from the allograft until the knee will come to full extension but not hyperextend with a 12-mm thick tibial component in place.

Bone cement is used to fix the revision femoral component to the allograft; however, the stem is press fit into the host femur. Morcellized autograft bone is added to the junction between the host and allograft bone. Onlay allograft struts from the unused portion of the allograft are attached with cerclage wire to the host-graft junction. These struts provide additional rotational stability.

Stability of the knee in flexion is restored when the host epicondyles are attached to the allograft. First, the epicondyles of the allograft must be excised. With the knee in 90° of flexion, the host epicondyles are attached to the allograft distal femur with #2 (or heavier) nonabsorbable sutures. The epicondyles should be brought as far anteriorly on the allograft as permitted by the tension in the collateral ligaments. Stability is first tested with a posterior-stabilized component. A varus-valgus-constrained insert should only be used if satisfactory stability is not achieved with a less-constrained insert after the epicondyles have been attached to the allograft.

The postoperative management of a type 3 bone defect reconstruction depends on the stability of the epicon-

dyles during knee flexion. Excellent stability is usually achieved when the host epicondyles are sutured to the allograft. In densely scarred knees, additional stability is often achieved when the capsular envelope of the knee is repaired. In these cases, a knee brace is not necessary postoperatively. However, if the epicondyles have not been rigidly attached to the allograft and motion between the host and graft is observed with knee flexion, a hinged knee brace should be used to limit knee flexion until the epicondyles have healed to the allograft.

Clinical Results: Revision Knee Arthroplasty With Large Bone Defects

The following options may be used for revising a failed knee arthroplasty associated with significant bone loss: (1) a primary component and cement to fill the bone defect; (2) a fixed- or rotating-hinged component; (3) a modified or custom component with stems and augments; or (4) a revision component with repair of the bone defects. The results of revisions involving these options are largely unreported in clinical studies of revision TKA because bone defects have not been categorized. However, we can gain insight into the efficacy of these options by looking at the results of revision knee surgery that involves large structural allografts to repair bone defects, or hinged implants that require removal of most of the metaphyseal bone for prosthesis insertion.

Primary Components—Hinged Components

The first option, using short-stemmed components and filling the bone defects with cement, is biomechanically unsound[5] (Fig. 7). The results have not been reported. Clinical results of the second option, the use of hinged implants, have not been good even when the implants were used as primary components in cases without bone defects.[2,3] Most of the failures resulted either from component loosening or from fracture of the femur at the tip of the femoral stem. Inglis and Walker[2] reported failure in 16 of 40 revisions that used fixed-axis hinges. Rerevision was required after an average 4.5 years.[2]

Rotating hinges were designed to address the problem of instability often associated with progressive bone loss and multiple revision surgeries. This type of implant allows axial rotation while providing varus-valgus and sagittal plane stability. However, in several studies, the clinical results have not been significantly better than with fixed-hinged components. Rand and associates[6] reported complications in over 50% of cases with the Kinematic Rotating Hinge (Howmedica, Rutherford, NJ). Progression of lucent lines was

seen in 42%, with probable loosening in 16%, and deep sepsis in 16% of cases.[6] Shaw and associates[7] reported aseptic progression of lucencies in 20% of revision cases when the same type of implant was used. The authors recommend and these studies confirm that the only indication for a mechanically linked prosthesis occurs when satisfactory stability cannot be achieved with a less-constrained prosthetic device.

Modified or Custom Components

The Total Condylar III (TC III, Johnson & Johnson, Raynham, MA) and Constrained Condylar Knee (CCK, Zimmer, Warsaw, IN) prostheses are nonlinked, semiconstrained prostheses that enhance varus-valgus stability with an enlarged tibial spine or post. These components were initially available with fixed stems of intermediate length for use in unstable knees. Donaldson and associates[8] reported satisfactory results with no failures of the TC III implant in 17 primary arthroplasties, but did observe a 36% failure rate from infection or aseptic loosening in 14 knee revision arthroplasties. Lachiewicz and Falatyn[9] similarly reported no mechanical failures with the TC III and CCK implants in 25 primary arthroplasties, but had 2 mechanical failures in 21 revision arthroplasties. In both of these studies, most of the component stems were fully cemented. There was no apparent difference in outcome when the bone defects were repaired either with augments or bone grafts. Rosenberg and associates[10] reviewed 36 knees revised with a TC III prosthesis at an average follow-up of 45 months. Although only 1 implant failed by aseptic loosening in this study, 16.7% demonstrated progressive radiolucencies on the tibial side. Eight patients who required

structural bone grafts showed no evidence of structural graft failure.[10]

Initially radiographs of the failed arthroplasty were used to custom design modified components. In most instances extended stems were attached to semiconstrained implants to manage bone and ligament damage. The surgeon selected variables such as the length and diameter of the stems as well as augment thicknesses. In most institutions, the clinical experience with custom implants is limited to a small number of cases. In 1991, Elia and Lotke[11] reported the most comprehensive study of a variety of modified implants, mostly with extended stems. In this series of 40 knees with bone defects deeper than 1 cm, the failure rate was 10% from loosening or instability at an average 41-month follow-up. No significant difference was found when the results of using cement, bone grafts, or custom components to manage bone defects were compared.

Stemmed Revision Implants With Augments or Cement: Bone Defects Not Classified

The evolution in prosthetic design to the modular revision prosthesis available today has been relatively recent; therefore there are only a few cases with adequate follow-up for study. In addition, most reports have been retrospective and have not categorized the extent of bone damage at the time of reconstruction. In one such study with a 3.5-year follow-up, metal wedges, augments, and cementless stems were used successfully in 84% of revision cases for aseptic loosening.[12] There was no difference between the 57 knees revised with a posterior-stabilized insert and the 19 with a condylar-constrained polyethylene. In another study, there was no apparent adverse effect of using cement to fill central bone defects in 40 long-stemmed Kinematic Stabilizer (Howmedica, Rutherford, NJ) revision cases or in using a fully cemented stem.[13] At an average follow-up of 56 months, only 1 case of aseptic loosening was identified.[13]

Stemmed Revision Components and Structural Allografts: Type 3 Bone Defects

The intermediate results of revision TKA involving structural allografts to repair massive bone defects (deficient bone/type 3 defects) are extensively reported. The bone defect repair consisted of femoral heads attached with screws or captured between the implant and host bone and stabilized with cement or with an allograft-prosthesis composite. Over 90% of the 131 reconstructions from a tabulation of cases from 8 different studies had not failed.[14-21] In the 2 largest series, the longest follow-up averaged 50 months.[14,20] Graft union and fixation stability were achieved most consistently when cementless, long intramedullary stems were used in the reconstruction. Axial loading of the host-graft junction prevented host-graft nonunion.

Large structural allografts used in revision TKA do not revascularize, resorb, or collapse.[22] From cadaveric retrievals, Parks and Engh[22] have demonstrated the ability of structural allografts to unite to host bone and provide structural support for a femoral or tibial component. Unlike acetabular bone grafts, the trabeculae of a femoral head allograft or a composite graft appears adequate for bone-defect reconstruction when used in conjunction with a long-stemmed component. More importantly, structural allografts appear to consistently heal to damaged host bone, including cortical bone in which it is difficult, if not impossible, to achieve good cement interdigitation.

Summary

Although the best method for managing large bone defects has not been established, the variables to consider are: (1) implant constraint (posterior-stabilized, varus-valgus-constrained, rotating hinge); (2) stem configuration (straight versus tapered, standard, or long-stemmed); (3) stem fixation (cement versus press-fit); and (4) method of bone-defect repair (cement, augments, bone graft). In principle, an implant with the least constraint required for satisfactory knee stability is selected to reduce stress on the implant-fixation interface with compromised bone. The severity of bone loss largely influences stem length. Canal-filling stems and cementless stem fixation are indicated when major structural allografts are used. Bone defects can be successfully and reliably repaired with metal augments, allograft bone, or cement, as long as long-stemmed components without excessive constraint are selected. Because structural allografts do not revascularize, the major advantage of the allograft, as compared to cement fill or augments, is the ability to unite to damaged host bone that has a poor cancellous structure.

References

1. Engh GA: Bone defect classification, in Engh GA, Rorabeck CH (eds): *Revision Total Knee Arthroplasty*. Baltimore, MD, Williams & Wilkins, 1997, pp 63–120.
2. Inglis AE, Walker PS: Revision of failed knee replacements using fixed-axis hinges. *J Bone Joint Surg* 1991;73B:757–761.
3. Jones EC, Insall JN, Inglis AE, Ranawat CS: GUEPAR knee arthroplasty results and late complications. *Clin Orthop* 1979;140:145–152.
4. Whiteside LA: Cementless reconstruction of massive tibial bone loss in revision total knee arthroplasty. *Clin Orthop* 1989;248:80–86.
5. Brooks PJ, Walker PS, Scott RD: Tibial component fixation in deficient tibial bone stock. *Clin Orthop* 1984;184:302–308.
6. Rand JA, Chao EY, Stauffer RN: Kinematic rotating-hinge total knee arthroplasty. *J Bone Joint Surg* 1987;69A:489–497.
7. Shaw JA, Balcom W, Greer RB III: Total knee arthroplasty using the kinematic rotating hinge prosthesis. *Orthopedics* 1989;12:647–654.
8. Donaldson WF III, Sculco TP, Insall JN, Ranawat CS: Total condylar III knee prosthesis: Long-term follow-up study. *Clin Orthop* 1988;226:21–28.
9. Lachiewicz PF, Falatyn SP: Clinical and radiographic results of the total condylar III and constrained condylar total knee arthroplasty. *J Arthroplasty* 1996;11:916–922.
10. Rosenberg AG, Verner JJ, Galante JO: Clinical results of total knee revision using the total condylar III prosthesis. *Clin Orthop* 1991;273:83–90.
11. Elia EA, Lotke PA: Results of revision total knee arthroplasty associated with significant bone loss. *Clin Orthop* 1991;271:114–121.
12. Haas SB, Insall JN, Montgomery W III, Windsor RE: Revision total knee arthroplasty with use of modular components with stems inserted without cement. *J Bone Joint Surg* 1995;77A:1700–1707.
13. Murray PB, Rand JA, Hanssen AD: Cemented long-stem revision total knee arthroplasty. *Clin Orthop* 1994;309:116–123.
14. Ghazavi MT, Stockley I, Yee G, Davis A, Gross AE: Reconstruction of massive bone defects with allograft in revision total knee arthroplasty. *J Bone Joint Surg* 1997;79A:17–25.
15. Tsahakis PJ, Beaver WB, Brick GW: Technique and results of allograft reconstruction in revision total knee arthroplasty. *Clin Orthop* 1994;303:86–94.
16. Mnaymneh W, Emerson RH, Borja F, Head WC, Malinin TI: Massive allografts in salvage revisions of failed total knee arthroplasties. *Clin Orthop* 1990;260:144–153.
17. Harris AI, Poddar S, Gitelis S, Sheinkop MB, Rosenberg AG: Arthroplasty with a composite of an allograft and a prosthesis for knees with severe deficiency of bone. *J Bone Joint Surg* 1995;77A:373–386.
18. Kraay MJ, Goldberg VM, Figgie MP, Figgie HE III: Distal femoral replacement with allograft/prosthetic reconstruction for treatment of supracondylar fractures in patients with total knee arthroplasty. *J Arthroplasty* 1992;7:7–16.
19. Mow CS, Wiedel JD: Structural allografting in revision total knee arthroplasty. *J Arthroplasty* 1996;11:235–241.
20. Engh GA, Herzwurm PJ, Parks NL: Treatment of major defects of bone with bulk allografts and stemmed components during total knee arthroplasty. *J Bone Joint Surg* 1997;79A:1030–1039.
21. Wilde AH, Schickendantz MS, Stulberg BN, Go RT: The incorporation of tibial allografts in total knee arthroplasty. *J Bone Joint Surg* 1990;72A:815–824.
22. Parks NL, Engh GA: Histology of nine structural bone grafts used in total knee arthroplasty. *Clin Orthop* 1997;345:17–23.

Cementless Fixation Issues in Revision Total Knee Arthroplasty

Leo A. Whiteside, MD

Introduction

Reconstitution of bone stock is a primary concern at revision surgery for failed total knee arthroplasty (Fig. 1). Fixation often is difficult because the cancellous bone has been depleted, so it may be tempting to cement the implant to diaphyseal cortical bone. However, revision with cement ultimately destroys more bone stock. Rather, cementless fixation techniques that use an uncemented stem to engage the isthmus and bone graft to fill the defects can provide adequate fixation as well as afford the opportunity to reconstruct the bone stock about the knee.[1–3]

The main concerns with massive bone grafting—vascularization and incorporation—remain significant issues in the knee,[4] and bone grafting with allograft still raises the question of immunocompatibility. Bone tissue itself is not highly immunogenic, but the marrow cells incite a vigorous immune response[5] and can create an inflammatory process that blocks ossification and incorporation of the graft.[6]

Early reports of allograft reconstruction in the tibia and cementless fixation of the tibial component have been encouraging,[1,2] and reconstruction of the femur with cementless components now has been well documented in the literature.[7,8] Loss of bone in the distal femur is a major problem after a cemented total knee arthroplasty has failed, and revision surgery with a cemented stem can cause even more bone loss. An effort has been made since 1984 to reconstruct bone defects with morcellized allograft bone and to fix the implants to the existing bone structure without cement. Initially it was thought that cementless fixation of the components would be tenuous and that repeat revision would be necessary to achieve durable fixation with the improved bone stock. However, durability of the construct has been surprisingly reliable and repeated revision due to failure of fixation has not been necessary.[3]

In cases of infected total knee arthroplasty, treatment regimens range from debridement and antibiotics to removal and fusion, but the standard treatment has been to remove the implants, treat with antibiotics for 6 weeks, and finally perform revision

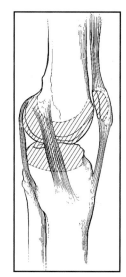

Fig. 1 Bone loss from the femur, tibia, and patella may be extensive in failed total knee arthroplasty, but the ligaments and capsule usually are competent. Cancellous bone stock is rarely intact. The shaded area represents loss of cortical wall and cancellous structure. The ligaments, capsule, and tendons usually are intact. (Reproduced with permission from Whiteside LA: Bone grafting in revision cementless total knee arthroplasty. *Tech Orthop* 1992;7:39–46.)

arthroplasty with antibiotic-impregnated cement.[9–12] However, cementless reconstruction is attractive for

This chapter has been adapted with permission from Whiteside LA: Results of cementless revision total knee arthroplasty, in Engh GA, Rorabeck CH (eds): *Revision Total Knee Arthroplasty*. Baltimore, MD, Williams & Wilkins, 1997, pp 444–459.

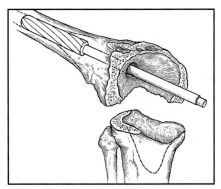

Fig. 2 Intramedullary alignment provides the only reliable landmarks for minimal resection. Recognizing that severe bone loss has occurred, the surgeon should resect only a small amount of bone to allow firm footing for the implant. (Reproduced with permission from Whiteside LA: Results of cementless revision total knee arthroplasty, in Engh GA, Rorabeck CH (eds): *Revision Total Knee Arthroplasty*. Baltimore, MD, Williams & Wilkins, 1997, pp 444–459.)

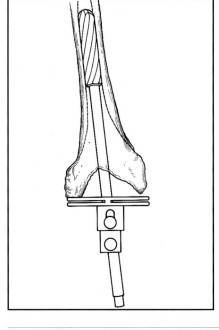

Fig. 3 Large cavitary and peripheral defects are present with failure of large implants. Intramedullary instruments provide the only reliable landmarks for resection. As little bone as possible is taken from the distal femur. (Reproduced with permission from Whiteside LA: Results of cementless revision total knee arthroplasty, in Engh GA, Rorabeck CH (eds): *Revision Total Knee Arthroplasty*. Baltimore, MD, Williams & Wilkins, 1997, pp 444–459.)

these revision cases because further bone destruction is avoided and bone stock can also be restored.[1,2,13,14] This chapter describes a technique for using bone graft to treat massive bone loss in cementless reconstruction of a failed total knee arthroplasty.

Bone Preparation Technique

Bone loss is one of the major problems in failed total knee arthroplasty, so minimal bone should be resected during preparation to preserve the remaining bone stock (Fig. 2). The amount of bone erosion makes complete seating of the component nearly impossible, so that augmented fixation with a stem almost always is necessary to achieve toggle control of the implant. This technique results in substantial, uncontained defects in both the femur and the tibia. Seating the implant on the existing bone stock controls axial migration, and the stem prevents the implant from tilting into the defect. Screw and peg fixation can add stability to the con-

struct, thereby allowing the cavitary deficiencies to be filled with morcellized bone. This bone grafting technique promotes rapid healing and reconstitution of bone stock without the technical difficulty and late collapse associated with massive allograft replacement.

Femoral Preparation

When bone destruction is assessed, the medial and lateral condyles usually are found to be partially intact. With intramedullary instrumentation as a guide, the distal surface of the femur is resected just enough to achieve firm seating of the femoral component on 1 side of the bone. Both sides may be engaged by the implant in some cases, but often only 1 of the 2 condyles can afford firm seating for the femoral component without excessive resection of the distal femur (Fig. 3). After all the cuts are made with the saw and all the surfaces are prepared (Fig. 4), the femoral component is partially inserted and the morcellized allograft is packed into the deficient areas. The

implant then is driven until it is fully seated, and then more bone graft can be packed tightly into the distal and posterior cavitary defects (Fig. 5). Prolonged protection from weight-bearing allows healing of bone into the cavitary defects for mediolateral and anteroposterior support of the implant.

Tibial Preparation

Reconstruction of massive tibial defects also relies upon rim support for axial loading and a stem to stabilize the implant. Screws can be used effectively in the tibial component to augment fixation, with nonstructural allograft filling the central and peripheral defects. Massive block allografting is feasible for these defects, but with long-stem and augmented fixation, morcellized cancellous allografting can reconstruct the proximal tibial bone with low failure and complication rates.[3]

The lateral tibial cortex usually is relatively well preserved, and the fibular head almost always is present. The fibular head can be used for

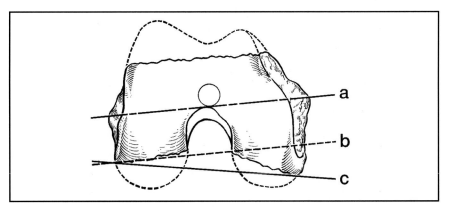

Fig. 4 A straight line through the medial and lateral femoral epicondyles provides correct rotational alignment. The dotted lines represent the original contours of the distal femur before total knee failure. Line a passes through the epicondyles. Line b represents the proper resection line for the posterior femoral condyles. If line c is followed, severe internal rotation of the femoral component will occur. (Reproduced with permission from Whiteside LA: Bone grafting in revision cementless total knee arthroplasty. *Tech Orthop* 1992;7:39–46.)

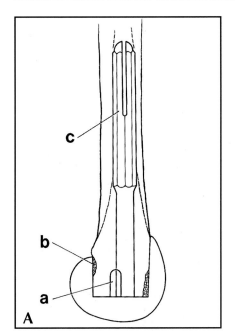
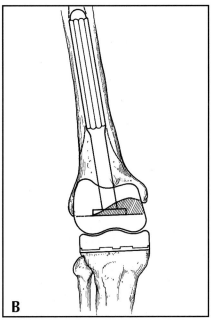

Fig. 5 A, Fixation of the femoral component into viable bone is achieved by means of a posterior stabilizing housing: (a) a peg driven into the distal femoral surface, (b) a thickened posterior surface, and (c) a long stem, which allows soft bone graft to be used. **B,** The stem fixed tightly in the diaphysis in combination with rim seating prevents the implant from migrating proximally and tilting into the defect. (Reproduced with permission from Whiteside LA: Results of cementless revision total knee arthroplasty, in Engh GA, Rorabeck CH (eds): *Revision Total Knee Arthroplasty.* Baltimore, MD, Williams & Wilkins, 1997, pp 444–459.)

proximal seating of the tibial component if the remaining tibial architecture is severely destroyed (Fig. 6). In the worst cases, all cancellous bone is gone, leaving a large cavitary defect and substantial deficiency of the tibial rim. Long-stem fixation is advised in these cases regardless of whether block allografting or morcellized allografting technique is used. When morcellized graft is used, the tibial tray should seat on the intact portion of the tibial rim, and the stem should engage the isthmus of the tibia. As with the femoral component, the tightly fit diaphyseal stem maintains stability and prevents tilting of the component so that massive defects may be filled with allograft and protected until healing and bone formation occur in the grafted area (Fig. 7).

Grafting Technique

Block allograft traditionally has been used for massive bone deficiencies, but the complication rate is high, and the destructive effects of allograft rejection can limit long-term success.[6,15] Large segments of allograft also heal slowly, are never replaced by new bone, and weaken as the ossification and vascularization front proceeds.[16,17] In contrast, morcellized allograft has proven structurally reliable for both small and large defects while supporting new bone formation.[18,19] Pieces of morcellized bone that are 1 cm in diameter maintain their integrity long enough to act as a substrate for new bone formation. Pieces smaller than 0.5 to 1 cm in diameter tend to be resorbed, and those larger than 1 cm incorporate slowly, if ever, and tend to collapse.

Rejection can be a major problem with allograft bone because marrow is immunogenic.[6,15] However, marrow elements can be thoroughly removed from morcellized allograft to prevent the inflammatory response and loss of graft, and to capitalize on the osteoconductive potential of the allograft. The allograft acts as scaffolding for new bone growth, and although it is not osteoinductive, demineralized bone, which is mildly osteoinductive, can be added to the allograft to enhance bone formation. The surrounding bone structure supplies most of the osteoinductive activity because metaphyseal

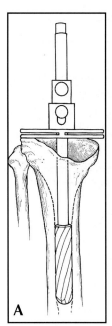

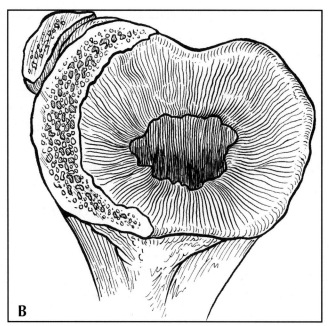

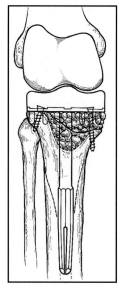

Fig. 6 A, Intramedullary instruments allow accurate alignment. Here a planer is used to trim the upper tibial rim. Minimal resection should be done, which may leave large rim defects. (Reproduced with permission from Whiteside LA: Results of cementless revision total knee arthroplasty, in Engh GA, Rorabeck CH (eds): *Revision Total Knee Arthroplasty*. Baltimore, MD, Williams & Wilkins, 1997, pp 444–459.) B, With long stem support of the tibial component, one quarter of the rim of the proximal tibia can be used to support the implant. The fibular head also may be used for tibial support. (Reproduced with permission from Whiteside LA: Bone grafting in revision cementless total knee arthroplasty. *Tech Orthop* 1992;7:39–46.)

Fig. 7 Fixation of the tibial component with rim contact on viable bone, screw fixation into the cortical shell, peg fixation into intact bone structure, and stem fixation into the diaphysis allows adequate stabilization until the grafted area can be incorporated. (Reproduced with permission from Whiteside LA: Results of cementless revision total knee arthroplasty, in Engh GA, Rorabeck CH (eds): *Revision Total Knee Arthroplasty*. Baltimore, MD, Williams & Wilkins, 1997, pp 444–459.)

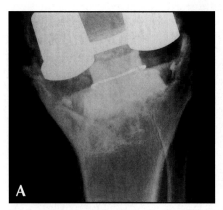

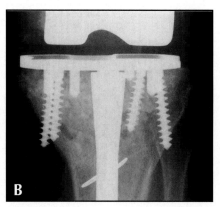

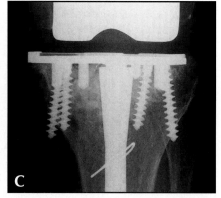

Fig. 8 A, Preoperative radiograph of a left knee with a failed cemented component. Massive central and peripheral bone loss has occurred. B, Radiograph of the same knee at 1 month postoperative. Tibial grafting with morcellized allograft fills the defect. The lateral edge of the tibial tray is resting on bone. The stem prevents the medial edge from sinking into the allograft. C, Radiograph of the same knee at 7 years postoperative. The graft has ossified and trabecular bone is evident along the medial side of the tibia.

bone has a rich blood supply and maintains the capacity to heal even after repeated failed arthroplasty.

Grafting Preparation and Placement
Pieces of morcellized fresh-frozen cancellous allograft measuring 0.5 to

1 cm in diameter are soaked for 5 to 10 minutes in normal saline solution that contains 500,000 units of

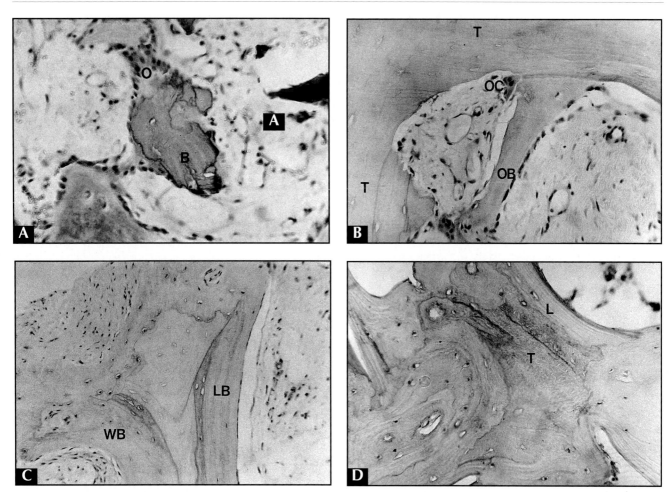

Fig. 9 A, Photograph of histologic section from the 3-week biopsy specimen. Granules of demineralized bone (B) are visible and are surrounded by plump osteoblasts (O) and new osteoid. Vascular stroma is present throughout the allografted area. There is no histologic evidence of bone resorption. (Stain, hematoxylin and eosin; original magnification, × 160.) **B,** Photograph of histologic section from the 3-month biopsy specimen. Dead trabeculae (T) are still abundant. Osteoclasts (OC) and new osteoid with osteoblasts (OB) are evident adjacent to the allograft. The allografted area contains multiple sites of bone resorption. New osteoid often is found on 1 surface of a trabecula and osteoclastic resorption on the opposite surface. Osteoblasts at this time interval are flatter and less numerous than in the 3-week biopsy specimen. (Stain, hematoxylin and eosin; original magnification, × 160.) **C,** Photograph of histologic section from the 21-month biopsy specimen. Mature lamellar bone (LB) and disorganized woven bone (WB) surround the allograft. The bone remodeling rate in the allografted area has decreased significantly. Trabeculae now are entombed completely by mature or woven bone. Bone remodeling has decreased and osteoblastic or osteoclastic activity is directed toward new bone, not toward allograft. (Stain, hematoxylin and eosin; original magnification, × 100.) **D,** Photograph of histologic section from the 37-month biopsy specimen. Entombed trabeculae (T) are present throughout the allograft biopsy. The visible allograft is completely encased by mature lamellar bone (L). Bone remodeling continues at normal levels; few osteoclasts are found, and there is minimal evidence of osteoblastic activity. (Stain, hematoxylin and eosin; original magnification, × 100.) (Reproduced with permission from Whiteside LA: Results of cementless revision total knee arthroplasty, in Engh GA, Rorabeck CH (eds): *Revision Total Knee Arthroplasty*. Baltimore, MD, Williams & Wilkins, 1997, pp 444–459.)

polymyxin, 50,000 units of bacitracin, and 1 g per liter of cephazolin. The fluid is removed and 10 cc of powdered demineralized cancellous bone is added to each 30 cc of the cancellous morcellized bone. Bone fragments and diaphyseal reamings are added to improve the osteoinductive potential. The medullary contents are aspirated into a mucous trap, the fat is allowed to rise to the surface and is suctioned off. Then the bone-cell-rich aqueous portion is added to the allograft bone mixture just prior to the grafting procedure. This mixture is packed into the bone defects, and the implants are then impacted so that they seat on the remnant of viable bone while compacting the morcellized bone graft.

Summary and Conclusion

Although massive solid allografts can be expected to vascularize and form new bone,[20] variable amounts of replacement as well as collapse and necrosis may be prominent features of these large block allografts.[16,17]

Immunocompatibility seems to be an important factor in allograft healing and incorporation. Large block allograft of the acetabulum appears to be more likely to succeed if autograft is used.[21] Rejection appears to be a significant factor in survival of large allografts.[6] Although bone itself is not highly immunogenic, the role of marrow elements in the cancellous bone graft may be crucial. When possible, marrow contents should be washed carefully from the interstices of cancellous bone to remove cellular elements that do not contribute to osteoinduction but do produce an inflammatory immune response that can compromise healing and bone formation. Washing and soaking the components in antibiotic solution has the additional benefit of making available a reservoir of antibiotic that is released slowly during the postoperative period.[22]

Morcellized cancellous bone, rather than finely ground bone which tends to be destroyed by phagocytosis, is the best available choice for reconstructing large volumes of deficient bone stock. Fixation is completely dependent on the existing bone, so that massive defects must be protected until sufficient rigidity develops in the grafted material to allow sharing of weightbearing loads.

Clinical experience has shown that migration of the tibial component after reconstruction with morcellized allograft is rare during the first 2 to 5 years after surgery (Fig. 8).[4] These results are surprising in light of reported experience with structural allografts of the acetabulum. Jasty and

Harris[19] reported loosening of acetabular components after 4 years in 32% of their cases. The biologic behavior of morcellized allograft differs from that of block allograft, however. Vascularization and ossification are rapid, and a permanent, competent loadbearing structure is achieved by filling large deficient areas.[1,2] The biologic response obtained with the correct technique appears to be early and vigorous. It does not seem likely that progressive collapse would occur after remodeling and healing have been established (Fig. 9).

Bone graft handling probably is crucial to the success of grafting of the knee. Antibiotic soaking and washing, removal of bone marrow, and adequate support of the implants are all necessary factors for consistent success of this technique. The results of this salvage procedure have been encouraging. The grafting technique appears to provide long-term support for the implants, so that repeat revision is unlikely.

Acknowledgment

The author thanks Charles D. Short, MD, and Michael G. Tanner, MS, for histologic analysis of bone graft specimens; and Diane J. Morton, MS, for editorial assistance with the manuscript.

References

1. Samuelson KM: Bone grafting and noncemented revision arthroplasty of the knee. *Clin Orthop* 1988;226:93–101.
2. Whiteside LA: Cementless reconstruction of massive tibial bone loss in revision total knee arthroplasty. *Clin Orthop* 1989;248:80–86.
3. Whiteside LA, Ohl MD: Tibial tubercle osteotomy for exposure of the difficult total knee arthroplasty. *Clin Orthop* 1990;260:6–9.
4. Wilde AH, Schickendantz MS, Stulberg BN, Go RT: The incorporation of tibial allografts in total knee arthroplasty. *J Bone Joint Surg* 1990;72A:815–824.
5. Goldberg VM, Powell A, Shaffer JW, Zika J, Bos GD, Heiple KG: Bone grafting: Role of histocompatibility in transplantation. *J Orthop Res* 1985;3:389–404.
6. Muscolo DL, Caletti E, Schajowicz F, Araujo ES, Makino A: Tissue-typing in human massive allografts of frozen bone. *J Bone Joint Surg* 1987;69A:583–595.
7. Whiteside LA: Treatment of infected total knee arthroplasty. *Clin Orthop* 1994;299:169–172.
8. Whiteside L: Radiological and histological analysis of morcellized bone grafting in revision total knee replacement. *Clin Orthop*, in press.
9. Booth RE Jr, Lotke PA: The results of spacer block technique in revision of infected total knee arthroplasty. *Clin Orthop* 1989;248:57–60.
10. Freeman MA, Sudlow RA, Casewell MW, Radcliff SS: The management of infected total knee replacements. *J Bone Joint Surg* 1985;67B:764–768.
11. Jacobs MA, Hungerford DS, Krackow KA, Lennox DW: Revision of septic total knee arthroplasty. *Clin Orthop* 1989;238:159–166.
12. Windsor RE, Insall JN, Urs WK, Miller DV, Brause BD: Two-stage reimplantation for the salvage of total knee arthroplasty complicated by infection: Further follow-up and refinement of indications. *J Bone Joint Surg* 1990;72A:272–278.
13. Whiteside LA: Bone grafting in revision cementless total knee arthroplasty. *Tech Orthop* 1992;7:39–46.
14. Whiteside LA: Cementless revision total knee arthroplasty. *Clin Orthop* 1993;286:160–167.
15. Friedlaender GE: Bone grafts: The basic science rationale for clinical applications. *J Bone Joint Surg* 1987;69A:786–790.
16. Gitelis S, Heligman D, Quill G, Plasecki P: The use of large allografts for tumor reconstruction and salvage of the failed total hip arthroplasty. *Clin Orthop* 1988;231:62–70.
17. Head WC, Malinin TI, Berklacich F: Freeze-dried proximal femur allografts in revision total hip arthroplasty: A preliminary report. *Clin Orthop* 1987;215:109–121.
18. Gerber SD, Harris WH: Femoral head autografting to augment acetabular deficiency in patients requiring total hip replacement: A minimum five-year and an average seven-year follow-up study. *J Bone Joint Surg* 1986;68A:1241–1248.
19. Jasty M, Harris WH: Salvage total hip reconstruction in patients with major acetabular bone deficiency using structural femoral head allografts. *J Bone Joint Surg* 1990;72B:63–67.
20. Kandel RA, Gross AE, Ganel A, McDermott AG, Langer F, Pritzker KP: Histopathology of failed osteoarticular shell allografts. *Clin Orthop* 1985;197:103–110.
21. Convery FR, Minteer-Convery M, Devine SD, Meyers MH: Acetabular augmentation in primary and revision total hip arthroplasty with cementless prostheses. *Clin Orthop* 1990;252:167–175.
22. McLaren AC: Antibiotic bone graft: Early clinical results. Proceedings of the American Academy of Orthopaedic Surgeons 57th Annual Meeting, New Orleans, LA. Park Ridge, IL, American Academy of Orthopaedic Surgeons, 1990, p 228.

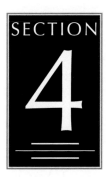
Knee: Sports Medicine

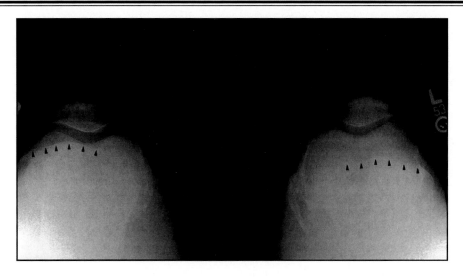

Factors Contributing to Function of the Knee Joint After Injury or Reconstruction of the Anterior Cruciate Ligament

Scott F. Dye, MD
Edward M. Wojtys, MD
Freddie H. Fu, MD
Donald C. Fithian, MD
Jan Gillquist, MD

Restoration of musculoskeletal function is a fundamental goal of orthopaedic treatment. Until now, clinical orthopaedic concepts of injury, repair, and restoration of function of musculoskeletal systems have been described and understood primarily in structural and biomechanical terms. This perception probably evolved because the structural characteristics are the most readily visualized factors, both in the clinical setting (for example, pathologic laxity due to a ruptured ligament or a fracture) and through the preponderance of structural and pathoanatomic data offered by most current imaging modalities. Structural characteristics are also the factors most directly altered by surgical intervention, such as stability following repair or reconstruction of a ligament or fixation of a fracture. It is a common belief that the restoration of measurable structural and biomechanical parameters to an injured joint, such as the knee, indicates the restoration of function to that system. We do not share this view.

In the past few years, emerging clinical and basic-science findings have indicated a much greater degree of underlying biologic complexity. Evidence suggests that the correction of identifiable structural abnormalities is often not sufficient to restore a joint to its full preinjury level of physiologic function. For example, replacement of a ruptured anterior cruciate ligament (ACL) with a graft does not necessarily prevent pain, swelling, or degenerative changes in the knee, even if the increased anterior-posterior laxity that had been present before the procedure is restored to normal. This observation indicates that factors other than anatomic and structural ones probably contribute to the restoration of joint function after injury. We believe that, although these other factors are less easily visualized, they play an important role in the ultimate functional status of an injured musculoskeletal system, such as the knee. The purpose of this chapter is to discuss the concept of musculoskeletal function and to consider the various factors that contribute to the restoration of knee function after injury or reconstruction of the ACL.

Restoration of Knee Function Following Anterior Cruciate Ligament Reconstruction

Reconstruction of the ACL is one of the most commonly performed orthopaedic procedures in the technologically advanced countries of the world. The primary goal of the reconstruction is to restore stability to the knee and thereby, presumably, to restore its function and allow the patient to return to normal activities, including sports. Another goal is to prevent early degenerative changes. In order to achieve these goals, the immediate objective of the surgery is to reduce abnormal laxity by replacing the injured ACL with a graft. Current methods for the objective assessment of the success of such reconstructive procedures most often involve evaluation of structural and biomechanical parameters, such as knee laxity as measured with instrumented testing and degenerative changes as estimated on plain radiographs.

Daniel and associates[1] used a metabolic study (technetium bone scintigraphy) as well as a structural study (plain radiography) to assess the development of degenerative changes in patients who had sustained an acute traumatic hemarthrosis of the knee. Although it was nonrandomized, their prospective study included a large number of patients who had an injury of the ACL and had been managed nonsurgically or with early or delayed surgical reconstruction. The study also included patients in whom the knee was stable on instrumented testing and who were thus presumed to have a normal ACL or only a partial tear. A disturbing finding of that study was that reconstruction of the ACL did not prevent the development of early degenerative changes in the knee despite the fact that ligamentous stability had been restored. In fact, 5 years after the injury the reconstructed knees showed markedly greater degenerative changes on technetium scintiscans and standard radiographs than did those that had been treated nonsurgically.

Follow-up studies by Daniel and associates[2] and Fithian[3] revealed that, an average of 10 years after the injury, the reconstructed knees continued to show greater degenerative changes on plain radiographs than did those that had been treated nonsurgically. This was attributed, in part, to the higher prevalence of meniscal surgery among patients who had a reconstruction. However, even when the knees that had had a meniscal procedure were excluded, more degenerative changes were seen in the reconstructed knees than in the knees that had been treated nonsurgically. It should be noted that the reconstructive procedures were of an earlier era and included open techniques followed by a period of immobilization. Nevertheless, the results indicate that surgery, which may restore mechanical normalcy, does not necessarily resolve all of the problems caused by associated pathologic

changes resulting from the original or subsequent trauma and, indeed, can represent an additional insult to the knee.

The main focus of ongoing work directed by one of us (D.C.F.) has been the analysis of patients with unstable knees who decided not to have ACL surgery.[3] In that study, the anterior-posterior laxity of the knee, which was used as an indicator of the structural integrity of the ACL, was measured with the KT-1000 device developed by Daniel and associates.[1] The early laxity grade was found to be predictive of the later laxity grade in knees that were not reconstructed.[3] Of 53 patients in whom the knee was classified as stable initially, 48 (91%) had a stable knee 10 years later. Of 111 patients in whom the knee was classified as unstable initially and who did not have a reconstruction, 93 (84%) had an unstable knee 10 years later. Despite the instability, less degenerative change was evident on the follow-up radiographs and bone scintiscans of these patients than on those of 84 patients in whom the ligament had been reconstructed. The activity level at the time of follow-up was similar for the patients who had had surgery and those who had not, and it was decreased in both groups compared with the level before the injury. The patients who had had a reconstruction had the greatest percentage reduction in the total number of hours of participation in sports. The changes in activity level, however, may have been made according to lifestyle choices that were unrelated to the functional capacity of the knee. The findings of the studies by Fithian[3] and by Daniel and associates[1] confirm that knees may remain free of degenerative changes in the presence of abnormal laxity secondary to injury of the ACL and that the restoration of certain

mechanical characteristics is not sufficient to restore the preinjury level of physiologic function.

In a review of the literature regarding reconstruction of the ACL,[4] one of us (J.G.) noted a trend toward a high prevalence of good or excellent results ranging from 66% (45 of 68) to 90% (37 of 41).[1,2,5-15] However, none of the investigators, with the exception of Daniel and associates,[1] analyzed the outcomes of surgical treatment relative to the results of nonsurgical treatment with a metabolic study in a large number of knees that had an injured ACL. Gillquist also observed that perhaps the only effect of reconstruction of the ACL in some individuals was to "give the patient enough security to go back to strenuous sports, and then (ruin) the knee." The results of the study by Daniel and associates and the observations by Gillquist, along with the experience of many orthopaedic surgeons, belie a current recommendation in the international sportsmedicine community that patients who have reconstruction of the ACL should be encouraged to return to sports, particularly the sport during which the index injury occurred. Frank and Jackson,[16] in a comprehensive review of the current state of reconstruction of the ACL, observed that few reconstructed knees are returned to normal and that no normal ligaments are being created surgically.

Concept of Joint Function

This apparent lack of full functional restoration after injury of the ACL is a cause for concern. Much of what may be considered important regarding the lack of restoration of joint function is derived from one's concept of the meaning of the term joint function. Function can be defined as the purpose for which an entity is specially fit.[17] A concept of joint function proposed by the senior one of us (S.F.D.)[18] in 1996 is that joints are systems that are designed to transmit mechanical loads between components and yet, by virtue of the fact that they are living structures, to maintain tissue homeostasis over a broad range of physical demands. In mechanical engineering, systems that are designed to transfer loads differentially between components are called transmissions. The knee can thus be viewed as a kind of living, metabolically active, biologic transmission whose function is to accept and redirect loads between and among the femur, tibia, patella, and fibula.[18] The cruciate ligaments in this analogy can be seen as nonrigid, sensate adaptive linkages within the transmission. The articular cartilages can be viewed as bearings and the menisci, as mobile sensate bearings[19] within the transmission. The muscles act not only as cellular engines that provide motive forces across the knee in concentric contraction but also as brakes and dampening systems that absorb shock loads in eccentric contraction.[18] Winter[20] revealed that the muscles about the knee actually absorb more than 3 times the energy that is generated in motive forces. The various components of a living joint are constantly metabolically active, with complex molecular and cellular mechanisms that are designed to maintain and restore tissue homeostasis under normal and injurious biomechanical conditions.[21] In our view, the concept of musculoskeletal function includes the capacity not only to generate, transmit, absorb, and dissipate loads but also to maintain tissue homeostasis while doing so.

Envelope of Function

The envelope of function[18] is a concept that was developed by the senior one of us as a simple method that incorporates and connects the concepts of load transference and tissue homeostasis in order to visually represent the functional capacity of the knee. It defines a range of loading that is compatible with, and probably inductive of, the overall tissue homeostasis of a given joint or musculoskeletal system. The concept, in its simplest form, is a load and frequency distribution that defines a safe range of loading (the envelope of function) for a given joint[18] (Fig. 1). The upper limit of the envelope represents a threshold between loads that are compatible with tissue homeostasis and loads that initiate the complex biologic cascade of trauma-induced inflammation and repair (Fig. 2). The area within the envelope is the zone of homeostasis or the zone of homeostatic loading. Loads that are beyond the threshold of the envelope but are lower than those that induce macrostructural failure of a component are in the area that can be termed the zone of supraphysiologic overload. Loading in this region can cause, for example, the painful osseous remodeling associated with the initial stages of a stress fracture, which is evident as increased activity on technetium scintiscans before any structural changes are noted on radiographs. These sites of increased osseous metabolic activity may return to homeostasis, as documented by normal scintigraphic activity, following nonsurgical treatment primarily involving a reduction of loading. If more energy is placed across a joint, a second threshold is reached: the lower limit of the zone of structural failure. Such high loads result in overt macrostructural failure of at least 1 component of a joint or musculoskeletal system, such as a rupture of the ACL or a fracture of the tibial plateau. A lengthy period of decreased loading, such as may be associated with prolonged bed rest or extended space travel in a microgravity environment, can result in a loss of homeostasis as evidenced by osteopenia and muscle atrophy. This lower-threshold limit demarcates the zone of subphysiologic underload. We believe that most, if not all, musculoskeletal systems respond to differential loading as depicted in these 4 regions.

Frost's work[22-29] regarding homeostatic properties and principles of musculoskeletal tissues, particularly bone, independently corroborates and complements the concept of the envelope of function. Frost's view of excessive microdamage corresponds to the loading of tissues within the zone of supraphysiologic overload. Too little loading over time, which results in disuse osteopenia, is reflected in his concept of minimum effective strain, or minimum effective signal, as a lower-threshold limit.

The capacity of a knee to transfer loads safely can vary greatly after injury of the ACL. Different envelope shapes can represent these changing capacities. An idealized preinjury normal envelope of function for a soccer player, for example, can be represented graphically (Fig. 3, A). A single high-load event, such as one causing acute rupture of the ACL, can result in marked and immediate diminution of the envelope of that knee (Fig. 3, B). With time and rehabilitation alone, the function of many knees may be partially restored to a level that is sufficient for the patient to participate in activities of daily living, swimming, and bicycling and that may be compatible with tissue homeostasis (Fig. 3, C). We believe that this restoration is probably to a large degree a result of the effect of complex neuromuscular mechanisms providing improved dynamic control of the injured knee, which can be achieved through training and conditioning, despite the

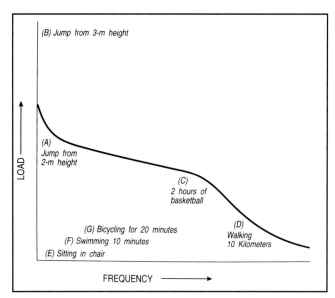

Fig. 1 Graph representing the envelope of function[18] for an athletically active young adult. The letters represent the loads associated with different activities. All of the loading examples, except *B*, are within the envelope for this particular knee. The shape of the envelope of function represented here is an idealized theoretical model. The actual loads transmitted across an individual knee under these different conditions are variable and are due to multiple complex factors, including the dynamic center of gravity, the rate of load application, and the angles of flexion and rotation. The limits of the envelope of function for the joint of an actual patient are probably more complex. (Reproduced with permission from Dye SF: The knee as a biologic transmission with an envelope of function: A theory. *Clin Orthop* 1996;325:10–18.)

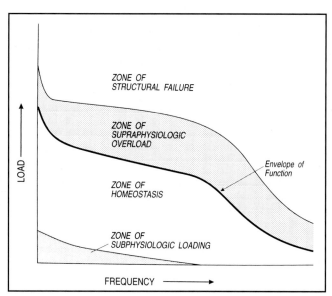

Fig. 2 Graph showing the 4 different zones of loading across a joint. The area within the envelope of function is the zone of homeostasis. The region of loading greater than that within the envelope of function but insufficient to cause macrostructural damage is the zone of supraphysiologic overload. The region of loading great enough to cause macrostructural damage is the zone of structural failure. The region of decreased loading over time resulting in a loss of tissue homeostasis is the zone of subphysiologic underload. (Adapted with permission from Dye SF: The knee as a biologic transmission with an envelope of function: A theory. *Clin Orthop* 1996;325:10–18.)

absence of the linkage provided by the ACL. However, it is possible that only a certain additional percentage of the preinjury envelope of function can be restored by reconstruction in such a patient, because the reconstruction may not correct all of the pathologic changes in the joint (Fig. 3, *D*). These changes often include damage of subchondral bone, articular cartilage, and menisci; synovitis; and injury of the components of the neuromuscular system and other static restraints. Thus, if the patient is encouraged to resume high-stress sports activity, the injured knee may be forced into its new lower zone of supraphysiologic overload. Such loading could result in increased subchondral micro-osseous

remodeling that is detectable scintigraphically in the presence of normal radiographic findings. If left unchecked, this process may eventually lead to overt degenerative changes. This sequence of changes in the functional envelope of an idealized knee after injury of the ACL provides a rational explanation for the findings of Daniel and associates[1] and Gillquist[4] as well as the observations of many practicing orthopaedic surgeons that are not explained from a purely structural and biomechanical perspective. The envelope of function[18] can also be represented in 3 mathematical dimensions or more by the addition of other variables, such as time or the degree of flexion (Fig. 4).

Factors Contributing to Joint Function

In addition to the general factors of age, gender, and nutrition, we believe that several categories of factors contribute to the functional capacity of any joint. Although many different methods could be devised to organize all of the possible factors and there may be factors that have not yet been determined, we have found it logical and useful, especially from a clinical perspective, to consider 4 categories of factors: anatomic, kinematic, physiologic, and treatment.

Anatomic Factors

Anatomic factors in joint function include the macromorphology and

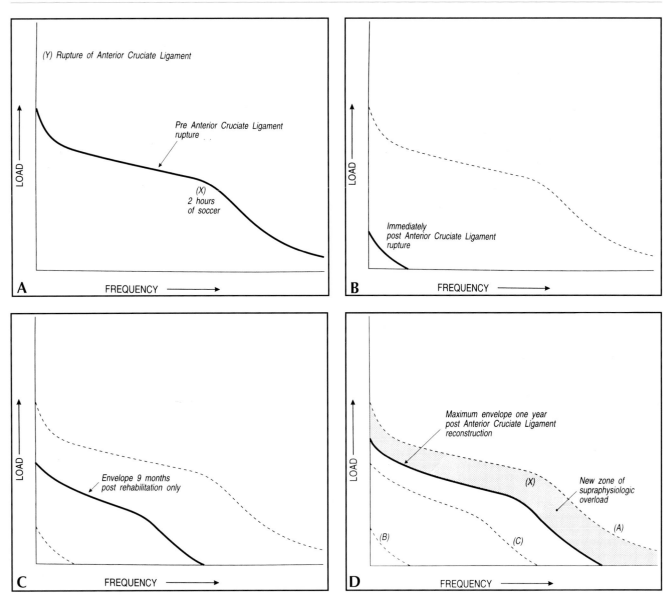

Fig. 3 Graphs demonstrating the dynamic character of the envelope of function of a knee with a rupture of the anterior cruciate ligament. (Reproduced with permission from Dye SF: The knee as a biologic transmission with an envelope of function: A theory. *Clin Orthop* 1996;325:10–18.) **A,** The preinjury envelope of function. Loading event X represents 2 hours of soccer and is within the preinjury envelope. Loading event Y represents a single load that is great enough to cause an acute rupture of the anterior cruciate ligament. **B,** The envelope of function immediately after rupture of the anterior cruciate ligament. **C,** The envelope of function 9 months after treatment with a rehabilitation program alone. The envelope has broadened sufficiently to include most activities of daily living and certain low-impact sports, such as bicycling. **D,** The envelope of function 1 year after reconstruction of the anterior cruciate ligament and postoperative rehabilitation. The envelope has not been fully restored to the preinjury status. The area between the postoperative and preinjury envelopes represents a new zone of supraphysiologic overload, which potentially extends to a zone of structural failure. If a patient returns to previous high-impact loading (X), which is now outside the postoperative envelope of function, the knee will be at risk for early degenerative changes and structural failure of the graft.

micromorphology, the resultant structural integrity, and the biomechanical characteristics of all components. In the knee, these include the ligaments, tendons, retinacula, muscles, menisci, articular cartilage, nerves, vessels, and bone. The alignment of the limb and the height and weight of the individual must also be considered. It is clear, from a review of the literature regarding the current state of anatomic restoration of

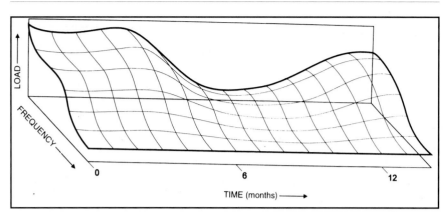

Fig. 4 A 3-dimensional representation of the dynamic changes in the envelope of function of an idealized injured joint with time. The variable of time, from 0 to 14 months, has been added on a third, Z, axis. The downward slope of the undulations in the envelope represents diminished load-acceptance capacity after injury, while the upward slope of the undulations represents increased capacity due to healing of joint and neuromuscular tissues. In this case, the maximum capacity has not returned to normal by 14 months.

the ACL after injury, that normal morphology is not being regained despite the use of various surgical techniques.[16] No current method of reconstruction recreates the complex fan morphology of the insertion of a normal ACL on the femur and tibia. Most reconstructions of the ACL are designed to mimic the anteromedial bundle of the ligament. The micro-anatomy of the ACL is complex. Electron microscopy studies[30–32] have shown that the normal pattern of mixed large and small fibrils is not achieved with current reconstructive procedures (Fig. 5). In addition, the normal complex insertion of the ligament through transition zones of fibrocartilage and calcified cartilage is not reproduced with current techniques.

Ligaments not only act as structural checkreins that restrict the movement of joints but also serve as sources of sensation for more proximal neural elements.[19,33–36] To our knowledge, restoration of normal neuromorphology and distribution has not been documented in the current literature on ACL reconstruc-

tion in humans, although Barrack and associates[37] recently demonstrated partial restoration of histologic neuromorphology as well as limited restoration of sensory-evoked potentials in canines. The increased laxity found in many knees after reconstruction of the ACL demonstrates that the strength of the ligamentous substitute is insufficient for the loads that are applied. As far as we know, no animal model has demonstrated restoration of normal anatomic or biomechanical characteristics after reconstruction of the ACL. As noted by one of us (J.G.)[4] and by van Rens and associates,[38] even reconstructions that have appeared to be excellent have failed at relatively low loads.

Kinematic Factors
Kinematic factors can be defined as those that determine the motion of a given joint or musculoskeletal segment under load. In the knee, these factors include the pattern of sequential tightening of the fibers of the ACL and the dynamic function of all of the complex neuromuscular con-

trol mechanisms, including neuro-proprioceptive output characteristics from the limb as well as cerebral and cerebellar sequencing of motor unit contractions, spinal reflex mechanisms, dynamic muscle strength, and endurance.[39–42]

The neuromuscular capability of the lower extremity after surgical or nonsurgical treatment of a ruptured ACL can be an important prognosticator of function of the knee.[43] The results of research have indicated the importance of eccentric muscle function in increased stiffness across the knee joint as well as the absorption of impact loads transmitted across the knee joint.[20] The importance of muscle tone for the protection of the static soft-tissue restraints of the knee has been demonstrated by a number of investigators. Wang and Walker[44] showed that a compressive force equal to approximately the body weight could decrease rotatory laxity by 80%. Markolf and associates[45] demonstrated the substantial protective effect of well-conditioned muscles in the lower extremities of athletes. Those authors showed a 10-fold increase in the stiffness of the knee joint with contraction of the muscles compared with the stiffness with the muscles in a relaxed state. Recent work has indicated that weakness of the quadriceps after reconstruction of the ACL primarily reflects a deficit in neural activator drive from the central nervous system rather than a pure muscle weakness.[46] In addition, several authors[43,47] have emphasized the importance of specific and exact temporal activation of muscle, as reflected by muscle reaction time and time to peak torque. Research by Wojtys and Huston,[48] who studied the effects of injury of the ACL and reconstruction of the patellar ligament with an autogenous graft as well as neuromuscular performance, indicated that

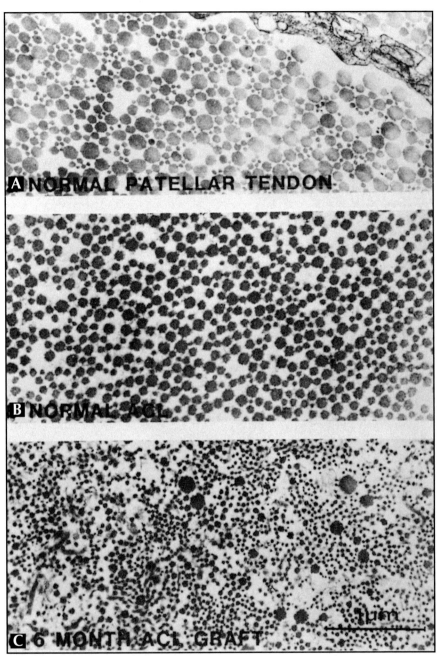

Fig. 5 Transverse-section electron microscopy studies. A normal patellar ligament from a human subject who was younger than 30 years of age (**A**) has a mix of large and small-diameter fibrils. A normal anterior cruciate ligament from a human subject who was younger than 30 years of age (**B**) has fibrils that are smaller than those in the patellar ligament. An anterior cruciate ligament-patellar ligament autogenous graft that had been in situ for 6 months after implantation in a human (**C**) shows a predominance of small fibrils and the remains of the larger fibrils from the donor patellar ligament (original magnifications, x 34,000). (Reproduced with permission from Oakes BW: Collagen ultrastructure in the normal ACL and in ACL graft, in Jackson DW (ed): *The Anterior Cruciate Ligament: Current and Future Concepts.* New York, NY, Raven Press, 1993, p 214.)

patients who underwent surgery did not regain the same functional performance as demonstrated by a group of age-matched controls. Those authors indicated that formal rehabilitation of the knee improved muscle strength, endurance, time to peak torque, and muscle reaction time but did not restore normal levels of performance. During isokinetic testing, the hamstrings reached peak torque before the quadriceps in the control subjects. However, the pattern was reversed in the patients who had been managed surgically; the hamstrings reached peak torque after the quadriceps even at 18 months postoperatively. Of interest is the fact that the untreated, contralateral limb of the patients who had had a reconstruction also showed the same abnormal recruitment pattern.

The importance of proprioceptive neuromuscular conditioning to the function of the knee was demonstrated by Caraffa and associates[49] in a prospective, controlled study of 600 soccer players on 40 teams. During 3 full seasons, the prevalence of injury of the ACL in 300 soccer players who participated in proprioceptive training was substantially lower (a mean of 0.15 injury per team) than that in a similar group of 300 players who did not participate in proprioceptive training (a mean of 1.15 injuries per team). The evidence strongly suggests that it is possible to prevent certain injuries of the ACL with simple enhancements of the neuromuscular control mechanisms.[49]

Physiologic Factors

Physiologic factors can be defined as the biochemical and metabolic processes that maintain and restore tissue homeostasis in joints and musculoskeletal components. The complex physiologic factors that determine homeostasis of musculoskeletal systems under normal conditions and

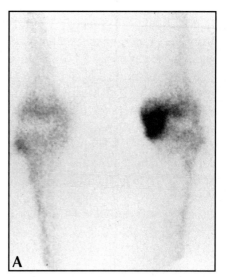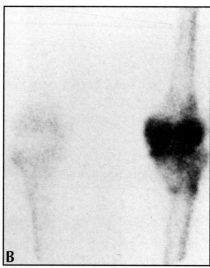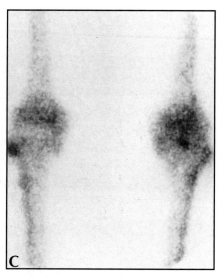

Fig. 6 Anteroposterior technetium scintiscans of the knees of a 32-year-old man, demonstrating restoration of osseous homeostasis after reconstruction of the ligament. (Reproduced with permission from Dye SF, Chew MH: Restoration of osseous homeostasis after anterior cruciate ligament reconstruction. *Am J Sports Med* 1993;21:749–750.) **A,** Preoperatively, there is intense uptake in the medial compartment of the left knee. **B,** Four months after the reconstruction and a partial medial meniscectomy, there is marked uptake in 3 compartments. **C,** Twenty-one months postoperatively, normal scintigraphic activity has been restored in the medial compartment, with mild residual uptake in the proximal part of the tibial tunnel.

after injury are becoming the focus of orthopaedic research worldwide.[50] The recent emphasis on these factors is shown by the distribution of the types of research presented at the meetings of the Orthopaedic Research Society. During the last decade, the emphasis has shifted from biomechanical and structural studies to the assessment of metabolic variables.

The loss of tissue homeostasis is often undetectable with the use of structural imaging studies, such as plain radiography and magnetic resonance imaging (MRI). This loss, which is demonstrated in bone by persistently abnormal technetium scintiscans after the injury, can be a prelude to the eventual development and progression of irreversible degenerative changes.[51–55] The capability of a scintiscan to demonstrate regions of eventual overt degenerative changes in a knee before radiographic changes are evident was validated in an animal model by McBride and associates.[56] Those authors created a posttraumatic

osteoarthrosis model by sectioning the ACL of rabbits. With use of sequential radiographs, technetium scintiscans, and histologic analysis, the authors found that the scintiscans showed increased osseous metabolic activity by 2 weeks, whereas radiographic changes could not be detected until the 8th week. Recent studies[53,57] have shown that the restoration of osseous homeostasis, as documented by normal findings on technetium scintiscans, is possible after reconstruction of the ACL with a bone-patellar ligament-bone autogenous graft followed by incremental rehabilitation (Fig. 6). Of interest is the finding that, 4 months after the reconstruction, the scintiscans demonstrated much greater activity, reflecting the fact that major surgery represents a serious yet reversible metabolic disturbance in the knee. Aglietti and associates[58] showed that some residual abnormal scintigraphic activity after reconstruction of the ACL, with uninjured or repaired menisci, is compatible with the ab-

sence of overt degenerative changes as many as 5 years postoperatively.

Compared with technetium scintigraphy, positron emission tomography with use of fluorine$_{18}$ is capable of much higher resolution of radiographically undetectable increased osseous metabolic activity in a chronically symptomatic knee after injury of the ACL.[59] This technique involves the production of short-half-life positron emitters, such as fluorine$_{18}$, generated in a cyclotron by the addition of a proton to the nuclei of a stable precursor. The added proton converts to a neutron by emitting a positron (an anti-particle of the electron). When a positron comes into contact with a nearby electron, a matter-antimatter annihilation event occurs, with the production of gamma radiation detectable with scintillation devices.[60,61] Fluorine$_{18}$ combines to sites of active turnover of bone, thereby localizing the process. This scintigraphic method is fundamentally different from the standard technetium scintiscan, which relies on the carrier molecule methylene diphosphonate. In 1 study,[53] a 34-year-old man with a unilateral chronically symptomatic injury of the ACL had increased osseous metabolic activity in 3 compartments on technetium bone scintigraphy. The positron emission tomography scan confirmed the intraosseous location of the increased osseous metabolic activity at high resolution (Fig. 7). With the use of different tracers and metabolites, positron emission tomography may be able to geographically demonstrate homeostatic characteristics of musculoskeletal soft tissue with high resolution.

Marks and associates[62] demonstrated the association between acute rupture of the ACL and impaction injuries of the anterior aspect of the lateral femoral condyle and the posterior aspect of the lateral tibial plateau with the use of technetium bone scintigraphy and MRI. The impaction injuries occurred secondary to failure of the ligament with transient rotatory subluxation of the lateral compartment (Fig. 8). The specific sites of these osseous injuries are commonly associated with acute rupture of the ACL.[63] Johnson and associates[64] noted metabolic and structural damage of articular cartilage on the anterior aspect of the lateral femoral condyle overlying a region of subchondral injury, as evidenced by death of chondrocytes in some patients after injury of the ACL (Fig. 9). It is likely that the capacity of such knees to transfer loads would be diminished compared with the capacity of knees with normal tissues.

In contradistinction to knees with the acute pattern of injury, chronically symptomatic knees with an injured ACL have demonstrated loss of osseous homeostasis primarily in the medial compartment, which is rarely involved in the index injury.[65,66] This

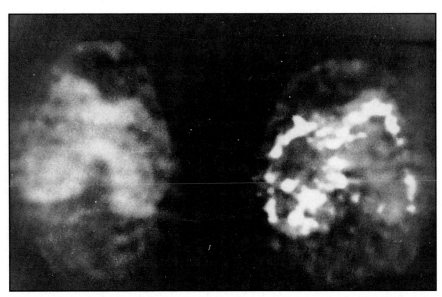

Fig. 7 Fluorine$_{18}$ positron emission tomography scan of the knees of a 34-year-old man who had an 8-year history of chronic injury of the anterior cruciate ligament of the right knee. The white areas indicate increased osseous metabolic activity in the distal aspect of the right femur. No fluorine$_{18}$ activity is noted in the left femur.

chronic pattern of increased scintigraphic activity in the medial compartment probably reflects a different underlying pathokinematic genesis than that involved in the acute pattern seen in the lateral compartment with an impaction injury. The medial compartment is anatomically more constrained than the lateral compartment;[67,68] therefore, it is probably subjected to greater forces with the increases in translation associated with the absence of a functional ACL. These greater forces can induce increased osseous metabolic activity, as shown on technetium scintigraphy (Fig. 6, A).

Recent basic-science research[69] has established that the mechanical environment affects, in addition to the homeostasis of bone, the homeostasis of soft tissues, including cartilage, ligaments, and tendons. For example, chondrocytes remodel the extracellular matrix in response to changes in cellular deformation secondary to load,[70–72] as demonstrated by increases

in proteoglycans, interstitial ion concentration, and pH. Micromanipulation of individual cartilage cells in vitro has been shown to increase the cytosolic calcium level,[73] which plays a role in the synthesis of DNA, the synthesis of extracellular matrix, and cellular differentiation.

The in vivo response of articular cartilage to differential loading was demonstrated by Kiviranta and associates[74] in a canine model. Those authors showed that moderate loading across the knee joint (as produced by the dogs running 4 km a day for 15 weeks) induced an increase in the thickness of the articular cartilage and an increase in the proteoglycan content, whereas excessive loading (as produced by the dogs running 20 km a day up a 15° grade for 40 weeks) resulted in quantitative decreases in the thickness of the cartilage and in the production of proteoglycans.

Tendons also appear to be quite sensitive to a differential range of loading. Arnoczky and associates[75] and

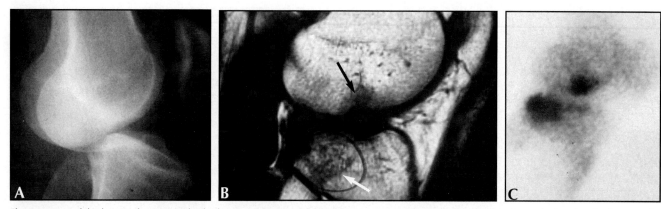

Fig. 8 Images of the knees of patients who had an acute rupture of the anterior cruciate ligament. A, Lateral radiograph showing the impact of the anterior aspect of the lateral femoral condyle on the posterior aspect of the lateral tibial plateau that occurs with acute rupture of the anterior cruciate ligament. (Courtesy of Paul H. Marks, MD) B, T1-weighted magnetic resonance image showing sites of osseous injury of the anterior aspect of the lateral femoral condyle (black arrow) and the posterior aspect of the lateral tibial plateau (white arrow). C, Technetium-99m methylene diphosphonate scintiscan showing regions of increased osseous metabolic activity at the sites of osseous impaction on the anterior aspect of the lateral femoral condyle and the posterior aspect of the lateral tibial plateau. (Reproduced with permission from Dye SF: The use of technetium scintigraphy in the assessment of musculoskeletal trauma, in *Recent Advances in Operative Orthopedics*. St. Louis, MO, Mosby-Year Book, 1995, vol 3, pp 183–216.)

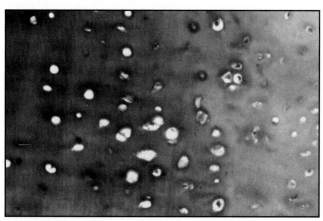

Fig. 9 Micrograph of articular cartilage from the anterior aspect of the lateral femoral condyle, 3 weeks after acute injury of the anterior cruciate ligament, revealing death of chondrocytes as evidenced by the absence of nuclear material in the empty lacunae. The more superficial layers of the articular cartilage are to the right, and the deeper layers are to the left (hematoxylin and eosin; original magnification, × 20). (Courtesy of Darren L. Johnson, MD)

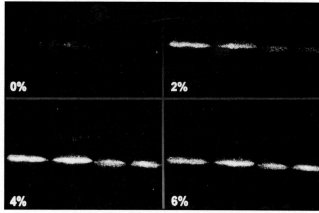

Fig. 10 Sequential images of living tenocytes, made with the use of confocal laser microscopy. A section of living tendon was put under 0, 2, 4, and 6% strain, and the intracellular cytosolic calcium concentration was assessed qualitatively. At 0% strain there was minimum cytosolic calcium concentration, at 2% strain there was increased calcium concentration, at 4% strain there was maximum calcium concentration, and at 6% strain there was decreased calcium concentration. (Courtesy of K. Shirakura, MD)

Shirakura and associates (personal communication, 1995) demonstrated that the cells within a tendon deform in response to tensile load, thus leading to a differential manifestation of metabolic characteristics. With use of confocal laser microscopy, both groups of authors determined that the deformation was nonlinear in response to load. They suggested that cell membranes do not deform beyond a certain degree because of the physical limitations imposed by the cell membrane or the local matrix. Like the deformation of cartilage cells, increased cytosolic calcium concentrations have been found in response to strain, which suggests a common pathway regulating the response of in situ cellular deformations of tenocytes. For example, Shirakura and associates showed that there was minimum cytosolic calcium concentration at 0% strain, the calcium concentration was increased

Table 1
Categorization of factors that contribute to the envelope of function in knees with an injury of the anterior cruciate ligament

Factors	History	Physical Examination	Instrumented Testing	Imaging
Anatomic	Sense of looseness	Positive Lachman test	Abnormal instrumented laxity testing	Radiographs, magnetic resonance imaging
Kinematic	Giving-way	Positive pivot-shift test	Abnormal instrumented six-degrees-of-freedom testing	Cine computed tomography, cine magnetic resonance imaging
Physiologic	Aching	Warmth and tenderness	Instrumented infrared temperature assessment	Technetium-99m methylene diphosphonate scintiscans, positron emission tomography

at 2% strain, it was maximum at 4% strain, and it started to decrease at 6% strain (Fig. 10).

The basic-science studies that we noted are beginning to define the upper-threshold limits of the envelope of function at the tissue and cellular levels. In other words, a certain degree of loading and resultant deformation is compatible with, and perhaps inductive of, homeostasis of musculoskeletal tissues. Forces beyond that degree of loading result in metabolic tissue failure, and sufficiently high or prolonged loads result in structural tissue failure. The studies that we discussed provide strong evidence linking differential loading and musculoskeletal tissue response.

Treatment Factors

Treatment factors include nonsurgical measures, such as restriction of load, neuromuscular training (muscle-strengthening and proprioceptive enhancements that increase force production, load absorption, coordination, and balance), bracing, and anti-inflammatory therapies (such as medication and tissue-cooling), as well as surgical procedures, including those involving the menisci and the articular cartilage and various techniques of repair or reconstruction of the ACL.

Indicators of Functional Restoration

Indicators that a joint is being loaded within its physiologic capacity—that is, within its envelope of function—include the absence of discomfort, of warmth, of swelling, and of functional instability as well as the presence of normal findings on long-term radiographs and a technetium scintiscan. Indicators that a joint is being loaded outside of its functional envelope include discomfort, warmth, swelling, instability, abnormally increased activity on a technetium scintiscan, and eventual development of radiographic degenerative changes. The various factors that contribute to joint function can be categorized on the basis of the history, physical examination, instrumented testing, and imaging (Table 1). In 1997, Marks[76] suggested the concept of the ACL risk equation, with which he attempted to detail and differentially weight the various factors that pertain to the knee.

We believe that the effects of all of the extant factors, including treatment factors, that contribute to joint function are summated at the cellular and tissue levels by the presence or absence of homeostasis. As Daniel and associates[1] showed, the knees of patients who had a structurally inadequate ACL demonstrated a positive

Lachman test and an abnormal instrumented laxity test on clinical examination but still functioned well, without the development of degenerative changes. This may have been the result of changes in lifestyle to allow for limitation of loading as well as excellent dynamic muscle-sequencing and robust metabolic maintenance and repair mechanisms, resulting in overall joint homeostasis as demonstrated in bone by technetium scintigraphy.[1]

Unlike most imaging studies that are currently available to orthopaedic surgeons, scintigraphic techniques allow for the geographic assessment of tissue homeostasis of osseous components about joints.[53,77] MRI, as currently configured, cannot reliably demonstrate sites of increased osseous metabolic activity[77] or even whether a given joint is in a living subject or from a cadaver.[78] Better methods of documenting and tracking the homeostatic characteristics of all musculoskeletal components, including soft tissues, may reveal a variety of underlying metabolic adaptive processes. These processes are at present mostly covert. Positron emission tomography[60,79] or other imaging technology, such as functional MRI,[61,80] may be able to provide this information in the future. Someday, orthopaedists and their patients may be able to view a 3-dimensional hologram of the knee or other musculoskeletal systems, with the differential degree of healing of various tissues represented by different colors and intensities.[81] When these underlying metabolic adaptive mechanisms can be easily visualized and tracked over time, insights may be gained that could result in different concepts of musculoskeletal injury and response. These insights may lead to currently unexpected therapeutic advances.

Overview

A knee with an injured ACL is an interesting representative of a damaged musculoskeletal system. The restoration of certain structural and biomechanical parameters alone does not ensure the restoration of physiologic function. We believe that it is important to consider the range of factors that contribute to the functional capacity of the knee, including kinematic and physiologic factors, when managing patients who have an injured ACL. The conceptualization of tissue damage and response after such an injury should be broadened to include the often complex associated pathologic changes noted in a variety of musculoskeletal components besides the ACL. The combination of osseous and cartilaginous damage and the disturbance of the neuromuscular control mechanisms, in addition to the damage to the ACL and other tissues, can result in diminution of the functional capacity of the entire joint to transmit load safely.

From our review of the current literature regarding reconstruction of the ACL, it seems clear that perfection—that is, full restoration of the preinjury status—often is not achieved and the long-term results are not completely satisfactory. However, the function of

knees that have been treated with modern reconstructive techniques along with incremental rehabilitation has been shown to approach normal, as documented on postoperative scintigraphic studies that showed no early degenerative changes.[53,57]

The goal of therapy after injury of the ACL should be the maximization of the load-transference capacity of the knee joint as safely and predictably as possible. Rehabilitative, nonsurgical management may be sufficient for many patients. Despite the best therapeutic efforts, however, it is likely that the full preinjury function of the joint will not be restored in most patients. The use of the envelope-of-function construct can thus be of value in educating patients by demonstrating, in simple graphic form, the estimated potential functional capacity of a joint at different stages in the treatment program. The envelope also demonstrates the activities that are more likely to be safe and therefore compatible with long-term function of the joint as well as the activities that may be associated with a risk of early degenerative changes.

We view with concern the continued presence of even mild discomfort, warmth, and swelling associated with certain loading activities in knees that have an injured or reconstructed ACL. These findings are a direct clinical manifestation of a loss of joint homeostasis. Patients who have these findings should be counseled to decrease, at least temporarily, the loading across the symptomatic joint. This decrease in loading, in combination with other nonsurgical means, should reverse the clinical signs toward homeostasis.

By recommending that patients decrease loading across the joint to a safe level that is compatible with the maintenance of tissue homeostasis

through avoidance of certain high-loading activities, we are not advocating a sedentary lifestyle. On the contrary, it is desirable that patients be as active as possible within the upper-threshold limits of their own specific functional envelope. Even a patient who has a severely damaged knee often can participate safely in an aerobic swimming or bicycling program that effectively maintains muscle strength and tone, flexibility of the joint, cardiovascular conditioning, and production of endorphins without supraphysiologic overload of the joint as a whole.[18]

Additional advances in the treatment of knees with injury of the ACL are likely to result not only from better techniques for recreating an internal structural linkage but also from methods to improve the neuromuscular control mechanisms, such as prevention of muscle atrophy and restoration of proprioception. Advances are also likely to come from improvements in the metabolic healing properties of all injured musculoskeletal tissues, perhaps through such techniques as genetic engineering. Therapeutic methods that are designed to work symbiotically with the patient's unique set of musculoskeletal characteristics are likely to result in successful orthopaedic treatment.

References

1. Daniel DM, Stone ML, Dobson BE, Fithian DC, Rossman DJ, Kaufman KR: Fate of the ACL-injured patient: A prospective outcome study. *Am J Sports Med* 1994;22:632–644.

2. Daniel DM, Fithian DC, Stone ML, Dobson BE, Luetzow WF, Kaufman KR: A ten-year prospective outcome study of the ACL-injured patient. Proceedings of the American Academy of Orthopaedic Surgeons 63rd Annual Meeting, Atlanta, GA. Rosemont, IL, American Academy of Orthopaedic Surgeons, 1996, p 77.

3. Fithian DC: The fate of the anterior cruciate ligament injured patient: Long-term follow-up: The San Diego Experience. Proceedings of the American Academy of Orthopaedic Surgeons 64th Annual Meeting, San Francisco, CA.

Rosemont, IL, American Academy of Orthopaedic Surgeons, 1997, p 123.

4. Gillquist JI: Repair and reconstruction of the
ACL: Is it good enough? *Arthroscopy* 1993;9:
68–71.

5. Aglietti P, Buzzi R, D'Andria S, Zaccherotti G:
Long-term study of anterior cruciate ligament
reconstruction for chronic instability using the
central one-third patellar tendon and a lateral
extraarticular tenodesis. *Am J Sports Med* 1992;
20:38–45.

6. Andersson C, Odensten M, Good L, Gillquist
J: Surgical and non-surgical treatment of acute
rupture of the anterior cruciate ligament: A
randomized study with long-term follow-up.
J Bone Joint Surg 1989;71A:965–974.

7. Bach BR Jr, Jones GT, Sweet FA, Hager CA:
Arthroscopy-assisted anterior cruciate ligament
reconstruction using patellar tendon substitution: Two- to four-year follow-up results. *Am J
Sports Med* 1994;22:758–767.

8. Fritschy D, Daniel DM, Rossman D, Rangger
C: Bone imaging after acute knee hemarthrosis.
Knee Surg Sports Traumatol Arthrosc 1993;1:20–27.

9. Howell SM, Taylor MA: Brace-free rehabilitation, with early return to activity, for knees
reconstructed with a double-looped semitendinosus and gracilis graft. *J Bone Joint Surg* 1996;
78A:814–825.

10. Johnson RJ, Eriksson E, Haggmark T, Pope
MH: Five- to ten-year follow-up evaluation
after reconstruction of the anterior cruciate ligament. *Clin Orthop* 1984;183:122–140.

11. Marcacci M, Zaffagnini S, Iacono F, Neri MP,
Petitto A: Early versus late reconstruction for
anterior cruciate ligament rupture: Results after
five years of followup. *Am J Sports Med* 1995;
23:690–693.

12. Noyes FR, Barber-Westin SD: Reconstruction
of the anterior cruciate ligament with human
allograft: Comparison of early and later results.
J Bone Joint Surg 1996;78A:524–537.

13. O'Neill DB: Arthroscopically assisted reconstruction of the anterior cruciate ligament: A
prospective randomized analysis of three techniques. *J Bone Joint Surg* 1996;78A:803–813.

14. Shelbourne KD, Klootwyk TE, Wilckens JH,
De Carlo MS: Ligament stability two to six
years after anterior cruciate ligament reconstruction with autogenous patellar tendon graft
and participation in accelerated rehabilitation
program. *Am J Sports Med* 1995;23:575–579.

15. Sommerlath K, Lysholm J, Gillquist J: The
long-term course after treatment of acute anterior cruciate ligament ruptures: A 9 to 16 year
followup. *Am J Sports Med* 1991;19:156–162.

16. Frank CB, Jackson DW: The science of reconstruction of the anterior cruciate ligament.
J Bone Joint Surg 1997;79A:1556–1576.

17. *Webster's Third New International Dictionary of the
English Language Unabridged.* Springfield, Massachusetts, Merriam-Webster, 1986, vol 1, p 920.

18. Dye SF: The knee as a biologic transmission
with an envelope of function: A theory. *Clin
Orthop* 1996;325:10–18.

19. Dye SF, Vaupel GL, Dye CC, et al: Conscious
neurosensory mapping of the internal structures of the human knee without intraarticular
anesthesia. *Orthop Trans* 1997;21:20.

20. Winter DA: Energy generation and absorption
at the ankle and knee during fast, natural, and
slow cadences. *Clin Orthop* 1983;175:147–154.

21. Guyton AC (ed): *Textbook of Medical Physiology*,
ed 7. Philadelphia, PA, WB Saunders, 1986.

22. Frost HM: A determinant of bone architecture:
The minimum effective strain. *Clin Orthop*
1983;175:286–292.

23. Frost HM: Editorial: Some ABCs of skeletal
pathophysiology: I. Introduction to the series.
Calcif Tissue Int 1989;45:1–3.

24. Frost HM: Editorial: Some ABCs of skeletal
pathophysiology: II. General mediator mechanism properties. *Calcif Tissue Int* 1989;45:68–70.

25. Frost HM: Editorial: Some ABCs of skeletal
pathophysiology: IV. The transient/steady state
distinction. *Calcif Tissue Int* 1989;45:134–136.

26. Frost HM: Editorial: Some ABCs of skeletal
pathophysiology: 5. Microdamage physiology.
Calcif Tissue Int 1991;49:229–231.

27. Frost HM: Editorial: Some ABCs of skeletal
pathophysiology: 6. The growth/modeling/
remodeling distinction. *Calcif Tissue Int* 1991;
49:301–302.

28. Frost HM: Editorial: Some ABCs of skeletal
pathophysiology: 7. Tissue mechanisms controlling bone mass. *Calcif Tissue Int* 1991;49:
303–304.

29. Frost HM: Editorial: Some ABCs of skeletal
pathophysiology: 8. The trivial/physiologic/
pathologic distinction. *Calcif Tissue Int* 1992;50:
105–106.

30. Neurath MF, Printz H, Stofft E: Cellular ultrastructure of the ruptured anterior cruciate ligament: A transmission electron microscopic and
immunohistochemical study in 55 cases. *Acta
Orthop Scand* 1994;65:71–76.

31. Oakes BW: Collagen ultrastructure in the normal ACL and in ACL graft, in Jackson DW,
Arnoczky SP, Woo SLY, Frank CB, Simon TM
(eds): *The Anterior Cruciate Ligament: Current and
Future Concepts.* New York, NY, Raven Press,
1993, pp 209–217.

32. Shino K, Oakes BW, Horibe S, Nakata K,
Nakamura N: Collagen fibril populations in
human anterior cruciate ligament allografts:
Electron microscopic analysis. *Am J Sports Med*
1995;23:203–208.

33. Goertzen M, Gruber J, Dellmann A, Clahsen
H, Schulitz KP: Neurohistological findings
after experimental anterior cruciate ligament
allograft transplantation. *Arch Orthop Trauma
Surg* 1992;111:126–129.

34. Johansson H, Sjolander P, Sojka P: Receptors in
the knee joint ligaments and their role in the
biomechanics of the joint. *Crit Rev Biomed Eng*
1991;18:341–368.

35. Johansson H, Sjolander P, Sojka P: A sensory
role for the cruciate ligaments. *Clin Orthop*
1991;268:161–178.

36. Schultz RA, Miller DC, Kerr CS, Micheli L:
Mechanoreceptors in human cruciate ligaments: A histological study. *J Bone Joint Surg*
1984;66A:1072–1076.

37. Barrack RL, Lund PJ, Munn BG, Wink C,
Happel L: Evidence of reinnervation of free
patellar tendon autograft used for anterior cruciate ligament reconstruction. *Am J Sports Med*
1997;25:196–202.

38. van Rens TJ, van den Berg AF, Huiskes R,
Kuypers W: Substitution of the anterior cruciate ligament: A long-term histologic and biomechanical study with autogenous pedicled
grafts of the iliotibial band in dogs. *Arthroscopy*
1986;2:139–154.

39. Grillner S: Neural networks for vertebrate
locomotion. *Sci Am* 1996;274:64–69.

40. Marr D: A theory of cerebellar cortex. *J Physiol
(Lond)* 1969;202:437–470.

41. Albus JS: A theory of cerebellar function. *Math
Biosci* 1971;10:25–61.

42. Schmahmann JD: An emerging concept: The
cerebellar contribution to higher function. *Arch
Neurol* 1991;48:1178–1187.

43. Wojtys EM, Huston LJ: Longitudinal effects of
ACL injury and patellar tendon autograft
reconstruction on neuromuscular performance.
Orthop Trans 1997;21:195.

44. Wang CJ, Walker PS: Rotatory laxity of the
human knee joint. *J Bone Joint Surg* 1974;56A:
161–170.

45. Markolf KL, Graff-Radford A, Amstutz HC: In
vivo knee stability: A quantitative assessment
using an instrumented clinical testing apparatus. *J Bone Joint Surg* 1978;60A:664–674.

46. Elmqvist LG, Lorentzon R, Johansson C, Fugl-
Meyer AR: Does a torn anterior cruciate ligament lead to change in the central nervous
drive of the knee extensors? *Europ J Appl
Physiol Occup Physiol* 1988;58:203–207.

47. Goldfuss AJ, Morehouse CA, LeVeau BF:
Effect of muscular tension on knee stability.
Med Sci Sports 1973;5:267–271.

48. Wojtys EM, Huston LJ: Neuromuscular performance in normal and anterior cruciate ligament-deficient lower extremities. *Am J Sports
Med* 1994;22:89–104.

49. Caraffa A, Cerulli G, Projetti M, Aisa G, Rizzo
A: Prevention of anterior cruciate ligament injuries in soccer: A prospective controlled study
of proprioceptive training. *Knee Surg Sports
Traumatol Arthrosc* 1996;4:19–21.

50. Fu FH: Physiologic/biologic factors in anterior
cruciate ligament reconstructed knees: Proceedings of the American Academy of Orthopaedic Surgeons 64th Annual Meeting, San
Francisco, CA. Rosemont, IL, American Academy of Orthopaedic Surgeons, 1997, p 123.

51. Dieppe P, Cushnaghan J, Young P, Kirwan J:
Prediction of the progression of joint space
narrowing in osteoarthritis of the knee by bone
scintigraphy. *Ann Rheum Dis* 1993;52:557–563.

52. Dye SF: The use of technetium scintigraphy in
the assessment of musculoskeletal trauma, in
Recent Advances in Operative Orthopedics. St.

Louis, MO, Mosby-Year Book, 1995, vol 3, pp 183–216.

53. Dye SF Chew MH: The use of scintigraphy to detect increased osseous metabolic activity about the knee. *J Bone Joint Surg* 1993;75A: 1388–1406.

54. Dye SF, Chew M, McBride J, Sostre G: Restoration of osseous homeostasis of the knee following mensical surgery. *Orthop Trans* 1992;16:725–726.

55. Egund N, Frost S, Brismar J, Gustafson T: Radiography and scintigraphy in the assessment of early gonarthrosis. *Acta Radiol* 1988;29: 451–455.

56. McBride JT, Rodkey WG, Brooks DE, Dye S, Cowan C: Early detection of osteoarthritis using technetium 99m MDP imaging, radiographs, histology and gross pathology in an experimental rabbit model. *Orthop Trans* 1991; 15:348–349.

57. Dye SF, Chew MH: Restoration of osseous homeostasis after anterior cruciate ligament reconstruction. *Am J Sports Med* 1993;21: 748–750.

58. Aglietti P, Zaccherotti G, De Biase P, Taddei I: A comparison between medial meniscus repair, partial meniscectomy, and normal meniscus in anterior cruciate ligament reconstructed knees. *Clin Orthop* 1994;307:165–173.

59. Dye SF, Herzog RJ, Marks PH, Nottage WM III: Current concepts in orthopaedic imaging: Knee and shoulder. Proceedings of the American Academy of Orthopaedic Surgeons 64th Annual Meeting, San Francisco, CA. Rosemont, IL, American Academy of Orthopaedic Surgeons, 1997, p 312.

60. Muehllehner G, Karp JS: Positron emission tomography imaging: Technical considerations. *Semin Nucl Med* 1986;16:35–50.

61. Mueller WM, Yetkin GZ, Hammeke TA, et al: Functional magnetic resonance imaging mapping of the motor cortex in patients with cerebral tumors. *Neurosurgery* 1996;39:515–520.

62. Marks PH, Goldenberg JA, Vezina WC, Chamberlain MJ, Vellet AD, Fowler PJ: Subchondral bone infractions in acute ligamentous knee injuries demonstrated on bone scintigraphy and magnetic resonance imaging. *J Nucl Med* 1992; 33:516–520.

63. Stoller DW, Cannon WD Jr, Anderson LJ: The knee, in Stoller DW (ed): *Magnetic Resonance Imaging in Orthopaedics and Sports Medicine*, ed 2. Philadelphia, PA, Lippincott-Raven, 1997, pp 203–442.

64. Johnson DL, Urban WP Jr, Caborn DNM, Vanarthros WJ, Carlson CS: Articular cartilage changes seen with magnetic resonance imaging-detected bone bruises associated with acute anterior cruciate ligament rupture. *Am J Sports Med* 1998;26:409–414.

65. Dorchak JD, Barrack RL, Alexander AH, Dye SF, Dresser TP: Radionuclide imaging of the knee with chronic anterior cruciate ligament tear. *Orthop Rev* 1993;22:1233–1241.

66. Dye SF, Andersen CT, Stowell MT: Unrecognized abnormal osseous metabolic activity about the knee of patients with symptomatic anterior cruciate ligament deficiency. *Orthop Trans* 1987;11:492.

67. Shapeero LG, Dye SF, Lipton MJ, Gould RG, Galvin EG, Genant HK: Functional dynamics of the knee joint by ultrafast, cine-CT. *Invest Radiol* 1988;23:118–123.

68. Thompson WO, Thaete FL, Fu FH, Dye SF: Tibial meniscal dynamics using three-dimensional reconstruction of magnetic resonance images. *Am J Sports Med* 1991;19:210–216.

69. Frank CB, Hart DA: The biology of tendons and ligaments, in Mow VC, Ratcliffe A, Woo SLY (eds): *Biomechanics of Diarthrodial Joints*. New York, NY, Springer-Verlag, 1990, pp 39–62.

70. Broom ND, Myers DB: A study of the structural response of wet hyaline cartilage to various loading situations. *Connect Tissue Res* 1980; 7:227–237.

71. Gray ML, Pizzanelli AM, Grodzinsky AJ, Lee RC: Mechanical and physiochemical determinants of the chondrocyte biosynthetic response. *J Orthop Res* 1988;6:777–792.

72. Guilak F, Mow VC: Determination of the mechanical response of the chondrocyte in situ using finite element modeling and confocal microscopy. *Adv Bioeng (ASME)* 1992;22:21–23.

73. Guilak F, Donahue H, Zell R, et al: Deformation-induced calcium signalling in articular chondrocytes, in Mow VC, Guilak F, Tron-Son-Tray R, Houchmuth RM (eds): *Cell Mechanics and Cellular Engineering*. New York, NY, Springer-Verlag, 1994, pp 380–397.

74. Kiviranta I, Tammi M, JurvelinJ, Arokoski J, Saamanen AM, Helminen HJ: Articular cartilage thickness and glycosaminoglycan distribution in the canine knee joint after strenuous running exercise. *Clin Orthop* 1992;283: 302–308.

75. Arnoczky SP, Hoonjan A, Whallon JH, Cloutier B: Cell deformation in tendons under tensile load: A morphological analysis using confocal laser microscopy. *Trans Orthop Res Soc* 1994;19:495.

76. Marks PH: The anterior cruciate ligament risk equation. Proceedings of the American Academy of Orthopaedic Surgeons 64th Annual Meeting, San Francisco, CA. Rosemont, IL, American Academy of Orthopaedic Surgeons, 1997, p 312.

77. Dye SF, Shifflett S, Bessolo R, Vaupel G: Comparison of magnetic resonance imaging and technetium scintigraphy in the detection of increased osseous metabolic activity about the knee of symptomatic adults. *Orthop Trans* 1993; 17:1060–1061.

78. Lang P, Jergesen HE, Genant HK, Moseley ME, Schulte-Monting J: Magnetic resonance imaging of the ischemic femoral head in pigs: Dependency of signal intensities and relaxation times on elapsed time. *Clin Orthop* 1989;244: 272–280.

79. Muehllehner G, Karp JS: A positron camera using position-sensitive detectors: PENN-PET. *J Nucl Med* 1986;27:90–98.

80. Moseley ME, deCrespigny A, Spielman DM: Magnetic resonance imaging of human brain function. *Surg Neurol* 1996;45:385–391.

81. Dye SF: The future of anterior cruciate ligament restoration. *Clin Orthop* 1996;325: 130–139.

The Posterior Cruciate Ligament Injured Knee: Principles of Evaluation and Treatment

Mark D. Miller, MD
John A. Bergfeld, MD
Peter J. Fowler, MD, FACSC
Christopher D. Harner, MD
Frank R. Noyes, MD

Introduction

Although our knowledge regarding the evaluation and treatment of the posterior cruciate ligament (PCL)-injured knee continues to lag far behind that of the anterior cruciate ligament (ACL)-injured knee, the PCL remains a major focus of ongoing sports medicine research. New surgical techniques continue to be developed that attempt to reproduce the anatomy and function of the PCL. However, substantial controversy exists over the natural history and surgical indications for PCL injuries. In this article we will begin with a review of the basic science of the PCL, discuss mechanisms of injury, and attempt to elucidate the natural history of the PCL-injured knee. We will then discuss the principles of evaluation and treatment of PCL injuries as well as review commonly accepted surgical indications. Finally, we will highlight some of the important rehabilitation principles and forecast future directions for further research.

Basic Science
Functional Anatomy

The PCL has two functional components, an anterolateral portion, and a

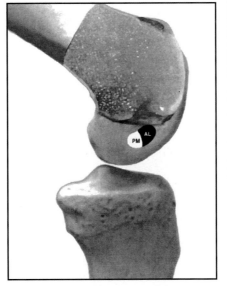
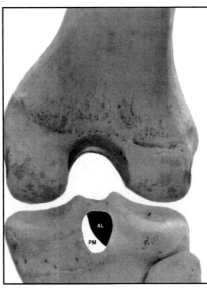

Fig. 1 Lateral and posterior views demonstrating the "footprints" of the anterolateral and posteromedial portions of the posterior cruciate ligament.

posteromedial portion (Fig. 1). These components, or "bundles," are named based on the femoral origin and tibial insertion. The anterolateral portion, which is tight in flexion, is biomechanically superior to the smaller posteromedial portion.[1] For this reason, most surgical "one bundle" techniques attempt to reproduce the anterolateral portion of the ligament. In addition, there are two variable

meniscofemoral ligaments (ligament of Humphry, anterior; and ligament of Wrisberg, posterior) that arise from the posterior horn of the lateral meniscus, run on either side of the PCL, and insert on the medial femoral condyle with the PCL. Although these ligaments are also biomechanically inferior to the anterolateral portion of the PCL,[1] they should be preserved whenever possible.

Ligament Biomechanics

The PCL is the primary restraint to posterior tibial translation, sustaining from 85% to almost 100% of the load at 90° of flexion.[2,3] The PCL is not twice as "strong" as the ACL, as was once believed.[4] It has an ultimate load capacity that only slightly exceeds that of the ACL.[5] However, as noted above, the stiffness, ultimate load, and modulus of elasticity are highly dependent on the portion of the ligament tested, with the anterolateral component exhibiting superior biomechanical properties.[1,6]

Mechanism of Injury

An acute injury to a static structure results from elongation of that structure beyond its elastic limits. This most often occurs as a result of joint distraction or dislocation, and it is resisted by the ligament itself and by other structures. The injury can occur as a result of passive (external) or active (internal) forces. PCL injuries are most often the result of passive forces. Perhaps the most common mechanism of injury to the PCL is an anterior blow to the proximal tibia (the so-called "dashboard" injury). Hyperflexion is the most common mechanism in sports-related injuries.[7] Other less common mechanisms of injury include hyperextension and quadriceps-active anterior knee dislocation.

Although most injuries are associated with midsubstance ruptures, flexion injuries have a tendency to be located on the tibial side of the ligament, and extension injuries are more commonly located on the femoral side.

Natural History

The natural history of the PCL-injured knee is one of the most controversial areas in sports medicine. It has long been purported that isolated PCL injuries do well,[8,9] and recent reports further support this precept.[10] It is important to note that a recent study[10] did not include advanced (grade 3) injuries. Other studies have identified a high incidence of late chondrosis of the medial femoral condyle and patellofemoral joint with nonsurgical treatment.[11–13] Another recent study substantiated this and also identified an increased incidence of meniscal tears associated with chronic PCL injuries.[14] These effects are likely a result of increased contact pressures that occur as a result of PCL deficiency.[15,16] Still other reports suggest that the prognosis of the PCL-injured knee is highly variable, and that there may be no way to predict long-term outcomes.[17] Perhaps the most commonly held belief is that degenerative change is probably inevitable, and that current surgical techniques cannot forestall it.[18,19] Nevertheless, PCL injuries may not be as benign as we previously thought, especially with advanced (grade 3) injuries.

Clinical Evaluation
Physical Examination

The most sensitive test for PCL injury is the posterior drawer test.[20] Perhaps the most important aspect of this test is to assess the translation from the normal starting point of the medial tibial plateau/medial femoral condyle position.[21] Although the classic 0 to 5 mm (grade 1), 5 to 10 mm (grade 2), and > 10 mm (grade 3) displacements are commonly used, it is perhaps more helpful to classify PCL injuries based on the medial tibial plateau/medial femoral condyle position. In this classification, grade 1 injuries preserve some anterior position of the tibia, grade 2 injuries occur when the tibia is "flush" with the medial femoral condyle, and grade 3 injuries allow displacement of the tibia posterior to the condyle (Fig. 2).

One of the authors (JAB) has found that the presence of decreased posterior laxity with internal rotation more often indicates a PCL injury that will do well with nonsurgical treatment. He believes that a PCL-injured knee with a positive posterior drawer test that does not decrease with internal tibial rotation usually requires PCL reconstruction.

A variety of other adjunctive tests for PCL injury have been described and have been summarized elsewhere.[22] These tests include the drop back or "sag" sign,[23] the posterior Lachman,[24] the prone drawer test,[25] the quadriceps active test,[26] and the dynamic posterior shift test.[27]

It is essential to perform a complete examination of the knee to include the menisci (joint line tenderness and McMurray testing), ACL (Lachman and Pivot shift tests), varus/valgus instability, and, perhaps most importantly, the posterolateral corner.

The association of PCL injuries with posterolateral corner (PLC) injuries is only now being understood. Much like in ACL/PLC injuries, PLC injuries may require early PCL and PLC reconstruction, which can affect the natural history of these combined injuries. The key examination feature to recognition of these previously misunderstood injuries is external rotation asymmetry. This examination is best performed with the patient prone. Asymmetry (an increase of > 10° to 15° of foot external rotation compared to the opposite, uninjured side) at 30° of knee flexion is associated with PLC injury. If there is asymmetry at both 30° and 90° of flexion, an injury to both the PCL and the PLC should be suspected.[28] Other adjunctive tests for PLC injury include the external rotation recurvatum test,[29] the posterolateral drawer test,[29] and the reversed pivot-shift test.[30] It should be noted, however, that these adjunctive tests may have a high false positive rate, and comparison with the opposite side is essential.[31]

Imaging Studies

Plain radiographs are often not helpful in the evaluation of acute PCL injuries. They should always be obtained, however, because bony avulsion can be identified, and there is little controversy that these bony injuries should be fixed.[32] Plain radiographs, particularly flexion weightbearing posteroanterior views[33] and patellar views, can be helpful in evaluating chondrosis in long-standing PCL injuries.

Recently, Professor Puddu, of Italy, described a plain radiographic view that may be helpful in the evaluation of PCL-injured knees (Puddu G, personal communication, 1997). The view (Fig. 3) is similar to the Laurin view for the patella,[34] except the patient is positioned supine with the knees flexed 70°. The resulting image is evaluated based on the location of the tibia in relation to the femur, and is compared with the normal side (taken simultaneously).

Stress radiographs can also be useful in the evaluation of PCL injury and treatment (Figs. 4 and 5). One recent study concluded that stress radiography is superior to both the arthrometer and clinical posterior testing for determining PCL status.[35] These investigators determined that 8 mm or more of increased posterior translation on stress radiographs was indicative of complete PCL rupture.

Radionuclide imaging (bone scans), which can identify the early chondrosis that can be associated with chronic PCL injury, may prove of use in following these injuries and their treatment. Magnetic resonance imaging (MRI) can be useful in confirming PCL injuries. One recent study

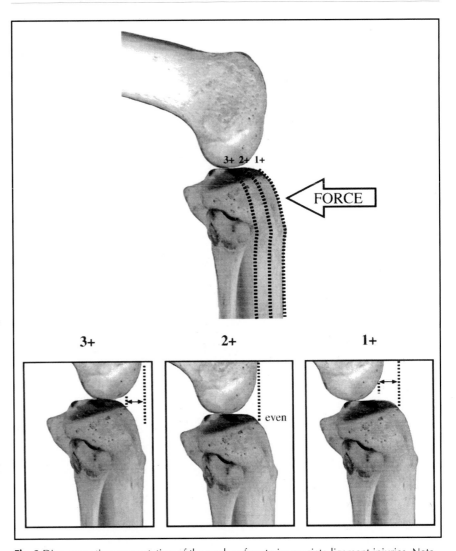

Fig. 2 Diagrammatic representation of the grades of posterior cruciate ligament injuries. Note that in grade 3 injuries, the tibia can be displaced posterior to the medial femoral condyle.

demonstrated that MRI had a 100% sensitivity and specificity in identifying complete tears of the PCL.[36] MRI may also be useful in the evaluation of the menisci and articular surfaces.

Examination Under Anesthesia

Examination under anesthesia can yield valuable information and aid in final planning prior to performing surgery. In addition to confirming that the PCL is injured (posterior drawer, Godfrey),[23] it is also critical for confirming the presence or absence of a PLC injury (external rotation asym-

metry, asymmetric posterolateral drawer/recurvatum/reversed pivot shift).

Diagnostic Arthroscopy

Diagnostic arthroscopy is useful as a final confirmation of PCL injury during the initial stages of PCL reconstruction. Often, upon initial inspection, the PCL may appear to be intact, however, it is critical to recognize that this ligament is encased in its own synovial sheath, and that injuries to the ligament often cannot be noted until the PCL itself is visualized.

Direct visualization of PCL in-

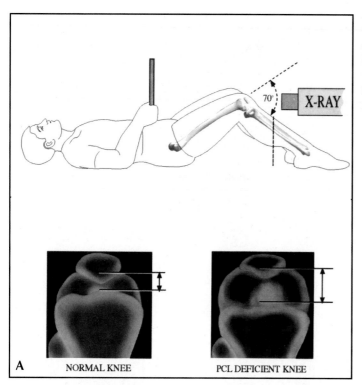

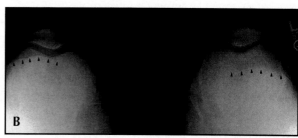

A — NORMAL KNEE   PCL DEFICIENT KNEE

Fig. 3 Puddu view for demonstration of posterior displacement of the tibia. **A,** Diagrammatic view of technique (top) and resultant image (bottom). **B,** Radiograph of a patient with a left knee posterolateral corner injury. Arrowheads outline the proximal tibia. Note posterior displacement of the injured left knee.

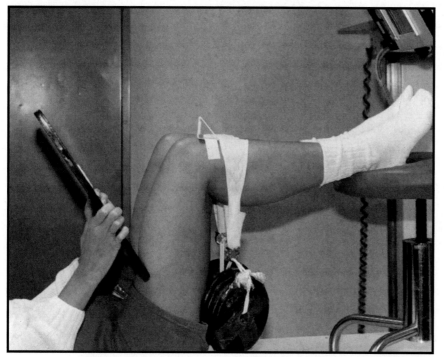

Fig. 4 Sunrise stress radiographic technique. An 89-N weight is suspended from each proximal tibia at the level of the tibial tubercle while the tibias are held in a horizontal plane approximately 2 to 3 cm apart. The X-ray beam is projected from the distal to proximal at a 30° angle while the patient holds a 14 × 17 inch radiographic cassette on the midportion of both thighs oriented at 90° to the X-ray beam.

juries can sometimes be accomplished by using a modified Gillquist view (Fig. 6, *A*) or by using the posteromedial portal for viewing (Fig. 6, *B*). Most often, however, the presence of a PCL injury is best noted with indirect signs.[37] These indirect signs include (1) the sloppy ACL sign (ACL pseudolaxity), (2) posterior displacement of the medial femoral condyle in relation to the medial meniscus, and (3) chondrosis of the medial femoral condyle and patellofemoral joint (late finding).

Perhaps the most important of these indirect signs is the first. In a PCL-injured knee, the ACL will often appear to be lax. If an anterior drawer force is placed on the knee, restoring the normal relationship of the medial tibial plateau and the medial femoral condyle, this laxity will resolve (Fig. 7). Failure to appreciate this pseudolaxity may encourage the unwary surgeon to perform

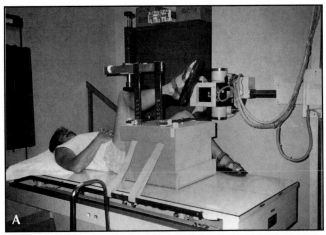
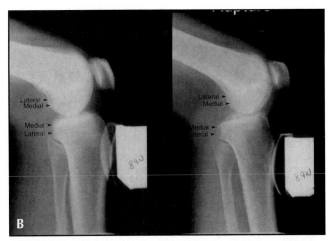

Fig. 5 A, Stress radiography testing with the modified X-Stress device (SAMSO, Bologna, Italy) is shown. An 89-N posterior load is applied to the anterior proximal tibia at the level of the tibial tubercle with the knee flexed to approximately 70°. The limb is positioned in neutral rotation with the tibia unconstrained and the quadriceps muscle completely relaxed. A lateral radiograph is taken of each knee from medial to lateral with a standard tube-to-cassette distance of 1 m. **B,** Resultant stress radiographs of a subject's intact (noninvolved) and posterior cruciate ligament (PCL)-deficient (complete PCL rupture) knees. The PCL-deficient knee demonstrated a 19-mm increase in posterior translation compared to the intact knee. Medial and lateral refer to the respective femoral condyle or tibial plateau. (Reproduced with permission from Hewett TE, Noyes FR, Lee MD: Diagnosis of complete and partial posterior cruciate ligament ruptures: Stress radiography compared with KT-1000 arthrometer and posterior drawer testing. *Am J Sports Med* 1997;25:648–655.)

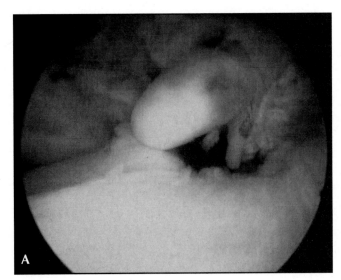
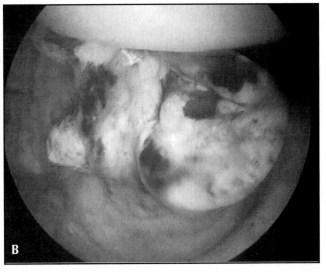

Fig. 6 Arthroscopic view of torn posterior cruciate ligament (PCL). **A,** Stump of PCL seen through modified Gillquist view. **B,** PCL remnants seen through a posteromedial portal.

an ACL reconstruction in an ACL-intact knee.

Surgical Indications
Given the controversy regarding the natural history of the PCL-deficient knee and historical inconsistencies in our ability to reconstruct this liga-ment, it is difficult to provide clear-cut recommendations regarding the indications for surgery. There is almost universal agreement that avulsion fractures of the PCL should be repaired primarily.[32,38,39] There is also general agreement that combined injuries, injuries to the PCL and ACL, the PCL and PLC, or to the PCL and medial collateral ligament, should also be surgically reconstructed.[40–42] Some authors recommend reconstruction in patients with PCL injuries and reparable meniscal tears or chondral injuries.[43] Outside of these parameters, there is little

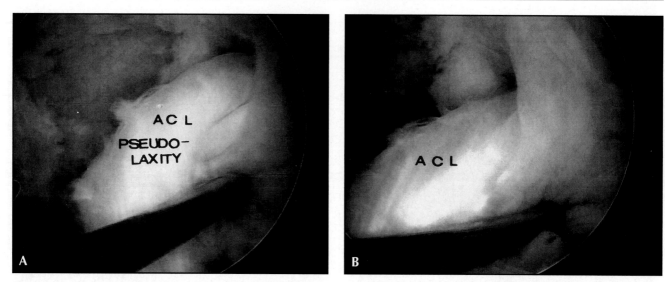

Fig. 7 Sloppy anterior cruciate ligament (ACL) sign, also known as ACL pseudolaxity, should not be mistaken for a torn ACL. **A,** Arthoscopic appearance of ACL pseudolaxity. **B,** Normal appearance of ACL with application of anterior drawer force.

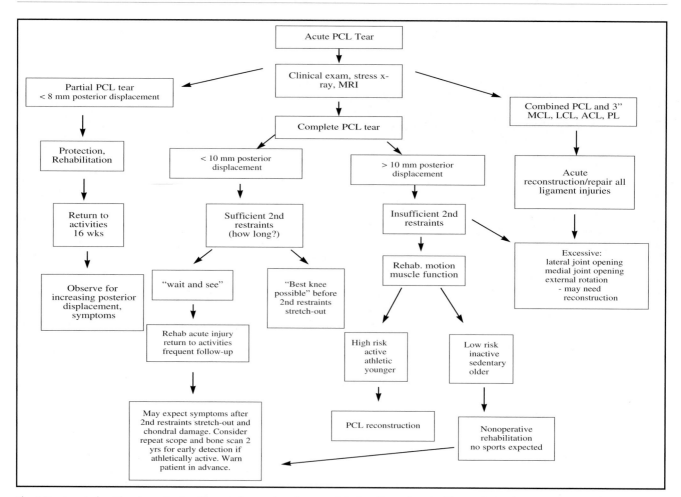

Fig. 8 Treatment algorithm for patients with posterior cruciate ligament injuries. (Reproduced with permission from Noyes FR, Barber-Westin SD: Treatment of complex injuries involving the posterior cruciate and posterolateral ligaments of the knee. *Am J Knee Surg* 1996;9:200–214.)

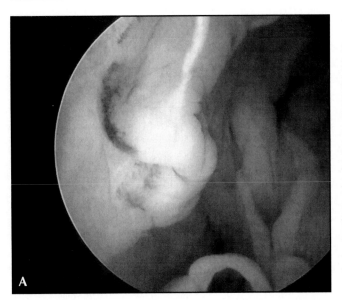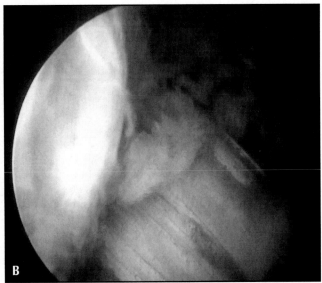

Fig. 9 A, Arthroscopic view (anterolateral portal) demonstrating a complete tear of the posterior cruciate ligament (PCL). **B,** Same arthroscopic view following PCL reconstruction with a bone-patella tendon-bone autograft.

consensus, even among the authors of this chapter. Most authors recommend PCL reconstruction in patients with grade 3 laxity early, and in patients with symptomatic grade 2 or 3 chronic laxity, but a great deal of controversy still exists. Perhaps further refinements in surgical techniques and a better understanding of the natural history of the PCL-deficient knee will expand these indications in the future.

One author's treatment rationale for patients with chronic PCL ruptures[44] is shown in Figure 8. When evaluating PCL injuries, it is important to determine if there is a varus malalignment of the knee. If so, a high tibial osteotomy should be performed prior to PCL reconstruction.[45] Finally, arthrosis rating is performed and knees with severe advance arthrosis are excluded from consideration for PCL reconstruction.

Surgical Techniques

A variety of surgical techniques for PCL reconstruction have been described. These are perhaps best con-

sidered in groups: (1) historical non-anatomic procedures, (2) arthroscopic anterior procedures, (3) posterior inlay procedures, (4) 2-bundle procedures, and (5) some combination of the above. Unfortunately, with the exception of the first group, there is a paucity of literature regarding surgical results for the various PCL reconstruction techniques. Nevertheless, it is important to note the differences between the groups for future comparison.

Historical Procedures

A variety of nonanatomic procedures have been described for reconstruction of the PCL. Perhaps the best known of these procedures include transfer of the medial head of the gastrocnemius (with or without a bone block),[46] popliteus dynamic transfer,[47] and semimembranosus reconstruction.[48] Unfortunately, all of these procedures ultimately failed and are no longer recommended.[49]

Arthroscopic Anterior Procedures

These procedures require that the tibial tunnel be drilled from anterior

to posterior. The graft (hamstring, patella tendon, Achilles tendon allograft, and others have been used) is then passed through the tibial tunnel and into the femoral tunnel. Unfortunately, the graft must negotiate a sharp "killer" turn (Friedman M, unpublished data, 1992), upon its exit from the tibial tunnel in order to be oriented towards the femoral tunnel. This turn has been implicated as a possible cause of late laxity with these procedures.[50]

Published results for arthroscopic PCL reconstructions are inconsistent. Better results have been reported with the use of patella tendon grafts,[11] and more discouraging results with hamstring grafts.[19,51] However, it appears that regardless of graft choice, the condition of most patients will improve, but the patients will develop some residual posterior laxity with these procedures.[52,53]

Posterior Inlay Procedures

This technique, first reported by Berg,[50] is appealing because it avoids the "killer" turn. The tibial side of the graft (patella tendon graft originally described, but quadriceps tendon and Achilles tendon grafts have also been used) is secured directly into a trough in the back of the tibia. The graft can then be directed straight to the femoral tunnel without an excessive bend. Modifications to the original technique to simplify the approach and graft passage have been described[54] (Fig. 9). **(CD–25.1)**

Two-Bundle Procedures

This technique attempts to reconstruct both portions of the PCL (anterolateral and posteromedial). Two separate grafts (eg, double hamstring grafts) or a split graft (eg, quadriceps tendon) are passed through a tibial tunnel, or secured on the back of the tibia and then passed through separate drill holes in the femur. The more anterolateral lateral portion of the graft is secured in flexion and the posteromedial portion is secured with the knee in extension. Two-bundle PCL grafts offer an attractive option; however, recommendations regarding the orientation and exact placement of these grafts will require further in vitro biomechanical studies.

Rehabilitation

Postoperative rehabilitation following PCL reconstruction is evolving. Most protocols emphasize the need for posterior support of the operative calf during nonbraced periods. The effect of gravity and the tendency for the tibia to displace posteriorly must be appreciated. Immediate postoperative care includes bracing the knee in full extension. This is believed to minimize the stress on the PCL.[55] Ambulation with weightbearing as tolerated is encouraged early, minimizing the effects of graft immobilization.[56] With simultaneous use of the hamstrings, quadriceps, and gastrocnemius during ambulation, the cruciates re-

main essentially unloaded.[57] Supported quadriceps exercises and ankle pumps are encouraged early. Bracing in extension is instituted for 6 weeks, and closed chain rehabilitative exercises are started shortly after this period. Proprioceptive training is usually initiated at 12 weeks. This is said to add further stability to the knee.[58] Hamstring exercises are delayed until the fourth postoperative month and light jogging is allowed at 6 months.

PCL functional braces are still under investigation. The theory is to position the tibia more anteriorly, which may counter the effect of gravity, reduce patellofemoral compression, and enhance the function of the quadriceps.

Conclusion

It is important for orthopaedic surgeons to be aware of new concepts in PCL injuries. A basic understanding of the anatomy and biomechanics is helpful in surgical planning. An appreciation of the mechanism of injury is useful in evaluating these injuries. The natural history of the PCL-injured knee continues to be a matter of intense debate, but we now understand that it may not be as benign as we once assumed. Clinical evaluation of PCL injuries is critical for all providers who take care of knee injuries. Surgical indications are also unclear in the literature, but it is hoped that they will expand with improved techniques. Surgical techniques should attempt to reproduce normal anatomy as much as possible, and results may be expected to improve with newer procedures. Rehabilitation should attempt to counter the normal effects of gravity, and posterior support should be included. In summary, the treatment of PCL injuries continues to evolve, and renewed emphasis on this problem may lead to new solutions.

References

1. Harner CD, Xerogeanes JW, Livesay GA, et al: The human posterior cruciate ligament complex: An interdisciplinary study. Ligament morphology and biomechanical evaluation *Am J Sports Med* 1995;23:736–745.

2. Butler DL, Noyes FR, Grood ES: Ligamentous restraints to anterior-posterior drawer in the human knee: A biomechanical study. *J Bone Joint Surg* 1980;62A:259–270.

3. Gollehon DL, Torzilli PA, Warren RF: The role of the posterolateral and cruciate ligaments in the stability of the human knee: A biomechanical study. *J Bone Joint Surg* 1987;69A:233–242.

4. Kennedy JC, Hawkins RJ, Willis RB, Danylchuck KD: Tension studies of human knee ligaments: Yield point, ultimate failure, and disruption of the cruciate and tibial collateral ligaments. *J Bone Joint Surg* 1976;58A:350–355.

5. Prietto MP, Bain JR, Stonebrook SN, Settlage RA: Tensile strength of the human posterior cruciate ligament (PCL) *Trans Orthop Res Soc* 1988;13:195.

6. Race A, Amis AA: The mechanical properties of the two bundles of the human posterior cruciate ligament: *J Biomech* 1994;27:13–24.

7. Fowler PJ, Messieh SS: Isolated posterior cruciate ligament injuries in athletes. *Am J Sports Med* 1987;15:553–557.

8. Parolie JM, Bergfeld JA: Long-term results of nonoperative treatment of isolated posterior cruciate ligament injuries in the athlete. *Am J Sports Med* 1986;14:35–38.

9. Torg JS, Barton TM, Pavlov H, Stine R: Natural history of the posterior cruciate ligament-deficient knee. *Clin Orthop* 1989; 246:208–216.

10. Shelbourne KD, Patel DV: The natural history of acute, isolated nonoperatively treated posterior cruciate ligament injuries of the knee: A prospective study. Proceedings of the American Academy of Orthopaedic Surgeons 64th Annual meeting, San Francisco, CA. Rosemont, IL, American Academy of Orthopaedic Surgeons, 1997, pp 77–78.

11. Clancy WG Jr, Shelbourne KD, Zoellner GB, Keene JS, Reider B, Rosenberg TD: Treatment of knee joint instability secondary to rupture of the posterior cruciate ligament: Report of a new procedure. *J Bone Joint Surg* 1983;65A:310–322.

12. Dejour H, Walch G, Peyrot J, et al: The natural history of rupture of the posterior cruciate ligament. *Fr J Orthop Surg* 1988;2:112–120.

13. Keller PM, Shelbourne KD, McCarroll JR, Rettig AC: Nonoperatively treated isolated posterior cruciate ligament injuries. *Am J Sports Med* 1993;21:132–136.

14. Geissler WB, Whipple TL: Intraarticular abnormalities in association with posterior cruciate ligament injuries. *Am J Sports Med* 1993;21:846–849.

15. Skyhar MJ, Warren RF, Ortiz GJ, Schwartz E, Otis JC: The effects of sectioning of the poste-

rior cruciate ligament and the posterolateral complex on the articular contact pressures within the knee. *J Bone Joint Surg* 1993;75A: 694–699.

16. MacDonald P, Miniaci A, Fowler P, Marks P, Finlay B: A biomechanical analysis of joint contact forces in the posterior cruciate deficient knee. *Knee Surg Sports Traumatol Arthroscopy* 1996;3:252–255.

17. Boynton MD, Tietjens BR: Long-term followup of the untreated isolated posterior cruciate ligament-deficient knee. *Am J Sports Med* 1996;24:306–310.

18. Cross MJ, Powell JF: Long-term followup of posterior cruciate ligament rupture: A study of 116 cases. *Am J Sports Med* 1984;12:292–297.

19. Lipscomb AB Jr, Anderson AF, Norwig ED, Hovis WD, Brown DL: Isolated posterior cruciate ligament reconstruction: Long-term results. *Am J Sports Med* 1993;21:490–496.

20. Grood ES, Stowers SF, Noyes FR: Limits of movement in the human knee: Effect of sectioning the posterior cruciate ligament and posterolateral structures. *J Bone Joint Surg* 1988; 70A:88–97.

21. Müller W (ed): *The Knee: Form, Function, and Ligament Reconstruction.* Berlin, Germany, Springer-Verlag, 1983.

22. Miller MD, Johnson DL, Harner CD, Fu FH: Posterior cruciate ligament injuries. *Orthop Rev* 1993;22:1201–1210.

23. Godfrey JD: Ligamentous injuries of the knee. *Curr Pract Orthop Surg* 1973;5:56–92.

24. Torg JS, Conrad W, Kalen V: Clinical diagnosis of anterior cruciate ligment instability in the athlete. *Am J Sports Med* 1976;4:84–93.

25. Whipple TL, Ellis FD: Posterior cruciate ligament injuries. *Clin Sports Med* 1991;10: 515–527.

26. Daniel DM, Stone ML, Barnett P, Sachs R: Use of the quadriceps active test to diagnose posterior cruciate-ligament disruption and measure posterior laxity of the knee. *J Bone Joint Surg* 1988;70A:386–391.

27. Shelbourne KD, Benedict F, McCarroll JR, Rettig AC: Dynamic posterior shift test: An adjuvant in evaluation of posterior tibial subluxation. *Am J Sports Med* 1989;17:275–277.

28. Veltri DM, Warren RF: Posterolateral instability of the knee, in Jackson DW: *Instructional Course Lectures 44.* Rosemont, IL, American Academy of Orthopaedic Surgeons, 1995, pp 441–453.

29. Hughston JC, Norwood LA Jr: The posterolateral drawer test and external rotational recurvatum test for posterolateral rotatory instability of the knee. *Clin Orthop* 1980;147:82–87.

30. Jakob RP, Hassler H, Staeubli HU: Observations on rotatory instability of the lateral compartment of the knee: Experimental studies on the functional anatomy and the pathomechanism of the true and the reversed pivot shift sign. *Acta Orthop Scand* 1981;191(suppl):1–32.

31. Cooper DE: Tests for posterolateral instability of the knee in normal subjects: Results of examination under anesthesia. *J Bone Joint Surg* 1991;73A:30–36.

32. Meyers MH: Isolated avulsion of the tibial attachment of the posterior cruciate ligament of the knee. *J Bone Joint Surg* 1975;57A:669–672.

33. Rosenberg TD, Paulos LE, Parker RD, Coward DB, Scott SM: The 45 degree posteroanterior flexion weight-bearing radiograph of the knee. *J Bone Joint Surg* 1988;70A:1479–1483.

34. Laurin CA, Dussault R, Levesque HP: The tangential x-ray investigation of the patellofemoral joint: X-ray technique, diagnostic criteria and their interpretation. *Clin Orthop* 1979; 144:16–26.

35. Hewett TE, Noyes FR, Lee MD: Diagnosis of complete and partial posterior cruciate ligament ruptures: Stress radiography compared with KT-1000 arthrometer and posterior drawer testing. *Am J Sports Med* 1997;25:648–655.

36. Gross ML, Grover JS, Bassett LW, Seeger LL, Finerman GA: Magnetic resonance imaging of the posterior cruciate ligament: Clinical use to improve diagnostic accuracy. *Am J Sports Med* 1992;20:732–737.

37. Fanelli GC, Giannotti BF, Edson CJ: The posterior cruciate ligament arthroscopic evaluation and treatment. *Arthroscopy* 1994;10:673–688.

38. Satku K, Chew CN, Seow H: Posterior cruciate ligament injuries. *Acta Orthop Scand* 1984; 55:26–29.

39. Richter M, Kiefer H, Hehl G, Kinzl L: Primary repair for posterior cruciate ligament injuries: An eight-year followup of fifty-three patients. *Am J Sports Med* 1996;24:298–305.

40. Sisto DJ, Warren RF: Complete knee dislocation: A follow-up study of operative treatment. *Clin Orthop* 1985;198:94–101.

41. Roman PD, Hopson CN, Zenni EJ Jr: Traumatic dislocation of the knee: A report of 30 cases and literature review. *Orthop Rev* 1987;16:917–924.

42. Plancher KD, Siliski JM, Ribbans W: Traumatic dislocation of the knee: Complications and results of operative and nonoperative treatment. Proceedings of the American Academy of Orthopaedic Surgeons 56th Annual Meeting, Las Vegas, NV. Park Ridge, IL, American Academy of Orthopaedic Surgeons, 1989, p 85.

43. Shino K, Horibe S, Nakata K, Maeda A, Hamada M, Nakamura N: Conservative treatment of isolated injuries to the posterior cruciate ligament in athletes. *J Bone Joint Surg* 1995;77B:895–900.

44. Noyes FR, Barber-Westin SD: Treatment of complex injuries involving the posterior cruciate and posterolateral ligaments of the knee. *Am J Knee Surg* 1996;9:200–214.

45. Noyes FR, Roberts CS: High tibial osteotomy in knees with associated chronic ligament deficiencies, in Jackson DW (ed): *Reconstructive Knee Surgery.* New York, NY, Raven Press, 1995, pp 185–210.

46. Hughston JC, Degenhardt TC: Reconstruction of the posterior cruciate ligament. *Clin Orthop* 1982;164:59–77.

47. McCormick WC, Bagg RJ, Kennedy CW Jr, Leukens CA: Reconstruction of the posterior cruciate ligament: Preliminary report of a new procedure. *Clin Orthop* 1976;118:30–31.

48. Southmayd WW, Rubin BD: Reconstruction of the posterior cruciate ligament using the semimembranosus tendon. *Clin Orthop* 1980;150: 196–197.

49. Roth JH, Bray RC, Best TM, Cunning LA, Jacobson RP: Posterior cruciate ligament reconstruction by transfer of the medial gastrocnemius tendon. *Am J Sports Med* 1988; 16:21–28.

50. Berg EE: Posterior cruciate ligament tibial inlay reconstruction. *Arthroscopy* 1995;11:69–76.

51. Barrett GR, Savoie FH: Operative management of acute PCL injuries with associated pathology: Long-term results. *Orthopedics* 1991;14: 687–692.

52. Maday M, Fu FH, Harner CD, Irrgang JJ: Posterior cruciate ligament reconstruction using fresh frozen allograft tissue: Indications, techniques, results, and controversies. Proceedings of the American Academy of Orthopaedic Surgeons 60th Annual Meeting, San Francisco, CA. Rosemont, IL, American Academy of Orthopaedic Surgeons, 1993, p 413.

53. Noyes FR, Barber-Westin SD: Posterior cruciate ligament allograft reconstruction with and without a ligament augmentation device. *Arthroscopy* 1994;10:371–382.

54. Miller MD, Olszewski AD: Posterior cruciate ligament injuries: New treatment options. *Am J Knee Surg* 1995;8:145–154.

55. Ogata K, McCarthy JA: Measurements of length and tension patterns during reconstruction of the posterior cruciate ligament. *Am J Sports Med* 1992;20:351–355.

56. Kasperczyk WJ, Bosch U, Oestern HJ, Tscherne H: Influence of immobilization on autograft healing in the knee joint: A preliminary study in a sheep knee PCL model. *Arch Orthop Trauma Surg* 1991;110:158–161.

57. O'Connor JJ: Can muscle co-contraction protect knee ligaments after injury or repair? *J Bone Joint Surg* 1993;75B:41–48.

58. Johansson H, Sjolander P, Sojka P: A sensory role for the cruciate ligaments. *Clin Orthop* 1991;268:161–178.

Reference to Video

Miller MD, Hinkin DT: *Posterior Cruciate Ligament and Posterolateral Corner Reconstruction Using Autograft Tissues: New Techniques.* Colorado, United States Air Force Academy, 1996.

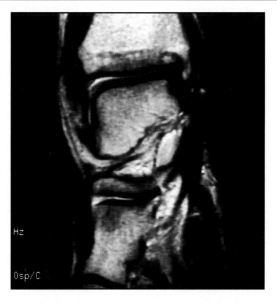

Disorders of the Achilles Tendon Insertion and Achilles Tendinitis

Mark S. Myerson, MD
William McGarvey, MD

Introduction

As a consequence of its size and unique functional anatomy, the Achilles tendon is susceptible to both acute and chronic injury. This chapter addresses some of these disorders, including the various forms of tendinitis, as well as the varied pain syndromes of the retrocalcaneal space, including retrocalcaneal bursitis and Haglund's deformity.

Functional and Gross Anatomy

The Achilles tendon is the continuation of the muscle of the triceps surae, which originates as the 2 heads of the gastrocnemius muscle from the medial and lateral femoral condyles. More distally, the gastrocnemius blends with the soleus muscle and forms the Achilles tendon, which then inserts into the middle third of the posterior tuberosity of the calcaneus. At the tendon-bone junction, the enthesis is composed of calcified and noncalcified cartilage. The paratenon that surrounds the tendon is able to stretch 2 to 3 cm with tendon movement, thereby allowing the Achilles tendon to glide smoothly. The tendon is vascularized via anterior muscular branches as well as osseous and periosteal vessels near the insertion site, and, although there is both a proximal and distal intratendinous vascular supply, con-

siderably fewer vessels are present 4 cm proximal to the calcaneus.[1-3] The region of the tendon 3 to 5 cm proximal to the insertion is a relatively avascular zone and, not surprisingly, is the area of the tendon most prone to various pathologies, including chronic tendinitis and rupture. One assumes that hypovascularity is at least 1 of the causes of rupture.

The Achilles tendon, posterior calcaneus, retrocalcaneal bursa, and pretendinous bursa are the anatomic structures comprising the posterior heel. The retrocalcaneal bursa lies anterior to the posterior superior calcaneal tuberosity of the calcaneus and lubricates the tendon anteriorly as well as the superior aspect of the calcaneus.[4] It is important to recognize that there is a normal communication between the posterior Achilles tendon and the retrocalcaneal bursa, and retrocalcaneal injection of steroid may adversely affect the Achilles tendon insertion. If the posterolateral and superior process of the calcaneus is enlarged, it is referred to as a Haglund's deformity.[5] The enthesis, the bursa, and the bursal walls form a complex insertional region protecting the Achilles and the posterior heel against wear and tear. The histopathology of the insertional region of the Achilles has been well studied by Rufai and associates.[6]

They found that in cadaver specimens with a prominent superior tuberosity, the walls of the bursa were fibrocartilaginous and replaced the calcaneal periosteum. If the tuberosity was not prominent, then the bursal fibrocartilages were absent. They concluded that these fibrocartilages could be implicated in retrocalcaneal bursitis.

From a functional standpoint, the gastrocnemius and the soleus muscles are important and strong muscles of plantarflexion of the foot, although due to its origin on the femoral condyles the gastrocnemius also flexes the knee. The gastrocnemius supplies the power for propulsion in walking, running, and jumping, whereas the soleus stabilizes the leg on the foot; the soleus is far more susceptible to immobilization by disuse atrophy. While running, the Achilles tendon is subject to forces that are 6 to 8 times body weight.[7] For example, hyperpronation of the foot during stance-phase activities may aggravate any underlying Achilles dysfunction, particularly tendinitis. Because the Achilles tendon inserts into the calcaneus, subtalar motion can place an uneven rotational force on the tendon fibers, which can lead to an imbalance at the tendon insertion, particularly with overuse. This is particularly noticeable in runners who over pronate, because excessive pronation of the foot during midstance causes an internal rotation force on the tibia. However, with knee extension, there is an external rotation force on the tibia, and these contradictory forces impart high stresses on the Achilles insertion.[8]

Achilles Tendinitis

Overuse injury of the Achilles tendon occurs commonly in individuals who are active and who subject the tendon to repetitive forces beyond its ability to heal. These injuries are noted in all athletes, not only runners. For those who regularly engage in other jumping activities, the forces may be normal in magnitude, but they are markedly increased in frequency, which increases the likelihood of injury. Achilles tendinitis does not represent a spectrum of disorders, and although acute and chronic inflammation may be present, it is more logical from a functional perspective to classify these disorders as those which either occur at the tendon insertion or more proximally, ie, insertional or noninsertional tendinitis.

The incidence of noninsertional Achilles tendinitis in runners is particularly high, occurring in approximately 10% of active runners,[9–12] and although tendinitis does occur in other athletic activities, such as ballet, tennis, soccer, and basketball, the pathogenesis of tendinitis is probably different in these individuals.[13] Noninsertional tendinitis occurs in more active athletes probably as a result of the repetitive stress of jumping, pushing off, and cutting activities, but this is in contrast to insertional tendinitis, which occurs in older, less athletic, and overweight individuals.

Noninsertional Achilles Tendinitis
We have found the histopathologic

classification system for noninsertional Achilles tendinitis developed by Puddu and associates[14] to be quite useful, because it separates tendinitis into 3 separate subgroups: paratendinitis, paratendinitis with tendinosis, and tendinosis. Paratendinitis is characterized by inflammation only of the tendon lining; tendinosis is a more advanced condition, with paratenon inflammation as well as intratendinous degeneration. Tendinosis is characterized by noninflammatory atrophic degeneration due to aging, microtrauma, or vascular compromise. The location of noninsertional Achilles tendinitis is generally in the hypovascular zone 4 cm proximal to the calcaneus, and the pathologic changes are the result of repetitive microtears that produce collagen degeneration, fibrosis, or even heterotopic ossification within the tendon.[15–17]

Perhaps the simplest explanation for the development of Achilles tendinitis is overuse associated with excessive forces on the Achilles tendon. There is a direct correlation between the incidence of Achilles tendinitis and the intensity of training and running activities.[18,19] Most athletes report a change in the duration, intensity, or frequency of their activities. However, one may not always find a marked alteration of physical activity, because the changes causing the inflammation may be the result of variations in the running surface or shoe wear. When acute, pain is present and associated with swelling, warmth, and tenderness 3 to 5 cm proximal to the insertion.

In acute paratendinitis, there is a diffuse fusiform, swelling, and the tenderness is present during active and passive dorsiflexion and plantarflexion. The pain is exacerbated by rubbing the tendon between the thumb and forefinger, and in doing so, thickening associated with crepi-

tus is noted when gliding the skin over the tendon. Rarely is any imaging study necessary, although if the diagnosis is in doubt, a magnetic resonance imaging (MRI) scan may be obtained, which is either normal, or associated with slight thickening of the paratenon.

In paratendinitis with tendinosis, there is more irregularity within the tendon and the thickening is quite diffuse and visible. Pain is marked, particularly when the tendon is squeezed.

In chronic tendinosis, in addition to the area of pain and thickening of the tendon, there is marked weakness and a decrease in push-off strength. As a result of the chronic degeneration, the tendon is not in functional continuity, the tendon elongates, and there is commonly an increase in passive dorsiflexion. MRI is not necessary to make the diagnosis, but may be of some benefit when planning surgical treatment.

Treatment is initiated with a modification of both the activity level and shoe wear. For any acute tendon inflammation, running should be curtailed; when activities are resumed, it is important to avoid climbing or running uphill. Sprinting and interval training should be temporarily discontinued. Stretching exercises are important, and these are performed by leaning forward and maintaining the stretch for 30 seconds. Shoe wear modifications are important (eg, a 1.5-cm heel lift), as are ice and a nonsteroidal anti-inflammatory medication. In severe cases, ultrasound and electrical stimulation, as well as a walking boot with a rocker-bottom-type sole worn for 6 weeks, is helpful. If passive dorsiflexion is limited, in addition to stretching the tendon complex, a night splint is useful to maintain and enhance passive stretching of the tendon. Corticosteroid injections are contraindicated. Once the acute phase is resolved, a gradual return to running follows, and an orthotic support can be prescribed if there appears to be a problem with excessive pronation.[20] During the ensuing phase of recovery, it is important to avoid reinjury that will occur with overtraining; cross-training with swimming and bicycling are very helpful.

Before resorting to surgery, patients with chronic refractory paratendinitis may be treated with injection of 2 ml of sterile saline into the tendon sheath. The goal of this injection is to lift the inflamed and adherent paratenon away from the tendon. If the inflammation persists beyond 6 months, surgical treatment may be indicated. The surgery is planned according to the extent of the pathologic process, because the technical aspects of the procedure and the recovery are considerably different. For surgical management of paratendinitis, the diseased and thickened paratenon is excised through a 4-cm medial incision centered over the maximum area of tenderness. The thickened paratenon is identified, and all adhesions of the paratenon are removed. A posterior splint is applied to maintain the foot in neutral dorsiflexion, and no weightbearing is permitted for 10 days, after which rehabilitation may commence. As an alternative to open removal of the inflamed paratenon, percutaneous vertical tenotomies of the tendon may be performed. A #15 knife blade is introduced into the tendon percutaneously in 4 positions (proximal, distal, medial, and lateral), and the ankle is passively plantar and dorsiflexed with each introduction of the knife. Maffulli and associates[21] reported their results of percutaneous tenotomy in 52 runners; 37 of 48 patients had a good result.

The surgical management of chronic tendinosis consists of debridement of the paratenon and removal of any degenerative necrotic tissue.[22,23] If minimal degeneration of the tendon is present after debridement, multiple 5-mm longitudinal fish-mouth incisions are made in the tendon to stimulate revascularization and healing. In patients with more tendon degeneration, the central fusiform thickened portion of the tendon must be excised, and the defect is primarily closed with a running 4-0 absorbable suture. More extensive degeneration of the tendon may require excision of the majority of the central tendon, which does not leave sufficient tendon for adequate healing or function, and this tendon defect must be augmented with additional tissue. For selected patients, the addition of a tendon transfer with the flexor hallucis longus will not only improve the strength of the deficient tendon, but the proximity of the flexor hallucis longus muscle to the Achilles tendon in all likelihood improves the blood supply to the degenerated Achilles tendon.

After surgery (whether debridement of tendinosis or a tendon transfer), the patient is not permitted to bear weight for 10 days; after 10 days, the patient is allowed to ambulate in a walker boot, commencing early range of motion and progressive weightbearing. The rehabilitation focuses on a gradual progression of resuming sporting activity, similar to that after acute rupture.

Outcomes with these procedures have been quite favorable, although the reported results of treating chronic paratendinitis have been better than those of tendinosis.[24-27] Kvist and Kvist[24] reported 96% good or excellent results after surgical treatment of paratendinitis. Although the reported results of surgical treatment for degenerative tendinosis are accep-

table, they are not as good as those for tendinitis, perhaps due to the pathology of ischemia and tendon degeneration. Recovery from surgical treatment for chronic Achilles tendinitis is not rapid, and we expect that patients will regain full function only after a year, particularly if more advanced degeneration of the tendon is present. Alfredson and associates[28] found that, at 6 months, patients still manifested substantial weakness of the affected limb compared with the opposite normal limb. Although their patients were immobilized in a short-leg cast for 6 weeks after surgery and although weightbearing and a functional stepwise recovery program was initiated, recovery was not as rapid as expected.

Insertional Achilles Tendinitis
Symptoms of insertional Achilles tendinitis are quite specific and revolve around pain at the bone-tendon junction that is frequently worse after exercise, but may ultimately become constant in nature. Although this is a fairly common finding in athletes, other conditions associated with posterior heel pain should be considered, including the various causes of insertional enthesopathy, the seronegative spondyloarthropathies, gout, systemic corticosteroids, oral fluoroquinolones, familial hyperlipidemia, sarcoidosis, and diffuse idiopathic skeletal hyperostosis.

The condition can be aggravated by uphill running or activities performed on hard surfaces. Frequently, a history of poor stretching, heel running, excessive mileage, or sudden increases in training intensity will be reported. The tenderness is quite specifically located at the Achilles tendon insertion, either directly posterior or posterolaterally. As increasing degeneration of the tendon occurs, a palpable defect in the substance of the tendon may be noted. Dorsiflexion is limited compared with the uninvolved side because of the relative tightness of the triceps surae. Heel pain is the cardinal complaint, and it is worsened by prolonged standing, walking, running uphill, or running on hard surfaces. The pain generally emanates from the posterior heel and is aggravated by either active or passive range of motion. Radiographs often demonstrate ossification in the most proximal extent of the insertion of the Achilles tendon or as a spur off the superior portion of the calcaneus. A radiograph does not accurately reflect the size of the osteophyte, because this structure has a very broad surface that extends across the central half of the tendon insertion. Although it would appear on radiographs that the osteophyte is located in the tendon that envelops the spur, the tendon is not actually attached to the spur, and the tendon insertion is continuous with the posterior wall of the calcaneus. Secondary imaging studies, such as MRI and ultrasonography, are not necessary to make the diagnosis or to plan treatment; on rare occasions, MRI may be of some help if extensive degeneration is encountered, because it may have some bearing on the choice of reconstructive procedure.

For most patients, nonsurgical management is initially successful.[29–31] Although many patients with insertional Achilles tendinitis are either sedentary or are recreational athletes, for those who are more active or competitive athletes, one should persevere with nonsurgical care. For the athlete, the use of modified training, ice, nonsteroidal anti-inflammatory medication, and heel lifts, in conjunction with stretching and strengthening exercises, are effective. Other simple measures,

such as widening or deepening the heel counter of the shoe, may also be effective, as can be pressure distribution using a silicon sleeve or pad in active and athletic patients. Various pads should be used to take the pressure off the Achilles insertion. A ¼- to ½-inch felt heel lift can be incorporated inside the shoe, although this may have a tendency to lift the heel out of the shoe. In the latter case, a heel wedge is added to the sole of the running shoe. A horseshoe-shaped felt pad is most effective and may be applied to either the shoe or the posterior heel. If these modalities are not effective, more aggressive stretching of the Achilles should be pursued, including use of a night splint to hold the foot in maximum dorsiflexion. If refractory, immobilization in a short leg walking cast or a walker boot may be used for 6 weeks.

After a period of rest from exercise, activities are gradually resumed, with incorporation of a good flexibility program with correction of any biomechanical abnormalities. Rest may be obtained not only by cessation, but also by diminution of the repetitive impact loading of the Achilles tendon. Cross-training may be useful after subsidence of the acute phase of this condition. Introduction of non-loading-type activities, such as swimming, bicycling, aqua jogging, or open chain kinetic-type weightlifting exercises, will permit athletes to keep in condition and have the added advantage of better compliance by allowing the athlete a training alternative. As always, ice, compression, and elevation are helpful in the early phases of this condition, as well as a short period of nonsteroidal anti-inflammatory medication. Physical therapy is sometimes employed in more resistant cases, with focus placed on hamstring and gastrocnemius-soleus complex flexibility as

well as modalities such as ultrasound and contrast baths to help control the pain and inflammation at the insertion site. Ultimately, when activity is resumed (particularly running), the mileage should be decreased and the running surface should be soft. Occasionally, a biomechanical abnormality, such as overpronation, is identified; a semirigid orthosis can help to control such a problem. It should be noted that in a pronated foot, slight undercorrection with an orthosis is better tolerated in runners than complete correction, and overcorrection is frequently intolerable. It is noted again that corticosteroid injections are contraindicated.

If the symptoms persist over time, and all nonsurgical treatments have been exhausted, surgery is indicated. We have found that for patients with degeneration of the insertion associated with ossification, a central heel-splitting incision is ideal because the pathologic process is easy to identify and treat. However, there are multiple surgical approaches to correct the problem, including isolated medial or lateral incisions, simultaneous medial and lateral incisions, posterior central splitting, and hockey stick and transverse incisions.[26,32] The surgical approach to treatment of this entity can therefore become quite confusing not only due to the plethora of the underlying diseases involving the Achilles insertion, but also to the varied incisions used to address the problem. Common to all procedures is resection of the inflamed retrocalcaneal bursa, removal of the prominent posterolateral bone, and debridement of the calcific and diseased tendon insertion. If the debridement of the involved tendon insertion causes a compromise in the integrity of the attachment to the posterior tuberosity, tendon reattachment or augmentation is necessary.

As noted above, the central heel-splitting incision has the advantage of direct visualization of the pathology, and ease of dissection of the torn portion of the tendon and removal of the bone spur. However, if the maximum pain is not located directly posteriorly, the incision should be located either medially or laterally because the torn portion of the tendon may not be visualized from the posterior incision. For any of these incisions, but in particular the central vertical incision, there should be absence of any skin pathology, normal potential for soft-tissue healing, and no previous scars in this location, which could create a hypertrophic scar. The potential for wound-healing problems and formation of a painful scar posteriorly directly over the heel, which would cause problems with shoe wear, must be taken into consideration.

The procedure is performed under local ankle block anesthesia with the patient in the prone position. A 4-cm vertical incision is made directly over the tendon, extending toward the plantar skin surface. The tendon is split longitudinally, maintaining full thickness of the incision down to bone inferiorly. Usually, the central portion of the tendon is the site of maximum degeneration, and this is therefore excised as a longitudinal ellipse. The hypertrophied osteophyte is identified anterior to the tendon, and it is removed completely with an osteotome. The posterior bone edge must be smoothed, removing any source of irritation to the Achilles tendon. Depending on the extent of degeneration and the amount of tendon resected, the tendon split is left open, repaired, or reattached to the calcaneus with a suture anchor. It is possible to remove one third of the tendon insertion without requiring reattachment to the calcaneus, although the exact

extent of dissection possible before rupture is not well understood.

After surgery, no weightbearing is permitted until full wound healing and perfect apposition of the skin edges are noted. By 3 weeks, most patients are full weightbearing either in a short-leg cast or a removable walker boot positioned in slight equinus. The duration of immobilization, determined by the extent of the tendon debridement, ranges from 4 to 8 weeks. This is followed by an aggressive course of therapy and rehabilitation, with the goal of improving strength and decreasing swelling and inflammation. Recovery after this surgery is slow, and it may take up to 12 months to return to normality, particularly for patients with seronegative spondyloarthropathy and insertional enthesopathy. The extent of disease and tendon involvement is much greater in patients older than 50 years of age.[33] The reported results of treatment of insertional tendinitis are satisfactory.[27,33,34]

Haglund's Deformity

The primary function of the retrocalcaneal bursa is to lubricate the tendon during walking or running. Irritation of the bursa may occur from a bone prominence; the bursa may enlarge, followed by impingement on the anterior distal tendon. The original description of the enlarged posterior superior and lateral calcaneal tuberosity was by Patrick Haglund in 1928;[5] it has since been associated with various shoe types, hence the names pump bump,[35] high heel,[36] and winter heel.[37] Haglund's disease occurs when this bursal projection is compressed with a poorly fitting shoe-heel counter that leads to subcutaneous irritation and bursitis in the adventitial bursa. In the case of an excessively large bursal projection, a reactive inflammation may ensue in

the retrocalcaneal bursal space, exacerbating symptoms of posterior heel pain. It should be emphasized that although Haglund's deformity may occur in up to 60% of patients with insertional Achilles tendinitis, Haglund's disease typically has no Achilles involvement whatsoever. The pump bump has a fairly innocuous presentation and, if symptomatic, should respond well to basic, simple interventions such as shoe modifications, pads, ice, and anti-inflammatory medication.

Patients who are treated for this typical superolateral bone prominence are younger, between 15 and 30 years old. The presentation is quite different from that of retrocalcaneal bursitis, although, as noted, these patients may experience acute retrocalcaneal bursitis in addition to the symptoms of pressure from the shoe. Symptoms arise from the bone prominence along the superior lateral margin of the calcaneus rubbing against the heel counter of the shoe. Skin irritation occurs, and these patients, often younger women, present with localized erythema and focal swelling. The etiology of this condition is usually developmental, aggravated by shoe wear patterns. Although trauma to the apophysis may occur in childhood, leading to the development of this bone prominence, this is unusual; more likely, there is a biomechanical cause for this condition that leads to mechanically induced posterior heel inflammation. The difficulties with diagnosis and treatment of retrocalcaneal pain are due partly to nomenclature inconsistencies, partly to anatomic discrepancies, and partly to the fact that it is difficult to accurately verify what exactly is the cause of pain. Even if it is assumed that the superolateral bone prominence is pathologic, there is no accurate and reproducible means of determining the extent of pathology, and how much bone to resect.

One should not become confused with the nomenclature of the numerous bumps on the posterior heel. As stated above, Haglund described the painful condition caused by bone prominence on the posterior superior lateral aspect of the calcaneus. Bone enlargement of the entire posterior aspect of the calcaneus may occur, whether this is directly posterior or slightly more inferiorly located at the insertion of the Achilles tendon. The patient with a symptomatic pump bump typically has a painful heel that is red and irritated, with a palpable and visible bony prominence on the posterolateral aspect. Frequently, the patient will have a high arched cavus foot with a particularly narrow heel. The condition is frequently worse in certain shoes, especially those that are described with a hard or irregularly shaped heel counter. A large, tender prominence is present on the lateral side of the Achilles insertion, but not directly on the central portion of the posterior tuberosity.

There are many radiographic measurements that attempt to identify the extent of Haglund's deformity, but none that we have found to be reliable or even helpful in planning treatment. Although there are many angles and lines that can be used to determine the presence of abnormal bone superiorly, none adequately portray the lateral bone prominence. The various measurements described include those by Fowler and Philip,[36] Steffensen and Evensen,[38] Pavlov and associates,[39] Chauveaux and associates,[40] and Sella and associates.[41] A Fowler angle >75° is supposedly diagnostic of an enlarged posterior calcaneus, although most other authors have found no correlation between the size of the angle and symptoms.[42–44] Pavlov and associates[39] believed that it was the height of the superior calcaneus that caused the symptoms, and not the angular relationships of the posterior calcaneus. They developed the parallel pitch line technique by drawing a line from the posterior superior articular facet to the posterior calcaneus, noting that the superior posterior calcaneus should be inferior to the superior line. The problem with this technique is that it measures neither the length nor the inclination of the calcaneus. Because pain may occur at the insertion of the Achilles tendon, an alternate measurement was described by Chauveaux and associates.[40] This angle is more relevant to other forms of posterior heel pain than it is to Haglund's deformity, because the pitch and length of the calcaneus are measured.

Conservative treatment for Haglund's disease is similar to that for insertional Achilles tendinitis, and is based on the relief of friction between the shoe counter, the heel, and particularly the inflamed bursa. Shoe wear adjustments can be made, with particular attention directed to the height of the heel, and rigidity and shape of its counter. Close-fitting rigid heel counters are to be avoided, so as to prevent irritation of the bursal projection. Use of a heel insert will elevate the heel from the shoe and may change the area of mechanical irritation at the upper edge of the heel counter. Heel height can sometimes be beneficial by decreasing the calcaneal pitch, which will essentially alleviate the bursal projection irritation by displacing the heel from the counter of the shoe. Patients who do not benefit from these measures, as well as the use of nonsteroidal anti-inflammatory medications, stretching exercises, and other therapeutic modalities, should be considered candidates for surgical intervention. Shoes with a moderate to high heel can actually reduce the amount of symptoms by reducing the calcaneal pitch angle and forcing the foot downwards and displacing it away from the heel counter.

Surgical intervention falls into 2 broad categories: resection of the bony prominence and displacement osteotomy. Resection of the prominent bone and bursa is most commonly performed and is the most reliable form of treatment. The key to a successful result is a sufficient resection of an appropriate amount of bone, which should include the entire bursal projection plus an additional 0.5 cm. We recommend a lateral incision immediately anterior to the Achilles insertion because the Achilles tendon itself is not usually involved in this condition, and the bursal projection is almost invariably on the lateral side.[45] If the symptoms warrant it, the retrocalcaneal bursa may be excised, although this is not usually necessary. The size of the ostectomy depends on the size of the bone prominence, although it is not necessary to remove a large amount of bone with this condition. It is important to use the described short vertical lateral incision for excision of a Haglund's deformity immediately anterior to the Achilles tendon, because there is less likelihood of injury to the sural nerve and the Achilles tendon itself. Other incisions that have been described for treating posterior heel pain are not indicated when resecting a superior lateral bone prominence.

The second method of treatment involves a dorsal closing wedge osteotomy, which realigns the prominent bursa by displacing it from the Achilles tendon. Zadek[46] and Keck and Kelly[47] have reported the results of a dorsally based osteotomy at the posterior calcaneus. Zadek believed that removal of the Achilles bursa alone would not be adequate, and he recommended calcaneal osteotomy to decrease the pressure on the posterior central heel without disrupting the insertion of the Achilles tendon. He recommended removal of a 0.6-cm wide wedge through the body of the calcaneus, leaving a plantar hinge intact, and use of chromic sutures to secure the osteotomy.[46] We do use this osteotomy for selected cases, using rigid internal fixation, but the osteotomy should be performed as a greenstick fracture of the interior cortex without completely detaching the bone. In this manner, there is less likelihood of any shift of the posterior tuberosity. The position of the closing wedge osteotomy is also critical, because placement too far anterior or posterior will compromise either the subtalar joint or the posterior attachment of the Achilles tendon. More problematic, however, seems to be the occurrence of a sharp bone projection on the inferior posterior aspect of the calcaneus as a result of the shifting away of the heel pad slightly posterior and cephalad. This causes a very painful prominence that is not easy to treat with padding, and may necessitate a second operation. One should recognize, however, that this osteotomy changes the shape of the posterior heel, and although the posterior bone prominence will be decreased in size, it has been our experience that the heel widens slightly. Theoretically, due to the change in the position of the insertion of the Achilles tendon, the kinematics of the posterior ankle may change; however, we have not noted that this is a clinically significant problem. Due to the increased morbidity of this procedure when compared with more simple superolateral ostectomy, this operation should not be per-

formed routinely, although there are certain patients for whom this may be indicated due to an abnormal shape of the posterior heel.

The results after resection of Haglund's deformity have not always been well received. Nesse and Finsen[48] reviewed their results of 35 heels, noting that persistent pain was present in 12 heels and additional various leg complications and complaints in 22 heels. They noted that the effect on heel pain was independent of the size of the resected bone, but that stiffness and ankle pain were much more commonly associated with large, rather than small, resections. It is for this reason that these and other authors[49] have recommended nonsurgical methods of treatment wherever possible. Other authors[50] have reported more favorably on surgical treatment, finding (as we have) that resection of the bursa is not necessary, and that preoperative planning is important to ensure removal of an adequate amount of bone, the key to a successful result. It has been our experience that failure after excision of a Haglund's deformity is due either to insufficient bone resected or to injury of a branch of the sural nerve.

Retrocalcaneal Bursitis

Patients with retrocalcaneal bursitis are typically older individuals and low-level recreational athletes or nonathletes—in fact, often sedentary and obese. The presentation of retrocalcaneal bursitis is typically acute, with deep pain and visible swelling in the posterior soft tissues. This swelling may be quite noticeable, with a bulge of the soft tissues medial and lateral to the tendon, and associated with warmth and increased pain with range-of-motion maneuvers. In particular, passive dorsiflexion is uncomfortable, and tenderness

is present medially or laterally, or both, just anterior to the Achilles tendon. Although radiographs can demonstrate the characteristically prominent superior calcaneal deformity on lateral projections of the calcaneus, they are generally not too helpful, and the clinical findings remain diagnostic. On the lateral radiograph, one may observe obliteration of the normal soft-tissue shadow of the retrocalcaneal space, and the bone projection superiorly and posteriorly.

These patients are treated similarly to those with other insertional Achilles tendon pathology: with rest, ice, a heel lift, and, in particular, an open-back shoe. If refractory to these treatments, a single corticosteroid injection may be used, although one must be aware of the potential for tendon rupture if repeated injections are administered. If a steroid injection is used, one may consider temporary immobilization of the limb in walking cast or a walker boot to protect the tendon. If these measures fail, surgery may be indicated and is easily performed through a short vertical lateral incision, although some prefer a medial incision, or both, if the bone prominence is particularly large. If the lateral incision is used, it should be made immediately anterior to the tendon to avoid the sural nerve more anteriorly. Generally, it is possible to resect the posterior superior calcaneus with osteotomy from the lateral incision, and to use a medial incision when bone is still present medially and cannot be resected from the lateral incision. A generous amount of the retrocalcaneal space should be decompressed by this osteotomy, after resection of the inflamed bursa. After surgery, patients are not permitted to bear weight for 1 week, followed by activity as tolerated either in a short-leg cast or a walker boot for 4 weeks.

The reported results of resection of the bursa and posterior calcaneus for correction of refractory bursitis are varied. Some authors[45,51] maintain they have good results, provided sufficient bone is resected and no nerve complications ensue. However, Angermann[52] found a "cure" rate of only 50% in a study of 40 heels with chronic retrocalcaneal bursitis and resection of the posterior superior aspect of the calcaneus. Interestingly, this author did not find any correlation between the size of the bone resection and the result of surgery.

A different version of this Instructional Course Lecture has been published in *The Journal of Bone and Joint Surgery*.

References

1. Carr AJ, Norris SH: The blood supply of the calcaneal tendon. *J Bone Joint Surg* 1989;71B: 100–101.

2. Lagergren C, Lindholm A: Vascular distribution in the Achilles tendon: An angiographic and microangiographic study. *Acta Chir Scand* 1959;116:491–495.

3. Schmidt-Rohlfing B, Graf J, Schneider U, Niethard FU: The blood supply of the Achilles tendon. *Int Orthop* 1992;16:29–31.

4. Frey C, Rosenberg Z, Shereff MJ, Kim H: The retrocalcaneal bursa: Anatomy and bursography. *Foot Ankle* 1992;13:203–207.

5. Haglund P: Beitrag zur Klinik der Achillessehne. *Z Orthop Chir* 1927;49:49–58.

6. Rufai A, Ralphs JR, Benjamin M: Structure and histopathology of the insertional region of the human Achilles tendon. *J Orthop Res* 1995;13:585–593.

7. Soma CA, Mandelbaum BR: Achilles tendon disorders. *Clin Sports Med* 1994;13:811–823.

8. James SL, Bates BT, Osternig LR: Injuries to runners. *Am J Sports Med* 1978;6:40–50.

9. Clancy WG Jr, Neidhart D, Brand RL: Achilles tendonitis in runners: A report of five cases. *Am J Sports Med* 1976;4:46–57.

10. Clement DB, Taunton JE, Smart GW: Achilles tendinitis and peritendinitis: Etiology and treatment. *Am J Sports Med* 1984;12:179–184.

11. Krissoff WB, Ferris WD: Runner's injuries. *Phys Sportsmed* 1979;7:55–64.

12. Leach RE, James S, Wasilewski S: Achilles tendinitis. *Am J Sports Med* 1981;9:93–98.

13. Kvist M: Achilles tendon injuries in athletes. *Ann Chir Gynaecol* 1991;80:188–201.

14. Puddu G, Ippolito E, Postacchini F: A classification of Achilles tendon disease. *Am J Sports Med* 1976;4:145–150.

15. Fox JM, Blazina ME, Jobe FW, et al: Degeneration and rupture of the Achilles tendon. *Clin Orthop* 1975;107:221–224.

16. Gould N, Korson R: Stenosing tenosynovitis of the pseudosheath of the tendo Achilles. *Foot Ankle* 1980;1:179–187.

17. Lotke PA: Ossification of the Achilles tendon: Report of seven cases. *J Bone Joint Surg* 1970; 52A:157–160.

18. Bovens AM, Janssen GM, Vermeer HG, Hoeberigs JH, Janssen MP, Verstappen FT: Occurrence of running injuries in adults following a supervised training program. *Int J Sports Med* 1989;10(suppl 3):S186–S190.

19. Scott SH, Winter DA: Internal forces of chronic running injury sites. *Med Sci Sports Exerc* 1990;22:357–369.

20. Mohr RN: Achilles tendonitis: Rationale for use and application of orthotics. *Foot Ankle Clin* 1997;2:439–456.

21. Maffulli N, Testa V, Capasso G, Bifulco G, Binfield PM: Results of percutaneous longitudinal tenotomy for Achilles tendinopathy in middle- and long-distance runners. *Am J Sports Med* 1997;25:835–840.

22. Backman C, Boquist L, Friden J, Lorentzon R, Toolanen G: Chronic Achilles paratenonitis with tendinosis: An experimental model in the rabbit. *J Orthop Res* 1990;8:541–547.

23. Kvist M, Jozsa L, Jarvinen MJ, Kvist H: Chronic Achilles paratenonitis in athletes: A histological and histochemical study. *Pathology* 1987;19:1–11.

24. Kvist H, Kvist M: The operative treatment of chronic calcaneal paratenonitis. *J Bone Joint Surg* 1980;62B:353–357.

25. Nelen G, Martens M, Burssens A: Surgical treatment of chronic Achilles tendinitis. *Am J Sports Med* 1989;17:754–759.

26. Schepsis AA, Leach RE: Surgical management of Achilles tendinitis. *Am J Sports Med* 1987;15: 308–315.

27. Schepsis AA, Wagner C, Leach RE: Surgical management of Achilles tendon overuse injuries: A long-term follow-up study. *Am J Sports Med* 1994;22:611–619.

28. Alfredson H, Pietila T, Lorentzon R: Chronic Achilles tendinitis and calf muscle strength. *Am J Sports Med* 1996;24:829–833.

29. Clain MR, Baxter DE: Achilles tendinitis. *Foot Ankle* 1992;13:482–487.

30. Parkes JC, II, Hamilton WG, Patterson AH, Rawles JG Jr: The anterior impingement syndrome of the ankle. *J Trauma* 1980;20:895–898.

31. Scioli MW: Achilles tendinitis. *Orthop Clin North Am* 1994;25:177–182.

32. Digiovanni BF, Gould JS: Achilles tendinitis and posterior heel disorders. *Foot Ankle Clin* 1997;2:411–428.

33. Gerken AP, McGarvey WC, Baxter DE: Insertional Achilles tendinitis. *Foot Ankle Clin* 1996;1:237–248.

34. Leach RE, DiIorio E, Harney RA: Pathologic hindfoot conditions in the athlete. *Clin Orthop* 1983;177:116–121.

35. Dickinson PH, Coutts MB, Woodward EP, Handler D: Tendo Achillis bursitis: Report of twenty-one cases. *J Bone Joint Surg* 1966;48A: 77–81.

36. Fowler A, Philip JF: Abnormality of the calcaneus as a cause of painful heel: Its diagnosis and operative treatment. *Br J Surg* 1945;32: 494–498.

37. Nisbet NW: Tendo Achillis bursitis ("winter heel"). *Br Med J* 1954;2:1394–1395.

38. Steffensen JCA, Evensen A: Bursitis retrocalcanea achilli. *Acta Orthop Scand* 1958;27: 228–236.

39. Pavlov H, Heneghan MA, Hersh A, Goldman AB, Vigorita V: The Haglund syndrome: Initial and differential diagnosis. *Radiology* 1982;144: 83–88.

40. Chauveaux D, Liet P, Le Huec JC, Midy D: A new radiologic measurement for the diagnosis of Haglund's deformity. *Surg Radiol Anat* 1991;13:39–44.

41. Sella EJ, Caminear DS, McLarney EA: Haglund's syndrome. *J Foot Ankle Surg* 1998;37: 110–114.

42. Fuglsang F, Torup D: Bursitis retrocalcanearis. *Acta Orthop Scand* 1961;30:315–323.

43. Heneghan MA, Pavlov H: The Haglund painful heel syndrome: Experimental investigation of cause and therapeutic implications. *Clin Orthop* 1984;187:228–234.

44. Vega MR, Cavolo DJ, Green RM, Cohen RS: Haglund's deformity. *J Am Podiatry Assoc* 1984;74:129–135.

45. Stephens MM: Haglund's deformity and retrocalcaneal bursitis. *Orthop Clin North Am* 1994;25:41–46.

46. Zadek I: An operation for the cure of Achillobursitis. *Am J Surg* 1939;43:542–546.

47. Keck SW, Kelly PJ: Bursitis of the posterior part of the heel: Evaluation of the surgical treatment of eighteen patients. *J Bone Joint Surg* 1965;47A: 467–471.

48. Nesse E, Finsen V: Poor results after resection for Haglund's heel: Analysis of 35 heels in 23 patients after 3 years. *Acta Orthop Scand* 1994;65:107–109.

49. Taylor GJ: Prominence of the calcaneus: Is operation justified? *J Bone Joint Surg* 1986;68B:467–470.

50. Pauker M, Katz K, Yosipovitch Z: Calcaneal ostectomy for Haglund disease. *J Foot Surg* 1992;31:588–589.

51. Jones DC, James SL: Partial calcaneal ostectomy for retrocalcaneal bursitis. *Am J Sports Med* 1984;12:72–73.

52. Angermann P: Chronic retrocalcaneal bursitis treated by resection of the calcaneus. *Foot Ankle* 1990;10:285–287.

Achilles Tendon Ruptures

Mark S. Myerson, MD

Acute Ruptures

Etiology and Epidemiology

Why do the majority of acute ruptures of the Achilles tendon occur in males? On evaluation of our institutional experience, the male-to-female ratio is 30:1, somewhat higher than that previously reported[1] where the ratio was noted to range between 2:1 and 19:1. This may reflect a difference in the sporting activity of our patient population, because it has been repeatedly documented that more than 75% of Achilles tendon ruptures occur during sports activity in patients between the ages of 30 and 40 years.[2] These statistics contrast with a more recent study from Copenhagen of 209 patients with Achilles tendon rupture over an 18-year period. In these patients there were ruptures in 55 women and 158 men, with a median age of 41 years.[3] Yet it should not be assumed that because ruptures occur predominantly during athletic activity that it is the latter which precipitates the rupture, because the incidence of Achilles tendon ruptures is much more common in industrialized countries, where lifestyles are generally sedentary and where the interest in recreational athletics has suddenly increased.[2,4] There appears to have been a dramatic change in the incidence of Achilles tendon ruptures over the past 40 years, but this increase has occurred predominantly

in developed countries. Interestingly, Achilles tendon ruptures are a rarity in developing countries, especially in Africa and East Asia. In Hungary, the number of patients with an Achilles tendon rupture increased 285% in men and 500% in women between two successive 7-year periods.[5] The stereotypical Achilles rupture therefore seems to occur in the adult male who is not well conditioned and does not participate regularly in sports, although rupture usually occurs during some athletic activity.

In addition to this epidemiologic data, there are likely biologic and mechanical events that precede rupture. Clearly, tendon degeneration occurs as a result of a combination of hypovascularity and repetitive microtrauma, resulting in diffuse tendon degeneration and ultimately rupture.[6,7] Regeneration with tendon healing cannot occur due to the recurrent microtrauma, and this condition is worsened by underlying hypovascularity, substantiated by the fact that the vast majority of ruptures occur 4 to 6 cm proximal to the insertion of the tendon, where the blood supply to the tendon is poor.[8] In addition to these underlying problems, a critical load must be applied to the tendon, resulting in rupture. This is well identified clinically, because the majority of ruptures occur during a sudden push-off during some sporting activity. Different stresses may precipitate

rupture, including pushing off with the weightbearing forefoot while extending the knee joint, as in sprinting, running, and jumping. Unexpected dorsiflexion of the ankle (which occurs, for example, when slipping is associated with a sudden deceleration when falling forward as well as more abrupt dorsiflexion on a plantarflexed foot when jumping from a height) will cause a rupture. The critical threshold for rupture, however, is not clear, although in addition to the factors identified above, genetics, the neuroendocrine environment, and growth factors also play a role. In addition, there are histopathologic changes, including hypoxic degeneration, mucoid degeneration, and calcifying tendinopathy, that occur in association with rupture. These factors may have some relevance for patients who sustain a rupture, because there is an increased likelihood of contralateral rupture when compared with the general population, and antecedent Achilles tendinitis occurs in 15% of patients who sustain a rupture.[9]

The use of corticosteroids, orally or injectable, has been associated with collagen necrosis and an increased incidence of rupture.[10] Despite this latter well-known fact, patients with various forms of Achilles tendinitis continue to receive steroid injection. In addition to corticosteroids, anabolic steroids and fluoroquinolone antibiotics have been shown to cause collagen dysplasia and reduced tensile strength of the Achilles tendon.[11] Other reported causes of tendon rupture include gout,[12] hyperthyroidism and renal insufficiency,[13] and arteriosclerosis.[14] It would be of some benefit to identify patients at risk for Achilles rupture, particularly those who experience chronic pain as a result of tendinitis. This pain is often a sign of progressive degeneration of the tendon, which can lead to its rupture. The clinical course and sonograms were studied prospectively in 36 patients with chronic degenerative tendinosis to find a prognostic parameter predictive of rupture. Analysis of the tendons that subsequently ruptured exhibited high-grade thickening, and these patients with sonographic findings had a worse clinical outcome after nonsurgical treatment. In this study, 28% of patients with thickening of the tendon associated with chronic pain had a spontaneous rupture.[15]

In summary, the Achilles tendon ruptures as a result of a sequence of events that is based on an underlying hypovascularity, resulting in localized degeneration and weakening of the tendon, which somehow lowers the tendon threshold for rupture. The precise position and load that causes the injury remains obscure, but it is probably a complex equation of neuromuscular control and external factors, including the applied load to the foot.

Diagnosis

Most patients present with a typical history, and describe an audible snap as if someone hit them in the back of the ankle. Although push-off strength is markedly compromised, the diagnosis of the acute rupture is surprisingly not always made, due in part to the strength of the remaining muscles

of plantarflexion. The combination of the use of all of the plantarflexor muscles, including the flexor hallucis longus (FHL) and flexor digitorum longus (FDL), and the posterior tibial and peroneal muscles, provides some strength for walking. Yet while patients are able to walk, and perhaps even function with respect to some activities of daily living, push-off strength is markedly compromised. Individuals are unable to perform a single or, even less likely, a repetitive heel rise, and activities that require greater amounts of push-off strength (including ascending and descending stairs, running, and jumping) are generally not possible. In addition to the acute pain and swelling, a limp and plantarflexion weakness are present on examination. The rupture commonly occurs approximately 4 cm proximal to the insertion of the tendon, and although avulsion of the calcaneus may occur, it is relatively uncommon unless antecedent insertional tendinitis has been present. A defect or indentation of the posterior tendon is either visible or palpable if there is not too much swelling of the limb present, and the diagnosis is always confirmed by a positive Thompson test.[16] In this test, the affected calf is squeezed, and a positive test indicates discontinuity of the muscle with the heel because loss of passive plantarflexion of the foot is present.

Imaging studies are not necessary as part of the diagnostic work-up for rupture. If one suspects an avulsion of the tendon off the insertion, a lateral radiograph may show a small fracture, and therefore may be helpful with respect to preoperative planning. Magnetic resonance imaging (MRI) is not necessary to make the diagnosis and does not seem to have a role in planning treatment. Ultrasonography has been used as a technique for defi-

nition of Achilles tendon pathology and rupture,[17] and although I have not found that this test is necessary to make the diagnosis, it may be useful when nonsurgical treatment is contemplated. Ultrasound can accurately determine the gap between tendon ends. The test is performed with the foot held in passive plantarflexion, noting whether the tendon ends approximate. If there is adequate apposition between the tendon ends, nonsurgical treatment may have a greater likelihood of success, and for the appropriately selected individual this remains a useful test. Richter and associates[18] demonstrated that functional treatment of the rupture in a brace without surgery is possible through careful sonographic analysis of the patients with Achilles rupture.

Treatment Alternatives

As part of the decision-making process for treatment, one should define the various functional goals and activities of daily living for each individual. While it may be argued that maximum and expeditious resumption of athletic activity may only reasonably be accomplished with surgical treatment, accurate parameters must be used to evaluate the success of treatment. To provide a valid means of comparison, all clinical parameters including pain, stiffness, muscle weakness, footwear restrictions, as well as range of motion of the ankle and isokinetic calf muscle strength, should be included as part of the patient evaluation process. The majority of these injuries occur in the setting of some athletic activity, and a prompt return to their sport may be important to the successful outcome of treatment. In 1993, Cetti and associates[19] showed that there were significantly fewer complaints 1 year after the injury in patients treated surgically. In a prospective randomized study of 111 patients with acute rupture, they found that those treated surgically had significantly higher rates of resuming sports activities at the same level, a lesser degree of calf atrophy, better ankle movement, and fewer complaints. Mandelbaum and associates[9] demonstrated a 92% return to sports by 6 months with a 2.6% deficit on isokinetic testing. Neumann and associates[20] demonstrated permanent kinematic and neuromuscular changes of the gait pattern after Achilles tendon rupture that was treated surgically but that included immobilization in a cast after surgery. Although these studies provide some insight into the outcome of treatment, a general lack of a standardized method for subjective and objective assessment of these injuries limits interpretation of the data reported in the literature. For the future, prospectively designed studies using standard and accepted tools will become most important to further assess patient selection for treatment protocols.

Nonsurgical Versus Surgical Management

The pendulum towards surgical or nonsurgical management of Achilles tendon ruptures has shifted repeatedly this century, and these swings are likely to continue.[21–24] Although there have been attempts to compare the results of patients treated surgically with those managed nonsurgically, the methods of patient evaluation have not been adequate, and, although many reports found that better results occurred in the surgical groups, the majority of studies were not randomized or carefully controlled.[25,26] Helgeland and associates[27] prospectively evaluated 38 patients with Achilles rupture whose treatment was randomized to surgical and nonsurgical treatment. They identified a markedly increased incidence of complications after nonsurgical treatment. In particular, they noted that for these patients the plantarflexion range was markedly reduced in the injured foot when compared with the opposite foot, and there were also reduced muscle strength and an increased rate of rerupture in those treated without surgery.[27]

The methods of immobilization and rehabilitation used after surgery or nonsurgical treatment generally involved the use of prolonged casting with limited bearing of weight. After long immobilization periods in equinus after surgical treatment of Achilles tendon rupture, long-lasting motor patterns in functional movement have been identified. Thermann and associates[28] identified, in a experimental biomechanical model in rabbits, the results of surgical compared with functional nonsurgical treatment in a specially designed orthosis taped to the limb of the rabbit. They found that there were no significant biomechanical differences after 3 months, and when compared with the results reported in the literature for cast immobilization, their functional treatment resulted in a significantly faster course of healing. Neumann and associates[20] documented alterations in gait pattern, noting kinematic and neuromuscular changes 1 year after surgery and neuromuscular deficits. As a result of the noted complications after surgery, various studies began to support nonsurgical management of Achilles ruptures,[25,26] culminating in an editorial in 1973 that stated, ". . . in view of the excellent results obtainable by conservative treatment, it is doubtful whether surgical repair in closed rupture of the Achilles tendon can be justified."[29] However, over the past decade, numerous advances have been made with respect to both surgical techniques and rehabilitation modalities in the entire field of sports-related injury. As a result of these technical and therapeutic improvements, studies began to demonstrate superior results with surgical repair.[19,30,31] During the last 20 years, as patient expectations and functional goals have increased, surgical options have gained acceptance and popularity. In keeping with these patient goals, the recent emphasis has focused on aggressive postoperative protocols after surgical treatment, with early weightbearing and controlled range-of-motion exercises. These latter postoperative treatment programs avoid cast immobilization and were found to be well tolerated, safe, and effective. Although these studies reported superior outcomes and demonstrated particular value for well-motivated patients and athletes, it is still unclear whether or not the results of these treatment protocols apply to all patients, or are limited to those who especially desire the highest functional outcome. Perhaps as improved methods of patient evaluation and the results of randomized prospective studies emerge, the pendulum will swing back toward nonsurgical methods of treatment. At the present time, however, it is our practice to limit nonsurgical treatment to the sick patient, the sedentary individual, or those with very limited functional and athletic goals.

The controversy regarding surgical and nonsurgical treatment alternatives does not end here, because, once a decision is made to perform surgery, it is necessary to choose from a plethora of technical alternatives for this repair. Any method of repair should perfectly restore continuity of the ruptured tendon ends, have them heal in a physiologic position, and restore normal dynamic muscle function. This goal is not always easy to accomplish, given the multiple strands of the tendon after the acute rupture, and this problem becomes more marked with percutaneous methods of repair. Perhaps the most important aspect of surgical repair, regardless of the method of suture used, is the accurate tensioning of the repair and establishing the exact dynamic resting length of the tendon. A repair may not be considered successful if the tendon-muscle-tendon unit is too short, and the foot is positioned in equinus. From a functional standpoint however, overlengthening of the Achilles is worse, and severely compromises push-off strength. It is for this reason that one must view the results of percutaneous methods of repair with some scepticism, because the tendon ends can never be accurately apposed.

Bunnell[32] and Kessler[33] were the first to popularize the end-to-end suture technique for ruptured tendons. In 1977, Ma and Griffith[34] described a percutaneous repair, and although this method remains popular, there is an unacceptable incidence of sural nerve injury, a less than anatomic positioning of the tendon, and a higher incidence of rerupture. Various other methods of suture have been advocated, including a 3-bundle suture technique,[12] a suture weave,[35] a 6-strand-suture technique,[36] and the use of external fixation techniques.[22]

In addition to direct repair of the tendon, various augmentation techniques have been described to supplement the strength of the repair using part of the gastrocnemius fascia or the plantaris tendon, if the latter is present. The gastrocnemius may be used as an aponeurosis flap, performed as a slide of the superficial fascia overlying the muscle,[21] or rotation of 1 or 2 central flaps of fascia.[37] The use of the plantaris makes sense when considering augmentation of a primary repair, because the direct repair may be followed by a weave of the plantaris through the Achilles tendon. Alternatively, the plantaris tendon may be used to prevent adhesion formation between the skin and the repaired tendon by fanning it out to use as a thin fascial membrane covering the repair.[37] All these methods aim to improve the continuity and strength of the repair construct, but in practice, the need for these augmentation procedures is not necessary to treat the acute rupture, because apposition of the tendon ends is always possible, and with appropriate suture techniques, reinforcement should not be required.

In addition to these methods of repair, more extensive techniques of reconstruction have been described using the fascia lata,[38] peroneus brevis,[39] FDL,[40] or FHL.[41] These reconstructive procedures are not necessary for treatment of the acute rupture, and they are discussed in more detail below with respect to management of chronic neglected ruptures. The use of various exogenous materials to reinforce the primary repair of the Achilles tendon have been reported, including carbon fiber,[42] marlex mesh,[14] dacron grafts,[43] and polypropylene braids,[44] but these are of historical interest only.

Surgical Technique

Regardless of the method of surgery selected, the surgeon should select a safe and effective procedure, one that will allow the patient to accomplish realistic goals in a timely manner. I prefer to delay surgery for approximately 1 week after rupture. The reduction of swelling prior to commencement of surgery is important in order to minimize the potential for problems with wound closure and infection. Not only does the swelling decrease by this time, but the apposition of the tendon ends becomes easier, because some consolidation of the tendon ends occurs during this time, making the repair technically easier. Before this time, although surgery may be performed and accomplished satisfactorily, the tendon ends are very frayed, and establishing the correct tension on the tendon ends may be difficult. Surgery is performed with the patient in the prone position, and although any anesthesia may be used, my preference is to administer local anesthesia. In most cases, both feet are prepared as part of the operative field to permit accurate side-to-side comparison of the resting dynamic tension of the repaired tendon. An anteromedial incision is made along the length of the paratenon and the Achilles tendon, extending to the musculotendinous junction. Each end of the tear is sutured with 1 or 2 strands of a #2 nonabsorbable material using a modified whip-suture technique. It is important not to include too much tendon in each pass of the suture, so as to avoid potential tendon compression and necrosis.

The most important aspect of surgical repair, regardless of the method of suture used, is to correctly tension the tendon, and this can be facilitated by carefully commencing the suture at the correct position on the tendon. Insertion of the suture should not begin at the end of the frayed portion of the tendon ends. The tendon should be laid down with the frayed ends apposed to get a sense of the correct position of the repair, and then the suture strands should be inserted. Before tying the sutures, each strand is pulled to obtain a sense of the correct tension, and then this position is compared with the opposite limb. It is for this reason that I find that it is useful to include the opposite limb in the operative field to allow adequate comparison of the resting tension on both tendons while in the prone position. The sutures are then tied, with the knots passed to the anterior aspect of the tendon and secured. Wound closure after Achilles repair is generally difficult, and it is worsened by the swelling and bulk of the repaired tendon in the subcutaneous position, which creates tension on the skin edges and increases the likelihood of wound complications. To minimize this tension, I perform a fasciotomy of the posterior compartment of the leg, which increases the horizontal or cross-sectional diameter of the subcutaneous tissues and facilitates skin closure. If the plantaris tendon is present, it is used to cover the tendon repair. I have not found that it is necessary to augment the repair; however, the plantaris can be unravelled and used to create a thin layer over the repair to prevent adhesion formation between the tendon and the skin. The paratenon should be closed with 4-0 absorbable suture, and the ankle is taken through a complete range of motion to evaluate the stability of the repair. The wound is closed with interrupted nylon mattress sutures, and a posterior splint is applied with the foot positioned in neutral dorsiflexion.

Rehabilitation After Surgery

Historically, prolonged cast immobilization was used to treat ruptures when either surgical or nonsurgical methods were used. However, the use of a cast increases the likelihood of muscle atrophy, joint stiffness, cartilage atrophy, degenerative arthritis, adhesion formation, and deep venous thrombosis. In contrast, limb and joint mobilization limits muscle atrophy,[45] promotes fiber polymerization to collagen,[46] fosters an increased organization of collagen in the repair site that leads to increased strength,[47] and increases tendon and muscle strength.[48] In addition to the biologic effects of immobilization, there are permanent deficits of the Achilles tendon, which can be demonstrated with isokinetic testing.[26,49–51] More recent work has emphasized early range of motion of the foot after surgery without the use of a cast. Mandelbaum and associates[9] reported on 29 athletes who were started early range-of-motion and conditioning programs postoperatively. By 6 weeks, 90% of the patients had full range of motion, and by 6 months, 92% returned to sports participation, and on isokinetic testing at 6 months these patients had no more than an average of 2.9% deficit in plantarflexion strength. Functional rehabilitation, which includes early motion and weightbearing, therefore appears to be safe and highly effective at returning athletes and other patients to activities of daily life and sport with the highest level of function. Other authors have since documented similar successes with immediate movement of the ankle and foot after surgical treatment, with no increase in wound complications, and a marked decrease in the formation of skin adhesions to the tendon scar. Motta and associates[52] reported on 78 physically active patients who were treated after surgery with early assisted movement of the ankle and foot with excellent results.

I therefore advocate initiation of weightbearing and range of motion once the sutures are removed, between 10 and 14 days after surgery, in a hinged range-of-motion walker boot that permits motion of the ankle. The hinge is set to permit full plantarflexion, but with a stop to dorsiflexion at the neutral position, and the boot is worn for 8 weeks. The therapy program begins almost immediately, permitting range of motion and progressive exercise with accelerated weightbearing. During the early phases of rehabilitation, patients are encouraged to increase weightbearing. Riding a bicycle is permitted at 3 weeks, exercise in a pool by 4 weeks, and by 8 weeks, push-off strengthening is started with a stair-climbing device. By the beginning of the third month, the patient begins single-toe heel rises, jogging, and a general increase in push-off strengthening activities. Because overuse and fatigue can occur at any time, attention to symptoms of overuse during the retraining phase is essential.

The technique described above applies to ruptures that occur proximal to the insertion, with a sufficient stump distally for suture. In those cases in which the tendon is avulsed from the calcaneus, the tendon is reattached to the bone with a suture anchor. There is generally sufficient tendon on the medial and lateral margins of the posterior calcaneus for additional insertion of sutures, but this should not be relied upon. The postoperative routine is similar after this method of repair, although it is necessary to be aware of the increased potential for failure of the suture construct.

Complications

The reported incidence of complications after Achilles tendon repair varies considerably, although the largest review included 775 ruptures treated surgically with an incidence of 20% of complications, many of which were quite minor.[24] Complications include skin necrosis, wound infection, sural neuroma, and adhesion of the skin to the repaired tendon. Although the reported incidence of rerupture of the tendon is considerably higher after nonsurgical treatment, in my experience, the incomplete return of function and performance is more common and problematic. Perhaps the single largest problem of nonsurgical treatment is the inability to establish functional continuity of the tendon with a normal dynamic resting length of the tendon maintained. Theoretically, many of the complications of cast immobilization may be eliminated by commencing early weightbearing in a functional boot, allowing some active and passive plantarflexion of the foot. The potential for failure of nonsurgical treatment must be weighed against the increased possibility of infection, anesthetic problems, and wound dehiscence after surgery.

Infection can be a disastrous complication because the options for soft-tissue coverage over the Achilles tendon are very limited.[53] The problem is that large skin and soft-tissue defects over the Achilles tendon are difficult to treat because of the relative avascularity of the adjacent tissue and the likelihood of exposed tendon. Split-thickness skin grafts rarely are suitable, because the take over the exposed tendon is unlikely. Although local flaps are described and possible, the donor site is often unsightly and associated with unacceptable scarring. If a wound problem is encountered, weightbearing should be limited, and the limb should be elevated to reduce tissue swelling. Oral antibiotics are invariably sufficient, and wound debridements should be kept to a minimum to avoid inadvertent exposure of the Achilles. I use Silvadene ointment applied liberally over the incision until granulation tissue is present, at which time wet-to-dry dressings with saline may be used. The patient may get the wound wet in a shower, but not soak the limb in a tub, and after cleansing with soap and

water, Silvadene is applied to cover the entire exposed tissue. Fortunately, this complication occurs relatively infrequently, yet even with exposed tendon, this method of wound care is effective, and rarely are local or free flaps necessary to solve the problem. When the defect is larger, a free microvascular flap will lead to acceptable coverage and function.[53] If a deep infection occurs, all the sutures must be removed, and hopefully some revascularization of the tendon will occur with healing, albeit in a compromised position. Other problems, such as scarring of the skin to the incision, have been minimized by the ambulatory program outlined above, but if problematic, various physical therapy modalities are used to decrease scarring and adhesion formation to the skin. If rerupture occurs, it is usually within the first 4 to 6 months after initiation of treatment. I have never encountered this problem with the surgical treatment and rehabilitation program outlined above, but the potential for complications exists and each requires special treatment, as described earlier.

Chronic Ruptures

Patients who sustain a rupture of the Achilles tendon are ideally treated expeditiously after injury, whether the treatment chosen is functional brace treatment or surgery.[25,30,31] Various terms, including the neglected or the missed rupture, have been applied to delayed diagnosis and treatment. As described above, I prefer to delay treatment for 1 or 2 weeks, when some fibrous reorganization of the tendon ends occur and there is less swelling present, before performing surgery. Certainly, if the rupture is diagnosed within the first few weeks of injury, this is not a neglected rupture, nor is it likely that any functional deficit will be experienced by this

minimal delay. Boyden and associates[54] compared the results of early and later repair of Achilles rupture in 21 patients, but did not find significant differences between the 2 groups, who were treated before or after 6 weeks following injury. However, substantial losses of function were noted in both groups on isokinetic and isometric testing, which were notably worse than those recently reported. It is difficult to draw a conclusion regarding the timing of surgery with respect to these patients because a functional method of recovery with early weightbearing and rehabilitation was not used for any of these patients.[54]

It is likely that if treatment is delayed for 6 weeks after rupture, the expected outcome cannot parallel the results had the repair been performed more expeditiously, although this depends on the extent of the gap between the tendon ends and the potential for muscle recovery. Two weeks after rupture, the gap between the torn tendon ends begins to fill with fibrous scar tissue, which does not have the same contractile strength as the normal tendon. The fibroblasts are disorganized and not longitudinally oriented, and this scar will gradually stretch and elongate because it is unable to withstand the tensile forces applied by the gastrocnemius-soleus complex. Although the tendon may occasionally heal in continuity, albeit in an elongated position, a long-standing rupture more commonly results in a gap, the length of which is determined by the amount of retraction of the proximal stump. The extent to which the patient perceives this as a problem depends on his or her activities of daily living, because some patients are able to ambulate without any functioning Achilles tendon. It is of interest that the clinical presentation of the neglected rupture is quite similar to that in patients who were treated with or without surgery but with subsequent elongation of the muscle-tendon unit.

Patient Evaluation

The strength of the gastrocnemius-soleus complex is established by observing ambulation, which should include the ability to walk on tiptoe or on the heels. The patient should be evaluated in the prone and seated positions, while testing maximum passive dorsiflexion. The prone dorsiflexion test is reliable, and although the extent of passive dorsiflexion varies for each individual, it is generally symmetrical for both extremities, which makes it possible to assess the extent of excessive dorsiflexion. Plantarflexion strength is further determined manually, and then with a double and single heel-rise test. Some patients can perform a single heel rise with no functional Achilles, but a repetitive heel-rise test is generally not possible. If a more accurate measure of strength is necessary, manual muscle testing is not sufficient, and isokinetic strength and power should be determined using machines, such as a dynamometer, that adequately document power and strength. This testing is performed through motions of dorsiflexion and plantarflexion and is analyzed as a percentage deficit relative to the opposite limb normalized for body weight. At 60 degree-seconds, these correlate with strength, and at 120 degree-seconds, they correlate with power parameters.

The size of the gap between the tendon ends must be carefully assessed, and although this can at times be assessed by palpation, if surgery is planned the method of reconstruction does depend on the extent of this gap, which should therefore be more accurately determined by MRI or ultrasound.

Management Options

Brace management is indicated for those patients who are not experiencing functional deficits as a result of the loss of push-off strength and who are not disabled in their activities of daily living. To this group should be added those who have potential problems with wound healing. Due to the magnitude of the dissection for correction of neglected ruptures, one must ensure that all potential for wound compromise is eliminated, including cigarette smoking, chronic dermatologic problems or chronic swelling of the limb, venous stasis, and arteriosclerosis causing lower limb ischemia. The brace options include a molded polypropylene ankle-foot orthosis (AFO), with or without a hinge at the ankle. A molded AFO is made, and the posterior ankle of the brace is transversely cut and reinforced by attaching a short piece of dense rubber to the medial and lateral margins of the brace. This AFO permits passive dorsiflexion with mild passive resistance, and the reinforced rubber contracts at the end point of dorsiflexion to forcibly plantarflex the foot. Some patients tolerate the brace well and find that it improves both stability and push-off strength such that surgery is not required.

Reconstruction of the Chronic Rupture

The ideal function of the gastrocnemius-soleus muscle can be regained only if the muscle is healthy, and without atrophy, both of which are unlikely if considerable time has elapsed since injury. Ideally, end-to-end tendon apposition of the tendon ends should be attempted, but this should be accomplished without placing the foot in marked equinus, which may not be possible if the gap between the tendon ends is great. For these reasons, many techniques for repair, reconstruction, or augmentation of the chronic Achilles tendon rupture have been proposed.[38,39,43,55–58] Many of these methods of reconstruction depend on harvesting avascular autologous tissue, such as multiple strips of fascia lata,[38] proximal Achilles turn-down flaps,[59] and the plantaris tendon.[56] The V-Y tendon advancement of the more proximal gastrocnemius muscle-tendon complex, as described initially, is generally avascular, but this depends on the method of muscle detachment and how it is advanced. These tendinous flaps are revascularized from the surrounding tissue or paratenon. However, it is possible to perform a substantial V-Y advancement while maintaining muscle integrity and continuity posteriorly, and this procedure has the potential of being vascularized.

The tendon transfers that are used to augment a deficient Achilles, ie, the peroneus brevis, FHL, or FDL, similarly are able to function despite a markedly compromised blood supply, although the muscle remains viable. When selecting either of these tendons, one must consider the donor morbidity and the strength of the transfer itself. Each of the described tendons used for transfer, ie, the peroneus brevis, the FHL, and the FDL, create some deficit that must be anticipated. For example, the peroneus brevis transfer as originally described by Turco and Spinella[58] is able to augment the Achilles, but this will inevitably compromise eversion strength. The balance of the muscles of eversion (the peroneus longus and brevis) and inversion (the posterior tibial, and to a lesser extent, the anterior tibial muscle) is therefore affected. One may anticipate the muscle deficit created by tendon transfer based on the percentages of total muscle force acting on the ankle.[60] The total strength of the peroneus longus and brevis (as a percentage of force on the ankle) is 7.1%, with the peroneus brevis accounting for 2.6%. The remaining available eversion force of 4.5% is insufficient to counteract the strength of the posterior tibial muscle, which accounts for 6.4% of the force across the ankle. The anterior tibial muscle may further add to some dynamic inversion, and the inversion/eversion balance is theoretically markedly compromised. This dynamic disruption of inversion and eversion does not occur with the use of either the FDL or the FHL, although these too have their drawbacks.[40,41,61,62]

I base the decision as to which technique to use for the neglected Achilles rupture on the distance between the tendon ends, the presence of gastrocnemius-soleus muscle atrophy, and the age and athletic activities of the patient. Generally, the reconstruction is planned according to the size of the defect between the tendon ends, and it is helpful to plan the extent of the surgery preoperatively. As with repair of an acute rupture, it is essential to obtain an anatomic end result, and this requires correct tensioning of the repair. A tourniquet is optional for all procedures. If used, it should be applied to the thigh and not the calf, to avoid tethering the gastrocnemius-soleus complex. If a more distal or calf tourniquet is used, tethering will prevent the proximal stump from being pulled distally. Wound closure after any of the procedures described below must be performed carefully to avoid subsequent skin necrosis. The paratenon should be repaired when possible to help maintain the blood supply to the tendon, followed by

wound closure in layers. After surgery, the lower leg is immobilized in a bulky dressing, incorporating splints to hold the ankle in a neutral position. A neutral position is preferred after all reconstructive procedures unless the ankle is intentionally placed in equinus to facilitate end-to-end repair of smaller gaps between the tendon ends. The postoperative course is the same for all the different procedures, because the need for functional rehabilitation with early mobilization and strengthening is identical to that after repair of an acute rupture. Postoperatively, patients are allowed to commence range-of-motion exercises once the sutures are removed, and weightbearing commences at about 2 weeks in a removable hinged range-of-motion walker boot that allows complete flexion of the ankle but has a dorsiflexion block that can be adjusted during the recovery process.

Defects of 1 to 2 cm

End-to-end anastomosis of the tendon ends is clearly optimum but may not be possible after neglected ruptures, although for this minimal defect, it is usually possible to accomplish the repair without any augmentation or reconstruction. The muscle can usually be mobilized and the repair performed with the foot held in mild equinus, and the foot gradually assumes a plantigrade position during rehabilitation. Exact end-to-end apposition of the tendon is important, and the repair is no different from that described above for management of the acute rupture. The success of this repair depends on an adequate suture fixation followed by aggressive rehabilitation to maximize isokinetic function. This procedure is easily accomplished if the gap is 1 cm or less. If the gap is greater, it is necessary to rely on the tensile properties of the muscle-tendon unit

to achieve end-to-end tendon apposition. The exposure and method of suture is identical to that described above, but, prior to tying the sutures, tension is applied for approximately 10 minutes to "stress relax" the myotendinous junction. This technique will gain up to 2 cm in length, depending on the extent of atrophy and the elastic properties of the tissue. The ankle is then placed in the desired amount of plantarflexion to achieve end-to-end repair, and after posterior compartment fasciotomy and skin closure, the lower limb is immobilized in a neutral position. Postoperative management is similar to that described above.

Defects of 2 to 5 cm

For these larger defects, I use a V-Y myotendinous lengthening, although this can occasionally be augmented with the FHL transfer described below. As originally described, this procedure reportedly corrected strength deficit when performed without the addition of the FHL transfer, and it relies on remaining muscle function, regardless of the length of time elapsed since injury. Theoretically, if the muscle is scarred this is not likely to work; however, this has not been my experience and that of others because, despite muscle atrophy, after tendon advancement, muscle strength and function seem to return. However, this procedure cannot be used if the muscle is severely atrophied and scarred as, for example, after infection. Although the FHL may be used as a sole transfer for these defects, this unnecessarily sacrifices a healthy functioning muscle, and if any function can be anticipated from the gastrocnemius, the V-Y advancement is preferable.

The procedure is performed with the patient in the prone position. A long incision is made, beginning proximal to the myotendinous junction in the midline, and gently curving immediately posteromedial to the Achilles tendon distally. After debridement of the tendon ends, an additional 1 cm of tendon length is further lost, necessitating careful planning of the length required of the proximal tendon flap. An inverted V incision is made in the fascia of the gastrocnemius, taking care to leave the underlying muscle attached to the anterior paratenon. The length of the arms of the inverted V should be twice as long as the defect, usually about 12 to 18 cm long. The planning of the flap is important in order to preserve the muscle attachment to the fascia and tendon posteriorly. Leave a margin of at least 1 cm on each side of the tendon flap proximally, although this is not possible distally where the incision is made into the tendon itself. The flap is then gently advanced by separating the muscle edges bluntly so as to preserve the posterior muscle tissue attached. For defects of up to 5 cm it is not difficult to advance the entire flap and preserve the muscle in continuity posteriorly. However, if the defect is larger, then the muscle posteriorly may become detached as the flap is advanced. An end-to-end repair is performed using a whip suture as described above. The Y is then closed with 2-0 nonabsorbable suture. Routine closure is performed and a bulky splint is applied in 10° to 20° of plantarflexion. Postoperative rehabilitation is performed as described above.

The results of the V-Y advancement for treatment of neglected Achilles tendon ruptures were reported recently by Us and associates.[63] These authors examined their patients with isokinetic testing and found a deficiency in peak torque ranging from 2% to 22% when compared to the unaffected limb. However, they noted that all patients were able to return to their preinjury activities, including sports. Other authors have reported similar success using the V-Y advancement procedure, with a 25% deficit in peak torque testing on Cybex postoperatively.[64]

Defects > 5 cm

For defects of this magnitude, rely on a tendon transfer either alone or in combination with a V-Y advancement of the gastrocnemius muscle and tendon. A turn-down flap of tendon may be used, but this is not my preferred method of reconstruction because of the bulk of the tendon at the point at which it is passed inferiorly. Although the peroneus brevis has been successfully used in these circumstances,[58] because this tendon is a weaker flexor, its use will compromise eversion, and I do not recommend it. The alternatives are to use either the FDL[40] or the FHL[62] as previously described. The use of either of these tendons retains its function as a plantarflexor of the foot, although neither approximates the strength of the gastrocnemius-soleus. Each of these procedures has its theoretical advantages and, of course, its proponents; however, due to the greater strength and the proximity of the muscle to the Achilles, I prefer to use the FHL. Although weak in comparison, the FHL is the second strongest plantarflexor next to the gastrocnemius-soleus complex, although it is less than one-tenth the power and strength of the latter muscle.[60]

The patient is positioned slightly laterally with the affected side down and the ipsilateral hip and knee flexed, or, if preferred, the prone position may be used. The skin marking for the incision on the foot corresponds to the talonavicular joint proximally and the mid-portion of the first metatarsal distally. The plane of the dissection is super-ficial to the abductor hallucis and flexor hallucis brevis, which are reflected dorsally or away from the first metatarsal. The FHL and FDL are identified, with the FHL being the more medial structure. The medial plantar branch of the medial plantar nerve can be damaged by this dissection, and it must be identified and retracted. To prevent proximal and distal retraction of the FHL tendon ends, two sutures are inserted into the FHL tendon, 1 cm apart, at the level at which the FHL is to be cut. The FHL is sutured by tenodesis of its distal stump to the FDL, while the ankle and toes are held in a neutral position. There are invariably cross-connections between the FHL and the FDL, and suture of the two tendons distally may not be necessary if the FHL is harvested proximal to these cross-connections. The range of motion of the hallux is assessed and, unless full dorsiflexion of the hallux is possible after the tenodesis, the sutures must be changed to adjust the tension on the stump of the FHL. More proximally, at the level of the foot where the FHL and FDL tendons cross each other (the Knot of Henry), there are multiple fibrous cross-connections between these tendons, and these usually need to be released for the FHL to be pulled into the proximal wound. A second incision is made along the medial border of the Achilles tendon from the myotendinous junction to 2 cm distal to the Achilles insertion. The deep posterior compartment of the leg is then opened longitudinally. The FHL muscle is identified, and its tendon is pulled into the proximal wound. At times, it is necessary to open the flexor retinaculum as far distal as the sustentaculum tali to permit the tendon to pass into the proximal wound. A 4.5-mm drill hole is made 1 cm distal to the

Achilles tendon insertion and 1.5 cm anterior to the posterior margin of the calcaneal cortex from medial to lateral. A 1-cm incision is made on the lateral posterior margin of the heel posterior to the sural nerve and immediately over the drill hole. The tendon is then passed from medial to lateral, and then back medially through a subcutaneous tunnel over the dorsal cortex of the calcaneus. In the past, I have tried drilling 2 holes, made at 90° to each other, but this construct seems too tenuous, because fracture of the calcaneus may occur. A suture passer may be used to pull the tendon of the FHL from proximal to distal through the drill hole. Alternatively, the end of a small metallic suction tip is passed from lateral to medial, and the suture on the FHL is sucked into the tip, facilitating passage of the tendon from medial to lateral. If the harvested FHL tendon is long, the FHL may be woven through the distal stump of the Achilles, although this does not appear to be necessary to obtain full function. The FHL is sutured in a side-to-side tenodesis manner to the Achilles with 2-0 nonabsorbable monofilament, and the muscle is sutured to the Achilles with 4-0 absorbable suture. The Achilles should be used in the final repair wherever possible, regardless of the length of time since rupture, in the hope that the gastrocnemius-soleus muscle strength will augment the transfer. The FHL, although strong, is markedly weaker than the gastrocnemius-soleus, and alone cannot be expected to return the patient to full activity. One must recognize, however, that the FHL is used here as a tendon transfer, and the strength and integrity of this transfer should not be compromised by a dead, atrophic, and nonyielding Achilles. If the proximal gastrocnemius-soleus mus-

cle has no contractility, a tenodesis of the FHL to the remaining Achilles may impair the ability of the FHL to function, and a tenodesis effect will occur.

The construct is tensioned with the ankle in neutral flexion. At the completion of the repair, the foot is taken through a full range of motion, and the ability of the construct to withstand dorsiflexion beyond neutral is carefully checked. The postoperative routine is identical to that described above for chronic rupture repair techniques.

Complications

The main complications associated with delayed repair of the Achilles tendon are wound necrosis, rerupture, infection, and inability to gain dorsiflexion. Wound-edge necrosis can best be avoided by using meticulous soft-tissue handling techniques, full-thickness flaps, and routine posterior fasciotomy. In addition, a bulky, cotton dressing with a posterior splint should be used to minimize initial motion pressure on the wound. Infection can be devastating if full-thickness necrosis occurs, exposing the tendon. In this case, the tendon must be kept constantly moist, to avoid desiccation, by using regular wet-dressing changes with oral antibiotics and permitting healing by secondary intention. An alternative method of wound management uses the application of Silvadene dressings followed by split-thickness skin grafting over the granulating surface.

Ankle stiffness can best be avoided by a regimented postoperative rehabilitation course and by ensuring that the repair does not require the ankle to be placed in excessive plantarflexion. Perhaps a more clinically significant complication is the lack either of free motion or of the ability to regain adequate push-off strength. Either of

these may be caused by incorrect tensioning of the repair or by elongation of the repair construct postoperatively. Ankle stiffness results from insufficient length because the repair must be made with the foot held in equinus. This position is far less compromising than repairs performed in a functionally elongated position. A patient with the latter repair never fully regains push-off strength.

The chronic or neglected Achilles tendon rupture poses a difficult problem for the orthopaedic surgeon. Most patients will complain of an inability to perform a single toe-stance or heel-rise, weakness at push-off of the gait cycle, and the inability to participate in recreational sports due to lack of strength. Bracing with a spring-loaded, hinged AFO can improve function and power at push-off, but will not permit the patient to perform toe rises.

The etiology of the chronic rupture can be multifactorial, including missed initial diagnoses, inappropriate treatment of an acute rupture, chronic Achilles tendinosis leading to microtears with subsequent lengthening, and ruptures associated with inflammatory disorders, such as rheumatoid arthritis and systemic lupus erythematosus. Ruptures in patients with inflammatory disorders can be very difficult to diagnose and treat. Such patients frequently have involvement of multiple joints (causing a decreased range of motion and weakness), are on multidrug regimens (often including steroids that can increase the risk of postoperative complications), and can sustain spontaneous ruptures that may be undetected for years. There does not seem to be a time limit beyond which a repair of a chronic rupture will not improve function. Regardless of the etiology, the size of the defect, and the time since rupture, the decision-making algorithm and repair techniques outlined above provide patients with improved strength, function, and power, and freedom from a brace. However, it must be remembered that the patient must be motivated toward an aggressive rehabilitation course and be compliant with such a regimen.

References

1. Carden DG, Noble J, Chalmers J, Lunn P, Ellis J: Rupture of the calcaneal tendon: The early and late management. *J Bone Joint Surg* 1987; 69B:416–420.

2. Jozsa L, Kvist M, Balint BJ, et al: The role of recreational sport activity in Achilles tendon rupture: A clinical, pathoanatomical, and sociological study of 292 cases. *Am J Sports Med* 1989;17:338–343.

3. Levi N: The incidence of Achilles tendon rupture in Copenhagen. *Injury* 1997;28:311–313.

4. Sun Y-S, Yen T-F, Chie LH: Ruptured Achilles tendon: Report of 40 cases. *Zhonghua Yixue Zazhi* 1977;57:94–96.

5. Jozsa L, Kannus P: Histopathological findings in spontaneous tendon ruptures. *Scand J Med Sci Sports* 1997;7:113–118.

6. Fox JM, Blazina ME, Jobe FW, et al: Degeneration and rupture of the Achilles tendon. *Clin Orthop* 1975;107:221–224.

7. Lagergren C, Lindholm A: Vascular distribution in the Achilles tendon: An angiographic and microangiographic study. *Acta Chir Scand* 1959;116:491–495.

8. Arner O, Lindholm A: Avulsion fracture of the os calcaneus. *Acta Chir Scand* 1949;117:258–260.

9. Mandelbaum BR, Myerson MS, Forster R: Achilles tendon ruptures: A new method of repair, early range of motion, and functional rehabilitation. *Am J Sports Med* 1995;23:392–395.

10. Mahler F, Fritschy D: Partial and complete ruptures of the Achilles tendon and local corticosteroid injections. *Br J Sports Med* 1992;26: 7–14.

11. Laseter JT, Russell JA: Anabolic steroid-induced tendon pathology: A review of the literature. *Med Sci Sports Exerc* 1991;23:1–3.

12. Beskin JL, Sanders RA, Hunter SC, Hughston JC: Surgical repair of Achilles tendon ruptures. *Am J Sports Med* 1987;15:1–8.

13. Cirincione RJ, Baker BE: Tendon ruptures with secondary hyperparathyroidism: A case report. *J Bone Joint Surg* 1975;57A:852–853.

14. Hosey G, Kowalchick E, Tesoro D, et al: Comparison of the mechanical and histologic properties of Achilles tendons in New Zealand white rabbits secondarily repaired with Marlex mesh. *J Foot Surg* 1991;30:214–233.

15. Nehrer S, Breitenseher M, Brodner W, et al: Clinical and sonographic evaluation of the risk of rupture in the Achilles tendon. *Arch Orthop Trauma Surg* 1997;116:14–18.

16. Thompson TC, Doherty JH: Spontaneous rupture of tendon of Achilles: A new clinical diagnostic test. *J Trauma* 1962;2:126–129.

17. Harcke HT, Grissom LE, Finkelstein MS: Evaluation of the musculoskeletal system with sonography. *Am J Roentgenol* 1988;150: 1253–1261.

18. Richter J, Josten C, David A, Clasbrummel B, Muhr G: Sports fitness after functional conservative versus surgical treatment of acute Achilles tendon ruptures. *Zentralbl Chir* 1994;119:538–544.

19. Cetti R, Christensen SE, Ejsted R, Jensen NM, Jorgensen U: Operative versus nonoperative treatment of Achilles tendon rupture: A prospective randomized study and review of the literature. *Am J Sports Med* 1993;21:791–799.

20. Neumann D, Vogt L, Banzer W, Schreiber U: Kinematic and neuromuscular changes of the gait pattern after Achilles tendon rupture. *Foot Ankle Int* 1997;18:339–341.

21. Christensen I: Rupture of the Achilles tendon: Analysis of 57 cases. *Acta Chir Scand* 1953;106: 50–60.

22. Nada A: Rupture of the calcaneal tendon: Treatment by external fixation. *J Bone Joint Surg* 1985;67B:449–453.

23. Quenu J, Stoianovitch: Les ruptures du tendon d'Achille. *Rev Chir (Paris)* 1929;67:647–678.

24. Wills CA, Washburn S, Caiozzo V, Prietto CA: Achilles tendon rupture: A review of the literature comparing surgical versus nonsurgical treatment. *Clin Orthop* 1986;207:156–163.

25. Lea RB, Smith L: Non-surgical treatment of tendo achillis rupture. *J Bone Joint Surg* 1972; 54A:1398–1407.

26. Nistor L: Surgical and non-surgical treatment of Achilles tendon rupture: A prospective randomized study. *J Bone Joint Surg* 1981;63A: 394–399.

27. Helgeland J, Odland P, Hove LM: Achilles tendon rupture: Surgical or non-surgical treatment. *Tidsskr Nor Laegeforen* 1997;117:1763–1766.

28. Thermann H, Frerichs O, Biewener A, Krettek C, Schandelmeier P: Functional treatment of acute rupture of the Achilles tendon: An experimental biomechanical study. *Unfallchirurg* 1995;98:507–513.

29. Achilles tendon rupture. *Lancet* 1973;1: 189–190.

30. Inglis AE, Scott WN, Sculco TP, Patterson AH: Ruptures of the tendo Achillis: An objective assessment of surgical and non-surgical treatment. *J Bone Joint Surg* 1976;58A:990–993.

31. Jacobs D, Martens M, Van Audekercke R, Mulier JC, Mulier F: Comparison of conservative and operative treatment of Achilles tendon rupture. *Am J Sports Med* 1978;6:107–111.

32. Bunnell S: Primary repair of severed tendons: The use of stainless steel wire. *Am J Surg* 1940; 47:502–516.

33. Kessler I: The "grasping" technique for tendon repair. *Hand* 1973;5:253–255.

34. Ma GW, Griffith TG: Percutaneous repair of acute closed ruptured Achilles tendon: A new technique. *Clin Orthop* 1977;128:247–255.

35. Cetti R: Ruptured Achilles tendon: Preliminary results of a new treatment. *Br J Sports Med* 1988;22:6–8.

36. Mortensen NH, Saether J: Achilles tendon repair: A new method of Achilles tendon repair tested on cadaverous materials. *J Trauma* 1991; 31:381–384.

37. Kirschenbaum SE, Kelman C: Modification of the Lindholm procedure for plastic repair of ruptured Achilles tendon: A case report. *J Foot Surg* 1980;19:4–11.

38. Bugg EI Jr, Boyd BM: Repair of neglected rupture or laceration of the Achilles tendon. *Clin Orthop* 1968;56:73–75.

39. Perez Teuffer A: Traumatic rupture of the Achilles tendon: Reconstruction by transplant and graft using the lateral peroneus brevis. *Orthop Clin North Am* 1974;5:89–93.

40. Mann RA, Holmes GB, Jr, Seale KS, Collins DN: Chronic rupture of the Achilles tendon: A new technique of repair. *J Bone Joint Surg* 1991;73A:214–219.

41. Wapner KL, Hecht PJ, Mills RH Jr: Reconstruction of neglected Achilles tendon injury. *Orthop Clin North Am* 1995;26:249–263.

42. Jenkins DH, Forster IW, McKibbin B, Ralis ZA: Induction of tendon and ligament formation by carbon implants. *J Bone Joint Surg* 1977;59B:53–57.

43. Levy M, Velkes S, Goldstein J, Rosner M: A method of repair for Achilles tendon ruptures without cast immobilization: Preliminary report. *Clin Orthop* 1984;187:199–204.

44. Giannini S, Girolami M, Ceccarelli F, Catani F, Stea S: Surgical repair of Achilles tendon ruptures using polypropylene braid augmentation. *Foot Ankle Int* 1994;15:372–375.

45. Booth FW: Physiologic and biochemical effects of immobilization on muscle. *Clin Orthop* 1987;219:15–20.

46. Pepels WRJ, Plasmans CMT, Sloof TJJH: Abstract: The course of healing of tendons and ligaments. *Acta Orthop Scand* 1983;54:952.

47. Gelberman RH, Manske PR, Vande Berg JS, Lesker PA, Akeson WH: Flexor tendon repair in vitro: A comparative histologic study of the rabbit, chicken, dog, and monkey. *J Orthop Res* 1984;2:39–48.

48. Enwemeka CS, Spielholz NI, Nelson AJ: The effect of early functional activities on experimentally tenotomized Achilles tendons in rats. *Am J Phys Med Rehabil* 1988;67:264–269.

49. Bradley JP, Tibone JE: Percutaneous and open surgical repairs of Achilles tendon ruptures: A comparative study. *Am J Sports Med* 1990;18: 188–195.

50. Inglis AE, Sculco TP: Surgical repair of ruptures of the tendo Achillis. *Clin Orthop* 1981; 156:160–169.

51. Shields CL Jr, Kerlan RK, Jobe FW, Carter VS, Lombardo SJ: The Cybex II evaluation of sur-

gically repaired Achilles tendon ruptures. *Am J Sports Med* 1978;6:369–372.

52. Motta P, Errichiello C, Pontini I: Achilles tendon rupture: A new technique for easy surgical repair and immediate movement of the ankle and foot. *Am J Sports Med* 1997;25:172–176.

53. Leppilahti J, Kaarela O, Teerikangas H, Raatikainen T, Orava S, Waris T: Free tissue coverage of wound complications following Achilles tendon rupture surgery. *Clin Orthop* 1996;328:171–176.

54. Boyden EM, Kitaoka HB, Cahalan TD, An KN: Late versus early repair of Achilles tendon rupture: Clinical and biomechanical evaluation. *Clin Orthop* 1995;317:150–158.

55. Howard CB, Winston I, Bell W, Mackie I, Jenkins DH: Late repair of the calcaneal tendon with carbon fibre. *J Bone Joint Surg* 1984;66B: 206–208.

56. Lynn TA: Repair of the torn Achilles tendon, using the plantaris tendon as a reinforcing membrane. *J Bone Joint Surg* 1966;48A:268–272.

57. Schedl R, Fasol P: Achilles tendon repair with the plantaris tendon compared with repair using polyglycol threads. *J Trauma* 1979;19: 189–194.

58. Turco VJ, Spinella AJ: Achilles tendon ruptures: Peroneus brevis transfer. *Foot Ankle* 1987;7:253–259.

59. Bosworth DM: Repair of defects in the tendo Achillis. *J Bone Joint Surg* 1956;38A:111–114.

60. Silver RL, de la Garza J, Rang M: The myth of muscle balance: A study of relative strengths and excursions of normal muscles about the foot and ankle. *J Bone Joint Surg* 1985;67B: 432–437.

61. Wapner KL, Hecht PJ: Repair of chronic Achilles tendon rupture with flexor hallucis longus tendon transfer. *Op Tech Orthop* 1994; 4:132–137.

62. Wapner KL, Pavlock GS, Hecht PJ, Naselli F, Walther R: Repair of chronic Achilles tendon rupture with flexor hallucis longus tendon transfer. *Foot Ankle* 1993;14:443–449.

63. Us AK, Bilgin SS, Aydin T, Mergen E: Repair of neglected Achilles tendon ruptures: Procedures and functional results. *Arch Orthop Trauma Surg* 1997;116:408–411.

64. Kissel CG, Blacklidge DK, Crowley DL: Repair of neglected Achilles tendon ruptures: Procedure and functional results. *J Foot Ankle Surg* 1994;33:46–52.

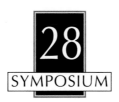

Ankle Arthritis: Emerging Concepts and Management Strategies

Charles L. Saltzman, MD
Joseph A. Buckwalter, MD

Advances in understanding of the special features of the ankle joint and of the pathogenesis of degenerative joint disease have led to new approaches to the treatment of ankle arthritis. Compared with other major lower extremity joints, the ankle joint possesses unique epidemiologic, anatomic, biomechanical, and biologic characteristics. Unlike the hip and knee, which are prone to development of primary osteoarthritis, ankle arthritis usually is the end result of a traumatic event. Ankle articular cartilage has characteristic differences from hip or knee cartilage that may protect the ankle from developing primary osteoarthritis. Ankle articular cartilage preserves its tensile stiffness and fracture stress better than hip articular cartilage. Metabolic differences between knee and ankle articular cartilage might further help to explain the relative rarity of primary ankle osteoarthritis. Recently, in developed nations, physicians have noted a progressive increase in the incidence of disabling ankle arthritis, an increase that may

in part be due to the combined effect of the widespread use of life-protecting thoracoabdominal level air-bag restraints and the general aging of the population. The increased incidence of painful post-traumatic ankle osteoarthritis has spurred interest in finding therapeutic solutions to this often functionally limiting problem.

In the following chapters, the unique aspects of ankle arthritis and emerging approaches for treatment are described. First, the distinctive characteristics of the ankle joint and ankle osteoarthritis are presented. Second, exciting work using joint distraction techniques to promote formation of a new articular surface in both in vitro and in vivo models is described. Third, a chapter is dedicated to explaining the current techniques for evaluating and treating malalignments of the lower extremities, causing focal increased ankle articular stress. Fourth, an arthroscopic approach for ankle fusion is described in a chapter dedicated to the use of arthroscopy in ankle arthritis. With the development of

arthroscopic techniques specific for the ankle joint, fusion rates have improved and immediate postoperative morbidity has diminished. Despite these technical improvements, ankle arthroscopic fusion is not appropriate for many patients, and ankle arthrodesis procedures still have problems with nonunion, malunion, infection, leg-length discrepancy, painful hindfoot motion, or neurovascular injury. The fifth chapter is devoted to the strategies to manage these challenging problems. Finally, a review of the state of the art of total ankle arthroplasty is presented. New designs have shown promising early results and the potential to avoid some of the late complications attributed to ankle arthrodeses.

The pathogenesis and optimal treatment of painful ankle arthritis is clearly different from that of hip or knee arthritis. We hope these chapters will stimulate interest in further study of ankle arthritis, and improved management of increasing numbers of patients with this clinical problem.

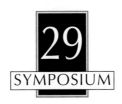

Ankle Osteoarthritis: Distinctive Characteristics

Joseph A. Buckwalter, MD
Charles L. Saltzman, MD

Because osteoarthritis causes similar symptoms of pain and loss of motion in different joints, few investigators have made an attempt to determine if osteoarthritis differs among joints in pathogenesis, clinical presentation, and response to treatment. The majority of clinical and basic scientific studies have focused on hip and knee osteoarthritis, and physicians have generally assumed that information developed from these studies applies equally well to other joints. Ankle osteoarthritis has received relatively little attention, making it difficult to identify and define differences between ankle osteoarthritis and osteoarthritis in other synovial joints. Nonetheless, review of available clinical and experimental studies shows that ankle osteoarthritis has characteristics that distinguish it from osteoarthritis occurring in other synovial joints, including the hip and knee, and that these distinctive characteristics result in differences in prevalence, clinical presentation, natural history, and, possibly, in results of treatment.

This chapter first reviews current understanding of the clinical syndrome of osteoarthritis and its relationship to joint degeneration. Subsequent sections consider the unique characteristics of the ankle joint, the prevalence and pathogenesis of ankle osteoarthritis, and the implications of the response of ankle osteoarthritis to

alterations in joint contact stress for understanding of the pathogenesis and treatment of ankle osteoarthritis.

Osteoarthritis

Osteoarthritis, also referred to as degenerative joint disease, degenerative arthritis, osteoarthrosis, or hypertrophic arthritis, is a clinical syndrome that results from degeneration of a synovial joint.[1,2] The critical feature of the joint degeneration responsible for osteoarthritis is a progressive loss of articular cartilage, accompanied by attempted repair of articular cartilage, remodeling, and sclerosis of subchondral bone.[1,2] In many instances, subchondral bone cysts and osteophytes form as part of the syndrome of osteoarthritis. However, subchondral bone cysts and osteophytes may form in the absence of clinically significant articular cartilage degeneration and, thus, in themselves are not diagnostic of osteoarthritis. Furthermore, in addition to degenerative changes in the synovial joint, the diagnosis of osteoarthritis requires the presence of symptoms that include joint pain and loss of joint function. Patients with osteoarthritis may also have restriction of joint motion, crepitus with joint motion, joint effusions, and deformity.

In most joints, osteoarthritis most commonly develops in the absence of a known cause, a condition referred to as primary or idiopathic osteoarthritis.

Less frequently, it develops as a result of joint injuries, infections, or a variety of hereditary, developmental, metabolic, and neurologic disorders, a group of conditions referred to as secondary osteoarthritis.[2] The age of onset of secondary osteoarthritis depends on the underlying cause. Thus, it may develop in young adults and even children as well as the elderly. In contrast, a strong association exists between the prevalence of primary osteoarthritis and age. The percentage of people with evidence of osteoarthritis in one or more joints increases from less than 5% of people between 15 and 44 years of age, to 25% to 30% of people 45 to 64 years of age, to more than 60% and in some populations as high as 90% of the people over 65 years of age.[3] Despite this strong association with age and the widespread view that primary osteoarthritis results from "wear and tear" of synovial joints, the relationships between age and osteoarthritis remain poorly defined. Furthermore, the changes observed in articular cartilage with aging differ from those observed in osteoarthritis, and normal lifelong joint use has not been shown to cause articular joint degeneration.[2,4–6] Thus, osteoarthritis is not simply the result of aging or of mechanical wear from normal joint use.

The joint degeneration responsible for osteoarthritis is not uniformly

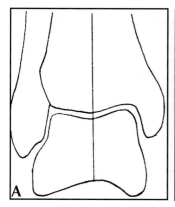
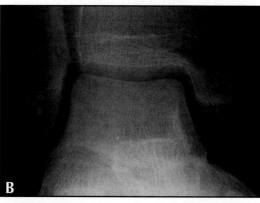

Fig. 1 Ankle joint structure. **A,** Drawing of the ankle joint showing how the talus fits in the mortise formed by the distal ends of the fibula and tibia. The medial malleolus and the medial surface of the talus form the opposing medial articular surfaces, the distal tibia and the superior talus form the opposing central articular surfaces, and the lateral malleolus and the lateral surface of the talus form the opposing lateral articular surfaces. Notice how the convexity of the distal tibial articular surface matches the concavity of the superior talar articular surface. The center of the matching convexity and concavity is used to divide the joint into medial and lateral compartments for study of joint loading and joint degeneration. **B,** Standing radiograph of the ankle joint showing the features outlined in the drawing.

progressive. Because repair and re-modeling reactions can alter the rate of progression of the disorder, the rate of joint degeneration varies considerably among individuals and among joints. Occasionally it occurs rapidly, but in most instances it progresses slowly over many years, although it may stabilize or even improve spontaneously, with at least partial restoration of an articular surface and a decrease in symptoms. This phenomenon of stabilization and even regression of the degenerative changes has been observed in almost every synovial joint, including the ankle.

Unique Characteristics of the Ankle Joint

The differences in anatomy and motion between the ankle joint and the other major joints of the lower limb, the hip and the knee, are readily apparent. Other differences, including the area of contact between opposing articular surfaces and articular cartilage thickness, tensile properties, and metabolism, are less apparent. Taken

together, the unique mechanical and biologic characteristics of the ankle affect the development, clinical presentation, and course of osteoarthritis and the response to treatment of osteoarthritis in this joint.

Anatomy and Motion

The bony anatomy of the ankle joint determines the planes and ranges of joint motion and confers a high degree of stability and congruence when the joint is loaded. The 3 bones that form the ankle joint, the tibia, fibula, and talus, support 3 sets of opposing articular surfaces. The tibial medial malleolus and the medial facet of the talus form the medial articular surfaces, the fibular lateral malleolus and the talar lateral articular surface form the lateral articular surfaces, and the distal tibia and the superior dome of the talus form the central articular surfaces (Fig. 1). The distal tibial articular surface has a longitudinal convexity that matches a concavity on the surface of the talus. The center of the matching convexi-

ty and concavity of the distal tibial and superior talar articular surfaces is used to divide the tibiotalar articulation into the medial and lateral compartments for evaluation of ankle loading and degenerative changes (Fig. 1, A). The distal tibia, including the medial malleolus together with the lateral malleolus form the ankle mortise, which contains the talus. Firm anterior and posterior ligaments bind the distal tibia and fibula together, forming the distal tibiofibular syndesmosis. Medial and lateral ligamentous complexes and the ankle joint capsule stabilize the relationship between the talus and the mortise.

The bony anatomy, ligaments, and joint capsule guide and restrain movement between the talus and the mortise so that the talus has a continuously changing axis of rotation as it moves from maximum dorsiflexion to maximum plantarflexion relative to the mortise. The talus and mortise widen slightly from posterior to anterior. Thus when the talus is plantarflexed, the narrowest portion of the talus sits in the ankle mortise and allows rotatory movement between the talus and mortise. When the talus is maximally dorsiflexed, the tibiofibular syndesmosis spreads and the wider portion of the talar articular surface locks into the ankle mortise, allowing little or no rotation between the talus and the mortise. In most normal ankles, the soft-tissue structures, including joint capsule, ligaments, and muscle tendon units that cross the joint, prevent significant translation of the talus relative to the mortise.

Articular Surface Contact Area

When loaded, the human ankle joint has a smaller area of contact between the opposing articular surfaces than the knee or hip. At 500 N of load, the contact area of the ankle joint averages 350 mm^2,[7,8] compared with 1,120 mm^2 for the knee[9] and 1,100 mm^2 for the hip.[10] Although in vivo contact stress has not been measured in the ankle, the smaller contact area must make the normal peak contact stress higher in the ankle than in the knee or hip.

Articular Cartilage Thickness and Tensile Properties

Ankle joint articular cartilage differs from that of the knee and hip in thickness and tensile properties. The thickness of ankle articular cartilage ranges from less than 1 mm to slightly less than 2 mm.[11,12] In contrast, the knee and hip joints have regions of articular cartilage that may be more than 6 mm thick and in most load-bearing areas the articular cartilage of these joints is at least 3 mm thick.[13] Work by Kempson[14] shows that the tensile properties of ankle and hip articular cartilage differ and that these differences increase with age (Figs. 2 and 3). In particular, the tensile fracture stress and tensile stiffness of ankle articular cartilage deteriorate less rapidly with age than hip articular cartilage tensile properties.[14] Although the tensile fracture stress of hip femoral articular cartilage is initially greater than the tensile fracture stress of talar articular cartilage, hip cartilage tensile fracture stress declines exponentially with age while talar articular cartilage tensile fracture stress declines linearly (Fig. 2). As a result of these aging changes, beginning in middle age, ankle articular cartilage can withstand greater tensile loads than hip articular cartilage, and this difference increases with increasing age. Age-related changes in hip and ankle articular cartilage tensile stiffness follow a similar pattern (Fig. 3). Presumably, age-related declines in articular cartilage tensile properties result from

progressive weakening of the articular cartilage collagen fibril network. The cause or causes of the age-related weakening of the articular cartilage matrix have not been explained, but age-related changes in articular cartilage collagen fibril structure and collagen cross-linking have been identified that may contribute to changes in matrix tensile properties.[4,5] Kempson has suggested that the differences in articular cartilage tensile properties may explain the apparent vulnerability of the hip and knee for the development of degenerative changes with increasing age, and the relative resistance of the ankle to the development of primary osteoarthritis.[14]

Articular Cartilage Metabolism

Ankle articular cartilage may differ from articular cartilage from other joints in expression of an enzyme that can degrade articular cartilage and in response to the catabolic cytokine interleukin-1. Recently Chubinskaya and associates[15] detected messenger RNA for neutrophil collagenase (MMP-8) in human knee articular cartilage chondrocytes, but not in ankle articular cartilage chondrocytes. Häuselmann and associates[16] have reported that the catabolic cytokine interleukin-1 inhibited proteoglycan synthesis by knee articular cartilage chondrocytes more effectively than it inhibited proteoglycan synthesis by ankle articular cartilage chondrocytes.[16,17] The difference in the response to interleukin-1 between knee and ankle articular cartilage chondrocytes appears to be caused by the greater number of interleukin-1 receptors in knee articular cartilage chondrocytes. These observations will need further study, but they suggest that there are metabolic differences between knee and ankle articular cartilage that might help explain

the relative rarity of primary ankle osteoarthritis.

Prevalence of Ankle Osteoarthritis

Determining the prevalence of ankle osteoarthritis is more difficult than it might at first seem. As in other joints, the correlation between degenerative changes in the joint and the clinical syndrome of osteoarthritis is not consistent.[18,19] In addition, it is extremely expensive and difficult to obtain and study unbiased samples of populations to determine the prevalence of osteoarthritis. For these reasons, studies of the prevalence of osteoarthritis by examination of autopsy specimens, evaluation of radiographs of populations of patients, and evaluation of patients presenting with symptomatic osteoarthritis have significant limitations.

Autopsy Studies

Despite their limitations, including relatively small numbers of joints examined and lack of random or systematic sampling of populations, studies of joints at autopsy can provide useful information concerning differences in prevalence of degeneration among joints. Meachim and Emery[20-23] examined knee, shoulder, and ankle joints at autopsies performed on adults. They found full-thickness chondral defects in 1 of 20 ankle joints from people older than 70 years of age.[22] Cartilage fibrillation was much more frequent than full-thickness defects in all joints. Huch and associates[17] resected 36 knees and 78 ankles from both limbs of 39 organ donors to evaluate the prevalence of ankle osteoarthritis. Joints were evaluated using a scale described by Collins: grade 0–normal gross appearance of a joint, grade I–fraying or fibrillation of the articular cartilage, grade 2–fibrillation and fissuring of

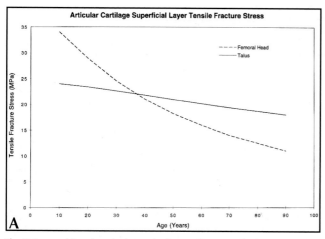

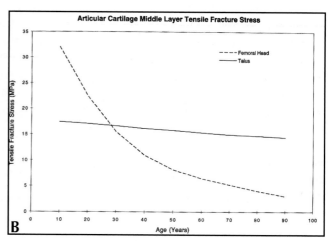

Fig. 2 Femoral head and talus articular cartilage tensile fracture stress versus age. **A,** Articular cartilage superficial layer tensile fracture stress versus age. **B,** Articular cartilage middle layer tensile fracture stress versus age. Notice that the tensile fracture stress of ankle articular cartilage is greater beginning in middle age than the tensile fracture stress of femoral head articular cartilage and that the difference increases with increasing age. These illustrations were developed from data reported by Kempson.[14]

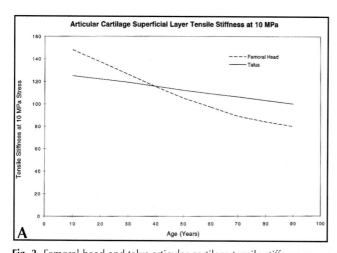

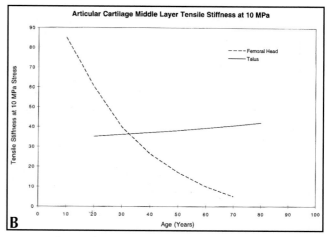

Fig. 3 Femoral head and talus articular cartilage tensile stiffness versus age. **A,** Articular cartilage superficial layer tensile stiffness versus age. **B,** Articular cartilage middle layer tensile stiffness versus age. Notice that the tensile stiffness of ankle articular cartilage is greater beginning in middle age than the tensile fracture stress of femoral head articular cartilage and that the difference increases with increasing age. These illustrations were developed from data reported by Kempson.[14]

the cartilage and osteophytes, grade 3–extensive fibrillation and fissuring with frequent osteophytes and 30% or less full-thickness chondral defects, grade 4–frequent osteophytes and greater than 30% full-thickness chondral defects.[17,24] In these studies, grades 3 and 4 were defined as osteoarthritis, and grade 2 was defined as early osteoarthritis.[17] However, the authors did not have information con-

cerning possible symptoms associated with the joints studied, so it is not certain if the degenerative changes they identified were associated with clinical osteoarthritis. Using the Collins grading scale, Huch and associates[17] found grades 3 and 4 degenerative changes in 5 of 78 (6%) ankle joints and in 9 of 36 (25%) knee joints (Fig. 4). Degenerative changes were most commonly found on the medial aspect of

the ankle. In another series of investigations Muehleman and associates[25] examined 7 joints, including the knee and ankle of both lower extremities in 50 cadavers.[17,25] The individuals studied ranged in age from 36 to 94 years, with a mean age of 76 years. Sixty-six percent of the knee joints had grades 3 and 4 degenerative changes, compared with 18% of the ankle joints (Fig. 4). Ninety-five percent of the knees had grade 2, 3, or 4 degenerative changes compared with 76% of the ankles. The authors also observed that the medial compartments of both the knees and the ankles were more frequently involved than the lateral compartments, and that radiographs often showed no evidence of degenerative changes when direct examination of the joint showed regions of full-thickness cartilage erosion. Overall, the autopsy studies demonstrate that advanced degenerative changes are at least 3 times more prevalent in the knee than in the ankle, and that the prevalence of degenerative changes in both joints increases with increasing age (Fig. 4).

Radiographic Evaluations

Although epidemiologic studies based on radiographic evaluations document a striking increase in the prevalence of degenerative changes of all joints, including those of the foot and ankle, with increasing age,[3] the reported studies have not focused on ankle osteoarthritis. Radiographic studies of ankle joint degeneration have important limitations because of the lack of a strong correlation between the formation of osteophytes and clinical osteoarthritis[19] (Fig. 5), and the difficulty in evaluating the thickness of ankle articular cartilage, particularly on radiographs that were not performed in a standardized fashion. Furthermore, ankle radiographs often do not show signs of joint degeneration even when the ankle joint has regions of full-thickness erosion of articular cartilage.[25] For these reasons, attempts to evaluate the prevalence of ankle degeneration and osteoarthritis by plain radiographs alone have limited value.

Clinical Studies

Very few studies of the prevalence of osteoarthritis have included patients

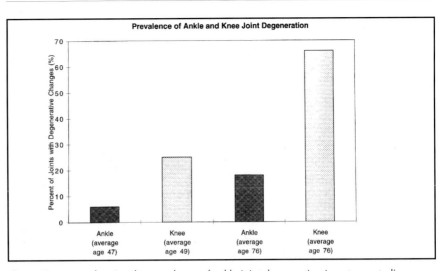

Fig. 4 Histograms showing the prevalence of ankle joint degeneration in autopsy studies reported by Huch and associates[17] and Muehleman and associates.[25] In these studies, the criteria for joint degeneration (osteoarthritis) were extensive articular cartilage fibrillation, osteophytes, and regions of full-thickness cartilage loss (Collins grades 3 and 4). Notice that joint degeneration was more than 3 times more common in the knee than in the ankle, and that the prevalence of joint degeneration in the knee and the ankle increased with age.

with ankle osteoarthritis. The available information suggests that knee osteoarthritis is 8 to 10 times more common than ankle osteoarthritis.[17,26–28] However, the best currently available estimates suggest that knee replacements are performed at least 25 times more frequently than ankle replacements and ankle fusions combined.[3] These observations, combined with the data from autopsy studies showing that advanced knee joint degeneration is about 3 to 5 times more common than advanced ankle joint degeneration, suggest that surgical procedures are performed less frequently for patients with advanced ankle osteoarthritis than for patients with advanced osteoarthritis of the knee. The reasons for this are unclear. It is possible that ankle joint degeneration and osteoarthritis cause less severe pain and functional limitation than knee degeneration and osteoarthritis. Lack of understanding of the evaluation and treatment of ankle osteoarthritis among physicians,

the efficacy of nonsurgical treatments for ankle osteoarthritis or the lack of effective and widely accepted surgical treatments for ankle osteoarthritis may also contribute to the apparent difference in the frequency of surgical treatment of ankle and knee osteoarthritis.

Pathogenesis of Ankle Osteoarthritis

Review of clinical experience and published reports of the treatment of ankle osteoarthritis indicates that primary ankle osteoarthritis is rare and that secondary ankle osteoarthritis that develops following ankle fractures or ligamentous injury is the most common cause of ankle osteoarthritis.[29–36] Patients with neuropathic degenerative disease of the ankle and degenerative disease following necrosis of the talus with collapse of the articular surface make up a small portion of the individuals with degenerative disease of the ankle.[32,37–39] Primary osteoarthritis is the most common diagnosis for patients treated with hip and knee

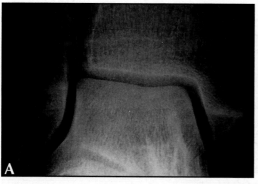
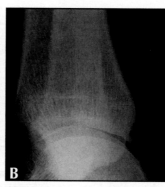

Fig. 5 Standing radiographs showing the ankle of a middle-age adult. **A,** Anteroposterior radiograph, and **B,** lateral radiograph. These studies were obtained to evaluate an acute ankle injury. The patient participated in a variety of athletic activities but she had no history of joint pain, swelling, crepitus or stiffness, and, therefore, she did not have osteoarthritis. The radiographs do not show a fracture or decreased articular cartilage thickness, but osteophytes are present at the tip of the medial malleolus (seen on the anteroposterior view) and the posterior edge of the tibia (seen on the lateral view).

Outline 1
Stages in development of posttraumatic ankle osteoarthritis

Stage I.   Increased Contact Stress Damages Articular Cartilage
             Disruption or alteration of the matrix macromolecular framework associated with an increase in water concentration may be caused by high levels of contact stress. At first, the type 11 collagen concentration remains unchanged, but the collagen meshwork may be damaged and the concentration of aggrecan and the degree of proteoglycan aggregation decrease.

Stage II.   Chondrocyte Response to Matrix Disruption or Alteration
             When chondrocytes detect a disruption or alteration of their matrix they respond by increasing matrix synthesis and degradation and by proliferating. Their response may restore the tissue, maintain the tissue in an altered state, or increase cartilage volume. They may sustain an increased level of activity for years.

Stage III.   Decline in the Chondrocyte Response
             Failure of the chondrocytic response to restore or maintain the tissue leads to loss of articular cartilage accompanied or preceded by a decline in the chondrocytic response. The causes for the decline in chondrocytic response remain poorly understood, but it may be partially the result of mechanical damage to the tissue with injury to chondrocytes and a down regulation of the chondrocytic response to anabolic cytokines.

---

replacements. In contrast, posttraumatic osteoarthritis is the most common diagnosis for patients treated with ankle arthrodesis or replacement. This observation raises the possibility that the ankle may be at least as vulnerable and perhaps more vulnerable than the hip and knee for the development of severe posttraumatic osteoarthritis. The relative rarity of primary osteoarthritis of the ankle may be the result of the congruency, stability, and restrained motion of the ankle joint, tensile properties of ankle articular cartilage, the metabolic characteristics of ankle joint articular cartilage, or a combination of these factors. The thinness of ankle articular cartilage and the small contact area leading to high peak-contact stresses may make the joint more susceptible to posttraumatic osteoarthritis. In particular, the thin-

ner, stiffer articular cartilage of the ankle may be less able to adapt to articular surface incongruity and increased contact stresses than the thicker articular cartilage of the hip and knee, and the contact stresses may be higher in the ankle.

Joint injuries can cause articular cartilage and subchondral bone damage that is not repaired, create articular surface incongruencies, and decrease joint stability. Long-term incongruency or instability can increase localized contact stress. The ankle osteoarthritis that occurs following joint injuries appears to follow a pattern consistent with the hypothesis that posttraumatic ankle osteoarthritis is a result of elevated contact stress that exceeds the capacity of the joint to repair itself or adapt. According to this hypothesis, the development of posttraumatic ankle osteoarthritis progresses through 3 overlapping stages: (1) articular cartilage injury, (2) chondrocyte response to tissue injury, and (3) decline in the chondrocyte response (Outline 1).

Neuropathies and necrosis of the talus that cause incongruity of the articular surface also lead to secondary ankle osteoarthritis. Patients with neuropathies can develop rapidly progressive joint degeneration following minimal injury or in the absence of a history of an injury. This may occur because the loss of positional sense leads to undetected ligamentous or articular surface injuries that create localized regions of increased contact stress. Articular surface incongruency caused by necrosis of the talus may have the same effect.

Consistent with the hypothesis that excessive contact stress leads to degeneration of ankle articular cartilage, significant residual joint incongruity and severe disruption of the ankle joint articular surface predictably lead to joint degeneration, commonly within 2 years of injury

(Fig. 6); but advanced joint degeneration also can develop within 2 years of injuries that cause relatively little apparent damage to the articular surface (Fig. 7). In some of these latter cases the joint surface many have sustained damage that is not apparent by radiographic evaluation. In others, joint instability caused by alteration of the anatomy of the mortise, like spreading of the distal tibiofibular syndesmosis or shortening and rotation of the fibula or capsular and ligamentous laxity, may be responsible for degeneration of the joint. However, some patients develop progressive joint degeneration following ankle injuries in the absence of apparent articular surface damage, alteration of the joint anatomy, or instability, and other patients with articular surface incongruity or joint instability do not develop progressive joint degeneration. Thus, the pathogenesis of posttraumatic ankle osteoarthritis is more complex than it appears, and needs extensive further study.

Effects of Decreased Joint Contact Stress on Ankle Osteoarthritis

A variety of treatments of ankle osteoarthritis, including weight reduction, shoe modifications, orthoses, joint distraction, osteotomies, and procedures intended to restore ligamentous stability, have been based on the assumptions that these treatments redistribute or decrease articular surface contact stresses and that decreasing or redistributing stress will decrease symptoms. Some authors have also suggested that decreasing joint contact stress may slow the progression of articular cartilage degeneration and possibly stimulate restoration of some form of articular surface. Several sets of experimental and clinical observations support these assumptions.

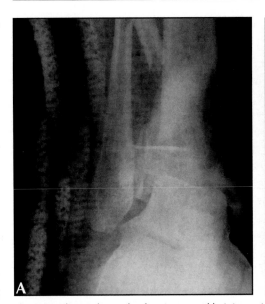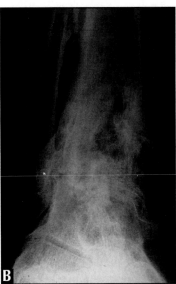

Fig. 6 Standing radiographs showing an ankle injury with extensive damage to the tibial articular surface. **A,** Anteroposterior radiograph showing almost complete disruption of the tibial articular surface and a fibula fracture immediately after the injury. **B,** Anteroposterior radiograph showing complete loss of articular cartilage less than 2 years after the injury.

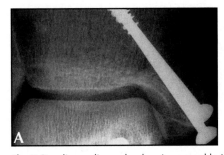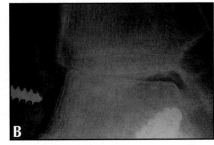

Fig. 7 Standing radiographs showing an ankle injury with relatively minor apparent damage to the tibial articular surface. **A,** Anteroposterior radiograph showing a medial malleolar fracture with minimal involvement of the tibial articular surface. The patient also had a fibula fracture and a talus fracture. The injuries were treated by internal fixation. **B,** Anteroposterior radiograph showing loss of articular cartilage less than 2 years after the injury.

Joint Distraction

Limited experimental studies indicate that joint distraction with external fixation devices promotes formation of a new articular surface.[40,41] Clinical studies of the effects of distraction of arthritic ankle joints using external fixators also suggest that decreasing joint contact stress can decrease symptoms and stimulate formation of a new articular surface.[42-44] In 1978, Judet and Judet[44] reported the results

of treating 16 patients with advanced ankle osteoarthritis by distraction and motion of the joint. They distracted the joints 4 to 8 mm while allowing motion for 6 to 12 weeks. Eight of their patients regained the ability to walk for unlimited distances and 13 of their patients had symptomatic improvement. More recently, van Valburg and associates[43] treated advanced posttraumatic osteoarthritis of the ankle with joint distraction in 11 patients. After application of an Ilizarov device, the authors distracted the joints 0.5 mm per day for 5 days and then maintained the distraction of the articular surfaces throughout the course of treatment. Patients were allowed to walk a few days after surgery, active joint motion was started between 6 and 12 weeks after surgery, and after 12 to 22 weeks the distraction device was removed. At an average of 20 months after treatment none of the patients had proceeded with an arthrodesis: all 11 patients had less pain, and 5 were pain free; 6 had more motion; and, 3 of 6 that had radiographic studies had increased joint space. The authors concluded that distraction of an osteoarthritic ankle joint delays arthrodesis, and that it may stimulate repair of osteoarthritic cartilage.

Osteotomies

Osteotomies of osteoarthritic hips and knees have been shown to decrease symptoms and stimulate formation of a new articular surface in some patients.[2] Osteotomies have not been widely used for the treatment of primary or posttraumatic ankle osteoarthritis, but in 1 study tibial osteotomies produced good or excellent results in 15 of 18 patients with primary ankle osteoarthritis.[45] Another report described significant improvement in ankle function and decreased pain in 8 patients with ankle osteoarthritis treated by tibial osteotomy.[46] The authors attributed the functional and symptomatic improvement to redistribution of pressure on the joint surface.

Ligament Reconstruction

Some patients with instability of the ankle due to laxity of the lateral ligaments develop osteoarthritis in the medial compartment of the joint,[31,33,35,47] possibly as a result of increased loading of the medial joint.[31,48] Harrington[31] studied 36 patients with a history of lateral ankle instability for more than 10 years. These patients had increasing ankle pain and radiographic evidence of degeneration of the medial joint compartment. In addition to demonstrating an association between chronic lateral ligamentous instability and development of medial compartment degeneration, he found that 14 of 22 ankles in patients with symptomatic ankle osteoarthritis had decreased symptoms and widening of the medial joint space following lateral ligament reconstruction. He concluded that restoration of lateral ligamentous stability has the potential to prevent progression of joint degeneration and, in selected patients, may reverse some of the degenerative changes.

Conclusion

The available evidence strongly suggests that ankle osteoarthritis has distinctive characteristics. This condition is less well understood and has been less thoroughly investigated than osteoarthritis of the knee, hip, and shoulder. Autopsy studies and clinical experience show that primary ankle degeneration and osteoarthritis occur less frequently than primary joint degeneration and osteoarthritis in other joints of the lower limb, including the knee. The reasons for this have not been clearly demonstrated, but relatively greater tensile strength of ankle articular cartilage in people of middle age and older may be partially responsible. Differences in articular cartilage metabolism may also contribute to the decreased susceptibility of the ankle for development of primary osteoarthritis. Perhaps because of the relative rarity of primary ankle osteoarthritis, a high proportion of the patients with ankle osteoarthritis have a history of ankle joint injuries including fractures, dislocations, or subluxations associated with fractures and capsular and ligamentous injuries. In these patients, the development of joint degeneration appears to result from increased joint contact stress that exceeds the capacity of the joint to repair itself or adapt to higher stress levels. The thinness of ankle articular cartilage and the small contact area of the ankle joint articular surfaces may increase the susceptibility of the joint to posttraumatic osteoarthritis. Other experimental and clinical evidence demonstrates that redistributing or decreasing joint contact stress has the potential to decrease symptoms of ankle osteoarthritis and, possibly, in some instances, restore a functional articular surface. These observations are necessarily speculative as a result of the lack of extensive study of ankle osteoarthritis. Nonetheless, they strongly suggest that ankle osteoarthritis has distinctive characteristics that need further investigation and that should guide treatment of this condition.

References

1. Buckwalter JA, Martin JA: Degenerative joint disease. *Clin Symp* 1995;47:1–32.

2. Buckwalter JA, Mankin HJ: Articular cartilage: Part II. Degeneration and osteoarthrosis, repair, regeneration, and transplantation. *J Bone Joint Surg* 1997;79A:612–632.

3. Praemer A, Furner S, Rice DP (eds): *Musculoskeletal Conditions in the United States*. Park Ridge, IL, American Academy of Orthopaedic Surgeons, 1992.

4. Buckwalter JA, Woo SL, Goldberg VM, et al: Soft-tissue aging and musculoskeletal function. *J Bone Joint Surg* 1993;75A:1533–1548.

5. Buckwalter JA, Mankin HJ: Articular cartilage: Part I. Tissue design and chondrocyte-matrix interactions. *J Bone Joint Surg* 1997;79A:600–611.

6. Newton PM, Mow VC, Gardner TR, Buckwalter JA, Albright JP: The effect of lifelong exercise on canine articular cartilage. *Am J Sports Med* 1997;25:282–287.

7. Beaudoin AJ, Fiore SM, Krause WR, Adelaar RS: Effect of isolated talocalcaneal fusion on contact in the ankle and talonavicular joints. *Foot Ankle* 1991;12:19–25.

8. Kimizuka M, Kurosawa H, Fukubayashi T: Load-bearing pattern of the ankle joint: Contact area and pressure distribution. *Arch Orthop Trauma Surg* 1980;96:45–49.

9. Ihn JC, Kim SJ, Park IH: In vitro study of contact area and pressure distribution in the human knee after partial and total meniscectomy. *Int Orthop* 1993;17:214–218.

10. Brown TD, Shaw DT: In vitro contact stress distributions in the natural human hip. *J Biomech* 1983;16:373–384.

11. Schenck RC Jr, Athanasiou KA: Biomechanical topography of human ankle cartilage. *Trans Ors* 1993;18:279.

12. Athanasiou KA, Niederauer GG, Schenck RC Jr: Biomechanical topography of human ankle cartilage. *Ann Biomed Eng* 1995;23:697–704.

13. Ateshian GA, Soslowsky U, Mow VC: Quantitation of articular surface topography and cartilage thickness in knee joints using stereophotogrammetry. *J Biomech* 1991;24:761–776.

14. Kempson GE: Age-related changes in the tensile properties of human articular cartilage: A comparative study between the femoral head of the hip joint and the talus of the ankle joint. *Biochim Biophys Acta* 1991;1075:223–230.

15. Chubinskaya S, Huch K, Mikecz K, et al: Chondrocyte matrix metalloproteinase-8: Up-regulation of neutrophil collagenase by interleukin-I beta in human cartilage from knee and ankle joints. *Lab Invest* 1996;74:232–240.

16. Häuselmann HJ, Flechtenmacher J, Gitelis SH, Kuettner KE, Aydelotte MB: Chondrocytes from human knee and ankle joints show differences in response to IL-1 and IL-1 receptor inhibitor. *Orthop Trans* 1993;17:710.

17. Huch K, Kuettner KE, Dieppe P: Osteoarthritis in ankle and knee joints. *Semin Arthritis Rheum* 1997;26:667–674.

18. Dieppe PA, Cushnaghan J, Shepstone L: The Bristol "OA500" study: Progression of osteoarthritis (OA) over 3 years and the relationship between clinical and radiographic changes at the knee joint. *Osteoarthritis Cartilage* 1997;5:87–97.

19. van-der-Schoot DK, Den Outer AJ, Bode PJ, Obermann WR, van Vugt AB: Degenerative changes at the knee and ankle related to malunion of tibial fractures: 15-year follow-up of 88 patients. *J Bone Joint Surg* 1996;78B:722–725.

20. Meachim G, Emery IH: Cartilage fibrillation in shoulder and hip joints in Liverpool necropsies. *J Anat* 1973;116:161–179.

21. Meachim G, Emery IH: Quantitative aspects of patello-femoral cartilage fibrillation in Liverpool necropsies. *Ann Rheum Dis* 1974;33:39–47.

22. Meachim G: Cartilage fibrillation at the ankle joint in Liverpool necropsies. *J Anat* 1975; 119:601–610.

23. Meachim G: Cartilage fibrillation on the lateral tibial plateau in Liverpool necropsies. *J Anat* 1976;121:97–106.

24. Collins DH (ed): *Osteoarthritis: The Pathology of Articular and Spinal Diseases*. London, England, Edward Arnold, 1949, pp 74–115.

25. Muehleman C, Bareither D, Huch K, Cole AA, Kuettner KE: Prevalence of degenerative morphological changes in the joints of the lower extremity. *Osteoarthritis Cartilage* 1997;5:23–37.

26. Cushnaghan J, Dieppe P: Study of 500 patients with limb joint osteoarthritis: I. Analysis by age, sex, and distribution of symptomatic joint sites. *Ann Rheum Dis* 1991;50:8–13.

27. Peyron JG: The epidemiology of osteoarthritis, in Moskowitz RW, Howell DS, Goldberg VM, Mankin HJ (eds): *Osteoarthritis: Diagnosis and Management*. Philadelphia, PA, WB Saunders, 1984, pp 9–27.

28. Wilson MG, Michet CJ Jr, Ilstrup DM, Melton LJ III: Idiopathic symptomatic osteoarthritis of the hip and knee: A population-based incidence study. *Mayo Clin Proc* 1990;65:1214–1221.

29. Demetriades L, Strauss E, Gallina J: Osteoarthritis of the ankle. *Clin Orthop* 1998;349: 28–42.

30. Wyss C, Zollinger H: The causes of subsequent arthrodesis of the ankle joint. *Acta Orthop Belg* 1991;57(suppl 1):22–27.

31. Harrington KD: Degenerative arthritis of the ankle secondary to long-standing lateral ligament instability. *J Bone Joint Surg* 1979;61A: 354–361.

32. Inokuchi S, Ogawa K, Usami N, Hashimoto T: Long-term follow up of talus fractures. *Orthopedics* 1996;19:477–481.

33. Schafer D, Hintermann B: Arthroscopic assessment of the chronic unstable ankle joint. *Knee Surg Sports Traumatol Arthrosc* 1996;4:48–52.

34. Taga I, Shino K, Inoue M, Nakata K, Maeda A: Articular cartilage lesions in ankles with lateral ligament injury: An arthroscopic study. *Am J Sports Med* 1993;21:120–126.

35. Rieck B, Reiser M, Bernett P: Post-traumatic arthrosis of the upper ankle joint in chronic insufficiency of the fibular ligament [German]. *Orthopade* 1986;15:466–471.

36. Leeds HC, Ehrlich MG: Instability of the distal tibiofibular syndesmosis after bimalleolar and trimalleolar ankle fractures. *J Bone Joint Surg* 1984;66A:490–503.

37. Slowman-Kovacs SD, Braunstein EM, Brandt KD: Rapidly progressive Charcot arthropathy following minor joint trauma in patients with diabetic neuropathy. *Arthritis Rheum* 1990; 33:412–417.

38. Cheng YM, Lin SY, Tien YC, Wu HS: Ankle arthrodesis. *Kao Hsiung I Hsueh Ko Hsueh Tsa Chih* 1993;9:524–531.

39. Buechel FF, Pappas MJ, Lorio LJ: New Jersey low contact stress total ankle replacement: Biomechanical rationale and review of 23 cementless cases. *Foot Ankle* 1988;8:279–290.

40. Krogsgaard MR, Blyme P: Formation of joint surfaces by traction. *Acta Orthop Scand* 1997; (suppl 274):46.

41. Van Valburg AA, Van Roermund PM, Van Roy HLAM, Verbout AJ, Lafeber FPJG, Bijlsma JWJ: Repair of cartilage by joint distraction, tested in the Pond-Nuki model for osteoarthritis. *Trans Orthop Res Soc* 1997;22:494.

42. Van Valburg AA, Van Roermund PM, Larnmens J: Promising results of Ilizarov joint distraction in the treatment of ankle osteoarthritis. *Trans Orthop Res Soc* 1997;22:271.

43. Van Valburg AA, Van Roermund PM, Lammens J, et al: Can Ilizarov joint distraction delay the need for an arthrodesis of the ankle? A preliminary report. *J Bone Joint Surg* 1995; 77B:720–725.

44. Judet R, Judet T: The use of a hinge distraction apparatus after arthrolysis and arthroplasty. *Rev Chir Orthop* 1978;64:353–365.

45. Takakura Y, Tanaka Y, Kumai T, Tamai S: Low tibial osteotomy for osteoarthritis of the ankle: Results of a new operation in 18 patients. *J Bone Joint Surg* 1995;77B:50–54.

46. Cheng YM, Chang JK, Hsu CY, Huang SD, Lin SY: Lower tibial osteotomy for osteoarthritis of the ankle. *Kao Hsiung I Hsueh Ko Hsueh Tsa Chih* 1994;10:430–437.

47. Lofvenberg R, Karrholm J, Lund B: The outcome of nonoperated patients with chronic lateral instability of the ankle: A 20-year follow-up study. *Foot Ankle Int* 1994;15:165–169.

48. Noguchi K: Biomechanical analysis for osteoarthritis of the ankle. *Nippon Seikeigeka Gakkai Zasshi* 1985;59:215–222.

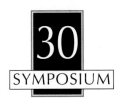

Arthroscopic Ankle Debridement and Fusion: Indications, Techniques, and Results

Timothy C. Fitzgibbons, MD

Introduction

Arthroscopy of the ankle is a commonly performed and accepted procedure for many of the afflictions that affect the ankle joint. The role of arthroscopy in patients with osteoarthritis of the ankle, however, is still in question. The purpose of this chapter is to discuss the role of arthroscopy in the treatment of arthritis of the ankle and, specifically, to discuss ankle debridement and arthroscopic ankle arthrodesis. This chapter is divided into two sections. The first section discusses general arthroscopic ankle debridement. It covers the specific entities of loose bodies, chondral lesions, and anterior ankle bony impingement. The second half of the chapter discusses arthroscopic ankle arthrodesis, with specific emphasis on the surgical technique that I use.

Arthroscopy of the Ankle: General Technique Principles

It is not the purpose of this chapter to discuss how to perform an arthroscopy of the ankle. However, I think it is important to mention briefly the general equipment and techniques used for the specific problems that have to do with arthritis of the ankle. This is especially important in arthroscopic ankle fusion. I refer the

readers to the discussion by Richard Ferkel for more specific details regarding arthroscopy of the ankle.[1]

It is my policy at the present time to perform arthroscopy of the ankle in a regular operating room on a regular operating room table, using a 2.7-mm 30° arthroscope. Small and large shaving systems are used, depending on the specific procedure. At the present time, distraction, either skeletal or soft tissue, is used only occasionally. Although a tourniquet is applied, it is used only when indicated. All patients are routinely injected with 0.25% Marcaine with epinephrine prior to the procedure for hemostasis and postoperative pain control. At the present time, the anteromedial and anterolateral portals are used 90% of the time.

Incisions are made with a #15 blade, not a #11 blade. Small hemostats are used to carefully dissect the skin and subcutaneous tissue and to spread the tissues down to the capsule to avoid injuries to the small sensory nerves. In the anterolateral portal the branches of the superficial peroneal nerve are in jeopardy. On the anteromedial portal the branches of the saphenous nerve are in jeopardy. Even with this careful dissection, however, all patients should be warned that they still may end up

with some temporary or permanent paresthesias that are unavoidable.

A recent article by Feiwell and Frey[2] noted how the various combinations of the anteromedial, anterolateral, and posterolateral portals allowed essentially complete access to all surfaces of the ankle joint. Therefore, we can state that "we have the technology but is it the prudent thing to do?"

Arthroscopic Ankle Debridement for Degenerative Joint Disease

Arthroscopic ankle debridement has paralleled the experience noted with arthroscopic debridement for other joints. As with other joints, there was an initial enthusiasm that arthroscopic debridement would be efficacious, only to find later that the long-term results were not acceptable. If one reviews the literature, the general consensus has normally been that patients with severe degenerative arthritis do not do well with arthroscopic debridement.[3–10] The general feeling has been that specific pathologic entities such as loose bodies, chondromalacia, and osteophytes, however, might occasionally be treatable in some patients with degenerative arthritis. A recent article by van Dijk and Scholte[11] concluded that arthroscopic surgery of the ankle joint was a successful procedure in the treatment

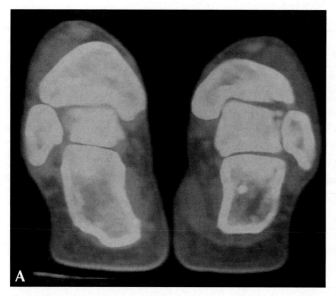 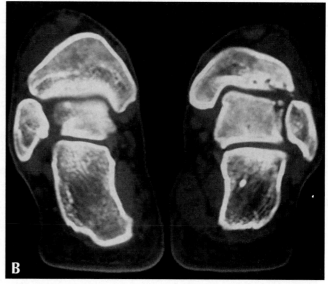

Fig 1 A, Computed tomography (CT) scan of patient with typical osteochondritis dissecans lesion. **B,** CT scan of patient with osteochondral defects involving both tibia and talus; prognosis much more severe than typical osteochondritis dissecans.

of impingement lesions, osteochondral defects, and removal of loose bodies. If this article is read critically, it does not appear that many of these patients had any evidence of severe degenerative arthritis. Amendola and associates[12] recently reported their experience with ankle arthroscopy in 79 patients. Their conclusion was that patients with degenerative joint disease (DJD), posttraumatic chondromalacia, or arthrofibrosis, and patients on workers' compensation did not do well with arthroscopic ankle debridement. In 1992, I reviewed my experience with ankle arthroscopy.[13] This retrospective study of 47 patients over an 8-year period revealed 16 patients with DJD, 14 patients with anterior tibial spurring, 7 patients with loose bodies, and 10 patients with so-called osteochondral lesions. The results showed that patients with degenerative changes uniformly did poorly after arthroscopic debridement. Patients with loose bodies without significant DJD did well. Patients with osteochondral lesions and anterior spurs with associated degenerative

arthritis did not do well.

The consensus in the literature today seems to be that arthroscopic ankle debridement for DJD is probably only appropriate in selective cases.

Loose Bodies

As noted above, my experience in the 1992 study was that essentially all patients with isolated loose bodies in the ankle had good to excellent results from arthroscopic removal of the loose body. However, those patients with degenerative arthritis and removal of loose body did not do well. I feel that this experience is consistent with the experience at other centers and therefore the consensus now appears to be that in those patients with significant degenerative arthritis of the ankle, arthroscopic debridement of the ankle and removal of loose bodies does not render any form of long-term satisfaction.

Osteochondral Defects

For purposes of this chapter the definition of an osteochondral defect associated with degenerative arthritis

of the ankle is that of articular cartilage loss on either the talus or tibia, with exposed eburnated bone. This must be differentiated from osteochondritis dissecans (osteochondral talar dome fracture), which is not a form of degenerative arthritis of the ankle and should not be considered in the discussion of arthroscopic debridement for ankle arthritis. Figure 1 shows the difference between the computed tomography (CT) scan of a patient with osteochondritis dissecans and a CT scan of a patient with an osteochondral defect involving both the talus and the tibia. The lesion associated with changes on both sides of the joint simply will not have the same prognosis as the osteochondritis dissecans lesion.

Treatment of osteochondral defects of the ankle has basically followed the guidelines for arthroscopic debridement for osteochondritis dissecans. The first stage is to debride all loose articular cartilage down to bleeding bone. It is important to note that all articular cartilage that remains is adherent to the deep bone. After the debridement, the base of the defect is drilled, either with multiple Kirschner wire insertions or, recently, the use of the microfracture technique. These patients are then kept nonweightbearing for as long as 8 weeks. A possible evolving treatment for osteochondral lesions of the ankle is that of "mosaicplasty."[14,15] This procedure involves the harvesting of osteocartilaginous plugs from the nonweightbearing aspects of the femoral condyle. These plugs are then transplanted into the area of the osteochondral defect. A recent report by Hangody and associates[15] reported on 11 cases in which this was performed in the ankle joint. It appeared, however, that these cases were all patients with osteochondritis dissecans. There is concern that the biochemical changes in the joint with osteoarthritis may affect the efficacy of this procedure.[16] It is also questionable whether this procedure can be performed arthroscopically, and more clinical experience is necessary before this can be advocated.

At the present time, I feel that arthroscopic debridement of osteochondral lesions in patients with severe degenerative arthritis probably will not effect the overall outcome. Only in those patients with isolated lesions and otherwise normal cartilage does it seem to make sense to consider this procedure.

Anterior Tibial Talar Spurs

In 1992, Scranton and McDermott[17] published an article comparing open versus arthroscopic debridement of anterior tibial talar impingement spurs. In that article they divided anterior impingement into 4 types, ranging from synovial impingement to anterior spurs in combination with severe DJD. It was their recommendation that those grade 4 patients with significant degenerative arthritis

should not have arthroscopic debridement but rather should have open debridement of the spurs. A review of the article raises questions as to whether even with open debridement these patients had much improvement. Three relatively recent articles describing the arthroscopic approach to anterior impingement have advocated this as a satisfactory procedure.[18–20] However, if one looks at these articles critically, all of these patients were young athletes and did not appear to have significant arthritis. A 1997 article by van Dijk and associates[21] further divided those patients with anterior impingement into those that had osteoarthritis. The types were graded from 0, which was a normal joint, to type 3, complete loss of joint space. Their conclusion was that those patients with loss of joint space and more degenerative arthritis simply did not do well with anterior tibial spur removal.

The arthroscopic approach to anterior spur removal has been well described.[1] It is important that a shaver be used initially to peel off the capsule from the anterior osteophyte. Subsequent to that the abrader can be inserted and the spur can be removed. If the capsule is not removed adequately then the spur is normally not adequately removed arthroscopically.

The consensus is that if significant joint space narrowing is present and significant DJD is present, then arthroscopic anterior spur debridement is probably not indicated.

Arthroscopic Ankle Arthrodesis

Arthroscopic ankle arthrodesis is a well-described procedure for the treatment of multiple forms of arthritis of the ankle.[22–33] Starting with Schneider's description of one case carrying through the mid 1990s, all authors have concluded that there is certainly an indication for arthro-

scopic ankle fusion. In the first 10 years, the consensus in the literature seemed to be that fusion rates were comparable to those achieved with open techniques. All authors felt that this was an in situ fusion and that no significant correction was possible. All authors seemed to emphasize the technical difficulty of the procedure and the steep learning curve. Most authors used skeletal or soft-tissue distraction. This procedure seemed indicated only in selective cases.

My experience began in 1989. Prior to that, the open technique was advocated by the late Kenneth Johnson, using the external Calandruccio clamp. I had been discouraged with the nonfusion rate and difficulty with alignment of the hindfoot due to gross instability produced by bone resection. The experience of this community has been described in the literature.[34,35] The initial arthroscopic technique used by the Creighton University/University of Nebraska Medical Center group was with external distraction. Although the initial arthrodesis rate was 93%, the overall complication rate was 55%. Almost all the complications that occurred were related in some way to the skeletal distraction pins. For that reason, from 1994 on, no skeletal distraction has been used. The arthrodesis rate at the most recent review was 93.3% and the complication rate has decreased dramatically. A recent classic "state of the art" article by Glick and associates[36] revealed a 97% fusion rate and an average time to fusion of 9 weeks. This was a multicenter study, which I believe demonstrates the success of arthroscopic ankle arthrodesis.

Another recent interesting article by Paremain and associates[37] described an ankle arthrodesis using "a mini arthrotomy technique." There is no question that the arthroscopic

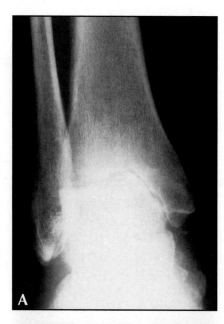

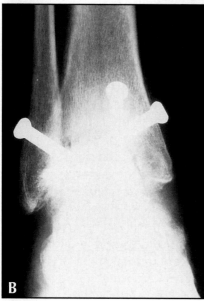

Fig. 2 A, Preoperative radiograph with notable talar tilt. **B,** Postoperative radiograph after arthroscopic fusion, note reasonably normal clinical alignment.

<table>
<tr><td>

Outline 1

Techniques for arthroscopic ankle arthrodesis

Operating room set up and equipment

Regular operating room and operating room table

    Supine position with bump under affected hip

    No distraction

    Hip/iliac crest prepped

    2.7-mm 30° arthroscope used (Fig. 3)

    Irrigation pump

    Tourniquet rarely used

    Preoperative injection with 0.25% Marcaine with epinephrine

    Curettes, pituitary rongeur, 5.0 full radius resectors and burrs used

Injections, incisions, and scope insertion

    Basically the same as for a routine arthroscopy of the ankle

    Standard anterolateral and anteromedial portals

    15-gauge scalpel with hemostat spreading of soft tissues to avoid injury to cutaneous nerves (Fig. 4)

Surgical technique

    Step 1: Initial arthroscopic soft-tissue resection

        Tedious and time consuming, but necessary

        Use full radius resector and pituitary rongeur

    Step 2: Removal of articular cartilage

        Under direct visualization remove articular cartilage with curettes, full radius resector, and burrs (Fig. 5)

        Important to remove articular cartilage from both gutters

    Step 3: Final feathering of the joint

        Most important part of procedure in my opinion

        We use small osteotome but burrs also acceptable (Fig. 6)

    Step 4: Bone marrow aspiration

        Demineralized bone matrix mixture (DBM) and injection of bone graft

        15 cc of bone marrow and 5 cc aliquots obtained with 11 gauge bone marrow aspiration needle and mixed with DBM and injected into ankle (Fig. 7)

    Step 5: Insertion of internal fixation

        Foot of bed dropped 90°, affected foot placed on padded Mayo stand, fluoroscopy utilized (Fig. 8)

        Technique of Hansen-Sangeorzan with 3 screws, (especially important "home run screw" 7.3-mm self-drilling self-tapping partially threaded cannulated AO screw is used) (Figs. 9 and 10)

    Step 6: Closure and postoperative care

        Robert Jones dressing with AO splints for 48 to 72 hours

        Short leg nonweightbearing fiberglass cast for 4 weeks

        Short leg fiberglass weightbearing cast for 4 weeks

        Weightbearing removable short leg brace for 4 weeks

</td></tr>
</table>

ankle arthrodesis at times, towards the end of the procedure, can become a "semi-open" technique. However, it is my opinion that there is no substitute for arthroscopic visualization of the entire joint.

The advantages to arthroscopic ankle fusion are that no gross insta-bility is produced at the ankle joint with removal of the articular cartilage, which makes it easier to maintain normal alignment. There is also no question that the patients have less pain and morbidity. Only if one has experienced how well these patients do postoperatively does one really appreciate how much less morbid this is to the patients. Now with equal or better fusion rates and few complications, the popularity of arthroscopic ankle fusion has increased. The disadvantages are that there is a moderately steep learning curve. Also, there is still no way to correct gross malalignment.

The specific indications for arthroscopic ankle fusion appear to be degenerative and rheumatoid arthritis. However, other forms of arthritis of the ankle can be approached arthroscopically. It is important that there be a reasonably normal alignment of the hindfoot, although some varus or valgus tilting can be excepted. Figure 2 shows notable tilting of the tibial talar joint, which in past years may have been construed as unacceptable for arthroscopic fusion. However, the patient had a clinically normally aligned hindfoot and the tibial talar tilting was simply caused by articular cartilage loss. Removal of the more normal articular cartilage allowed satisfactory realignment and a satisfactory arthroscopic arthrodesis was performed.

The important point here is that if the patient has reasonably normal clinical alignment, I do not consider tilting of the tibial talar joint to be a contraindication for arthroscopic ankle fusion. Contraindications for arthroscopic ankle fusion would be Charcot arthropathy and active infection.

Author's Technique for Arthroscopic Ankle Arthrodesis

The technique described in Outline 1 and Figures 3 through 10 is an evolution of a surgical technique first developed by Dr. Lynn Crosby and myself. Although our initial techniques were similar, they were not performed exactly the same. Since the initial days, this technique has been modified multiple times. The technique described represents modifications made by both of us and also by Dr. Scott McMullen. It should be noted that a description of the screw insertion technique has been published.[38]

Summary

The use of the arthroscope in arthritis of the ankle has been well described and there is no question that it is a significant part of the armamentarium for the orthopaedic surgeon dealing with these patients. Unfortunately, those patients with advanced arthritis and loss of joint space do not respond well to traditional arthroscopic debridement, removal of loose bodies, debridement and drilling of osteochondral lesions, and removal of anterior osteophytes. These pro-

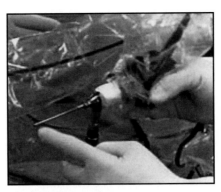

Fig. 3 2.7-mm 30° arthroscope.

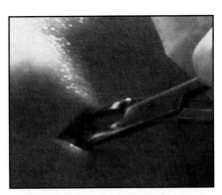

Fig. 4 15-gauge scalpel with hemostat spreading of soft tissues.

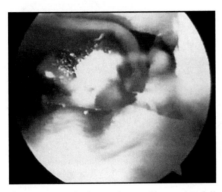

Fig. 5 Removal of articular cartilage using full radius resector.

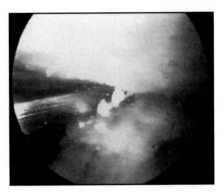

Fig. 6 Final feathering of distal tibia with arthroscopic use of osteotome.

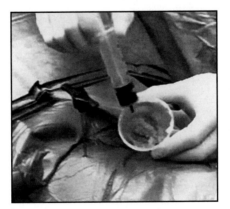

Fig. 7 Aspiration of bone marrow from iliac crest and mixing with demineralized bone matrix.

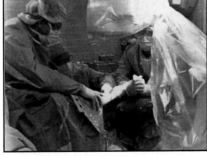

Fig. 8 Foot of bed dropped 90° with the foot on Mayo stand.

cedures should only be used on those patients with minimal to no degenerative arthritis. Arthroscopic ankle arthrodesis is becoming more of the accepted primary procedure for most cases of arthritis of the ankle, in my opinion. Some varus or valgus tilting of the tibial talar joint can be accepted if clinical alignment is relatively normal. Significant malalignments cannot be corrected with arthroscopic fusion.

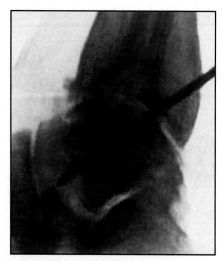

Fig. 9 Insertion of guide pin for "home run" screw, through posterior tibia down neck of talus.

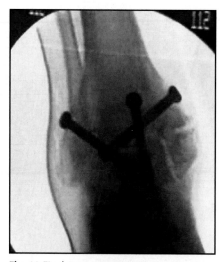

Fig. 10 Final 3-screw construct.

References

1. Ferkel RD, Whipple TL (eds): *Arthroscopic Surgery: The Foot & The Ankle*. Philadelphia, PA, Lippincott-Raven, 1996.

2. Feiwell LA, Frey C: Anatomic study of arthroscopic debridement of the ankle. *Foot Ankle Int* 1994;15:614–621.

3. Martin DF, Baker CL, Curl WW, Andrews JR, Robie DB, Haas AF: Operative ankle arthroscopy: Long-term follow-up. *Am J Sports Med* 1989;17:16–23.

4. Ferkel RD, Fischer SP: Progress in ankle arthroscopy. *Clin Orthop* 1989;240:210–220.

5. Biedert R: Anterior ankle pain in sports medicine: Aetiology and indications for arthroscopy. *Arch Orthop Trauma Surg* 1991;110:293–297.

6. Demaziere A, Ogilvie-Harris DJ: Operative arthroscopy of the ankle: 107 cases. *Rev Rhum Mal Osteoartic* 1991;58:93–97.

7. Feder KS, Schonholtz GJ: Ankle arthroscopy: Review and long-term results. *Foot Ankle* 1992;13:382–385.

8. Jerosch J, Schneider T, Strauss JM, Schurmann N: Arthroscopy of the upper ankle joint: List of indications from the literature: Realistic expectations, complications. *Unfallchirurg* 1993;96:82–87.

9. Loong TW, Mitra AK, Tan SK: Role of arthroscopy in ankle disorder: Early experience. *Ann Acad Med Singapore* 1994;23:348–350.

10. Ogilvie-Harris DJ, Sekyi-Otu A: Arthroscopic debridement for the osteoarthritic ankle. *Arthroscopy* 1995;11:433–436.

11. van Dijk CN, Scholte D: Arthroscopy of the ankle joint. *Arthroscopy* 1997;13:90–96.

12. Amendola A, Petrik J, Webster-Bogaert S: Ankle arthroscopy: Outcome in 79 consecutive patients. *Arthroscopy* 1996;12:565–573.

13. Miller BH, Fitzgibbons TC: Abstract: Arthroscopy of the ankle joint: Is it truly useful? *Foot Ankle* 1992;13:296.

14. Hangody L, Kish G, Karpati Z, Szerb I, Udvarhelyi I: Arthroscopic autogenous osteochondral mosaicplasty for the treatment of femoral condylar articular defects: A preliminary report. *Knee Surg Sports Traumatol Arthrosc* 1997;5:262–267.

15. Hangody L, Kish G, Karpati Z, Szerb I, Eberhardt R: Treatment of osteochondritis dissecans of the talus: Use of the mosaicplasty technique. A preliminary report. *Foot Ankle Int* 1997;18:628–634.

16. Minas T, Nehrer S: Current concepts in the treatment of articular cartilage defects. *Orthopedics* 1997;20:525–538.

17. Scranton PE Jr, McDermott JE: Anterior tibiotalar spurs: A comparison of open versus arthroscopic debridement. *Foot Ankle Int* 1992;13:125–129.

18. Ogilvie-Harris DJ, Mahomed N, Demaziere A: Anterior impingement of the ankle treated by arthroscopic removal of bony spurs. *J Bone Joint Surg* 1993;75B:437–440.

19. Reynaert P, Gelen G, Greens G: Abstract: Arthroscopic treatment of anterior impingement of the ankle. *Foot Ankle Int* 1996;17:129.

20. van Dijk CN, Verhagen RA, Tol JL: Arthroscopy for problems after ankle fracture. *J Bone Joint Surg* 1997;79B:280–284.

21. van Dijk CN, Tol JL, Verheyen CC: A prospective study of prognostic factors concerning the outcome of arthroscopic surgery for anterior ankle impingement. *Am J Sports Med* 1997;25:737–745.

22. Schneider D: Arthroscopic ankle fusion. *Arth Video J* 1983;3.

23. Morgan CD: Arthroscopic tibiotalar arthrodesis, in McGinty JB, Caspari RB, Jackson RW, Poehling GG (eds): *Operative Arthroscopy*. New York, NY, Raven Press, 1991, pp 695–701.

24. Myerson MS, Allon SM: Arthroscopic ankle arthrodesis. *Contemp Orthop* 1989:19:21–27.

25. Myerson MS, Quill G: Ankle arthrodesis: A comparison of an arthroscopic and an open method of treatment. *Clin Orthop* 1991;268:84–95.

26. de Waal Malefijt MC, van Kampen A: Arthroscopic ankle arthrodesis: A new technique. *Ned Tijdschr Geneeskd* 1992;136:2585–2588.

27. Ogilvie-Harris DJ, Lieberman I, Fitsialos D: Arthroscopically assisted arthrodesis for osteoarthrotic ankles. *J Bone Joint Surg* 1993;75A:1167–1174.

28. Dent CM, Patil M, Fairclough JA: Arthroscopic ankle arthrodesis. *J Bone Joint Surg* 1993;75B:830–832.

29. Fleiss DJ: Letter: Arthroscopically assisted arthrodesis for osteoarthrotic ankles. *J Bone Joint Surg* 1994;76A:1112.

30. Bresler F, Mole D, Schmidt D: A tibiotalar arthrodesis under arthroscopy. *Rev Chir Orthop Reparatrice Appar Mot* 1994;80:744–748.

31. Bonnin M, Carret JP: Arthrodesis of the ankle under arthroscopy: Apropos of 10 cases reviewed after a year. *Rev Chir Orthop Reparatrice Appar Mot* 1995;81:128–135.

32. Corso SJ, Zimmer TJ: Technique and clinical evaluation of arthroscopic ankle arthrodesis. *Arthroscopy* 1995;11:585–590.

33. Turan I, Wredmark T, Fellander-Tsai L: Arthroscopic ankle arthrodesis in rheumatoid arthritis. *Clin Orthop* 1995;320:110–114.

34. Crosby LA, Formanek TS, Fitzgibbons TC: Arthroscopic ankle fusion utilizing demineralized bone matrix and bone marrow grafting. Proceedings of the American Academy of Orthopaedic Surgeons 59th Annual Meeting, Washington, DC. Park Ridge, IL, American Academy of Orthopaedic Surgeons, 1992, p 309.

35. Crosby LA, Yee TC, Formanek TS, Fitzgibbons TC: Complications following arthroscopic ankle arthrodesis. *Foot Ankle Int* 1996;17:340–342.

36. Glick JM, Morgan CD, Myerson MS, Sampson TG, Mann JA: Ankle arthrodesis using an arthroscopic method: Long-term follow-up of 34 cases. *Arthroscopy* 1996;12:428–434.

37. Paremain GD, Miller SD, Myerson MS: Ankle arthrodesis: Results after the miniarthrotomy technique. *Foot Ankle Int* 1996;17:247–252.

38. Holt ES, Hansen ST, Mayo KA, Sangeorzan BJ: Ankle arthrodesis using internal screw fixation. *Clin Orthop* 1991;268:21–28.

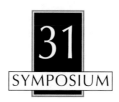

Joint Distraction as Treatment for Ankle Osteoarthritis

Peter M. van Roermund, PhD
Floris P.J.G. Lafeber, PhD

Osteoarthritis

The patient with ankle osteoarthritis has to cope with progressive pain, stiffness, and functional impairment. There is an ongoing deterioration of the joint cartilage due to rupture of the collagen network, loss of matrix molecules, mostly proteoglycans and collagen fragments, and, as a result, loss of the mechanical properties of the cartilage.[1] As a consequence of these mechanical and biochemical changes of the cartilage matrix, normal joint use will further increase cartilage damage. Chondrocytes sense these changes in the damaged matrix and will attempt to repair the matrix.[2] Finally, these chondrocytes lose their phenotype and dedifferentiate. They start to proliferate and produce inappropriate types of matrix molecules,[3] catabolic cytokines, and matrix proteases, damaging the cartilage further.[4] Bone is characteristically altered by sclerosis, and osteophytes are formed, possibly in an attempt to stabilize the joint, minimizing mechanical impact on the cartilage. Both for patient and physician the main question to be answered is: how can this process of progressive cartilage damage be stopped? How can a complete destruction of the joint be prevented? At present, severe osteoarthritis cannot be stopped. The only really effective procedures in treatment of

severely painful osteoarthritic ankle joints are ankle arthrodesis or arthroplasty. However, both of these procedures cause the patient to lose the joint. So the basic problem is that no proven effective remedy for osteoarthritis exists.

Attempts to treat osteoarthritis are numerous. Pain may be effectively treated with medication, possibly by suppression of mild secondary inflammation, which partly might delay destruction of articular cartilage.[5] Alternative nonmedicinal and noninvasive treatments, such as electromagnetic stimulation, acupuncture, diathermy, or yoga, may relieve pain but have never been proven to be effective in repair of joint destruction.[6,7] Much effort is put into the development of new modalities to treat moderate to severe cases of osteoarthritis. Only a limited number of reports on clinical application of these new approaches are available at present. In autologous chondrocyte transplantation,[8] healthy cartilage is taken from uninvolved areas of an injured joint during arthroscopy. Chondrocytes are isolated, cultured ex vivo, and then injected in the area of the defect. Results are not yet conclusive.[9] Further advances in the procedures of cell isolation, multiplication, and retransplantation will be required to improve the technique.

This technique may be specifically useful in repair of deep isolated cartilage defects, which are a precursor of osteoarthritis. Results of arthroscopic debridement of osteoarthritic joints, especially in the late stages of osteoarthritis, are reported to be unpredictable, and, if beneficial, lasting for an uncertain period of time. Laser-assisted arthroscopic debridement[10] is used to remove osteophytes, to reshape cartilage surface, and to remove inflamed synovial tissue. It has been suggested that this method offers an advantage over conventional debridement. However, further research is required to investigate possible adverse effects on articular chondrocytes, which may counteract the positive effects of laser debridement. Several clinical studies have evaluated the use of intra-articular injections of hyaluron,[11] a viscous substance important in joint lubrication. It may be questioned whether the minor effects justify serial intra-articular injections. Although this treatment is gaining acceptance for treatment of osteoarthritis, further evidence of efficacy and utility is required to determine whether hyaluron will become an established form of treatment. Osteochondral retransplantation[12] of intact tissue taken from nonweight-bearing areas to chondral defects seems promising judging from animal

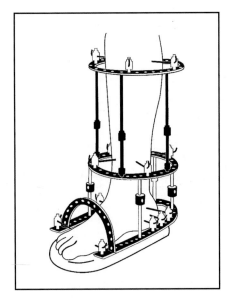

Fig. 1 Schematic drawing of the Ilizarov fixation used for ankle distraction.

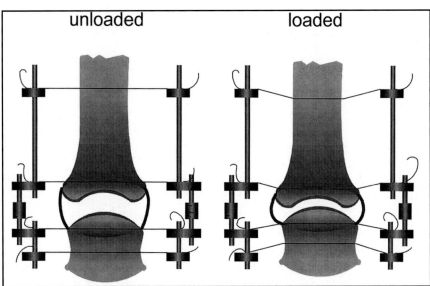

Fig. 2 Schematic depiction of the intra-articular intermittent fluid pressures during walking due to the axial flexibility in the Ilizarov external fixation.

studies, but clinical studies have still to be reported on.

Joint Distraction: A Relatively New Approach in the Treatment of Osteoarthritis

This technique is based on the hypothesis that osteoarthritic cartilage has some reparative activity if it is mechanically unloaded and if the intermittent synovial fluid flow and fluid pressure, essential for the nutrition of cartilage, is maintained. The aim is to achieve a temporary (about 3 months) release of mechanical stress on articular cartilage by a distraction of the articular surfaces combined with continuation of intra-articular intermittent fluid flow/fluid pressure (Fig. 1). This strategy was the basis for a study on the effects of joint distraction in treatment of severe ankle osteoarthritis, including the repair capacity of cartilage under these conditions, as reported by van Valburg.[13]

Apart from unloading the osteoarthritic cartilage, another characteristic of joint distraction is the maintenance of intra-articular intermittent fluid flow. Absence of mechanical contact between both degenerative articular surfaces is achieved by distraction of the joint by means of an external fixation frame. Intermittent fluid flow/fluid pressure can be maintained by the use of hinges in the distraction frame. Such an articulating distraction has been used for the osteoarthritic hip.[13] Intermittent intra-articular fluid flow can also be obtained by the use of an Ilizarov frame with thin (1.5 mm) Kirshner wires (K-wires), tensioned to external rings (Fig. 1). Loading and unloading of the joint in such a distraction frame will result in intermittent intra-articular fluid pressure/fluid flow due to the flexibility of the K-wires[14] (Fig. 2).

The Technique of Distraction

Distraction of the ankle joint is done by using Ilizarov ring fixation consisting of 2 rings around the leg, 1 half ring around the heel, and 2 long plates at both sides of the foot at the front connected by a half ring (Fig. 1). Two K-wires are drilled through the proximal and distal part of the tibia and fixed under 12 N to 2 external rings, both connected by screw-threaded rods. Two wires with olives are drilled through the calcaneus and fixed under 5 N tension to a half ring, 1 wire without tension through the talus and 1 wire under 9 N with an olive wire medial through the forefoot (Fig. 1). It is important to drill a pin through the talus, otherwise the subtalar joint is distracted as well, which is not preferred. Distraction is subsequently carried out for 0.5 mm twice daily until a total distraction of 5 mm is achieved. The absence of mechanical loading of both degenerative articular surfaces of tibia and talus, checked by radiograph under joint loading, is maintained for about 3 months, during which time full weightbearing is allowed. Intermittent changes in ankle joint fluid pressure during loading and unloading under distraction were measured in patients by the use of a pressure sensitive catheter placed intra-articularly. On average it appeared that intra-articular fluid pressure changed from 3 to 10 kPa during loading and unloading, with a frequency of around 0.5 Hz during walking.[14] A representative measurement is shown in Figure 3.

Clinical Experiences
A Retrospective Study

Eleven relatively young (35 ± 15 years) patients with severe posttraumatic ankle osteoarthritis had been treated with Ilizarov joint distraction for 3 months. The osteoarthritis was so painful that an arthrodesis was indicated but refused. Mean follow-up of these patients at the time of evaluation was 20 ± 6 month (ranging from 1 to 5 years). The retrospective data, collected from charts before and after treatment, were surprisingly good and revealed a prolonged relief of pain and unchanged or increased joint mobility. The radiographic joint space, initially narrowed because of osteoarthritis, was unchanged or had remained widened after distraction in 50% of the cases. Such data are inspiring and strongly suggest that joint distraction is a promising approach in treatment of severe ankle osteoarthritis. The observed prolonged clinical improvement and the joint space widening suggest that joint distraction has a beneficial effect on cartilage metabolism.

A Prospective Uncontrolled Study

Between 1993 and 1997, 26 patients were treated. In 16 cases the follow-up was 1 year, in 12 cases, 2 years, in 4 cases there was a follow-up of 3 years, and in a single case there was a follow-up of 4 years. Five had a follow-up of less than 1 year and 5 were failures in the first year and were treated with an arthrodesis. As in the retrospective evaluation, patients were relatively young, 39 years (range, 17 to 53 years), and mostly male. In most cases, the osteoarthritis was posttraumatic. Inclusion criterion was a severely painful ankle for

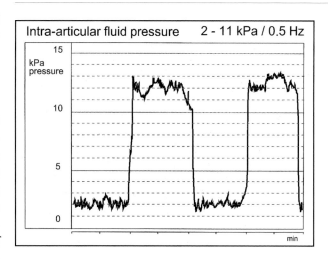

Fig. 3 Representation of an intra-articular pressure measurement in an ankle joint during Ilizarov distraction. During loading intra-articular fluid pressure increases, and there is a subsequent decrease during unloading.

which an arthrodesis was considered. If needed, osteophytes were removed arthroscopically to place and fix the foot into a plantigrade position. The 5-mm distraction for 3 months was carried out as described above. The clinical status, evaluated by measurement of pain, crepitus, and swelling, was expressed as a percentage of the maximum score. After removal of the external fixation frame, the scores remained initially high because of persisting swelling and crepitus, but they improved after 1 year and in the following years (Fig. 4). Functional loss was assessed by a questionnaire, a modification of the functional index for hip and knee osteoarthritis.[15] Function improved significantly after 1 year and this improvement continued (Fig. 4). Pain was measured by use of a box-scale, ranging from 10 (unbearable pain) to 0 (pain free). After 1 year there was a significant relief of pain, with a further improvement in the following years. Ankle mobility was measured by the range of motion. Joint mobility was maintained during the entire follow-up, showing a small improvement in the years after joint distraction. Moreover, radiographic measurements demonstrated an increase in joint space width (Fig. 5). All data

were comparable to the data from the retrospective study. Our conclusion is that Ilizarov joint distraction of a painful osteoarthritic ankle joint can result in clinical improvement after a year, and that this improvement continues for a significant period of time. Although we do not know at present how long these effects may last, in most patients, an arthrodesis could at least be delayed for several years.

Possible Underlying Mechanisms

A 3-month distraction period might be just enough to give the dedifferentiated chondrocytes in the osteoarthritic cartilage the opportunity to redifferentiate, to stop proliferation, and to create an appropriate matrix around them. In the follow-up after distraction, matrix repair might be continued, as is suggested by the slow but progressive increase in joint space widening in the years after distraction. Matrix repair may be facilitated by diminished mechanical impact on the cartilage during revalidation in the first months after distraction, a period of walking with crutches and low impact joint loading. We found a reduction of subchondral sclerosis and bone density in the tibial shaft as a result of the distraction. Bone den-

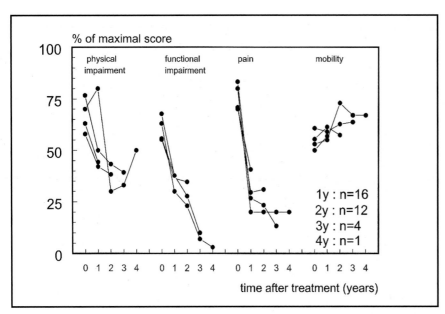

Fig. 4 Average scores for clinical impairment, functional impairment, pain, and joint mobility before Ilizarov joint distraction and after 1, 2, 3, and 4 years of follow-up. Data are presented as a percentage of the maximum score being: 10 points for clinical impairment; 30 points for functional impairment, and 10 points for pain. Mobility is presented as percentage from the contralateral control joint.

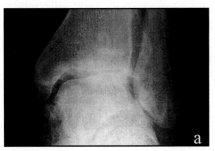
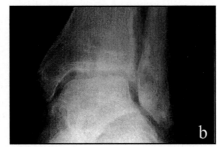

Fig. 5 Radiographs of a tibiotalar joint before (**A**) and 3 years after (**B**) joint distraction. Joint space was widened compared to the condition before distraction.

sity was restored within 1 year after distraction, but subchondral sclerosis remained reduced for more than 2 years (personal communication, AC Marÿnissen, 1998). This result of the distraction may improve shock absorption by the bone, diminishing the impact on the cartilage. The idea of actual repair of cartilage, however, remains difficult to prove in patients. Magnetic resonance imaging (MRI) and radiographs will not provide us with the proper data. More funda-

mental approaches, such as cultures of human articular cartilage and animal models for osteoarthritis, are needed to unravel the actual mechanisms behind possible cartilage repair as a result of joint distraction.

Does Joint Distraction Result in Cartilage Repair?
An Experimental In Vitro Study
Mild to moderate human preclinical osteoarthritic knee cartilage was subjected to the characteristics of joint

distraction: absence of mechanical loading and the presence of intermittent fluid pressure. This type of cartilage shows histologic changes of osteoarthritis comparable to clinically defined osteoarthritis.[16] In general, all changes observed in osteoarthritic joints are, to a lesser extent, observed in the joints with preclinical osteoarthritic cartilage and are significantly different from joints with normal cartilage. This type of osteoarthritic cartilage, normal healthy knee cartilage, and inflammatory cells (mononuclear cells) from the osteoarthritic synovial fluid were used to investigate the in vitro effects on articular cartilage of intermittent fluid pressures (0 to 13 kPa; 0. 33 Hz) as measured in the patients, in absence of mechanical stress. Cartilage and mononuclear cells were cultured both separately and together (coculture). Intermittent fluid pressure was applied via a pressure chamber to which a computer-controlled pressure system was connected (Fig. 6). Controls were placed in an identical chamber at ambient pressure. Cartilage matrix (proteoglycan) synthesis was stimulated by about 50% by intermittent fluid pressure in osteoarthritic cartilage; normal cartilage was not affected.[17] No effects on proteoglycan release were detected. Inhibition of proteoglycan synthesis, induced by osteoarthritic synovial fluid mononuclear cells in coculture, was reduced when cultures had been exposed to intermittent fluid pressure. Analysis of conditioned media of osteoarthritic synovial fluid cells revealed that the beneficial effect of intermittent fluid pressure was accompanied by a decrease in production of the catabolic cytokines interleukin-1 (IL-1) and tumor necrosis factor-alpha (TNFα), cytokines involved in upregulation of matrix-destructive metalloproteinase activity. Thus, low levels of intermittent fluid pressure as occurring in vivo during joint distraction may have beneficial effects on joint tissue in osteoarthritis, indicating that this factor could be involved in actual repair of cartilage.

A Canine In Vivo Model

Intermittent fluid pressure in absence of mechanical stresses in vitro strongly suggests that joint distraction can provide structural beneficial changes in osteoarthritic cartilage. Unfortunately, actual repair of osteoarthritic cartilage in patients is difficult to study. Evaluation of cartilage by MRI or histologic evaluation of cartilage biopsies after arthroscopy have their restrictions (not representative or too little material, no quantitative measures).[18,19] For this reason, an animal model was used to study the effects of joint distraction on the early changes in articular cartilage and on secondary inflammation in osteoarthritis. In beagle dogs, experimental osteoarthritis was induced by anterior cruciate ligament transection (ACLT) in 1 knee joint, with subsequent instability. The other knee served as internal control. Eleven weeks later, the ACLT dogs were randomly divided into 2 groups. One group was treated with articulating joint distraction (Fig. 7); the other dogs received no treatment after ACLT (osteoarthritic controls). The aim of distraction was to achieve the absence of mechanical stresses on the articular cartilage in combination with intra-articular intermittent fluid pressure, as observed during clinical treatment. Because the dogs did not load their treated joint significantly, changes in intra-articular fluid pressure were generated by motion of the joint. These changes in intra-articular fluid pressure, measured by means of a pressure transducer connected to an intra-articularly positioned catheter, revealed that flex-

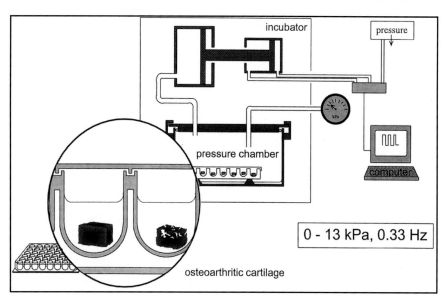

Fig. 6 Schematic drawing of the in vitro pressure device. Microtiter plates (96-well) with normal and osteoarthritic cartilage are placed in a pressure chamber to which a computer controlled pressure system is connected. Control cultures are carried out in an identical chamber under ambient pressure.

ion and extension of the canine knee joint, under distraction without joint loading, resulted in pressure levels from 3 ± 2 to 12 ± 5 kPa. The absence of mechanical contact between both articulating surfaces was demonstrated radiographically (Fig. 7). Dogs were exercised in a group twice a day for half an hour on a patio. Twenty-five weeks after ACLT all dogs were killed, and both cartilage and synovium of all knee joints were analyzed according to standard procedures.

Histologic gradation of inflammation of the synovial tissue revealed a mild degree of inflammation in the osteoarthritic control group which was significantly reduced by joint distraction. This corroborates the in vitro findings, showing that the absence of mechanical stress combined with intermittent fluid pressure decreases the secondary inflammatory features present in human osteoarthritis. In addition, joint distraction results in normalization of

cartilage matrix turnover. Changes in proteoglycan synthesis and release, characteristic for early osteoarthritis, were completely normalized in the osteoarthritic joints treated with distraction. Effects were observed in femoral as well as tibial cartilage. The decreased proteoglycan content, as a characteristic of osteoarthritis, was not improved by joint distraction. It is likely that a subsequent follow-up period is needed after removal of the fixation frame. In patients, clinical improvement, including joint space widening, was experienced gradually after removal of the distraction frame. In the presently used animal model, such a follow-up is impossible, because joint instability caused by ACLT remains a trigger for osteoarthritis. In conclusion, joint distraction, a combination of unloading of degenerative cartilage in the presence of intermittent fluid pressures, induces reduction of inflammation and normalization of matrix turnover. Both in vivo and in vitro experiments

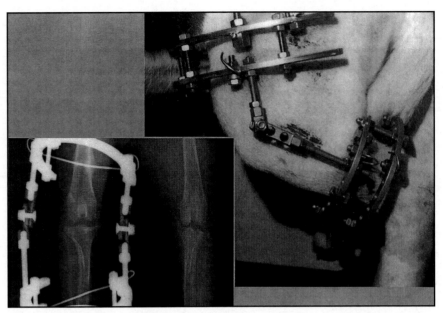

Fig. 7 Illustration of joint distraction of the dog knee joint. Half pins are drilled into the femur and connected with half oval rings around the upper limb. Kirschner wires are drilled through the tibia and connected to rings around the lower limb. Distraction of the femoral and tibial fixations is carried out by use of screw-threaded rods with hinges. The radiograph shows joint space widening as a control for the absence of mechanical stress during distraction.

suggest that the promising clinical results of ankle distraction are accompanied by actual changes in cartilage.

What is the Future for Joint Distraction as a Treatment for Osteoarthritis?

Evidence that ankle distraction results in cartilage repair and may be advocated as a remedy for osteoarthritis is still circumstantial. Nevertheless, the results of clinical, in vitro, and animal studies as described are hopeful. The clinical study has to be controlled, although such a set-up will be difficult. Animal studies that allow a prolonged follow-up after temporary joint distraction must be initiated to evaluate if there is real cartilage repair. The importance of the transient reduction of bone density in the tibial shaft after ankle distraction and the prolonged diminished subchondral sclerosis should also be investigated. Although the reported distraction technique can be applied to many other joints,[20] its effect on osteoarthritis in particular joints must be studied separately. In other words, many more studies are needed before we can conclude that joint distraction is a remedy for osteoarthritis.

References

1. Buckwalter JA, Mankin HJ: Articular cartilage: Part I. Tissue design and chondrocyte-matrix interactions. *J Bone Joint Surg* 1997;79A:600–611.

2. Lafeber FP, van Roy H, Wilbrink B, Huber-Bruning O, Bijlsma JW: Human osteoarthritic cartilage is synthetically more active but in culture less vital than normal cartilage. *J Rheumatol* 1992;19:123–129.

3. Lafeber FP, van der Kraan PM, van Roy HL, et al: Local changes in proteoglycan synthesis during culture are different for normal and osteoarthritic cartilage. *Am J Pathol* 1992;140: 1421–1429.

4. Buckwalter JA, Mankin HJ: Articular cartilage: Part II. Degeneration and osteoarthrosis, repair, regeneration, and transplantation. *J Bone Joint Surg* 1997;79A:612–632.

5. March LM, Brooks PM: Clinical trials in osteoarthritis. *Ann Rheum Dis* 1996;55:491–493.

6. Puett DW, Griffin MR: Published trials of non-medicinal and noninvasive therapies for hip and knee osteoarthritis. *Ann Intern Med* 1994; 121:133–140.

7. Takeda W, Wessel J: Acupuncture for the treatment of pain of osteoarthritic knees. *Arthritis Care Res* 1994;7:118–122.

8. Buckwalter JA, Lohmander S: Operative treatment of osteoarthrosis: Current practice and future development. *J Bone Joint Surg* 1994;76A: 1405–1418.

9. Breinan HA, Minas T, Hsu HP, Nehrer S, Sledge CB, Spector M: Effect of cultured autologous chondrocytes on repair of chondral defects in a canine model. *J Bone Joint Surg* 1997;79A:1439–1451.

10. Zangger P, Gerber BE: Use of laser in arthroscopy of the ankle: Indications, method, first results [German]. *Orthopade* 1996;25:73–78.

11. Lohmander LS, Dalen N, Englund G, et al: Intra-articular hyaluronan injections in the treatment of osteoarthritis of the knee: A randomised, double blind, placebo controlled multicentre trial. Hyaluronan Multicentre Trial Group. *Ann Rheum Dis* 1996;55:424–431.

12. Bobic V: Arthroscopic osteochondral autograft transplantation in anterior cruciate ligament reconstruction: A preliminary clinical study. *Knee Surg Sports Traumatol Arthrosc* 1996;3: 262–264.

13. van Valburg AA: *Ilizarov Joint Distraction in Treatment of Osteoarthritis*. Elinkwijk, Utrecht, University Medical Centre of Utrecht, The Netherlands. Thesis.

14. van Valburg AA, van Roermund PM, Lammens J, et al: Can Ilizarov joint distraction delay the need for an arthrodesis of the ankle? A preliminary report. *J Bone Joint Surg* 1995;77B:720–725.

15. Lequesne MG, Mery C, Samson M, Gerard P: Indexes of severity for osteoarthritis of the hip and knee: Validation. Value in comparison with other assessment tests. *Scand J Rheumatol* 1987;65(suppl):85–89.

16. van Valburg AA, Wenting MJ, Beekman B, Te Koppele JM, Lafeber FP, Bijlsma JW: Degenerated human articular cartilage at autopsy represents preclinical osteoarthritic cartilage: Comparison with clinically defined osteoarthritic cartilage. *J Rheumatol* 1997;24:358–364.

17. Lafeber F, Veldhuijzen JP, Vanroy JL, Huber-Bruning O, Bijlsma JW: Intermittent hydrostatic compressive force stimulates exclusively the proteoglycan synthesis of osteoarthritic human cartilage. *Br J Rheumatol* 1992;31:437–442.

18. Brandt KD, Fife RS, Braunstein EM, Katz B: Radiographic grading of the severity of knee osteoarthritis: Relation of the Kellgren and Lawrence grade to a grade based on joint space narrowing, and correlation with arthroscopic evidence of articular cartilage degeneration. *Arthritis Rheum* 1991;34:1381–1386.

19. Martel W, Adler RS, Chan K, Niklason L, Helvie MA, Jonsson K: Overview: New methods in imaging osteoarthritis. *J Rheumatol* 1991;27(suppl):32–37.

20. van Roermund PM, van Valburg AA, Duivemann E, et al: Function of stiff joints may be restored by Ilizarov joint distraction: Three case reports. *Clin Orthop* 1998;348:220–227.

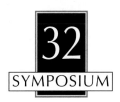

Arthrodesis of the Ankle: Technique, Complications, and Salvage Treatment

Harold B. Kitaoka, MD

Introduction

In recent years, advances have been made in the management of arthritis of the ankle. Clinical results with longer duration of follow-up of ankle reconstruction techniques such as arthrodesis and arthroplasty are now available. Techniques for managing limited arthritis such as cheilectomy and low tibial osteotomy are gaining favor. Other techniques, such as distraction arthroplasty, are promising alternatives that demand further investigation. Information regarding the efficacy of managing specific complex problems that affect the ankle is now available.

Ankle Arthritis and Treatment

Painful, disabling arthrosis of the ankle may occur following trauma or chronic instability, or it may be related to rheumatoid arthritis, degenerative joint disease, synovial osteochondromatosis, osteochondritis dissecans, talar osteonecrosis, tumors, hemophilia, infection, or neuropathy.

Evaluation of the painful or malaligned ankle joint begins with a thorough history and physical examination. Questions concerning a previous history of trauma, instability episodes, swelling, fever, night pain, or progressive sensory changes of the foot should all be addressed to the patient in an attempt to delineate an underlying disease process. In addition, the patient's response to previous forms of therapy should be assessed. Each joint of the lower extremity should be examined, documenting range of motion, painful motion, localized tenderness, swelling, stability, and alignment. Selective lidocaine injection into a specific joint may aid localization of the most symptomatic joint.

For assessment of ankle and hindfoot disorders, plain film radiography should be performed with standing anteroposterior and lateral views of the ankle as well as standing anteroposterior and oblique views of the foot. A mortise view is also useful for evaluating the ankle. Ankle and hindfoot alignment while weightbearing may be assessed with a standing tibiocalcaneal view (modified Cobey or Morrey view). Sometimes plain tomograms or computed tomography (CT) scans oriented parallel and perpendicular to the longitudinal axis of the foot are useful in delineating ankle and hindfoot pathology such as arthritis, tumors, and fractures. Technetium and indium bone scans are helpful in evaluating the likelihood of infection, stress fracture, bone tumor, or inflammatory disease, and for localizing an area of pathology that is not apparent on plain radiographs. Occasionally, a magnetic resonance imaging (MRI) scan is indicated to evaluate such painful ankle conditions as tendon disorders, osteonecrosis, stress fractures, infections, and soft-tissue tumors. In patients suspected of having inflammatory arthritis, testing may include blood count, blood chemistry group, rheumatoid factor, antinuclear antibody, sedimentation rate, and HLA-B27.

In general, most patients with ankle arthritis should initially receive nonsurgical treatment. Nonsurgical management of the ankle includes oral nonsteroidal anti-inflammatory medications, judicious use of intra-articular corticosteroid injections, footwear modifications, and bracing. Modifying the shoe with a rocker bottom sole and a solid ankle cushion heel may provide some relief for the stiff, arthritic ankle. This may not be adequate and immobilization with a laced ankle support or a polypropylene ankle foot orthosis should be considered. The ankle foot orthosis provides stability to ankle and hindfoot and therefore is applicable for patients with combined ankle and hindfoot arthrosis and for patients who are not candidates for surgery due to either local or general conditions.

Ankle cheilectomy is useful in selected patients who develop symptomatic anterior ankle osteophytes.

These osteophytes usually affect the distal tibia, but they may also occur on the talus and restrict ankle dorsiflexion. Patients may recognize the limitation of dorsiflexion with stair climbing and complain of anterior ankle pain. On examination, restriction of dorsiflexion, tenderness of the anterior joint line, pain with passive dorsiflexion of the ankle, and the presence of anterior osteophytes on the lateral radiograph of the ankle are consistent with this disorder. The osteophytes may be palpable. It is important to distinguish this condition from other disorders, as it is not unusual to observe anterior ankle osteophytes radiographically in patients who are asymptomatic. Nonsteroidal oral anti-inflammatory medications are useful, and if these do not provide adequate relief, surgery such as cheilectomy may be indicated. This is easily accomplished through an ankle arthrotomy and there are also advocates of the arthroscopic technique. While there are some potential advantages of arthroscopy for this condition, rare complications, such as dorsal foot numbness, have been reported.

For advanced arthrosis of the ankle, refractory to nonsurgical treatment efforts, ankle reconstruction operations may be considered. Several authors recently presented good results with total ankle replacement with limited (less than 5 year) follow-up, but nearly all reports of long-term results cited problems of recurrent pain, stiffness, component migration, loosening, and malalignment.[1-3] There are newer designs of total ankle replacement prostheses under investigation, which have the potential of addressing some of the deficiencies of previous designs. Until more critical analysis of these devices is available (such as long-term clinical and radiologic results,

gait analysis, mechanical testing) most would agree that the current standard treatment for advanced ankle arthrosis is arthrodesis. Distraction arthroplasty of the ankle and low tibial osteotomy have also been performed for ankle arthritis, with success in selected patients.

Ankle Arthrodesis

Posttraumatic arthritis is the most common indication for ankle fusion. Ankle fusion is also indicated in arthritis and in deformities resulting from rheumatoid arthritis, degenerative arthritis, osteonecrosis of the talus, neuromuscular conditions, and failed operations, such as total ankle arthroplasty. Arthrodesis of the ankle should rarely be performed in patients with neuropathic (Charcot) arthropathy secondary to a sensory neuropathy, because many of these patients have limited symptoms, and high complication and failure rates have been reported. With current methods of open reduction and internal fixation, acute ankle trauma is rarely treated by primary arthrodesis.

Each year new variations of ankle arthrodesis methods are reported and in general the results are good (approximately 90% union rate) when applied to patients with isolated ankle arthrosis uncomplicated by neuropathy, infection, multiple joint involvement, severe malalignment, severe bony deficiency, or major soft-tissue problems. In adults, rigid fixation is necessary. Internal fixation using compression screws has become a standard method in the past decade. There are variations in surgical approach, screw types, number of screws, and screw placement, but most authors recommend at least two screws for fixation, and some advocate adding an onlay fibular graft.

In recent years, there have been additional publications relating to

specific complex ankle problems such as salvage of ankle arthrodesis nonunion, management of infected nonunion, arthrodesis in patients with major bony deficit (eg, from failed total ankle replacement, infection, or tumor), arthrodesis in patients with sensory neuropathy, arthrodesis in patients with ongoing sepsis, severe osteopenia, and combined ankle and hindfoot arthrosis.[1,4-10] Because of the complexity of these disorders, it is suggested that a number of different arthrodesis methods be available in a surgeon's armamentarium, including external fixation techniques.

Regardless of the fixation methods, alignment is critical. Preferred alignment is neutral flexion-extension, hindfoot valgus of 5° to 10°, external rotation of 5° to 10°, neutral medial-lateral displacement, and posterior translation of the talus with respect to the tibia of between 0 and 1 cm. This posterior translation is designed to decrease the anterior lever arm of the foot, which reduces the overloading of the intact midfoot joints. The malleoli may need to be excised or shaved to prevent painful impingement against the upper margin of the counter of the shoe.

Approaches to the ankle include the anteromedial, anterolateral, posterior, and combined medial and lateral approaches. The combined medial and lateral transmalleolar approach consists of hockey stick-shaped incisions over the medial malleolus and anterior margin of the distal fibula respectively. Dissection is carried out over the malleoli, taking care to protect the superficial peroneal nerve laterally and the saphenous nerve medially. The fibula is transected obliquely 4 to 6 cm proximal to the tip with an oscillating saw and can be used as an onlay graft, preserving soft-tissue attachment to the malleolus. Dissection along the anterior ankle further exposes the joint for resection and realignment.

The anteromedial incision is longitudinally oriented medial to the anterior tibial tendon and centered over the ankle. The anterolateral approach is lateral to the extensor digitorum longus and peroneus tertius tendons and centered over the ankle. The posterior approach is generally along the lateral margin of the Achilles tendon, taking care to protect the sural nerve. The interval between the flexor hallucis longus and the peroneal tendons is developed. The Achilles tendon can be divided to maximize the exposure but should be repaired.

Methods of preparing the joint for arthrodesis include osteotomies of the distal tibia and talar dome perpendicular to the long axis of the tibia producing flat, parallel surfaces. This results in limited shortening (1 cm) of the extremity. Others prefer to remove the remaining articular cartilage while preserving the subchondral bone and bony contour or to use chevron-shaped osteotomies to maximize bony contact and stability. Simply removing the articular cartilage with or without the underlying subchondral bone minimizes shortening of the extremity and has the potential of improving stability (compared to flat parallel cuts), but this method is not applicable when there is substantial deformity to be corrected. Cartilage removal can be accomplished with the standard arthrotomy or arthroscopically.

Fusion may also be accomplished by bridging the ankle joint with an onlay or inlay graft. The inlay graft may be constructed from the distal anterior tibia, sliding the graft distally into the neck of the talus. This technique, popularized by Blair, is useful in ankle arthrosis with talar

osteonecrosis. The distal fibula may be used as an onlay graft. Combined intra-articular and extra-articular arthrodesis is another option, performed posteriorly by creating a trough in the distal tibia, talus, and calcaneus, which is then packed with morcellated iliac crest bone graft. With each of these methods some form of fixation is recommended.

Methods of ankle arthrodesis fixation include internal compression screws, external fixation devices, internal fixation with plates and screws or staples, percutaneous pins, and intramedullary nailing (Fig. 1). Large (6.5 mm or 7.0 mm) cancellous screws may be effective, but care must be taken not to violate the subtalar joint. Intraoperative radiographs are helpful to assess fixation placement, bony apposition, and alignment. Most authors agree that the internal compression arthrodesis technique with at least two screws is necessary for adequate fixation. Supplemental fibular onlay grafting has been shown to add stability to the screw fixation in cadaveric testing.[11]

External fixation devices, such as the Calandruccio triangular external fixation device or small wire ring fixators, may also be used. They play an important role in patients with open wounds or active infection or with a failed ankle arthrodesis. These devices are also useful in patients with severe talar bone deficiency or severe osteopenia, where adequate purchase with compression screws is not possible. Complications such as pin tract infections may occur and are normally successfully managed by oral antibiotics. Because neuromas can occur with external fixation, pins should be carefully placed.

Fixation with a plate and screws or a blade plate through a posterior approach has been described with

high union rates. Arthrodesis of the ankle with two longitudinally placed Steinmann pins in patients with rheumatoid arthritis has also been shown to be successful, as has fixation with a locked intramedullary nail passed from the plantar hindfoot and spanning the subtalar and ankle joints. The latter procedure should be reserved for the rare patient who has both ankle and subtalar arthritis.

Arthrodeses are usually united by 4 months postoperatively, and most patients obtain full clinical benefit of an ankle fusion by approximately 6 to 8 months postoperatively. Long-term studies of ankle fusion results report satisfactory clinical results in over 80% of patients. Following ankle fusion, gait is normal in the majority of patients, although it has been shown that walking speed is decreased because of a shortened stride length. Motion through Chopart's (talonavicular and calcaneocuboid) and Lisfranc's (tarsometatarsal) joints allows residual tibiopedal motion approximately 30% to 40% of normal. Subtalar motion following ankle fusion is often diminished, but many of these patients have some degree of subtalar joint stiffness before surgery. Some longer-term follow-up studies demonstrated degenerative changes at Chopart's and Lisfranc joints, but most of these radiologic abnormalities were asymptomatic.

Complications and Failures

Common reasons for failures of ankle arthrodesis are nonunion, malunion, infection, leg length discrepancy, painful hindfoot motion, and neurovascular injury. While nonunion was a frequent complication with older techniques, modern compression techniques commonly have union rates of approximately 90%. Ankle arthrodesis nonunion

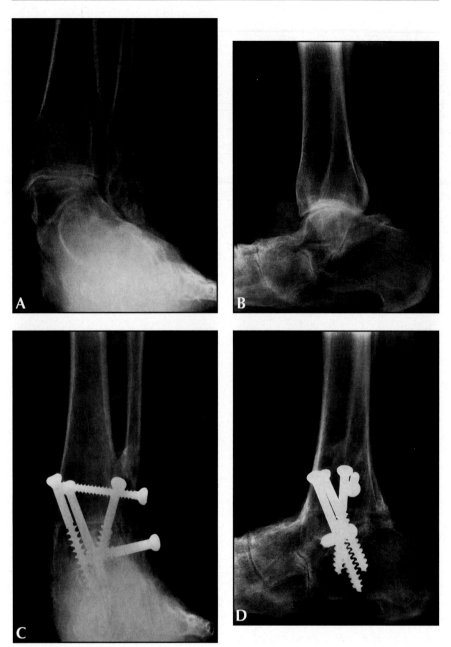

Fig. 1 Radiographs of a 40-year-old woman with rheumatoid arthritis of the ankle and hindfoot, valgus deformity at both the ankle and hindfoot levels, and ankylosed subtalar joint; anteroposterior (**A**) and lateral (**B**) radiographs. Patient underwent arthrodesis with internal fixation with screws, and lateral malleolar only graft. Valgus malalignment was improved by correction of ankle valgus, internal rotation of foot, and medial displacement of foot. Anteroposterior (**C**) and lateral (**D**) radiographs 2.7 years postoperatively with good clinical and radiologic results. (Reproduced with permission from Felix N, Kitaoka HB: Ankle arthrodesis in patients with rheumatoid arthritis. *Clin Orthop* 1998;349:58–64.)

surgeons advocated postponing arthrodesis until the patient has discontinued tobacco use.

Special Reconstruction Problems
Arthrodesis for Rheumatoid Arthritis
Rheumatoid arthritis may involve the ankle joint.[5,8] The early stage of the disease is characterized by painful synovitis, and treatment may include appropriate drug therapy, corticosteroid joint injection, immobilization in a splint, brace, or cast, and (rarely) synovectomy. Later stages of the disease are characterized by arthritis and deformity for which arthrodesis of the affected joints may be indicated.

Rheumatoid arthritis affecting the ankle may be a challenge to manage because of the frequency with which complicating factors occur, such as malalignment, hindfoot joint involvement, severe osteopenia, advanced joint erosive changes with loss of bone stock, and poor soft-tissue envelope about the ankle. The standard surgical treatment for the ankle is arthrodesis. A recently published series had a 96% union rate, and complications were comparable to other reports of arthrodesis in nonrheumatoid patients using either internal or external fixation.[5] Because of the osteopenia, some authors recommend the use of longitudinal Steinmann pins. Based on a laboratory study, the fixation stability of the internal compression arthrodesis technique with screws may be improved with the addition of a fibular onlay graft.

Arthrodesis in Patients with Ongoing Sepsis
Arthrodesis in patients with ongoing sepsis may be addressed by debridement, antibiotics, revision arthrodesis with external fixation, and soft-tissue coverage as needed.[4,6] It is important in these patients to define any local or

may be successfully salvaged by revision arthrodesis using external fixation and supplemental bone graft (Fig. 2).[7] In selected cases, internal fixation may be used. Arthrodesis of the ankle in patients who smoke is associated with a higher incidence of pseudoarthrosis; therefore, some

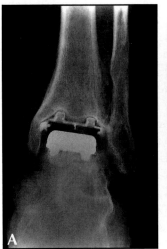 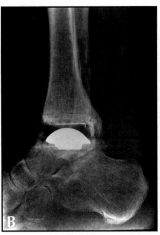 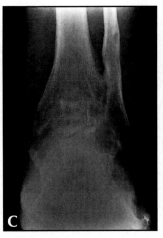 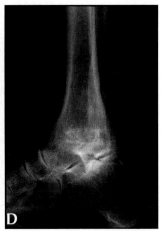

Fig. 2 Radiograph of a patient with a painful total ankle replacement. Anteroposterior (**A**) and lateral (**B**) radiographs demonstrate loosening of both tibial and talar components, subsidence, and malleolar impingement. Anteroposterior (**C**) and lateral (**D**) radiographs 14.5 years later, following modified Chuinard arthrodesis with intercalated iliac crest bone graft and external fixation. Patient had a good clinical and radiologic result, with preservation of ankle height and hindfoot joints. (Reproduced with permission from Kitaoka HB, Romness DW: Arthrodesis for failed ankle arthroplasty. *J Arthroplasty* 1992;7:277–284.)

systemic factors compromising the results, as well as the degree and distribution of bony involvement in order to predict the likelihood of success. Either locally or systemically compromised hosts with diffuse bony involvement (especially central column deficiency) have a much higher failure rate.

Arthrodesis in the Setting of Talar Osteonecrosis

Conventional ankle arthrodesis techniques for arthrosis associated with talar osteonecrosis may fail, as union to necrotic bone may not occur.[1] When osteonecrosis of the entire talar body leads to segmental collapse, arthrosis of both ankle and subtalar joints may occur, requiring arthrodesis with bone graft spanning both levels. In cases in which there is partial body necrosis and only ankle arthrosis (not subtalar), a conventional joint resection arthrodesis may be appropriate, bone grafting the defect.

If there is ankle arthrosis and talar body osteonecrosis without subtalar

arthrosis, other operations, such as the Blair anterior distal tibial sliding bone graft technique, are preferred. The sliding graft technique involves arthrodesis between the anterior tibia to the talar head and neck, which has more viable bone than the talar body. The ankle is approached anteriorly through the interval between the extensor digitorum longus and extensor hallucis longus tendons. The deep dissection requires careful retraction of neurovascular structures (deep peroneal nerve and anterior tibial artery) medially and is carried down to the ankle joint. A rectangular tibial graft measuring 2 to 2.5 cm in width and 3.5 to 5 cm in length is cut with an oscillating saw. A slot is cut into the talar neck about 2 cm in depth to accept the sliding tibial graft. A compression screw is used to fix the proximal graft to the tibia; a longitudinal Steinmann pin through the calcaneus into the tibia may be used for additional stabilization. It is usually not necessary to resect the entire talar body.

Arthrodesis in the Setting of Major Bony Deficit

Large defects resulting from debridement of infected bone, tumor resection, arthrodesis nonunion, or failed ankle replacement present a difficult reconstruction problem.[9] A massive residual defect may be addressed by achieving direct bony apposition, but this results in considerable shortening of the extremity. Intercalated tricortical iliac crest bone graft may be fashioned to fill the defect in order to preserve length. Union rates of up to 89% were reported in a large series of patients with failed ankle replacement. Vascularized fibula transfer and Ilizarov external fixation methods may also have application in selected cases of patients with large bony defects.

Ankle Arthrodesis Malunion

Malposition of the ankle in excessive equinus makes it difficult for the foot to clear the floor while walking. Patients may compensate by externally rotating the extremity. Genu recurvatum may occur resulting from the chronic "back-knee" gait or laxity of the medial collateral ligament from the repetitive valgus stress to the knee. Equinus alignment may cause metatarsalgia and excessive loading of the midfoot joints, with subsequent pain and/or arthrosis. Residual varus or excessive valgus can result in the formation of painful calluses under the fifth or first metatarsals, respectively, and may lead to subtalar arthrosis. Anterior translation of the talus relative to the tibia will cause excessive loading of the midtarsal joints as well. Revision arthrodesis with realignment may be successfully performed.

Arthrodesis of Neuropathic Ankle

Ankle arthrodesis in the neuropathic joint, as in patients with diabetes mellitus, could be considered for carefully selected patients. Neuropathic arthropathy can occur in patients with a subclinical disease without the loss of superficial and deep pain sensation. Typical radiologic features of neuropathic arthropathy may not present. Unfortunately, complications and failures are common following arthrodesis in these patients, with union rates much lower than normal. There may be a role for surgical treatment in patients who fail brace immobilization, or who have intractable ulcers or recurrent infection. Careful assessment of the vascular condition before surgery is essential.

Multiple Joint Disease

Patients with longstanding ankle disorders often develop stiffness of the subtalar joint, which may or may not be associated with pain.[7] It is tempting to extend the arthrodesis across both ankle and subtalar joints in order to eliminate the possibility of late symptoms at the subtalar level,

but it is generally advisable to limit the arthrodesis to the symptomatic joint or joints.

Tibiotalocalcaneal Arthrodesis In patients with arthrosis affecting the ankle and hindfoot, tibiotalar arthrodesis may not be appropriate if there is a high likelihood of residual hindfoot pain.[5,7,11,12] Differential joint injection of a local anesthetic agent may help clarify the contribution of a particular joint to a patient's symptoms and therefore may help the surgeon decide whether to extend the arthrodesis to include the hindfoot. Severe bony (talar) deficiency or selected cases of talar osteonecrosis may also necessitate extension of the arthrodesis due to the limited potential for union of the isolated tibiotalar arthrodesis in these patients. Tibiotalocalcaneal arthrodesis is indicated for symptomatic ankle and subtalar arthrosis unresponsive to bracing, injections, and nonsteroidal anti-inflammatory medications. This may be accomplished in one stage with fusion rates approximating those for primary tibiotalar arthrodesis. The operation may be accomplished through medial and lateral incisions with the patient supine on the operating table. As with the isolated ankle arthrodesis, the ankle joint is resected using an oscillating saw to make 2 parallel cuts, with care taken to minimize the degree of bony resection. Residual articular cartilage and subchondral bone are removed at the subtalar level and fixation applied across both ankle and subtalar levels. Different fixation methods have been used with success, but a commonly performed technique involves multiple cancellous screws placed from proximal to distal extending across both ankle and subtalar levels. A fibular onlay graft may be applied with screw fixation into the tibia and the calcaneus. As an alternative, ex-

ternal fixation may be used, with pins placed transversely in the tibia and the calcaneus. Some investigators use a posterior approach with the patient positioned prone, with fixation consisting of either a posterior plate or external fixator. Achieving appropriate alignment is critical with this operation, particularly with respect to varus-valgus position, as there is limited compensation from the adjacent unfused joints for even small degrees of malalignment. Malalignment in the varus-valgus plane will often result in a painful, intractable plantar keratosis under the medial or lateral plantar forefoot.

Tibiocalcaneal Arthrodesis When the talar body is either deficient, infected, or osteonecrotic, tibiocalcaneal arthrodesis could be considered.[12] If it is determined that the little remaining talar body is not salvageable, the remaining fragments of talar body may be removed and arthrodesis of the distal tibia directly to the calcaneus may be performed with internal or external fixation. As with the tibiotalocalcaneal arthrodesis, appropriate alignment is crucial. Although this procedure may have acceptable clinical results, the operation has the inherent disadvantage of creating considerable shortening of the extremity. The malleoli may be resected to prevent impingement from footwear.

Pantalar Arthrodesis The indications for pantalar arthrodesis are very limited, but its use has been reported to treat severe rheumatoid arthritis involving the ankle and hindfoot.[8] Occasionally, patients who undergo triple arthrodesis and develop subsequent ankle arthrosis require extension of the arthrodesis across the ankle, which results in a pantalar arthrodesis. The operation can be performed either in a one-stage or two-stage procedure.

References

1. Kitaoka HB, Johnson KA: Ankle replacement arthroplasty, in Morrey BF, An KN (eds): *Reconstructive Surgery of the Joints*, ed 2. New York, NY, Churchill Livingstone, 1996, pp 1757–1769.

2. Kitaoka HB, Patzer GL: Clinical results of the Mayo total ankle arthroplasty. *J Bone Joint Surg* 1996;78A:1658–1664.

3. Kitaoka HB, Patzer GL, Ilstrup DM, Wallrichs SL: Survivorship analysis of the Mayo total ankle arthroplasty. *J Bone Joint Surg* 1994;76A:974–979.

4. Cierny G III, Cook WG, Mader JT: Ankle arthrodesis in the presence of ongoing sepsis: Indications, methods, and results. *Orthop Clin North Am* 1989;20:709–721.

5. Felix NA, Kitaoka HB: Ankle arthrodesis in patients with rheumatoid arthritis. *Clin Orthop* 1998;349:58–64.

6. Johnson EE, Weltmer J, Lian GJ, Cracchiolo A III: Ilizarov ankle arthrodesis. *Clin Orthop* 1992;280:160–169.

7. Kitaoka HB, Anderson PJ, Morrey BF: Revision of ankle arthrodesis with external fixation for non-union. *J Bone Joint Surg* 1992;74A:1191–1200.

8. Kitaoka HB: Rheumatoid hindfoot. *Orthop Clin North Am* 1989;20:593–604.

9. Kitaoka HB, Romness DW: Arthrodesis for failed ankle arthroplasty. *J Arthroplasty* 1992;7:277–284.

10. Russotti GM, Johnson KA, Cass JR: Tibiotalocalcaneal arthrodesis for arthritis and deformity of the hind part of the foot. *J Bone Joint Surg* 1988;70A:1304–1307.

11. Thordarson DB, Markolf KL, Cracchiolo A III: Arthrodesis of the ankle with cancellous-bone screws and fibular strut graft: Biomechanical analysis. *J Bone Joint Surg* 1990;72A:1359–1363.

12. Kitaoka HB, Patzer GL: Arthrodesis for the treatment of arthrosis of the ankle and osteonecrosis of the talus. *J Bone Joint Surg* 1998;80A:370–379.

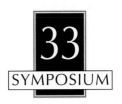

Total Ankle Arthroplasty: State of the Art

Charles L. Saltzman, MD

Introduction

Initial results with total ankle arthroplasty were disappointing for both patients and surgeons. In the search for a workable ankle arthroplasty, a number of different designs have been tried. Most clinical series include 20 to 40 patients followed for an average of 5 years or less (Table 1). Only general observations can be made from the published data.

Patient satisfaction with first generation, cemented ankle implants has ranged from 19% to 81%.[1-8] Length of follow-up was a major factor with patient satisfaction, as patients with longer follow-up generally had declining degrees of satisfaction. The rates of radiographic loosening with these early implants were quite substantial, ranging from 22% to 75%.[2-5,7-10] The major factors implicated with loosening were highly constrained designs and cement fixation. It is not known whether the use of cement alone or the combination of the use of cement and the need to create adequate space for cementation was the chief contributing factor to increased loosening rates.

Total ankle arthroplasty has also been plagued with unusually high wound problems. The soft tissues around the ankle region, especially in rheumatoid and elderly patients, provide a relatively thin envelope for arthroplasty containment. Problems with superficial and deep infections,

resection arthroplasties, attempted reimplantations or arthrodeses and, occasionally, below-knee amputations have dampened the enthusiasm of many of the orthopaedic surgeons who are involved with total ankle replacement.

Indeed, the cumulative experience of many centers has suggested little role for total ankle arthroplasty in treatment of patients with end-stage ankle arthritis. After reviewing the large Mayo Clinic experience with Dr. Stauffer's Mayo ankle implant, Kitaoka and Patzer[8] stated, "We no longer recommend ankle arthroplasty with the constrained Mayo implant for rheumatoid arthritis or osteoarthrosis of the ankle." Similarly, after reviewing the London Hospital's experience with their ankle implant, Bolton-Maggs and associates[10] stated,

"In view of the high complication rate and the generally poor long-term clinical results, we recommend arthrodesis as the treatment of choice for the painful, stiff arthritic ankle regardless of the underlying, pathological process." After publication of these types of reports, most orthopaedic surgeons have recommended ankle arthrodesis as the treatment of choice for end-stage ankle arthritis.

Arthrodesis Results

Today, virtually all major orthopaedic textbooks, course manuals, and review publications state that ankle arthrodesis is the surgical treatment of choice for end-stage ankle arthritis. Most ankle arthrodeses do relieve pain, at least in the short term. However, the operation is not without complication, and the long-term

Table 1

Good-to-excellent satisfaction rates after total ankle replacements (older designs)

Device	Reference	No. Ankles	Average Follow-up (in months)	Satisfaction Rate (%)
Smith	Dini and Bassett[1]	21	27	46
ICLH	Goldie and Herberts[2]	18	36	60
TPR	Jensen and Kroner[3]	23	59	69
Bath + Wessex	Carlsson et al[4]	52	60	81
TPR	Das[5]	37	60	52
LCS	Buechel et al[6]	40	72	85
Smith	Kirkup[7]	18	84	61
Mayo	Kitaoka and Patzer[8]	160	108	19

(ICLH = Imperial College, London Hospital; TPR = Thomson-Parkridge-Richards; LCS = low contact stress)

results are still incompletely understood.[11,12] There are a few very encouraging reports of the intermediate term results of ankle fusions, performed at an average of greater than 7 years after surgery. However, there are also several reports that describe both short- and long-term problems with ankle fusions.[13] The common problems described are eventual development of subtalar and midtarsal degenerative joint disease, pain with walking or standing, need for ambulatory aids, and need for permanent shoe modifications. Although the short-term results and complication rates have been markedly improved by modern techniques of limited periosteal stripping, rigid internal fixation, and meticulous attention to alignment/position, the long-term effects of these improved approaches are still unknown. Several orthopaedic surgeons believe the rates of problems related to arthrodeses to be unacceptably high, and have continued to search for a workable ankle arthroplasty for selected circumstances.[14–18]

Agility Ankle

The Agility Ankle (DePuy, Inc, Warsaw, IN; FDA Class II) was designed by Dr. Frank Alvine (Fig. 1). A unique feature of the implant design involves incorporation of a syndesmosis fusion to improve stability of the tibial component. Another unusual feature is that the tibial component implant is placed in approximately 22° of external rotation to allow for the natural outward positioning of the transmalleolar ankle axis. This noncemented implant uses porous, coated beads. The implant is inserted after the talus has been aligned under the tibia and distracted with an external fixator.

The first 100 patients who underwent total ankle arthroplasty using an Agility Ankle were reviewed independent of the surgeon.[19] Of those 100 patients, 45 had a diagnosis of posttraumatic degenerative joint disease, 26 had a diagnosis of primary osteoarthrosis, 26 had a diagnosis of rheumatoid arthritis, 2 had a diagnosis of septic arthritis, and 1 had a diagnosis of psoriatic arthritis. No patient was involved with a workmens' compensation claim. The mean age at surgery was 63 years old (range, 28 to 81 years). The average length of follow-up was 4.8 years (range, 2.8 to 12.3 years). Of these 100 patients, 2 died within 2 years, and radiographic evaluation was available on the remaining 93 patients (98 ankles). Twelve patients (14 ankles) with greater than 2-year follow-up were deceased at the time of the study. The study group thus was comprised of 83 patients (86 ankles) who completed a questionnaire, and 54 patients (56 ankles) who returned for independent clinical evaluation.

There were 5 complications in the initial series, involving 3 talar component revisions, 1 tibial component revision, and 1 total ankle resection with arthrodesis. There were 2 superficial wound infections and no deep infections. At follow-up, 54% of the patients had no pain, 29% had mild pain, 16% had moderate pain, and no patients had severe pain. Most patients were satisfied with the results, with 79% rating their satisfaction level as extremely satisfied, 13% rating their satisfaction level at satisfied, and 8% rating their satisfaction as indifferent or disappointed/unhappy.

Seventy-two percent of the patients reported an increase in their level of function, 10% had a noticeable limp, 6% used a cane regularly, and 4% required an ankle/foot arthrosis to control valgus deformity. Postoperatively, the mean range of dorsiflexion-plantarflexion at follow-up was 36° (range 10° to 64°). Fifty percent of patients had a plantarflexion contracture averaging 7°, and 67% felt more comfortable walking in a shoe with a slight heel.

The radiographic results suggest the importance of successful, early syndesmosis fusion. Sixty-two percent had early union, defined as radiographic union by 6 months. Of the remaining patients, 29% had a delayed union, defined as a union occurring after 6 months postoperatively, and 9% had a nonunion. There were 19 cases of component migration, with 12 tibial components and 7 talar components demonstrating radiographic migration. Eight of the 12 (67%) ankles with tibial component migration were associated with delayed or nonunion of the syndesmosis. Talar component migration was independent of syndesmosis union.

The radiographs were evaluated for evidence of circumferential lucencies. Circumferential lucencies around the tibial component were present in 20% of the lateral radiographs; circumferential lucencies of the talus were present on 1% of the lateral radiographs. When the circumferential lucencies were stratified by the presence of tibial/fibular syndesmosis union, they appeared to occur more frequently with nonunion (42%) than with delayed union (7%) or early union (2%). Thirty-eight percent of all cases showed evidence of lysis. The time course of lysis suggested that this was not a particulate debris lysis but rather was caused by wear of the component at the bone/component interface. All of the syndesmosis nonunion cases showed lysis, whereas only 64% of the syndesmosis delayed union cases and 28% of the early union cases showed lysis.

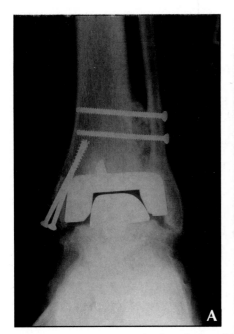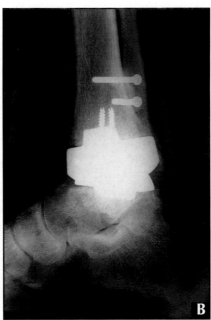

Fig. 1 A, Anteroposterior and **B,** lateral view of the Agility Ankle 4 years after implantation in a 78-year-old male with osteoarthrosis. This implant design incorporates a syndesmosis fusion, and cementless bead fixation. In this case, the medial malleolar screws were used to fix an intraoperative fracture.

The results of this study suggest that the use of the Agility Ankle with good syndesmosis fusion resulted in reliable, good function and radiographic stability in most patients, at an average of 5 years follow-up. Delayed or nonunion of the syndesmosis was associated with component migration, circumferential lucencies, and lysis.

Howmedica Ankle

Dr. Theodore Waugh, who helped design the Howmedica Total Ankle (Howmedica Inc, Rutherford, NJ; FDA Class II), has recently reported his long-term follow-up on the original design, as well as his intermediate-term follow-up on a modified design with sintered bead coating. In the original series,[20] Waugh followed 50 patients prospectively for 15 to 19 years after total ankle replacement. Of these 50 patients, 18 replacements were considered successful, 23 implants were considered unsuccessful, 4 were lost to follow-up, and 5 were deceased. The average age at implantation for men was 49 years and for women was 58 years. The average age of unsuccessful replacement for men was 43 years and for women was 47 years. Of the 23 failures, approximately 50% were attributable to loosening of the prosthesis. Usually loosening was seen within 4 years of the time of surgery, and was more common in higher-demand patients. Survivorship analysis has shown that there has been little change between 6 and 15 years after surgery, with an average survivorship of approximately 60% during this time. More recently, Dr. Waugh has used the Howmedica Total Ankle implant with a sintered bead coating on both metal components. Of the 20 sintered ankle prostheses (FDA "customized" Class III) inserted without cement in the past 8 years, followed for over 5 years, he reports no cases of loosening or sinkage. The improved results with the cementless approach also reflect a progressive shift in the surgical indications toward lower activity, older patients with polyarticular disease (TR Waugh, personal communication, 1997).

TNK Ankle

In Nara, Japan, Dr. Yoshino Takakura has been working towards developing an improved ankle prosthesis. His original design involved the use of a metal and polyethylene implant. The results of 30 metal and polyethylene implants with an average of 8.8 follow-up years have been reported, with loosening and sinking of the prosthesis recognized in all cases from 5 years after replacement.[21] Further follow-up of 23 cases, at an average of approximately 14 years, included 9 cases with the ankle intact, 7 revisions, and 7 patients deceased. Of the 9 intact cases, 2 were rated as good, 4 were rated as fair, and 3 were rated as poor.

Takakura and associates[22] also reported 9 cases using a ceramic prosthesis with cement, with an average follow-up of 6.7 years. In this small group of patients, they noted increased loosening and sinking as compared to 30 cases of ceramic prostheses used without cement, followed up for an average of 4.1 years. In the uncemented group, the authors identified loosening and sinking beginning to appear in some cases 3 years after the surgery, and this worsened with time. In response to this observation, Takakura modified his prosthesis in 1991 to include beads, coated hydroxyapatite, and use of screw fixation for the tibial component (Fig. 2). In early follow-up of 18 cases using the new modified ceramic prosthesis, Takakura has noted good or excellent results, with new bone

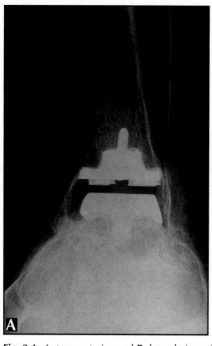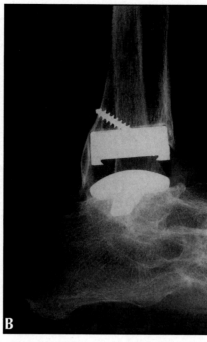

Fig. 2 A, Anteroposterior and **B,** lateral view of the TNK ankle 3.5 years after implantation in a 56-year-old female with rheumatoid arthritis. The TNK is a 2-component, uncemented ceramic implant with screw fixation, and bead and hydroxyapatite coating (Courtesy of Dr. Yoshino Takakura).

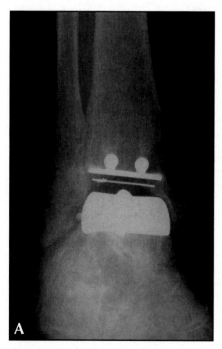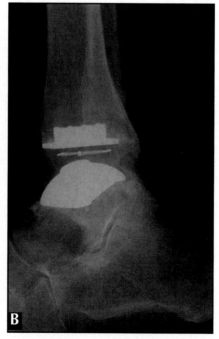

Fig. 3 A, Anteroposterior and **B,** lateral view of the STAR ankle 7 years after implantation in a patient with ankle arthritis secondary to hemochromatosis. This 3-component design involves a floating polyethylene meniscus (marked by the thin wire) and cementless hydroxyapatite fixation (Courtesy of Dr. Hakon Kofoed).

formation integrated into the prosthesis. In summary, Takakura's implant (FDA Class III) has evolved from a cement-fixated, metal/polyethylene implant through a cemented ceramic implant, then to an uncemented ceramic implant, and now to an uncemented ceramic implant with screw fixation, and bead and hydroxyapatite coating. Longer-term follow-up is needed to determine whether the more recent changes in design will result in a more durable operative outcome.

Buechel-Pappas Ultra Total Ankle Replacement

The Buechel-Pappas Ultra Total Ankle Replacement (FDA Class III) incorporates a meniscal bearing design. Originally, these investigators developed a mobile bearing prosthesis (New Jersey LCS Total Ankle, Endotec, South Orange, NJ). This design was found occasionally to result in mechanical bearing subluxation, fracture of the tibial plate, fracture of the meniscal bearing, and irreducible dislocation. The design was modified in the current implant to include a deeper talar sulcus for containing the bearing component, an additional talar fixation fin, and porous coating covered by a titanium-nitride thin film ceramic.

Intermediate term results of the Buechel-Pappas cementless total ankle arthroplasty have been reported recently by independent examiners. In this series, 30 of 38 ankles were followed up for an average of 4.5 years (range, 2 to 8 years). Mean age of patients at surgery was 49 years (range, 25 to 81 years). There were 12 complications, including 6 wound healing problems, 2 cases of subtalar degenerative joint disease secondary to osteonecrosis and component collapse, 2 revisions (1 talar component, 1 tibial component), 1 arthrodesis for pain, and 1 malleolar nonunion. At follow-up, 5 patients had no pain, 11 patients reported slight pain, and 8 patients reported moderate pain. Six patients required use of a cane. Range of motion averaged 5° of dorsiflexion and 16° of plantarflexion. Overall, the results were rated as excellent in 13 patients, good in 6, fair in 6, and poor in 5. All 3 patients with osteonecrosis had a poor result.

Scandinavian Total Ankle Replacement

The Scandinavian Total Ankle Replacement (STAR), in its current form (FDA Class III), is a 3-component arthroplasty consisting of a flat tibial guide plate, a talar component cap, and a sliding polyethylene meniscus (Fig. 3). A hydroxyapatite coating is used for component fixation. It evolved from a previous, 2-component system, which was initially cemented; then a 3-component system, which was initially cemented, and now the current 3-component, uncemented system. Kofoed and associates[23,24] have reported the results of the use of this prosthesis in several separate series. Most recently, they reported the results of 52 ankles (25 osteoarthrosis, 27 rheumatoid arthritis) with an average age at surgery of 58 years. All implants were cemented. Between 1981 and 1985, they used the 2-component prosthesis; between 1986 and 1989, they used the 3-component prosthesis. They reported that all patients had pain relief and improved functional mobility. During follow-up, they found that patients with osteoarthrosis did not develop subtalar degenerative joint disease. A survivorship analysis revealed that at an average of 10 years, they had an approximately 70% survival, with confidence intervals from approximately 50% to 96%. This report pooled outcome data from both the 2-compo-

nent and 3-component designs and does not give any insight into the difference in outcomes of a 2-component versus a 3-component cemented STAR ankle arthroplasty. The intermediate term results of the cementless STAR prosthesis used for treatment of ankle osteoarthrosis have been reported for 31 ankles, followed for an average of 3.5 years (range, 1 to 8 years). In this series, there was only 1 revision, which was performed for malalignment. All patients were clinically improved as a result of the operation, and had no evidence of component loosening or subsidence. The authors believe that the cementless design is improved as compared to the cemented design, and that the complication rates are reduced with use of this implant.

Summary

Total ankle arthroplasty results from the 1970s and 1980s were comparatively poor. The outcomes of these surgeries deteriorated rather dramatically with time. Causes of failure were multifactorial, but the 2 features that seemed central to implant failure were constrained designs and cement fixation. Total ankle operations are considered technically demanding procedures, with relatively high early postoperative complication rates.

As yet, the ideal total ankle patient remains to be defined. With the current implant results as a guide, the optimal patient is an older person who is low demand and has multiple joint problems involving either the ipsilateral foot or knee or contralateral ankle. Good alignment and ligamentous stability are essential. Osteonecrosis and profound osteoporosis are associated with poor results due to problems with bony fixation. Patients should be advised that the implant may fail, and that this may require further surgery, including the potential need for an ankle fusion or below-knee amputation.

The results of ankle fusions, although usually initially good, seem to deteriorate with time (Table 2). Not uncommonly, patients develop either transverse tarsal or subtalar degenerative joint disease several years after an ankle arthrodesis. Because of the associated pain and functional limitations that can follow ankle fusion, efforts to develop a workable total ankle replacement continue. At present, the long-term results of most new designs are unknown. Today, total ankle arthroplasty probably should be limited to centers where surgeons have the volume of patients to master the demanding techniques needed for

Table 2
Radiographic loosening after total ankle replacement (older designs)

Device	Reference	No. Ankles	Average Follow-up (in months)	Loosening (%)
ICLH	Goldie and Herberts[2]	18	36	22
ICLH	Helm and Stevens[9]	14	54	57
TPR	Jensen and Kroner[3]	23	59	52
Bath + Wessex	Carlsson et al[4]	52	60	67
TPR	Das[5]	37	60	26
ICLH	Bolton-Maggs, et al[10]	41	66	32
Smith	Kirkup[7]	18	84	39
Mayo	Kitaoka and Patzer[8]	160	108	75

(ICLH = Imperial College, London Hospital; TPR = Thomson-Parkridge-Richards)

these operations and conduct prospective clinical trials to determine what factors lead to successful and unsuccessful outcomes.

References

1. Dini AA, Bassett FH III: Evaluation of the early result of Smith total ankle replacement. *Clin Orthop* 1980;146:228–230.

2. Goldie IF, Herberts P: Prosthetic replacement of the ankle joint. *Reconstr Surg Traumatol* 1981; 18:205–210.

3. Jensen NC, Kroner K: Total ankle joint replacement: A clinical follow-up. *Orthopedics* 1992;15:236–239.

4. Carlsson AS, Henricson A, Linder L, Nilsson JA, Redlund-Johnell 1: A survival analysis of 52 Bath and Wessex ankle replacements: A clinical and radiographic study in patients with rheumatoid arthritis and a critical review of the literature. *Foot* 1994;4:34–40.

5. Das AK Jr: Total ankle arthroplasty: A review of 37 cases. *J Tenn Med Assoc* 1988;81:682–685.

6. Buechel FF, Pappas MJ, Iorio LJ: New Jersey low contact stress total ankle replacement: Biomechanical rationale and review of 23 cementless cases. *Foot Ankle* 1988;8:279–290.

7. Kirkup J: Richard Smith ankle arthroplasty. *J R Soc Med* 1985;78:301–304.

8. Kitaoka HB, Patzer GL: Clinical results of the Mayo total ankle arthroplasty. *J Bone Joint Surg* 1996;78A:1658–1664.

9. Helm R, Stevens J: Long-term results of total ankle replacement. *J Arthroplasty* 1986;1:271–277.

10. Bolton-Maggs BG, Sudlow RA, Freeman MA: Total ankle arthroplasty: A long-term review of the London Hospital experience. *J Bone Joint Surg* 1985;67B:785–790.

11. Morgan CD, Henke JA, Bailey RW, Kaufer H: Long-term results of tibiotalar arthrodesis. *J Bone Joint Surg* 1985;67A:546–550.

12. Glick JM, Morgan CD, Myerson MS, Sampson TG, Mann JA: Ankle arthrodesis using an arthroscopic method: Long-term follow-up of 34 cases. *Arthroscopy* 1996;12:428–434.

13. Morrey BF, Wiedeman GP Jr: Complications and long-term results of ankle arthrodeses following trauma. *J Bone Joint Surg* 1980;62A:777–784.

14. Ahlberg A, Henricson AS: Late results of ankle fusion. *Acta Orthop Scand* 1981;52:103–105.

15. Mazur JM, Schwartz E, Simon SR: Ankle arthrodesis: Long-term follow-up with gait analysis. *J Bone Joint Surg* 1979;61A:964–975.

16. Boobbyer GN: The long-term results of ankle arthrodesis. *Acta Orthop Scand* 1981;52:107–110.

17. Said E, Hunka L, Siller TN: Where ankle fusion stands today. *J Bone Joint Surg* 1978;60B: 211–214.

18. Lynch AF, Bourne RB, Rorabeck CH: The long-term results of ankle arthrodesis. *J Bone Joint Surg* 1988;70B:113–116.

19. Pyevich MT, Alvine FG, Saltzman CL, Callaghan JJ: Total ankle arthroplasty: A unique design (2 to 11-year follow-up). *J Bone Joint Surg* 1998;80A, in press.

20. Waugh TR, Evanski PM, McMaster WC: Irvine ankle arthroplasty: Prosthetic design and surgical technique. *Clin Orthop* 1976;114: 180–184.

21. Takakura Y, Tanaka Y, Sugimoto K, Tamai S, Masuhara K: Ankle arthroplasty: A comparative study of cemented metal and uncemented ceramic prostheses. *Clin Orthop* 1990;252: 209–216.

22. Takakura Y, Tanaka Y, Akiyama S, Tamai S: Results of total ankle arthroplasty. *J Foot Surg* 1996;11:9–16.

23. Kofoed H, Danborg L: Biological fixation of ankle arthroplasty: A sequential consecutive prospective clinico-radiographic series of 20 ankles with arthrosis followed for 1-4 years. *Foot* 1995;5:27–31.

24. Kofoed H, Sorensen TS: Ankle arthroplasty for rheumatoid arthritis and osteoarthritis: Prospective long-term study of cemented replacements. *J Bone Joint Surg* 1998;80B:328–332.

Surgical Treatment for Neuropathic Arthropathy of the Foot and Ankle

Jeffrey E. Johnson, MD

Nonsurgical treatment with use of a total-contact cast followed by appropriate bracing and footwear is the so-called gold standard for the treatment of most neuropathic (Charcot) fractures and dislocations of the foot and ankle. However, surgical treatment is indicated for chronic recurrent ulceration, joint instability, or, in some instances, pain that has not responded to nonsurgical treatment. Acute fractures may also be treated surgically if the patient is seen before demineralization of bone and inflammation of soft tissue have occurred. The goals of surgical treatment are to preserve function with the aid of appropriate footwear or bracing and to avoid the need for amputation. These goals are achieved through restoration of the contour or alignment of the affected segment of the foot and ankle. Despite the potential for major surgical complications, successful limb salvage and reconstruction was achieved in 124 (87%) of 143 patients in 8 clinical series.[1–7]

Natural History and Clinical Presentation

Neuropathic (Charcot) osteoarthropathy is a noninfective, destructive lesion of a bone and joint resulting from a fracture or dislocation, or both, in a patient who has peripheral neuropathy. Diabetes is the most common cause of these deformity-causing fractures in the United States, and they were reported in 101 (0.1%) of 68,000 patients who had diabetes mellitus.[8] There are an estimated 16 million diabetic individuals in the United States.[9] Because of improvements in the treatment of diabetes, diabetic patients are living longer. Therefore, neuropathic arthropathy, a late effect of peripheral neuropathy of the foot and ankle, continues to be a problem that is seen in orthopaedic practices.

Frequently, a Charcot fracture or dislocation is caused by a minor acute injury, such as a sprain of the ankle or foot, or by an overuse syndrome resulting from repetitive minor injuries. However, it may also be the result of an acute traumatic event, such as a fall from a height or a motor-vehicle accident.

The etiology and pathophysiology of neuropathic destruction of bones and joints are poorly understood. However, the stages of bone and joint destruction, followed by fracture-healing and remodeling, were described by Eichenholtz.[10] The Eichenholtz classification is based on the characteristic clinical and radiographic changes that occur with neuropathic destruction or fracture of a joint over time and is therefore a temporally based classification. As shown in Table 1, these changes progress from the acute phase (dissolution), through the healing phase

Table 1
Classification System of Eichenholtz[10]

Stage	Radiographic Features	Clinical Features
I—Dissolution	Demineralization of regional bone, periarticular fragmentation, dislocation of joint	Acute inflammation (easily confused with infection): swelling, erythema, warmth
II—Coalescence	Absorption of osseous debris in soft tissues, organization and early healing of fracture fragments, periosteal new-bone formation	Less inflammation, less fluctuation in swelling, increased stability at fracture site
III—Resolution	Smoothing of edges of large fragments of bone, sclerosis, osseous or fibrous ankylosis	Permanent enlargement of foot and ankle, fixed deformity, minimum daily swelling or activity-related swelling, normalization of skin temperature

(Adapted with permission from Johnson JE: Surgical reconstruction of the diabetic Charcot foot and ankle. *Foot Ankle Clin* 1997;2:39–40.)

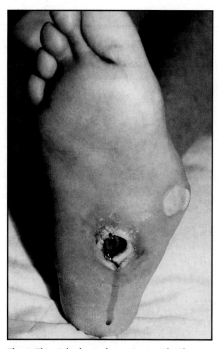

Fig. 1 The right foot of a patient with Charcot arthropathy who had collapse of the midfoot and abduction of the forefoot after a fracture-dislocation of the midfoot, which resulted in ulceration of the medial and plantar aspects of the foot.

(coalescence), to the resolution phase. The timing and selection of a reconstructive procedure for a patient who has a neuropathic joint should be made with a clear understanding of the natural history of a Charcot joint and the temporal stage of the neuropathic process. Different classifications for the characteristic patterns of neuropathic destruction of bones and joints have been described by other investigators.[11–13] An understanding of these patterns is helpful when making the diagnosis and planning treatment for patients who have occult neuropathy.

Deformities of the foot and ankle resulting from a neuropathic fracture or dislocation cause difficulty with shoe-fitting and marked alteration in the load applied to various parts of the plantar surface of the foot during weightbearing. These changes lead to an increased propensity for ulceration in high-pressure areas (Fig. 1). These ulcers may become a portal of entry for bacteria and thus may result in superficial or deep infection. A deformity may also be associated with joint instability, which is accentuated by weightbearing, especially with involvement of the hindfoot or ankle. These changes result in loss of the plantigrade position of the foot and the development of progressive varus, valgus, equinus, or calcaneus deformity.

Nonsurgical Treatment

Nonsurgical treatment is indicated for most Charcot deformities of the foot and ankle. Most deformities are treated with immobilization in a total-contact cast to allow healing and stabilization of the fracture. If the ankle or hindfoot joints are involved, prolonged immobilization in an ankle-foot orthosis for 12 to 18 months, or indefinitely, is often indicated. Involvement of the midfoot and forefoot is typically treated with appropriate extra-depth footwear and custom total-contact inserts.

Surgical Treatment

Surgical treatment is indicated when a patient has a severe deformity of the foot and ankle that is not amenable to management with a custom brace or custom footwear, marked instability (usually involving the hindfoot and ankle), or recurrent ulceration. A markedly unstable Charcot joint may be associated with pain; however, unlike painful osteoarthrosis, a painful Charcot joint is rarely the sole reason for surgical treatment.

The Goals of Surgery

One goal of surgical treatment of a Charcot foot and ankle is to restore the stability and alignment of the foot and ankle so that footwear and a brace can be worn. For most patients who have a deformity that is severe enough to necessitate surgical treatment, a partial amputation of the foot or a below-the-knee amputation is usually the only alternative treatment option. Therefore, an additional goal of surgical intervention is to prevent the inevitable amputation of a limb that is destined to have recurrent ulceration.

Patients who have a moderate-to-severe deformity resulting from neuropathic arthropathy need special footwear with custom total-contact inserts and, sometimes, a custom brace to prevent recurrent ulceration and progressive deformity. Therefore, the decision is not between surgery or the use of prescription footwear and bracing but rather between surgery followed by prescription footwear and bracing or prescription footwear and bracing alone. Therefore, surgery is indicated primarily to make these patients better candidates for prescription footwear and bracing. Although some patients who have a solid fusion after a realignment arthrodesis may eventually be weaned from the ankle-foot orthosis, weaning is an unrealistic goal for many patients and may lead to recurrent ulceration or stress fractures of the tibia.[14]

Timing of Surgery

Surgical treatment of a Charcot foot is usually carried out in the quiescent (resolution) phase of the fracture pattern (Eichenholtz stage III) after the use of a cast, prescription footwear, or a brace, or all 3, have failed. An acute fracture associated with neuropathic arthropathy may be treated with open reduction and fixation if treatment is performed early, before neuropathic inflammation of the soft tissue occurs and while bone stock is still sufficient for rigid fixation. However, most patients are not seen for treatment early enough for this approach. When the acute (dissolution) phase (Eichenholtz stage I) has begun, the demineralization of regional bone and swelling make surgical management of the fracture difficult, leading to a higher rate of failure of fixation, recurrent deformity, and infection.

An ulcer of the foot that is associated with a neuropathic deformity is treated, until it has healed (if possible), with use of a total-contact cast so that the incision for the reconstructive procedure may be made through intact skin to reduce the possibility of postoperative infection. If underlying osteomyelitis is suspected in association with a neuropathic fracture, imaging with a combined technetium-99m bone scan and indium-111-labeled white blood cell scan with use of the dual-window technique helps to confirm or rule out this suspicion.[15,16] If osteomyelitis is present, it is treated with appropriate debridement and antibiotic therapy until the wound has healed and the infection has resolved. Then, the choice with regard to surgical or nonsurgical treatment of the remaining deformity can be made.

Treatment of an Acute Fracture Associated With Neuropathic Arthropathy

The most important factor in the successful treatment of an acute fracture in a patient who has neuropathic arthropathy is the recognition of the fact that the patient has a severe peripheral neuropathy. A series of small monofilament nylon rods (Semmes-Weinstein monofilaments) can be used to determine the severity and location of the sensory neuropathy.[17] If sensory testing with Semmes-Weinstein monofilaments shows loss of protective sensation, it is important to alter the typical treatment regimen to help prevent subsequent Charcot

destruction of the joint. It is also important to warn the patient about the potential risk of Charcot involvement of the joint, whether or not surgical treatment of the fracture is undertaken.

The first step in the treatment of an acute fracture is to determine whether it is associated with neuropathic changes (that is, Eichenholtz stage I) or with peripheral neuropathy but not yet with neuropathic changes. This differentiation often can be made on the basis of the medical history. For example, when a patient has had a relatively minor injury followed by several days or weeks of erythema and swelling and has a displaced fracture on presentation, the fracture is usually treated as an Eichenholtz stage I injury with use of a total-contact cast. However, a patient with severe diabetic peripheral neuropathy who has sustained an acute displaced fracture may be managed with the same orthopaedic principles as would be followed for a patient who does not have neuropathy (if seen acutely), except that a higher rate of complications would be expected and a prolonged postoperative period of nonweightbearing and immobilization in a total-contact cast followed by use of a brace would be indicated. If treatment after the fixation of a fracture does not include rigid external immobilization and a prolonged period of nonweightbearing, the fixation may fail before the fracture has healed (Fig. 2).

Acute fractures of the ankle, talus, or midfoot may be treated with use of the same indications for open reduction and internal fixation, assuming that the patient is medically fit, the vascular status is adequate, there is minimum swelling, and the skin is in good condition. Patients who have an acute fracture that is already Eichenholtz stage I, with early dem-

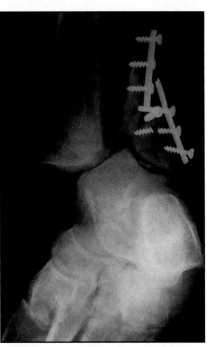

Fig. 2 Postoperative radiograph, made 4 weeks after open reduction and internal fixation of a fracture of the distal part of the fibula with injury of the deltoid ligament, demonstrating valgus displacement and failure of the plate and screws in the fibula. The patient had been managed with a prefabricated removable brace for postoperative immobilization and was allowed toe-touch weightbearing.

ineralization and soft-tissue inflammation, are poorer candidates for surgical treatment. Internal fixation of an ankle fracture is augmented by the addition of 1 or 2 Steinmann pins across the ankle and subtalar joints to prevent hardware failure and joint deformity (Fig. 3). The pins are cut off below the level of the plantar skin and are removed 6 to 8 weeks postoperatively at the time of a cast change.

It is important to extend the duration of immobilization for a fracture in a patient with peripheral neuropathy to approximately double the normal period of time that a patient without neuropathy would be non-

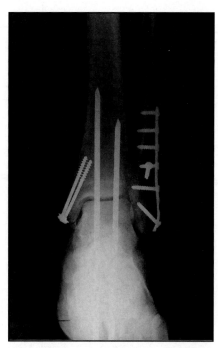

Fig. 3 Anteroposterior radiograph showing percutaneously placed smooth Steinmann pins that were used to augment the internal fixation of a bimalleolar fracture of the ankle until the fracture healed.

weightbearing. Therefore, a patient with neuropathy who has a typical fracture of the ankle is managed with nonweightbearing for approximately 3 months (compared with 6 weeks for a patient without neuropathy), and a cast is worn until approximately 4 to 5 months after the injury, at which time the patient is able to walk while wearing a weightbearing cast and the fracture has united. A brace is then worn for 1 year after the injury to prevent late development of a Charcot joint. A patient who is doing well 12 to 18 months after the injury may be weaned from the brace and subsequently managed with use of extra-depth footwear with custom-molded total-contact inserts. During this period, the patient is carefully monitored for the development of a Charcot joint.

The prolonged duration of immo-

bilization in this protocol may be excessive for patients in whom a Charcot joint is not destined to develop. However, there are no known factors that predict which fracture will progress to a Charcot joint in a patient who has a neuropathy. Therefore, in order to prevent severe deformity, it seems prudent to manage every patient who has loss of protective sensation as if a Charcot joint will develop.

Types of Reconstructive Procedures for Neuropathic Deformity
Ostectomy
The midfoot is the most common location for neuropathic destruction.[18] The apex of the rocker-bottom deformity of the foot that results from this neuropathic destruction is a frequent cause of recurrent ulceration because of the prominence at the apex in the sole of the foot. The most common surgical procedure to treat a neuropathic deformity that causes recurrent ulceration and difficulty with footwear is the removal of the osseous prominence on the medial, lateral, or plantar aspect of the foot.

The first step in the surgical treatment of any neuropathic deformity is to obtain closure of the overlying ulcer, if possible, so that the incision to remove the osseous prominence can be made through intact skin. An alternative technique is to excise the ulcer through a plantar, longitudinal, elliptical incision made directly over the prominence. However, this technique exposes a large amount of underlying cancellous bone to the open ulcer with a potential for bacterial colonization of the underlying superficial bone.

A preferred method (Fig. 4) is to obtain closure of the ulcer with a series of total-contact casts so that the incision can be made through intact

skin on the medial or lateral border of the foot closest to the osseous prominence.[11,19] The skin incision is made as a full-thickness flap down to the osseous prominence. A periosteal elevator is used to separate the overlying soft tissue from the protuberant bone. A small power saw or an osteotome is used to resect the bone surface, which is then rasped to provide a smooth broad surface in the weightbearing area. Major tendon attachments, such as the peroneus brevis, anterior tibial tendon, posterior tibial tendon, and Achilles tendon, should be preserved and reattached to bone if they are detached. Resection of a large prominence in the medial part of the midfoot involving the medial cuneiform should include reattachment of the anterior tibial tendon through holes drilled into the remaining bone. Many patients have a coexistent contracture of the Achilles tendon, and percutaneous lengthening of the Achilles tendon is frequently performed at the time of plantar ostectomy.[20]

The skin is closed over a suction drain, which is left in place for 24 hours with a compression splint. The next day, a total-contact cast is applied to stabilize the soft tissues, promote wound healing, and allow the patient limited weightbearing. It is especially important to avoid excessive bone resection in the midfoot, where removal of the plantar ligaments may cause progression of the rocker-bottom deformity. An ostectomy of the plantar aspect of the midfoot is more successful when the neuropathic deformity is stable in the sagittal and transverse planes.

The sutures are removed when the incision has healed, usually 2 to 3 weeks after the procedure. At the time of 1 of the cast changes, a mold of the foot is made for a total-contact insert so that the appropriate footwear and a custom insert will be

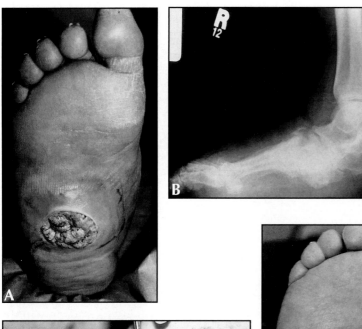

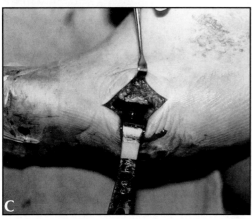

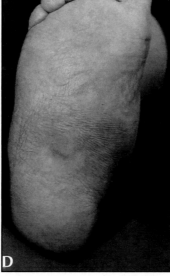

Fig. 4 A patient who had a chronic recurrent plantar ulcer beneath a rocker-bottom deformity. **A,** Photograph of the plantar aspect of the foot, made before treatment with a total-contact cast, which allowed the ulcer to heal before ostectomy. **B,** Lateral radiograph demonstrating a neuropathic rocker-bottom deformity of the midfoot with a large plantar prominence. Note the equinus position of the hindfoot secondary to contracture of the Achilles tendon. **C,** Intraoperative photograph demonstrating the incision, made lateral to the healed ulcer, for the resection of the plantar prominence, which was a portion of the cuboid bone. Percutaneous lengthening of the Achilles tendon was also performed. **D,** Postoperative photograph made 6 months after the plantar ostectomy, demonstrating the healed ulcer. Postoperatively, the patient was managed with a double-upright calf-lacer ankle-foot orthosis attached to an extra-depth shoe with a custom total-contact insert.

other reasonable option for treatment. The goal of surgery is to restore the alignment and stability of the foot so that the patient can use a brace and special footwear. This surgery is not intended to substitute for appropriate footwear or use of a brace.

The contraindications to arthrodesis include: (1) infection of the soft tissue or bone except when the arthrodesis is performed as a staged procedure after the infection has been treated, all osteomyelitic bone has been resected, and the soft tissues have healed; (2) a fracture that is in the acute (dissolution) phase of the neuropathic disease process (Eichenholtz stage I); (3) uncontrolled diabetes or malnutrition; (4) peripheral vascular disease; (5) insufficient bone stock to obtain rigid fixation; and (6) the inability of the patient to comply with the postoperative regimen (because of mental illness).

Technique Preoperatively, a total-contact cast is used until the acute phase of the Charcot fracture process has subsided and the skin is intact. Extensive longitudinal incisions are used with full-thickness skin flaps to bone. If the deformity is mild to moderate and is limited to the ankle and subtalar joints, tibiotalocalcaneal arthrodesis may be performed through a posterior approach.[21] For correction of a severe deformity, exposure is enhanced by making medial and lateral incisions over the ankle rather than a posterior incision. Bone is resected to allow correction of the deformity and to provide apposition of stable bleeding bone surfaces to promote successful fusion. A contracture of the Achilles tendon is corrected with percutaneous lengthening especially when a midfoot or hindfoot arthrodesis is performed. Autologous bone grafting is used to fill any defects and to provide both an intra-articular and an extra-articular arthrodesis when

ready for use when healing has occurred and the cast is removed.

Realignment and Arthrodesis
Severe Charcot deformity or instability of the foot and ankle is treated

with realignment of the involved joint and stabilization by arthrodesis (Fig. 5). Most patients considering this surgery have had a failure of treatment with a brace and special footwear, and amputation is the only

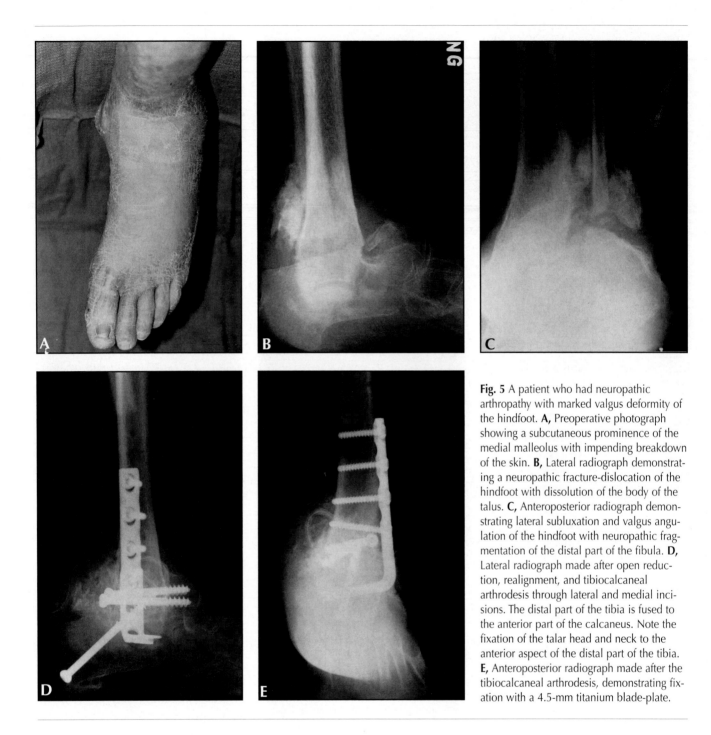

Fig. 5 A patient who had neuropathic arthropathy with marked valgus deformity of the hindfoot. **A,** Preoperative photograph showing a subcutaneous prominence of the medial malleolus with impending breakdown of the skin. **B,** Lateral radiograph demonstrating a neuropathic fracture-dislocation of the hindfoot with dissolution of the body of the talus. **C,** Anteroposterior radiograph demonstrating lateral subluxation and valgus angulation of the hindfoot with neuropathic fragmentation of the distal part of the fibula. **D,** Lateral radiograph made after open reduction, realignment, and tibiocalcaneal arthrodesis through lateral and medial incisions. The distal part of the tibia is fused to the anterior part of the calcaneus. Note the fixation of the talar head and neck to the anterior aspect of the distal part of the tibia. **E,** Anteroposterior radiograph made after the tibiocalcaneal arthrodesis, demonstrating fixation with a 4.5-mm titanium blade-plate.

possible. Morcellized pieces of resected tibial and fibular bone may also be used when bone grafting is needed primarily for extra-articular application. Large, threaded Steinmann pins, compression blade-plates, or custom intramedullary rods are used in whatever combination provides adequate rigid internal fixation (Figs. 6 and 7).

Use of a plate on the plantar aspect of the medial column of the midfoot has been advocated to enhance the rigidity of an arthrodesis of the midfoot.[22] External fixation provides adequate stability, but positioning of the foot and ankle is more difficult with an external fixator; such fixation is reserved for patients who have an

open wound and need osseous stabilization. Problems at the pin sites may also force early removal of the fixator, leading to nonunion or malunion.

Long-term immobilization is crucial for achieving union. In general, the duration of immobilization after an arthrodesis for patients who have neuropathic arthropathy is twice as long as that for patients who do not have neuropathic arthropathy. The postoperative regimen includes 3 months of nonweightbearing in a total-contact cast followed by 1 to 2 months in a weightbearing total-contact cast. The patient then is managed with a bivalved ankle-foot orthosis with a rocker sole added to the footplate until the use of footwear and a definitive brace is possible. Bracing is continued for 12 to 18 months postoperatively, as in the treatment of a neuropathic fracture. After an arthrodesis of the midfoot, an extra-depth shoe with an extended steel shank and a rocker sole may be used if there is little swelling and the fusion is solid. For patients who have involvement of the hindfoot and ankle, this type of shoe is attached either to a double-upright calf-lacer or a patellar-ligament-bearing ankle-foot orthosis (Figs. 8 and 9). A custom-molded polypropylene ankle-foot orthosis may be used inside a shoe with a rocker sole if the deformity of the foot is not severe.

When there is a severe deformity of the foot, it is preferable to use whatever shoe-and-foot-orthosis combination accommodates the foot deformity and then to have the shoe attached to a double-upright brace. A custom-molded polypropylene ankle-foot orthosis that extends into the foot region takes up space in the shoe and may not adequately accommodate a severe deformity of the foot, thereby causing a recurrent ulcer. After an arthrodesis of the midfoot, hindfoot, or ankle, use of a brace is necessary for at least the first 12 to 18 months, to allow complete healing and a return to weightbearing. Arthrodesis of the ankle, hindfoot, or midfoot at the level of the talonavicular joint is prone to either recurrent Charcot changes at adjacent joints or stress fractures[14] and should be protected with use of a brace indefinitely. After an arthrodesis

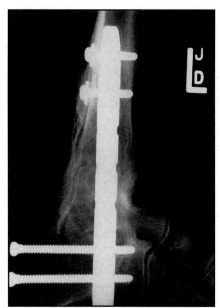

Fig. 6 Lateral radiograph made 7 months after a tibiotalocalcaneal arthrodesis through a posterior approach, showing fixation with a retrograde locked intramedullary nail.

of the midfoot distal to the level of the talonavicular joint, stability of the site is provided with use of an extra-depth shoe with a total-contact insert, an extended steel shank, and a rocker sole.

The choice of whether to wean a patient from the ankle-foot orthosis at 12 to 18 months after an arthrodesis depends on multiple factors, including union and stability at the site of the arthrodesis, the location of the arthrodesis, and the reliability as well as the activity level of the patient. After an arthrodesis of the hindfoot involving the tibiotalocalcaneal joint, active patients may be prone to stress fractures in the distal part of the tibia when a brace is not used for strenuous activities because the foot acts as a long, rigid lever arm that places stresses on the tibia[14] (Fig. 7).

Results of Reconstruction of a Charcot Joint

The rates of union reported after arthrodesis of the foot and ankle for

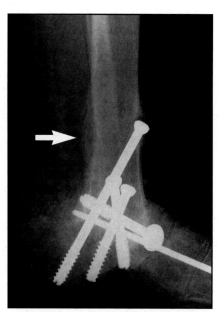

Fig. 7 Radiograph made after a tibiotalocalcaneal arthrodesis that was stabilized with multiple partially threaded cannulated screws augmented with a single threaded Steinmann pin. Note the healed stress fracture (arrow) through the proximal screw-hole in the tibia, which had occurred when the patient walked without a brace 7 months postoperatively. The fracture was treated for 12 weeks with a total-contact cast followed by resumption of the use of a brace. This stress fracture might have been prevented by the insertion of a more distal screw, avoiding the crest of the tibia, and if the patient had complied better with the postoperative use of the brace.

the treatment of neuropathic deformity in 143 patients in 8 clinical series averaged 70% (range, 54% to 100%).[1-7] However, the goal of achieving a stable foot on which a brace or a shoe, or both, could be worn was attained for 87% (124) of the patients after the initial surgical procedure, regardless of whether or not a solid union or a stable nonunion had been achieved.[1-7] Complications that may lead to failure of the procedure and necessitate a repeat procedure include a deep wound infection, an unstable nonunion, and a malunion.

Although authors of earlier reports

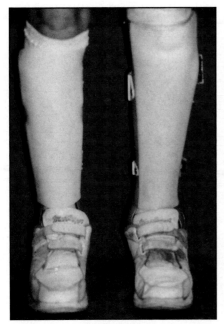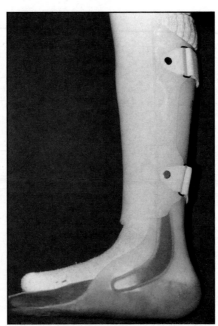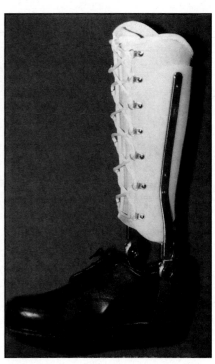

Fig. 8 The 2-piece polypropylene clamshell-type ankle-foot orthosis used for immobilization of an Eichenholtz stage-II or stage-III neuropathic fracture or after arthrodesis of the hindfoot for the treatment of a neuropathic deformity.

Fig. 9 Double-upright modified calf-lacer ankle-foot orthosis attached to an extra-depth shoe with an extended steel shank and a rocker sole. This style of orthosis is used when there is a severe deformity of the foot that needs to be accommodated by specialized footwear.

have expressed caution with respect to the performance of an arthrodesis for the treatment of neuropathic arthropathy,[6,23] modern techniques of internal fixation and prolonged immobilization have substantially increased the rate of union and decreased the rate of complications. The rate of satisfaction with these procedures is high, in large part because pain is not a major factor.[1,2,4,5,24] Most patients are grateful if the ability to walk in an appropriate shoe or brace is restored and an amputation is avoided.

In a recent study, 32 arthrodeses were performed for the treatment of neuropathic deformities of the foot and ankle; the series included 27 feet (25 patients) (unpublished data, 1996). Five of these procedures had been preceded by an initial attempt at realignment arthrodesis; 2 were repeat arthrodeses, and 3 were plantar ostectomies. Including the reoperations, 26 (96%) of the 27 feet were eventually rendered stable and the

patient was able to wear a brace. The goals of surgery were not met in 1 patient, who developed a deep infection requiring transtibial amputation.

The Dilemma Concerning Reconstructive Procedures in Patients Who Have Charcot Arthropathy

Because of the technical difficulty involved in managing patients who have Charcot arthropathy as well as the potential complications and the prolonged duration of treatment that is required, some practitioners may offer an amputation rather than reconstruction to treat a neuropathic deformity that does not allow use of a brace. Previous studies on energy expenditure according to level of amputation have demonstrated that the more distal the level of the amputation, the less energy expended during walking.[25] Therefore, it would be logical that a patient with a Charcot deformity who has been managed

with reconstruction would expend less energy during walking and may have a higher level of function than would a patient who has been managed with an amputation, especially a patient who has limited cardiovascular reserves.

Perhaps the most compelling reason for limb salvage is the long-term uncertainty about the status of the other foot. Peripheral vascular disease or an ulcer on the contralateral foot may lead to a deep wound infection, necessitating an amputation in the future. Reconstruction instead of amputation for the treatment of a neuropathic deformity in a patient who is a candidate for reconstruction may allow the patient to avoid eventual bilateral amputation.

Overview

Reconstruction of the Charcot foot and ankle is a valuable technique for the management of a patient who has a severe deformity that cannot be treated with use of appropriate footwear and a brace. The goals of surgery are to allow the patient to wear a shoe and a brace and to prevent amputation. Despite complications, the overall rate of success is more than 80%.[1-7] Stability and appropriate alignment are more important than union for achieving a successful result. Meticulous handling of the soft tissues and rigid internal fixation with use of bone-grafting are important parts of the surgical technique. Prolonged immobilization is necessary. Limb salvage with realignment and arthrodesis of a severely deformed foot and ankle allows most patients to avoid amputation and probably provides a more functional limb. Use of these surgical indications and techniques results in a high degree of patient satisfaction.

References

1. Alvarez RG, Barbour TM, Perkins TD: Tibio-calcaneal arthrodesis for nonbraceable neuropathic ankle deformity. *Foot Ankle Int* 1994;15: 354–359.

2. Bono JV, Roger DJ, Jacobs RL: Surgical arthrodesis of the neuropathic foot: A salvage procedure. *Clin Orthop* 1993;296:14–20.

3. Early JS, Hansen ST: Surgical reconstruction of the diabetic foot: A salvage approach for midfoot collapse. *Foot Ankle Int* 1996;17:325–330.

4. Papa J, Myerson M, Girard P: Salvage, with arthrodesis, in intractable diabetic neuropathic arthropathy of the foot and ankle. *J Bone Joint Surg* 1993;75A:1056–1066.

5. Sammarco GJ, Conti SF: Surgical treatment of neuroarthropathic foot deformity. *Foot Ankle Int* 1998;19:102–109.

6. Stuart MJ, Morrey BF: Arthrodesis of the diabetic neuropathic ankle joint. *Clin Orthop* 1990; 253:209–211.

7. Tisdel CL, Marcus RE, Heiple KG: Triple arthrodesis for diabetic peritalar neuroarthropathy. *Foot Ankle Int* 1995;16:332–338.

8. Sinha S, Munichoodappa CS, Kozak GP: Neuro-arthropathy (Charcot joints) in diabetes mellitus. *Medicine* 1972;51:191–210.

9. American Diabetes Association: *Diabetes: 1996 Vital Statistics.* Alexandria, VA, American Diabetes Association, 1996, p 13.

10. Eichenholtz SN (ed): *Charcot Joints.* Springfield, IL, CC Thomas, 1966.

11. Brodsky JW, Rouse AM: Exostectomy for symptomatic bony prominences in diabetic Charcot feet. *Clin Orthop* 1993;296:21–26.

12. Cofield RH, Morrison MJ, Beabout JW: Diabetic neuroarthropathy in the foot: Patient characteristics and patterns of radiographic change. *Foot Ankle* 1983;4:15–22.

13. Harris JR, Brand PW: Patterns of disintegration of the tarsus in the anaesthetic foot. *J Bone Joint Surg* 1966;48B:4–16.

14. Mitchell JR, Johnson JE, Collier BD, Gould JS: Stress fracture of the tibia following extensive hindfoot and ankle arthrodesis: A report of three cases. *Foot Ankle Int* 1995;16:445–448.

15. Johnson JE, Kennedy EJ, Shereff MJ, Patel NC, Collier BD: Prospective study of bone, indium-111-labeled white blood cell, and gallium-67 scanning for the evaluation of osteomyelitis in the diabetic foot. *Foot Ankle Int* 1996;17:10–16.

16. Schauwecker DS, Park HM, Burt RW, Mock BH, Wellman HN: Combined bone scintigraphy and indium-111 leukocyte scans in neuropathic foot disease. *J Nucl Med* 1988;29: 1651–1655.

17. Mueller MJ: Identifying patients with diabetes mellitus who are at risk for lower-extremity complications: Use of Semmes-Weinstein monofilaments. *Phys Ther* 1996;76:68–71.

18. Brodsky JW: The diabetic foot, in Mann RA, Coughlin MJ (eds): *Surgery of the Foot and Ankle,* ed 6. St. Louis, MO, Mosby-Year Book, 1993, pp 877–958.

19. Johnson JE: Surgical reconstruction of the diabetic Charcot foot and ankle. *Foot Ankle Clin* 1997;2:37–55.

20. Myerson MS, Henderson MR, Saxby T, Short KW: Management of midfoot diabetic neuroarthropathy. *Foot Ankle Int* 1994;15:233–241.

21. Russotti GM, Johnson KA, Cass JR: Tibiotalocalcaneal arthrodesis for arthritis and deformity of the hind part of the foot. *J Bone Joint Surg* 1988;70A:1304–1307.

22. Schon LC, Marks RM: The management of neuroarthropathic fracture-dislocations in the diabetic patient. *Orthop Clin North Am* 1995; 26:375–392.

23. Cleveland M: Surgical fusion of unstable joints due to neuropathic disturbance. *Am J Surg* 1939;43:580–584.

24. Myerson MS, Alvarez RG, Brodsky JW, Johnson JE: Symposium: Neuroarthropathy of the foot. *Contemp Orthop* 1993;26:43–64.

25. Pinzur MS, Gold J, Schwartz D, Gross N: Energy demands for walking in dysvascular amputees as related to the level of amputation. *Orthopedics* 1992;15:1033–1036.

35

Periarticular Osteotomies: The Importance of Limb Alignment

Haemish A. Crawford, MBChB, FRACS
Annunziato Amendola, MD, FRCSC

Introduction

The role of the periarticular osteotomy in the ankle is to restore the mechanical alignment of the lower limb and to normalize the joint contact forces across the ankle joint as much as possible. In the lower limb, the planning, surgical techniques, and clinical outcomes of periarticular osteotomies of the hip and knee have been reported extensively. However, few papers have addressed the role of osteotomy in the treatment of osteoarthritis of the ankle,[1–3] perhaps because of the very low incidence of primary osteoarthritis in the ankle compared with the other joints.[1] Malalignment can lead to increased point contact forces across the joint and result in osteoarthritis in the affected "compartment" of the joint[4–6] (Fig. 1). Chronic compensation of a joint to adjacent malalignment can lead to joint overload and secondary osteoarthritis. Not only can malalignment of a long bone lead to osteoarthritis as in Figure 1, but, fusing a joint in a malreduced position can lead to premature osteoarthritis in adjacent joints of the same limb. In malunited ankle fractures, often correction of the malunion is all that is necessary. However, axial alignment must be assessed and corrected to prevent failure of the reconstructive procedure (Fig. 2).

Etiology of Osteoarthritis

Trueta[7] showed that osteoarthritis was a result of biochemical changes in the deep chondral layers of the cartilage and in the subchondral bone. With malalignment of the limb, the uneven contact pressures cause a vascular change in this area, leading to poor nutrition and subsequent death in the deep chondral cells, which results in fibrillation and subsequent degeneration of the cartilage. In addition to the increased point contact stress with malalignment, there is also an increased shear force on the cartilage if the joint surface is no longer perpendicular to the long axis of the bone.[8] An assumption often made in realigning a deformed limb is that in the new position "normal" cartilage will be loaded; however, this cartilage may have an underlying biologic derangement as in primary osteoarthritis or have been damaged in the same preceding trauma.

Both the proximity of the angular deformity to the joint and the position the joint is in contribute to the contact area and subsequent forces across the joint. In cadaver studies, it has been shown that a substantial decrease in tibiotalar contact area occurs when there is a distal tibial fracture angulated in recurvatum or antecurvatum.[4,5,9] An even smaller area of contact is present when the foot is placed in plantarflexion or dorsiflexion as well. A more proximal tibial fracture has its greatest effect on the knee, while middle third angulations in the tibia cause a minimal change in contact pressures in the knee or ankle. The subtalar joint may protect the ankle joint from premature osteoarthritis due to limb malalignment.[6] The ankle joint is most congruent in the neutral position, and the orientation of the subtalar joint axis helps maintain this congruency during the gait cycle. Inman[10] was the first to show that the subtalar joint compensates for tibial varus and valgus deformities and, more recently, cadaver studies have shown that the greatest decreases in contact area in the tibiotalar joint occur when the angulated tibia is loaded in the presence of a fixed subtalar joint.[6] The downside of these compensatory changes in the subtalar joint is that premature arthritis may occur in this joint as a result of altered forces across the joint.

Staging

The optimum time for intervention in the osteoarthritic ankle is difficult to ascertain, because the natural history of early changes in the tibiotalar

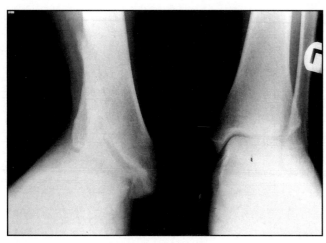
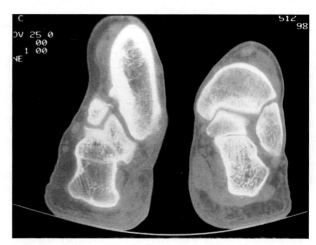

Fig. 1 Residual valgus deformity of the ankle joint and congenital tibial pseudoarthrosis. Although the hindfoot is in neutral through the subtalar joint, the obliquity of the ankle joint precludes long-term success.

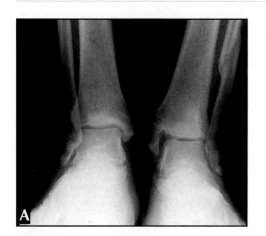
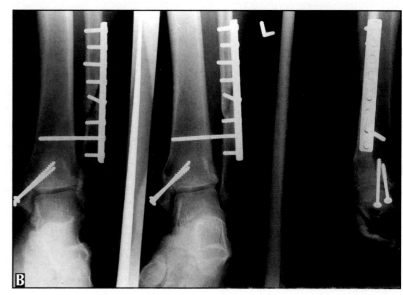
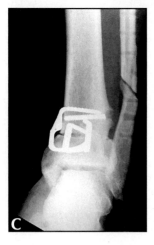

Fig. 2 A, A malunited AO Type C fibular fracture and medial malleolar fracture. **B,** A corrective osteotomy to realign the fracture fails due to failure to address the mechanical axis. **C,** Mechanical axis correction through distal tibial osteotomy using staples for fixation.

joint associated with malalignment is not clearly determined. The classification system produced by Takakura and associates[1] (Table 1) for primary osteoarthritis is useful in considering the surgical options for a patient with an arthritic ankle.[1] Stage 4 can usually be treated by arthrodesis and stage 1 by nonsurgical means. However, stages 2 and 3 present the most challenging decision making to the orthopaedic surgeon. It is in these lower

Table 1
Classification of ankle arthritis from weightbearing radiographs

Stage 1	No joint space narrowing; early sclerosis and osteophyte formation
Stage 2	Medial joint space narrowing
Stage 3	Joint space obliterated with subchondral bone contact medially
Stage 4	Whole joint space obliterated with complete bone contact

stages that periarticular osteotomy of the ankle may have some role in trying to prevent progression of the arthritis. More frequent use of ankle arthroscopy and magnetic resonance imaging (MRI) may help provide a more accurate assessment of the articular surface and influence the indications for osteotomy (Fig. 3).

Assessment of Limb Alignment

The assessment of limb alignment is difficult, because mechanical axis deviation accounts for all types of deformity: rotation, angulation, and translation. Not only is the overall limb alignment important (the mechanical axis) but the orientation of each joint to the anatomic axis of the individual bones also needs to be assessed. The most common way of assessing overall limb alignment is a standing long leg radiograph of both legs with the X-ray beam centered on the knee (Fig. 4). This examination is useful as it allows comparison of one limb to the other. However, it does not address the mechanical axis during the single leg stance phase of gait; which a single standing radiograph of each individual limb achieves. These radiographs should be taken with the patella facing directly forward equally centered between the femoral condyles, which characteristically results in a mortise view of the ankle joint.[11] These radiographs have been developed primarily for assessing the mechanical axis of the limb to assist

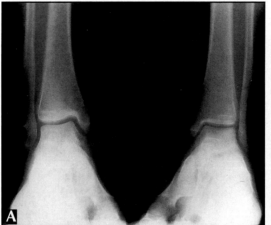
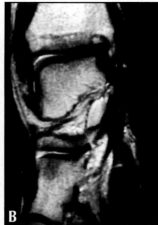
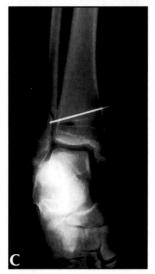
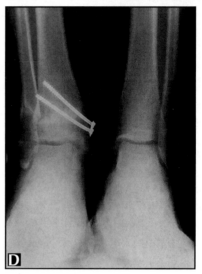

Fig. 3 A, Malunited bimalleolar fracture. **B,** MRI evaluation can be valuable to confirm medial overload. **C,** Intraoperative technique using fluoroscopic guidance for the fibular osteotomy and the opening wedge osteotomy of the tibia. **D,** Fixation is necessary on the tibial side.

in the preoperative planning of knee surgery.[12–14] The ankle joint is usually found right at the bottom edge of the radiograph, often with the subtalar joint missing and with the X-ray beam centered on the knee, which makes it difficult to calculate the tibiotalar angle. Any deformity distal to the ankle joint must also be recorded with the radiograph.

There is variation in the literature as to which bony landmark should be used to measure the tibiotalar angle. Either a line at a tangent to the dome of the talus or a line at a tangent to

the tibial diaphysis has been used.[1,13,15–17] Despite these variations, a number of authors have calculated the lateral distal tibial angle (LDTA) in representative samples of the normal population (Table 2).

In assessing deformity, the routine procedure is to take anteroposterior (AP) and lateral radiographs of the affected limb. However, these projections do not always lie in the plane of maximum deformity, and therefore may underestimate the degree of malalignment. In order to assess the deformity in more detail, further

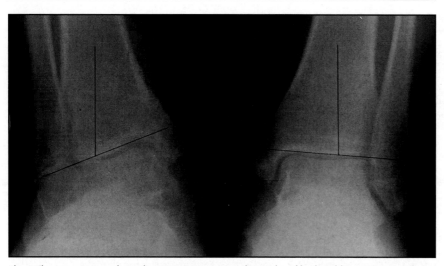

Fig. 4 The importance of standing anteroposterior radiographs of both ankles to measure the weightbearing deformity in the ankle joint.

Table 2 The variation in the lateral distal tibial angle (LDTA)	
Moreland[13]	89.8° +/-2.7° valgus
McKie[15]	91.4° +/-3.8° varus
Chao[16]	92.9° +/-3.3° varus
Takakura[2]	91° varus

radiographs can be taken at different angles, or else sophisticated algebraic equations can be used to determine the exact deformity.[18-20] As well as the angulation and translation deformity seen on plane radiographs, consideration must also be given to any rotational deformity that may co-exist.[21] Computed tomography (CT) scanning is an accurate way of measuring rotation.[22] If the patient does not move while being scanned, the resultant scan is not limb position dependent or technician dependent (Fig. 5). The published results of tibial rotation measured by CT scanning vary because of the definition of the reference axis chosen by the authors.[22-24] Eckhoff and Johnson[24] showed in a cadaver model that significant variation and tibial version existed between their 5 specimens, with a range of 15° to 30°. They used a reference axis of the proximal tibia as a line joining the posterior bony prominences of the tibia at least 2 mm distal to the articular surface but no more than 20 mm distal to the joint line. The reference axis of the distal tibia was a line joining the 2 most distal points of the malleoli.

Preoperative Planning

Before discussing the actual techniques for periarticular osteotomies of the ankle joint, it is necessary to consider the principles of correcting lower limb malalignment.[23] Before any surgical correction, there must be an adequate soft-tissue envelope, ankle joint stability, and sufficient joint motion to allow a functional range of motion after the osteotomy. The general medical condition of the patient must also be considered, especially any underlying vascular disease or diabetes mellitus. Once surgery has been decided on, the deformity has to be defined as part of the preoperative planning so that the appropriate procedure will be carried out. In most cases in the ankle joint, the deformity is a result of trauma to the distal tibia, physeal arrest in the growth plate at some time in childhood, or, rarely, because of idiopathic osteoarthritis. Consideration must be given to the whole limb alignment, as there may be a multilevel deformity, requiring a 2-level correction. Paley and associates[25] defined the center of rotation and angulation (CORA) as being the intersection point of the

proximal and distal mechanical or anatomic axis in the tibia. If there is a single level deformity, these 2 axes will intersect at the apex of the deformity. If they do not intersect here, then a multiplanar deformity or translation component must also be present. The orientation of the ankle joint to the mechanical or anatomic axis is calculated so that any rotational malalignment can also be corrected. One deformity often overlooked is leg-length inequality secondary to trauma or growth arrest. If this coexists with the malalignment, it can be corrected with an opening wedge osteotomy, if it is a small deformity, or by distraction osteogenesis, if greater length is required. If 2-level deformity is present, ie, varus gonarthrosis of the knee and ankle, then the proximal deformity should be addressed first. The reasons for this approach are twofold. First, it is difficult to assess the effect of proximal tibial osteotomy on the ankle alignment, and second, the proximal realignment may resolve some or most of the symptoms. If an arthrodesis of the ankle or foot is planned, proximal alignment correction should be carried out before any arthrodesis to avoid malposition of the fixed arthrodesis.

Because the mechanical axis is drawn from a point in the center of the femoral head to the center of the ankle joint, deformities in the femoral neck or tibial plafond may result in very little overall limb malalignment but marked joint malorientation. In these cases, it is necessary to calculate

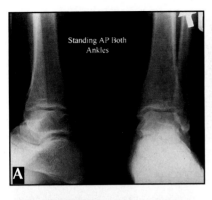

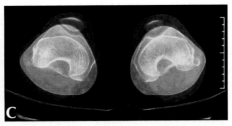

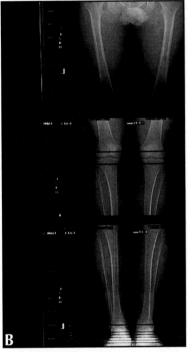

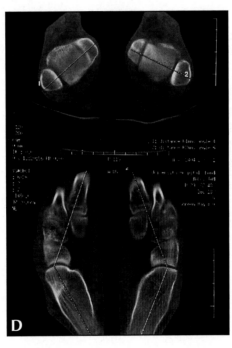

Fig. 5 A case of idiopathic tibial rotation deformity. **A,** Standing anteroposterior radiograph demonstrates the abnormal rotation in the right ankle. **B,** To assess the degree of rotation superimposed computed tomography (CT) at the hip, knee, ankle, and foot are used. **C,** No rotational deformity at the level of the knee. **D,** The rotational deformity can be seen at the ankle and foot levels.

the lateral distal tibial angle (LDTA) from the contralateral normal limb to help plan the amount of correction necessary.[25] The above has only outlined malalignment and malorientation in the sagittal plane. Malalignment in the coronal (lateral plane) is also calculated so that it can be corrected at the time of the osteotomy. Takakura and associates[2] found that the angle of the tibial joint surface on

the lateral view (TLS) indicated the amount of anterior opening of the joint, and they were able to correct this approximately 6° in the posttraumatic cases by doing an appropriate opening wedge osteotomy.

Technique

An opening medial wedge osteotomy is used to correct a varus ankle joint, and a closing medial wedge osteotomy

is used for a valgus ankle. The medial side is much easier to approach and less destructive. The advantages of a closing wedge osteotomy are that it offers more inherent stability and does not require a bone graft. However, it does shorten the limb. An opening wedge osteotomy, on the other hand, usually requires internal fixation and structural bone graft, which results in lengthening of the shortened limb (Fig. 6). The opening wedge valgus osteotomy is performed at the level of the deformity or, if this is not possible, 4 cm proximal to the ankle joint line. If the distal tibial growth plate is still open, the osteotomy should be performed at least 3 cm proximal to the epiphyseal plate. An oblique osteotomy of the fibula is performed first at the same level as the site of the tibial osteotomy to allow angulation of the fibula. The tibial malalignment is corrected, which prevents deformation of the tibiofibular syndesmosis. An incomplete horizontal osteotomy is made through the tibia parallel to the distal tibial joint line, using the lateral tibial cortex as a fulcrum for the correction. The preplanned correction can then be performed and checked with the image intensifier before tricortical bone graft from the iliac crest is impacted into the bony defect. The use of rigid internal fixation, as shown in Figure 7, allows early weightbearing and movement of the ankle joint, which may avoid the postoperative stiffness that can occur when Kirschner wires alone are used.

Primary osteoarthritis of the ankle is a rare condition in which the deformity is characteristically in varus, with increased anterior opening of the tibiotalar joint. The condition has its highest incidence in Japanese women and is thought to be caused by the way they sit cross-legged. If the varus

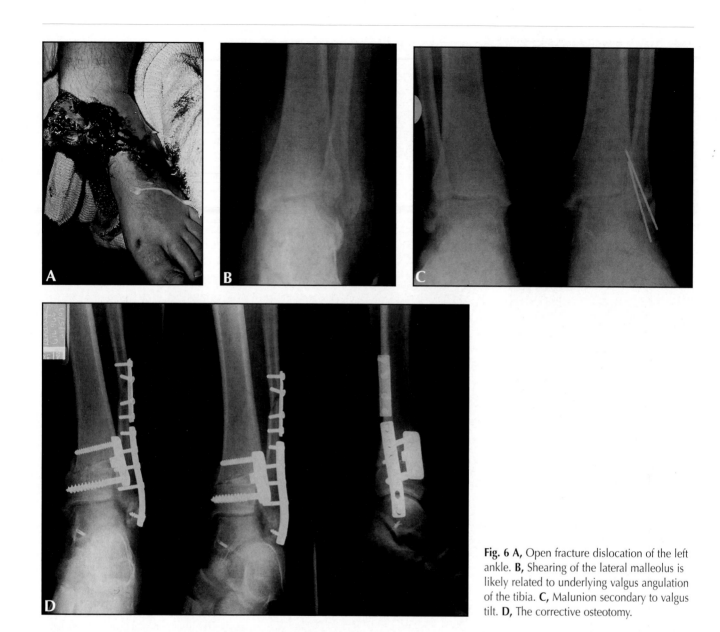

Fig. 6 A, Open fracture dislocation of the left ankle. **B,** Shearing of the lateral malleolus is likely related to underlying valgus angulation of the tibia. **C,** Malunion secondary to valgus tilt. **D,** The corrective osteotomy.

Fig. 7 A and **B,** Medial compartment osteoarthritis secondary to tibial malunion in the AP and lateral planes. **C,** Correction of distal tibial deformity in 2 planes.

deformity of the ankle is so great that the subtalar joint cannot compensate for it, osteoarthritis may develop on the medial side of the joint. After arthroscopic evaluation, Takakura and associates[1] performed distal tibial opening wedge osteotomies on 18 patients, with an excellent result in 6 cases, good in 9, fair in 3, and poor in none after an average follow-up of 6 years, 9 months.

The timing of the surgery is one of the crucial decisions in all osteotomies. The natural history of osteoarthritis of the ankle is not well defined, as it is in the hip or the knee, which makes the decision of when to operate difficult. A high risk patient, as outlined earlier, who has a coronal deformity close to the joint and a stiff subtalar joint but no symptoms or radiographic changes may benefit from a prophylactic osteotomy. On the other hand, the patient with pain, varus alignment and radiographic and arthroscopic changes on the medial side of the joint may benefit from an opening wedge osteotomy, to unload this area and transfer the forces through the lateral compartment. Advanced osteoarthritis that requires arthrodesis, in which varus and valgus coexist, usually requires an osteotomy at the time of the arthrodesis to correct the alignment appropriately rather than attempt to correct the alignment through the ankle arthrodesis alone (Fig. 6).

Achieving correct limb alignment is most important in the success of any reconstructive procedure. Corrective osteotomy has a definite place in the treatment of ankle osteoarthritis.

References

1. Takakura Y, Tanaka Y, Kumai T, Tamai S: Low tibial osteotomy for osteoarthritis of the ankle: Results of a new operation in 18 patients. *J Bone Joint Surg* 1995;77B:50–54.

2. Takakura Y, Takaoka T, Tanaka Y, Yajima H, Tamai S: Results of opening wedge osteotomy for the treatment of a post-traumatic varus deformity of the ankle. *J Bone Joint Surg* 1998; 80A:213–218.

3. Graehl PM, Hersh MR, Heckman JD: Supramalleolar osteotomy for the treatment of symptomatic tibial malunion. *J Orthop Trauma* 1987; 1:281–292.

4. Tarr RR, Resnick CT, Wagner KS, Sarmiento A: Changes in tibiotalar joint contact areas following experimentally induced tibial angular deformities. *Clin Orthop* 1985;199:72–80.

5. Wagner KS, Tarr RR, Resnick C, Sarmiento A: The effect of simulated tibial deformities on the ankle joint during the gait cycle. *Foot Ankle* 1984;5:131–141.

6. Ting AJ, Tarr RR, Sarmiento A, Wagner K, Resnick C: The role of subtalar motion and ankle contact pressure changes from angular deformities of the tibia. *Foot Ankle* 1987;7: 290–299.

7. Trueta J: Studies on the etiopathology of osteoarthritis of the hip. *Clin Orthop* 1963;31:7–19.

8. Radin EL, Burr DB, Caterson B, Fyhrie D, Brown TD, Boyd RD: Mechanical determinants of osteoarthrosis. *Semin Arthritis Rheum* 1991;21(3 suppl 2):12–21.

9. McKellop HA, Llinas A, Sarmiento A: Effects of tibial malalignment on the knee and ankle. *Orthop Clin North Am* 1994;25:415–423.

10. Inman VT (ed): *The Joints of the Ankle.* Baltimore, MD, Williams & Wilkins, 1976.

11. Wright JG, Treble N, Feinstein AR: Measurement of lower limb alignment using long radiographs. *J Bone Joint Surg* 1991;73B:-721–723.

12. Bauer M, Bergstrom B, Hemborg A: Arthrosis of the ankle evaluated on films in weight-bearing position. *Acta Radiol (Stockh)* 1979;20:88–92.

13. Moreland JR, Bassett LW, Hanker GJ: Radiographic analysis of the axial alignment of the lower extremity. *J Bone Joint Surg* 1987;69A: 745–749.

14. Hsu RW, Himeno S, Coventry MB, Chao EY: Normal axial alignment of the lower extremity and load-bearing distribution at the knee. *Clin Orthop* 1990;255:215–227.

15. Tetsworth K, Paley D: Malalignment and degenerative arthropathy. *Orthop Clin North Am* 1994;25:367–377.

16. Chao EY, Neluheni EV, Hsu RW, Paley D: Biomechanics of malalignment. *Orthop Clin North Am* 1994;25:379–386.

17. Paley D, Tetsworth K: Mechanical axis deviation of the lower limbs: Preoperative planning of uniapical angular deformities of the tibia or femur. *Clin Orthop* 1992;280:48–64.

18. Green SA, Green HD: The influence of radiographic projection on the appearance of deformities. *Orthop Clin North Am* 1994;25:467–475.

19. Bar HF, Breitfuss H: Analysis of angular deformities on radiographs. *J Bone Joint Surg* 1989; 71B:710–711.

20. Ries M, O'Neill D: A method to determine the true angulation of long bone deformity. *Clin Orthop* 1987;218:191–194.

21. Eckhoff DG: Effect of limb malrotation on malalignment and osteoarthritis. *Orthop Clin North Am* 1994;25:405–414.

22. Jakob RP, Haertel M, Stussi E: Tibial torsion calculated by computerized tomography and compared to other methods of measurement. *J Bone Joint Surg* 1980;62B:238–242.

23. Jend HH, Heller M, Dallek M, Schoettle H: Measurement of tibial torsion by computer tomography. *Acta Radiol (Stockh)* 1981;22: 271–276.

24. Eckhoff DG, Johnson KK: Three-dimensional computed tomography reconstruction of tibial torsion. *Clin Orthop* 1994;302:42–46.

25. Paley D, Herzenberg JE, Tetsworth K, McKie J, Bhave A: Deformity planning for frontal and sagittal plane corrective osteotomies. *Orthop Clin North Am* 1994;25:425–465.

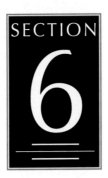

SECTION

6

Foot

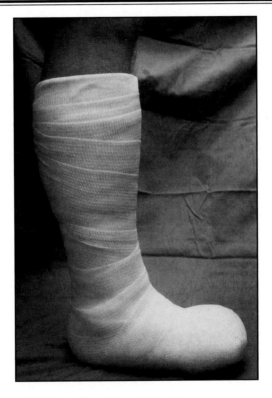

Evaluation of the Diabetic Foot

James W. Brodsky, MD

Introduction

It has been over 5 years since the last presentation of a course on the diabetic foot in the Instructional Course Lectures. In that interval, much additional knowledge, research, and practical strategies for treatment and diagnosis have evolved. The burgeoning interest in the diabetic foot has been manifested by work published in the literature of many different and diverse medical specialties, including orthopaedic surgery. The current Instructional Course on the diabetic foot was revised and expanded 4 years ago in response both to the growth in information that needs to be conveyed on this complex subject and to a rising interest among orthopaedic surgeons in surgical and nonsurgical problems of the diabetic foot.

The increasing interest of orthopaedists reflects a natural predilection of that specialty for understanding the pathology of and treating the lesions of the insensitive foot. Most of the lesions of the diabetic foot are related in some way to areas of abnormal pressure under or on the foot and/or to biomechanical abnormalities of the foot, ankle, and leg. As extremity specialists, and as specialists in the musculoskeletal system, it is gratifying to see both orthopaedic clinical practice and orthopaedic

research resources turned to the problems of the enlarging diabetic population in this and other developed countries.

In the current milieu of managed care in this country, orthopaedic surgeons are further motivated to provide comprehensive lower extremity care. The vast spectrum of disease, disorders, and injuries of the lower limb make it imperative that the principles of diabetic foot care form an integral part of our teaching literature. In this expanded format, authors expound on the diabetic foot according to the following topics: Outpatient diagnosis and management, James W. Brodsky, MD; Total contact casts, Stephen A. Conti, MD; Infections, Charles Saltzman, MD; Charcot joints, Jeffrey E. Johnson, MD; and Amputations of the foot, Douglas A. Smith, MD. My thanks to each of my fellow contributors for making this a successful teaching effort.

The Problem

Patients with diabetes have become an increasingly familiar part of the orthopaedic patient population. The number of diabetics in the United States has continued to increase, not only by virtue of increased numbers, but also as a result of greater recognition of a portion of the millions of undiagnosed patients. Estimates by

the American Diabetes Association are that the prevalence of diabetes totals 15.7 million people today (5.9% of the American population). Of these, fully one third are undiagnosed. The incidence of diabetes is high in our population as a whole, with variations noted among different ethnic and socioeconomic groups. More than half of the lower limb amputations in this country are performed in patients with diabetes. With greater longevity, the number of complications of the diabetes and the number of patients with multisystem complications continues to increase. Patients with unrelated trauma or degenerative musculoskeletal conditions are noted ever more frequently also to have diabetes and its complications. Infection, deformity, and dysfunction of the lower extremity that result from the effects of diabetes pose threats to other orthopaedic interventions. For example, patients with total knee or total hip arthroplasty are at risk from infected foot wounds because the distal lesions could seed the implants. Fractures of the ankle, even nondisplaced fractures, can become disasters of deformity and joint destruction in diabetics with peripheral neuropathy. Failure to recognize the loss of protective sensation that results from diabetic peripheral neuropathy, and, therefore, the increased risk of developing a neuropathic joint after fracture has produced countless cases of unhappy, even litigious patients. Knowledge of these complications is an important tool that enables the orthopaedic surgeon to inform the patient of the risks to the foot and ankle in diabetes. Moreover, orthopaedic surgeons are uniquely qualified to manage these complex musculoskeletal problems because of their training and experience in treating a wide range of lower limb problems and trauma, of prescribing shoes, and of comprehending the issues of gait and stability as they relate to the function of the entire lower limb. At times it can be a confusing, even a daunting, task to determine the proper specialty or combination of specialists to care for the multiple systems involved in the acutely or chronically ill patient with diabetes. These chapters on the diabetic foot should assist the reader in forming a treatment plan for patients who present with an acute diabetic foot problem.

Diabetic foot problems are estimated to account for approximately 25% of all diabetic hospital admissions. The economic impact of diabetic foot problems was estimated to reach $98 billion in the United States in 1997, representing $44 billion in actual medical costs and $54 billion in expenses related to disability and mortality. Although these statistics attempt to include the costs of lost productivity of workers with diabetes, the human impact on daily routines of family life, of work, and of recreation is truly widespread and inestimable. The American Diabetes Association noted 88 million disability days lost from work in 1997 as a result of diabetes. Early recognition of diabetic foot problems, prompt and proper diagnosis, patient education, and preventive care have been shown to be effective measures for reductions in morbidity and in cost to individuals, families, and society.[1]

Pathophysiology of the Diabetic Foot

Many factors contribute to the altered physiology and the pathologic states of the lower limb of diabetics. The major factors are neuropathy, vascular disease, deformity, immune abnormalities, gait and pressure abnormalities, local tissue factors, and systemic abnormalities.

Neuropathy

The primary cause or source of the vast majority of diabetic foot and ankle lesions, problems, and complications is diabetic peripheral neuropathy. Although they are not exclusively the effect of sensory neuropathy, most problems arise because the foot, leg, or parts thereof, are wholly or partially insensate.[2,3] Vascular disease and vascular abnormalities are common in diabetics and well recognized as a part of the complex combination of systemic influences on the feet of diabetic patients, but it is clear that most diabetic problems begin as a result of local trauma and tissue damage caused by the loss of or diminution of protective sensation. Injury to the bones and joints can occur following repetitive trauma, trivial trauma, or no recognized trauma at all. Most ulcers and infections are the result of a break in the soft-tissue envelope caused by unrecognized (unperceived) pressure.

This simple concept of the central, key role of neuropathy is frequently overlooked. Because the neuropathy cannot be reversed or ameliorated, most orthopaedic surgical and nonsurgical interventions are aimed at accommodating areas of pressure and compensating for the loss of protective sensation by substituting other methods of injury prevention, such as cushioning shoewear and insoles and routines for daily inspection of feet and of shoes.

Laboratory studies have demonstrated that repetitive low-level trauma to soft tissue can produce tissue inflammation and, ultimately, tissue necrosis, if sufficient cycles of trauma were applied to the limb. Even if each repetition is well below the threshold for tissue damage, the cumulative effect exceeds that threshold, resulting in ulceration. Histologic documentation of the progressive stages of cellular infiltrates of inflammation and necrosis have been demonstrated. In the final stage, tissue necrosis leads to tissue loss, ie, ulceration.[4] The same mechanism occurs in the diabetic foot, in which pressure under or over a bony prominence may not be particularly great, but eventually leads to soft tissue loss as a result of the many repetitions of the mechanical cycle of gait.

The most dramatic component of diabetic peripheral neuropathy is the sensory loss, but there are 3 different aspects of neuropathy. These are sensory, autonomic, and motor neuropathies.

Sensory Neuropathy Sensory neuropathy is the most important of the 3 forms of peripheral neuropathy, because it is most directly related to trauma to the lower extremity. Sensory neuropathy is the most critical contributing factor to neuropathic fractures, ulcerations, and skin breakdown. The absence of protective sensation leads to small injuries, catastrophic injuries, or a cumulative set of injuries to the foot. The neuropathy typically occurs in a stocking distribution, ie, it tends to be below the knee. It is progressively more dense as the examination progresses distally on the lower limb. This is consistent with the fact that ulcerations and infections over the toes and under the metatarsals are far more common than similar lesions around the ankle.

Testing for diabetic neuropathy is critical, even if the testing is very basic. To begin, a specific history inquiring about previous neuropathic events is essential. The examination for sensation can be brief. Even in the emergency department, one can test for light touch, pinprick, and position sense. The key is first to recognize the need to include this information in the orthopaedic history and physical, and second, to document the findings in the patient's record. Failure to identify the neuropathy in a patient with a fractured ankle can have long-reaching medical and even medicolegal ramifications if the otherwise appropriately treated fracture fails to heal and drifts into a neuropathic varus or valgus deformity.

The simplest, most reproducible, and currently most widely used method of testing for neuropathy is to use the Semmes-Weinstein monofilaments.[5,6] The monofilaments are relatively inexpensive, and are easy to use. They are graded on a logarithmic scale of the pressure that the filament applies, which is a function both of the cross-sectional area of the filament and of its stiffness (Fig. 1). The thicker, stiffer monofilaments require greater force to bend them. The monofilaments, made of a plastic filament embedded in a handle, are employed by holding the monofilament perpendicular to the skin. Pressure is applied through the handle on the tip until the filament begins to bend (Fig. 2). The patient, whose eyes are closed, registers whether or not the pressure is felt, ie, it is a threshold test. A small map can be constructed of the level and pattern of sensation from the knee and the toes. Most published investigations have indicated that the ability to

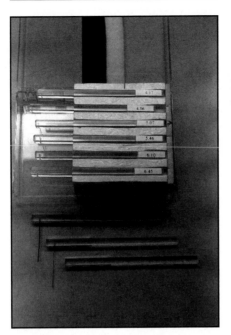

Fig. 1 Semmes-Weinstein monofilaments. Filaments are graded on a logarithmic scale. This set has a wide range.

feel the 5.07 monofilament correlates reasonably to a protective level of sensation in the majority of patients. However, a significant amount of work remains to be done on this subject, to refine the techniques and to define those patients who are exceptions to these guidelines. Moreover, significant variations in applied pressure occur with small variations in the angle of the filament to the skin. Despite these limitations, the Semmes-Weinstein monofilaments remain the most practical and clinically reproducible method currently available both for screening for neuropathy and for quantifying the density of peripheral neuropathy in the lower limbs of diabetics.

Autonomic Neuropathy Autonomic neuropathy is an "unseen" but very significant component of neuropathy. It is a major etiologic factor in the development of both soft-tissue and bony lesions. Autonomic neuropathy leads to abnormalities of

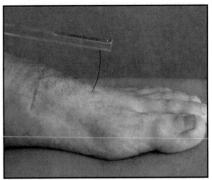

Fig. 2 Semmes-Weinstein monofilament is a threshhold test. Pressure is applied perpendicular to the skin until the filament begins to bend. The patient, with eyes closed, is asked to identify the touch of the monofilament.

regulation of skin temperature and sweating. The skin of the foot becomes dry and scaly. As it stiffens, it may crack easily, opening a portal in the dermis for bacteria to enter, the first step in infection. Fissures in the typical thick calluses on the plantar surface propagate through the skin.

The autonomic neuropathy plays an important role in neuroarthropathy, or Charcot joints. This effect has been likened by some authors to the effects of a severe autosympathectomy. The resulting loss of autoregulation in blood flow causes increased flow to the area. This hyperemia has been clinically noted by numerous studies of the Charcot foot in diabetes, and documentation of the lack of ischemia has been demonstrated.[7] Weakening of the tissues is postulated to occur from this hyperemia, leading to weakening or dissolution of the periarticular tissues, followed by joint collapse.

Motor Neuropathy Motor neuropathy contributes to deformity by way of the contractures that occur as a result of the dysfunction and scarring of the intrinsic muscles of the foot. This contracture leads to claw toe deformities. As the metatar-

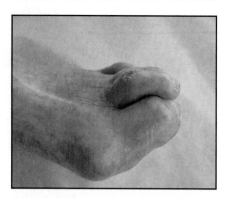

Fig. 3 The MTP joint hyper-extension deformity causes increased weightbearing pressure under the metatarsal head. He associated PIP joint flexion increases pressure over the dorsum of PIP joint, where it rubs against the shoe.

sophalangeal joints hyperextend, the base of the proximal phalanx migrates proximally and depresses the distal metatarsalgia (Fig. 3). This increases the mechanical pressure under the metatarsal head, leading to the classic metatarsal "mal perforans" ulceration on the plantar forefoot. The reciprocal flexion contracture at the interphalangeal joints creates dorsal prominences that rub against the toe box of the shoe, which lead to ulceration as well. Peroneal mononeuropathy is a special form of combined motor and sensory neuropathy that occurs occasionally. A foot drop, either unilateral or bilateral, is the motor result of the lesion.

Peripheral Vascular Disease

Peripheral vascular disease, in fact, all forms of atherosclerotic cardiovascular disease, are more prevalent, more severe, and occur at an earlier age in the diabetic compared to the nondiabetic population. The distribution throughout the extremity is more diffuse, particularly in the lower limb, and it can be rapidly progressive. It affects diabetic women more than women in the population in general. The lesions occur in the large vessels of the aortoiliac and femoral regions, but also have a wide distribution and peculiar characteristics in the infrapopliteal arterial tree.

Treatment of the proximal vascular lesions is an important part of the program for healing the diabetic foot. These patients will experience major improvement in the viability of the foot once the large, proximal lesions are treated with endarterectomy or a bypass procedure. Frequently, these proximal procedures are essential to overcome the distal ischemia of the foot and ankle.

Distal lesions of the arterial tree in the lower leg are characterized by diffuse involvement of all 3 of the vessels of the popliteal trifurcation, the anterior tibial, posterior tibial, and peroneal arteries. The lumenal narrowing is ragged and widespread, unlike the limited, discrete atherosclerotic lesions in the nondiabetic with vascular occlusive disease, which seldom occur below the knee. Histologically, diabetic and nondiabetic lesions differ in the location of the calcification, which is in the intimal layer in nondiabetics, but in the media in the arteries of diabetics. The latter leads to the pipe-like radiographic appearance of vessels on plain radiographs.

Treatment of distal arterial lesions usually requires a distal bypass procedure to whichever of the vessels is patent at or below the level of the ankle. Balloon angioplasty, selectively used in some medical centers, is applicable only in cases of a relatively isolated and discrete lesion, which, as noted above, is more the exception than the rule. The distal bypass procedures frequently use in situ saphenous vein grafts in which the venous valves have been cut, avoiding the need to reverse the vein within the limb. Salvage of a foot is frequently a function of the combined teamwork of the orthopaedic and vascular surgeons, who represent only two of the members of the multidisciplinary team required to treat the diabetic patient with foot problems.

Much has been discussed about the supposed "small vessel disease" in diabetics, but the anatomic lesion of this purported condition remains unidentified, and its very existence has been challenged by more than one author.[8–10] Changes in the capillary permeability and basement membrane thickening are well described, but there is no proof of a small vessel occlusive lesion, and the connection between these capillary changes and the occurrence of infection or ulceration remains unproved.[11] Blood flow in diabetics has been demonstrated to be the same as in other patients with peripheral neuropathy from other causes. Thus the cause of diabetic ulcerations cannot scientifically be ascribed to microvascular disease. Neuropathy continues to be a sufficient and pathophysiologically accurate explanation for most lesions.

Vascular disease has a large role in the presence of pain in the lower extremity of diabetic patients with neuropathic foot disease. This is separate and distinct from the pain of Charcot joints and the pain of the neuropathy itself. Contrary to the conventional wisdom that Charcot joints present with classical "painless swelling," previous studies have documented that about half of all patients with Charcot joints present with a chief complaint of pain;[7] although the pain is not commensurate with the degree of osseous destruction, as it would be felt in a nonneuropathic patient.

Paradoxically, the peripheral neuropathy of diabetes (and other etiologies as well), which produces a loss of sensory capacity, can, at the same time, cause painful dysesthesias. The treatment of dysesthesias usually consists of medication. The most commonly employed regimen is low-dose or medium-dose amitriptylline or nortriptylline, taken at bedtime. The medication is difficult to administer and difficult to take. The dosage must be slowly increased to titrate it to the level of the patient's symptoms while minimizing the frequent side effects of drowsiness and lethargy. Other medications used include other neuroleptics, such as hydantoin or tegretol, as well as mexitilene.[12,13] Some patients obtain relief from the use of topical capsaicin-containing creams. These nonprescription derivatives of chili peppers produce a burning sensation initially, but paradoxically reduce the burning and other dysesthesias after continued use. Intractable cases require consultation with a neurologist or pain management specialist. Painful dysesthesias remain a vexing chronic problem for which no treatment is uniformly applicable or wholly successful.

Most diabetic patients with neuropathy treated by the orthopaedic surgeon have altered but not absent sensation. As noted above, both Charcot arthropathy and peripheral neuropathy can cause pain. However, the most serious cause of pain is ischemia. The doctor (the whole health care team, actually) needs to be wary of the patient who complains of a painful distal lesion on the foot, the most common example of which is the "painful ingrown toenail." In patients with neuropathic ulcerations, it is unlikely that they have sufficient sensation to report pain from the nail or other distal source. In most instances, what is mistakenly reported as a painful nail or painful ulcer is actually the pain of distal ischemia. This rest ischemia is char-

acterized by a history of pain that is felt at night, often waking the patient from sleep, and is relieved by standing, or walking about. The dependent position of the lower limb increases the arterial flow to the foot through the marginal effect of gravity. Thoughtless but aggressive nail trimmings have resulted in below-knee amputations when the pain of ischemia is unrecognized. If the vascular status of the limb is uncertain, and if there are questionable pulses or no palpable pulses, then vascular testing must be undertaken before even the simplest procedure, such as nail trimming.

Deformity

Deformity of the foot and ankle, whether gross or subtle, usually leads to an area or areas of increased bony prominence. These areas produce various problems, including localized areas of pressure, gait abnormalities, and biomechanical malalignment of the limb. The diagnosis and treatment of these deformities is one aspect of the management of the diabetic foot that is particularly within the expertise of the orthopaedic surgeon.

The most common deformity, the clawed toe, is actually a combination of flexion deformities at the interphalangeal joints and extension deformity at the metatarsophalangeal joints. The severity is a function of the stiffness and irreducibility of the deformities. While hammertoes and clawtoes occur in the nonneuropathic population, the incidence appears to be higher in diabetics. The stiffness may be a function of the duration of the diabetes, the severity of the neuropathy, or the chronic level of elevated glucose (level of control of diabetic hyperglycemia). Limited joint mobility syndrome has been described in diabetics. It affects mul-

tiple joints, is not localized preferentially to the lower limb, and is caused by stiffening of the periarticular soft tissue. This stiffening is believed to occur as a result of glycosylation of the collagen in those tissues.[14,15]

Other deformities include local prominences of a Charcot joint, equinus deformities at the ankle and/or transverse tarsal joints, and varus and valgus deformities of the hindfoot and of the ankle. Dr. Johnson discusses Charcot deformities in detail in Chapter 34. These deformities can be the result of prolonged bedrest due to other medical conditions or can be caused by peroneal mononeuropathy. An equinus contracture can obviously cause dramatic abnormalities of gait. But the equinus can also be responsible for plantar metatarsal ulcerations caused by rigid pressure on the forefoot. It is important to identify proximal deformities that increase midfoot and forefoot pressures in order to properly diagnose the source of the pressure and take appropriate therapeutic steps. Another example would be recurrent ulceration under the lateral border of the foot at the base of the fifth metatarsal, in the presence of a varus hindfoot deformity due, for example, to a Charcot deformity in the subtalar joint. Resection of the base of the metatarsal may be insufficient to relieve the pressure borne on this spot, and it may be necessary to realign the hindfoot out of the varus deformity in order to solve the forefoot problem. Still, this example remains consistent with the principle of identifying the source of the pressure in neuropathic ulcerations. That source can be local, or augmented by proximal deformity.

Identification of deformity is an integral part of comprehending the primary formula for the development of neuropathic ulceration in the diabetic foot. While mildly oversimplified, it is accurate to say that all neuropathic ulceration requires the combination of 2 factors, insensitivity (caused by neuropathy) and pressure (usually caused by bony prominences). Patients without neuropathy who have deformity, such as a hammertoe or hallux valgus, report pain, but do not ulcerate because their intact sensibility of the foot protects them by causing pain at the site of the deformity. The opposite is also true. That is, patients with peripheral neuropathy generally do not ulcerate, especially over the midfoot and forefoot, in the absence of a source of pressure, either internal or external. The internal source would be the bony prominence and the external source would be either pressure from a shoe or applied trauma to the soft tissue. Ulcerations in the plantar arch are uncommon because there is no source of pressure in this area unless the patient has a type 1 midfoot Charcot breakdown, with collapse or reversal of the bony arch.[16] Thus, the most common sites of diabetic foot ulceration in the absence of a Charcot joint are under the metatarsal heads, the medial sesamoid, the dorsum of the interphalangeal joints of the toes, the navicular tuberosity, and the base of the fifth metatarsal.

Despite the central role of mechanical pressure in the development of neuropathic ulceration, it still remains ignored or unrecognized, especially by other medical specialists who participate in the care of the diabetic foot. Reduction or elimination of pressure is a fundamental role for the orthopaedic surgeon in the diabetic foot care team. Regardless of what kind of control we exert on local or systemic factors; regardless of the types of dressings we apply, or the choice of antibiotics, if we fail to treat the underlying pressure, the ulcera-

tions will either recur or will fail to heal primarily. Orthopaedic decision making with regard to the diabetic foot often involves the decision between external pressure relief, with casts, braces, shoes, and insoles, versus internal pressure relief, with bone resection or realignment.

The notable exception to this rule is the ulceration over the heel, especially the posterior aspect of the heel. These ulcers tend to be predominantly vascular in origin. Clinical experience has shown that they respond poorly to the weight-relieving measures, such as total contact casts, that are so effective in the forefoot and midfoot; because the source is not primarily mechanical. Patients with ulcerations over any portion of the heel—posterior, sides or plantar—need expeditious vascular evaluation. The fat pad under the heel is relatively vascular tissue. When a heel ulcer occurs, frequently there is occlusion, or stenosis of the arterial branches to the heel that arise from the posterior tibial artery, and revascularization must take priority consideration.

Immune Abnormalities

Diabetics do not necessarily have an increased susceptibility to bacterial infection, but once infection is present, many diabetic patients appear to have abnormalities in combating the infection. Laboratory studies have demonstrated the altered chemotaxis of polymorphonuclear leukocytes. Capillary abnormalities affect white cell migration as well.[17]

Gait Abnormalities

Numerous studies have documented gait abnormalities and increased pressures under the feet of diabetic patients with neuropathy.[18–21] These contribute to our understanding of the etiology of ulceration in patients with advanced neuropathy, and cor-

respond to the role of pressure in the development of ulceration in neuropathic feet. More work remains to be done to investigate gait abnormalities in diabetic patients.

Local Tissue Factors

Local tissue factors are conditions that may change the nutrition or perfusion of the soft tissue. They include edema of the tissue, callus formation, fungal colonization of the skin, or hyperkeratotic lesions.

Systemic Abnormalities

Systemic factors, apart from neuropathy and vasculopathy, that affect healing of lesions of the diabetic foot include control of diabetic hyperglycemia and the nutritional status of the patient. Several authors have stated that better control of the primary abnormality of the diabetes, hyperglycemia, resulted in better healing of the wounds of the lower limb.[22] Conversely, infection, including foot infection, is commonly recognized to be a source of sudden worsening in glucose control, with erratic and marked elevation of serum glucose. The surgical literature is replete with studies that point to the need for adequate nutrition for healing of surgical wounds. The same is true for healing of diabetic ulcers. The simple indices of nutrition that indicate whether or not the patient has adequate nutrition for wound healing are total lymphocyte count of $> 1500/ml$, total protein > 6.2 gm/dl, and albumin > 3.5 gm/dl.[23]

Diagnosis: Practical Evaluation of the Diabetic Foot and Diabetic Patient
History
A thorough history is the first step in diagnosis of this uniquely unpredictable and diversely manifest disease. It is particularly important to

include specific information needed to assess risk in the diabetic patient, including knowledge of a previous history of a neuropathic event, such as ulceration, Charcot joint, or extensive infection from minor injury. We need to know date of onset, and duration of diabetes; types of diabetes therapy, ie, insulin dependent or non-insulin dependent; duration of insulin therapy; frequency of blood glucose testing, and whether it is recorded; and visual function. Can the patient see well enough to use a glucometer, and to inspect his/her own feet and shoes? It is also helpful to inquire about flexibility (can the patient flex the hip and knee sufficiently to touch and see his/her own sole?); about mobility (use of walking aids such as crutches, walker, or wheelchair); about the distance the patient can walk, and symptoms of claudication with walking. We need to know the dates and nature of previous hospitalizations and surgeries for the feet, and the history of systemic disorders such as hypertension, renal disease, atherosclerotic heart disease, retinal surgery or corneal implants, and kidney or pancreas organ transplant. It is important to list immunosuppressive medications.

Physical Examination

Examination of the foot and ankle includes the following 6 areas of concern. Vascular testing includes capillary refill, color, warmth, and hair growth. Sensory testing includes light touch, pinprick and/or position sense, and Semmes-Weinstein monofilament testing. Testing of joints checks range of motion, and looks for contractures or deformities. Tendons are tested for equinus, Achilles contracture, and flexor and extensor contractures. Bones are examined for changes in arch, unusual bony prominences, and any change in shape or orientation

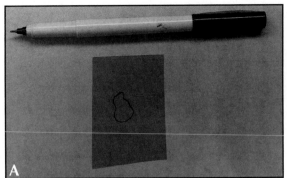
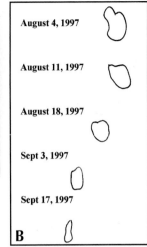

Fig. 4 A, The ulcer is traced on a clear film, and then, **B**, the ulcer outlined is traced into the chart to keep an accurate chronological record of ulcer size and shape.

of the foot. The skin is checked for breaks in the skin, onychomycosis, ingrown nails, and paronychia. Ulcerations, if present, are examined to determine site, depth, presence of granulation, exposed deep structures, surrounding cellulitis, proximal lymphangitis. Ulcers are traced onto clear film (Fig. 4, *A*) and the tracings are needed sequentially into the chart with date and orientation to give a chronologic record of ulcer size (Fig. 4, *B*).

Radiographs

Radiographs should be done standing, when possible. Standing films provide a technique that is easier to reproduce by different technologists or by the same technologist at different times. Some conditions, either local to the foot (such as a recent fracture) or systemic in the patient (poor balance, or an open plantar wound), may preclude the use of standing films. In these instances, a sitting film that places the foot plantigrade on or next to the radiographic cassette is preferable to films taken in the supine position, which have a rather unpredictable outcome. Interpretation of the films should include inspection for fractures and dislocations (either

recent or remote), deformity, Charcot joints, bone erosion in an area of a soft-tissue wound, and arterial calcification.

Vascular Studies

Laboratory evaluation of the vascular status of every diabetic patient is not necessary. Many, if not most, patients will present with strong and palpable pulses. In this situation, it is rarely necessary to incur the expense of conducting noninvasive vascular testing. However, when the patient clearly has diminished pulses, or pulses that cannot be felt at all, then vascular testing is most certainly indicated, particularly if the patient has a concurrent problem with the foot, such as a nonhealing ulcer, or a progressive infection. Vascular insufficiency should be suspected in nonhealing ulcers in which appropriate pressure-relieving measures have failed to produce significant improvement. The level of vascularity necessary to maintain the uninjured foot is much less than that required to heal the injured one. That is, any trauma (such as infection, ulcers, or surgery) increases the metabolic requirements of the foot and limb. In a foot that has marginal perfusion, any trauma (including surgi-

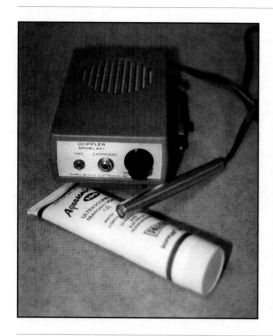

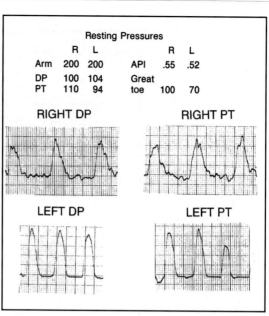

Resting Pressures

	R	L		R	L
Arm	200	200	API	.55	.52
DP	100	104	Great		
PT	110	94	toe	100	70

RIGHT DP   RIGHT PT

LEFT DP   LEFT PT

Fig. 5 Doppler arterial pulse-volume recording. (Reproduced with permission from Brodsky JW: Outpatient diagnosis and care of the diabetic foot, in Heckman JD (ed): *Instructional Course Lectures 42.* Rosemont, IL, American Academy of Orthopaedic Surgeons, 1993, pp 121–139.)

cal intervention) can push the patient over the edge of this fine balance, resulting in a nonhealing wound, or even gangrene.

Vascular evaluation usually begins with noninvasive testing. In patients who test positive and who have a clinical problem related to the arterial insufficiency (a nonhealing wound or osteomyelitis that requires debridement or partial foot amputation), consultation with a vascular surgeon is recommended. If reconstruction of the ischemia is considered, the vascular surgeon will usually order arteriography to demonstrate the lesions, their location, and severity.

There are several types of noninvasive vascular testing, but the 2 most commonly employed are arterial Doppler ultrasound and transcutaneous oxygen tension (TcPO$_2$) measurement. Multiple studies have been done evaluating both methods as predictors of amputation healing, that is, the ability to determine viable amputation levels preoperatively.[21] Fewer studies have been done evaluating these studies as predictors of healing of ulcerations. The literature suggests

that they are approximately equivalent in accuracy, although some advocates believe that the TcPO$_2$ measurement is more accurate. It is also somewhat more cumbersome and time-consuming and is somewhat temperature dependent. TcPO$_2$ measurement is not applicable distal to the midfoot, so it offers no equivalent to toe pressures with the Doppler technique. Arterial Doppler ultrasound has the advantage of being less expensive, less cumbersome, but more of an extrapolation, rather than direct data on blood flow. Arterial Dopplers are based on the assumption that flow in the vessel is proportionate to the amount of pressure required to compress the vessel to the point of occlusion. This is the same physiologic assumption on which the measurement of arterial blood pressure at the antecubital fossa is based. These blood pressures are taken in the same manner, with the exception of the use of an ultrasonic probe instead of a stethoscope. In noncalcified vessels, these assumptions are dependable, and the data is accurate relative to the established norms. The

ratio between the ultrasound-determined ankle arterial pressure and the same pressure method measuring at the antecubital fossa has been widely used. It has been referred to as the ankle-brachial index (ABI) or the ankle pressure index (API). Earlier references referred to this number as a reliable predictor of healing.[24,25] However, falsely elevated pressures are obtained when the Doppler technique is applied to the limb with arterial calcification, because greater pressures are necessary to occlude the stiffened, noncompliant vessel. Because vessel calcification is common in diabetes, it is necessary to look to additional information beyond the numbers and their ratios. Two more reliable forms of ultrasound information are toe plethysmography pressures and pulse-volume waveform recordings (Fig. 5). Toe pressures have been demonstrated to be a more accurate predictor of healing than ankle/arm ratios. Toes with an arterial pressure of 40 mm Hg or greater were shown to be most likely to heal. Below this level, healing was much less likely.[26] These pressures are measured using a small toe cuff. The vessels in the digits are less susceptible to the changes of calcification than those more proximal in the limb. Pulse volume recordings (PVRs) are tracings done on graph paper, similar to an electrocardiogram, which show the pattern of flow at a given level of ultrasound evaluation. PVRs demonstrate the quality of vessel compliance and whether or not there is pulsatile flow at a given level of the lower limb. The tracings demonstrate the pattern of the flow, which is related both to the compliance and patency of the vessel. Normal flow is triphasic (Fig. 5, *top right*) as demonstrated with the first and largest peak representing systole, the negative curve below baseline representing diastole, and the secondary smaller positive peak representing the contracture of the vessel walls. Biphasic and monophasic flow patterns demonstrate progressive loss of the normal resilience of the vessel wall (Fig. 5, *bottom left* and *right*). Both $TcPO_2$ and Doppler arterial ultrasound are screening techniques. The arteriogram is definitive, but not without its own risks, especially that of acute tubular necrosis from the contrast material. This risk is elevated if the patient is dehydrated.

The goal of vascular evaluation, and when needed, vascular reconstruction, is to provide adequate perfusion to the limb so that it can survive both injury and surgery. In nonemergent situations, revascularization by the vascular surgeon should precede orthopaedic surgery. In addition to aggressive debridement of infection and the use of partial foot amputation rather than below knee amputation where applicable, revascularization is a major factor in limb salvage surgery in the diabetic.

Laboratory Studies

Laboratory studies of the blood may be helpful in the presence of a severe

Table 1
The depth/ischemia classification of diabetic foot lesions

Grade	Definition	Treatment
Depth Classification		
0	The "at risk" foot. Previous ulcer, or neuropathy with deformity that may cause new ulceration	Patient education Regular examination Appropriate shoewear and insoles
1	Superficial ulceration, not infected	External pressure relief: Total contact cast, walking brace, special shoewear, etc
2	Deep ulceration exposing tendon or joint (with/without superficial infection)	Surgical debridement → wound care → pressure relief if closes and converts to grade 1 (PRN antibiotics)
3	Extensive ulceration with exposed bone, and/or deep infection: ie, osteomyelitis or abscess	Surgical debridements → ray or partial foot amputations → IV antibiotics → pressure relief if wound converts to grade 1
Ischemia Classification		
A	Not ischemic	Adequate vascularity for healing
B	Ischemia without gangrene	Vascular evaluation (Doppler, $TcPO_2$, arteriogram, etc.) → vascular reconstruction PRN
C	Partial (forefoot) gangrene of foot	Vascular evaluation → vascular reconstruction (proximal and/or distal bypass or angioplasty) → partial foot amputation
D	Complete foot gangrene	Vascular evaluation → major extremity amputation (BKA, AKA) with possible proximal vascular reconstruction

PRN, as needed; IV, intravenous; $TcPO_2$, transcutaneous oxygen pressure; BKA, below-knee amputation; AKA, above-knee amputation

(Reproduced with permission from Brodsky JW: The diabetic foot, in Mann RA, Coughlin MJ (eds): Surgery of the Foot and Ankle, ed 6. St. Louis, MO, Mosby Year Book, 1993, pp 1361–1467.)

infection in the foot of a diabetic. However, the white blood cell count (WBC), in particular, can be misleading in the presence of a major infection. Diabetics may fail to mount a febrile response, even in the presence of deep and extensive infection. This is even more true in the ever-increasing population of diabetics who have received kidney or combined kidney-pancreas transplants and are on life-long immunosuppressive drug regimens. When

there is clearly elevated WBC and local cellulitis, studies have documented the improvement in surgical outcome if the local and systemic parameters for infection are made to recede with wound care and intravenous antibiotics prior to performing definitive surgical resection and closing.[27]

Imaging Studies

Imaging studies can be a helpful part of the diagnostic evaluation of the diabetic foot. They should not be used routinely, but rather they are used to find occult fracture and early Charcot deformities (prior to radiographic changes), and to look for infection. Dilemmas arise, not infrequently, regarding the presence and extent of infection. It is critical to keep in mind that not all radiographic bone changes are caused by osteomyelitis. In fact, osteomyelitis is rarely seen in the diabetic foot unless there is or has been a contiguous break in the soft tissue. By contrast, diabetic osteopathy can include neuropathic fractures, spontaneous resorption of phalanges and distal portions of metatarsals, and extensive periosteal elevation along the tibia as a result of chronic venous stasis.

Cellulitis is far more common than abscess formation. If the latter is suspected, magnetic resonance imaging (MRI) is very helpful, as well as cost effective[28] for detecting deep infection. While MRI is a relatively expensive procedure, early application in suspected deep infection is a cost-saving strategy, because it can allow rapid decision-making with regard to surgical debridement. Early intervention may yield better results and reduce length of hospital stay by answering the diagnostic question.

However, it is important to understand the limitations of MRI. MRI has been shown to be extremely sensitive to changes in the bone, even more sensitive than a technitium-99 bone scan early in the disease process.[29] What the MRI has in sensitivity, it lacks in specificity with regard to imaging of the bone. Any disease process affecting the bone, or even adjacent to the bone, will cause a change in the bone signal because of edema (increased water content) of the marrow. This is not specific for osteomyelitis, which cannot be distinguished from trauma or fracture by MRI signal alone. However, in most medical centers and in the community, it is generally more cost-effective, if an occult fracture, or other bone process is suspected, to screen with a bone scan rather than with MRI. MRI is uniquely valuable in the detection and definition of the extent of soft-tissue lesions, such as abscess formation in the diabetic foot.

Once an area of suspected bone injury or occult Charcot process is identified, details of the exact nature and extent of the process should be obtained by complex motion tomography or computed tomography, which can then be directed to the area identified by the screening test. The classic example is the hot, red, swollen foot which is suspicious for abscess and appears cellulitic, in a patient who is afebrile and appears well systemically. While it is important to remember that the systemic response to infection in the extremity can often be blunted or absent in diabetic patients, the other diagnostic possibility is that this is the acute inflammation of a Charcot foot prior to the appearance of radiographic changes.

Even more confusing can be the case of a patient with a chronic Charcot foot that has collapsed, producing a bony prominence leading to ulceration. The patient presents with infection in the foot, but it is not clear whether the infection is confined to the soft tissues, or whether it involves the bone (osteomyelitis). In this situation combined, simultaneous Tc-99 bone scan and Indium-labeled white blood cell scan can sometimes make this distinction.[30] However, this technique also has its drawbacks and limitations. First, it is cumbersome and time-consuming, and it requires an experienced team to administer and properly time the 2 separate administrations of radionu-clides, because this is a test that spans 24 to 30 hours. Second, the interpretation of the Indium study can be frustrating or inconclusive because the low level of counts produce poor spatial resolution, and make interpretation difficult in a substantial number of cases.

Wound Classification

Wound classification of the diabetic foot began with the landmark system developed by Wagner and Meggitt at Rancho Los Amigos in the 1970s. In the Wagner-Meggitt classification,[24] there were 5 grades, which described the wound and also the condition of the entire foot. The depth of the wound, the association with infection, and the vascular status of the wound are all included in this classification. It has been the standard by which description of diabetic soft-tissue lesions could be compared throughout the world, and it is one of the most frequently cited works in the field of the diabetic foot. Because the Wagner-Meggitt classification was the earliest classification system, several other wound and foot wound classifications have emerged in recent years to advance our ability to describe the lesions and conditions of the diabetic foot, excluding, on the whole, the conditions and stages of Charcot joints.[31]

The Depth-Ischemia Classification (Table 1), a modification of the Wagner classification, has several advantages. It is simple and easy to remember, and its principles are familiar. It addresses the viability and condition of the foot by separately describing the wound and the underlying vascular status of the foot.

In the Depth-Ischemia Classification each foot is assigned a number, which represents the status or depth of the wound, and a letter, which represents the vascular status of the foot.

The justification for this is that the old Wagner classification allowed a number of confusing combinations of lesions and, in certain instances, incorrectly represented the true condition of the foot by the assigned grade. For example, if a foot had forefoot ischemia with uninfected soft tissues and a superficial ulcer under one of the lesser metatarsal heads, it is inadequately descriptive for it to be classified as a grade 1 lesion (superficial ulcer), but it is exaggerated to call it a grade 4 lesion (partial forefoot gangrene). The Depth-Ischemia classification is more concise and practical and separates the two concepts of wound severity and ischemia, which are not related, as was implied by the old classification. Moreover, in the original classification, a grade 1 lesion (superficial ulcer) clearly could be seen to progress to a grade 2 (deep ulcer) and then to a grade 3 (osteomyelitis or abscess). However, there is no logical progression from osteomyelitis (grade 3) to forefoot gangrene (grade 4). The original Wagner classification showed a reversibility between and among some lesions that was not possible, such as the reversion from grade 4 (gangrene) to grade 3 (osteomyelitis).

The Depth-Ischemia classification is represented in Table 1. There are four levels in each part of the classification. In the depth portion, grade 0 is the foot at risk. This foot has no current ulceration or wound, but is classified as at risk because of a history of a previous ulceration or because of the presence of sensory neuropathy, especially with deformity in the toes or foot.

Grade 1 is a superficial ulcer, which is neither infected nor has exposed at its base any deep structure (Fig. 6). Grade 2 is a deep ulcer, which has exposed a deep structure of tendon or joint, but not bone (Fig.

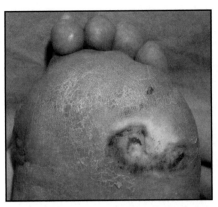

Fig. 6 Grade 1A diabetic ulcer. The wound is relatively superficial.

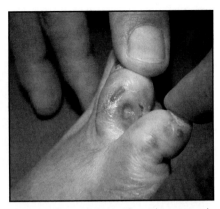

Fig. 7 Grade 2A diabetic ulcer. The proximal interphalangeal joint capsule is exposed.

7). A grade 2 lesion may or may not have superficial infection. A grade 3 lesion is extensive ulceration with exposure of the bone and/or deep infection. If the bone is palpated through the ulcer with a sterile, blunt instrument, it is grade 3, and probably has osteomyelitis[32] (Fig. 8). The deep infection can be osteomyelitis and/or abscess.

The first of the four levels in the "Ischemia" portion of the classification is grade A, which represents the foot that is not ischemic. There is sufficient vascularity for healing of the wound. No diagnostic or therapeutic vascular intervention is required. Grade B is a level of ischemia that may impair healing, but has not yet led to gangrene. This is clearly a wide band on the spectrum; but as a classification group it is justified by the corresponding treatment, vascular evaluation, and possible vascular reconstruction. A large group of lesions of the diabetic foot fall in this category. Grade C is partial gangrene of the foot. This level also requires vascular evaluation and possible reconstruction, but these feet are evaluated and treated for the best level of amputation that can be healed. This grade denotes the fact that partial foot salvage is now

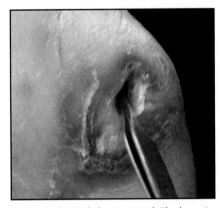

Fig. 8 Grade 3B diabetic wound. The bone is palpable at the depth of the ulcer. Radiographs demonstrate early osteomyelitis.

the best possible outcome. Grade D is complete gangrene of the foot. While this patient also requires vascular evaluation and possible proximal vascular bypass, the goal is no longer foot salvage, but rather limb salvage. Determination of the level of amputation, either above the knee amputation or below the knee amputation, is now the question.

Clinical Problems and Outpatient Treatments

Although it may seem that a host of indescribable problems assail the diabetic foot, these can be categorized into the 5 major areas, vascular disease, ulcerations, infections, Charcot

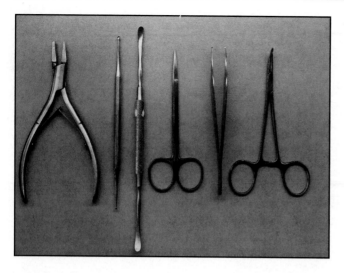

Fig. 9 Basic nail care instruments for the clinic.

Outline 1
Nail care instruments

Double-action bone rongeur
Anvil nail splitter
Freer elevator
Hemostat for nail removal
Cotton-tipped swabs
Nail currette
Pointed iris scissors and Adson's forceps
Hobby drill with sanding disks/drums

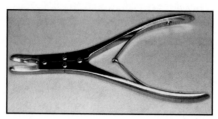

Fig. 10 Double-action rongeur for nail trimming.

joints, and amputations. These chapters on the diabetic foot reflect the design of the course itself over the last 4 years in the division of the lectures according to these subjects. Vascular disease has been discussed above. In the following lectures, Dr. Conti will discuss ulcerations, in particular the use of total contact casts in outpatient treatment; Dr. Saltzman will discuss infection and its treatment; Dr. Johnson will discuss the outpatient and inpatient management of Charcot joints; Dr. Smith discusses the criteria and techniques for amputation and foot salvage. Three treatment areas, wound care, skin and nail care, and patient education, are discussed below.

Wound Care

Innovations in the treatment of diabetic foot wounds, especially plantar ulcers, continue to be sought and found by many researchers in different fields. These innovations include the use of hyperbaric oxygen, platelet-derived and other topical wound-healing factors, and skin substitutes. A number of these new developments hold promise of improved wound healing, but as many questions have been raised as have been answered. First, what is the goal? Is it to achieve closure of a wound that otherwise would not have healed? Most uninfected wounds fail to heal because of ischemia or persistent pressure on the soft tissue. If that is the case, will a topical or local modality supercede the import of the basic principles of adequate perfusion and relief of pressure? If, as is likely, these modalities do not supercede these 2 principles, then what advantage is sought? In many

studies, the goal sought, or at least the result gained, is more rapid healing of the wound. A few excellent studies have demonstrated quicker wound healing, but data are still lacking to conclude that the reduced days or weeks of treatment represent a clinically significant improvement in outcome. While some of these modalities have succeeded in achieving more rapid wound healing, are they sufficiently better, qualitatively or quantitatively, to justify the costs, especially in this cost-conscious era? We must still investigate how long the healed feet remain healed and whether these modalities add anything to our typical prescription of shoes and insoles. On the other hand, if ease of treatment is greatly enhanced, such innovations may well prove to be keys to an overall higher level of care of the diabetic foot by all specialties of medicine.

Skin and Nail Care

Routine skin and nail care in the diabetic patient is an unglamorous but essential part of both treatment and prevention. Most of the routine work is done by a nurse, physician's assistant, or other trained medical affiliate, but the orthopaedic surgeon must still know and understand enough to direct these activities. It is essential to be willing to deal with these small problems properly in order to give both correct and complete care, and to prevent escalation of small problems to larger ones.

The basic instruments for the care of the nails in the clinic or office are shown in Figure 9 and are listed in Outline 1. The single most useful tool is a double action rongeur, such as the one depicted in Figure 10. This powerful bone-cutting instrument provides the safest method for trimming a thickened, onychomycotic nail that defies cutting with ordinary nail clippers (Fig. 11). It can generate

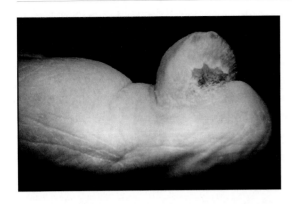

Fig. 11 A thickened, hypertrophic, onychomycotic great toe nail. (Reproduced with permission from Brodsky JW: Outpatient diagnosis and care of the diabetic foot, in Heckman JD (ed): *Instructional Course Lectures 42*. Rosemont, IL, American Academy of Orthopaedic Surgeons, 1993, pp 121–139.)

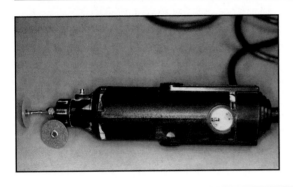

Fig. 12 Electric hobby drill for sanding down calluses and nails in diabetic patients.

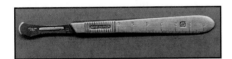

Fig. 13 The No. 17 blade, designed specifically for callus and ulcer trimming. Note the rounded shape.

sufficient force to nibble away the nail without twisting, elevating, or avulsing it. The rounded beaks protect the surrounding soft tissue and can be used to carefully push the soft tissue away. The nail should be trimmed in multiple small bites, not sheared in a single stroke. In grossly thickened nails, the nail can be thinned somewhat, as well as shortened. The edges are then smoothed with the electric sander (Fig. 12).

The electric sander is the safest instrument for smoothing and reducing calluses and nails. It works rather slowly on very thick, fungal nails; therefore, it is more efficient to

trim them first. However, if the personnel doing this task are not highly skilled with the rongeur, or if the patient has severe or unreconstructable peripheral vascular disease, it is safer to use the sander alone. The primary danger is that the sanding disk can become a rotating blade when turned sideways. Sanding drums as well as disks can be used. The sander should be used on the slowest speed. When used to reduce calluses, the skin temperature should be tested intermittently with the examiner's fingertip to guard against overheating and burning the skin, because the patient may not feel it.

To trim calluses, as well as the hyperkeratotic borders of ulcers, the number 17 scalpel blade is ideally suited (Fig. 13). It has a double edge, but a rounded shape, which reduces the risk of nicking the patient. It fits a regular scalpel handle.

Autonomic neuropathy can cause the skin of the feet to be excessively

dry and scaly. As the skin loses its normal compliance, it tends to crack and fissure, leading to infection. Patients with these skin problems should be instructed in the use of a skin moisturizing routine to keep the skin pliable. Various moisturizing creams and lotions are acceptable. One practical and inexpensive routine is to have the patient spread a thin layer of petroleum jelly on the feet after the shower or bath to seal in the water absorbed by the skin. Reduction of the calluses themselves also helps to prevent cracking.

In addition to routine trimming, nail care includes treatment of infected and uninfected ingrown nails. Most ingrown nails occur in the hallux. It is not the distal corner alone that becomes ingrown, rather the entire side of the nail. Infection follows ingrowing, and similarly begins along medial or lateral borders, or both. In order to cure the infection, it is necessary to decompress the area by removing the nail margin, allowing drainage. It is imperative to assure that the patient has adequate perfusion before this very distal procedure is performed. If necessary, the patient is first sent to the vascular laboratory for evaluation. Some procedures are delayed because of the newfound need for vascular reconstruction.

The anvil-type nail splitter is the ideal method for this procedure, which is usally done under digital block anesthesia. The lower jaw of the splitter is flat and separates the nail from the nail bed. The upper jaw of the splitter is triangular in cross-section and it splits the nail as it comes down on the flat lower blade (Fig. 14). The split-off section of the nail is then elevated with the blunt end of a Freer or other elevator. The nail section is removed with a clamp, and the resulting pocket is gently,

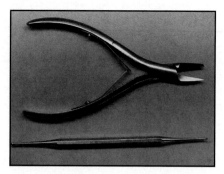

Fig. 14 Nail splitter, ("nail anvil") has a flat lower jaw to slide between the nail bed and the nail plate. The upper jaw is sharp and splits the nail against the lower jaw, protecting the nail bed.

superficially explored and gently debrided with a curette to remove fibrous material, but not to remove the matrix itself. This nail splitter is safer to use than a scalpel, because it prevents laceration of the nail bed. The nail bed is a very thin layer directly over the phalanx, and bone involvement, with infection, is possible. It is safer, more effective, and more reliable to use the phenol to ablate the matrix cells than to use the curette to remove the matrix, which is seldom, if ever, complete.

If the ingrown nail is a recurring problem, in addition to removal of the nail margin, ablation of the corresponding margin of the matrix and nail bed is required. After removal of the nail under the ischemia of a digital tourniquet (made of a 2.5-inch penrose drain), phenol is applied to ablate the cells of the nail matrix and nail bed. I have found that 2 applications of 90 seconds duration is successful, with each application followed by an alcohol rinse. Prior to applying the phenol each time, the nail bed must be thoroughly dried. Application is done with cotton-tipped swabs.

Patient Education

Patient education is said to be important in all medical problems, but in the diabetic patient, it is critical. Prevention of diabetic foot problems remains the very best treatment, and the patient must take the responsibility for prevention through a self-care program. Much has been done to set the stage. Many clinics and hospitals offer diabetic education. The American Diabetes Association has great resources available for patient education and teaching. The American Association of Diabetic Educators is dedicated to the enormous task of teaching diabetic patients about all aspects of their care, including glucose testing, insulin administration, and many other parts of the disease, in addition to inspection of the feet.

We, too, must encourage a program of daily or twice daily foot and shoe inspection. Patients and/or family members must be taught to shake out shoes before donning to remove any foreign objects. They must look all around and over the feet for signs of erythema, discoloration, or breaks in the skin. Many of our patients cannot do this for themselves. They may be too stiff or arthritic to position the foot for viewing, or they may have impaired vision from diabetic retinopathy. Use of a mirror can be handy. Most often the help of a family member or friend must be enlisted. The goal is to build daily inspection into the routine of bathing and dressing. Allied medical professionals can teach these techniques to the patient.

References

1. *Diabetes: 1997 Vital Statistics*. Alexandria, VA, American Diabetes Association, 1997.

2. Delbridge L, Ctercteko G, Fowler C, Reeve TS, Le Quesne LP: The aetiology of diabetic neuropathic ulceration of the foot. *Br J Surg* 1985;72:1–6.

3. Masson EA, Hay EM, Stockley I, Veves A, Betts BP, Boulton AJ: Abnormal foot pressures alone may not cause ulceration. *Diabet Med* 1989;6:426–428.

4. Brand PW: The insensitive foot (including leprosy), in Jahss MH (ed): *Disorders of the Foot and Ankle: Medical and Surgical Management*, ed 2. Philadelphia, PA, WB Saunders, 1991, vol 3, pp 2170–2186.

5. Gelberman RH, Szabo RM, Williamson RV, Dimick MP: Sensibility testing in peripheral-nerve compression syndromes: An experimental study in humans. *J Bone Joint Surg* 1983;65: 632–638.

6. Levin S, Pearsall G, Ruderman RJ: Von Frey's method of measuring pressure sensibility in the hand: An engineering analysis of the Weinstein-Semmes pressure aesthesiometer. *J Hand Surg* 1978;3A:211–216.

7. Brodsky JW, Chambers R, Kwong PK, Wagner FW: Abstract: Patterns of disintegration in the Charcot tarsus of diabetes and relation to treatment. *Foot Ankle* 1986;6:323–324.

8. Chantelau E, Ma XY, Herrnberger S, Dohmen C, Trappe P, Baba T: Effect of medial arterial calcification of O2 supply to exercising diabetic feet. *Diabetes* 1990;39:938–941.

9. Irwin ST, Gilmore J, McGrann S, Hood J, Allen JA: Blood flow in diabetics with foot lesions due to "small vessel disease." *Br J Surg* 1988;75:1201–1206.

10. LoGerfo FW, Coffman JD: Vascular and microvascular disease of the foot in diabetes. Implications for foot care. *N Engl J Med* 1984; 311:1615–1619.

11. Louie TJ, Bartlett JG, Tally FP, Gorbach SL: Aerobic and anaerobic bacteria in diabetic foot ulcers. *Ann Intern Med* 1976;85:461–463.

12. Oskarsson P, Ljunggren JG, Lins PE: Efficacy and safety of mexiletine in the treatment of painful diabetic neuropathy: The Mexiletine Study Group. *Diabetes Care* 1997;20:1594–1597.

13. Stracke H, Meyer UE, Schumacher HE, Federlin K: Mexiletine in the treatment of diabetic neuropathy. *Diabetes Care* 1992;15: 1550–1555.

14. Delbridge L, Perry P, Marr S, et al: Limited joint mobility in the diabetic foot: Relationship to neuropathic ulceration. *Diabet Med* 1988;5: 333–337.

15. Fernando DJ, Masson EA, Veves A, Boulton AJ: Relationship of limited joint mobility to abnormal foot pressures and diabetic foot ulceration. *Diabetes Care* 1991;14:8–11.

16. Brodsky JW: The diabetic foot, in Mann RA, Coughlin MJ (eds): *Surgery of the Foot and Ankle*, ed 6. St. Louis, MO, CV Mosby, 1993.

17. Bagdade JD, Root RK, Bulger RJ: Impaired leukocyte function in patients with poorly controlled diabetes. *Diabetes* 1974;23:9–15.

18. Bauman JH, Girling JP, Brand PW: Plantar pressures and trophic ulceration. *J Bone Joint Surg* 1963;45B:652–673.

19. Boulton AJ, Betts RP, Franks CI, Newrick PG, Ward JD, Duckworth T: Abnormalities of foot pressure in early diabetic neuropathy. *Diabetic Med* 1987;4:225–228.

20. Ctercteko GC, Dhanendran M, Hutton WC, Le Quesne LP: Vertical forces acting on the feet

of diabetic patients with neuropathic ulceration. *Br J Surg* 1981;68:608–614.

21. Duckworth T, Boulton AJ, Betts RP, Franks CI, Ward JD: Plantar pressure measurements and the prevention of ulceration in the diabetic foot. *J Bone Joint Surg* 1985;67B:79–85.

22. Rayfield EJ, Ault MJ, Keusch GT, Brothers MJ, Nechemias C, Smith H: Infection and diabetes: The case for glucose control. *Am J Med* 1982;72:439–450.

23. Dickhaut SC, DeLee JC, Page CP: Nutritional status: Importance in predicting wound-healing after amputation. *J Bone Joint Surg* 1984;66A: 71–75.

24. Wagner FW Jr: Part II: A classification and treatment program for diabetic, neuropathic and dysvascular foot problems, in Cooper RR (ed): American Academy of Orthopaedic Surgeons *Instructional Course Lectures XXVIII*. St. Louis, MO, CV Mosby, 1979, pp 143–165.

25. Wagner FW Jr: The dysvascular foot: A system for diagnosis and treatment. *Foot Ankle* 1981; 2:64–122.

26. Apelqvist J, Castenfors J, Larsson J, Stenstrom A, Agardh CD: Prognostic value of systolic ankle and toe blood pressure levels in outcome of diabetic foot ulcer. *Diabetes Care* 1989;12: 373–378.

27. Bessman AN, Wagner W: Nonclostridial gas gangrene: Report of 48 cases and review of the literature. *JAMA* 1975;233:958–963.

28. Morrison WB, Schweitzer ME, Wapner KL, Hecht PJ, Gannon FH, Behm WR: Osteomyelitis in feet of diabetics: Clinical accuracy, surgical utility, and cost-effectiveness of MR imaging. *Radiology* 1995;196:557–564.

29. Yuh WT, Corson JD, Baraniewski HM, et al: Osteomyelitis of the foot in diabetic patients: Evaluation with plain film, 99mTc-MDP bone scintigraphy, and MR imaging. *Am J Roentgenol* 1989;152:795–800.

30. Splittgerber GF, Spiegelhoff DR, Buggy BP: Combined leukocyte and bone imaging used to evaluate diabetic osteoarthropathy and osteomyelitis. *Clin Nucl Med* 1989;14:156–160.

31. Pecoraro RE, Reiber GE: Classification of wounds in diabetic amputees. *Wounds* 1990; 2:65–73.

32. Grayson ML, Gibbons GW, Balogh K, Levin E, Karchmer AW: Probing to bone in infected pedal ulcers: A clinical sign of underlying osteomyelitis in diabetic patients. *JAMA* 1995; 273:721–723.

Total Contact Casting

Stephen F. Conti, MD

Introduction

In the early 1930s, Drs. Milroy Paul and Joseph Kahn, working in Ceylon, India, conceptualized the idea of using casting for trophic ulceration secondary to Hansen's disease.[1] They described an ambulatory technique to treat leprosy patients as an alternative to prolonged and expensive periods of bed rest in the hospital. In the 1960s, Paul Brand[2,3] who had worked in India in the early 1950s, adopted the same casting technique in the United States at the Gillis W. Long Hansen's Disease Center in Carville, Louisiana, to treat patients afflicted with Hansen's disease and diabetes mellitus.

Brand and his colleagues noted one significant problem with the casting technique as used in India. This problem, which was also noted by other clinicians, was that as the padding in the cast became compressed over time, it allowed the foot to move within the cast, creating new ulcers. Brand began to construct his casts without padding, in order to allow the cast material to conform exactly to the shape of the foot and leg. Currently, the term total contact cast refers to a composite, anatomically conforming, below-knee cast that is applied over minimal padding, often enclosing the toes. The use of total contact casting as an ambulatory treatment for plantar ulceration in leprosy has since been further expanded to include a variety of other conditions involving insensitivity of the feet, including diabetes mellitus, tabes dorsalis, Charcot-Marie-Tooth disease, syringomyelia and chronic alcoholism, and ulcerations due to idiopathic peripheral neuropathy. Total contact casts are also used to treat neuroarthropathy (Charcot fractures and joints) and to provide immobilization following surgery in patients with sensory neuropathy.

Pathophysiology of Foot Ulceration

A brief review of the factors that can contribute to plantar ulceration in patients with diabetes mellitus is necessary to understand the rationale behind the use of casts to treat this condition. The primary factor in the cause of diabetic foot ulceration is the presence of peripheral neuropathy, leading to diminished or absent sensation. Insensitivity allows excessive and prolonged pressures to occur over the skin, which eventually results in tissue breakdown and ulcer formation.[2,4] In addition to peripheral neuropathy, mechanical factors, such as foot deformities (including clawtoes, midfoot collapse, and hindfoot subluxation), loss of intrinsic muscle function, abnormal load distribution in the forefoot, shear forces, vascular insufficiency, poor skin quality, and infection can contribute to the formation of plantar ulcerations.[2,5,6]

Classification of Diabetic Foot Ulcerations

It is necessary to have a thoughtful classification scheme for foot ulcers in order to develop a rational treatment program and decide on the appropriate use of total contact casting. Many classification systems have been proposed. Wagner proposed a classification of foot ulcerations, which is widely accepted because of its longevity and ease of use[7] (Table 1).

Brodsky has proposed a depth/ischemia classification system that lends itself to a more refined treatment protocol[7] (Table 2). This scheme recognizes ulcer depth and circulation to the foot as separate entities rather than parts of a continuum as in the Wagner classification.

Proposed Mechanisms of Action of Casts

Four mechanisms have been proposed to explain how casts function to heal plantar ulcers. They include protection from trauma, immobilization of skin edges, reduction of edema, and reduction of pressure over the ulcers. Limb immobilization decreases the spread of local infection and, by limiting the stress on granulation tissue and skin edges, protects the foot from further trauma. In 36 to 48 hours, swelling is reduced and the resultant decrease in interstitial fluid pressure leads to improved microcirculation and, the-

Table 1
Wagner classification and recommended management

Stage	Classification	Recommendations
0	Pressure area on foot aggravated by footwear	Footwear modification
I	Open but superficial ulceration	Local treatment
		Footwear modification
II	Full thickness ulceration	Occlusive cast
		Footwear modification
III	Full thickness ulceration with secondary infection	Debridement
		Antibiotics
IV	Local gangrene	Antibiotics
		Local amputation
		Hyperbaric O_2
V	Extensive gangrene, entire foot	Regional amputation
		Antibiotics
		Rehabilitation

oretically, ulcer healing. Casts have been shown to reduce edema; however, this has not been correlated with improved wound healing. (Marzano R, Kay D, 1995, unpublished data.) The widely accepted rationale for how total contact casting functions to heal diabetic ulcers is that the cast reduces pressure over the wound by redistributing the weightbearing load over a greater plantar surface area.

In 1985, Birke and associates[8] reported a 75% to 84% reduction in peak pressure at the first and third metatarsal heads, respectively, when subjects walked in a cast. In this study, the right feet of 6 normal subjects were tested, using 4 relatively thick sensors, which could have possibly altered the pressures beneath them. However, because the great toe and the metatarsal head region are prone to develop ulceration in the diabetic patients[3] this simple study was significant, being the first to suggest that casts did function to reduce pressure in certain areas.

Using a more sophisticated plantar pressure measuring system, Conti and associates[6] and Martin and Conti[9] examined plantar pressures in casts in subjects with normal arches

and with midfoot collapse and rocker bottom deformity. The conclusion of these studies was that casts function by increasing the plantar weightbearing surface area, thereby lowering plantar pressures. Both short leg casts and total contact casts reduced midfoot pressure, but only total contact casts significantly lowered forefoot pressure. Neither type of cast reduced heel pressure. An average reduction of pressure over the ulcer site of 42% to 46% was achieved through casting. The authors believed that molding the cast to the bottom of the foot allows the entire sole to participate in force distribution, thereby resulting in lower pressures.

Shaw and associates[10] further refined the mechanism of reduction of forefoot pressures in total contact casts. By studying ground reaction forces, in addition to plantar pressures, they concluded that approximately one third of the total load is carried by the wall of the cast instead of being transmitted through the plantar surface. This study supports the concept that a cast that is intimately molded to the leg is better at reducing forces on the ulcer than a cast that is loosely applied. It also

highlights the potential differences between total contact casts and removable walker boots that are purported to be as effective at plantar pressure reduction.

The advantages of total contact casts over strict nonweightbearing ambulation are as follows: (1) A cast maintains the ambulatory status of the patient. Patients with diabetes, who have poor vision, balance problems, weakness, and limited cardiac reserve are significantly limited in their ability to use crutches or a walker. Also, lengthy and expensive hospital stays as well as the potential problems of prolonged bed rest can be avoided. Sedentary workers can return to their jobs without any income loss. (2) A cast reduces edema and plantar pressure. (3) A cast protects the foot from further trauma. (4) A cast requires less patient compliance than nonweightbearing crutch ambulation. There is no need for daily dressing changes or specialized wound care.

The disadvantages and/or complications of total contact casting are as follows: (1) Prolonged immobilization in a cast can cause joint stiffness and muscle atrophy. Diabetic tissue is normally less pliable, due to nonenzymatic glycosylation of collagen, and the superimposed stiffness from the cast can be significant. (2) Poor cast application and removal can cause new ulceration and skin breakdown. This can be minimized by using a skillful cast application technique and by regular monitoring at frequent office follow-up visits. Even with proper precautions, skin abrasion[11,12] and fungal infection have been reported. New skin breakdown can be treated by discontinuing use of the cast for a few days until the new ulcer has healed. Fungal infection, reported in 15% of all casted patients, can be treated with local application of antifungal cream after the cast is no longer needed. Rarely is casting interrupted due to fungal infection. (3) Because the casts have little padding, cast saw cuts can occur during removal. It is crucial to prevent this complication by using meticulous technique. Health care personnel should have special instruction on proper cast removal.

Pathophysiology of Neuroarthropathic Fractures

The second major indication for total contact casting is in the treatment of acute Charcot fractures secondary to diabetic neuropathy. Again, an understanding of the pathophysiology of Charcot fractures is necessary to conceptualize the role of total contact casts in their treatment. In 1936, William Jordan[13] first described the occurrence of neuropathic arthropathy of the foot and ankle in diabetic patients. Many similar reports have followed.[14–16] The prevalence of neuropathic arthropathy in patients with diabetes mellitus has been reported in the literature to be from 0.08% to 7.5%.[17–19] The most common areas of neuroarthropathy are the midfoot and hindfoot.[20,21]

Newman[22] stated that the earliest changes in neuroarthropathic joints occurred in the soft tissue surrounding the joints. In those cases of neuropathic osteoarthropathy that do not begin with spontaneous fractures, he postulated that gross neuropathic changes in the ligaments were responsible for spontaneous dislocation of the foot. Ligaments and joint capsules are thought to be stretched by the abnormal stress applied to the joint, leading to hypermobility, eventual joint dislocation, and subsequent fragmentation. Hyperemic resorption through osteoclastic activities can alter ligamentous insertion into the bone and

Table 2
The depth/ischemia classification of diabetic foot lesions

Grade	Definition	Treatment*
Depth Classification		
0	The "at risk" foot. Previous ulcer, or neuropathy with deformity that may cause new ulceration	Patient education Regular examination Appropriate shoewear and insoles
1	Superficial ulceration, not infected	External pressure relief: Total contact cast, walking brace, special shoewear, etc
2	Deep ulceration exposing tendon or joint (with/without superficial infection)	Surgical debridement → wound care → pressure relief if closes and converts to grade 1 (PRN antibiotics)
3	Extensive ulceration with exposed bone, and/or deep infection: ie, osteomyelitis, or abscess	Surgical debridements → ray or partial foot amputations → IV antibiotics → pressure relief if wound converts to grade 1
Ischemia Classification		
A	Not ischemic	Adequate vascularity for healing
B	Ischemia without gangrene	Vascular evaluation (Doppler, TcPO$_2$, arteriogram, etc.) → vascular reconstruction PRN
C	Partial (forefoot) gangrene of foot	Vascular evaluation → vascular reconstruction (proximal and/or distal bypass or angioplasty) → partial foot amputation
D	Complete foot gangrene	Vascular evaluation → major extremity amputation (BKA, AKA) with possible proximal vascular reconstruction

PRN, as needed; IV, intravenous; TcPO$_2$, transcutaneous oxygen pressure; BKA, below-knee amputation; AKA, above-knee amputation

(Reproduced with permission from Brodsky JW: The diabetic foot, in Mann RA, Coughlin MJ (eds): Surgery of the Foot and Ankle, ed 6. St. Louis, MO, Mosby Year Book, 1993, pp 1361–1467.)

may be another contributing factor for dislocation. Multiple other factors appear to contribute to the development of bone and joint destruction in patients with diabetes mellitus;[23] however, a detailed discussion of all these factors is beyond the scope of this chapter.

Norman and associates[24] also classified neuropathic joints as acute or chronic, based on the suddenness of their onset and speed of development. The acute phase of neuropathy

is often precipitated by minor trauma and is characterized by swelling, erythema, a local increase in temperature, joint effusion, ligament laxity, and bone resorption. Early clinical and radiographic signs may resemble those of osteoarthritis and infection. The similarity between infection and neuroarthropathy can delay the diagnosis and treatment of early subluxation, especially when radiographs are normal. The early recognition and immobilization of the neuroarthropathic foot must be the goal of any treatment algorithm.

Radiographic Staging and Treatment of Neuropathic Joints

Eichenholtz[25] described 3 distinct radiologic stages of neuroarthropathy. These are (1) stage of development, (2) stage of coalescence, and (3) stage of reconstruction.

The stage of development represents an acute, destructive period associated clinically with joint effusion, soft-tissue edema, subluxation, intra-articular fractures, and fragmentation of bone. This stage is usually induced by minor trauma and aggravated by persistent ambulation on an insensitive foot. The process induces a hyperemic response, leading to bone resorption and progressive deterioration. Clinically, this may present with painless, unilateral warmth and swelling, with normal radiographs. It may continue for as little as a few hours or as long as several weeks before there is radiographic evidence of joint fragmentation. Early recognition is imperative for successful treatment, because aggressive cast immobilization can prevent late deformity. Nonweightbearing total contact casting should be initiated during the acute phase of the disease.

The second stage, the stage of coalescence, can be identified clinically by a lessening of edema, reduction of skin temperature, resorption of fine debris, and healing of fractures. This phase indicates the beginning of the reparative phase. Partial weightbearing total contact casting is the recommended treatment in this phase. The use of a bivalved ankle-foot orthosis (AFO) or Charcot restraint orthotic walker (CROW) brace is an alternative.

In the third and final stage, the stage of reconstruction, further repair and remodeling of the bone takes place. This stage can be recognized clinically by the absence of edema and local warmth and radiographically by increased bone density and sclerosis. At this stage, it is recommended to wean the patient into a double upright calf lacing brace with appropriate total contact orthoses and soft leather depth shoes with rocker soles. Depending on joint stability, the patient may remain in the brace indefinitely or move to footwear alone. Chronic or late neuropathic bone and joint changes are problematic but can be managed effectively with shoe modifications and, in selective cases, by reconstructive surgery.

Indications for Total Contact Casts

There are 3 indications for total contact casts. The first is ambulatory treatment of uninfected superficial forefoot and midfoot plantar ulcerations, including Wagner grade 1 and 2 ulcers or Brodsky grade 1 ulcers. Heel ulcers are often the result of ischemia combined with osteomyelitis, and because total contact casts do not unload the heel, casting is not indicated for plantar heel ulcerations. Deeper ulcers with exposed tendon or bone require surgical debridement and local wound care to convert them to superficial ulcers before total contact casting is undertaken. Casting is not recommended for dorsal foot or leg ulcers. The second indication is for treatment of Eichenholtz stage 1 or 2 neuroarthropathic fractures, and the third is for postoperative immobilization, following either open reduction and internal fixation of acute foot or ankle fractures or reconstructive surgery for late deformity.

Contraindications for Total Contact Casts

The 4 absolute contraindications are as follows: (1) Deep infection in the form of deep abscess, osteomyelitis or gangrene should not be casted. Excessive drainage from the ulcer is clinical justification to assess for underlying osteomyelitis or abscess. Antibiotic therapy and bed rest or nonweightbearing on the limb until the acute infection has subsided has been recommended.[25] If the ulcer is deeper than it is wide, it should be surgically debrided and opened to allow the deeper layers to heal and prevent premature superficial healing. (2) Poor skin quality is a contraindication to casting. Patients who are on chronic corticosteroids or those with stasis ulcers are most likely to develop skin breakdown with total contact casting. (3) Severe arterial insufficiency is another contraindication. Although most diabetic patients have some atherosclerotic vascular insufficiency, only those with pregangrenous feet are at risk of developing a catastrophic ischemic event from the circular bandage of the cast. A clinical examination suggesting ischemia, ankle/brachial index less than 0.45, Doppler toe pressures less than 30 mm Hg, or a transcutaneous pressure of oxygen ($TcPO_2$) less than 30 warrant special attention. (4) The final absolute contraindication is poor patient compliance. Patients who are unable to keep regularly scheduled follow-up visits and are unable to follow the cast precautions and instructions should not be casted.

In addition to these absolute contraindications there are 2 relative contraindications. (1) Fluctuating edema of the limb, which occurs, for example, in some dialysis patients, may be a relative contraindication for total contact casting. Total uniform contact between the cast and the limb is the essential element to success. If the limb becomes loose in the cast, shear forces caused by movement of skin in the cast can delay healing or cause skin breakdown. (2) The use of total contact casting in blind, ataxic, or obese patients is another relative contraindication. Some additional precautions or alternative methods of therapy may be necessary to prevent falls.

Cast Application

There is no universally accepted technique or single method of applying a total contact cast that is exclusively effective. In fact, multiple variations on the themes that follow are successful. The goal is to obtain an intimate fit of the cast around the foot and leg through meticulous molding. One method of doing this is to apply plaster directly to the skin without padding. However, as noted previously, standard short leg casts made of 3 layers of padding have been shown clinically and experimentally to reduce plantar pressure and allow acceptable rates of ulcer healing. Another controversy is over foot position in the cast, the question being whether a patient with a forefoot ulcer should be casted in slight dorsiflexion in an attempt to further unload that area during ambulation. Finally, the physician must decide whether to leave the toes exposed or enclose them in the cast. The claimed advantage of open toes is the ability to check circulation and for evidence of erythema. The more obvious disadvantages are that the toes are unprotected and exposed to trauma, objects may find their way into the cast through the opening, and the possibility of iatrogenic ulcer formation is increased. This last complication is of significant practical concern. Finishing the cast at the metatarsal heads can allow the end of the cast to press on the dorsal surface of the foot as it is forced down during the end of midstance and toe-off, and this pressure can cause ulceration in some patients.

Wound assessment is the first step in cast application. The ulcer surface may require mechanical debridement of the exudate that sometimes covers it. This is best accomplished with a sterile cotton swab or gauze sponge. Use of antiseptics that contain iodine, alcohol, or peroxide is not indicated, because these substances are toxic to granulating tissue and can delay wound healing. Antibiotic soaps, which are rinsed off with saline after use, can be used for this purpose. Usually, sharp debridement of the ulcer base is performed. The hypertrophic marginal callus that forms around the ulcer should be sharply excised until this area is level with the adjacent normal skin. Theoretically, pressure on the callused area during weightbearing will cause marginal ischemia that will delay wound healing. After the callous is trimmed, the ulcer may then be covered with a sterile nonadhesive dressing and one or two 2 × 2-in gauze sponges.

Skin preparation is accomplished by first washing the skin with mild soap and water if necessary. A hypoallergenic moisturizer is then applied to the skin everywhere except at the web spaces between the toes, which have an antifungal powder applied sparingly as needed. Single 2 × 2-in gauze sponges are then placed between the toes (Fig. 1). A square piece of foam padding is positioned around the toes and trimmed (Fig. 2). For midfoot ulcers, the foam is placed around the toes only. In patients with forefoot ulcers, the foam is extended proximally just behind the metatarsal heads to create a well under the metatarsal heads once the cast is applied, allowing pressure reduction. Next, the leg is wrapped with a single layer of 3 or 4-inch cast padding from the tibial tubercle to just beyond the tips of the toes, with each layer overlapped by

50%. A 0.25-in thick strip of medical grade felt is cut approximately 4 cm wide and positioned from just distal to the tibial tubercle to just proximal to the ankle joint along the crest of the tibia. Additional 0.125-in thick felt strips, made by splitting the 0.25-in felt in half, are positioned over the medial and lateral malleoli (Fig. 3).

Traditional casting technique would then involve molding a single layer of conforming plaster wrap over the entire leg, followed by 2 layers of fiberglass casting tape. The toes are completely enclosed (Fig. 4). Patients then remain nonweightbearing for 24 hours, to allow the plaster to dry thoroughly, after which they are allowed to ambulate. Using plantar pressure analysis, it has been shown that equivalent plantar pressure reductions are achieved by simply wrapping the leg with the fiberglass tape without the plaster underlayer (unpublished data). Intimate molding, especially through the longitudinal arch and around the leg, is stressed in both techniques (Fig. 5). A rocker bottom cast boot is attached to aid in gait, to protect the bottom of the cast, and to keep the cast clean. Patients can then leave the office ambulating weightbearing as tolerated if their condition permits. If the patient has a significant amount of swelling, the involved extremity is elevated for 10 minutes prior to cast application. I prefer to cast the foot with the ankle in a neutral position relative to the leg regardless of the site of the ulcer, because slight dorsiflexion or plantarflexion makes walking in the cast difficult. Plantarflexion can cause increased pressure on the anterior edge of the cast just below the knee or along the shin, producing a secondary ulcer.

Postcasting Care

Most patients are brought back after 5 to 7 days for the first cast change.

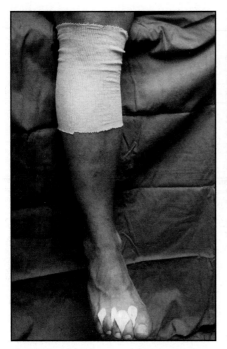

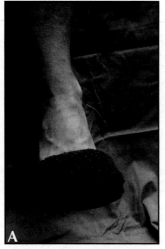

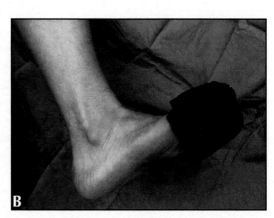

Fig. 2 A, A piece of foam is cut and placed around the toes. **B,** The plantar aspect of the foam is beveled just proximal to the metatarsal heads.

Fig. 1 After debridement of the ulcer and preparation of the skin, the stockinette is applied to the proximal leg and the gauze sponges placed between the toes.

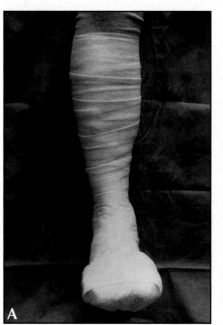

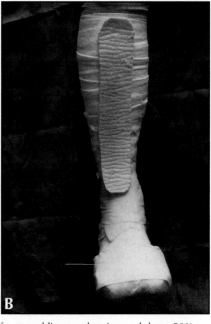

Fig. 3 A, The leg is wrapped with a single layer of cast padding overlapping each layer 50%. **B,** An anterior felt pad is positioned over the tibial crest. The foam absorbs the pressure of the anterior cast against the leg as the patient walks over the cast from midstance to toe-off.

Rapid edema reduction can make the cast loose, resulting in possible skin irritation or ulceration. Patients are brought back every 2 weeks thereafter for cast changes. Specific precautions and cast care instructions are reinforced at each visit. A handout is used to remind patients about the details of cast care (see Appendix). In the case of plantar ulcerations, casting is discontinued when the ulcer is healed and appropriate footwear is available to the patient. For casts used to treat Charcot fractures, the casting is discontinued when edema is reduced, the temperature difference between the 2 feet is within 2°C (no perceptible difference to the examiner), and radiographs show consolidation and healing of fractures.

Appropriate footwear must be available to patients immediately after cast removal. The basic principles in the pedorthic management of plantar ulcers are the even distribution of plantar pressure by transfer from areas of high pressure, such as metatarsal heads, to areas of lower pressure; shock absorption; reduction of friction and shear by limitation of tissue motion; and accommodation of deformities.[26] Prescription footwear should not be considered a primary treatment for ulcers, rather such care is intended as a long-term management technique for maintaining healed areas and preventing further ulceration.

Shoe modifications should be done according to the needs of the patient.

Important characteristics for shoes used in the pedorthic management of plantar ulcers include: a long medial counter to control the heel and medial arch, a Blucher opening to allow easy entry into the shoe, a shock-absorbing sole to reduce impact shock, and a low heel to decrease pressure on the metatarsal heads and the toes.

External shoe modifications include the rocker sole, the shape and position of which varies according to the patient's specific foot problems, and sole flares and stabilizers. A flare is an extension to the heel and/or sole of the shoe, and it can be placed medially or laterally to stabilize hindfoot, midfoot, or forefoot instability. An extended offset heel is an additional extension added to the side of the shoe, including both the sole and upper, to stabilize severe hindfoot or midfoot instabilities. The addition of an extended steel shank in the rocker sole can further prevent the shoe from bending, limiting toe and midfoot motion and aiding in propulsion on toe-off. Total contact orthoses are very effective in the distribution and transfer of plantar pressure and in reduction or elimination of weightbearing from problem areas. Custom-made shoes are indicated only for extremely severe deformities and for feet that cannot be fit with depth shoes, even with extensive modifications.

Alternatives to Total Contact Casting

Currently, total contact casting remains the gold standard for the treatment of diabetic foot ulceration. Some alternatives to total contact casting that have been reported in the literature will be discussed.

Standard below knee walking casts have been used to promote healing of neuropathic plantar ulcers in patients with diabetes and Hansen's disease since the 1930s. Reduction of plantar

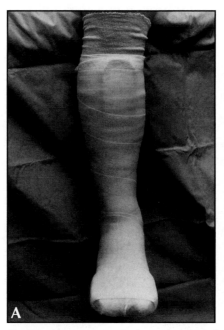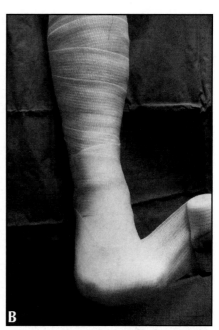

Fig. 4 A, After wrapping the leg with a single layer of gauze the fiberglass casting material is wrapped around the leg. The first layer should be applied and molded to the leg and arch area as it is hardening. This increases the contact of the skin with the cast and promotes all the functions of the cast. **B,** The toes are included in the fiberglass wrapping.

pressure over the ulcer site is the goal. Pollard and Le Quesne[27] demonstrated that conventional walking casts reduce plantar foot pressure. Birke and associates[8] demonstrated equal plantar distribution in short leg casts and total contact casts. Conti and associates[6] have shown that the 2 types of casts are similar; however, they warned that compression over time of the multilayered cast padding in a standard cast may significantly alter those results. They also felt that casts made of fiberglass without plaster were as efficacious as more traditional plaster and fiberglass composite casts. Huband and Carr[28] demonstrated ulcer healing in 12 patients using standard short leg walking casts. They showed that plaster or fiberglass casting tape was equally efficacious. The open toe design of a standard cast may predispose to iatrogenic dorsal foot ulceration and foreign body entrance into

the cast and, therefore, the closed toe design of the total contact cast is superior. As with total contact casting, a standard walking cast is indicated only for the management of patients with superficial forefoot or midfoot plantar ulcerations. Heel ulcers are not unloaded by either cast.

The bivalved AFO walker or the CROW brace[29] is a total contact orthosis that approximates the fit of a well-molded plaster cast. Conventional AFO braces had been used after cast treatment prior to the development of the CROW. Persistent anterior edema with the AFO was managed with the addition of an anterior shell. However, patients had difficulty fitting the brace into a shoe. This lead to the development of the full foot enclosure. In the CROW, a custom foot orthosis is manufactured to accommodate for bone deformity. A rocker bottom sole facilitates ambulation, and a ventilation hole is

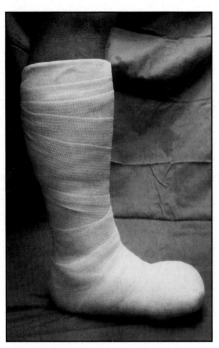

Fig. 5 Final view of total contact cast.

provided for increased comfort. The anterior and posterior shells make the CROW easy to wear. They are primarily used for patients who have a plantar ulcer associated with fluctuating edema in the foot and leg or in patients who are being weaned from a total contact cast following treatment for neuroarthropathy. The CROW continues to control edema, allows ambulation, and provides satisfaction to the patient. Few reports are available describing successful treatment with the CROW.

A commercial prefabricated walking brace[7] can be used for both diabetic ulcer care and in the management of neuroarthropathy. Diabetic ulcers must be protectively padded and closely monitored. The typical posttrauma cam walker can be modified with pads and used for this purpose. Recently, a new design in cast bracing has become available that has a closed padded heel. The fixed ankle heel control type cast brace may be modified for use in diabetic foot

ulcers. This cast brace is designed to control heel position and foot motion. With this device, use of a custom-made insole is necessary for satisfactory ulcer treatment and prevention. The cast braces offer an advantage over plaster type casts in that they may be removed for wound care, and they allow easy, frequent inspection of suspected infections. They also provide better hygiene and greater patient comfort. Disadvantages include lack of objective quantification of plantar pressure reduction. Also, because the device cannot achieve an intimate contour with the leg, it cannot unload the foot as effectively as a total contact cast.

The IPOS postoperative shoe (IPOS, Niagara Falls, NY) can be used to treat patients with superficial plantar forefoot ulcers. It is designed with 10° of dorsiflexion and a heel that is elevated 4 cm to avoid any forefoot contact with the ground. The distal edge of the shoe ends at the proximal metatarsals. Needleman[30] reported 77% of patients with Wagner grade 1 and 2 forefoot ulcers healed in an average of 8 weeks and there was a 78% compliance rate. The advantages include expected high patient compliance, ability for bipedal ambulation, ability to evaluate the foot frequently for infection, and relatively low cost. This treatment method may be more acceptable to patients who live long distances from the treating physician and who would find regular cast changes to be burdensome. Disadvantages include problems with balance and the potential for forming new ulcers on other parts of the foot due to increased load and the fact that it is indicated only for forefoot ulcerations.

Discussion

Diabetes mellitus and its complications represent a significant expense

to the health care system. The concept of disease state management includes teaching patients and physicians to use appropriate resources to prevent many of these complications. Preventing and healing neuropathic plantar ulcerations can be frustrating, time consuming, and expensive. Questions of efficacy and cost of treatment become important in this disease. There are questions about the cost of healing foot ulcers versus amputation. Costs following the successful healing of plantar ulcerations have also been raised. In a report[31] in 1995, the total cost to the system was calculated for 3 years following the successful healing of a foot ulcer either by nonsurgical treatment or amputation. The total cost for patients who were without ischemia who healed their ulcer primarily was $16,100. The total cost for the same period in patients who underwent major amputation to heal their ulcer was $63,100. It would seem that healing a plantar ulceration and salvaging a limb results in a cost savings over amputating the limb even after the acute treatment is over.

Sinacore and associates[32] described the effectiveness of total contact casting in their reports of patients who had chronic plantar ulcers for an average of 11 months (ranging from 1 week to 13 years) despite other forms of treatment, such as daily dressing changes, antibiotic therapy, frequent callus shaving and debridement, and multiple skin grafts. They noted healing in 82% of 33 ulcers after an average of 44 days in a total contact cast. Helm and associates[33] reported a 73% rate of healing in 22 patients, with an average time to healing of 38 days. Boulton and associates[11] found healing in 100% of 7 patients treated with a total contact cast for an average of 6 weeks. Walker and associates[34] reported a 71% healing rate in an average of 35.8 days in a series of 77 diabetic patients with neuropathic ulceration of the foot. Myerson and associates[35] confirmed the effectiveness of total contact casting in their series of 71 neuropathic ulcers of the foot in 66 patients. They reported 64 of 71 (90%) ulcers were healed at a mean of 5.5 weeks (range 1 to 14 weeks). Mueller and associates,[12] in their first reported controlled clinical trial study, described an ulcer healing rate of 90% (19 of 21 patients) with a mean time of healing of 42 ± 29 days (range 8 to 91 days). The combined results of these studies yield an average rate of successful healing of 84.3% in an average time of 39.9 days in the cast.

Time to healing has been shown to vary depending on the site of the ulcer. The time period for the healing of plantar ulcers on the forefoot by total contact casting varies from ulcers elsewhere on the foot. Walker and associates[34] reported in their study that forefoot ulcers (metatarsal heads and toe) healed in an average of 30.6 days compared to nonforefoot ulcers (dorsum of the foot, heel, plantar arch, ankle, medial aspect of the metatarsal and toe, or transmetatarsal amputation sites) which healed in an average of 42.1 days. My experience is comparable, in that forefoot ulcerations treated by total contact casting take relatively less time to heal compared to the nonforefoot ulcerations.

Although most ulcers are the result of neuropathy, the evaluation of the vascular status of the limb plays an important role in the overall management of foot ulcers in patients with diabetes mellitus. In addition to small-vessel disease, there is a significant incidence of large-vessel disease, especially below the level of the trifurcation of the popliteal artery. Sinacore and associates[32] suggested

that total contact casting was effective even for ischemic ulcers. A report by Laing and associates[36] contradicts that belief. They treated 36 diabetic patients with neuropathic ulcers, 28 healed in an average of 6.3 weeks. Eight of the ulcers failed to heal. Six of these were in ischemic limbs, with average Doppler Ankle/Brachial (A/B) index of 0.61 (range 0.44 to 0.81). By contrast, the average A/B index in the healed diabetic ulcers was 1.2 (range 0.7 to 2). Myerson and associates[35] found that most ulcers will heal in a reasonable period of time regardless of the marginal pressure indices on Doppler testing. They recommend vascular consultation only for those patients who have marginal circulation and fail to heal after an appropriate time in a total contact cast. I believe that all painless neuropathic ulcers should receive a trial of total contact casting prior to vascular evaluation. The only exceptions are obvious painful, ischemic ulcers or those that have severe ischemia with gross trophic changes suggesting impending gangrene. Alternative healing strategies should be employed pending vascular evaluation. Vascular insufficiency should be considered in cases of recalcitrant ulcerations.

There are several other reasons for failure of an ulcer to heal with total contact casting. Patient noncompliance due to absence of pain in the feet is often a factor. Although casting is an ambulatory treatment option, patients are asked to restrict their activity to one-third normal while in the cast. Appropriate counseling is often all that is necessary to achieve compliance. Severe deformity that is not accommodated by the cast is another problem. This is especially common in the case of midfoot collapse. Exostectomy, Achilles tendon lengthening, or more extensive reconstructions may be necessary to

reduce excessive pressures. Underlying osteomyelitis, especially in the forefoot and heel, is also a reason for failure of casting. Excessive drainage is often the only clinical clue to the diagnosis. Appropriate radiologic testing can confirm the diagnosis and assess the extent of the infection. Antibiotics may suppress the drainage temporarily. Occasionally, the physician may prescribe antibiotics and casting, which allows an ulcer to close, only to find that the entire foot has become cellulitic. An expeditious workup for osteomyelitis should be undertaken in this situation. Patients who are casted and have dormant osteomyelitis will often heal superficially, but breakdown occurs soon after casting is discontinued.[4,37]

Recurrent ulceration is usually caused by noncompliance with prescription footwear or by failure of footwear to reduce pressure. Significant deformity may not be sufficiently unloaded in the shoe. Plantar pressure measurement made in the shoe may help to assess if footwear is optimal. Helm and associates[38] in a 6-year research project, found that patient compliance and deformities secondary to Charcot changes were the major causes for ulcer recurrence. They reported a recurrence rate of 19.4% in their study of 102 patients. Myerson and associates[35] described a recurrence rate of 31.1% in their study of 71 neuropathic ulcers. We have used an inshoe pressure-measuring device for several years and have found that 50% of recurrent ulcerations can be prevented by modifying the footwear based on the test results.

Current research is investigating the role of topical wound healing agents on ulcer healing. The use of platelet-derived growth factor has been found effective in 3 separate published clinical trials.[39-41] These studies demonstrated that the combination of aggressive revascularization and debridement, infection control and unloading of plantar ulcers, along with the use of PDWHF (platelet-derived wound-healing factor), was effective in ulcer healing. However, the role of PDWHF apart from other aspects of an overall wound-healing regimen is not entirely clear. Results of 2 other clinical trials that used recombinant growth factors in patients with pressure sores and split thickness skin grafts have been recently published.[23,42] To date, there have been no other published studies on recombinant growth factors and diabetic ulcer healing. The next logical step in ulcer healing will be to combine FDA approved growth factor preparations with removable ambulatory pressure relieving devices. Care must be taken to evaluate these devices fully before use. Currently, total contact casting is the gold standard by which all other devices must be assessed.

References

1. Khan JS: Treatment of leprous trophic ulcers. *Leprosy India* 1939;11:19–21.

2. Brand PW: The insensitive foot (including leprosy), in Jahss MH (ed): *Disorders of the Foot.* Philadelphia, PA, WB Saunders, 1982, vol 2, pp 1266–1286.

3. Brand PW: The diabetic foot, in Ellenberg M, Rifkin H (eds): *Diabetes Mellitus: Theory and Practice,* ed 3. New Hyde Park, NY, Medical Examination Publishing, 1983, pp 829–849.

4. Bauman JH, Girling JP, Brand PW: Plantar pressures and trophic ulceration: An evaluation of footwear. *J Bone Joint Surg* 1963;45B:652–673.

5. Coleman WG, Brand PW, Birke JA: The total contact cast: A therapy for plantar ulceration of the insensitive feet. *J Am Podiatry Assoc* 1984;74:548–552.

Appendix
Total Contact Cast Instructions

You have had a total-contact cast applied to your foot for the purpose of healing the ulcer (sore) on your foot. These ulcers do not heal because of the extremely high pressures on the sole of the foot during walking. The cast was made to decrease the pressure on the ulcer, thereby allowing the ulcer to heal. In addition to the pressure relief, the cast is designed to be very snug fitting, with the toes enclosed for protection.

For the total contact cast to be effective, you must know how to take care of your cast. The following is a list of what to do and not to do.

Do not bear weight or walk on your cast until you are told to do so by the person putting the cast on your foot.

We recommend you limit your walking and standing to one third of the normal daily routine or walking distance.

Never use the cast to strike or hit objects. Dents, cracks or softened areas of the cast may cause excessive pressure on your foot in the cast and should be reported immediately.

Keep the cast dry at all times. Water will destroy your cast. Sponge bathing is recommended instead of showering while in your cast. Use a rubberized short leg disposable sleeve to protect the cast when bathing. DO NOT submerge your cast in water. If the cast does become wet, dry it immediately with a towel or hair dryer set to "cool". If it rains, cover the cast with a plastic bag.

Your cast may be inconvenient, and you may have difficulty sleeping. This is not uncommon. You may try wrapping the cast in a towel or placing it on a pillow while in bed.

After you have been wearing the cast several days, perspiration and dirt may cause itching of the skin inside the cast. This is common. You must ignore it. Do not stick pencils, coat hangers, or other objects in the cast to scratch the skin.

Inspect the entire cast daily. Look and feel for deep cracks or soft spots on the cast. use a small hand mirror to inspect the sole of the cast or have a family member check the sole of the cast.

Never attempt to remove your cast by yourself.

Removing Your Cast

We have a specially designed saw to remove the cast with little discomfort. It should be removed only by a health care professional. After removal, your skin may be flaky and dry, and your joint may feel stiff. Apply a thick cream or oil for several days to moisten and soften the skin.

You will need to have your specially made shoes ready to wear immediately after the cast is removed to prevent your foot form getting another ulcer.

Warning Signs

If any of the following signs or symptoms occur call (physician phone number).

Excessive swelling of the leg or foot if the cast becomes too tight.

The cast becomes too loose and your leg can move up or down in the cast greater than 1/4 inch.

The cast has any deep cracks or soft spots.

Any drainage of pus or blood on the outside of the cast. This will appear brownish or dark yellow.

Any foul-smelling odor from the cast.

You experience any excessive tenderness in your groin or the casted foot.

Any excessive leg pain or annoying pressure in the ankle or foot which will not go away.

You notice any sudden onset of fever or an unusual elevation in your blood sugar. We highly recommend daily self-monitoring of your blood glucose during casting if you are not already doing so.

If any of the above conditions exist, do the following:

Notify appropriate professional personnel at once.

Do not walk on your cast. Keep your leg elevated.

Use crutches or a walker and keep the casted foot off the ground until seen by professional personnel.

6. Conti SF, Martin RL, Chaytor ER, Hughes C, Luttrell L: Plantar pressure measurements during ambulation in weightbearing conventional short leg casts and total contact casts. *Foot Ankle Int* 1996;17:464–469.

7. Brodsky JW: The diabetic foot, in Mann RA, Coughlin MJ (eds): *Surgery of the Foot and Ankle*, ed 6. St. Louis, MO, Mosby-Year Book, 1993, vol 2, pp 977–957.

8. Birke JA, Sims DS Jr, Buford WL: Walking casts: Effect on plantar foot pressures. *J Rehabil Res Dev* 1985;22:18–22.

9. Martin RL, Conti SF: Plantar pressure analysis of diabetic rockerbottom deformity in total contact casts. *Foot Ankle Int* 1996;17:470–472.

10. Shaw JE, Hsi WL, Ulbrecht JS, Norkitis A, Becker MB, Cavanagh PR: The mechanism of plantar unloading in total contact casts: Implications for design and clinical use. *Foot Ankle Int* 1997;18:809–817.

11. Boulton AJ, Bowker JH, Gadia M, et al: Use of plaster casts in the management of diabetic neuropathic foot ulcers. *Diabetes Care* 1986;9:149–152.

12. Mueller MJ, Diamond JE, Sinacore DR, et al: Total contact casting in treatment of diabetic plantar ulcers: controlled clinical trial. *Diabetes Care* 1989;12:384–388.

13. Jordan WR: Neuritic manifestations in diabetes mellitus. *Arch Intern Med* 1936;57:307–366.

14. Clohisy DR, Thompson RC Jr: Fractures associated with neuropathic arthropathy in adults who have juvenile-onset diabetes. *J Bone Joint Surg* 1988;70A:1192–1200.

15. Clouse ME, Gramm HF, Legg M, Flood T: Diabetic osteoarthropathy: Clinical and roentgenographic observations in 90 cases, *Am J Roentgenol Radium Ther Nucl Med* 1974;121:22–34.

16. Sinha S, Munichoodappa CS, Kozak GP: Neuro-arthropathy (Charcot joints) in diabetes mellitus: Clinical study of 101 cases. *Medicine* 1972;51:191–210.

17. Bailey CC, Root HF: Neuropathic foot lesions in diabetes mellitus. *N Engl J Med* 1947;236:397–401.

18. Forgacs S: Clinical picture of diabetic osteoarthropathy. *Acta Diabetol Lat* 1976;13:111–129.

19. Pogonowska MJ, Collins LC, Dobson HL: Diabetic osteopathy. *Radiology* 1967;89:265–271.

20. Anania WC, Rosen RC, Wallace JA, Weinblatt MA, Gerland JS, Castillo J: Treatment of diabetic skin ulcerations with povidone-iodine and sugar: Two case reports. *J Am Podiatr Med Assoc* 1985;75:472–474.

21. Holstein P, Larsen K, Sager P: Decompression with the aid of insoles in the treatment of diabetic neuropathic ulcers. *Acta Orthop Scand* 1976;47:463–468.

22. Newman JH: Spontaneous dislocation in diabetic neuropathy: A report of six cases. *J Bone Joint Surg* 1979;61B:484–488.

23. Robson MC, Phillips LG, Thomason A, Robsosn LE, Pierce GF: Platelet-derived growth factor BB for the treatment of chronic pressure ulcers. *Lancet* 1992;339:23–25.

24. Norman A, Robbins H, Milgram JE: The acute neuropathic arthropathy: A rapid, severely disorganizing form of arthritis. *Radiology* 1967;90:1159–1164.

25. Eichenholtz SN (ed): *Charcot Joints*. Springfield, IL, Charles C Thomas, 1966.

26. Chantelau E, Breuer U, Leisch AC, Tanudjaja T, Reuter M: Outpatient treatment of unilateral diabetic foot ulcers with "half shoes." *Diabet Med* 1993;10:267–270.

27. Pollard JP, Le Quesne LP: Method of healing diabetic forefoot ulcers. *Br Med J* 1983;286:436–437.

28. Huband MS, Carr JB: A simplified method of total contact casting for diabetic foot ulcers. *Contemp Orthop* 1993;26:143–147.

29. Morgan JM, Biehl WC III, Wagner FW Jr: Management of neuropathic arthropathy with the Charcot Restraint Orthotic Walker. *Clin Orthop* 1993;296:58–63.

30. Needleman RL: Successes and pitfalls in the healing of neuropathic forefoot ulcerations with the IPOS postoperative shoe. *Foot Ankle Int* 1997;18:412–417.

31. Apelqvist J, Ragnarson-Tennvall G, Larsson J, Persson U: Long-term costs for foot ulcers in diabetic patients in a multidisciplinary setting. *Foot Ankle Int* 1995;16:388–394.

32. Sinacore DR, Mueller, MJ, Diamond JE, Blair VP III, Drury D, Rose SJ: Diabetic plantar ulcers treated by total contact casting: A clinical report. *Phys Ther* 1987;67:1543–1549.

33. Helm PA, Walker SC, Pullium G: Total contact casting in diabetic patients with neuropathic foot ulcerations. *Arch Phys Med Rehabil* 1984;65:691–693.

34. Walker SC, Helm PA, Pullium G: Total contact casting and chronic diabetic neuropathic foot ulcerations: Healing rates by wound location. *Arch Phys Med Rehabil* 1987;68:217–221.

35. Myerson M, Papa J, Eaton K, Wilson K: The total contact cast for management of neuropathic plantar ulceration of the foot. *J Bone Joint Surg* 1992;74A:261–269.

36. Laing PW, Cogley DI, Klenerman L: Neuropathic foot ulceration treated by total contact casts. *J Bone Joint Surg* 1992;74B:133–136.

37. Levin ME: Medical evaluation and treatment, in Levin ME, O'Neal LW (eds): *The Diabetic Foot*. St. Louis, MO, CV Mosby, 1983, pp 1–60.

38. Helm PA, Walker SC, Pullium GF: Recurrence of neuropathic ulceration following healing in a total contact cast. *Arch Phys Med Rehabil* 1991;72:967–970.

39. Fylling CP, Knighton DR, Gordinier RH: The use of a comprehensive wound care protocol including topical growth factor therapy in treatment of diabetic neuropathic ulcers, in Ward J, Goto Y (eds): *Diabetic Neuropathy*. Chichester, England, John Wiley & Sons, 1990, pp 567–578.

40. Knighton DR, Ciresi K, Kiegel VD, Schumerth S, Butler E, Cerra F: Stimulation of repair in chronic, nonhealing, cutaneous ulcers using platelet-derived wound healing formula. *Surg Gynecol Obstet* 1990;170:56–60.

41. Knighton DR, Fylling CP, Fiegel VD, Cerra F: Amputation prevention in an independently reviewed at-risk diabetic population using a comprehensive wound care protocol. *Am J Surg* 1990;160:466–471.

42. Brown GL, Nanney LB, Griffen J, et al: Enhancement of wound healing by topical treatment with epidermal growth factor. *N Engl J Med* 1989;321:76–79.

Diabetic Foot Infections

Charles L. Saltzman, MD
Walter J. Pedowitz, MD

Scope of the Problem

Trivial infections in diabetic feet can have disastrous effects. The monetary and human impact of these infections is staggering. The infected foot is one of the most common causes of admission of diabetic patients to the hospital, often requiring prolonged care. Infection is also a major pathway to ultimate amputation. The incidence of amputation in patients with diabetes is approximately 5%, 40 times that of the nondiabetic population.[1]

Pathophysiology

The pathophysiology of diabetic foot infection is complex. Patients with long-standing disease and multiple secondary complications are most prone to develop serious infections. Once initiated, both host and microbiologic factors impact the aggressiveness of the infection. The host factors that have been shown to result in an increased risk of amputation are diabetes mellitus for longer than 10 years, chronic hyperglycemia, impaired vision or joint mobility (required to perform preventive foot care), lack of knowledge about preventive foot care, increasing age, nephropathy, single/widowed/separated or divorced persons, alcohol use, nonwhites, males, and a history of previous amputation. Events leading to serious, limb-threatening infections typically involve an initial episode of minor trauma (eg, shoe-related repetitive pressure, accidental cuts or wounds, thermal trauma, and/or decubitus ulceration), cutaneous ulceration, and failure to heal. Other causal factors found to impact the outcome of a local foot infection are edema, impairing cutaneous blood flow; noncompliance in medical recommendations; negligent self-care; and inadequate social support.

The etiology of foot ulcers is clearly multifactorial, including neuropathy, vascular disease, infection, delayed wound healing, and, sometimes, development of gangrene. In large studies, the absence of protective sensation has been found to be the primary related factor for the development of ulcers and infection. The absence of protective sensation typically causes a distal, symmetric, "stocking" distribution of sensory loss mostly confined below the knees. Patients may initially experience a constant burning type of pain, which is worse at night. With further progression of the sensory neuropathy, they may develop unrecognized injury, ulceration, fracture, and foot deformity.

Concomitant with the development of sensory neuropathy, many patients also acquire either motor and/or autonomic neuropathy. The motor neuropathy manifests itself with claw-toe deformities caused by atrophy of the foot intrinsic muscles. Claw-toe deformities expose bony prominences on the dorsum of the toe to increased pressure from normal shoe wear. They also result in migration of the metatarsal fat pad, with plantar loss of cover of the metatarsal heads, loss of toe weightbearing during terminal stance, and increased pressure on exposed metatarsal heads. Some patients will also develop mononeuropathies causing focal deficits, such as foot drop from an anterior tibial mononeuropathy, recurrent ankle sprains from peroneal weakness, or flatfoot deformity from posterior tibialis denervation.

Although less prevalent, autonomic neuropathy can create vexing epidermal problems from diminished sweating. This may result in the drying of epidermal keratin, cracking and fissuring of noncompliant skin, and increased susceptibility to infection. Arteriovenous shunting secondary to autonomic neuropathy further compromises the ability of skin to heal minor ulcerations and deliver antibiotics peripherally.

The vascular disease that occurs secondary to diabetes mellitus usually involves all 3 major arterial supplies to the leg and foot. Decreased blood flow compromises the host's ability to heal and fight infection. Furthermore, these patients often have decreased local immune response. Basement membrane thickening has been proposed as a basic factor responsible for hampering leukocyte migration to the infection site. Laboratory studies show that phagocytic activity is impaired by hyperglycemia, and that neutrophils do not function properly in this environment.

In summary, the host factors that result in clinically significant diabetic foot infections are complex. Due to sensory neuropathy, visual or physical impairments, and frequent social isolation, many patients fail to recognize ulceration or infection early on. Lack of vascular nutrition, either due to autonomic arteriovenous shunting or from vascular insufficiency, further confounds the ability of the host to fight infection. The cellular response is often weak and insufficient to successfully eradicate invading microbiologic flora. Malnutrition, hyperglycemia, decreased peripheral microvasculature, anaerobic metabolism, and poor wound healing all help to create a hospitable environment for the bacteria.[2]

Infectious Agents

Most often, infections of the diabetic foot are polymicrobial. On average, 3 to 5 organisms are cultured from the moderately to severely infected foot. The type of organism(s) present may be gram-positive cocci and/or gram-negative rods, and anaerobes, with the latter seen more often in infections of increasing severity. The gram-positive organisms include *Staphylococcus aureus, Staphylococcus epidermidis, group B Streptococcus,* and *enterococci.* The gram-negative organisms may include *Proteus, Escherichia coli* or *Pseudomonas.* Among the anaerobes, *Bacteroides* is the most common infecting agent.[2]

Diagnosis of Cellulitis and/or Osteomyelitis

A complete history and physical examination are essential first steps. Local signs of infection, including erythema, swelling, and purulent drainage, should be noted. Foul-smelling drainage usually suggests an anaerobic infection. The examiner should try to probe to bone, using a sterile cotton swab. In this setting, the ability to probe to bone has an 80% positive predictive value of underlying osteomyelitis. The scope of the work-up depends on the level of clinical infection, but it usually includes obtaining a set of vital signs, temperature, a spot glucose test, and a white blood cell count with differential. These results must be interpreted with caution, because absence of fever or leukocytosis may be the result of diabetic immunosuppression, which can hide the serious underlying nature of the disease. Two thirds of patients with limb-threatening infection do not demonstrate fever of greater than 100° F. Half do not demonstrate leukocytosis.

Ulcers can be classified in various ways.[1,2–4] Probably the most common method used is that proposed by Wagner. In this classification scheme, ulcers are graded from 0 to 5 according to the depth of the ulcer, whether there is exposed tendon or bone, and whether there is an abscess or gangrene present. This system may be good to help guide surgical decisions, but it is not particularly helpful for clinical microbiologic purposes.

A more relevant system for guiding therapy is based on determining the aggressiveness of infection in the limb. Infections are classified as mild, moderate, or severe. Mild infections involve superficial ulceration, purulent discharge, minimal/absent cellulitis, and no osteomyelitis or systemic toxicity. Moderate-to-severe infec-

tions (potentially limb-threatening) involve ulcerations to deep tissues, purulent discharge, cellulitis, systemic toxicity, and mild-to-moderate necrosis, with or without osteomyelitis. Severe (potentially life-threatening) infections involve ulceration to deep tissues; purulent discharge; cellulitis; systemic toxicity, including septic shock, marked necrosis, or gangrene; and bacteremia, with or without osteomyelitis. Some of the moderate-to-severe infections that may require emergent surgical intervention are crepitant anaerobic cellulitis, non-clostridial/clostridial myonecrosis, or synergistic necrotizing fasciitis. This system of classifying infections according to whether they are local, limb-threatening, or life-threatening (mild, moderate, or severe) is helpful in determining appropriate treatment.

Culture/Biopsy

Our understanding of the need for culture or biopsy continues to evolve. Superficial cultures are rarely of value. Deep tissue cultures correlate poorly with superficial cultures, which tend to over-represent pathogens. The general consensus is to avoid superficial cultures.

The importance and need for deep cultures has changed with the emergence of better and more broad-spectrum antibiotics. Culture-specific treatment has not been shown to have better results than empiric treatment with broad-spectrum coverage. At present, it seems reasonable to perform bone biopsies or deep cultures at the time of surgical treatment, or in situations in which empiric therapy is failing. If empiric therapy results in an improved clinical condition, the authors recommend continuing that therapy rather than changing to a more culture-specific and narrower-spectrum antibiotic, because there are notorious problems with false-negative cultures in diabetic foot infections.

Imaging

The two clinical indications for imaging the diabetic foot are osteomyelitis and abscess formation. Osteomyelitis takes 10 to 21 days to become apparent on plain films, because a period of time is required before there is enough bone resorption to be radiographically apparent. In a diabetic patient with a poor vascular blood supply, bone resorption can take a considerably longer time than in a patient with an adequate blood supply.[5]

More sophisticated imaging modalities include the use of a technetium-labeled bone scan combined with indium-111 leukocyte scans, or magnetic resonance imaging (MRI) investigations. Because of the relative ease of use, MRI has become far more popular than the combined scan approach. Compared to the nuclear medicine scans, MRI will better delineate anatomy, especially abscess cavities and marrow involvement. MRI scans, however, tend to over-represent the amount of involved bone, and surgeons must be cautious when deciding the extent of osteomyelitis based on an MRI scan alone. Johnson and associates[6] have advocated the use of the indium-labeled scans to follow up negative plain films because the indium scan will not be false-positive from Charcot osteoarthropathy (as will the MRI), and when the indium scan is negative, the clinician can feel comfortable that there is little likelihood of ongoing infection.

Treatment

Most ulcers in diabetic patients are not infected, but are rather due to tissue necrosis from unrecognized elevated pressure.[1,2] Ulcers can occur anywhere on the foot. Plantar ulcers are best treated with total contact casting. Reports on total contact casting for plantar ulceration in noninfected diabetic feet are extremely encouraging. Within 5 weeks, 90% of ulcers will heal.[7]

For mild infections, patients usually are treated as outpatients with oral antibiotic coverage for *Staphylococcus aureus*, *Staphylococcus epidermidis*, and *Streptococcus*. Many different medications can be used. The most common ones are dicloxacillin, first-generation cephalosporins, clindamycin, and amoxicillin-clavulanic acid. The patient is brought back in 2 to 3 days for reevaluation. If the patient is not responding, the medication should be changed to another oral agent. If the condition is getting worse, the clinician may consider switching to IV therapy. Typically, mild infections are treated with local wound care, using wet-to-dry dressing changes or Silvadene, and pressure relief modalities, such as the use of crutches, custom-made orthotics with cut-outs, postoperative shoes with the forefoot removed, or healing sandals. After a 2 to 3 week course of antibiotics, if the infection is completely abated, the antibiotics are usually discontinued.

Moderate infections that are limb threatening are often caused by a synergistic combination of gram-positive and gram-negative aerobes and anaerobes. At the present time, to effectively treat these problems, IV antibiotics are required. The most common strategies are to use ampicillin-sulbactam, ticarcillin-clavulanate, piperacillin-tazobactam, or a fluocinolone with clindamycin (for penicillin-allergic patients). If present, abscesses are drained or excised, and necrotic bone is debrided. All patients should be assessed for the potential need for distal revascularization. The length of the IV course is typically 4 to 6 weeks, unless all infected bone and tissue has been removed. Recently, the earlier switch from IV therapy to an oral fluocinolone has been recommended.[8] More studies on the value of the newer oral fluocinolone are needed before a major change in treatment strategy can be advised.

For severe infections, the clinician must stabilize the patient and debride, drain, or amputate the infected part as is clinically necessary. In life-threatening infections, broad-spectrum antibiotics should be used. Imipenem-cilastatin is one of the more-powerful broad-spectrum antibiotics that can be used in this setting. Similarly, a combination of vancomycin, metronidazole, and aztreonam can be considered. If ampicillin-sulbactam is initiated, it should be started with an aminoglycoside to cover aggressive gram-negative organisms. If the patient is not responding to the regimen, an infectious disease consultation may be necessary.

Surgical Treatment of Infection

Appropriate antibiotics are no substitute for proper wound care and adequate surgical debridement. Patients with moderate-to-severe infections should receive early and aggressive drainage and debridement of all necrotic tissue. If the infection has significantly destroyed the function of the foot and/or endangers the patient's life, guillotine amputation to control sepsis may be indicated.

Some basic rules help in most circumstances. These rules include: (1) Debride all necrotic tissue and do not leave any dead tissue behind. (2) All surfaces should be bleeding at the end of the operation. (3) Check the histopathology of residual margins for evidence of residual infection. (4) If the initial debridement is uncertain, pack the wound open and repeat the surgery within a few days, if necessary. (5) Try to achieve an eventual closure, even if it means removal of more bone. (6) When closed, wound edges must be well perfused.

Postoperatively, the foot should not be allowed to dangle for excessive periods of time to avoid potential complications of venous stasis and wound dehiscence. The failure of a wound to heal may indicate vascular compromise. Reevaluate and restore circulation, if possible. If not possible, resect back to a viable level. These wounds heal slowly; in general, the sutures should be left in at least 3 weeks.

Improved results in the care of the diabetic foot have resulted from an aggressive approach to wound management, antibiotic coverage, revascularization when necessary, improved perioperative management, and a general team approach to the care of the patient. Relapses are more common in the diabetic foot than for other infections, and the clinician must attempt to educate the patient and the family about how to avoid unrecognized injury and how to recognize the early signs of infection.

References

1. Grayson ML: Diabetic foot infections: Antimicrobial therapy. *Infect Dis Clin North Am* 1995;9:143–161.

2. Frykberg RG, Veves A: Diabetic foot infections. *Diabetes Metab Rev* 1996;12:255–270.

3. Hass DW, McAndrew MP: Bacterial osteomyelitis in adults: Evolving considerations in diagnosis and treatment. *Am J Med* 1996;101:550–561.

4 van der Meer JW, Koopmans PP, Lutterman JA: Antibiotic therapy in diabetic foot infection. *Diabet Med* 1996;13(suppl 1):S48–S51.

5. Newman LG: Imaging techniques in the diabetic foot. *Clin Podiatr Med Surg* 1995;12:75–86.

6. Johnson JE, Kennedy EJ, Shereff MJ, Patel NC, Collier BD: Prospective study of bone, indium-111-labeled white blood cell, and gallium-67 scanning for the evaluation of osteomyelitis in the diabetic foot. *Foot Ankle Int* 1996;17:10–16.

7. Smith AJ, Daniels T, Bohnen JM: Soft tissue infections and the diabetic foot. *Am J Surg* 1996;172:7S–12S.

8. Lipsky BA, Baker PD, Landon GC, Fernay R: Antibiotic therapy for diabetic foot infections: Comparison of two parenteral-to-oral regimens. *Clin Infect Dis* 1997;24:643–648.

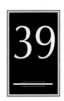

Principles of Partial Foot Amputations in the Diabetic

Douglas G. Smith, MD

Introduction

Lower extremity amputations are performed because of gangrene, severe infection, ischemia, or severe deformity of the diabetic foot. In the years 1988 to 1992 there were an estimated 130,000 amputations performed each year in the United States. This number comes from the National Hospital Discharge Survey's (NHDS) estimate of 110,000 amputations annually, the Department of Veterans Affairs Hospital's estimate of 17,000 amputations annually, and the unknown, but lesser number estimated from the military, private charitable, and Indian Health Services Hospitals.[1] Even though persons with diabetes represent only about 3% of the total US population, 51% of the discharge diagnosis for amputation also listed the diagnosis of diabetes. Using this number, approximately 65,000 individuals with diabetes undergo lower extremity amputations per year.[1]

Table 1 shows the estimated breakdown by surgical amputation level of the percentage of lower extremity amputations performed for persons with and without diabetes, based on the NHDS data. Many physicians believe that the rate of transfemoral amputations has decreased dramatically in the last 20 years, but statistics from the NHDS indicate that overall, more transfemoral amputations are done each year than transtibial amputations. The data do show that in persons with diabetes the ratio of transtibial to transfemoral amputations is slightly more favorable, but closer than many expect[1] (Table 1).

Decision Making

In diabetes, tissue loss, deep infection, especially osteomyelitis, chronic ulceration, or ischemia are the most frequent reasons for amputation. The preoperative evaluation of these patients includes the clinical examination and evaluation of the tissue quality, level of tissue necrosis from infection, perfusion, nutrition, immune status, and functional abilities. Preoperative screening tests to directly or indirectly measure perfusion can be helpful, but no single test is 100% accurate. Clinical judgment is still an extremely important factor in preoperative assessment of diabetic patients. Although much attention is given to circulation, perfusion pressures, and oxygen diffusion, blood flow is not the only issue.

Table 1
Lower extremity amputations by amputation level and presence of diabetes (NHDS 1989-92)[20]

Amputation Level	Diabetes		No Diabetes		Total	
	No.	%	No.	%	No.	%
Toe	21,671	40.3	12,427	24.1	34,098	32.3
Foot/ankle	7,773	14.5	2,967	5.8	10,740	10.2
Transtibial	13,484	25.1	11,048	21.4	24,527	23.3
Knee disarticulation	704	1.3	778	1.5	1,482	1.4
Transfemoral	8,612	16.0	20,028	38.8	28,640	27.2
Hip/pelvis	87	0.2	386	0.7	473	0.5
Not specified	1,378	2.6	3,971	7.7	5,349	5.1
Total	53,709	100.0	51,605	100.0	105,309	100.0

This chapter was adapted with permission from Smith DG: Principles of partial foot amputations in the diabetic. *Foot Ankle Clin* 1997;2:171–186.

If blood flow to the involved extremity is poor and cannot be improved with angioplasty or vascular bypass, then partial foot amputation is not feasible. Attention needs to be directed at choosing the wisest proximal amputation for that particular patient's clinical situation and rehabilitation goals. For the diabetic patient who is a candidate for partial foot amputation, either the patient with adequate perfusion to the foot, or the patient with reconstructable vascular disease, the surgeon needs to ask the question: "Is this foot worth saving?" All too often, after the patient has already undergone vascular bypass surgery, the team realizes that the foot is not really salvageable and a higher level amputation is required. Some of the other factors besides blood flow that are extremely important in the decision process include the soft-tissue envelope, deformities, sensation, contractures, and rehabilitation goals.

The question regarding the soft-tissue envelope is, "Will the ulcer heal, will it stay healed, or will new ulcers form?"

Deformities, including claw toes, bunion deformity, peritalar subluxation, Charcot collapse, and other bony prominence can impact new ulcer formation and function.[2] "Can these deformities be corrected?"

Regarding sensation, the surgeon must ask, "Is there any sensation to protect the foot after salvage? Are shoe modifications available that might help protect the foot without sensation?"

Contractures, such as Achilles tendon, knee, and toe contractures are common. "How will the contractures impact the function and durability of the salvaged foot? Can the contractures be corrected?"

Questions about rehabilitation goals are: "Does or will the patient ambulate? How will the patient transfer safely? Can this patient use special devices or a prosthesis safely?"

The answers to these questions, whether to proceed with an amputation, and at what level the amputation should be performed, should be considered for every patient during the decision-making process.

Most of the Time: The Goal is to Salvage Part of the Foot

Patients with partial foot amputations require less energy to ambulate than if amputation was performed at the transtibial or transfemoral levels.[3] Even in patients who are marginal ambulators, the improved ability to transfer independently can make a tremendous difference in lifestyle. Often it is not whether a person ambulates with a prosthesis that makes the difference between returning home or requiring nursing supervision, but rather whether they can transfer safely and independently. Most physicians underemphasize the importance of independent transfer ability.

Occasionally: The Most Distal Amputation is Not the Wisest Amputation

Occasionally it is predicted that the patient will function better with the higher level amputation. Special conditions that warrant this radical type of thinking might include nonambulatory patients, patients with spasticity, and patients with severe contractures. For nonambulatory patients, the goals are not simply to obtain wound healing, but to minimize complications, improve sitting balance, transfers, and nursing care. Thus, occasionally, a more proximal amputation might more successfully meet all of the goals. A good example is the bedridden patient with a knee-flexion contracture, who might be better served with a knee disarticulation than a below-knee amputation, even if the biologic factors are present to allow the more distal amputation to heal.

Another example is the patient with a severe equinovarus deformity of the ankle presenting with an ulcer down to bone over the fifth metatarsal head from walking on the lateral border of the foot. A ray amputation without correction of the ankle deformity will result in rapid recurrent ulceration. Either the deformity must be corrected, or a transtibial amputation considered. Preoperative assessment of the patient's potential to be a prosthetic user, the specific needs to maintain independent transfers, or the best weight distribution for seating can also help direct level selection and postoperative rehabilitation wisely.

Surgical Level

The surgical amputation level must be the balance of biology and function. Outline 1 lists considerations in determining the biologic healing level, and the functional level. The biologic healing level is determined to try and predict the most distal amputation level that has a reasonable probability to heal. The functional level is the amputation level at which the patient will probably function best. Occasionally, if the clinical examination, ischemic index, transcutaneous oxygen tension measurement ($TcPO_2$), temperature of the skin, or nutrition indicate that there is little chance of distal wound healing, then biology determines the surgical level and one must do a very high amputation, even if only a toe or forefoot is infected and gangrenous.

Multiple surgeries in the elderly are not desirable. It is not acceptable to have the attitude that we can try the distal amputation, even if there is no reasonable chance of healing, and can amputate higher next time. Each surgery will decrease nutritional reserves and decrease the chance of wound healing. The longer patients are in bed, the more deconditioned they become, and the harder it is to rehabilitate and resume walking. The more surgeries, the higher the risk of problems such as deep venous thrombosis, pulmonary embolism, pneumonia, urinary tract infections, infected intravenous sites, and skin pressure sores. Careful selection of the initial amputation level is essential.

Comments on Adjuncts for Evaluation and Decision Making

Doppler ultrasound blood pressure assessment is the most readily available objective measurement of limb blood flow and perfusion. Arterial wall calcification increases the pressure needed to compress these vessels, often giving an artificially elevated reading. Low pressures are indicative of poor perfusion. Normal and high pressures can be confusing because of vessel wall calcification, and are not predictive of normal perfusion or of wound healing. Digital vessels are not usually calcified, and toe blood pressures appear to be more predictive of healing than ankle pressures.[4,5]

$TcPO_2$ are noninvasive and becoming more readily available in many vascular laboratories.[6] These tests measure the partial pressure of oxygen diffusing through the skin with a special temperature-controlled oxygen electrode. The ultimate reading is based on several factors, including the oxygen delivery to the tissue, the oxygen use by the tissue, and the diffusion of the gas through the skin. Cellulitis and edema can increase use and decrease diffusion, thereby giving lower values. Caution in interpretation of $TcPO_2$ during acute cellulitis or edema is warranted. Also, a

---

Outline 1
Considerations in determining functional and biologic healing

Biologic Healing Level
Trying to predict the most distal level that has a reasonable chance to heal
1. Clinical examination
2. Skin temperature–a line of demarcation is often an excellent indicator of healing level
3. Tissue quality–all necrotic and infected tissue must be removed
4. Nutrition–often accessed by using albumin and total lymphocyte count
5. Ischemic index = arm BP/ankle BP
6. Toe blood pressure–70 to 80 mm Hg is normal
7. $TcPO_2$ = transcutaneous pressure of oxygen at that site, a measure of oxygen delivered to the skin; swelling, cellulitis, venous stasis skin changes will all lower toe $TcPO_2$

Functional Level
The amputation level the patient will function the best with
1. Previous level of ambulation
2. Intelligence
3. Cognitive skills
4. Motivation
5. Cardiopulmonary capacity
6. Spasticity or contractures
7. Rehabilitation goals

BP, blood pressure

---

paradoxical response of $TcPO_2$ to warming on the plantar foot skin has been recently reported, and warrants caution in interpreting plantar foot $TcPO_2$ values.[7] $TcPO_2$ has been shown to be statistically accurate in predicting amputation healing, but false negatives still exist, and many patients' measurements fall into a gray zone for predicting healing.

Xenon 133 skin clearance has been used successfully in the past to predict healing of amputations, but the preparation of the xenon 133 gas/saline solution and the application of this test are highly technician dependent, expensive, and time consuming. A small amount of prepared xenon 133/saline solution is injected intradermally at various sites, and the rate of washout is monitored by gamma camera. After conducting a prospective trial, one previously enthusiastic author is no longer convinced of xenon 133's predictive value, and believes that $TcPO_2$ and $TcPCO_2$ are more predictive and readily available.[8]

Arteriography has not been helpful in predicting successful healing of amputations, and this invasive test is probably not indicated solely for the purpose of level selection. Arteriography is indicated if the patient is truly a candidate for arterial reconstruction or angioplasty.

Nutrition and immunocompetence have been shown to correlate directly with amputation wound healing. Many laboratory tests are available to assess nutrition and immunocompetence, and some are quite expensive. Albumin and total lymphocyte count (TLC) are readily available and inexpensive screening parameters. Several studies have shown increased healing of amputations in dysvascular patients who had a serum albumin level of at least 3.0 or 3.5 grams/deciliter, and TLC > 1,500 cells per cubic millimeter.[9,10] Preoperative nutritional screening is recommended to allow nutritional improvement preoperatively, or consideration of a higher level amputation.

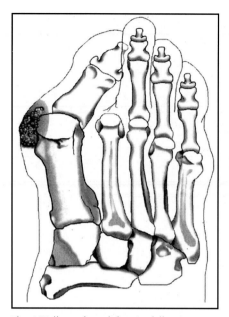

Fig. 1 Hallux valgus deformity following second toe amputation. (Reproduced with permission from the Prosthetics Research Study, Seattle, WA.)

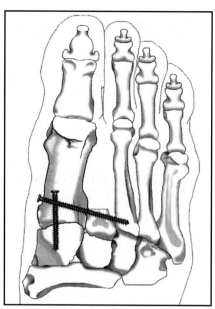

Fig. 2 Second ray amputation with screw fixation to narrow the foot. (Reproduced with permission from the Prosthetics Research Study, Seattle, WA.)

Activity level, ambulatory potential, cognitive skills, and overall medical condition must be evaluated to determine if the most distal level is really appropriate for the patient. In patients who are likely to remain ambulatory, the goal is to achieve healing at the most distal level that can be fit with a prosthesis, and to successful rehabilitate the patient. Recent series of diabetic patients demonstrate that successful wound healing can be achieved in 70% to 80% of these patients at the below-knee or more distal amputation levels. This is in sharp contrast to 25 years ago when, because of a fear of wound failure, surgeons elected to perform 80% of all lower extremity amputations at the above-knee level.

Foot Amputation Levels
Toe Amputations
Toe amputations are common, accounting for 24% of all amputations in diabetic patients.[1] The importance of obtaining successful wound healing and minimizing complications from this often minimized procedure cannot be underestimated. Technically, toe amputations can be performed with side-to-side or plantar-to-dorsal flaps to use the best available soft tissue. The bone should be shortened to a level that allows adequate soft-tissue closure without tension, either disarticulated or metaphyseal. Durable, tension-free soft-tissue padding is much more important than the amount (if any) of phalangeal bone that remains.

In great toe amputations, if the entire proximal phalanx is removed, the sesamoids will often retract, exposing the keel-shaped plantar surface of the first metatarsal to weightbearing. This can lead to high local pressures, callous formation, and ulceration. The sesamoids can be stabilized in position for weightbearing by leaving the base of the proxi-

mal phalanx intact or by tenodesis of the flexor hallucis brevis tendon.

Beware of isolated second toe amputations, because severe hallux valgus deformity of the first toe commonly results (Fig. 1). There is no single solution for every patient. This deformity may possibly be prevented by second ray amputation, first metatarsophalangeal fusion, or considering amputation of both the first and second toes. I prefer second ray amputation and surgical narrowing of the foot with screw fixation when possible (Fig. 2). For the metatarsophalangeal joint level amputation, transferring the extensor tendon to the capsule can help to elevate the metatarsal head and maintain an even distribution for weightbearing. Prosthetic replacement is not required after toe amputations. However, custom-molded insoles and extra-depth shoes are indicated for diabetic patients who have required toe amputation.

Ray Amputations
A ray amputation removes the toe and all or some of the corresponding metatarsal. Isolated ray amputations can be durable; however, multiple ray amputations, especially in dysvascular patients, can narrow the foot excessively. After ray amputation, the body weight must be born by the remaining metatarsal heads. The amount of force that is borne by one or more of the remaining metatarsal heads can increase dramatically. This increased pressure can lead to new areas of callus and ulceration.

Surgically, it is often difficult to close the ray amputation wounds primarily. More skin is usually required than is readily apparent. Instead of closing these wounds under tension, it is usually advisable to leave a portion of the wound open and allow secondary healing, or to consider a transmetatarsal amputation.

The fifth ray amputation has been the most useful of all the ray amputations (Fig. 3). Plantar-lateral ulcers around the fifth metatarsal head are common, and often lead to exposed bone and osteomyelitis. A fifth ray amputation allows the entire ulcer to be excised and the wound closed primarily. A racquet-shaped incision is used to remove the fifth toe and the ulcer, a straight lateral incision extends toward the base of the fifth metatarsal to allow division of the fifth metatarsal near the base. The base of the fifth metatarsal is preserved to keep the attachment of the peroneus brevis tendon. If the entire fifth metatarsal needs to be excised, the peroneus brevis tendon is reattached locally to help preserve eversion of the foot.

All viable skin is retained because, as stated previously, more skin is usually required than is apparent. In the first or fifth ray amputations, any redundant skin helps by providing more padding of the remaining medial or lateral border of the foot, and this skin should be retained. In general, for more extensive involvement of the foot, which would require multiple-ray amputations, a transverse amputation at the transmetatarsal level will be more durable. Prosthetic requirements after ray amputations include extra-depth shoes with custom-molded insoles.

Midfoot Amputations

The transmetatarsal and Lisfranc amputations are reliable and durable. Surgically, a healthy, durable soft-tissue envelope is more important than a specific bone length. The bones should be shortened to allow soft-tissue closure without tension, rather than transected at a specific predetermined anatomic bone level. A long

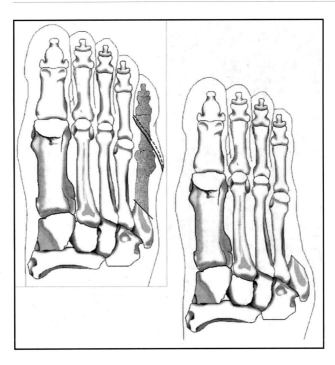

Fig. 3 Fifth ray amputation for fifth metatarsal head ulcer. (Reproduced with permission from the Prosthetics Research Study, Seattle, WA.)

plantar flap is preferable, but equal dorsal and plantar flaps work well and are often the only available option, especially for metatarsal head ulcers.

Muscle balance around the foot should be carefully evaluated preoperatively with specific attention to heel cord tightness, anterior tibialis, posterior tibialis, and peroneal muscle strength. Midfoot amputations significantly shorten the lever arm of the foot; therefore, Achilles tendon lengthening is almost always necessary (Fig. 4). Tibial or peroneal muscle insertions should be reattached locally if their attachments are released during bone resection.

The Achilles tendon lengthening is usually done using 3 percutaneous hemitendon sections. The distal and proximal cuts transect the medial half of the tendon, and the middle cut transects the lateral half of the tendon. Gentle force lengthens the tendon. In theory, this placement of cuts leaves the Achilles tendon with a more lateral attachment and tendency against the varus, which can occur

following midfoot amputations.

Postoperative casting prevents deformities, controls edema, and speeds rehabilitation. The foot should be casted in 5° to 10° of dorsiflexion. Prosthetic requirements can vary widely. During the first year following amputation, many patients benefit from an ankle-foot orthosis with a long foot plate and a toe filler. This orthosis should be worn at all times, except when bathing, in order to prevent an equinus deformity from developing. Later, a custom in-shoe orthotic device with a toe filler can be used with an extra-depth shoe for some patients.

Hindfoot Amputations

A Chopart amputation removes forefoot and midfoot, saving only the talus and calcaneus. Rebalancing procedures are required to prevent equinus and varus deformities. Complete Achilles tenotomy and transfer of the anterior tibialis, extensor digitorum longus, or peroneal tendons through a drill hole in the talus or calcaneus

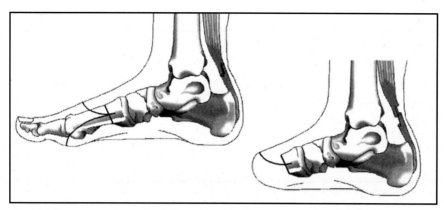

Fig. 4 Midfoot amputation and Achilles tendon lengthening. (Reproduced with permission from the Prosthetics Research Study, Seattle, WA.)

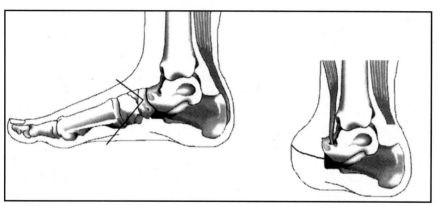

Fig. 5 Hindfoot amputation with anterior tibialis tendon transfer and Achilles tendon tenotomy. (Reproduced with permission from the Prosthetics Research Study, Seattle, WA.)

are an important part of this rebalancing (Fig. 5). Postoperative casting is also a must in order to prevent the strong tendency towards equinus. If a deformity can be prevented, patients with both a Chopart and a Syme's amputation prefer the Chopart level.

The Boyd hindfoot amputation is a talectomy and calcaneotibial arthrodesis after forward translation of the calcaneus. The Pirogoff hindfoot amputation is a talectomy with calcaneotibial arthrodesis after vertical transection of the calcaneus through the midbody, and a forward rotation of the remaining posterior process of the calcaneus under the tibia. These latter 2 amputations are done mostly in children to preserve length and growth centers, prevent heel pad migration, and improve socket suspension.[11] These amputation levels have generally not been used for patients with diabetes. The added length often complicates prosthetic fitting, compared to a Syme's amputation.

The hindfoot prosthesis for a Chopart amputation requires more secure stabilization than a midfoot prosthesis, in order to keep the heel from pistoning during gait. An anterior shell usually must be added to an ankle foot orthosis- (AFO-) style prosthesis, or, alternatively, a posterior opening socket prosthesis can be used. The ability to laminate a foot plate of carbon fiber directly to the undersurface of the prosthetic socket

can now result in a hindfoot prosthesis with minimal added height. However, with this construct there is no room to add a heel cushion, and some patients find this prosthesis too rigid at heel strike. The ankle region of this prosthesis remains very bulky and cosmetically dissatisfying to some patients. For patients whose main goals are to maintain independent transfers, the hindfoot amputations can be a very good level. For patients who ambulate with higher functional activity, a more proximal amputation, such as the Syme's or transtibial amputation, might be wiser.

Partial Calcanectomy

Partial calcanectomy, which involves excision of the posterior process of the calcaneus, should be considered an amputation of the back of the foot. In select patients with large heel ulceration or calcaneal osteomyelitis, this can be a very functional alternative to a below-knee amputation.[12] The local soft-tissue flap requires that the foot have reasonable good perfusion for healing and durability.

Surgically, the ulcer is excised, and longitudinal extensions of the incision up along the Achilles tendon and distally onto the plantar aspect of the foot allow access to dissect the posterior process of the calcaneus and the insertion of the Achilles tendon. The entire posterior process of the calcaneus is removed from the posterior edge of the posterior facet of the subtalar joint along a straight line to the inferior corner of the calcaneocuboid joint. All necrotic Achilles tendon is debrided, and no reattachment of this tendon is usually possible because of the extent of debridement (Fig. 6). Removing this large bony prominence allows for fairly large soft-tissue defects to be closed primarily over suction drainage. Splinting the foot in the equinus position relaxes the soft tissues and keeps tension off the closure during healing. Long-term equinus deformity is not a problem because of the Achilles tendon resection.

Discussing this procedure with patients as an amputation of the back of the foot helps emphasize the cosmetic and functional deformity. Because the posterior process of the calcaneus and the Achilles tendon attachment are both removed, a rigid AFO-style partial foot prosthesis with a cushion heel is required.

Syme's Amputations

The Syme's amputation is an ankle disarticulation in which the calcaneus and talus are removed while carefully dissecting on bone to preserve the heel skin and fat pad to cover the distal tibia.[13–15] The malleoli must be removed and contoured. Controversy exists as to whether to remove the malleoli initially or at a second-stage operation 6 to 8 weeks later. An advantage of 2 stages might be improved healing in dysvascular patients. Disadvantages include the second surgical procedure and a delay in rehabilitation because of the inability to bear weight until after the second stage. I believe that with careful surgical technique, the Syme's amputation can be performed safely in 1 stage, even for diabetic patients.[16]

A late complication of the Syme's amputation is the posterior and medial migration of the fat pad. Options to stabilize the fat pad include tenodesis of the Achilles tendon to the posterior margin of the tibia through drill holes; transferring anterior tibialis and extensor digitorum tendons to the anterior aspect of the fat pad; or removing the cartilage and subchondral bone to allow scarring of the fat pad to bone, with or without pin fixation. My preference is to perform tenodesis of the Achilles tendon to the

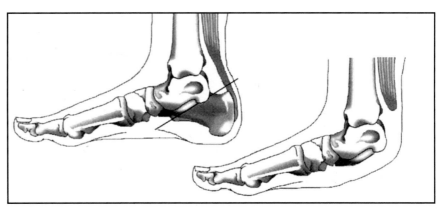

Fig. 6 Partial calcanectomy for large heel ulceration. (Reproduced with permission from the Prosthetics Research Study, Seattle, WA.)

posterior tibia[17] (Fig. 7). Careful casting postoperatively can also help keep the fat pad centered under the tibia during healing.

The Syme's amputation is an end-bearing level. Retaining the smooth, broad surface of the distal tibia and the heel pad allows direct transfer of weight from the end of the residual limb to the prosthesis. Below-knee or above-knee amputations do not allow this direct transfer of weight. Because of the ability to end bear, the amputee can occasionally ambulate without a prosthesis in emergency situations, or for bathroom activities. The socket design can take advantage of this end bearing to optimize a comfortable fit with a lower socket profile proximally.

The Syme's prosthesis is wider at the ankle level than a below-knee prosthesis. This cosmetic concern is occasionally bothersome. Use of newer materials and surgical narrowing of the malleolar flair have lessened this concern. Because of the low profile of some newer elastic response feet, the Syme's amputee can now benefit from energy-storing technology. Sockets do not need the high contour of a patellar-tendon bearing design because of the end-bearing quality of the residual limb.

The socket can be windowed either posteriorly or medially if the limb is bulbous, or a flexible socket-within-a-socket design can be used if the limb is less bulbous. Because of the tibial flare, the Syme's socket is usually self suspending.

Transtibial Amputations

The transtibial amputation is the most commonly performed major limb amputation. The long posterior flap technique has become standard, and good results can be expected even in a majority of dysvascular patients.[18] Anteroposterior, sagittal, and skewed flaps have all been described and are occasionally useful in specific patients. The level of tibial transection should be as long as possible between the tibial tubercle and the junction of the middle and distal thirds of the tibia, based on the available healthy soft tissues. Historically, it was taught that the tibia should always be transected 6 inches (15 cm) from the knee joint line, but the trend in recent years is toward longer transtibial amputations. Amputations in the distal third of the tibia should be avoided, because they have poor soft-tissue padding and are more difficult to fit comfortably with a prosthesis.

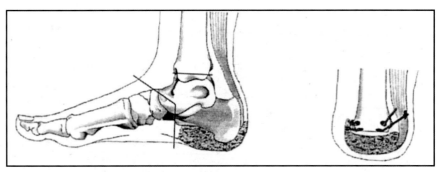

Fig. 7 Syme's amputation and stabilization of the heel pad with Achilles tenodesis to the tibia. (Reproduced with permission from the Prosthetics Research Study, Seattle, WA.)

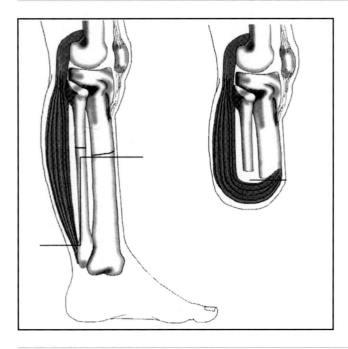

Fig. 8 Below-knee amputation with long posterior flap technique. (Reproduced with permission from the Prosthetics Research Study, Seattle, WA.)

The surgical goals are a cylindrically shaped residual limb with muscle stabilization, distal tibial padding, and a nontender and nonadherent scar. The long posterior flap length is equal to the diameter of the limb at the level of bone transection plus 1 cm. The fibula is transected 1 to 2 cm shorter than the tibia. The sural nerve should be identified, drawn down 5 to 10 cm, resected, and allowed to retract, to avoid a painful neuroma in the posterior flap. The posterior fascia should be myodesed to periosteum or to drill holes in the tibia to prevent retraction (Fig. 8).

Distal tibiofibular synostosis, the Ertl procedure, is not commonly performed. The principle, to create a broad bone mass terminally to improve the distal end-bearing property of the limb, is rarely achieved. The complication of a painful nonunion can be difficult to treat. Distal tibiofibular synostosis may be indicated in a wide traumatic diastasis to improve stabilization of the bone and soft tissues, but it is rarely indicated in dysvascular or diabetic patients.

The transtibial amputation is especially well suited to rigid dressings and immediate postoperative pros-

thetic management.[19,20] Protocols for weightbearing in these casts continue to be debated. My protocol for diabetic patients is to apply a cast in the operating room, but not initiate weightbearing until after the first cast change at 5 to 7 days. This first cast functions to help prevent knee flexion contractures, to decrease pain, and to control edema. If wound healing appears to be progressing well at the first cast change, a pilon and foot are added to the second cast, and 20 to 30 lbs of weightbearing is begun. The cast is changed weekly, and the weightbearing is advanced to 100 lbs over 4 weeks. After 4 to 6 weeks of casting, the first prosthesis is fabricated. The socket on this first prosthesis often needs to be changed 1 or 2 times in the first year, as atrophy of the residual limb occurs.

Pain Issue

Phantom sensation, a sense that all or some of the amputated part is still present, is very common following amputation.[21] This phantom sense is usually not bothersome to the patient, especially in diabetic patients with neuropathy. True phantom pain, a sensation in the amputated part that is described using words descriptive of pain, is fortunately rare. I believe that real phantom pain occurs less often in diabetic patients than in patients with traumatic amputations. The study of phantom pain is extremely interesting, and new research suggests that mechanisms designed to block the pain pathways around the time of amputation surgery do reduce the need for opioid medication in the hospital period, and may decrease the incidence of chronic phantom pain.[8,22–25]

When pain remains a serious problem, the best management is nonsurgical. Local physical measures, including massage, cold, and exercise are often effective. Other measures, such as acupuncture and regional sympathectomy, may under given circumstances have a place in therapy when the pain is intractable. Although transcutaneous electrical nerve stimulators (TENS) have been used with moderate short-term success, it is rare to see a patient who has continued to use a TENS unit for more than 1 year. Pharmacologic treatment has been reasonably successful with several oral agents, including amitriptyline, carbamazepine, dilatin, and, more recently, mexiletine. The appropriate use of an intravenous lidocaine challenge has been shown to be predictive of a favorable response to oral mexiletine. Unfortunately, we have not found good indicators to predict who will respond to treatment with amitriptyline, carbamazepine, or dilatin. Psychologic support can be beneficial, particularly when personality problems seem to accentuate the occurrence of pain. The individual needs patience and reassurance that the discomfort will improve over time, especially when a supportive social environment is present.

Summary

Unfortunately, amputation surgery is still a very important part of the treatment for diabetic foot problems. The decision-making process must be done thoughtfully, remembering that blood flow is not the only issue. Many factors enter into the decision to perform a partial foot amputation or to perform a more proximal level amputation. Adherence to good surgical principle, proven techniques, and gentle soft-tissue handling can make the difference between a successful and durable amputation or continued complications and frustrations.

Acknowledgement

A special thank you to Kathleen J. Ponto for providing the illustrations.

References

1. Reiber GE, Boyko EJ, Smith DG: Lower extremity foot ulcers and amputations in diabetes, in National Diabetes Data Group (eds): *Diabetes in America*, ed 2. Bethesda, MD, NIH, 1995.

2. Smith DG, Barnes BC, Sands AK, Boyko EJ, Ahroni JH: Prevalence of radiographic foot abnormalities in patients with diabetes. *Foot Ankle Int* 1997;18:343–346.

3. Waters RL, Perry J, Antonelli D, Hislop H: Energy cost of walking of amputees: The influence of level of amputation. *J Bone Joint Surg* 1976;58A:42–46.

4. Bone GE, Pomajzl MJ: Toe blood pressure by photoplethysmography: An index of healing in forefoot amputation. *Surgery* 1981;89:569–574.

5. Ramsey DE, Manke DA, Sumner DS: Toe blood pressure: A valuable adjunct to ankle pressure measurement for assessing peripheral arterial disease. *J Cardiovasc Surg (Torino)* 1983; 24:43–48.

6. Burgess EM, Matsen FA III, Wyss CR, Simmons CW: Segmental transcutaneous measurements of PO2 in patients requiring below-the-knee amputation for peripheral vascular insufficiency. *J Bone Joint Surg* 1982;64A:378–382.

7. Smith DG, Boyko EJ, Ahroni JH, Stensel VL, Davignon DR, Pecoraro RE: Paradoxical transcutaneous oxygen response to cutaneous warming on the plantar foot surface: A caution for interpretation of plantar foot TcPO$_2$ measurements. *Foot Ankle Int* 1994;16:787–791.

8. Malone JM, Anderson GG, Lalka SG, et al: Prospective comparison of noninvasive techniques for amputation level selection. *Am J Surg* 1987;154:179–184.

9. Dickhaut SC, DeLee JC, Page CP: Nutritional status: Importance in predicting wound-healing after amputation. *J Bone Joint Surg* 1984;66A: 71–75.

10. Pinzur M, Kaminsky M, Sage R, Cronin R, Osterman H: Amputations at the middle level of the foot: A retrospective and prospective review. *J Bone Joint Surg* 1986;68A:1061–1064.

11. Greene WB, Cary JM: Partial foot amputations in children: A comparison of the several types with the Syme amputation. *J Bone Joint Surg* 1982;64A:438–443.

12. Smith DG, Stuck RM, Ketner L, Sage RM, Pinzur MS: Partial calcanectomy for the treatment of large ulcerations of the heel and calcaneal osteomyelitis: An amputation of the back of the foot. *J Bone Joint Surg* 1992;74A: 571–576.

13. Harris RI: The history and development of Syme's amputation. *Artif Limbs* 1961;6:4,443.

14. Harris RI: Syme's amputation: The technique essential to secure a satisfactory end-bearing stump: Part I. *Can J Surg* 1963;6:456–469.

15. Harris RI: Syme's amputation: The technique essential to secure a satisfactory endbearing stump: Part II. *Can J Surg* 1964;7:53–63.

16. Pinzur MS, Smith D, Osterman H: Syme ankle disarticulation in peripheral vascular disease and diabetic foot infection: The one-stage versus two-stage procedure. *Foot Ankle Int* 1995; 16:124–127.

17. Smith DG, Sangeorzan BJ, Hansen ST Jr, Burgess EM: Achilles tendon tenodesis to prevent heel pad migration in the Syme's amputation. *Foot Ankle Int* 1994;15:14–17

18. Pinzur MS, Gottschalk F, Smith D, et al: Functional outcome of below-knee amputation in peripheral vascular insufficiency: A multicenter review. *Clin Orthop* 1993;286:247–249.

19. Burgess EM, Romano RL, Zettl JH (eds): *Management of Lower-Extremity Amputations: Surgery, Immediate Postsurgical Prosthetic Fitting, Patient Care*. Washington, DC, Prosthetic and Sensory Aids Service, Veterans Administration, 1969.

20. Mooney V, Harvey JP Jr, McBride E, Snelson R: Comparison of postoperative stump management: Plaster vs. soft dressings. *J Bone Joint Surg* 1971;53A:241–249.

21. Melzack R: Phantom limbs. *Sci Am* 1992;266: 120–126.

22. Bach S, Noreng MF, Tjellden NU: Phantom limb pain in amputees during the first 12 months following limb amputation, after preoperative lumbar epidural blockade. *Pain* 1988; 33:297–301.

23. Elizaga AM, Smith DG, Sharar SR, Edwards WT, Hansen ST Jr: Continuous regional analgesia by intraneuralh block: Effect on postoperative opioid requirements and phantom limb pain following amputation. *J Rehabil Res Dev* 1994;31:179–187.

24. Fisher A, Meller Y: Continuous postoperative regional analgesia by nerve sheath block for amputation surgery: A pilot study. *Anesth Analg* 1991;72:300–303.

25. Malawer MM, Buch R, Khurana JS, Garvey T, Rice L: Postoperative infusional continuous regional analgesia: A technique for relief of postoperative pain following major extremity surgery. *Clin Orthop* 1991;266:227–237.

40

Complications After Hallux Valgus Surgery

E. Greer Richardson, MD

Complications after hallux valgus surgery can occur even after detailed physical and radiographic evaluations, excellent surgical technique, and careful postoperative care.[1-4] Recurrence of the original deformity or development of the opposite deformity, hallux varus; clawed hallux; and transfer keratotic lesions that cause intractable discomfort beneath the lesser metatarsal heads all can compromise the results of surgery[5-7] (Fig. 1).

Prevention of Complications

Careful preoperative evaluation can identify factors that influence both the choice of surgical procedure and the results of treatment (Outline 1). For example, although a bunion typically is present with hallux valgus deformity, this is not always true (Fig. 4); neither is first metatarsal varus always present. The capsulosesamoid apparatus must be evaluated.[3,8-10]

Physical Examination

The feet should be examined with the patient sitting, standing, lying supine, and lying prone, unless there is some reason for not putting the patient in one or more of these positions. Recurrence of hallux valgus deformity is more likely when subluxation or dislocation of the first metatarsophalangeal joint is present. Pronation of the hallux (frequently an indication of severe deformity),

dislocation of the sesamoids laterally, fixed deformity, pes planus, joint hypermobility, and a tight heel cord may contribute to the likelihood of recurrence of the deformity after hallux valgus repair.

Radiographic Evaluation

Not enough emphasis can be placed on a concise, detailed evaluation of the weightbearing radiographs in the preoperative planning of procedures to correct hallux valgus deformity. As in the physical examination, radiographic examination of the feet is incomplete without weightbearing views. The difference in the magnitude of the deformity on nonweightbearing and weightbearing views often is striking.[11-15]

Weightbearing Anteroposterior View On a weightbearing anteroposterior view, the alignment of the first ray should be carefully evaluated and the following noted:[16] (1) varus of the first metatarsal (normal intermetatarsal angle is 9° or less), (2) severity of hallux valgus (normal hallux valgus angle is 15° or less), (3) congruity or incongruity of the first metatarsophalangeal joint (hallux valgus deformity can exist even in a congruous joint), (4) length of the first metatarsal relative to the second (is the second metatarsal more than 6 to 7 mm longer than the first?), (5) subluxation of the sesamoid bones (if present, to what extent?), (6) well-

developed facet between the first and the second metatarsals, suggesting difficulty displacing the first metatarsal laterally at the first metatarsocuneiform joint, (7) sloping of the first metatarsocuneiform articulation laterally to medially at a severe angle, (8) degenerative arthritic changes at the interphalangeal, metatarsophalangeal, or metatarsocuneiform articulations, (9) hallux valgus interphalangeus of 10° or less in neutral flexion and extension of the interphalangeal joint, (10) excessive distal metatarsal articular angle (normal distal metatarsal angle is 15° or less), (11) convex medial bowing of the proximal phalanx.[17]

Weightbearing Lateral View On the weightbearing lateral view of the foot, the following should be evaluated: (1) collapse deformity of the metatarsocuneiform, cuneiform-navicular, or naviculotalar articulation, (2) increased talocalcaneal angle, suggesting a valgus posture of the hindfoot, (3) calcaneal inclination angle (10° or more is normal; a reduced angle is indicative of a valgus hindfoot and possibly pes planus), (4) dorsiflexion of the first metatarsal, indicating incongruous reduction into concavity of the base of the proximal phalanx, (5) angle between the diaphysis of the proximal phalanx and the diaphysis of the first metatarsal (20° or more is normal), (6) delineation of the cortical

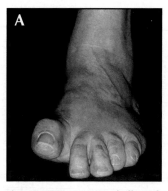 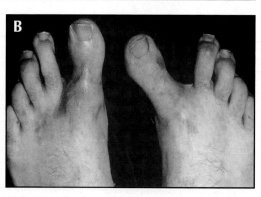

Fig. 1 A, Intrinsic minus hallux (clawtoe deformity) after failed distal metatarsal osteotomy. **B,** Severe hallux varus after a failed McBride bunionectomy and fibular sesamoidectomy.

Outline 1

Clinical considerations in the treatment of hallux valgus deformity

1. Pronation of the hallux and its part in the overall deformity.
2. The location of the sesamoid bones and if and where they are palpable.
3. Large callus formation on the tibial side of the hallux interphalangeal joint.
4. Pronation of the metatarsal head in tandem linkage with the hallux.
5. Pronation of the entire foot and correction of this hallucal pronation.
6. Passive correction of the deformity. If the valgus deformity is not correctable passively, measurement of the degree to which it can be corrected.
7. Passive weightbearing correction compared with passive nonweightbearing correction.
8. Active and passive ranges of motion of the first metatarsophalangeal joint with the hallux congruously reduced on the first metatarsal head and when the hallux deformity is not corrected.
9. Collapsed deformity at the mid- or hindfoot.
10. Contraction of the heel cord.
11. Asymmetry with weightbearing posture of the 2 feet even though both feet have a hallux valgus deformity. Is the prognosis the same after hallux valgus repair for both feet (Fig. 2)?
12. Prominence of the bursa over the medial aspect of the first metatarsal head.
13. With palpation of the medial eminence through the skin, determination of interposition of the capsule between skin and bone.
14. Hypermobile first ray compared with the other foot if the deformity is not bilateral. Can the first metatarsal passively be pushed towards the second metatarsal without restriction?
15. Hypermobility in all the joints of the foot and ankle.
16. First metatarsal head prominence dorsally with weight.
17. Clinical conditions of the lesser toes, particularly the second toe. (A fixed hammer deformity of the second toe with extensor posture of the toe at the second metatarsophalangeal joint or a second toe overlapping the hallux may create a space into which the hallux may rapidly return after hallux valgus repair.) The necessity of second toe realignment to obviate this potential problem (Fig. 3).
18. Previous surgeries that failed to correct the deformity.
19. Condition of the soft tissue.
20. Mobility of the first metatarsophalangeal joint.
21. Crepitance of the first metatarsophalangeal joint.
22. Palpable pedal pulses.
23. Intact sensory and motor components of the nerve supply to the foot.

---

outlines of the fifth, fourth, and third metatarsals even if overlapped (if the fifth and fourth metatarsal cortical borders are not clearly outlined on the weightbearing lateral radiograph, pronation of the foot should be suspected).

These observations help determine the degree of valgus thrust on the hallux metatarsophalangeal joint during the stance phase of gait, which influences treatment decisions. For example, correction of a recurrent valgus deformity in a patient with posterior tibial tendon insufficiency may require an arthrodesis. The lateral weightbearing radiograph also is invaluable in evaluating a flat, pronated, valgus foot.[15]

Nonweightbearing Medial Oblique View The nonweightbearing medial oblique view may show arthritic changes in the first metatarsal-medial cuneiform articulation or a calcaneonavicular tarsal coalition, changes that are not visible on other views. Either of these conditions may compromise surgery because they limit midtarsal and subtalar joint motion, increasing the strain on the capsular repair at the metatarsophalangeal joint and the stress across the first metatarsophalangeal and first metatarsal medial cuneiform articulations.

Weightbearing Sesamoid View The weightbearing sesamoid view (Fig. 5) is especially useful in the evaluation of recurrent hallux valgus deformity. Determining where the sesamoid bones lie in relation to their facets on the first metatarsal head often is difficult on an anteroposterior view; the sesamoids may appear markedly subluxed laterally on an anteroposterior view, while a sesamoid view shows them in anatomic position in their facets. Training our technicians to reliably and reproducibly obtain this view has been worth the effort. Repositioning the intrinsic and extrinsic muscles and the capsulosesamoid apparatus into their anatomic positions is the key to correction, and the weightbearing sesamoid view is helpful in planning the best means to accomplish this.[15]

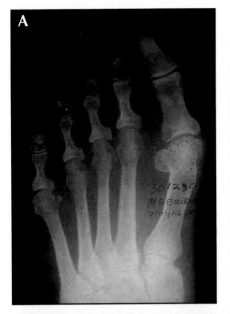

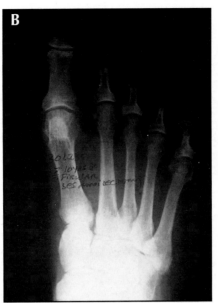

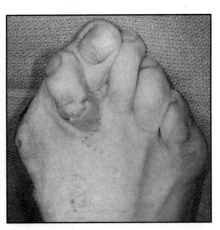

Fig. 3 Hallux valgus with cross-over deformity of the second toe.

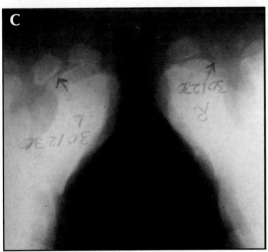

Fig. 2 Bilateral hallux valgus. **A,** Severe hallux valgus deformity failed after McBride procedure. **B** and **C,** Hallux valgus deformity treated with fibular sesamoidectomy. Greater correction is obtained but there is a higher risk for developing hallux varus.

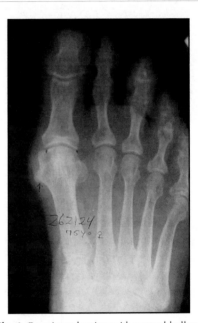

Fig. 4 Prominent bunion with normal hallux valgus angle.

Specific Complications
Recurrent Deformity
Recurrent Valgus Deformity With Normal Distal Metatarsal Articular Angle After Soft-Tissue Procedure Soft-tissue repair alone, given the fact that medial eminence removal is intrinsic to any "bunion repair," is not frequently performed, and its usefulness is controversial.[14,19-23] A first web space dissection and lateral release are essential elements of any soft-tissue repair.

To avoid recurrence of the deformity after simple bunionectomy (medial eminence excision and capsular imbrication) the procedure should be avoided, except in elderly patients who have impending skin breakdown over the medial eminence. Except in these patients, this procedure should not be considered even if the hallux is congruously reduced on the first metatarsal head and the hallux valgus and intermetatarsal angles are normal. Although it is tempting to do a minor procedure for a minor deformity, this is an error of judgment. A first web space dissection and lateral release should be performed with medial eminence removal and medial capsular imbrication.

The magnitude and rigidity of the recurrent deformity are guides to treatment. As a rule, a deformity that occurred after a soft-tissue procedure should not be treated with another soft-tissue procedure unless the deformity is completely flexible (the hallux can be easily reduced into varus and the first metatarsal freely translates laterally by

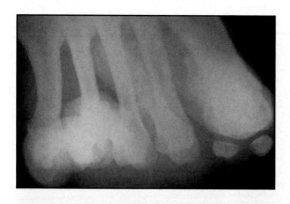

Fig. 5 Weightbearing sesamoid view.

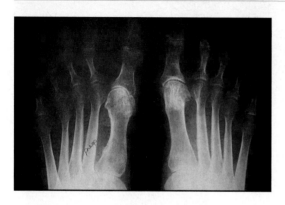

Fig. 6 Increased distal metatarsal articular angle and incongruent first metatarsophalangeal joint after basilar metatarsal osteotomy. Note degenerative changes.

manual pressure). First web space dissection, lateral release, and repeat medial capsular imbrication with manual medial displacement of the first metatarsal are recommended in patients with mild, flexible deformity that is symptomatic despite appropriate shoewear.[15,18,19] The indications include (1) an intermetatarsal 1-2 angle of 13° or less; (2) a hallux valgus angle of 30° or less; (3) a normal distal metatarsal articular angle (less than 10° to 15°); (4) minimal degenerative changes at the first metatarsophalangeal joint; (5) 50° to 60° of passive motion of the first metatarsophalangeal joint; (6) subluxation but not complete dislocation of the sesamoid bones; (7) ability to displace the first metatarsal laterally at the metatarsocuneiform joint from its abnormal varus inclination; (8) some degree of longitudinal arch present when weightbearing, determined clinically and radiographically. If the arch is improved with passive dorsiflexion of the hallux while standing, the patient does not have fixed, structural pes planus, and a soft-tissue repair is likely to endure.

Recurrent Hallux Valgus Deformity With Abnormal Distal Metatarsal Articular Angle After a Soft-Tissue Procedure When an increased distal metatarsal articular angle is present in recurrent hallux valgus, reducing the hallux will place the metatarsophalangeal joint incongruously on the metatarsal head (Fig. 6). The phalanx will rest in varus on the first metatarsal head and will leave the lateral aspect of the first metatarsal head uncovered. Correction of this deformity is accomplished with medial capsulorrhaphy, distal metatarsal displacement osteotomy (chevron), and first web space dissection with lateral soft-tissue release. Osteonecrosis of the first metatarsal head is a risk with distal metatarsal osteotomy and lateral release (Fig. 7), but the extent of necrosis and its clinical significance are unknown.[15,17]

Malunion After Chevron Osteotomy Malunion after a chevron osteotomy (Fig. 8) is uncommon if 3 steps in operative technique are followed: (1) the osteotomy is internally fixed and manually tested, and fixation is changed or augmented with a pin or small fragment screw if any movement occurs; (2) the distal fragment is placed plantar or inferior to the proximal fragment after internal fixation; and (3) weightbearing is guarded if fixation is not rigid.[15,24–27]

The difficulty in correcting a dorsal malunion after chevron osteotomy is preserving length. The initial chevron osteotomy often shortens the hallux 4 to 6 mm, and impaction and necrosis at the osteotomy site can decrease length another 4 to 6 mm, resulting in 1 to 1.5 cm of shortening that causes transfer metatarsalgia beneath the second metatarsal head or prevents relief of existing metatarsalgia. Varus or valgus malunion can occur after a chevron osteotomy, but this is not as common as dorsal malunion. Varus or valgus malunion of a chevron osteotomy, even with mild to moderate incongruity of the first metatarsophalangeal joint, is tolerated better by the patient than a dorsal malunion with transfer metatarsalgia. Regardless of the plane(s) of the malunion, the surgical technique to correct the deformity is basically the same.

Technique for Correcting Distal Malunion After Failed Chevron Osteotomy

The distal metatarsal is exposed from the junction of the middle and distal thirds to the base of the proximal phalanx. The previous osteotomy is inspected, but its "limbs" should not predetermine the plane(s) of the corrective osteotomy. With a 2-mm drill bit (even smaller if available), a semicircle of unicortical holes is made from dorsal to plantar adjacent to or within the previous osteotomy site (an arc of approximately 60°). These holes are connected by using only the corner of a 5- to 6-mm sharp, straight osteotome as a cutting edge. Care should be taken not to penetrate the lateral cortex with the osteotome. Using the 2-mm (or less) drill bit, numerous holes are made in the lateral cortex and the osteotomy is completed with a thin (1 mm × 9 mm) blade on a small power saw. This technique reduces the amount of shortening. The head is manually rotated plantarward until the dorsal cortex of the capital (distal) fragment is inferior (plantar) to the dorsal cortex of the shaft (proximal) fragment. This will slightly plantarflex the first metatarsal head, allowing it to assume more of the weightbearing load across the metatarsal heads. If the capital fragment has healed in varus or valgus, the deformity is reversed until the capital fragment is reduced to normal anatomic alignment with the shaft. Of course the malunion may be in 2 or more planes, but this "broomstick" osteotomy will allow correction of all planes of deformity. Internal fixation with Kirschner wires (K-wires), small screws, or absorbable pins is necessary. Interfragmentary wires are technically difficult to use in this location but are not contraindicated.

Postoperative Care

Depending on the rigidity of fixation and body habitus of the patient, as well as compliance by the patient, protected weightbearing can begin immediately. A short leg cast that extends distal to the toes and crutches or a walker may be necessary. The patient should be told before surgery that permanent loss of some metatarsophalangeal joint motion can be

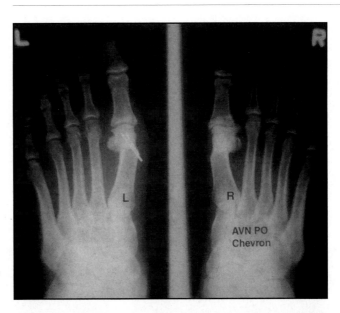

Fig. 7 Osteonecrosis after a distal metatarsal osteotomy (chevron).

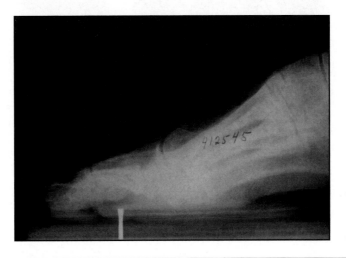

Fig. 8 Dorsal malunion after chevron osteotomy with intractable plantar keratosis beneath the second metatarsal.

expected, but that function should not be compromised. Full unprotected weightbearing is allowed when union of the osteotomy is apparent both clinically and radiographically. Final range of motion is not known until 12 to 18 months postoperatively.

Recurrent Hallux Valgus Deformity After Basilar Metatarsal Osteotomy and First Web Space Dissection or Release Recurrent deformity after basilar metatarsal osteotomy and first web space dissection or release should be treated with a second basilar metatarsal osteotomy, medial capsular imbrication of the

first metatarsophalangeal joint, and first web space dissection with release of the contracted lateral structures.[28-34] Indications for this procedure include: (1) an intermetatarsal angle of 14° or more; (2) hallux valgus angle of more than 30°; (3) normal distal metatarsal articular angle (10° to 15°); (4) splayed forefoot; (5) minimal to mild osteoarthritic changes at the first metatarsophalangeal joint (arthrodesis is indicated if the articular cartilage is damaged); (6) markedly subluxed or dislocated sesamoid bones; (7) 50° to 60° of passive range of motion of the first metatarsopha-

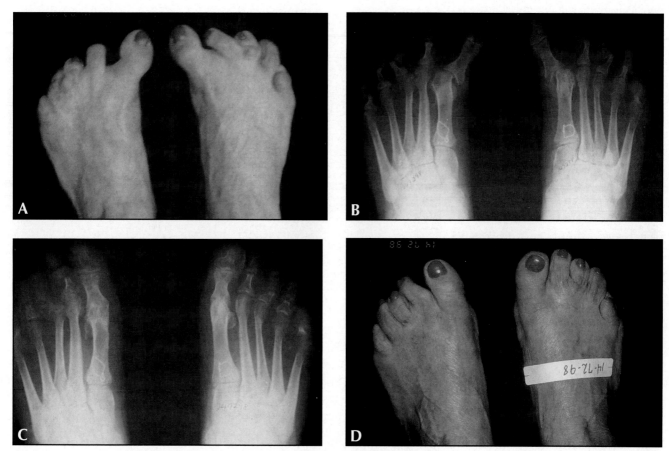

Fig. 9 A and **B,** Severe hallux varus in a 45-year-old woman after basilar metatarsal osteotomy. **C** and **D,** After fusion of first metatarsophalangeal joints.

langeal joint; and (8) arch structures that increase valgus stress on the metatarsophalangeal joint.

A combination of chevron and Akin osteotomies can be used for greater correction of valgus deformity.[15,35,36] Although Mitchell and Baxter[36] reported satisfactory results with this combined procedure, they caution that it should not be used if sesamoid subluxation and a wide intermetatarsal angle are present.

For severe recurrent deformity, arthrodesis of the first metatarsophalangeal joint often is the most appropriate operation[29,37,38] (Fig. 9). The surgical technique varies according to the type of osteotomy and the kind of fixation used.[39] Nonunion, malunion, and degenerative arthritis of

the interphalangeal joint of the hallux are the most frequent complications after arthrodesis of the first metatarsophalangeal joint. Accurate positioning of the hallux is essential during the procedure. Lapidus recommended combining arthrodesis of the first metatarsal medial cuneiform joint with distal soft-tissue release for severe recurrent deformities.[40–42]

Resection and Replacement Arthroplasty of the First Metatarsophalangeal Joint Resection (Keller) arthroplasty can be used for correction of recurrent deformity in elderly patients who have limited physical demands on their feet and who have some degree of osteoarthritis at the first metatarsophalangeal joint.[5,43–56] Its usefulness may be

expanded if the hallux, after resection of its base, is internally fixed to the first metatarsal before it is secured with 2 K-wires.

The results of replacement arthroplasty of the first metatarsophalangeal joint for correction of recurrent hallux valgus have varied[57] (Fig. 10). Cracchiolo and associates[58] recommended replacement arthroplasty of the first metatarsophalangeal joint in patients with rheumatoid arthritis and severe destruction of the metatarsophalangeal joints, but in most patients, resection of the base of the proximal phalanx, temporary internal fixation, and soft-tissue repair provide just as good results as replacement arthroplasty, with less expense and fewer complications (Fig. 11).

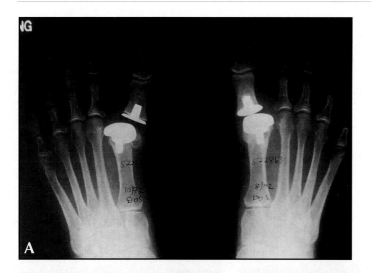

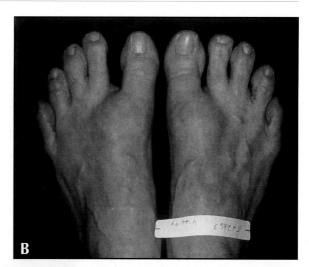

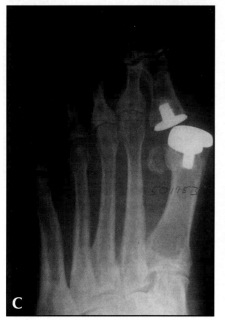

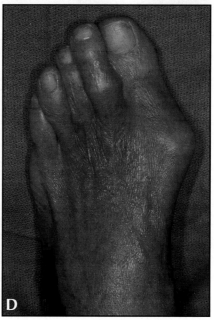

Fig. 10 A and **B,** Hallux varus deformity after replacement arthroplasty. **C** and **D,** Hallux valgus deformity after failed replacement arthroplasty.

Acquired Hallux Varus

Hallux varus[59–64] was not recognized as a complication of hallux valgus surgery until McBride[19] reported this deformity in 5.1% of patients treated with his procedure for hallux valgus (medial eminence removal, medial capsulorrhaphy, and fibular sesamoidectomy). Since then, many authors have reported this complication, with incidences varying from 2% (Peterson and associates[65]) to 17% (Trnka and associates[66]). Surprisingly, few patients with hallux varus complain about appearance (only if varus is greater than 10° to 15°) or discomfort (rare and usually associated with degenerative changes of the first metatarsophalangeal joint).[21]

Hawkins classified hallux varus into two types: static and dynamic.[3,15] Static deformities are uniplanar; dynamic deformities are multiplanar.

Static (Uniplanar) Hallux Varus

Supple, uniplanar, passively correctable hallux varus usually is asymptomatic and is mainly a cosmetic complication[21] (Fig. 12). When the foot is viewed in a weightbearing position, the hallux rests in varus, the metatarsophalangeal joint rests in a normal position in the sagittal plane (10° to the plantar surface of the foot or 20° to 25° to the first metatarsal), and the interphalangeal joint is in a normal position. Most often the hallux is not rotated abnormally in an axial plane and does not assume a "snake-in-the-grass" appearance in the frontal plane.[4] All the deformity occurs at the metatarsophalangeal joint, but only in

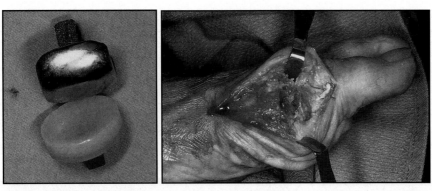

Fig. 11 Large size of prostheses required for replacement arthroplasty leaves large gap, making arthrodesis difficult.

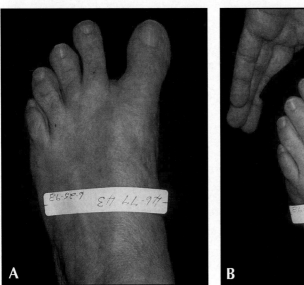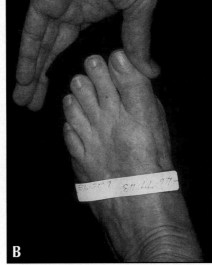

Fig. 12 A and **B,** Passively correctable hallux varus (static deformity).

the transverse or frontal plane. Uniplanar deformity most commonly occurs when a mild to moderate hallux valgus deformity is treated with a lateral soft-tissue release combined with medial capsular imbrication and medial eminence excision. According to Trnka and associates,[66] excising too much of the medial eminence (within or immediately lateral to the sagittal groove) is a major contributing factor to hallux varus. Excision of the fibular sesamoid and overcorrection of the first intermetatarsal angle to less than 5° also may be causes of hallux varus uniplanar deformity. Normally, the hallux rests on the first metatarsal head in about 10° of valgus. If the intermetatarsal angle is reduced to less than 5° and the hallux is reduced congruously on the metatarsal head, the necessary valgus angulation must be 15° (5° varus of the first metatarsal plus 10° distal metatarsal articular angle). Often the hallux is aligned parallel to the second toe if that toe is straight, or to the medial border of the foot if it is not, but this clinically straight posture actually places the hallux into varus in relation to the articular surface of the first metatarsal head. When the lateral restraining

structures are released and the medial eminence is removed, the hallux is at risk of drifting farther into varus. Overcorrection of the intermetatarsal angle and removal of the medial eminence at the sagittal groove instead of medial to it may contribute to the development of hallux varus deformity.

The surgical treatment of this deformity is straightforward and results are predictable. A static deformity is easier to correct than a dynamic one[1,3,67] (Fig. 13).

Soft-Tissue Correction
Technique

An incision is made on the medial side of the hallux at the midline in the internervous plane. The incision should extend from the midportion of the diaphysis of the proximal phalanx to 4 to 5 cm proximal to the metatarsophalangeal joint. The dorsal skin flap (on the capsule) is raised 4 to 5 mm, and the plantar flap is raised 2 to 3 mm. Care should be taken not to injure the dorsal sensory nerve near the medial eminence and first metatarsal.

A capsular incision is made in the midline medially. The dorsal and plantar capsular flaps are elevated until the dorsomedial corner of the first metatarsal and the tibial sesamoid plantarward are clearly exposed. After the hallux is adducted to the midline, the first metatarsophalangeal joint is flexed and extended. The soft-tissue release is carried dorsally and plantarward until the hallux can be placed into 10° to 15° of valgus on the metatarsal. The hallux is flexed and extended and passively dorsiflexed 40° to 50° in this valgus position. A small osteotome or periosteal elevator is placed between the articular surface of the tibial sesamoid and the first metatarsal head. If the tibial sesamoid slides back into its facet on

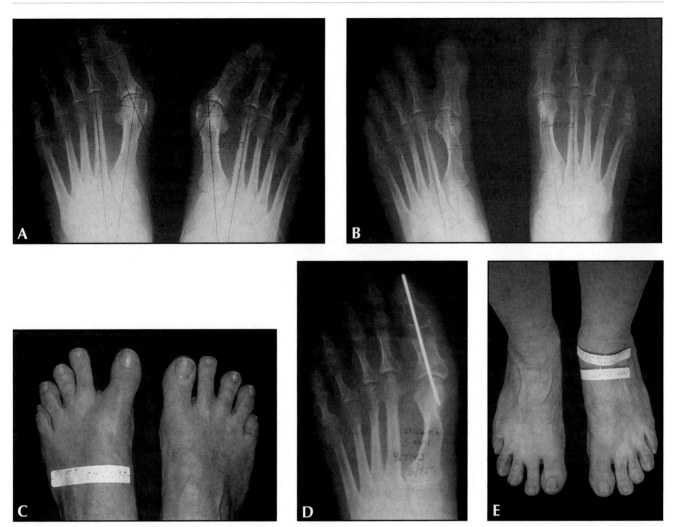

Fig. 13 A, Bilateral hallux valgus in a 62-year-old woman. **B** and **C,** Hallux varus developed after distal metatarsal osteotomy from a valgus malution and increased distal metatarsal articular angle. **D** and **E,** After medial capsulotomy and tibial sesamoid reduction for varus deformity. Pin remained for 5 weeks.

the metatarsal head with passive valgus of the hallux or requires only gentle levering and pushing to reduce and maintain it, the correction will be long-lasting.

With the hallux positioned in 15° valgus, 10° extension, and neutral rotation, a 0.062-in K-wire is placed obliquely from distal medial in the proximal phalanx to proximal lateral in the first metatarsal, starting at the metaphyseal-diaphyseal flair of the proximal phalanx. The wire is cut off beneath the skin where it can be removed in the office under local

anesthesia. The tourniquet is released and hemostasis obtained. The capsule should not be closed. The skin is closed with permanent 4-0 monofilament nylon suture. Simple stitches are placed near the wound margins, because the skin is under tension and mattress sutures could further compromise the blood supply to the skin margins. Because neither capsular nor subcutaneous sutures are used, the skin must be closed with more stitches than usual; gaps left between the stitches could cause a synovial fistula or an infection. A forefoot dressing is

applied. The dressing does not have to help maintain the reduced position of the hallux because this is done by the articular wire.[15]

Postoperative Care

The patient is allowed touch-down weightbearing in a removable boot with crutches for 3 weeks and then weightbearing to tolerance without crutches for an additional 3 weeks. In the first 3 weeks, the boot can be removed at night and for bathing. The wire is removed in the office in 4 to 6 weeks (6 weeks if the reduction was difficult). If it is necessary to remove the wire earlier than 3 weeks after surgery, the hallux should be taped to the second and third toes until it has no tendency to drift medially.

Although soft-tissue repair generally is a reliable procedure that does not markedly reduce range of motion of the first metatarsophalangeal joint and has minimal perioperative morbidity, occasionally tendon transfer or arthrodesis may be required for severe hallux varus deformity. I prefer arthrodesis to tendon transfer, although Johnson, Mann, Myerson, and others have reported favorable results after tendon transfer or tenodesis.[6,21,68–70]

Transfer of Extensor Hallucis Longus With Arthrodesis of the Interphalangeal Joint of the Hallux [4,6,71]

A dorsal curvilinear incision is made, starting just lateral to insertion of the extensor hallucis longus tendon, and is gently carried laterally toward the first web space in the interval between the first and second metatarsals. The incision is then inclined medially, ending along the lateral aspect of the extensor hallucis longus tendon at the first metatarsocuneiform joint. The extensor hallucis longus tendon is detached distally, and the surfaces of the interphalangeal joint are removed. After the distal phalanx is drilled from its articular surface, the arthrodesis site is placed together, and the drill bit is inserted through the end of the toe into the proximal phalanx. A 4.0-mm, small fragment, partially threaded, cancellous bone screw of the appropriate length is then inserted and the arthrodesis is compressed. A 2-0 absorbable suture is placed through the mobilized extensor hallucis longus tendon. A hole is drilled from dorsal to plantar in the lateral aspect of the base of the proximal phalanx. The drill bit is increased from a 2.5 mm to

3.5 mm. Curettes are used to further enlarge the hole if necessary. Since the "pulley" is the transverse intermetatarsal ligament, the tendon is pulled plantar to it through the drill hole in the proximal phalanx in a plantar to dorsal direction. A K-wire is used to hold the toe in the proper position, and the tendon is reattached so that it is taut. This holds the great toe in proper valgus and plantar alignment.

Dynamic (Multiplanar) Hallux Varus

Dynamic hallux varus is a multiplanar deformity that may rapidly become fixed. Multiplanar deformities often are symptomatic and difficult to correct surgically. I prefer the descriptive term "intrinsic minus deformity of the hallux with a varus component," which emphasizes that the varus is only one part of the deformity. This is an intrinsic-extrinsic muscle imbalance or an intrinsic minus hallux. In this type of hallux varus, the first metatarsophalangeal joint is hyperextended (usually with some degree of fixed soft-tissue contracture) and the interphalangeal joint is acutely flexed. The hallux is rotated and its varus and extension posture makes shoe wear difficult. The most common complaint is that the toe box of the shoe rubs on the dorsomedial surface of the interphalangeal joint. Patients frequently complain of a keratotic lesion beneath the first metatarsal head caused by the extended hallux pushing the first metatarsal head plantarward. Hammertoe deformities develop in the lesser toes (usually 2 and 3) and metatarsalgia develops as the hallux assists less and less in the stance phase of the gait cycle.[72]

Anatomy and Pathogenesis
The intrinsic muscles balance the hallux on the first metatarsal head,

while the extrinsic muscles add gross balance and greatly increase the mobility of the hallux.[3,4,58,73–75] The first metatarsophalangeal joint is a shallow, ball-in-socket joint with little stability from bony configurations. The location of the tendon insertions of the abductor-adductor hallucis, the flexor hallucis brevis (both components), and the extensor hallucis brevis balance the hallux congruently on the first metatarsal head. If the positions of these tendon insertions are altered relative to the axis of rotation in flexion or extension at the metatarsophalangeal joint, this balance is disrupted. In intrinsic minus-varus hallux, the ability of the flexor hallucis brevis to flex the metatarsophalangeal joint is decreased. The abductor hallucis, unencumbered by its antagonist (adductor), pulls the hallux medially, uncovering the metatarsal head laterally. The extensor hallucis brevis hyperextends the hallux against a weakened flexor hallucis brevis, and, as the hallux drifts medially and dorsally, the extrinsic muscle-tendon units begin to exacerbate the deformity. The flexor hallucis longus further flexes the interphalangeal joint, and the forces of the extensor hallucis longus and the extensor hallucis brevis increase the extension deformity. The sesamoid bones sublux medially, carrying the plantar plate, flexor hallucis brevis, and adductor and abductor hallucis tendons of insertion with them, thereby contributing to the pattern and rigidity of the deformity. The components of this deformity quickly become fixed, making passive correction impossible and surgical correction difficult and multifaceted.

Bony and Soft-Tissue Correction
Technique A midline medial incision is made and the metatarsal head is exposed by incising the capsule 2 to 3 mm plantar to where the skin inci-

sion was centered. The capsule is elevated from the head of the metatarsal and the base of the proximal phalanx dorsally and plantarward. The tibial sesamoid is exposed. If the deformity is fixed in extension at the metatarsophalangeal joint, a wider resection of the soft tissue is needed up to the junction of the neck and shaft of the first metatarsal. The hallux is manually reduced into a valgus position and then released to evaluate the tightness. The articular surfaces are examined, and if the head of the first metatarsal shows loss of articular cartilage or unhealthy appearing articular cartilage, presumably from chronic pressure placed against it, then an arthrodesis is indicated. If the articular cartilage appears reasonably normal, then the hallux is held in 10° of valgus and a 0.062-in K-wire is placed across the joint obliquely from the base of the proximal phalanx medially to the head and neck junction of the first metatarsal laterally. The sesamoids are placed beneath the head of the metatarsal. The interphalangeal joint contracture is released through a dorsal inverted L-incision with the transverse limb across the dorsum of the interphalangeal joint and the proximal limb extending 2 to 3 cm proximally along the dorsolateral border of the head and neck of the proximal phalanx.

If the metatarsophalangeal joint requires arthrodeses, the interphalangeal joint flexion contracture should be corrected by releasing the plantar plate and both collateral ligaments, bringing the interphalangeal joint into a corrected position, and holding it with a 0.062-in K-wire. If the metatarsophalangeal joint does not require arthrodeses, the articular surfaces of the interphalangeal joint are removed in preparation for an arthrodesis. This serves two purposes: it will correct a fixed deformity of

the interphalangeal joint, or, if the deformity is supple, it will allow relative shortening of the extensor and flexor hallucis longus muscle-tendon units, thereby decreasing their deforming forces.

The interphalangeal joint arthrodesis is fixed with crossed K-wires or a small intramedullary fragment screw. The technique of Johnson is recommended if a screw is used. A hole is drilled into the distal phalanx from the articular surface through the tip of the hallux just beneath the nail, and then the drill bit is reversed into the proximal phalanx. Usually a 4.0-mm partially threaded, cancellous, small fragment screw (40 to 50 mm) is used. I prefer Kirschner wires, but either technique is acceptable. The tourniquet is removed, and the hallux is held in 10° to 15° of valgus with the interphalangeal joint arthrodesed in neutral position, while the skin is closed with simple, interrupted, small sutures. The stitches are placed close to the skin edge, because bringing the hallux from a varus to a valgus posture places the skin under tension. Some wound necrosis medially frequently occurs after hallux varus repair, and the patient should be advised of this. A forefoot dressing is applied.

Postoperative Care The patient is encouraged to rest and elevate the foot above heart level for several days. For the first 3 weeks after surgery, only nonweightbearing ambulation on crutches is allowed. If the patient is allowed to bear weight, a short leg cast that extends past the toes is recommended. Weightbearing to tolerance in a removable walking boot is allowed for the next 3 weeks. The K-wire is removed between the fourth and sixth weeks, depending on how difficult it was to correct the deformity: the more difficult the deformity correction, the longer the fixation should remain.

References

1. Donley BG: Acquired hallux varus. *Foot Ankle Int* 1997;18:586–592.

2. Edelman RD: Iatrogenically induced hallux varus. *Clin Podiatr Med Surg* 1991;8:367–382.

3. Hawkins F: Acquired hallux varus: Cause, prevention and correction. *Clin Orthop* 1971;76:169–176.

4. Johnson KA, Saltzman CL, Friscia DA: Hallux varus, in Gould JS, Thompson FM, Cracchiolo A III, et al (eds): *Operative Foot Surgery*. Philadelphia, PA, WB Saunders, 1994, pp 28–35.

5. Johnson KA, Saltzman CL: Complications of resection arthroplasty (Keller) and replacement arthroplasty (silicone) procedures. *Contemp Orthop* 1991;23:139–147.

6. Johnson KA, Spiegl PV: Extensor hallucis longus transfer for hallux varus deformity. *J Bone Joint Surg* 1984;66A:681–686.

7. Joseph B, Jacob T, Chacko V: Hallux varus: A study of thirty cases. *J Foot Surg* 1984;23:392–397.

8. McElvenny RT: Hallux varus. *Quart Bull Northwest Univ Med Sch* 1941;15:277–280.

9. Antrobus JN: The primary deformity in hallux valgus and metatarsus primus varus. *Clin Orthop* 1984;184:251–255.

10. Scranton PE Jr, Rutkowski R: Anatomic variations in the first ray: Part I. Anatomic aspects related to bunion surgery. *Clin Orthop* 1980;151:244–255.

11. Austin DW, Leventen EO: A new osteotomy for hallux valgus: A horizontally directed "V" displacement osteotomy of the metatarsal head for hallux valgus and primus varus. *Clin Orthop* 1981;157:25–30.

12. Carr CR, Boyd BM: Correctional osteotomy for metatarsus primus varus and hallux valgus. *J Bone Joint Surg* 1968;50A:1353–1367.

13. Clark HR, Veith RG, Hansen ST Jr: Adolescent bunions treated by the modified Lapidus procedure. *Bull Hosp Jt Dis Orthop Inst* 1987;47:109–122.

14. Mann RA: Decision-making in bunion surgery, in Greene WB (ed): *Instructional Course Lectures XXXIX*. Park Ridge, IL, American Academy of Orthopaedic Surgeons, 1990, pp 3–13.

15. Richardson EG: Disorders of the hallux, in Crenshaw AH (ed): *Campbell's Operative Orthopaedics*, ed 8. St. Louis, MO, Mosby-Year Book, 1992, vol 4, pp 2615–2692.

16. Shereff MJ, Johnson KA: Radiographic anatomy of the hindfoot. *Clin Orthop* 1983;177:16–22.

17. Richardson EG, Graves SC, McClure JT, Boone RT: First metatarsal head-shaft angle: A method of determination. *Foot Ankle* 1993;14:181–185.

18. Hansen CE: Hallux valgus treated by the McBride operation: A follow-up. *Acta Orthop Scand* 1974;45:778–792.

19. McBride ED: The conservative operation for "bunions": End results and refinements of technique. *JAMA* 1935;105:1164–1168.

20. Coughlin MJ: Juvenile bunions, in Mann RA, Coughlin MJ (eds): *Surgery of the Foot and Ankle,* ed 6. St. Louis, MO, Mosby-Year Book, 1993, pp 297–339.

21. Mann RA, Coughlin MJ: Adult hallux valgus, in Mann RA, Coughlin MJ (eds): *Surgery of the Foot and Ankle,* ed 6. St. Louis, Mosby-Year Book, 1993, pp 167–296.

22. Franco MG, Kitaoka HB, Edaburn E: Simple bunionectomy. *Orthopedics* 1990;13:963–967.

23. Johnson JE, Clanton TO, Baxter DE, Gottlieb MS: Comparison of chevron osteotomy and modified McBride bunionectomy for correction of mild to moderate hallux valgus deformity. *Foot Ankle* 1991;12:61–68.

24. Hattrup SJ, Johnson KA: Chevron osteotomy: Analysis of factors in patients' dissatisfaction. *Foot Ankle* 1985;5:327–332.

25. Johnson KA: Chevron osteotomy of the first metatarsal: Patient selection and technique. *Contemp Orthop* 1981;3:707–711.

26. Meier PJ, Kenzora JE: The risks and benefits of distal first metatarsal osteotomies. *Foot Ankle* 1985;6:7–17.

27. Pochatko DJ, Schlehr FJ, Murphey MD, Hamilton JJ: Distal chevron osteotomy with lateral release for treatment of hallux valgus deformity. *Foot Ankle Int* 1994;15:457–461.

28. Coughlin MJ: Proximal first metatarsal osteotomy, in Johnson KA (ed): *The Foot and Ankle.* New York, NY, Raven Press, 1994, pp 85–105.

29. Fitzgerald JA: A review of long-term results of arthrodesis of the first metatarsophalangeal joint. *J Bone Joint Surg* 1969;51B:488–493.

30. Mann RA, Rudicel S. Graves SC: Repair of hallux valgus with a distal soft-tissue procedure and proximal metatarsal osteotomy: A long-term follow-up. *J Bone Joint Surg* 1992;74A: 124–129.

31. Stokes IA, Hutton WC, Stott JR, Lowe LW: Forces under the hallux valgus foot before and after surgery. *Clin Orthop* 1979;142:64–72.

32. Thordarson DB, Leventen EO: Hallux valgus correction with proximal metatarsal osteotomy: Two-year follow-up. *Foot Ankle* 1992;13: 321–326.

33. Trethowan J: Hallux valgus, in Choyce CC (ed): *A System of Surgery.* New York, NY, PB Hoeber, 1923.

34. Truslow W: Metatarsus primus varus or hallux valgus? *J Bone Joint Surg* 1925;7:98–108.

35. Mitchell CL, Fleming JL, Allen R, Glenney C, Sanford GA: Osteotomy-bunionectomy for hallux valgus. *J Bone Joint Surg* 1958;40A:41–60.

36. Mitchell LA, Baxter DE: A Chevron-Akin double osteotomy for correction of hallux valgus. *Foot Ankle* 1991;12:7–14.

37. Henry AP, Waugh W, Wood H: The use of footprints in assessing the results of operations of hallux valgus: A comparison of Keller's

operation and arthrodesis. *J Bone Joint Surg* 1975;57B:478–481.

38. Coughlin MJ, Mann RA: Arthrodesis of the first metatarsophalangeal joint as salvage for the failed Keller procedure. *J Bone Joint Surg* 1987;69A:68–75.

39. Mann RA, Thompson FM: Arthrodesis of the first metatarsophalangeal joint for hallux valgus in rheumatoid arthritis. *J Bone Joint Surg* 1984; 66A:687–692.

40. Lapidus PW: A quarter of a century of experience with the operative correction of the metatarsus varus primus in hallux valgus. *Bull Hosp Joint Dis* 1956;17:404–421.

41. Lapidus PW: The author's bunion operation from 1931 to 1959. *Clin Orthop* 1960;16: 119–135.

42. Mauldin DM, Sanders M, Whitmer WW: Correction of hallux valgus with metatarso-cuneiform stabilization. *Foot Ankle* 1990;11: 59–66.

43. Keller WL: The surgical treatment of bunions and hallux valgus. *NY Med J* 1904;80:741–742.

44. Ford LT, Gilula LA: Stress fractures of the middle metatarsals following the Keller operation. *J Bone Joint Surg* 1977;59A:117–118.

45. Friend G: Sequential metatarsal stress fractures after Keller arthroplasty with implant. *J Foot Surg* 1981;20:227–231.

46. Frisch EE: Technology of silicones in biomedical applications, in Rubin LR (ed): *Biomaterials in Reconstructive Surgery.* St. Louis, MO, CV Mosby, 1983, pp 73–90.

47. Johnson KA, Buck PG: Total replacement arthroplasty of the first metatarsophalangeal joint. *Foot Ankle* 1981;1:307–314.

48. Love TR, Whynot AS, Farine I, Lavoier M, Hunt L, Gross A: Keller arthroplasty: A prospective review. *Foot Ankle* 1987;8:46–54.

49. Merkle PF, Sculco TP: Prosthetic replacement of the first metatarsophalangeal joint. *Foot Ankle* 1989;9:267–271.

50. Rogers W, Joplin R: Hallux valgus, weak foot and the Keller operation: An end-result study. *Surg Clin North Am* 1947;27:1295–1302.

51. Shiel WC Jr, Jason M: Granulomatous inguinal lymphadenopathy after bilateral metatarsophalangeal joint silicone arthroplasty. *Foot Ankle* 1986;6:216–218.

52. Turner RS: Dynamic post-surgical hallux varus after lateral sesamoidectomy: Treatment and prevention. *Orthopedics* 1986;9:963–969.

53. Swanson AB, de Groot Swanson G, Maupin BK, et al: The use of a grommet bone-liner for flexible hinge implant arthroplasty of the great toe. *Foot Ankle* 1991;12:149–155.

54. Thomas FB: Keller's arthroplasty modified: A technique to ensure postoperative distraction of the toe. *J Bone Joint Surg* 1962;44B:356–365.

55. Vallier GT, Petersen SA, LaGrone MO: The Keller resection arthroplasty: A 13-year experience. *Foot Ankle* 1991;11:187–194.

56. Maschas A, Cartier P: Radiological results of the Keller operation. *Rev Chir Orthop Reparatrice Appar Mot* 1974;60(suppl 2):146–149.

57. Swanson AB: Implant arthroplasty for the great toe. *Clin Orthop* 1972;85:75–81.

58. Cracchiolo A III, Swanson A, Swanson GD: The arthritic great toe metatarsophalangeal joint: A review of flexible silicone implant arthroplasty from two medical centers. *Clin Orthop* 1981;157:64–69.

59. Banks AS, Ruch JA, Kalish SR: Surgical repair of hallux varus. *J Am Podiatr Med Assoc* 1988; 78:339–347.

60. Granberry WM, Hickey CH: Idiopathic adult hallux varus. *Foot Ankle Int* 1994;15:197–205.

61. Miller JW: Acquired hallux varus: A preventable and correctable disorder. *J Bone Joint Surg* 1975;57A:183–188.

62. Mills JA, Menelaus MB: Hallux varus. *J Bone Joint Surg* 1989;71B:437–440.

63. Thomson SA: Hallux varus and metatarsus varus: A five-year study (1954-1958). *Clin Orthop* 1960;16:109–118.

64. Sloane D: Congenital hallux varus: Operative connection. *J Bone Joint Surg* 1935;17:209–211.

65. Peterson DA, Zilberfarb JL, Greene MA, Colgrove RC: Avascular necrosis of the first metatarsal head: Incidence in distal osteotomy combined with lateral soft tissue release. *Foot Ankle Int* 1994;15:59–63.

66. Trnka H-J, Zettl R, Hungerford M, Mühlbauer M, Ritschl P: Acquired hallux varus and clinical tolerability. *Foot Ankle Int* 1997;18:593–597.

67. Tourné Y, Saragaglia D, Picard F, De Sousa B, Montbarbon E, Charbel A: Iatrogenic hallux varus surgical procedure: A study of 14 cases. *Foot Ankle Int* 1995;16:457–463.

68. Juliano PJ, Myerson MS, Cunningham BW: Biomechanical assessment of a new tenodesis for correction of hallux varus. *Foot Ankle Int* 1996;17:17–20.

69. Myerson M: Hallux varus, in Myerson M (ed): *Current Therapy in Foot and Ankle Surgery.* St. Louis, MO, Mosby-Year Book, 1993, pp 70–73.

70. Myerson MS, Komenda GA: Results of hallux varus correction using an extensor hallucis brevis tenodesis. *Foot Ankle Int* 1996;17:21–27.

71. Skalley TC, Myerson MS: The operative treatment of acquired hallux varus. *Clin Orthop* 1994;306:183–191.

72. Poehling GG, DeTorre J: Hallux varus and hammertoe deformity. *Orthop Trans* 1982;6:186.

73. Albreckht E: Pathology and treatment of hallux valgus. *Russki Vrach* 1911;10:14.

74. Jahss MH: Spontaneous hallux varus: Relation to poliomyelitis and congenital absence of the fibular sesamoid. *Foot Ankle* 1983;3:224–226.

75. Reverdin J: Anatomie et operation de l'hallux valgus. *Trans Int Med Cong* 1881;2:408-412.

Arthroscopy of the Great Toe

Carol Frey, MD
C. Niek van Dijk, MD

Open surgery about the first metatarsophalangeal (MTP) joint can result in stiffness, prolonged swelling, poor wound healing, and trouble with shoewear. However, advancements in small joint instrumentation and arthroscopic technique have expanded the application of arthroscopy in the first MTP joint and helped improve the treatment of many forefoot disorders. Along with the advancements in technique, however, it is important that the surgeon understand the pertinent gross and arthroscopic anatomy of the first MTP joint. A better understanding of the difficult anatomy surrounding the forefoot should help in the performance of arthroscopic surgery as well as in proper recognition of abnormal pathology when present. It should also be recognized that arthroscopy of this joint is a relatively new application, therefore, indications for the procedure are still developing, and no long-term clinical studies have been published. For these reasons, the procedure should be considered investigational at this time.

Gross Anatomy and Biomechanics

Minimal stability is provided by the shallow ball and socket articulation between the proximal phalanx and the metatarsal head. The soft tissues, including the capsule, ligaments, and musculotendinous structures, provide most of the support to the first MTP joint.

The extensor hallucis longus tendon divides the dorsum of the first MTP joint in half. The branches of the deep peroneal nerve innervate the lateral half and the branches of the superficial peroneal nerve innervate the medial half of the joint. The terminal branches of the saphenous nerve innervate the medial aspect of the great toe (Fig. 1).

On the plantar aspect of the first MTP joint, the sesamoids are within the medial and lateral portions of the flexor hallucis brevis tendon. The sesamoids are enveloped by the split tendon of the flexor hallucis brevis, which sends fibers to the plantar plate and subsequently attaches to the proximal aspect of the proximal phalanx. The plantar plate is a strong fibrous structure that inserts on either side of the MTP joint. The flexor hallucis longus tendon is both superficial and between the 2 heads of the flexor hallucis brevis tendon (Fig. 2).

Biomechanically, the instant centers of motion for the first MTP joint fall within the metatarsal head. Motion occurs between the metatarsal head and the proximal phalanx via a sliding action at the joint surface. In full extension or flexion, this sliding action gives way to compression of the dorsal or plantar articular surfaces of the metatarsal head and the proximal phalanx.

Arthroscopic Anatomy and Portals

The dorsal medial, dorsal lateral, and straight medial portals are the most commonly used portals for arthroscopy of the first MTP joint (Fig. 3). The dorsal medial and dorsal lateral portals are placed at the joint line and on either side of the extensor hallucis longus tendon. The straight medial portal is placed through the medial capsule midway between the dorsal and plantar aspect of the joint, usually under direct visualization.

Intra-articular examination includes visualization of 10 major areas: the lateral gutter; the lateral corner of the metatarsal head; the central portion of the metatarsal head; the medial corner of the metatarsal head; the medial gutter; the medial portion of the proximal phalanx; the central portion of the proximal phalanx; the lateral portion of the proximal phalanx; the medial sesamoid; and the lateral sesamoid.

Technique

The patient is placed in the supine position on the operating room table. General, spinal, epidural, or local

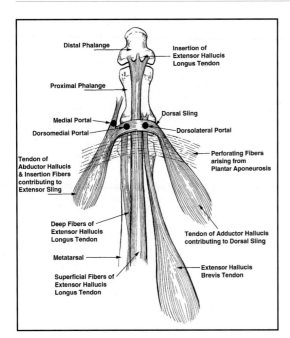

Fig. 1 Musculotendinous anatomy surrounding the first metatarsophalangeal joint. (Reproduced with permission from Frey C: Gross and arthroscopic anatomy of the foot, in Guhl J (ed): *Foot and Ankle Arthroscopy*, ed 3. New York, NY, Springer-Verlag, in press.)

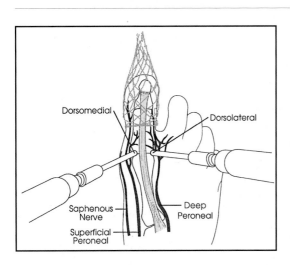

Fig. 2 Anatomic structures at risk with portal placement for first metatarsophalangeal joint arthroscopy. (Reproduced with permission from Frey C: Arthroscopy of the great toe, in Chow J (ed): *Advanced Arthroscopy*. New York, NY, Springer-Verlag, in press.)

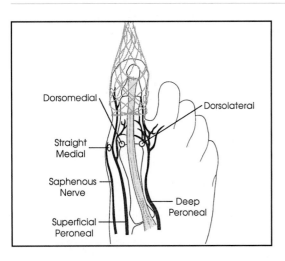

Fig. 3 The dorsal medial, dorsal lateral, and straight medial portals are the most commonly used portals for arthroscopy of the first metatarsophalangeal joint. (Reproduced with permission from Feder K: Arthroscopy and endoscopy of the foot, in Pfeffer G, Frey C (eds): *Current Practices in Foot and Ankle Surgery*. New York, NY, McGraw-Hill, 1994, vol 2.)

anesthesia can all be used. A sterile finger trap is placed on the toe to suspend the lower extremity, with traction applied at the level of the ankle if necessary (Fig. 4).

The dorsal medial or dorsal lateral portal is established first. The joint line is palpated just medial or lateral to the extensor hallucis longus tendon. A 19-gauge spinal needle is used to inflate the MTP joint with 5 ml of normal saline. A 4-mm longitudinal skin incision is made, the subcutaneous tissue is spread with a mosquito clamp to prevent neurovascular injury, and the joint is entered with an interchangeable cannula with a semiblunt trochar. Once visualization of the joint is accomplished through the initial portal, the remaining 2 portals can be established with a spinal needle under direct vision. Use of interchangeable cannulas allows rotation of the video arthroscope and instrumentation so that the entire joint and its pathology can be fully evaluated and treated.

The arthroscopic examination of the great toe is performed through the dorsal lateral portal. The dorsal medial portal provides superior visualization of the dorsal aspect of the metatarsal head and proximal phalanx. The medial and lateral sesamoids can be well visualized from the medial portal (Figs. 5 through 7).

Indications

Indications for surgical arthroscopy of the first MTP joint include osteophytes, hallux rigidus, chondromalacia, osteochondritis dissecans, loose bodies, arthrofibrosis, and synovitis secondary to hyperextension and hyperflexion injuries of the great toe. Evolution of surgical arthroscopic techniques may soon allow arthrodesis of the first MTP joint. Diagnostic arthroscopy may be indicated in cases of recurrent swelling and locking, persistent pain, and stiffness recalci-

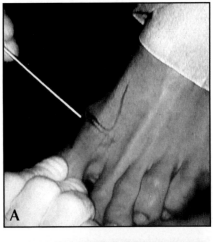
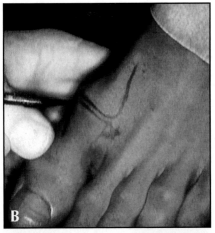
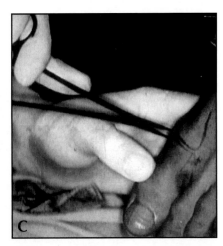
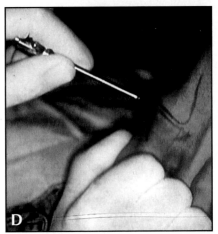
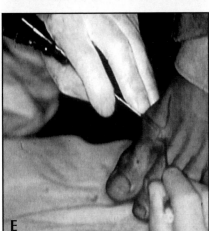

Fig. 4 Using manual traction or a sterile finger trap, the first metatarsophalangeal (MTP) joint can be palpated and a spinal needle introduced through the anteromedial portal site (**A**). Once the joint space is located, a longitudinal skin incision is made through the skin (**B**). Blunt dissection with a hemostat is used to enter the first MTP joint (**C**). The arthroscope with a blunt trocar is introduced through the anteromedial portal (**D**). The location of the anterolateral portal is made under direct visualization by introducing a spinal needle through the portal site (**E**). A skin incision is made for the anterolateral portal and the arthroscope is introduced. (Courtesy of C. Niek van Dijk.)

trant to a full regimen of conservative treatment.

The most common indications for arthroscopy of the great toe include treatment of hallux rigidus with a dorsal osteophyte, and chondromalacia. Dorsal osteophytes may be removed if they are mild to moderate in size. If the osteophyte is large, an open cheilectomy is recommended.

An arthroscopic cheilectomy can be performed through 2 or 3 portals. The arthroscopic shaver and burr are placed in the dorsal medial or medial portal and the arthroscope is placed in the dorsal lateral portal. The osteophyte is removed from distal to proximal and medial to lateral. Up to one third of the articular surface may be removed using this technique and

will help improve range of motion. If a finger trap is used for distraction, it is best to release it prior to removing the osteophytes because the traction may cause the capsule to pull tightly against the osteophyte. Postoperatively, the patient is placed on crutches for 5 days and range of motion exercises begun immediately.

In the presence of chondromalacia or osteochondral lesions, the pathology may be evaluated, loose fragments excised, and bone drilled or abraded to a bleeding surface. The patient is not allowed to bear weight for 2 weeks postoperatively, and early range of motion is encouraged at 5 days.

For evaluation and surgery of the medial sesamoid, the dorsal lateral portal is used for the arthroscope and

the instrumentation is placed in the medial portal. For the lateral sesamoid, the arthroscope is introduced through the dorsal medial portal and the instrumentation is placed in the dorsal lateral portal. To evaluate the sesamoid compartment, it is helpful to release the toe traction and place the great toe in plantar flexion.

Postoperative Care and Rehabilitation

Small portal wounds are closed with interrupted nylon sutures. To prevent fistula formation, a bulky compression dressing is applied for 4 to 7 days. Direct weightbearing is avoided. Sutures are removed at approximately 7 to 10 days after surgery and the patient is started on range of motion

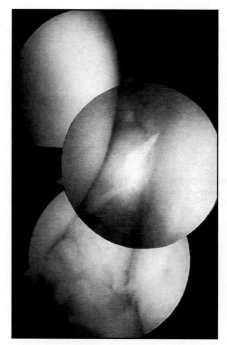

Fig. 5 The arthroscope is viewing from the anteromedial portal. The metatarsal head is on the left side, the base of the proximal phalanx is on the right side. Between the 2 structures is the plantar capsule and synovium. (Courtesy of C. Niek van Dijk.)

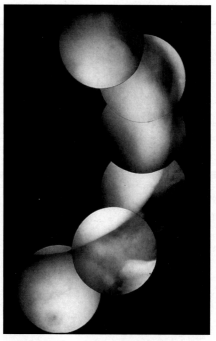

Fig. 6 The arthroscope is viewing from the medial portal. The metatarsal head is to the left and the medial sesamoid is seen plantar to the metatarsal head.

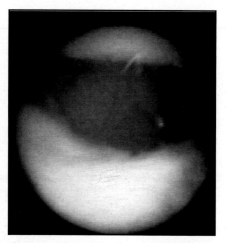

Fig. 7 An arthroscopic view of the lateral sesamoid. At the top is the plantar surface of the metatarsal head and on the bottom is the plantar capsule and the middle part of the lateral sesamoid. (Courtesy of C. Niek van Dijk.)

and strengthening exercises. A wooden shoe is used until postoperative swelling and pain have resolved.

Results

In 1972, Watanabe described the first arthroscopic examination of the MTP joint.[1] In 1986, Yovich and McIlwraith[2] showed that osteochondral fractures of the first MTP (fetlock) joint of the horse could be successfully treated with arthroscopic debridement. In the podiatric literature, Lundeen[3] reported the performance, but no clinical results, of 11 great toe arthroscopies. In 1988, Bartlett[4] reported his technique of first MTP joint surgical arthroscopy and the successful treatment of osteochondritis dissecans of the first metatarsal head. Ferkel and Van Breuken reviewed 12 surgical arthroscopies of the great toe in 1991 (personal communication, San Diego, 1991). The series treated multiple types of pathology of the MTP joint, and good results were reported in 83%.

Summary

The few available reports of arthroscopic treatment of the first MTP joint in the literature indicate favorable outcome. However, arthroscopy of the great toe is an advanced technique and should only be undertaken by experienced surgeons.

References

1. Watanabe M: *Selfox-Arthroscope (Watanabe No 24 Arthroscope)*. Tokyo, Japan, Teishin Hospital, 1972.
2. Yovich JV, McIlwraith CW: Arthroscopic surgery for osteochondral fractures of the proximal phalanx of the metacarpophalangeal and metatarsophalangeal (fetlock) joints in horses. *J Am Vet Med Assoc* 1986;188:273–279.
3. Lundeen RO: Arthroscopic approaches to the joints of the foot. *J Am Podiatr Med Assoc* 1987;77:451–455.
4. Bartlett DH: Arthroscopic management of osteochondritis dissecans of the first metatarsal head. *Arthroscopy* 1988;4:51–54.

Shoulder and Elbow

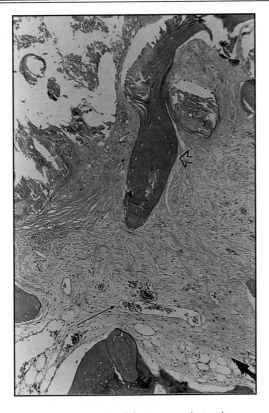

Osteonecrosis of the Humeral Head

Mark I. Loebenberg, MD
Ann Marie Plate, MD
Joseph D. Zuckerman, MD

Introduction

Osteonecrosis of the humeral head presents both diagnostic and therapeutic challenges to the treating orthopaedic surgeon. Although osteonecrosis of the humeral head is much less common than osteonecrosis of the hip, the humeral head remains the second most common site of this condition.[1-3] Matsen and associates[4] reported that 4.6% of patients with glenohumeral arthritis developed this condition secondary to osteonecrosis of the humeral head. The fact that the shoulder rarely serves as a weightbearing joint may result in a later diagnosis for this condition, often precluding effective conservative management. The key element in the successful treatment of this disease remains the identification of those patients who are at risk for osteonecrosis. A full and early diagnostic evaluation may make it possible to use less invasive modalities, which attempt to reverse the condition or stop its progression before the onset of significant arthrosis. Although prosthetic arthroplasty remains the mainstay in the treatment of osteonecrosis of the humeral head, this chapter will review the indications and efficacy of alternative procedures in addition to a summary of recent advances in the diagnostic workup. With an increased understanding of the etiology of this disorder, new opportunities for early identification and intervention will proliferate.

Etiology

At its core, osteonecrosis, wherever it is located, remains a disease process that results directly from damage to the vascular supply of the involved bone. This is certainly the case for the humeral head. A variety of underlying systemic disorders are closely associated with the development of osteonecrosis of the humeral head. In one form or another, all of these conditions compromise the natural blood supply to the humeral head. Aside from systemic etiologies, trauma remains a major cause of humeral osteonecrosis, although it is also understood to act through vascular compromise. Similarly dysbarism, which occurs in deep-sea divers or others exposed to compressed air environments, causes vasocongestion and ischemia. An understanding of the conditions associated with osteonecrosis is a critical factor in the differential diagnosis of nonspecific shoulder pain.

Corticosteroid Use

The majority of reported cases of humeral head osteonecrosis are secondary to systemic corticosteroid use.[5-7] Several theories have attempted to explain the relationship between exogenous corticosteroids and osteonecrosis. Alterations in fat metabolism lead to a fatty liver and hyperlipidemia.[8] Fat emboli have been shown to deposit in the subchondral regions leading to bone and marrow death in the area.[9] Other studies have demonstrated an increase in the intraosseous lipocyte size and resultant ischemia secondary to increased intraosseous pressures.[10]

Sickle Cell Disease

Osteonecrosis of the humeral head has been demonstrated to be present in 3.25% of patients with sickle cell anemia. Concomitant hemiglobinopathies raise the incidence to 4.85%.[11] Worldwide, sickle cell disease is the most common cause of osteonecrosis.[12] The pathologic process is believed to be secondary to increased blood viscosity and higher hematocrit levels.[11] Bilateral disease occurs in more than 67% of those patients with sickle cell disease who develop osteonecrosis. Only 22% of these patients develop symptoms of pain or restricted range of motion. Treatment of patients with this condition is particularly difficult,

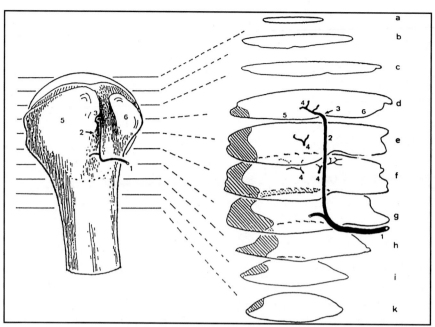

Fig. 1 Gerber and associates[16] demonstrated the blood supply of the humeral head. 1 = anterior circumflex artery (ACA); 2 = anterolateral branch of the ACA; 3 = entry of anterolateral branch of the ACA into humeral head; 4 = lesser tuberosity; 5 = greater tuberosity. Hatched areas are not supplied by the ACA. (Adapted with permission from Gerber C, Schneeberger AG, Vinh TS: The arterial vascularization of the humeral head: An anatomic study. *J Bone Joint Surg* 1990;72A:1486–1494.)

(Fig. 1). The primary vascular supply of the articular surface of the humeral head is derived from the anterior circumflex humeral artery, which continues into the arcuate artery once it enters the bone. Disruption of the anterior circumflex humeral artery mandates a dependence on collateral vascularization from the posterior humeral circumflex artery. The richness of this collateral circulation usually prevents the development of osteonecrosis when isolated greater or lesser tuberosity fractures compromise either of the major arteries. In the face of some 3-part and many 4-part fractures, both the primary and collateral vascularization are compromised. Several studies have demonstrated a wide range of resultant osteonecrosis after 4-part fractures, ranging from 26%[17] to 75%.[18] The observation that severe 3- and 4-part fractures do not always result in osteonecrosis may have a possible explanation in recent studies, which suggest a second anastomotic system supplied by posteromedial branches of the posterior circumflex humeral artery along the inferomedial capsule.[19] The tenuous blood supply of the humeral head can be further compromised by the large dissections often associated with traditional methods of open reduction and internal fixation. Therefore, many surgeons advocate minimally invasive techniques of open reduction and limited internal fixation[20] or pecutaneous fixation[21] to preserve any remaining vascular support.

Pathology

It is widely understood that the pathologic process of osteonecrosis of the humeral head is quite similar to that seen in the hip. Much of the pathophysiologic understanding of humeral head osteonecrosis has been

because prosthetic replacement has been associated with a very high rate of complication, most often severe prosthetic loosening.[12]

Gaucher's Disease

Small increases in intraosseous pressure can occlude susceptible subchondral microvasculature. Gaucher's disease, which causes an abnormal accumulation of glucocerebroside, often results in osteonecrosis. In addition to the increased intraosseous pressures, angiospasm resulting from damaged macrophages may also contribute to the development of osteonecrosis.[13]

Alcoholism/Cigarettes

Chronic alcohol use has a variety of systemic effects, including fatty changes in the liver. Fat emboli originating in the liver and increasing plasma fats may accumulate in the

humeral head causing effects similar to those induced by chronic corticosteroid use.[14] Smoking has been reported to increase the risk of osteonecrosis fourfold, most likely secondary to vascular spasm.[15]

Trauma

After posttraumatic stiffness and malunion, osteonecrosis is the next most common complication. A variety of different fracture patterns have resulted in the development of osteonecrosis, and these results can usually be explained on the basis of direct disruption of the vascular architecture of the proximal humerus. Anatomic studies on the vascular supply of the humeral head by Gerber and associates[16] have helped define the association between specific fracture patterns and an increase in the incidence of osteonecrosis

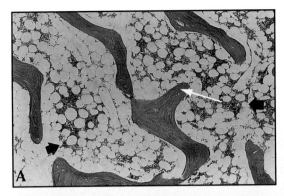
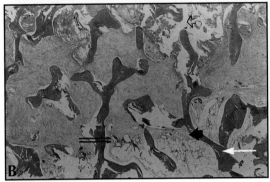
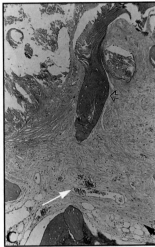

Fig. 2 A, A photomicrograph of normal cancellous trabeculae and marrow. Note the osteocytes in their lacunae (white arrow) and the fatty vascular marrow (wide black arrows). **B,** A photomicrograph of a humeral head demonstrating osteonecrosis. The lacunae are now empty (white arrow) and the cancellous bone is fragmented (open arrow). The wide black arrow shows the transition between normal cellular marrow and the fibrous marrow resulting from fibroblastic migration. Note the new vessels infiltrating the periphery of the fibrous marrow (double black arrow). **C,** A high-power view of the photomicrograph shown in **B.** The transition between fibrous marrow and normal marrow is seen at the bottom of the figure (wide black arrow). Neovascularization is noted (white arrow) within the fibrous marrow. Again, the trabeculae are necrotic with empty lacunae (open arrow).

extrapolated from the larger numbers of patients affected by osteonecrosis of the femoral head. Once ischemic bone injury occurs, it is followed by vascular ingrowth at the periphery of the lesion and the migration of undifferentiated mesenchymal cells (osteoprogenitor cells) into the necrotic cancellous bone.[11] Some of these cells proliferate into fibroblasts and form a layer of dense fibrous tissue in which macrophages resorb dead osteocytes and necrotic trabeculae (Fig. 2). Other cells differentiate into osteoblasts and lay down new bone on the remains of the dead trabeculae.[1] Thickening trabeculae result in

increased radiodensity at the margins of the lesion.[22] These radiodense areas are interspersed among areas of relative osteopenia caused by neovascularization and bone resorption.

The restoration of normal bone architecture through osteogenic remodelling often fails to keep pace with the ingrowth of mesenchymal tissue and the resorption of necrotic bone. Resorption continues until the majority of the necrotic haversian bone has been reabsorbed, resulting in weak and attenuated areas in the subchondral bone, areas that are unable to withstand the normal stresses of joint motion.[10] Microfractures occur, and

the cancellous bone beneath the articular surface begins to collapse, beginning at roughly 18 to 24 months after the onset of necrosis, because it takes that long to resorb enough bone for a pathologic fracture to occur[23] (Fig. 3). The articular surface, supported by subchondral bone, often fails to maintain its original contour. Arthrosis develops once the subchondral bone fatigues, leading to the characteristic flattening deformity. The resulting joint incongruity may, at a later date, even progress to degenerative changes on the glenoid surface.

Classification

Accurate radiographic staging of the osteonecrotic progression allows for a more consistent assessment of the efficacy of various treatment options. Prior staging studies have adapted the Ficat-Arlet classification system for osteonecrosis of the femoral head.[24] The humeral head modification by Cruess[2] has become the most widely used (Fig. 4). The staging is assessed solely on the basis of radiographic evidence obtained from a complete series of standard radiographs, including anteroposterior oblique views in internal and external rotation, in addition to an axillary lateral and scapular Y lateral view. It does not use any assessment of function or pain.

Stage I Stage I is the stage before any evidence of change can be seen on standard radiographs. Pathologic changes can be seen only with magnetic resonance imaging (MRI), which demonstrates necrotic areas where there is not enough bone loss to demonstrate osteopenia on plain films.

Stage II Stage II is first stage with radiographic changes. Usually, sclerotic changes in the superior central portion of the humeral head appear with maintenance of the sphericity of the humeral head. Mottled sclerosis may appear throughout the involved

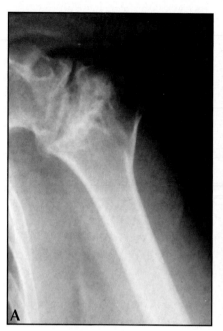
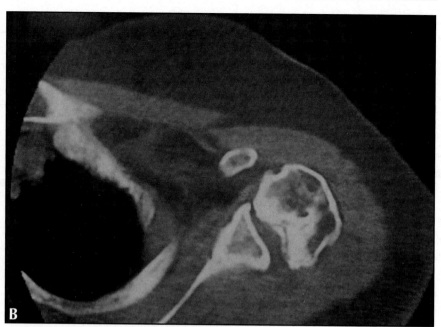

Fig. 3 The anteroposterior radiograph (**A**) and computed tomography scan (**B**) of a 54-year-old woman with advanced collapse of the articular surface of her left nondominant shoulder. Two years earlier, she had sustained a nondisplaced fracture of her proximal humerus, which subsequently developed osteonecrosis.

area of the humeral head.

Stage III Collapse or fracture of the subchondral bone results in the classic "crescent" sign, which characterizes this stage (Fig. 5). Mild flattening of the articular surface may occur without significant deformation of the articular surface.

Stage IV This stage is characterized by significant collapse of the articular surface, with accompanying loss of the integrity of the joint surface. Osteonecrotic fragments may become displaced and symptomatic loose bodies. Degenerative joint disease may develop, with loss of the joint space and further degeneration of the entire articular surface of the humeral head.

Stage V Stage V is the final stage, with degenerative joint disease extending across the joint space to include the surface of the glenoid.

Natural History

The natural history of osteonecrosis of the humeral head is quite variable. It is difficult to predict which patients will progress to severe arthrosis. The prognosis is somewhat related to the etiology of the osteonecrosis. Patients who have sickle cell disease tend not to progress to the point of arthroplasty.[12] This may be secondary to chronic pain in other joints, in addition to sickle cell crises which de-emphasize symptoms in the nonweightbearing shoulder. Patients with steroid-induced osteonecrosis are far more likely to progress in the severity of their symptoms. Cruess,[25] in his experience with 22 patients with corticosteroid-related osteonecrosis of the humeral head, classified progression into 3 groups. Seven patients did not progress to significant symptoms or deformity. The osteosclerotic lesions healed without fragmentation or collapse. In the second group, 8 of the 22 patients developed significant radiologic deformity, with restricted ranges of motion. These patients received no therapy and generally stabilized without further deterioration. The final 7 patients progressed to severe symptoms of pain and loss of range of motion, which resulted in the need for prosthetic arthroplasty.

Rutherford and Cofield[3] followed the natural history of the disease. Eleven patients (16 shoulders) presented with mild pain and were followed without intervention for an average period of 4.5 years. Only 2 of 11 patients with stage II or III disease had clinical progression. The 5 patients with stage IV or V disease all symptomatically worsened, but not to the extent of requiring surgical care. These authors also examined a second group of patients who presented with severe pain. Of the 17 shoulders included in this group, 11 had a proximal humeral replacement and 6 had a total shoulder arthroplasty, depending on the degree of glenoid involvement. Of these patients, 94% had no

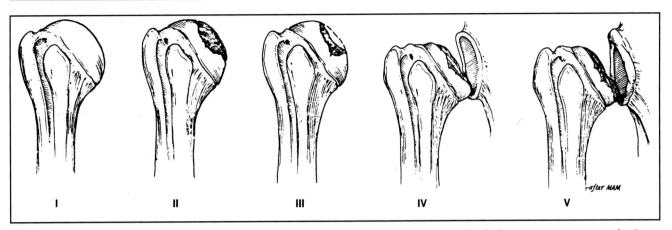

Fig. 4 The modified Cruess classification for osteonecrosis of the humeral head. Stage I: no radiographic findings. Stage II: First stage of radiographic changes with sclerosis in spherical humeral head. Stage III: The classic crescent sign appears with collapse or fracture of the subchondral bone. Stage IV: Characterized by significant collapse of the articular surface. Stage V: Degenerative joint disease extending across the joint surface to include the glenoid. (Reproduced with permission from Cushner MA, Friedman RJ: Osteonecrosis of the humeral head. *J Am Acad Orthop Surg* 1997;5:339–346.)

pain or only mild pain after arthroplasty, with significant improvements in their ranges of motion.

In 1996, L'Insalata and associates[26] published their experience with 42 patients (65 shoulders) treated for osteonecrosis. Most of these patients had steroid-induced osteonecrosis. In 71%, eventual progression of disease resulted in severe pain and disability or arthroplasty. Of the 65 shoulders, 35 (53%) required replacement within 2 years after initial presentation. Only 15 of the 30 shoulders treated nonsurgically had satisfactory results. As expected, poorer results were associated with stage III or more advanced disease.

Evaluation

Because the shoulder is less constrained than the hip joint and, under normal circumstances, is not a weightbearing joint, continued function remains possible despite a greater degree of deformity. For this reason, patients who have osteonecrosis of the humeral head often present later in the course of their disease. Nonetheless, any treatment plan

short of prosthetic arthroplasty is predicated on the early diagnosis of osteonecrosis. A careful history should make the treating physician aware of any associated conditions that might raise the suspicion of osteonecrosis in the diagnosis of new shoulder pain. Patients who have osteonecrosis of the humeral head typically present with shoulder pain before a significant loss of range of motion. More than 70% reported some difficulty sleeping comfortably, and only 21% were able to perform their usual work in a normal manner at the time of presentation. These patients have more difficulty with overhead activity than do other patients with glenohumeral arthritis. The area of the humeral head that is in contact with the glenoid at 60° of forward elevation corresponds to the region of the humeral head most often affected by flattening and collapse.[10] Passive range of motion in early osteonecrosis is normal and pain free. Functional motion is usually maintained until the development of more progressive degenerative joint disease.[2]

Standard radiographs are critical for the evaluation and classification of this condition. Patients who present relatively early may not have any radiographic evidence of the disease process. MRI, however, is capable of revealing the early hyperemia that occurs with neovascularization. Because the signal intensity of MRI is based on the water content of the tissues, scans show a change in the normal marrow signal, defining the extent and location of the lesion. MRI has a 91% sensitivity in the identification of both early and advanced disease. It is currently the accepted standard for the noninvasive diagnosis of osteonecrosis.[27] Bone scanning and tomography may also identify early osteonecrosis, but without the accuracy of MRI, which has, for the most part, replaced these modalities. Biopsy is rarely necessary for diagnosis.

Treatment

It is quite difficult to prevent the onset of osteonecrosis. Its association with serious systemic disorders and the corticosteroids often necessary for the treatment of these disorders

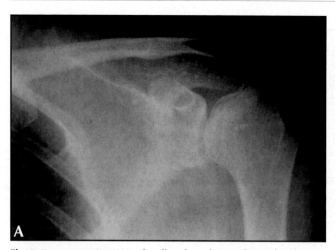
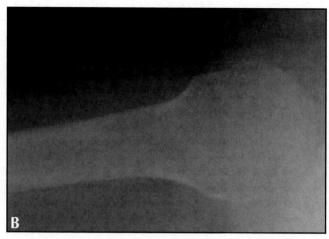

Fig. 5 Anteroposterior (**A**) and axillary lateral (**B**) radiographs of a 32-year-old woman who developed corticosteroid-induced osteonecrosis of her left shoulder during treatment of an ovarian carcinoma. The crescent sign denoting Stage III osteonecrosis is present in the superior central portion of the articular surface.

makes the humeral head an unfortunate casualty of a more central disease process. Any offending substances, such as cigarettes, alcohol, or elective corticosteroid use, should be discontinued. This may not slow the disease process, but it should serve to lower the future risk to other joints.

The 3 primary treatment objectives remain (1) to maintain current shoulder function, (2) to halt progression, and (3) to decrease patient symptoms. The stage of the disease at presentation often dictates the success of these objectives. It is important to maintain the range of motion and to prevent disuse-related stiffness.[28] Analgesic medications may provide varying degrees of relief. A physical therapy program should be undertaken to maintain full passive range of motion while restricting active overhead activities. Patients should not perform activities above shoulder height (abduction greater than 90°), because this position causes the greatest reaction forces across the joint. A therapy program is often adequate treatment for patients with stage I or II disease, resulting in minimal progression of symptoms. Healing usual-ly occurs without significant deformity, and most patients are able to return to normal activities.[2,3]

Several surgical options aside from prosthetic arthroplasty have been investigated in recent years. Arthroscopy has been used for the debridement of symptomatic joints with some success. A report in the literature of a single case of arthroscopic debridement and removal of loose bodies resulted in a complete resolution of symptoms for longer than 20 months.[29] No larger, controlled studies are available for a more definitive assessment of its efficacy. Similarly, a case report from Finland documented the effective use of a vascularized deltoid pedicle graft in a patient with stage III osteonecrosis of the humeral head.[30] The patient reported some resolution of symptoms at 18 months of follow-up. Although vascularized pedicle grafts have been found effective in the treatment of osteonecrosis of the femoral head, their value in the shoulder remains unproven.

Core decompression has been used on a limited basis in the shoulder. The procedure is designed to decompress the diseased area of the head by decreasing the intraosseous pressure, thereby improving blood flow and preventing further disease progression. Several studies have demonstrated only moderate success with this procedure. In the largest published study, Mont and associates[31] presented a series of 30 shoulders treated with core decompression with an average follow up of 5.5 years. Of the 30 shoulders, 22 showed excellent results; however, all of these patients had stage I or II disease at the time of surgery. The remaining 8 shoulders, with stage II disease or greater, did not show any improvement in symptoms. All of these patients eventually progressed to shoulder arthroplasty.[31] Because the natural history of osteonecrosis in the shoulder has shown that stages I and II often have a favorable outcome with conservative measures alone, the benefit of core decompression remains ambiguous. Urquhart and associates[32] demonstrated similar results and concluded that core decompression is an acceptable treatment for stage I, II, and III osteonecrosis. L'Insalata and associates[26] reported on 5 patients with stage III disease who underwent core decompression. All of these patients developed clinical and radiographic evidence of disease progression, and all of them did poorly, with 3 undergoing arthroplasty within 1 year and 1 within 3 years. The remaining patient had arthroplasty scheduled at 4 years. At our institution, the senior author of this chapter has used core decompression with moderate success. The difficulty remains in identifying patients early enough in the disease process for them to benefit from this procedure. The overwhelming majority of patients present at a point when collapse and incongruity at the articulation jeopardize the success of symptom resolution through decompression or revascularization.

Prosthetic arthroplasty, either proximal humeral replacement or total shoulder replacement, remains the most reliable surgical procedure for the relief of pain and stiffness associated with osteonecrosis of the humeral head. The indications for this procedure are similar to those for all joint replacement procedures. The patient must demonstrate significant pain, often accompanied with a marked functional deficit. The patient should have failed a sincere attempt at conservative management with analgesics and physical therapy. Cortisone injections into the glenohumeral joint may give transient relief and help delay arthroplasty on a short-term basis. Arthroplasty must be undertaken with caution, particularly because osteonecrosis of the humeral head tends to occur in a younger population than other forms of glenohumeral arthritis. It is critical to counsel patients not to return to all of their prior activities after surgery.

Radiographic criteria should not always serve as the primary indication for humeral head replacement.

Patients may complain of severe pain in spite of relative preservation of the joint space or localized collapse. This pain may be caused by loose bodies or by painful articular flap detachments from the affected necrotic bone (Fig. 6). In light of the youth of many of these patients, several important factors must be taken into consideration. We recommend the use of a press-fit humeral component. Good bone stock will allow for the necessary bone ingrowth mandated by these prostheses. Significant soft-tissue releases are usually not necessary, but attention must be paid to soft-tissue balancing. The rotator cuff should be inspected and repaired in the event of a tear. The humeral component should be carefully placed to allow for anatomic replacement of the articular surface, in order to minimize the risk of postoperative impingement or instability. Most cases of prosthetic loosening in total shoulder arthroplasty occur on the glenoid side. As such, the glenoid should only be resurfaced in patients with obvious stage V degeneration. As with degenerative osteoarthritis, the need for glenoid resurfacing has varied among surgeons. L'Insalata and associates[26] reported that 54% of their patients who underwent arthroplasty required a glenoid component. Rutherford and Cofield[3] reported a need for total shoulder replacement in 37% of their patients. We have not found it necessary to resurface the glenoid in the majority of our patients. If the patient is young and in need of a glenoid component, we strongly consider the use of an uncemented glenoid component.

Postoperative management consists of standard arthroplasty protocols, including immediate passive range of motion exercises. The amount of external rotation obtained after repair of the subscapularis

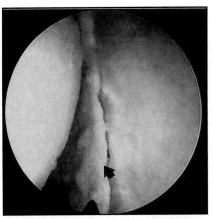

Fig. 6 Intraoperative photograph of a 60-year-old woman with progressive degeneration of the humeral head secondary to osteonecrosis. Arthroscopic evaluation demonstrated a large chondral flap lifting off of the articular surface of the humerus. The flap was debrided and resulted in only moderate, transient relief of symptoms. Six months later, the patient underwent hemiarthroplasty.

should be noted and reported to the physical therapist. Postoperative rupture of the subscapularis must be avoided. Passive exercises are maintained for 6 weeks, after which active strengthening of the deltoid and rotator cuff musculature is begun. Results of this procedure have been quite satisfactory. In addition to the aforementioned 94% relief of pain, Rutherford and Cofield reported an average range of motion of active abduction of 161° in hemiarthroplasty and 150° for total shoulder arthroplasty. External rotation averaged 77° and 67°, respectively.

Complications of arthroplasty for osteonecrosis are not common and, when they occur, are often related to the systemic disorder associated with osteonecrosis. More postoperative stiffness and a poorer general result have been associated with posttraumatic osteonecrosis.[33] Infection has been reported in an isolated case,[25] and, on occasion, postoperative rotator cuff tears have required surg-

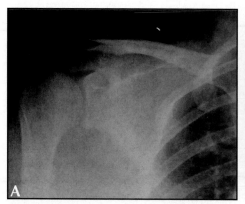

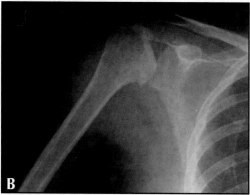

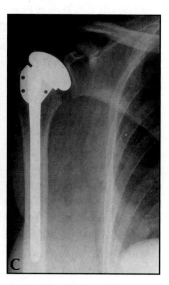

Fig. 7 Radiographs of a 49-year-old woman with osteonecrosis of her dominant right shoulder. There was no clear etiology of her osteonecrosis. Radiographs **A** and **B** chronicle the typical progressive nature of this condition, which often necessitates arthroplasty. The glenoid surface is often well preserved and hemiarthroplasty (**C**) usually provides adequate relief of symptoms.

ical repair.[3] Superior subluxations, brachial plexopathy, and secondary distal clavicle excisions have also been reported.[34]

Recommendations

The best prognosis for patients afflicted with osteonecrosis of the humeral head is associated with early diagnosis. A keen awareness of the conditions associated with this condition and a careful medical history will provide the treating physician with the best opportunity for early intervention. Depending on the patient's symptoms, treatment may consist of careful observation and follow-up, including regular standard radiographs and MRI to follow disease progression. Initial treatment should always be conservative in the early stages of the disease. Patients with stage I and II pathology should receive analgesic medications and activity modifications in addition to physical therapy for the restoration and preservation of maximum ranges of motion. These patients may require core decompression if symptoms persist or there is radiographic evidence of progression. This procedure should be undertaken prior to the onset of articular collapse or incon-

gruity. Regardless of radiographic findings, the symptoms of osteonecrosis are often successfully managed without arthroplasty. When patients with stage III, IV, or V disease continue to demonstrate significant functional deficits in addition to pain, prosthetic arthroplasty should be recommended. Hemiarthroplasty is usually an adequate procedure with excellent, reproducible results (Fig. 7). Resurfacing of the glenoid is occasionally necessary, and the treating surgeon must be prepared to proceed to total shoulder arthroplasty if indicated. As researchers gain a greater understanding of the etiology of this condition, newer, earlier, less invasive modalities may arise. Until then, prosthetic replacement will remain the most reliable method to restore range of motion and provide adequate pain relief.

References

1. Usher BW Jr, Friedman RJ: Steroid-induced osteonecrosis of the humeral head. *Orthopedics* 1995;18:47–51.

2. Cruess RL: Experience with steroid-induced avascular necrosis of the shoulder and etiologic considerations regarding osteonecrosis of the hip. *Clin Orthop* 1978;130:86–93.

3. Rutherford C, Cofield RH: Osteonecrosis of the shoulder. *Orthop Trans* 1987;11:239.

4. Matsen FA, Rockwood CA, Wirth MA, Lippett SB: Glenohumeral arthritis and its management, in Rockwood CA (ed): *The Shoulder*, ed 2. Philadelphia, PA, WB Saunders, 1998, pp 840–964.

5. Frich LH, Sojbjerg JO, Sneppen O: Shoulder arthroplasty in complex acute and chronic proximal humerus fractures. *Orthopedics* 1991;14:949–954.

6. Cofield R, Becker DA: Shoulder arthroplasty, in Morrey B (ed): *Reconstructive Surgery of the Joints*. New York, NY, Churchill Livingstone, 1996, pp 753–771.

7. Cruess RL: Steroid-induced avascular necrosis of the head of the humerus: Natural history and management. *J Bone Joint Surg* 1976;58B:313–317.

8. Patterson R, Bickel WH, Dahlin DC: Idiopathic avascular necrosis of the head of the femur: A study of 52 cases. *J Bone Joint Surg* 1964;46A:267.

9. Jones JP Jr, Sakovich L, Anderson CE: Experimentally produced osteonecrosis as a result of fat embolism, in Beckman EL, Elliott DH, Smith EM (eds): *Dysbarism-Related Osteonecrosis*. HEW Pub 75-153 (NIOSH), Washington, DC, US Government Printing Office, 1974, pp 117–132.

10. Jones JP Jr, Engleman EP, Najarian JS: Systemic fat embolism after renal homotransplantation and treatment with corticosteroids. *N Engl J Med* 1965;273:1453–1458.

11. Milner PF, Kraus AP, Sebes JI, et al: Osteonecrosis of the humeral head in sickle cell disease. *Clin Orthop* 1993;289:136–143.

12. David HG, Bridgman SA, Davies SC, Hine AL, Emery RJ: The shoulder in sickle-cell disease. *J Bone Joint Surg* 1993;75B:538–545.

13. Mankin H, Doppelt SH: Metabolic bone disease in patients with Gaucher's disease, in

Avioli LV, Krane SM (eds): *Metabolic Bone Disease and Clinically Related Disorders,* ed 2. Philadelphia, PA, WB Saunders, 1990.

14. Hungerford DS, Zizic TM: Alcoholism associated ischemic necrosis of the femoral head: Early diagnosis and treatment. *Clin Orthop* 1978;130:144–153.

15. Satterlee CC: Osteonecrosis and other noninflammatory degenerative diseases of the glenohumeral joint including Gaucher's disease, sickle cell disease, hemochromatosis, and synovial osteochondromatosis, in Norris TR (ed): *Orthopaedic Knowledge Update: Shoulder and Elbow.* Rosemont, IL, American Academy of Orthopaedic Surgeons, 1997, pp 233–242.

16. Gerber C, Schneeberger AG, Vinh TS: The arterial vascularization of the humeral head: An anatomic study. *J Bone Joint Surg* 1990;72A: 1486–1494.

17. Darder A, Darder A Jr, Sanchis V, Gastaldi E, Gomar F: Four-part proximal humeral fractures: Operative treatment using Kirschner wires and a tension band. *J Orthop Trauma* 1993;7:497–505.

18. Neer CS II: Displaced proximal humerus fractures: II. Treatment of three-part and four-part displacement. *J Bone Joint Surg* 1970;52A:1090–1103.

19. Brooks CH, Revell WJ, Heatley FW: Vascularity of the humeral head after proximal humeral fractures: An anatomic cadaver study. *J Bone Joint Surg* 1993;75B:132–136.

20. Flatow EL, Cuomo F, Maday MG, Miller SR, McIlveen SJ, Bigliani LU: Open reduction and internal fixation of two-part displaced fractures of the greater tuberosity of the proximal part of the humerus. *J Bone Joint Surg* 1991;73A: 1213–1218.

21. Jaberg H, Warner JJ, Jakob RP: Percutaneous stabilization of unstable fractures of the humerus. *J Bone Joint Surg* 1992;74A:508–515.

22. Steinberg M, Steinberg DR: *The Hip and Its Disorders.* Philadelphia, PA, WB Saunders, 1991.

23. Ostrum RF, Chao EYS, Bassett CAL, et al: Bone injury, regeneration, and repair, in Simon SR (ed): *Orthopaedic Basic Science.* Rosemont, IL, American Academy of Orthopaedic Surgeons, 1994, pp 277–323.

24. Ficat P, Arlet J: Necrosis of the femoral head, in Hungerford D (ed): *Ischemia and Necroses of Bones.* Baltimore, MD, Williams & Wilkins. 1980, pp 53–75.

25. Cruess RL: Corticosteroid-induced osteonecrosis of the humeral head. *Orthop Clin North Am* 1985;16:789–796.

26. L'Insalata J, Pagnani MJ, Warren RF, Dines DM: Humeral head osteonecrosis: Clinical course and radiographic predictors of outcome. *J Shoulder Elbow Surg* 1996;5:355–361.

27. Chang CC, Greenspan A, Gershwin ME: Osteonecrosis: Current perspectives on pathogenesis and treatment. *Semin Arthritis Rheum* 1993;23:47–69.

28. Cushner MA, Friedman RJ: Osteonecrosis of the humeral head. *J Am Acad Orthop Surg* 1997;5:339–346.

29. Hayes JM: Arthroscopic treatment of steroid-induced osteonecrosis of the humeral head. *Arthroscopy* 1989;5:218–221.

30. Rindell K: Muscle pedicled bone graft in revascularization of aseptic necrosis of the humeral head. *Ann Chir Gynaecol* 1987;76:283–285.

31. Mont MA, Maar DC, Urquhart MW, Lennox D, Hungerford DS: Avascular necrosis of the humeral head treated with core decompression: A retrospective review. *J Bone Joint Surg* 1993;75B:785–788.

32. Urquhart M, Mont MA, Maar DC, Lennox DW, Krackow KA, Hungerford DS: Abstract: Results of core decompression for avascular necrosis of the humeral head. *Orthop Trans* 1992;16:780.

33. Tanner MW, Cofield RH: Prosthetic arthroplasty for fractures and fracture-dislocations of the proximal humerus. *Clin Orthop* 1983;179: 116–128.

34. Hattrup SJ: Indications, technique, and result of shoulder arthroplasty in osteonecrosis. *Orthop Clin North Am* 1998;29:445–451.

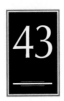

Complications of Shoulder Surgery

Thomas J. Gill, MD
Russell F. Warren, MD
Charles A. Rockwood, Jr, MD
Edward V. Craig, MD
Robert H. Cofield, MD
Richard J. Hawkins, MD

Introduction

This chapter will discuss some of the common and more serious complications associated with surgery around the shoulder. It is arranged in a case presentation format that is similar to that used in the symposium. Topics for discussion include complications related to instability surgery, rotator cuff surgery, arthroplasty, and fracture surgery, with special sections on arthrodesis (versus resection arthroplasty) and arthroscopy. Miscellaneous topics such as frozen shoulder and hardware complications are also presented.

Complications of Open Surgery for Instability

In treating shoulder instability, the 3 aims of reconstructive surgery are to restore stability, maintain pain-free mobility, and avoid complications. In the past, surgeons have concentrated on stability, selecting the simplest procedures by which to achieve that objective with a low recurrence rate.[1] More recent studies have demonstrated that patients are more concerned with full mobility and function, even to the exclusion of absolute stability.[2] Complications after surgical stabilization may imply that the direction of the instability was not recognized, that an anterior repair may be too tight, and that pain after stabilization may be caused by impingement.[1]

Loss of Motion Without Arthrosis

A 24-year-old man had a repair for anterior instability of his shoulder. Six months postoperatively, he still has some pain and there is only 0° of external rotation despite rigorous rehabilitation. Radiographs are normal, but the patient is unhappy with the functional outcome.

Loss of external rotation is a complication that is seen with stabilizations for anterior instability. A loss of rotation at 0° abduction with good rotation at 90° implies that the limitation in external rotation rests with the subscapularis, which moves above the center of joint rotation at 90° of abduction. Loss of external rotation at both 0° and 90° of abduction indicates that the capsule is tight as well. The choice of approach depends on the previous procedure. If the patient still cannot perform external rotation past 0° after 6 months of rehabilitation from a Bankart-type repair with capsular or rotator interval tightening, an arthroscopic capsular release and subacromial debridement should be performed. A wait longer than 6 months increases the risk of glenohumeral arthrosis from increased glenohumeral contact pressure, sometimes with posterior subluxation of the head. Arthroscopic release of the anterior capsule, including the subscapularis, until the desired amount of external rotation is achieved was the preferred approach. Releasing the inferior capsule arthroscopically does endanger the axillary nerve, although by staying sufficiently lateral in the pouch, injury to this nerve is rare.

An open Z-lengthening of the subscapularis should be considered if rotation is still restricted following the arthroscopic release, or if the surgeon prefers an open release. In general, 20° of rotation is gained for every 1 cm of lengthening. At least 30° of external rotation and 50° of elevation can typically be gained using this approach. If not, the subdeltoid and subcoracoid spaces should also be released. Leaving the patient with an internal rotation contracture will increase the joint compressive forces with attempted rotation while causing posterior translation of the humeral head over time. Such a combination often leads to degenerative wear in the posterior aspect of the joint and/or posterior instability in rare instances. The goals of performing a capsular release as early as 6 months postoperatively are relief of pain, improved function, and prevention of osteoarthrosis. Arthroscopic releases are preferred, but those less familiar with applications of the arthroscope prefer an open approach.

Loss of Motion With Glenohumeral Arthrosis

A 48-year-old man had a repair for anterior instability 10 years ago. He now has a significant internal rotation deformity of his arm. Although the patient's other motions are acceptable, pain persists and radiographs show osteoarthritis.

Glenohumeral arthrosis following surgery for instability is the result of excessively tight reconstructions. Samilson and Prieto[3] correlated limitation of external rotation with severity of arthrosis after surgical stabilization. Another cause of arthrosis following instability surgery has been malplacement or loosening of hardware.[3-7] Bone transplants at the anterior glenoid rim have also been associated with arthrosis,[8,9] as have osteotomies that enter the joint.

Osteoarthrosis of the glenohumeral joint is particularly common after a Putti-Platt capsulorrhaphy or Bristow procedure.[8,10] It has also been described after the Magnuson-Stack and duToit procedures.[9] In fact, arthrosis may result from any procedure that makes the shoulder too tight and limits motion. Following a Putti-Platt procedure, disabling pain is typically seen 10 to 13 years post-operatively in association with substantial limitation of motion.[9-12] The limitation of motion is frequently disabling, and is often as much as a 30° to 40° internal rotation contracture. Treatment of this complication depends on the degree of functional limitation, the amount of pain, and the extent of the arthrosis. Mild symptoms and mild arthrosis are treated with an alteration in activities, physiotherapy, and anti-inflammatory medications. If the symptoms and arthrosis are moderate, an arthroscopic anterior release or open Z-plasty lengthening of the subscapularis and capsule can be performed, as previously described.[10,11] Arthroscopic releases can be very successful under these circumstances, helping to diminish pain, increase function, and slow the progression of the arthrosis.

Marked joint degeneration (as seen on an axillary radiograph) or failure of soft-tissue release are indications for prosthetic replacement. A soft-tissue procedure to increase rotation must be performed at the same time as the arthroplasty. Options include an anterior Z-plasty lengthening, a 360° release, and/or an anterior interval release. The use of a smaller prosthetic humeral head and more medial reattachment of the subscapularis and capsule can also improve motion. Anteroposterior radiographs alone frequently underestimate the extent of joint space narrowing.

Hemiarthroplasty is performed if the glenoid is concentric, moderately degenerative, and the humeral head is centered on the axillary radiographic view. If the glenoid is flattened with posterior erosion, a hemiarthroplasty or, more commonly, a total shoulder arthroplasty might be performed with a posterior capsular plication and less retroversion than normal. The osteoarthrosis that results from the limitation of external rotation is likely the result of increased joint contact pressures and shear forces with continued attempts at rotation.

Late degenerative arthrosis has been documented following Bankart reconstruction.[2,4] In 1 study,[4] 14 of 33 shoulders had minimal changes, 3 had moderate changes, and 1 had severe changes at 15-year follow-up. There was a relationship between degenerative radiographic changes, length of follow-up, and restriction of external rotation with the arm abducted 90°.

Of the various options for open surgical anterior stabilization, Bankart reconstruction appears to have the lowest incidence of osteoarthrosis. In a long-term outcome study, Gill and associates[2] described a single case of osteoarthrosis in a group of 60 shoulders at 12 years follow-up. As with other techniques, the arthrosis was associated with a substantial postoperative loss of external rotation. Regardless of the instability procedure performed, preservation of motion is not only critical to the functional outcome and satisfaction of the patient, but it appears to be important in the prevention of arthrosis.

Complications of Hardware and Osteoarthrosis

A 46-year-old woman who underwent a Bristow procedure for recurrent anterior instability 3 years ago now complains of pain and limited motion. Although the patient has not experienced any instability since surgery, she has never been pain-free.

Complications of failed Bristow procedures include recurrent painful anterior instability, articular degeneration, nonunion of the coracoid transfer, loosening of the screw fixation, neurovascular injury, and posterior instability, with an overall complication incidence ranging from 14% to 48%.[7,8,13–15] Articular damage may be the result of direct contact of the humeral head with the transferred coracoid and screw. The screw may be found intra-articularly or impinging on the humeral head with motion. The risk of complications is lowered with proper technique for placement of the coracoid transplant.[15] As a result, the Bristow procedure is not recommended for the primary treatment of symptomatic anterior instability.[8]

The placement of hardware near the glenohumeral joint should be performed with caution. Screws and staples can produce complications that require reoperation and are capable of causing a permanent loss of joint function. Zuckerman and Matsen[7] identified 4 implant-related complications: (1) incorrect placement; (2) migration after placement; (3) loosening; and (4) breakage of the device. Patients with implant-related complications present with anterior shoulder pain, stiffness, crepitus, or radiating paresthesias. The average time from the original operation to the onset of symptoms averaged 16 months in 1 study. Staples are not recommended for rotator cuff repair because of their tendency to migrate. There is often a considerable delay in the diagnosis of implant-related complications. Adequate surgical exposure and careful placement of the implant are essential when these devices are used around the shoulder.

If at all possible, hardware should not be used around the glenohumeral joint. If complications do occur in this instance, the implant should be removed and the joint debrided. If significant osteoarthrosis has resulted from the use of hardware, an arthroplasty may be performed.

Neurovascular Injury

A 23-year-old woman complains of limited motion following a Putti-Platt procedure. Physical examination reveals full passive elevation, abduction, and rotation, but marked weakness in forward elevation and abduction.

Brachial plexus injuries have been sustained during Putti-Platt and Bristow procedures.[13] Suture material has been retrieved from around or within the musculocutaneous, ulnar axillary, and median nerves. Lacerations to the axillary artery have also been reported. These complications are caused by inadequate knowledge of regional anatomy, blind clamping of vascular lacerations, and the use of axillary incisions with limited exposure. During a Putti-Platt repair, abduction should be minimized and sutures placed under direct vision to avoid neurovascular injury.

A Bristow procedure presents a slightly different situation. The musculocutaneous nerve is at risk with the coracoid transfer, and it has been suggested that the musculocutaneous nerve be identified and mobilized.

Once an injury is discovered following a stabilization procedure, the indication for immediate exploration is the surgeon's decision based on knowledge of the events of the procedure. Most neurologic injuries following such surgery spontaneously resolve. A musculocutaneous injury following a Bristow procedure may be an indication for immediate surgical exploration. The neurologic structures involved should be explored at 3 to 6 months if there is no recovery by clinical and electromyographic examination, because there is a high likelihood of structural neurologic injury.[13] In general, good recovery of motor function with variable sensory return can generally be expected following nerve surgery.

Subscapularis Ruptures

A 19-year-old man who is a college football player underwent open Bankart repair for recurrent anterior instability 6 months ago. He complains of instability and pain during tackling drills with the affected arm.

Recurrent instability following a stabilization procedure may be related to several factors. First, a new traumatic event can precipitate a "new" instability, even after an effective previous repair. Second, rupture of the subscapularis can lead to recurrent anterior instability and weakness in internal rotation. Third, the previous procedure can fail. Fourth, there may have been a failure to identify an associated posterior or multidirectional component to the previous instability for which an anterior stabilization was performed.

It is important to identify the cause of the recurrent instability before surgical treatment is attempted. If an arthroscopic Bankart repair has failed with minimal new trauma, consideration should be given to performing a revision open Bankart procedure. If an open Bankart procedure fails after a new traumatic event, a second revision open Bankart procedure could be performed. Arthroscopic examination prior to the open procedure can confirm that a new Bankart lesion is the cause of the instability. The results following revision Bankart procedures are very good, with over 85% good and excellent results to be expected. If the recurrent instability is a result of previously missed posterior or multidirectional pathology, these other directions should be addressed at the time of the revision stabilization.

In the case presented, the subscapularis had torn. This diagnosis can be suggested on physical examination by the presence of increased external rotation compared to the opposite shoulder, weak internal rotation, and a positive lift-off test. Magnetic resonance imaging (MRI) can confirm the diagnosis. Rupture of the subscapularis can occur when the tendon has been released from the lesser tuberosity for surgical exposure in Bankart reconstruction; this is particularly true when the subscapularis and capsule are released together as a single flap. Tendon rupture can lead to recurrent instability, weakness, and pain. In order to prevent this complication, a meticulous repair of the subscapularis should be performed during the closure. The tenotomy should be made at least 10 to 15 mm from the insertion at the lesser tuberosity to allow an adequate soft-tissue stump for later repair. Strong nonabsorbable sutures should be used for repair, and external rotation should be limited to neutral for the first 2 weeks postoperatively in order to minimize stress on the healing anterior tissues.

Early repair of a torn subscapularis tendon is important. If the diagnosis of a torn subscapularis is made late, or if there is a delay of several months before the patient is taken to surgery, the subscapularis may be retracted far medially. This may be the reason that only 2 out of 3 subscapularis repairs appear to do well. If the tendon is not repairable or is of poor quality, a pectoralis transfer can be performed. It is important to ensure that the pectoralis is transferred under tension by placing the tendon lateral to the bicipital groove if stability and internal rotation are to be restored.

Failed Surgery for Multidirectional Instability

A 27-year-old woman who has had 4 previous stabilizations performed for multidirectional instability complains of severe pain with scapular winging. Electromyograms are negative, and translational testing in all 3 directions

reveals instability, with a reproduction of the patient's symptoms.

Failed surgery for multidirectional instability poses a difficult therapeutic dilemma. It is important to spend time getting to know these patients and understanding their emotional and physical condition. Assuming there are no psychiatric issues, the previous surgeries and surgical reports should be reviewed to determine what approaches (anterior versus posterior) and what soft tissues were used.

Typically, the results of surgery for multidirectional instability are poor, with less than a 50% success rate. An examination under anesthesia and arthroscopic examination may be helpful to determine the extent of shoulder instability, and whether there are any structural problems, such as a Bankart lesion, that can be addressed. Further attempts at stabilization must be made cautiously. If the patient's clinical complaints become life-altering, glenohumeral arthrodesis may be considered. Some surgeons have noted that patients may still complain of instability even after a successful fusion, although this was not our experience.

Complications of Rotator Cuff Surgery

Complications can be minimized during rotator cuff surgery by following several basic principles. One of the most important aspects of rotator cuff surgery is preservation of the deltoid origin. Deltoid detachment can be minimized by avoiding extensive coronal detachments. The axillary nerve is protected by limiting the deltoid split to 5 cm or less.[16] A simple longitudinal split with medial and lateral subperiosteal elevation allows a strong side-to-side closure with braided, nonabsorbable suture, and avoids the need for reattachment

through drill holes. If the deltoid muscle does pull off during the postoperative period, it should be reattached immediately in order to salvage the function of the muscle. Once the avulsed muscle has retracted, repair is almost impossible.

The acromion should not be shortened in order to maintain the proper fulcrum for deltoid function. Only the required amount of the anterior/inferior acromion should be resected to relieve impingement, with particular attention paid to any bone spurs present. Not only will deltoid dysfunction be minimized, but acromial fracture will be prevented as well. A strong, tension-free repair of the cuff tissue, including intimal tears, is important. To achieve this, fixation to bone is almost always required. Finally, the question remains as to how "heroic" we should be in trying to repair massive rotator cuff tears, with most of us agreeing that there is more reticence to attempts at a massive repair than in the past.

Failed Cuff Repair

A 67-year-old man complains of decreased motion and weakness 6 months after having undergone a rotator cuff repair. The patient denies any new trauma or acute onset of pain.

One of the most common complications of rotator cuff surgery is rerupture of the cuff, especially following a large or massive repair. Rerupture can occur even after the most technically well-performed reconstructions. Even so, several technical points should be considered. Although arthroscopic rotator cuff repairs are slowly becoming more popular, we decided to use an open approach with heavy, nonabsorbable sutures (#2 or #3 Ethibond sutures using a Mason-Allen or similar technique) that are then brought through drill holes into a bony trough. Suture anchors, although growing in popularity, had not as yet been used by any of us. Hypertrophied bursal tissue should not be mistaken for rotator cuff tissue when performing the repair. If the repair is believed to have excessive tension, an abduction pillow may be used for 4 to 6 weeks, allowing passive motion above the pillow. Early passive motion can be achieved in this manner and postoperative stiffness can be minimized, even for massive tears.

The results following revision cuff repairs are variable and depend on the size of the tear, quality of the tissue, and chronicity of the rupture. Other factors influencing the outcome following cuff repair include a high-riding humeral head and greater than 50% fatty infiltration of the cuff muscles. MRI can show whether the cuff muscles have been replaced by fat or are significantly retracted. If so, rehabilitation alone may be the best option. If the tear cannot be repaired at the time of revision, clinical improvement can sometimes be obtained by performing a simple debridement and removal of bone spurs followed by an appropriate postoperative rehabilitation program.

Rotator cuff repairs or revisions should not be performed under excessive tension. A methodical mobilization of tissue can be performed by releasing the coracohumeral ligament and subdeltoid adhesions. If further release is needed, the superior capsule can be sharply released and elevated from the superior glenoid neck above the origin of the long head of the biceps in order to free the supraspinatus. In general, the supraspinatus should not be advanced more than 2 cm to prevent injury to the suprascapular nerve. A Bankart lesion can be made to mobilize the subscapularis

or release the capsule off the glenoid neck outside the labrum.

The results following revision rotator cuff repair depend on the initial procedure and how it was done. If a patient had done well for 2 years following repair and rerupture occurs, a revision rotator cuff repair can be expected to have a good outcome. If the patient had never had good results after the first procedure, a favorable outcome can be expected less often. If the original procedure was not done adequately (eg, failing to secure the cuff to a bony trough using a strong suturing technique), revision cuff repair may be helpful.

Rotator Cuff Infection
A 60-year-old man who underwent reconstruction of a 5-cm tear 3 weeks ago has had increasing pain, fever, chills, and a draining incision.

One of the most serious complications following repair of large and massive cuff tears is postoperative infection. There must be a high index of suspicion for infection in the patient who returns with pain and limited mobility following this procedure. Early identification and treatment is the best chance for a reasonable functional outcome. Aspiration may be helpful, as are routine laboratory tests. An MRI may be helpful to identify any sequestered areas outside of the joint. If there is any doubt, surgical exploration and debridement should be performed as soon as possible, especially in the setting of a draining wound.

Once a thorough lavage and debridement are completed, every attempt should be made to repair the torn cuff as soon as possible, even at the primary debridement. Repairs done more than several days later are less likely to be possible because of the presence of muscle retraction, scarring, and adhesions. Multiple

debridements over several days may be required, depending on the chronicity of the infection and the organism involved. Primary closure of the wound should be done and it should not be left to granulate.

Intravenous antibiotics are generally used for 4 to 6 weeks with an indwelling catheter, followed by oral antibiotics for 2 weeks. The functional outcome is quite variable, but a fair outcome with minimal pain can generally be expected if the infection is treated early. If continued pain and functional disability result, arthrodesis is a consideration.

Perhaps even more important than repairing the rotator cuff is maintaining a functional deltoid. Patients with an irreparable cuff after debridement for an infection can still have a functional shoulder if the deltoid can be salvaged.

Loss of Motion
A 60-year-old woman has a stiff shoulder 8 months after rotator cuff repair.

A captured shoulder is a potential complication of rotator cuff surgery[17] and is characterized by subdeltoid adhesions and capsular scarring. The normal rolling motion of the humeral head on the glenoid is restricted, while the contribution of the supraspinatus in shoulder abduction is magnified, compressing the humeral head against the glenoid and possibly resulting in chondral wear. A lengthy period of rehabilitation is indicated, given the potential to rupture the cuff with a manipulation. An arthroscopic release may be safer than a manipulation, especially during the first 6 months following repair. Arthroscopy should also be used for recalcitrant cases. Treatment involves arthroscopic release of the subdeltoid adhesions, capsular releases, and appropriate soft-tissue debridement.

Arthroplasty

Total shoulder arthroplasty is associated with numerous complications. In order of frequency, these include prosthetic loosening, glenohumeral instability, rotator cuff tears, periprosthetic fracture, infection, implant failure or dissociation, deltoid dysfunction, and neurovascular injury.[18] Coupled with the fact that the average age of patients who have a total shoulder arthroplasty is the lowest among those for all major joint replacements, a thorough understanding of the biomechanical and technical considerations that pertain to shoulder replacement surgery is important.

The rate of complications inherent to historically applied constrained total shoulder arthroplasty ranges from 8% to 100%.[19,20] Complications have been the result of biomechanical considerations, including mechanical loosening, instability, and implant fracture, deformation, or dissociation.[18] These problems are the result of fundamental design flaws, and a lack of understanding of forces around the shoulder. These forces approximate body weight during unrestricted active elevation of the shoulder. Because of this fact, Wirth and Rockwood[18] question the use of constrained systems even as a salvage procedure. Currently, do not use constrained systems.

Complications such as loosening, instability, infection, and periprosthetic fracture are less common after unconstrained total shoulder arthroplasty. According to Neer and associates,[21] 4 factors must be addressed to minimize complications: (1) osseous deficiency of the humeral head or glenoid; (2) defective rotator cuff; (3) deficient/dysfunctional deltoid muscle; and (4) chronic instability.

Glenoid Loosening

A 71-year-old man who underwent a total shoulder arthroplasty 5 years ago now complains of increasing pain and decreased motion.

Radiographic loosening of the glenoid or humeral component is common and represents nearly one third of all complications associated with total shoulder arthroplasty.[18] Most cases of clinically significant loosening involve the glenoid. The diagnosis can be difficult, with a differential diagnosis that includes cuff tears, subscapularis ruptures, instability, infection, and even fracture. To complicate the matter, radiolucent lines are frequently seen after surgery as a result of suboptimal cementing technique. Torchia and Cofield[22] reported an 84% rate of glenoid radiolucencies at 12 years, with 44% definite radiologic loosening. Clinical loosening is less common,[21,23–25] with most series reporting a glenoid revision rate of less than 2%. Even so, the high incidence of radiographic glenoid loosening has led some authors to recommend primary hemiarthroplasty for glenohumeral osteoarthrosis.[26]

A variety of methods can be used to diagnose a loose glenoid component. Physical examination is very helpful, with patients reporting increased pain on motion testing, a restricted arc of motion, and the occasional presence of a "clunk" with motion. Sequential radiographs and/or arthrograms may document a change in position of the component, while fluoroscopically positioned spot views of the glenoid can show the bone-cement interface quite accurately. More recently, arthroscopy is becoming the procedure of choice to assess the stability of the glenoid.

Once it has been determined that the glenoid is loose, it should be removed. Bony defects in the glenoid may be grafted. The decision whether to reimplant a glenoid must be made on an individual basis. In general, the glenoid can be left out with a conversion to a hemiarthroplasty. The grafting procedure will permit the rare insertion of the glenoid in the future if symptoms dictate.

Several technical modifications can improve fixation and durability of the glenoid component.[18] The subchondral plate should be preserved using concentric spherical reaming for optimum osseous support,[27] new glenoid designs and biomaterials[28] are available, and mismatching of the diameters of the glenoid and humeral head[29,30] may be advantageous. The use of cemented, pegged polyethylene glenoid components is preferred. Epinephrine-soaked thrombin sponges are placed prior to cementing to keep the bony surface as dry as possible for interdigitation of the cement.

Humeral loosening is rarely a problem. Cofield[24] reported that lucent lines around a humeral prosthesis do not indicate future clinical problems. Radiolucent lines have been more frequently reported around uncemented humeral components. However, clinical loosening is rare.[24,31] A press-fit of the humeral component in the medullary canal is preferred. Occasionally, bone graft from the humeral head can be used to help fill a capacious canal. Cement is reserved for cases in which a stable press-fit cannot be obtained, or in fracture management (for example, 4-part fractures).

Arthroplasty Instability

A 56-year-old woman who underwent a total shoulder arthroplasty 7 months ago now complains of instability and pain.

Glenohumeral instability is the second most common complication following total shoulder arthroplasty, ranging from 0%[32] to 29%.[22] Anterior instability is usually the result of humeral component malrotation, anterior deltoid dysfunction,[26] or rupture of the repaired subscapularis.[33] Clinically obvious anterior subluxation or dislocation does not occur without an incompetent subscapularis or coracoacromial arch.[18,26] Disruption of the subscapularis repair can result from poor surgical technique, poor tissue quality, inappropriate physical therapy, or the use of oversized components. When performing the subscapularis tenotomy, an adequate stump of tendon left laterally is helpful for reattachment. The repair is later performed using interrupted, heavy, nonabsorbable sutures. Medializing the subscapularis and capsule to the osteotomy cut requires meticulous tendon to bone suturing, and can be quite difficult. In order to protect the subscapularis repair, external rotation may be restricted for the first 3 weeks.

Superior instability is associated with rotator cuff dysfunction, failed cuff repair, rotator cuff rupture, an incompetent coracoacromial arch, and an excessive acromioplasty. It is not directly related to the development of discomfort or impending component failure.[34] However, the potential for glenoid loosening is certainly increased because of edge loading at the superior glenoid rim.[23] Anterosuperior instability is a nearly unsolvable problem. Attempts to reconstruct the coracoacromial ligament or obtain coverage of the humeral component have limited success.

Posterior instability is typically associated with a glenoid component that is retroverted more than 20°, or a humeral component that is retroverted more than 45°.[18,25] A tight anterior closure or posterior glenoid erosion can also lead to posterior instability, as can arthroplasty for locked posterior dislocations. Chronic osteoarthrosis frequently causes erosion of the posterior aspect of the glenoid. If unrec-

ognized at surgery, the component can be inserted with excessive retroversion. Minor bony deficiencies can be compensated for by careful reaming of the anterior rim, or by alteration of the humeral version so that the combined glenohumeral retroversion equals 30°. For example, in the presence of a chronic, locked posterior dislocation, neutral version may be needed to prevent posterior instability. Severe deficiencies may require posterior bone grafting.[35] Computed tomography is helpful to assess the extent of bony deficiency. Posterior capsulorrhaphy is helpful to prevent posterior instability in this setting.

Inferior instability is typically found after arthroplasty for proximal humeral fractures, revision arthroplasty procedures, or previous osteosynthesis.[18,21,36] Inferior subluxation impedes the ability to elevate the arm because of shortening of the humerus and subsequent weakening of the deltoid. The resting tension of the deltoid and rotator cuff must be preserved during shoulder arthroplasty. In general, the head of the humeral component should be higher than the greater tuberosity after insertion. In cases of severe comminution, indirect reduction of the fracture fragments with longitudinal traction can temporarily restore humeral length to allow proper positioning of the humeral component to be assessed and marked prior to insertion.

If inferior instability does occur, several treatments can be attempted. Inferior subluxation caused by muscle atony presents the most difficult challenge, and is generally addressed through rehabilitation. A Kenny Howard sling can be used in cases of prolonged inferior instability in order to maintain reduction. The neurologic status of the deltoid and brachial plexus should be assessed. An inferior capsular shift and superior recon-

struction may be attempted if nonsurgical measures are unsuccessful.

Recurrent Cuff Tear
One year after undergoing a total shoulder arthroplasty, a 64-year-old man complains of pain, decreased motion, and weakness in his shoulder.

Postoperative tearing of the rotator cuff occurs in 1% to 13% of cases.[18,26] The natural history is similar to that seen in the general population, and pain is not a universal feature.[26] The diagnosis can be difficult. MRI may not be helpful, and arthrograms and arthroscopy are usually not. Surgical exploration following a high index of suspicion is the best method of diagnosis. Surgical cuff repair following arthroplasty poses a significant challenge. Emphasis should be placed on rehabilitation of the deltoid, the remaining cuff, and scapular stabilizers.

Periprosthetic Fracture
A 75-year-old man who underwent a total shoulder arthroplasty 6 years ago falls while walking down the stairs and sustains a fracture at the tip of the humeral prosthesis.

Periprosthetic fracture has been reported in 3% of shoulder arthroplasties,[18,26,37] and accounts for 20% of all complications.[38] Intraoperative fractures are the result of excessive and/or maldirected reaming, forceful humeral component insertion, or manipulation of the humerus during surgery to enhance exposure.[39] It is important during patient positioning to ensure that the arm is free to extend over the side of the table in order to facilitate humeral preparation. A bone hook is used to dislocate the humeral head to minimize the torque and forces necessary to deliver the humeral head. Power reamers are avoided, particularly in osteopenic bone. The humeral component is placed from a superolateral position to allow direct insertion into the humeral canal. Adequate surgical exposure and retractor placement also avoids the need for excessive humeral manipulation for visualization during glenoid preparation. If an intraoperative fracture does occur, immediate open reduction and internal fixation is recommended. Cerclage wiring with possible exchange of the humeral component to a long-stem prosthesis may be performed. Bone grafting is optimal.

Postoperative fractures also occur following total shoulder arthroplasty. Advocates of immediate open reduction and internal fixation[39,40] point out that the advanced age of many patients, marked osteopenia, and poor soft-tissue quality make nonsurgical treatment less attractive. In addition, a faster return to function has been reported with immediate fixation. Others believe that nonsurgical treatment with bracing can be successful.[18,37] If satisfactory alignment and/or healing cannot be obtained in a brace, open reduction and internal fixation with grafting as needed should be performed. **(CD-43.1)**

Infection

A 58-year-old man who underwent total shoulder arthroplasty 3 weeks ago now has increasing pain, fever, and chills. Infection following total shoulder arthroplasty is a rare but serious complication. The presence of comorbidities such as diabetes mellitus, rheumatoid arthritis, collagen vascular disorders and previous surgeries will increase the chance of infection.[18] The use of immunosuppressive drugs such as corticosteroids has also been associated with an increased risk of sepsis.

Laboratory tests such as a complete blood count, an erythrocyte sedimentation rate, and a C-reactive protein may help to confirm the diagnosis, but cannot definitively rule out infection. Radioisotope scanning and joint aspiration may also be helpful. In reality, sepsis becomes a clinical diagnosis based on a detailed history and physical examination. Once a diagnosis is made, options for treatment include antibiotic suppression, irrigation and debridement, removal of the implant with reimplantation, resection arthroplasty, and possible arthrodesis.

The type of treatment depends on the length of time from the index arthroplasty, the virulence of the offending organism, the stability of the implants, and the comorbidities of the patient. An aggressive approach to suspected infections is recommended. Early surgical exploration is performed, and appropriate cultures are taken. Frozen tissue sections can give additional information. In the absence of obvious purulence with a stable prosthesis, an extensive debridement with copious antibiotic irrigation is performed, and the implant retained.

If the implant is loose or a gram-negative organism is isolated, the implant is removed and antibiotic beads are placed. One-stage reimplantation is seldom indicated. Parenteral antibiotics are generally administered for 4 weeks, followed by 3 weeks of oral therapy. Staged reimplantation can be done at about 3 months. Consideration can be given to converting a total shoulder arthroplasty to a hemiarthroplasty at that time. If the organism was virulent, gram-negative, and debridements have failed, resectional arthroplasty may be the treatment of choice. Following resectional arthroplasty, pain relief can be expected in two thirds of patients, and active elevation of 70° can be achieved. Arthrodesis is also an option in this setting, but the huge amount of bone loss and graft that would be needed make it a less attractive alternative.

Neurologic Injury

A 41-year-old woman with rheumatoid arthritis has no biceps function with an absent biceps reflex on the first day after a total shoulder arthroplasty.

Nerve injury following total shoulder arthroplasty is rare, with an incidence ranging from less than 1%[25] to 4%.[41] The upper and middle trunks of the brachial plexus are most commonly affected. The long deltopectoral approach leaving the deltoid attached to the clavicle has been found to be associated with nerve injury, as have shorter surgical times and the use of methotrexate.[41] Most complications involving peripheral nerves in total shoulder arthroplasty are neurapraxias caused by compression or traction. Laceration of an axillary nerve has been reported.[42]

All patients should have a careful neurologic examination following total shoulder arthroplasty. When a deficit is noted, there is little indication for immediate exploration unless an intraoperative incident that could be related to the deficit is suspected. Otherwise, passive motion should be maintained during the recovery period. Temporary static splinting may be helpful. If a hematoma is suspected, an MRI scan may be helpful. If there is no improvement after 6 weeks, electromyography is performed to help determine whether the injury is to an isolated peripheral nerve (the musculocutaneous in this case) or to the brachial plexus. In addition, an electromyogram can assess the extent and degree of injury, that is, whether the injury is complete or incomplete. Surgical exploration should be performed in the rare event that there is no spontaneous improvement by clinical or electromyographic examination after 3 to 6 months. Neurologic injury after total shoulder arthroplasty has little effect on the long-term result.[41]

Miscellaneous Complications of Arthroplasty

A variety of complications related to the prosthesis have been reported in total shoulder arthroplasty (SD Martin, MD, CB Sledge, MD, WH Thomas, MD, TS Thornhill, MD, 1995, unpublished data). These include dissociation of modular humeral components,[43] dissociation of the polyethylene liner from its metal-backed glenoid component,[44,45] fracture of the glenoid keel or metal-backing,[44] and fracture of the glenoid fixation screws.[46]

Neer and Kirby[47] reported on the complications associated with revision shoulder arthroplasty. The most common causes of failure were preoperative conditions such as neuromuscular problems, infection, or systemic arthritis; surgical complications such as detachment of the deltoid muscle, nonunion of the greater tuberosity, or loosening/breakage of the components; and postoperative problems such as glenohumeral instability and insufficient rehabilitation. Loss of external rotation was also common. The results of revision arthroplasty were inferior to the results of primary arthroplasty.

There are many factors that contribute to a favorable outcome following total shoulder arthroplasty. Perhaps the most important element is maintenance of good deltoid function, which is essential to the success of total shoulder arthroplasty.[18]

Complications of Fracture Management

A variety of complications have been reported to follow closed or open treatment of proximal humeral fractures.[48,49] These include infection, neurovascular injury, malunion, nonunion, hardware failure, joint stiffness, heterotopic ossification, and cuff deficiency. Osteonecrosis is a specific complication of displaced proximal humerus fractures.[48] Infection occurs infrequently after open reduction and internal fixation of proximal humerus fractures because of an excellent vascular supply with good soft-tissue coverage.

The rate of nonunion is dependent on the fracture pattern, but is significantly increased with excessive soft-tissue stripping at surgery. Joint stiffness following surgery can be minimized by avoiding prolonged immobilization and prominent hardware. Heterotopic ossification is minimized by avoiding repetitive forceful attempts at closed reduction, operating within 7 days of injury, and the use of adequate irrigation during surgery to debride bone fragments.

Neurovascular Injury

A 31-year-old man collides with a tree while skiing and sustains a 3-part proximal humerus fracture. Evaluation in the emergency department reveals that the patient is neurologically intact. Open reduction and internal fixation are performed, but biceps function is absent in the recovery room.

Neurovascular injury following open reduction of proximal humeral fractures has been reported, with an incidence of axillary artery compromise up to 5% and a 6% incidence of brachial plexus injuries.[50,51] Vascular injuries are generally the result of the initial trauma and typically occur at the junction of the anterior humeral circumflex and axillary arteries. However, the axillary artery can be injured during open reduction through manipulation of the fracture fragments as well. The axillary nerve is vulnerable at the inferior aspect of the capsule, where it can be closely adherent with the altered fracture anatomy, or with excessive deltoid-splitting for exposure.[52] If the location of the nerve is unclear, it should be explored and protected. Overzealous retraction of the conjoined muscle to gain exposure can injure the musculocutaneous nerve as well.

In this case, it is not completely clear whether the musculocutaneous injury was caused in the operating room or at the time of the initial trauma, although intraoperative retraction is the most likely source. An electromyogram may be obtained at 6 weeks to document the extent and degree of injury. If there is no evidence of functional or electromyographic return, the nerve may be explored at 3 to 6 months.

Osteonecrosis

A 46-year-old woman who has a 3-part proximal humerus fracture undergoes open reduction and internal fixation using plates and screws. The fracture pattern was difficult to assess and reduce, and wide exposure was necessary to perform the internal fixation. One year later, the patient has shoulder pain and increased humeral head density on radiographs.

Osteonecrosis is one of the most severe complications following some 2-part fractures, displaced 3-part fractures, and 4-part fractures. The incidence ranges from 3% to 25% in 3-part fractures, and is as high as 90% in 4-part fractures.[48,53] The incidence of osteonecrosis is higher in patients who undergo open reduction and internal fixation than those treated closed.

In order to minimize this complication, a technique of open reduction and internal fixation that involves minimal soft-tissue stripping is recommended. After the superficial dissection, exposure of the entire proximal humerus is not performed. Instead, visualization and anatomic landmarks can be obtained through the fracture lines themselves. Indirect reduction through longitudinal traction while using a Freer elevator for gentle fragment manipulation is often all that is necessary to perform an adequate reduction. A tension-band wire technique[54] can be used for fracture fixation of 3-part and some 4-part fractures that minimizes soft-tissue stripping and provides adequate support for early postoperative motion.

If osteonecrosis does develop, a correlation with patient symptoms must be assessed, because not all osteonecrosis causes pain. Hemiarthroplasty can be performed in the setting of painful osteonecrosis, following open reduction and internal fixation of a proximal humerus fracture. A glenoid component may be necessary in long-standing cases if secondary destruction of the glenoid has occurred.

Cuff-Tuberosity Failure

A vigorous 69-year-old man falls and sustains a 4-part fracture of the proximal humerus. A hemiarthroplasty is performed. Postoperatively, the patient continues to complain of limited motion and pain despite months of appropriate rehabilitation. Range of motion testing reveals pain with active elevation to 80°. Radiographs show inferior subluxation of the humeral head with the tuberosities above the level of the prosthetic head.

Immediate prosthetic replacement for 4-part fractures has met with varied success and a host of complications. Neer[48] reported consistently good and excellent results, whereas the results of other authors have been less favorable.[55] Failures are generally the result of an inability to reconstruct the rotator cuff, failure to

obtain bony union (not soft-tissue attachment) of the tuberosities to the shaft, failure to reproduce the anatomic humeral offset and length that provides the necessary lever arm for the rotator cuff and deltoid muscles, and failure to recreate the appropriate glenohumeral retroversion to help insure joint stability. Axillary nerve palsy has been reported, as has instability of the implant.[56]

A good functional result following prosthetic replacement is directly related to the surgeon's ability to obtain union of the rotator cuff and its attached tuberosities to the humeral shaft. Techniques that can enhance this outcome include: (1) the use of cement, placing the humeral prosthesis in the appropriate resting length with 30° to 40° of retroversion; (2) secure fixation of the tuberosities to the humeral shaft (not the prosthesis); and (3) bone graft underneath the tuberosities, as needed.[56] If there is difficulty assessing the version of the prosthesis, a simple test can determine its accuracy. The hand and forearm should be placed in neutral rotation with the elbow adducted at the side. In this position, the humeral head should point to the glenoid. If the bicipital groove can be found, the lateral flange should be placed 7 mm posterior to it. Failure to achieve union of the tuberosities to the shaft results in a cuff-deficient shoulder. Early reconstruction allows the best chance at salvaging shoulder function. Late reconstruction is extremely challenging.

In the case presented, the humeral component has been placed in an inferior position. Humeral length has not been reestablished, and impingement is resulting from the tuberosities that have been repaired in a position superior to the humeral head. If the patient is able to live with the pain and limited motion, further

rehabilitation is all that should be done. If not, consideration might be given to a revision arthroplasty using a cemented humeral prosthesis to regain humeral length.

Application of Arthrodesis for Complications of Shoulder Surgery

Glenohumeral arthrodesis is indicated for the multiply operated rotator cuff patient with pain who remains disabled, and the multiply operated instability patient who remains unstable with recalcitrant, chronic pain that has not responded to more traditional measures. Failed and/or infected total shoulder arthroplasties can also be considered for arthrodesis, although resection arthroplasty may be the preferred option in these cases because of the technical challenge and generally poor outcomes that follow attempts at arthrodesis. Arthrodesis is a late salvage procedure in the patient with an extremely painful shoulder and without any other surgical options. Under such circumstances, patients will usually opt to live with the pain, and this may be the best option. A trial of immobilization for 1 to 2 weeks that greatly diminishes pain might suggest the outcome from glenohumeral fusion. Resection arthroplasty as an alternative to arthrodesis may be a better option following arthroplasty failure.

Malrotation of the Arthrodesis

A 27-year-old woman has an arthrodesis of her dominant shoulder for intractable multidirectional instability despite repeated attempts at surgical stabilization. The surgeon tells the patient that the arthrodesis was "successful" at 6 months because of radiographic evidence of union at the glenohumeral joint. However, the patient is functionally disabled, and is unable to feed herself, use a computer, or perform rectal hygiene.

The most common complication following glenohumeral arthrodesis is malrotation of the shoulder.[57] Nonunion, wound infection, iliac crest wound hematomas, and fracture below the implant also occur. Malposition is defined as fusion in more than 15° of flexion or abduction, or rotation of less than 40° or more than 60°. If the shoulder is in excessive abduction or flexion, it cannot hang comfortably when the arm is at the side. The scapula becomes medially or posteriorly rotated, resulting in periscapular muscle strain and chronic pain. Rotation must allow the patient to reach his or her mouth and opposite axilla, the front of his or her shirt, belt buckle, and buttocks. Reconstructive osteotomy as described by Groh and associates[57] is the procedure of choice to eliminate pain and improve function.

Frozen Shoulder

A 38-year-old woman in whom impingement is the diagnosis has an arthroscopic subacromial decompression. Four months later, there is global loss of motion in all planes with a firm endpoint on passive testing. The patient complains of pain, insomnia, and an inability to perform activities of daily living.

Frozen shoulder can be a postoperative complication rather than a primary, idiopathic condition. In this setting, a specific diagnosis as to the cause of the motion loss must be made. Typically, motion is restricted more in one plane than others. For example, loss of external rotation following instability surgery is generally caused by tight anterior soft tissues. In this setting, manipulation is not likely to be helpful. Arthroscopic release or an open release with subscapularis lengthening would be appropriate. In contrast, loss of elevation following an acromioplasty is

more often the result of subacromial and/or subdeltoid adhesions, and should be treated with an appropriate release or manipulation.

The diagnosis of frozen shoulder must be differentiated from true adhesive capsulitis. True adhesive capsulitis is a primary pathology of the joint capsule that typically results in a global loss of motion in all planes. The treatment of this condition involves rehabilitation with terminal stretch exercises. Manipulation under anesthesia is a useful adjunct in expediting the return to motion, especially if no improvements in motion are seen after 3 weeks of therapy. If a full range of motion is not restored at the time of closed manipulation, arthroscopic release is indicated.[58] A global release can be performed, beginning at the rotator interval and continuing anteriorly and inferiorly through the anterior capsule and subscapularis. The axillary pouch and posterior capsule are released as well, with care taken inferiorly to avoid the axillary nerve. Results following this treatment have been excellent.

Complications of manipulation include humeral fracture, dislocation, rotator cuff tearing, or rarely, neurovascular injury. Excessive force should be avoided during manipulation. If motion does not return using a judicious amount of force, arthroscopic release is generally a safer option.

Arthroscopy

In general, arthroscopy of the shoulder is a safe procedure. Of 21 experienced arthroscopists polled, only 9 complications were revealed out of over 1,100 cases.[59] Staple capsulorrhaphy had the highest complication rate (3.3%). Major complications, such as neurologic and vascular injuries, were extremely rare. Less common general complications included severe iatro-

genic cartilage damage during instrument insertion, instrument breakage, and reflex sympathetic dystrophy.[60]

Septic arthritis following shoulder arthroscopy is rare. Reported rates range from 0.04% to 3.4%.[61,62] The use of perioperative antibiotics has been reported to be beneficial, with up to a 4-fold reduction in infection rates.[61,63] Strict adherence to antiseptic techniques and the reduction of surgical time are also important.

Patient Positioning

A 21-year-old man has an arthroscopic Bankart procedure performed for anterior instability. A general anesthetic is used. The patient is noted to have a musculocutaneous nerve palsy in the recovery room.

Patient positioning, particularly of the head in the beach chair position, must be checked before and during any arthroscopic procedure. All bony prominences must be well padded. An axillary roll can help prevent compression of the brachial plexus against the thorax by the humeral head.[64] Excessive extension, rotation, and lateral flexion of the neck toward either side should be avoided to minimize tension on the plexus. Allowing the arm to hang off the table increases strain on the plexus by placing the arm in an abducted, externally rotated and extended position, as can happen with the use of an oversized shoulder roll. Adduction of the arm keeps the axillary and musculocutaneous nerves more medial with respect to the shoulder, thus allowing a safer area of instrumentation lateral to the coracoid. Traction with forward flexion of 20° minimizes plexus strain. Extreme arm extension and abduction should be avoided.

Proper patient positioning is essential to lessen the potential for pressure and traction neuropraxias.[60] Brachial plexus injury caused by malpositioning of the patient during surgery is a rare but documented complication.[64] In the lateral decubitus position, brachial plexus strain is most common. Although this is generally considered a rare complication, an incidence as high as 30% has been reported, with resolution of symptoms occurring in 6 to 12 weeks.[65,66] Pitman and associates[66] demonstrated that the incidence of subclinical neurapraxias is high, most likely related to arm positioning, joint distension, and traction. The musculocutaneous nerve was most vulnerable as it enters the conjoined muscles, particularly with the combination of traction and abduction. While in the lateral decubitus position, the patient's dependent arm should be placed anterior to the thorax and a roll placed in the axilla to avoid plexus compression. Balanced longitudinal skin traction not to exceed 10 to 15 lb should be anchored on the operating table instead of a fixed point on the floor.[64] The arm should be flexed 10° to 20° with no more than 70° of abduction. Some authors[60,67] have advocated the beach chair position to reduce the incidence of traction neurapraxias.

Once a neurologic injury is documented, it is almost always a neurapraxia. Full recovery is generally seen with expectant treatment.

Fluid Extravasation
A surgeon is performing an arthroscopic subacromial decompression when the surgical field becomes filled with blood. The surgeon increases the pressure of the arthroscopic pump in order to obtain hemostasis. Once the field clears, the pressure is left elevated. The procedure has been going on for over 90 minutes when the assistant notices that the patient's shoulder is greatly swollen. The surgery is rapidly completed and the arthroscope removed.

Extravasation of fluid can complicate shoulder arthroscopy.[60] All landmarks and portals should be marked prior to inserting the arthroscope to facilitate proper orientation if edema does occur. The pressure sensor should be attached to the arthroscope, and the pump pressure closely monitored. If extravasation does occur, it seldom poses a risk to the patient. Ogilvie-Harris and Boynton[68] demonstrated that the pressure in the deltoid muscle drops to baseline levels minutes after finishing a procedure with no clinical or electromyographic evidence of muscle damage. This is in direct contrast to arthroscopy of the knee, where extravasation of fluid can cause a compartment syndrome. Therefore, if extravasation does occur, turn off the fluid for 10 minutes. If the swelling persists, expedite the completion of the procedure.

Intraoperative bleeding can be minimized during shoulder arthroscopy by maintaining irrigation fluids at the recommended height or pressure, using a solution containing 10 ml of epinephrine (1:300,000 to 1:3,000,000) diluted in a 3-l bag, infiltrating portals with a marcaine and epinephrine solution, and the use of hypotensive anesthesia.[60] Hypotensive anesthesia is especially helpful during subacromial decompressions to prevent bleeding from the bursal capillaries as well as the exposed cancellous bed of the acromion. The use of electrocautery devices prior to and during shaving in the subacromial space is also recommended to prevent excessive soft-tissue bleeding. If a bleeding vessel is identified, it should be cauterized.

Complications Related to Subacromial Space Procedures
A 32-year-old man who is a football player has an arthroscopic subacromial decompression for impingement.

He returns to contact drills at 6 weeks postoperatively, and notices sharp pain in his shoulder and a return of his impingement symptoms after practice. Radiographs demonstrate a displaced acromial fracture.

Arthroscopic subacromial space procedures are generally safe, with favorable short-term results and a complication rate less than 1%.[59,60,69–71] Complications include intraoperative bleeding, instrument breakage, transient neurapraxias, and acromial fracture. Proper patient selection is essential.

Acromial burring should be performed cautiously to avoid fracture resulting from aggressive resection. If there is any doubt regarding the adequacy of resection, the lateral portal can be extended by 1 to 2 cm to allow digital palpation of the subacromial space. Any remaining bony prominences, particularly at the anterolateral corner of the acromion, can be identified and resected without removing more bone from adequately decompressed areas. This is especially helpful early in the learning curve with this procedure. The incidence of failure resulting from inadequate decompression can be minimized by using this technique without introducing any added morbidity. The presence of partial- or full-thickness rotator cuff tears can also be assessed using digital palpation. If a displaced fracture involving a significant portion of the acromion occurs as in this case, open reduction internal fixation using a tension-band technique should be performed.

Other complications of subacromial decompression include hematoma and traction neuropathy,[69] infection, acromial fracture,[72] reflex sympathetic dystrophy,[72,73] and instrument breakage. Heterotopic bone was reported postoperatively in 10 cases in 1 series,[74] with recurrent impingement occurring in 8. Patients at risk, such as those with hypertrophic pulmonary arthropathy, obesity, or diabetes, should be considered for heterotopic ossification prophylaxis. An increased rate of complications can be expected in patients with additional preoperative pathologic conditions, such as neck pain or restricted motion, and in a workers' compensation population.[73]

Complications Related to Arthroscopic Instability Surgery

A 25-year-old woman undergoes an arthroscopic Bankart procedure performed for recurrent anterior instability. Six months postoperatively, she returns to competitive kayaking, but sustains a dislocation in the high-post position (abduction, external rotation).

For an arthroscopic stabilization procedure to be accepted, it must parallel the results obtained with open stabilization of the same problem. Aside from high failure rates with arthroscopic stabilizations, the possibility of nerve injury may be greater.[75,76] In fact, the highest complication rate (3.2%) in shoulder arthroscopy has been reported with staple capsulorrhaphy,[59] and recurrence is more likely than with open repairs. Migration of hardware and articular damage is not uncommon.[7] As a result, we do not perform this procedure for the treatment of instability of the glenohumeral joint.

The approach to arthroscopic stabilization procedures has changed significantly over the past 2 years since the introduction of laser and heat probe techniques. In the past, a contributing factor to the high rate of unsuccessful arthroscopic Bankart procedures was a failure to address the capsular redundancy that typically accompanies traumatic Bankart lesions. Although this redundancy is able to be successfully addressed during open Bankart repairs,[2] simply suturing the anterior capsule/labrum back to the glenoid rim arthroscopically does not achieve the same goal. In order to address this problem, an anterior thermal capsulorrhaphy can be added to the vast majority of arthroscopic Bankart procedures. Postoperative stability is generally excellent, and has paralleled the results of open reconstructions at short-term follow-up. Restriction of motion has been minimal with this technique, averaging about 5° less external rotation on the operated shoulder. Complications with this technique have been minimal.

For glenohumeral instability without a Bankart lesion, a thermal capsulorrhaphy rather than an open inferior capsular shift can be considered. As with the arthroscopic Bankart procedures, early results have been very encouraging. Mild to moderate instabilities are immobilized for 1 week following the procedure, reserving 2- to 3-week immobilizations for severe unidirectional and most multidirectional instabilities. Altough anecdotal reports of axillary nerve injuries have been reported following thermal shrinkage of the axillary pouch, this complication has not been seen by us.

Even so, nerve injury can occur during arthroscopic procedures.[66,77,78] The suprascapular nerve is vulnerable with transglenoid techniques as it descends in the posterior aspect of the glenoid neck. The axillary nerve is at risk with thermal shrinkage of the inferior aspect of the axillary pouch, or with inferior instrument placement. A recent anatomic study has demonstrated a margin of safety of 1 cm with surgery to the inferior capsule (CL Eakin, MD, RJ Hawkins, MD, 1997, unpublished data). The axillary nerve is also vulnerable from a low posterior portal placement. The cannula should not be placed lower than 2 cm from the posterolateral border of the acromion to avoid damage to the nerve.[79] Finally, the musculocutaneous nerve can be damaged by placing an anterior portal too low or too medial. In general, the anterior portal must not be placed inferior or medial to the coracoid process.

Correct portal placement is essential to avoid nerve injury. The posterior portal is located approximately 2 cm distal and 1 cm medial to the posterolateral corner of the acromion. Distal placement can injure the axillary nerve. The cannula is inserted in the direction of the coracoid. More medial insertion can injure the suprascapular neurovascular bundle. The anterior portal is placed just distal to the acromioclavicular joint. It must remain lateral and proximal to the coracoid process. It can be established under direct visualization using a spinal needle, or via a Wissinger rod passed through the posterior cannula positioned in the superior interval. Passage of the rod below the subscapularis can injure the brachial plexus and axillary sheath. The musculocutaneous nerve is at risk of injury because of an excessively medial anterior portal placement. The lateral portal is placed 2 cm from the lateral border of the acromion. Inferior placement can damage the axillary nerve.

Nerve injuries during shoulder arthroscopy can also occur during joint distension, fluid extravasation, positioning, manipulation, excessive traction,[66] and portal placement.[80] Traction can be applied either parallel or perpendicular to the long axis of the arm. Perpendicular traction minimizes abduction and therefore neurapraxias.[81] In general, no more than 10 to 15 lb of traction is necessary and it should be attached to the operating table rather than applied by a fixed object. An assistant can also be used. The brachial plexus is at risk because it is attached at 2 points along its course (the prevertebral fascia at the transverse processes and the axillary fascia in the arm). As longitudinal traction increases the distance between these 2 fixed points, injury can occur. The freely moving humeral head and clavicle can also cause injury with malpositioning.

In general, proper patient selection and attention to technical detail will decrease the incidence of complications in shoulder arthroscopy. Careful patient and extremity positioning lessens the potential for pressure and traction neurapraxias. Electrosurgical instruments and adequate distension pressure helps to minimize intraoperative bleeding and improves visualization.

Conclusion

In general, the results following shoulder surgery are somewhat more variable than those obtained in other aspects of orthopaedic surgery. A significant reason for this is the failure to establish an accurate diagnosis prior to surgery. Seldom should the surgeon be in a position where the joint is being 'explored' in order to determine the source of pain. Diagnoses such as instability, impingement, acromioclavicular arthritis, and biceps tendinitis can rarely be made in this fashion. Instead, a careful history and physical examination coupled with appropriate imaging and laboratory tests will generally reveal the source of pathology. The difficulty in diagnosis around the shoulder is compounded by the fact that many problems, such as rotator cuff disease and instability, exist along a spectrum of severity, and are not mutually exclusive of other pathology. By having a clear understanding of the pathophysiology that affects the shoulder and making carefully selected surgical decisions, the incidence of complications surrounding surgery to the shoulder can be significantly diminished.

Once the decision to perform surgery has been made, knowledge of potential intraoperative and postoperative complications can significantly lower their incidence. For example, the use of hand reamers instead of power reamers and minimizing rotational torque during humeral preparation in total shoulder arthroplasty can minimize the potential for fracturing the humerus. The clinician should have a high index of suspicion when evaluating for potential postoperative complications such as infection. Early recognition and aggressive treatment will allow the optimal functional outcome. Lastly, the surgeon must know what can and cannot help. Surgery for a failed Bankart procedure can yield excellent results, but attempting to operate on superior instability following total shoulder arthroplasty is more likely to be futile.

References

1. Hawkins RH, Hawkins RJ: Failed anterior reconstruction for shoulder instability. *J Bone Joint Surg* 1985;67B:709–714.

2. Gill TJ, Micheli LJ, Gebhard F, Binder C: Bankart repair for anterior instability of the shoulder: Long-term outcome. *J Bone Joint Surg* 1997;79A:850–857.

3. Samilson RL, Prieto V: Dislocation arthropathy of the shoulder. *J Bone Joint Surg* 1983;65A:456–460.

4. Rosenberg BN, Richmond JC, Levine WN: Long-term followup of Bankart reconstruction: Incidence of late degenerative glenohumeral arthrosis. *Am J Sports Med* 1995;23:538–544.

5. O'Driscoll SW, Evans DC: Long-term results of staple capsulorrhaphy for anterior instability of the shoulder. *J Bone Joint Surg* 1993;75A:249–258.

6. Sisk TD, Boyd HB: Management of recurrent anterior dislocation of the shoulder: Du Toit-type or staple capsulorrhaphy. *Clin Orthop* 1974;103:150–156.

7. Zuckerman JD, Matsen FA III: Complications about the glenohumeral joint related to the use of screws and staples. *J Bone Joint Surg* 1984;66A:175–180.

8. Young DC, Rockwood CA Jr: Complications of a failed Bristow procedure and their management. *J Bone Joint Surg* 1991;73A:969–981.

9. Lusardi DA, Wirth MA, Wurtz D, Rockwood CA Jr: Loss of external rotation following anterior capsulorrhaphy of the shoulder. *J Bone Joint Surg* 1993;75A:1185–1192.

10. Hawkins RJ, Angelo RL: Glenohumeral osteoarthrosis: A late complication of the Putti-Platt repair. *J Bone Joint Surg* 1990;72A:1193–1197.

11. MacDonald PB, Hawkins RJ, Fowler PJ, Miniaci A: Release of the subscapularis for internal rotation contracture and pain after anterior repair for recurrent anterior dislocation of the shoulder. *J Bone Joint Surg* 1992;74A:734–737.

12. Leach RE, Corbett M, Schepsis A, Stockel J: Results of a modified Putti-Platt operation for recurrent shoulder dislocations and subluxations. *Clin Orthop* 1982;164:20–25.

13. Richards RR, Hudson AR, Bertoia JT, Urbaniak JR, Waddell JP: Injury to the brachial plexus during Putti-Platt and Bristow procedures: A report of eight cases. *Am J Sports Med* 1987;15:374–380.

14. Hill JA, Lombardo SJ, Kerlan RK, et al: The modified Bristow-Helfet procedure for recurrent anterior shoulder subluxations and dislocations. *Am J Sports Med* 1981;9:283–287.

15. Hovelius L, Korner L, Lundberg B, et al: The coracoid transfer for recurrent dislocation of the shoulder: Technical aspects of the Bristow-Latarjet procedure. *J Bone Joint Surg* 1983;65A:926–934.

16. Post M: Complications of rotator cuff surgery. *Clin Orthop* 1990;254:97–104.

17. Mormino MA, Gross RM, McCarthy JA: Captured shoulder: A complication of rotator cuff surgery. *Arthroscopy* 1996;12:457–461.

18. Wirth MA, Rockwood CA Jr: Complications of total shoulder-replacement

arthroplasty. *J Bone Joint Surg* 1996;78A:
603–616.

19. Laurence M: Replacement arthroplasty of
the rotator cuff deficient shoulder. *J Bone
Joint Surg* 1991;73B:916–919.

20. Post M: Constrained arthroplasty of the
shoulder. *Orthop Clin North Am* 1987;18:
455–462.

21. Neer CS II, Watson KC, Stanton FJ: Recent experience in total shoulder replacement. *J Bone Joint Surg* 1982;64A:319–337.

22. Torchia ME, Cofield RH: Long-term
results of Neer total shoulder arthroplasty.
Orthop Trans 1994;18:977.

23. Barrett WP, Franklin JL, Jackins SE, Wyss
CR, Matsen FA III: Total shoulder arthroplasty. *J Bone Joint Surg* 1987;69A:865–872.

24. Cofield RH: Total shoulder arthroplasty
with the Neer prosthesis. *J Bone Joint Surg*
1984;66A:899–906.

25. Hawkins RJ, Bell RH, Jallay B: Total
shoulder arthroplasty. *Clin Orthop* 1989;
242:188–194.

26. Wirth MA, Rockwood CA Jr: Complications of shoulder arthroplasty. *Clin Orthop*
1994;307:47–69.

27. Collins D, Tencer A, Sidles J, Matsen F
III: Edge displacement and deformation
of glenoid components in response to
eccentric loading: The effect of preparation of the glenoid bone. *J Bone Joint Surg*
1992;74A:501–507.

28. Wirth MA, Basamania C, Rockwood CA
Jr: Fixation of glenoid component: Keel
versus pegs. *Op Tech Orthop* 1994;4:
218–225.

29. Harryman DT, Sidles JA, Harris SL,
Lippitt SB, Matsen FA III: The effect of
articular conformity and the size of the
humeral head component on laxity and
motion after glenohumeral arthroplasty: A
study in cadavera. *J Bone Joint Surg* 1995;
77A:555–563.

30. Severt R, Thomas BJ, Tsenter MJ,
Amstutz HC, Kabo JM: The influence of
conformity and constraint on translational
forces and frictional torque in total shoulder arthroplasty. *Clin Orthop* 1993;292:
151–158.

31. Brenner BC, Ferlic DC, Clayton ML,
Dennis DA: Survivorship of uncon-
strained total shoulder arthroplasty. *J Bone
Joint Surg* 1989;71A:1289–1296.

32. McCoy SR, Warren RF, Bade HA III,
Ranawat CS, Inglis AE: Total shoulder

arthroplasty in rheumatoid arthritis.
J Arthroplasty 1989;4:105–113.

33. Moeckel BH, Altchek DW, Warren RF,
Wickiewicz TL, Dines DM: Instability of
the shoulder after arthroplasty. *J Bone Joint
Surg* 1993;75A:492–497.

34. Boyd AD Jr, Thomas WH, Scott RD,
Sledge CB, Thornhill TS: Total shoulder
arthroplasty versus hemiarthroplasty:
Indications for glenoid resurfacing.
J Arthroplasty 1990;5:329–336.

35. Neer CS II, Morrison DS: Glenoid bone-
grafting in total shoulder arthroplasty.
J Bone Joint Surg 1988;70A:1154–1162.

36. Frich LH, Sojbjerg JO, Sneppen O:
Shoulder arthroplasty in complex acute
and chronic proximal humeral fractures.
Orthopedics 1991;14:949–954.

37. Groh GI, Heckman MM, Curtis RJ,
Rockwood CA Jr: Treatment of fractures
adjacent to humeral prosthesis. *Orthop
Trans* 1994;18:1072.

38. Wirth MA: Part I: Periprosthetic fractures
of the upper extremity, in Rockwood CA
Jr, Green DP, Bucholz RW, Heckman JD
(eds): *Rockwood and Green's Fractures in
Adults*, ed 4. Philadelphia, PA, Lippincott-
Raven, 1996, pp 540–576.

39. Bonutti PM, Hawkins RJ: Fracture of the
humeral shaft associated with total shoulder replacement arthroplasty of the shoulder: A case report. *J Bone Joint Surg* 1992
;74A:617–618.

40. Boyd AD Jr, Thornhill TS, Barnes CL:
Fractures adjacent to humeral prostheses.
J Bone Joint Surg 1992;74A:1498–1504.

41. Lynch NM, Cofield RH, Silbert PL,
Hermann RC: Neurologic complications
after total shoulder arthroplasty. *J Shoulder
Elbow Surg* 1996;5:53–61.

42. Cofield RH: Unconstrained total shoulder prostheses. *Clin Orthop* 1983;173:
97–108.

43. Cooper RA, Brems JJ: Recurrent disassembly of a modular humeral prosthesis:
A case report. *J Arthroplasty* 1991;6:
375–377.

44. Cofield RH, Daly PJ: Total shoulder
arthroplasty with a tissue-ingrowth glenoid component. *J Shoulder Elbow Surg*
1992;1:77–85.

45. Driessnack RP, Ferlic DC, Wiedel JD:
Dissociation of the glenoid component in
the Macnab/English total shoulder arthroplasty. *J Arthroplasty* 1990;5:15–18.

46. McElwain JP, English E: The early results
of porous-coated total shoulder arthroplasty. *Clin Orthop* 1987;218:217–224.

47. Neer CS II, Kirby RM: Revision of
humeral head and total shoulder arthroplasties. *Clin Orthop* 1982;170:189–195.

48. Neer CS II: Displaced proximal humeral
fractures: Part II. Treatment of three-part
and four-part displacement. *J Bone Joint
Surg* 1970;52A:1090–1103.

49. Schlegel TF, Hawkins RJ: Displaced proximal humerus fractures: Evaluation and
treatment. *J Am Acad Orthop Surg* 1994;2:
54–66.

50. Stableforth PG: Four-part fractures of the
neck of the humerus. *J Bone Joint Surg*
1984;66B:104–108.

51. Zuckerman JD, Flugstad DL, Teitz CC,
King HA: Axillary artery injury as a complication of proximal humeral fractures:
Two case reports and a review of the literature. *Clin Orthop* 1984;189:234–237.

52. Flatow EL, Cuomo F, Maday MG, Miller
SR, McIlveen SJ, Bigliani LU: Open
reduction and internal fixation of two-
part displaced fractures of the greater
tuberosity of the proximal part of the
humerus. *J Bone Joint Surg* 1991;73A:
1213–1218.

53. Hägg O, Lundberg BJ: Aspects of prognostic factors in comminuted and dislocated proximal humeral fractures, in
Bateman JE, Walsh RP (eds): *Surgery of the
Shoulder*. Philadelphia, PA, BC Decker,
1984, pp 51–59.

54. Hawkins RJ, Bell RH, Gurr K: The
three-part fracture of the proximal part of
the humerus: Operative treatment. *J Bone
Joint Surg* 1986;68A:1410–1414.

55. Tanner MW, Cofield RH: Prosthetic
arthroplasty for fractures and fracture-dislocations of the proximal humerus. *Clin
Orthop* 1983;179:116–128.

56. Hawkins RJ, Switlyk P: Acute prosthetic
replacement for severe fractures of the
proximal humerus. *Clin Orthop* 1993;289:
156–160.

57. Groh GI, Williams GR, Jarman RN,
Rockwood CA Jr: Treatment of complica-
tions of shoulder arthrodesis. *J Bone Joint
Surg* 1997;79A:881–887.

58. Warner JJP: Frozen shoulder: Diagnosis
and management. *J Am Acad Orthop Surg*
1997;5:130–140.

59. Small NC: Complications in arthroscopic surgery performed by experienced arthroscopists. *Arthroscopy* 1988;4:215–221.

60. Bigliani LU, Flatow EL, Deliz ED: Complications of shoulder arthroscopy. *Orthop Rev* 1991;20:743–751.

61. D'Angelo GL, Ogilvie-Harris DJ: Septic arthritis following arthroscopy, with cost/benefit analysis of antibiotic prophylaxis. *Arthroscopy* 1988;4:10–14.

62. Johnson LL, Shneider DA, Austin MD, Goodman FG, Bullock JM, DeBruin JA: Two percent glutaraldehyde: A disinfectant in arthroscopy and arthroscopic surgery. *J Bone Joint Surg* 1982;64A:237–239.

63. Neu HC: Cephalosporin antibiotics as applied in surgery of bones and joints. *Clin Orthop* 1984;190:50–64.

64. Cooper DE, Jenkins RS, Bready L, Rockwood CA Jr: The prevention of injuries of the brachial plexus secondary to malposition of the patient during surgery. *Clin Orthop* 1988;228:33–41.

65. Klein AH, France JC, Mutschler TA, Fu FH: Measurement of brachial plexus strain in arthroscopy of the shoulder. *Arthroscopy* 1987;3:45–52.

66. Pitman MI, Nainzadeh N, Ergas E, Springer S: The use of somatosensory evoked potentials for detection of neuropraxia during shoulder arthroscopy. *Arthroscopy* 1988:4:250–255.

67. Skyhar MJ, Altchek DW, Warren RF, Wickiewicz TL, O'Brien SJ: Shoulder arthroscopy with the patient in the beach-chair position. *Arthroscopy* 1988;4:256–259.

68. Ogilvie-Harris DJ, Boynton E: Arthroscopic acromioplasty: Extravasation of fluid into the deltoid muscle. *Arthroscopy* 1990;6:52–54.

69. Ellman H: Arthroscopic subacromial decompression: Analysis of one- to three-year results. *Arthroscopy* 1987;3:173–181.

70. Altchek DW, Warren RF, Wickiewicz TL, Skyhar MJ, Ortiz G, Schwartz E: Arthroscopic acromioplasty: Technique and results. *J Bone Joint Surg* 1990;72A:1198–1207.

71. Gartsman GM: Arthroscopic acromioplasty for lesions of the rotator cuff. *J Bone Joint Surg* 1990;72A:169–180.

72. Esch JC: Arthroscopic subacromial decompression and postoperative management. *Orthop Clin North Am* 1993;24:161–171.

73. Hawkins RJ, Chris T, Bokor D, Kiefer G: Failed anterior acromioplasty: A review of 51 cases. *Clin Orthop* 1989;243:106–111.

74. Berg EE, Ciullo JV, Oglesby JW: Failure of arthroscopic decompression by subacromial heterotopic ossification causing recurrent impingement. *Arthroscopy* 1994;10:158–161.

75. Matthews LS, Vetter WL, Oweida SJ, Spearman J, Helfet DL: Arthroscopic staple capsulorrhaphy for recurrent anterior shoulder instability. *Arthroscopy* 1988;4:106–111.

76. Morgan CD, Bodenstab AB: Arthroscopic Bankart suture repair: Technique and early results. *Arthroscopy* 1987;3:111–122.

77. Committee on Complications of the Arthroscopy Association of North America: Complications in arthroscopy: The knee and other joints. *Arthroscopy* 1986;2:253–258.

78. Andrews JR, Carson WG: Shoulder joint arthroscopy. *Orthopedics* 1983;6:1157–1162.

79. Bryan WJ, Schauder K, Tullos HS: The axillary nerve and its relationship to common sports medicine shoulder procedures. *Am J Sports Med* 1986;14:113–116.

80. Matthews LS, Zarins B, Michael RH, Helfet DL: Anterior portal selection for shoulder arthroscopy. *Arthroscopy* 1985;1:33–39.

81. Stanish WD, Peterson DC: Shoulder arthroscopy and nerve injury: Pitfalls and prevention. *Arthroscopy* 1995;11:458–466.

Reference to Video

Wirth MA, Rockwood CA: Revision Shoulder Arthroplasty. San Antonio, TX, University of Texas Health Science Center, 1997.

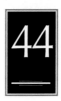

Epicondylitis in the Athlete

Michael G. Ciccotti, MD

In a simple letter published in *Lancet* in 1882, Henry J. Morris[1] introduced a previously undescribed entity, which he appropriately termed "lawn tennis arm". That brief description has since prompted the mind and pen of numerous orthopaedic researchers, resulting in a vast array of detailed diagnostic and therapeutic reports. However, many questions still remain unanswered with respect to this enigmatic entity called epicondylitis. Most simply defined, it is generally agreed to be an overuse injury of the musculotendinous origins of either the medial or lateral elbow. From that point on, however, debate and speculation continue with respect to many aspects of this disorder.

Etiology

The bulk of the literature on epicondylitis suggests that repetitive stress or overuse is the primary etiology of this disorder.[2–5] However, the occurrence of epicondylitis has also been documented in patients, athletes and nonathletes, after a single traumatic event.[4,5] No definitive etiology has been determined, and it would seem that either mode of injury might lead to this disorder. Epicondylitis has most commonly been associated on the lateral elbow with tennis and on the medial elbow with golf, but a host of sports (base-ball, javelin throwing, fencing) and occupational activities (carpentry, plumbing, meat cutting) have also been identified as possible causes.

A variety of risk factors have been proposed for epicondylitis. Because our understanding of these risk factors comes from the study of tennis, they are most often discussed in terms of racquet sports. Improper techniques, such as leading on the groundstroke with a flexed elbow and hitting the ball off center on the racquet, may enhance the occurrence of tennis elbow.[2,6,7] It has been shown that epicondylitis is most common in recreational tennis players, not in elite players, which suggests that technique may very well be a risk factor.[3] The use of poorly sized or inappropriate equipment may also be a key risk factor for epicondylitis.[2,6] Choosing the appropriately sized tennis racquet, golf club, bat, or other equipment has been successful in returning athletes to their sports after being treated for epicondylitis, indicating that inappropriate equipment is also an etiologic risk factor. Certainly, lack of experience has also been identified as a risk factor for this disorder, because a variety of epidemiologic studies of tennis elbow suggest that this entity occurs 7 to 10 times more frequently in less experienced players.[3] This higher rate may be related to improper technique or the choice of poorly fitting equipment. Certainly, there are a variety of risk factors for epicondylitis, all of which lead to repetitive stress or overuse as the most common etiology for this disorder.

Pathophysiology

Since the earliest description of epicondylitis, an abundance of literature has been devoted to its precise pathophysiology, resulting in numerous proposed theories. Early reviews consistently describe this entity as a purely inflammatory process involving such structures as the periosteum, synovium and annular ligament.[8–10] More recently, however, Nirschl and Pettrone[2] and Regan[11] have confirmed histologically that the normal parallel orientation of collagen fibers is disrupted by an invasion of fibroblasts and vascular granulation-like tissue, with a paucity of acute or chronic inflammatory cells. It may very well be that the early stages of epicondylitis have an inflammatory or synovitic component, which in later stages parallels the degenerative changes in the tendon substance. These degenerative changes, which have been identified as possible microtearing, with a subsequent, aborted neurovascular response, have been termed "angiofibroblastic hyperplasia" by Nirschl and Pettrone[2] and occur either medially or laterally. On the lateral side, they have most often been identified within the substance of the extensor carpi radialis brevis. On the medial side, these changes have been noted within the flexor carpi radialis or pronator teres. Thus, although no distinct, universal pathophysiology has been determined for epicondylitis, it is generally agreed that this entity represents a microtearing of either the medial or lateral tendon origin, with a subsequent failed healing response that alters the normal musculotendinous biomechanics.

Diagnosis

Epicondylitis is characterized by pain at either the lateral or medial epicondyle, which often radiates into the forearm. The severity of this pain varies greatly from patient to patient. Range of motion is most often full except in chronic severe cases, in which patients may lack full extension. The neurovascular status of the upper extremity is normal in pure epicondylitis.

Lateral epicondylitis results in tenderness over the conjoined tendon origin, most often localized to the extensor carpi radialis brevis. The area of maximum tenderness lies approximately 5 mm distal and anterior to the midpoint of the lateral epicondyle, and the pain is worsened with resisted wrist extension while the elbow is in full extension. This tenderness is in contradistinction to that seen with posterior intraosseous nerve syndrome (PIN) or intra-articular radiocapitellar disease (arthrosis/osteochondritis dessicans). PIN, an entrapment of the posterior interosseous branch of the radial nerve at the arcade of Frohse, may be confused with epicondylitis. The discomfort noted with PIN is more diffuse, and it usually occurs anterolaterally. It is worsened by resisted forearm supination and is rarely identifi-

able by electromyography or nerve conduction velocity testing. Intra-articular disease involving the radiocapitellar joint usually results in pain and clicking with elbow motion. Swelling of the joint is often present, and plain radiographs, computed tomography, or magnetic resonance imaging (MRI) will identify the lesion.

Medial epicondylitis results in tenderness most often over the flexor carpi radialis and pronator teres origins. The area of maximal tenderness is approximately 5 mm distal and anterior to the midpoint of the medial epicondyle, and the pain is worsened by resisted wrist flexion and forearm pronation. In cases of suspected medial epicondylitis, it is essential to consider primary ulnar neuropathy or medial collateral ligament instability. Ulnar neuritis can be identified by the elbow flexion test. This test is performed by placing the elbow in maximum flexion and the wrist in extension for approximately 30 to 60 seconds, resulting in medial elbow pain and numbness or tingling in the ring and little fingers. Ulnar collateral ligament instability is best identified with valgus stress testing at 30°, which produces pain along the course of the ligament, or by the milking test, which is performed by pulling on the thumb with the elbow flexed the and forearm supinated and which illicits pain along the medial collateral ligament.

Radiographs of the affected elbow are usually normal, but 20% to 25% of patients may have soft-tissue calcification about the epicondyle.[2] On the lateral side, this calcification appears to have no prognostic implications, but on the medial side this calcification, if present within the ulnar collateral ligament, may suggest concomitant instability. MRI may show increased signal within the

musculotendinous structures but rarely adds to the diagnostic or therapeutic decision-making process. An MRI, however, may be of use in diagnosis of the throwing athlete with confounding lateral or medial symptoms, for more precise identification of the source of pathology.

These straightforward principles suggest that epicondylitis should pose no diagnostic dilemma, however, as with any disorder, a multitude of other conditions may mimic epicondylitis. The most common or challenging ones include posterior interosseous nerve syndrome and radiocapitellar articular disease on the lateral elbow and ulnar neuropathy and medial collateral ligament instability on the medial elbow. It is also essential to consider cervical disease with radiculopathy in the differential diagnosis.

Nonsurgical Treatment

Certainly, consensus would suggest that nonsurgical treatment is the cornerstone of care for epicondylitis, because volumes of orthopaedic articles have proposed the success of nonsurgical measures for this disorder. But what exactly constitutes nonsurgical treatment? A closer look at the literature available indicates that this aspect of epicondylitis is also controversial and that there are a wide range of nonspecific measures. The general principles of nonsurgical treatment include initial relief of pain, followed by guided rehabilitation and return to previous activities.

Initial Phase

Relief of pain is the primary goal of the first phase of nonsurgical treatment. If a particular activity can be identified as causing the epicondylitis, this activity should be either modified or avoided. Complete inactivity or immobilization, however, should be discouraged to avoid disuse atrophy, which can compromise later rehabilitation. Ice is recommended for its local vasoconstrictive and anesthetic effects. An oral anti-inflammatory medication is often administered for a 10 to 14 day period, if the patient has no medical contraindication to the use of such drugs. But if one assumes that epicondylitis is a degenerative process and not inflammatory, why is there benefit from use of anti-inflammatory medications? It has been proposed that because this disorder often results in an accompanying synovitis, the anti-inflammatory medication may be effective in relieving the pain associated with the synovitis. If the patient does not respond to these initial therapeutic measures or if night pain is present, use of a corticosteroid injection has traditionally been proposed. As with the oral anti-inflammatory medications, the benefits of corticosteroid are most likely related to the accompanying synovitis that occurs with epicondylitis. The choice of dose and steroid preparation have remained arbitrary, because no carefully controlled prospective comparison of commonly used agents has been carried out.[12] The appropriate technique of injection requires instilling the mixture deep to the extensor carpi brevis on the lateral side and the flexor pronator mass on the medial side. Care should be taken to avoid injection into the superficial tissues, which may result in subcutaneous atrophy, or into the tendon, which may result in irreversible ultrastructural tendon changes. Is there therapeutic benefit from corticosteroid injections? Several short-term studies have indicated that pain relief occurs in 55% to 59% of patients receiving these injections, but recurrence of symptoms has been noted in 18% to 54% of those who initially experienced relief.[12]

In addition to oral and injectable anti-inflammatory medications, a variety of physical therapy modalities, such as ultrasound and high voltage galvanic stimulation, have been used to relieve the pain of epicondylitis. Although reports exist citing the success of each of these modalities, no prospective, randomized, controlled studies exist to demonstrate their efficacy. Therefore, although these modalities are recommended as part of the initial nonsurgical program, they should be discontinued if symptomatic relief is not obtained soon after their initiation.[13]

What treatment for sports-related injury would be complete without some form of bracing? Counterforce bracing was first introduced by Ilfeld in 1965. Theoretically, this type of brace inhibits full muscular expansion and thus decreases the force experienced by sensitive or injured muscular tissue proximal to the brace. Several studies have indicated that there is some benefit to the use of these supportive devices. Groppel and Nirschl[14] demonstrated with 3-dimensional cinematography and surface electromyography that lower extensor muscle activity was produced by the use of counterforce bracing during the tennis serve and one-handed tennis backhand. Snyder-Mackler and Epler,[15] using the more sensitive indwelling electromyographic technique, noted a significant reduction in muscle activity in the extensor carpi radialis brevis and extensor digitorum communis of healthy subjects during maximum voluntary isometric contraction while using an airbladder type of brace. Thus, if the athlete does not find these braces too cumbersome or too restrictive, they seem to have the benefit of decreasing symptoms during the athlete's return to activity.

Second Phase

Once the pain and discomfort of epicondylitis is eased by oral anti-inflammatory medications, injections, modalities, and counterforce bracing, a rehabilitation program is carried out for the involved arm. This begins with wrist extensor or flexor stretching and progressive isometric exercises. Initially these exercises may be done with the elbow flexed to minimize pain, then, as symptoms allow, the exercises are done with the elbow in progressively greater extension. As flexibility and strength improve, concentric and eccentric resistive exercises are performed. When the patient is capable of sprint repetitions to fatigue without significant elbow pain, a sports stimulation is staged. If successfully completed, the patient is reinitiated into his or her sport by gradually increasing the duration and intensity of exposure.

Upon return to sport, it is essential that the athlete and the athlete's coaches or trainers identify any inadequacies in equipment that may have led to the development of epicondylitis. The proper equipment, especially in the racquet sports, is essential to allow athletes to return to their sport and prevent subsequent episodes of epicondylitis.[16] Proper racquet grip size is assessed by measuring from the proximal palm crease to the tip of the ring finger, along its radial border. Lighter racquets, though providing less momentum, allow ease of positioning for impact. Frames of low vibration materials, such as graphite and epoxies, dampen impact forces imparted to the flexor and extensor origins. Using racquets that are less tightly strung or that have a higher string count per unit area and playing on slower surfaces, such as clay courts, will diminish the loads transmitted to the elbow. In golf, selection of clubs with proper weight, length, and grip can also significantly reduce the forces generated in the elbow.

As with equipment, proper technique is essential to allow the athlete to return to his or her sport safely.[16] If the athlete uses aberrant techniques in the sport, these should be identified and corrected through the guidance of coaches and trainers. For example, in tennis, the forehand stroke should allow the player to hit the ball in front of the body with the wrist and elbow extended. This allows the torso and the upper arm, rather than the wrist extensors, to provide most of the stroke power. The two-handed backhand stroke allows a distribution of forces between the upper extremities, and thus greatly diminishes force at the leading lateral epicondyle.[16]

As the athlete returns to sport, the conditioning of the involved elbow as well as the entire body is essential. Conditioning is best carried out with a slow, structured interval program that allows the athlete to return to the sport under the guidance of the coach, trainer, and physician. This conditioning should include flexibility, strength, and endurance training.

Although most authors report that the majority of patients with epicondylitis respond to nonsurgical care, there is a true paucity of clinical data on the long-term outcome of nonsurgical treatment. The available literature suggests that 5% to 15% of patients will suffer a recurrence of symptoms, but the majority of these patients with relapses will not have been fully rehabilitated or will have prematurely discontinued the preventive measures suggested.[16] In one such prospective review of nonsurgical treatment, Binder and Hazleman[13] noted that 26% of patients had a recurrence of symptoms, and over 40% had prolonged minor discomfort. Consequently, the previously documented rates of 85% to 90% for successful nonsurgical treatment may be somewhat optimistic, and persistent or recurrent symptoms may occur more frequently than has been reported in the past. Nonetheless, most clinical reports agree that nonsurgical management remains the mainstay of treatment for epicondylitis.

Surgical Treatment

The main indications for surgical treatment of epicondylitis include: (1) persistent, severe pain at the epicondylar region, (2) no response to a well-coordinated nonsurgical program spanning a minimal of 3 to 6 months, and (3) the exclusion of other diagnoses.

Historical Treatment

Historically, the surgical treatment for epicondylitis spans nearly three quarters of a century. For lateral epicondylitis, a host of techniques varying in popularity have been proposed, ranging from release of the extensor aponeurosis,[10] through transection of the annular ligament,[10,17] to open Z-plasty lengthening of the distal extensor carpi radialis brevis tendon.[18] Historically, very little has been written on the surgical treatment of medial epicondylitis. Various techniques, from percutaneous epicondylar release to epicondylectomy, have been vaguely reported.[16] Currently, the most widely accepted surgical procedure for lateral or medial epicondylitis involves: (1) excision of the pathologic portion of the tendon, (2) repair of the resulting defect, and (3) a firm reattachment of any elevated tendon origin back to the epicondyle.

Technique for Lateral Epicondylitis

With the patient supine and the arm supported on an arm board, a tourniquet is applied to the upper arm. A 5 to 7 cm oblique incision centered just anterior to the lateral epicondyle is created. The interval between the extensor carpi radialis longus and the extensor communis is identified and entered, revealing the underlying extensor carpi radialis brevis origin (Fig. 1, A). This origin is split longitudinally, and the area of pathology is carefully identified and then sharply debrided (Fig. 1, B). The lateral epicondyle is then rongeured to remove any fibrous tissue and to provide a bleeding surface for extensor reattachment. Although the extensor carpi radialis brevis is intimately attached to the underside of the longus, it is felt that adequate debridement may necessitate elevation of the majority of the brevis attachment from the epicondyle, and that a firm reattachment should be carried out. This is done by using a 5/64-inch drill bit to create a V-shaped tunnel, drilled perpendicular to the long access of the extended arm (Fig. 1, C). A heavy suture is then passed through the posterior leaf of elevated extensor tendon, through the bony tunnel from posterior to anterior, and then through the anterior leaf of elevated extensor tendon (Fig. 1, D). A side-to-side repair of the remaining extensor tendon is performed (Fig. 1, E). Routine subcutaneous and skin closures are carried out.

Technique for Medial Epicondylitis

With patient supine and the arm resting on an arm board, a tourniquet is applied. A 5 to 7 cm oblique incision is made centered just anterior to the medial epicondyle. The common flexor origin is incised at the pronator teres-flexor carpi radialis interval, either longitudinally (if the pathology is well localized) or transversely (if the tendon changes are diffuse or not easily identifiable) (Fig. 2, A). The

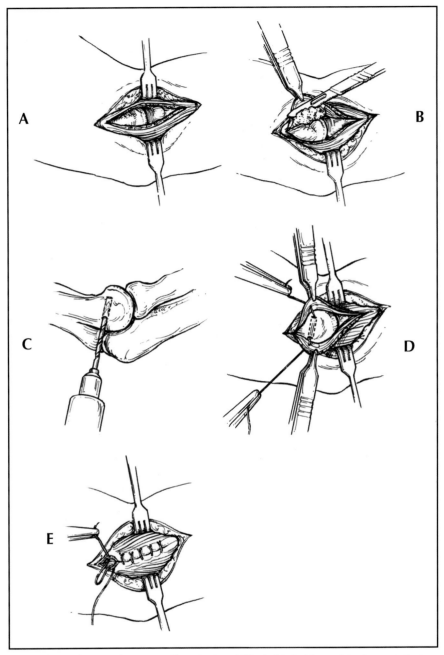

Fig. 1 Technique for surgical treatment of lateral epicondylitis. **A,** Skin incision and development of extensor interval. **B,** Excision of pathologic tissue. **C,** Drilling of lateral epicondylar bone tunnel. **D,** Reattachment of extensor origin to lateral epicondyle. **E,** Side-to-side repair of extensor origin. (Reproduced with permission from Ciccotti MG, Lombardo SJ: Lateral and medial epicondylitis, in Jobe FW (ed): *Operative Techniques in Upper Extremity Injuries in Sports.* St. Louis, MO, CV Mosby, 1996, pp 431–446.)

medial collateral ligament and the ulnar nerve are identified, assessed for pathology, and protected during the procedure. The pathologic tissue is then sharply excised, and the epi-condyle is prepared by rongeuring any fibrous tissue (Fig. 2, *B*) and by drilling small multiple holes in the medial epicondyle to create a vascular bed. The common flexor pronator origin is then reattached to the bleeding surface with interrupted sutures (Fig. 2, *C*). Routine subcutaneous and skin closures are carried out.

Postoperative Care

The postoperative care is similar for both lateral and medial epicondylitis. A posterior plaster splint is applied in the operating room. The splint and skin sutures are removed at 7 to 10 days postoperatively. Gentle passive and active elbow, wrist, and hand exercises are begun. Gentle isometrics are initiated at 3 to 4 weeks postoperatively, and more vigorous resistive exercises, including resisted wrist extension for lateral epicondylitis and resisted wrist flexion and forearm pronation for medial epicondylitis, are begun at 6 weeks postoperatively. A progressive strengthening program follows, and return to activity is generally attained by 3 to 4 months postoperatively.

Surgical Results

Of patients who undergo surgical treatment of lateral epicondylitis, 85% to 90% return to full activity without pain.[2,16] Approximately 10% to 12%, however, are noted to have some improvement but still have pain during aggressive activities. In approximately 2% to 3%, no appreciable improvement is obtained. In those patients with persistent symptoms, the other previously mentioned causes of lateral elbow pain should be pursued again. At the Kerlan-Jobe Orthopaedic Clinic,[4,16] 1,140 of 1,200 patients (95%), in whom lateral epicondylitis was diagnosed over a 10-year period, were successfully treated with nonsurgical measures. Sixty patients (5%) were unresponsive to nonsurgical treatment, and subsequently underwent extensor debridement and repair. Thirty-nine of these

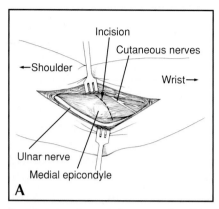
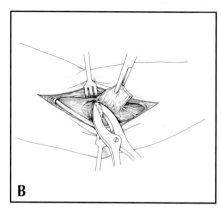
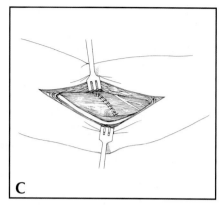

Fig. 2 Technique for surgical treatment of medial epicondylitis. **A,** skin incision and intended incision of common flexor-pronator origin. **B,** Distal reflection of common flexor-pronator origin with debridement of pathologic tissue. **C,** reattachment of common flexor-pronator origin to medial epicondyle. (Reproduced with permission from Jobe FW, Ciccotti MG: Lateral and medial epicondylitis of the elbow. *J Am Acad Orthop Surg* 1994;2:1–8.)

patients (65%) were seen 2.5 to 10 years after the procedure. Ninety-four percent of the patients reported dramatic improvement in symptoms. The objective outcome measures showed that 36% had limitations with heavy lifting, 50% had grip-dynamometer deficits, and 100% had some degree of isokinetic deficit. In our review at the Rothman Institute and Thomas Jefferson University, 24 patients were treated surgically for recalcitrant lateral epicondylitis over a 5-year period. Ninety-six percent showed overall good to excellent results with respect to pain relief and return to functional activity. All patients had significant strength improvement postoperatively as compared to preoperative hand grip-dynamometer measurements, but 12% were noted to have up to a 15% residual strength deficit. All athletes in the study returned to their preinjury level of sports competition within 6 months postoperatively.

With respect to medial epicondylitis, Vangsness and Jobe[19] reviewed 35 patients with recalcitrant medial epicondylitis treated surgically; they noted 97% good or excellent results and 98% subjective pain relief.

Eighty-six percent had no limitation in the use of the elbow. Grip-strength testing revealed no significant side-to-side differences postoperatively. All of the 20 athletically active patients returned to their sport. In general, surgical treatment of epicondylitis results in high patient satisfaction with reliable pain relief. Some residual strength deficits may exist, but these do not seem to interfere with functional activities.

Arthroscopy

Does arthroscopy have a place in the surgical treatment of epicondylitis? Several authors have proposed that an adequate arthroscopic debridement of the extensor carpi radialis brevis with subsequent decortication of the lateral epicondyle can be performed.[20] This procedure uses standard elbow arthroscopic techniques and has been previously described. Opponents have suggested that this technique may not allow thorough debridement and decortication of the epicondyle, that the lateral ulnar collateral ligament is at risk for detachment during the procedure, and that the released extensor carpi radialis brevis, which is not reattached by this

arthroscopic technique, may produce a functional deficit in the athlete's arm. Baker and Cummings[20] have shown in a cadaveric study that adequate decortication and debridement of the extensor carpi radialis brevis, without violation of the later ulnar collateral ligament, can be carried out arthroscopically. Their clinical results also suggest a high rate of success with this arthroscopic technique.[20] However, because of the paucity of clinical data available on arthroscopic treatment of epicondylitis, this technique remains controversial and has not yet gained wide support.

Summary

Since the first description of epicondylitis of the elbow in 1882, there have been volumes of descriptive, diagnostic, and therapeutic reports detailing every aspect of this entity. It is now known that epicondylitis can be caused both by occupational and sports-related activities, that its diagnosis may be confused with a variety of other pathologic entities affecting the elbow, that the majority of patients will respond favorably to well-guided nonsurgical treatment, and that in those patients whose persistent symptoms make them unable to return to their activities, surgical treatment results in reliable pain relief and return to preinjury level of activity.

References

1. Morris H: The rider's sprain. *Lancet* 1882;2:133–134.

2. Nirschl RP, Pettrone FA: Tennis elbow: The surgical treatment of lateral epicondylitis. *J Bone Joint Surg* 1979;61A:832–839.

3. Gruchow HW, Pelletier D: An epidemiologic study of tennis elbow: Incidence, recurrence, and effectiveness of prevention strategies. *Am J Sports Med* 1979;7:234–238.

4. Ciccotti MG, Lombardo SJ: Lateral and medial epicondylitis of the elbow, in Jobe FW, Pink MM, Glousman RE, Kvitne RS, Zemel NP (eds): *Operative Techniques in Upper Extremity Sports Injuries.* St. Louis, MO, Mosby-Year Book, 1996, pp 431–446.

5. Leach RE, Miller JK: Lateral and medial epicondylitis of the elbow. *Clin Sports Med* 1987;6:259–272.

6. Bernhang AM, Dehner W, Fogarty C: Tennis elbow: A biomechanical approach. *J Sports Med* 1974;2:235–260.

7. Kelley JD, Lombardo SJ, Pink M, Perry J, Giangarra CE: Electromyographic and cinematographic analysis of elbow function in tennis players with lateral epicondylitis. *Am J Sports Med* 1994;22: 359–363.

8. Runge F: Zur genese und behandlung des Schreibekrampfes. *Berliner Klin Wochenschr* 1873;10:245–248.

9. Trethowan WH: Editorial: "Tennis elbow." *Br Med J* 1929;2:1218–1224.

10. Bosworth DM: The role of the orbicular ligament in tennis elbow. *J Bone Joint Surg* 1955;37A:527–533.

11. Regan W, Wold L, Coonrad R, Morrey B: Microscopic histopathology of chronic refractory lateral epicondylitis. *Am J Sports Med* 1992;20:746–749.

12. Price R, Sinclair H, Heinrich I, Gibson T: Local injection treatment of tennis elbow: Hydrocortisone, triamcinolone and lignocaine compared. *Br J Rheumatol* 1991;30: 39–44.

13. Binder AI, Hazleman BL: Lateral humeral epicondylitis: A study of natural history and the effect of conservative therapy. *Br J Rheumatol* 1983;22:73–76.

14. Groppel JL, Nirschl RP: A mechanical and electromyographical analysis of the effects of various joint counterforce braces on the tennis player. *Am J Sports Med* 1986;14:195–200.

15. Snyder-Mackler L, Epler M: Effect of standard and Aircast tennis elbow bands on integrated electromyography of forearm extensor musculature proximal to the bands. *Am J Sports Med* 1989;17:278–281.

16. Jobe FW, Ciccotti MG: Lateral and medial epicondylitis of the elbow. *J Am Acad Orthop Surg* 1994;2:1–8

17. Newman JH, Goodfellow JW: Fibrillation of head of radius as one cause of tennis elbow. *Br Med J* 1975;2:328–330.

18. Garden RS: Tennis elbow. *J Bone Joint Surg* 1961;43B:100–106.

19. Vangsness CT Jr, Jobe FW: Surgical treatment of medial epicondylitis: Results in 35 elbows. *J Bone Joint Surg* 1991;73B:409–411.

20. Baker CL Jr, Cummings PD: Arthroscopic management of miscellaneous elbow disorders. *Op Tech Sports Med* 1998;6:16–21.

Medial Collateral Ligament Instability and Ulnar Neuritis in the Athlete's Elbow

Michael G. Ciccotti, MD
Frank W. Jobe, MD

Overhand or throwing athletes are at increased risk for developing a variety of elbow injuries. Whether it be while serving a volleyball, throwing a football, pitching a baseball, or climbing a mountain, these afflictions have challenged numerous orthopaedists to define, image, classify, and certainly treat. The voluminous literature available is testimony to this challenge. And yet, if one sifts through that information, one of several truths that hold steadfast is that anatomic form and biomechanical function are intimately related at the elbow joint. This symphony of form and function are ever so clearly epitomized by the overhand or throwing activity. This fluid, powerful motion includes rapid forceful extension, accompanied by valgus stress and pronation of the forearm often exceeding 300° per second. And yet, the velocity, power, and repetitiveness of these movements all contribute to the spectrum of elbow injuries seen in the overhand athlete. Two injuries that are commonly noted and often interrelated include medial collateral ligament instability and ulnar neuritis.

Medial Elbow Instability

Medial elbow instability can result from the sudden traumatic force generated by a single event such as javelin throwing or the chronic repetitive stress elicited in such activities as pitching.[1,2] The ligamentous anatomy of the elbow has been thoroughly described by a variety of authors and is quite familiar to orthopaedists, and yet several aspects warrant emphasis. Laboratory studies by Morrey and An[3] and Schwab and associates,[4] among others, have shown that elbow stability is primarily a function of the congruous bony articulation between the olecranon portion of the ulna and the trochlea of the humerus. Soft-tissue stability is primarily provided by the medial collateral ligament and less so by the anterior capsule, the lateral collateral ligament complex, and the flexor and extensor muscle masses. Morrey and An's cadaveric studies[3] have illustrated the sequential tightening of the medial collateral ligament fibers that progresses posteriorly as the elbow flexes. They have demonstrated that the medial collateral ligament consists of anterior, posterior, and transverse bands. Within the anterior band, there are 2 bundles: an isometric, inferior (or posterior) bundle and a nonisometric superior (or anterior) bundle. The isometric (posterior) bundle of the anterior band is the primary stabilizer of the medial elbow. The transverse band does not cross the joint but exists as a thickening of the caudalmost portion of the joint capsule to expand the greater sigmoid notch. Regan and associates[5] have documented the greater load to failure, stiffness, and cross-sectional area of the anterior band of the collateral ligament components.

The biomechanics of the throwing mechanism have been most thoroughly described in the baseball pitch, and an understanding of this mechanism sheds light on the pathophysiology of medial elbow instability. Various authors[1,6] have described the phases of wind-up, cocking, acceleration, deceleration, and follow through (Fig. 1). It is primarily during the cocking and acceleration phases that the peak angular velocity of the elbow joint is generated and valgus force exceeding the tensile strength of the ulnar collateral ligament may be produced.[6,7] With the proper mechanics, conditioning, and warm-up, most athletes are able to tolerate these forces. However, poor mechanics, conditioning, flexibility, or fatigue, can have an additive effect that results in muscle strain and allows further stress to be transmitted to the medial collateral ligament. If continued repeated stress is applied at a rate that is greater than the rate of

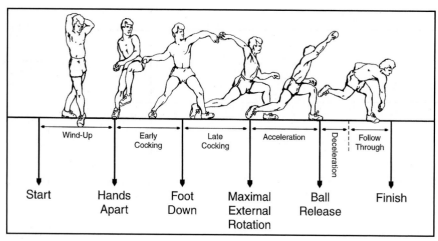

Fig. 1 The phases of the throwing mechanism: wind-up, early cocking, late cocking, acceleration, deceleration, and follow-through. (Reproduced with permission from DiGiovine NM, Jobe FW, Pink M, et al: An electromyographic analysis of the upper extremity in pitching. *J Shoulder Elbow Surg* 1992;1:15–25.)

tissue repair, then progressive microscopic damage occurs. This microscopic injury occurs initially as edema and inflammation within the ligament substance, followed by scarring and fiber dissociation, then progressing to ligament calcification and finally ossification. The resultant pathologic tissue within the ligament acts as a stress riser altering the normal biomechanics of the ligament and promoting further damage.[6] This can result in attenuation of the medial collateral ligament leading to a cascade of pathologic changes: valgus instability with radiocapitellar overload and subsequent degenerative changes. The olecranon is also allowed to ride medially, impinging on the trochlea and olecranon fossa, causing spur formation.[1]

Diagnosis

A history of repetitive overhand or throwing activities with pain along the medial elbow during the late cocking or acceleration phases is consistent with medial elbow instability. Patients may also describe a sensation of elbow "opening" while throwing,

and they may recall previous low-grade elbow discomfort with a single episode of giving way or "snapping," which probably represents the final injury to the ligament. Ulnar nerve symptoms may also be present with chronic instability because of compression from extensive inflammation about the ligament within the tunnel, friction from nerve subluxation, abrasion on osteophytes, or traction with repeated valgus loading of throwing.

On examination, these patients will have tenderness most often at the distal insertion of the medial collateral ligament on the ulna, which is worsened by valgus stress.[8] Valgus instability can be detected by securely holding the patient's wrist and hand between the examiner's elbow and trunk and flexing the patient's elbow 20° to 30° to unlock the olecranon from its fossa. Valgus stress is applied while simultaneously palpating the ligament with the thumb. The amount of medial laxity is then compared to the contralateral elbow. This test detects laxity in the anterior bundle of the anterior band of the medial collateral ligament. The milking sign[9]

detects laxity in the more functionally important posterior bundle of the anterior band of the medial collateral ligament. This test is performed by pulling on the thumb, and palpating along the medial collateral ligament while the elbow is flexed, forearm supinated, and shoulder extended. This generates a sense of laxity in the medial elbow as well as pain along the medial collateral ligament. The ulnar nerve should also be examined, as often those athletes with chronic medial instability will develop tenderness along the ulnar nerve (Tinel's sign), less frequently will have tingling or numbness in the ring or little finger, and rarely motor weakness in the intrinsics of the hand. Subluxation of the ulnar nerve with elbow flexion should be ruled out.

Radiographically, plain films, stress views, and magnetic resonance imaging (MRI) have all been used to aid in the diagnosis of medial collateral ligament injury. Plain films, though not diagnostic, will often illustrate associated abnormalities such as marginal osteophytes, loose bodies, ligamentous calcification, or heterotopic bone formation at the tip of the olecranon or in the fossa. Gravity valgus stress testing or stress radiographs compared with the contralateral elbow can often document excessive laxity even when clinical findings are equivocal. MRI has been used to evaluate elbow collateral ligament pathology and may illustrate soft-tissue ligamentous abnormalities including edema, partial tearing, or full-thickness tearing. Though the radiographs may be helpful, the keys to diagnosis of medial collateral ligament instability are a precise history and thorough physical examination.

Nonsurgical Treatment

Nonsurgical treatment is pursued initially in the majority of patients.

When begun early, nonsurgical treatment can be successful if the appropriate program is initiated. This regimen includes rest for approximately 2 to 4 weeks during which time heat and ice contrast as well as nonsteroidal anti-inflammatory agents are initiated. Physical therapy modalities such as phonophoresis, iontophoresis, or electrical stimulation may be used to diminish swelling and promote more rapid healing. Active elbow range of motion (ROM) is begun when the patient is pain-free, followed soon after by a strengthening program. A throwing program begins at approximately 3 months if the athlete has full ROM and symmetric strength compared to the contralateral elbow. This program begins with a short toss, long toss routine and progresses to pitching from a mound at submaximal velocity and increasing ultimately to full velocity. Such a nonsurgical program can be highly successful in returning the athlete to sports activity, especially if the medial injury is diagnosed expeditiously, a thorough nonsurgical program is initiated, and if a complete tear of the medial collateral ligament has not occurred.

Surgical Treatment

Surgical treatment for medial collateral ligament instability is indicated for the acute, complete rupture of the medial collateral ligament in throwers, and chronic pain or symptomatic instability without improvement after a minimum of 3 months nonsurgical treatment.[6,8,10,11] The goal of surgical treatment is to reestablish valgus stability in the presence of acute or chronic symptomatic functional laxity. A variety of surgical techniques have been proposed ranging from medial epicondylar relocation to direct suture repair;[12,13] however, reconstruction of the medial

collateral ligament using a free autogenous graft as described by Jobe and associates[10] in 1986 and subsequently by Conway and associates[8] in 1992 is now considered the paradigm of surgical treatment.

Surgical Technique

Reconstruction of the medial collateral ligament is performed under general anesthesia with the patient supine and the arm placed on an arm board. Following an examination, a pneumatic tourniquet is applied to the upper arm and both the surgical site and the graft harvest site are made sterile and are prepped and draped. After exsanguination of the limb and inflation of the cuff, a small towel is placed beneath the extended elbow and the forearm is supinated to apply a consistent valgus stress. A skin incision extending 3 to 5 cm both proximally and distally is then made over the medial epicondyle. Dissection is continued down to the muscle fascia with care to protect all sensory branches of the medial antebrachial cutaneous nerve. The medial epicondyle is then located and a longitudinal incision is made in the common flexor mass at its posterior third near the flexor carpi ulnaris (Fig. 2). With a periosteal elevator, the flexor mass is then separated from the medial collateral ligament–capsular complex. The medial collateral ligament is then inspected and palpated as a valgus stress is applied. A longitudinal split is made in the medial collateral ligament, allowing inspection of the underlying joint. The joint is evaluated for synovitis, loose bodies, or degenerative changes and the quality, length, and tension of the ligament are assessed while the valgus force is reapplied. At this point, a V-shaped bone tunnel is created using a 3.2-mm drill bit in the ulna located at the level of the

tubercle of the coronoid process (Fig. 3). Drill holes are then made within the medial epicondyle of the humerus at the level of the anatomic origin of the anterior bundle of the ligament, midway between the base and the tip of the medial epicondyle (Fig. 3). A single entrance hole is created with a 4.5-mm drill bit that then diverges anterosuperiorly in order to avoid penetration of the posterior cortex and possible injury to the ulnar nerve within the cubital tunnel. The flexor pronator mass is then split just proximal to the medial epicondyle (Fig. 2) in a longitudinal fashion in order to facilitate drilling the diverging exit tunnels using a 3.2-mm drill bit (Fig. 3).

At this point, the tendon graft is harvested. The palmaris longus tendon can be obtained from either upper extremity, though it is most often harvested from the ipsilateral arm (it is essential to document the presence of the palmaris longus preoperatively). The palmaris longus is harvested through a series of small transverse incisions beginning at the distal flexor crease of the wrist. The median nerve and its palmar cutaneous branch are protected as the tendon is isolated and followed to the palmar fascia, where it is released. Additional skin incisions are made at 7.5 and 15 cm from the wrist (Fig. 4), exposing the entire length of the palmaris longus. With tension applied distally, the tendon is divided at its musculotendinous junction and passed through the distal skin incisions where finally it is detached from its palmar fascial insertion, providing a free graft approximately 15 cm in length. These skin incisions are then irrigated and closed routinely. If a palmaris longus tendon is not present, alternate autogenous graft sources include the plantaris tendon or a 3- to 5-mm medial strip of

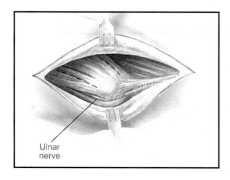

Fig. 2 The exposed flexor-pronator muscle origin on the medial epicondyle of the elbow. The dotted lines indicate the sites of incision through the flexor pronator muscle mass. (Reproduced with permission from Kvitne RS, Jobe FW: Ligamentous and posterior compartment injuries, in Jobe FW (ed): *Operative Techniques in Upper Extremity Sports Injuries*. St. Louis, MO, CV Mosby, 1996, pp 411–430.)

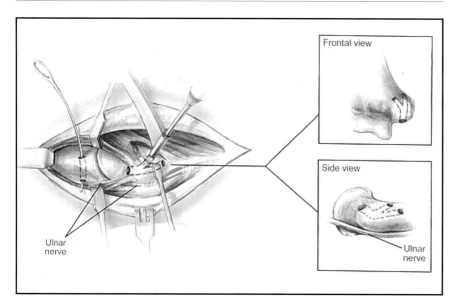

Fig. 3 The site of bone tunnel placement in the proximal ulna and the medial epicondyle of the humerus. Inset, Y-shaped tunnel within the medial epicondyle to avoid penetration of posterior cortex and injury of ulnar nerve in cubital tunnel (frontal and side views). (Reproduced with permission from Kvitne RS, Jobe FW: Ligamentous and posterior compartment injuries, in Jobe FW (ed): *Operative Techniques in Upper Extremity Sports Injuries*. St. Louis, MO, CV Mosby, 1996, pp 411–430.)

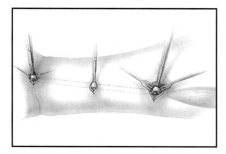

Fig. 4 Harvesting of palmaris longus tendon. (Reproduced with permission from Kvitne RS, Jobe FW: Ligamentous and posterior compartment injuries, in Jobe FW (ed): *Operative Techniques in Upper Extremity Sports Injuries*. St. Louis, MO, CV Mosby, 1996, pp 411–430.)

Achilles tendon. The graft is then prepared by removing all remaining muscular tissue. A No. 1 nonabsorbable suture is then placed in each end of the graft. A flexible suture passer is then used to thread the tendon through the bone tunnels within the proximal ulna and the medial epicondyle, creating a figure-of-8 configuration. This is done by passing the graft from anterior to posterior in the proximal ulna, then through the epicondylar entrance tunnel and out the anterior proximal humeral tunnel, then into the posterior proximal humeral tunnel and out the single distal medial epicondylar tunnel, then posterior to anterior through the ulnar tunnel and then finally into the single distal humeral medial epicondylar tunnel (Fig. 5). Care is taken to place both ends of the graft within a bony tunnel. With the elbow then held in a neutral varus-valgus position and at 45° of elbow flexion, the graft is pulled tautly and sutured to itself with the No. 1 nonabsorbable stitch (Fig. 6). The bundles of the graft are then sutured to one another and the remaining ligament capsule complex with absorbable stitches. The elbow is then brought through a full passive ROM to verify isometry and stability of the ligament reconstruction.

If motor ulnar nerve symptoms are present preoperatively, and significant scarring of the ulnar nerve is identified at the time of exposure, then transposition is necessary. The flexor pronator tendon origin is incised transversely between the anterior longitudinal split and the posterior longitudinal split and is then elevated distally, leaving a fringe of tendinous origin in order to facilitate later reattachment. The ulnar nerve is then dissected carefully and mobilized approximately to the level of the arcade of Struthers. A 2- to 3-cm portion of the medial intra-muscular septum is then excised in order to prevent any tethering with the anterior nerve transposition. Distal mobilization of the nerve involves carefully splitting the intra-muscular septum between the ulnar and humeral heads of the flexor carpi ulnaris, 2.5 cm beyond the medial epicondyle. The branches of the ulnar nerve to the flexor carpi ulnaris are carefully preserved and the accompanying vasculature is meticulously maintained in order to avoid any segmental devascularization of the nerve. The ulnar nerve is then transposed and positioned anterior to the medial epicondyle overlying the reconstructed medial collateral ligament. The common flexor pronator mass is then reattached with figure-of-8 absorbable stitches. The tourniquet is then released and hemostasis is obtained with electrocautery. Routine subcutaneous and skin closures are then carried out over a surgical drain. A long-arm posterior plaster splint is then applied with the elbow in 90° of flexion and neutral forearm rotation, leaving the hand and wrist free.

The key technical points of ulnar collateral ligament reconstruction include: (1) removal of all calcification from the ligament; (2) placing the humeral and ulnar tunnels in isometric positions; (3) removal of any bony prominences so that the graft does not abrade on either the humeral epicondyle or the ulna; (4) placement of the graft in a figure-of-8 fashion in order to insure strength and approximate the original ligament's biomechanics; (5) incorporation of the remaining medial collateral ligament with the graft; (6) placement of the ends of the tendon graft in the bony tunnels; and (7) meticulous handling of the medial antebrachial cutaneous and ulnar nerves, their branches, and their vasculature in order to avoid neural injury or segmental devascularization.

Postoperative Rehabilitation

The postreconstruction rehabilitation is initiated on postoperative day 1 with the use of a squeeze ball in the

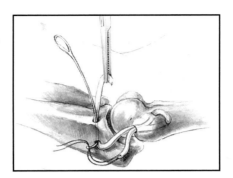
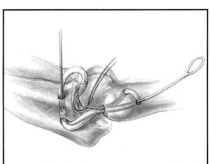

Fig. 5 Passage of tendon graft through bone tunnels in a figure-of-8 fashion. (Reproduced with permission from Kvitne RS, Jobe FW: Ligamentous and posterior compartment injuries, in Jobe FW (ed): *Operative Techniques in Upper Extremity Sports Injuries*. St. Louis, MO, CV Mosby, 1996, pp 411–430.)

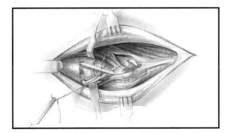
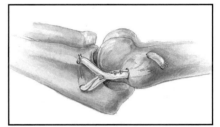

Fig. 6 Suture fixation of tendon graft. (Reproduced with permission from Kvitne RS, Jobe FW: Ligamentous and posterior compartment injuries, in Jobe FW (ed): *Operative Techniques in Upper Extremity Sports Injuries*. St. Louis, MO, CV Mosby, 1996, pp 411–430.)

ipsilateral hand. The postoperative splint is removed 10 to 14 days after surgery and gentle ROM is initiated. Wrist and elbow strengthening begin at 4 and 8 weeks, respectively, after surgery. Upper extremity muscle strengthening progresses through the first 4 months postoperatively. A short toss, long toss program begins at 4 months and progresses to pitching from the mound at 75% speed by 8 to 10 months. Pitching at full speed for 1 to 2 innings per outing is achieved by 1 year, and over the following 6 months, the duration of each outing is increased until full return of strength is accomplished.

Surgical Results

Conway and associates[8] reported on 56 overhand athletes undergoing medial collateral ligament recon-

struction of the elbow with an average follow-up of 6.3 years. Eighty-seven percent were found to have a midsubstance tear at the time of surgery. Forty-five patients (80%) were noted to have good or excellent results. Thirty-eight (68%) returned to the previous level of sports participation. Twelve of the 16 Major League baseball players who had a reconstruction as their primary operation (no previous elbow surgery) were able to return to their sport. Previous elbow surgery, however, was noted to decrease the chance of return to previous sport level. The most significant complication involved postoperative ulnar neuropathy in 12 patients (21%). In 5 patients, the condition was transient with symptoms resolving within 1 to 11 months, and 7 required nerve revision; 2 of these patients (3%) were most likely prevented from returning to their sport by ulnar nerve symptoms after the reconstruction. A subsequent review of 83 patients treated with medial collateral ligament reconstruction without ulnar nerve transposition at the Kerlan and Jobe Clinic has shown 94% good or excellent results (WH Thompson, MD, FW Jobe, MD, LA Yocum, MD, 1997, unpublished data.). The mean time of return to full competitive throwing was 13 months (range, 6 to 18 months). Transient postoperative ulnar nerve symptoms were seen in 4 patients (5%); 3 of these had paresthesias that resolved within 6 weeks, and 1 had motor difficulty that resolved in 6 months. This significant reduction in postoperative ulnar nerve symptoms seen with the modified medial collateral ligament reconstruction and avoidance of ulnar nerve transfer has prompted us to recommend this modified technique unless ulnar nerve symptoms are identified preoperatively.

Ulnar Neuritis

The ulnar nerve is the nerve most commonly injured about the elbow during sports activities.[14,15] Anatomically the serpiginous pathway of this nerve at the elbow makes it particularly susceptible to injury during overhand sports. Along its course, several sites of possible impingement exist. In the mid upper arm, it pierces the medial intermuscular septum and emerges from beneath the arcade of Struthers. This arcade is located approximately 8 cm above the medial epicondyle. The nerve then runs anterior to the medial head of the triceps and posterior to the intermuscular septum on its way toward the cubital tunnel. The boundaries of this tunnel include the posterior band of the medial collateral liga-

ment, the medial edge of the trochlea, the medial epicondylar groove, and the arcuate ligament, which represents the tendinous arch of the humeral and ulnar insertions of the flexor carpi ulnaris. With elbow flexion, Vanderpool and associates[16] noted that the arcuate ligament stretches approximately 5 mm for each 45°, thus narrowing the tunnel. Curtis[17] documented that also during flexion, the medial collateral ligament bulges medially, further decreasing the tunnel's size. The neurotopography of the ulnar nerve within the cubital tunnel has been described by several authors.[15,16] The intrinsic motor and sensory fibers of the nerve lie most superficial and are, therefore, most vulnerable to injury. The motor fibers to the extrinsic muscles (the flexor carpi ulnaris and the ulnar half of the flexor digitorum profundus) lie deeper and thus protected. Distal to the elbow, the nerve continues in the forearm between the humeral and ulnar heads of the flexor carpi ulnaris.

Three basic types of pathologic stress to the ulnar nerve have been identified: compression, friction, and traction. Compression of the ulnar nerve may occur in association with several conditions: (1) physiologic hypertrophy of the medial head of the triceps or the flexor carpi ulnaris in the elite athlete;[14] (2) thickening of the arcuate ligament, the so-called Osborne lesion;[18] and (3) intrinsic masses within the tunnel, such as lipomas or ganglion cysts. Pechan and Julis[19] have demonstrated that wrist extension, elbow flexion, and shoulder abduction, such as that which occurs in the early stages of the overhand pitching maneuver, can elevate intraneural pressures in the cubital tunnel 6 times that in the relaxed nerve. Friction neuritis commonly results from subluxation or disloca-

tion of the ulnar nerve anterior to the medial epicondyle. Childress[20] noted that 16% of the population demonstrate recurrent dislocation of the ulnar nerve as the elbow moves from complete extension to full flexion. This hypermobility is often secondary to congenital or developmental laxity of the soft-tissue constraints that normally maintain the ulnar nerve within the groove. Traction neuritis may develop subsequent to an attenuation or rupture of the medial collateral ligament, which allows excessive valgus stress to occur at the medial elbow.[8,15] Normally, the ulnar nerve is free to move in the groove both longitudinally and medially. Any restriction of this movement at any point along the nerve's course may lead to neural traction during the act of throwing.

Diagnosis

Clinically, the throwing athlete with ulnar neuritis initially presents with the insidious onset of pain along the medial elbow that seems to be exacerbated by overhand activities. The condition is commonly associated with intermittent paresthesias in the ring and little fingers. Medial elbow achiness or tingling radiating distally may also be present. The athlete may describe a clumsiness or heaviness of the hand and fingers, especially during throwing. When a subluxating ulnar nerve is present, there may also be a snapping sensation at the elbow with flexion and extension.

On physical examination, tenderness directly along the course of the ulnar nerve is noted, especially within the cubital tunnel and its passage into the flexor carpi ulnaris (Tinel's sign). The elbow flexion test described by Buehler and Thayer[21] may confirm the diagnosis of ulnar neuritis. This test involves maximally flexing the elbow while extending the wrist for

30 seconds or longer and if positive, pain, numbness, and tingling will occur along the ulnar nerve distribution. It is essential to rule out medial collateral ligament instability and medial epicondylitis when evaluating for ulnar neuritis in the athlete. Tenderness along the medial collateral ligament exacerbated by valgus stress or tenderness at the flexor pronator muscle mass worsened by resisted wrist flexion and forearm pronation should help to identify these other sources of medial elbow pain. Additional disorders to be considered in the differential diagnosis include cervical radiculopathy (particularly C-8), thoracic outlet syndrome, and ulnar nerve injury distal to the elbow (Guyon's canal or double crush syndromes).

Radiographic imaging of the elbow may help to identify calcification within the ulnar collateral ligament or intra-articular disorders; however, these areas are often normal in cases of pure ulnar neuritis. Electrodiagnostic studies are helpful when positive, but they may be negative and do not rule out the diagnosis of ulnar neuritis. Electromyography is frequently negative in the early stages of neuritis. It can, however, help to localize the site of the lesion and is useful for the differential diagnosis. Nerve conduction velocity testing should be carried out both above and below the elbow and may be used as an indicator of nerve recovery after injury or surgery.

Nonsurgical Treatment

Nonsurgical treatment of ulnar neuritis in the throwing athlete should consist initially of rest from throwing. A brief period of immobilization may also be prescribed in addition to nonsteroidal anti-inflammatory agents and ice massage. Upon resolution of symptoms, the patient is placed on a progressive rehabilitation program, including elbow ROM, strengthening and endurance exercises, and finally, return to athletic activity. In the general population, nonsurgical treatment may be successful upward of 86% to 90% of the time.[22,23] In throwing athletes, however, success rates are lower because of the likelihood of concomitant medial collateral ligament laxity.[15]

Surgical Treatment

The surgical treatment of ulnar neuritis has gradually evolved over nearly a century, resulting in a host of techniques. In situ decompression has been proposed because of its simplicity, low risk of impairing the blood supply of the ulnar nerve,[24] and lack of resulting scar.[25] A variety of reports on this procedure show successful results in patients with minimal compressive lesions characterized by mild pain and mild dysesthesias.[26,27] This procedure may be successful in the general population; however, it is not recommended in the overhand athlete because it does not eliminate the traction forces on the ulnar nerve associated with the throwing motion and may not address pathology within the cubital tunnel. Medial epicondylectomy has been proposed by a variety of authors as treatment for ulnar neuritis.[28-30] Again, successful results have been noted in the general population; however, this procedure is also not recommended for the athlete because the origin of the flexor pronator mass is significantly altered and subsequent strength deficits may result. The ulnar nerve is also destabilized, allowing it to ride anteriorly and making it susceptible to direct trauma[27] and friction neuritis. Heterotopic bone formation has also been seen after medial epicondylectomy. In addition, the medial collateral ligament may be injured at its origin on the medial epicondyle, resulting in medial elbow instability. Overall, the recurrence rate after medial epicondylectomy is the highest of all reported surgical techniques.[31] Anterior subcutaneous transposition has been employed for the general population.[32,33] The advantages of subcutaneous transposition include a relatively simple dissection with lack of scar formation; however, a less direct route of transposition may increase the likelihood of kinking at both the entry and exit points of the transposed nerve, and hypermobility of the nerve can result. There is minimal protection from direct trauma in the subcutaneous position, a situation that may be even more problematic in the thinner athlete. With these disadvantages in mind, this technique is not generally recommended in the overhand athlete or the athlete involved in contact sports. Anterior intramuscular transposition has been proposed by several authors;[20,34] however, it has been noted to result in significant neural scarring within the flexor pronator mass, which may tether the nerve. This scarring may cause nerve traction because of the significant flexor pronator muscle activity with the overhand mechanism.[15,35] Anterior submuscular transposition has been proposed by several authors as the best alternative for the overhand athlete.[14,15,31,35] The nerve's deep submuscular placement protects it from external trauma and also creates a nearly straight line course from the upper arm to the forearm, thereby avoiding any kinking or tension forces with throwing. In addition, the exposure allows inspection of the medial collateral ligament and direct treatment of intra-articular loose bodies or osteophytes if present.

Surgical Technique

The preferred surgical technique in athletes is Learmonth's submuscular

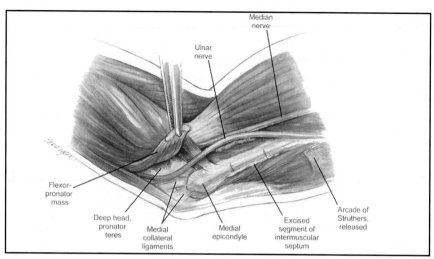

Fig. 7 Anterior submuscular transposition of the ulnar nerve. (Reproduced with permission from Boatwright JR, D'Alessandro DF: Nerve entrapment syndromes at the elbow, in Jobe FW (ed): *Operative Techniques in Upper Extremity Sports Injuries*. St. Louis, MO, CV Mosby, 1996, pp 518–537.)

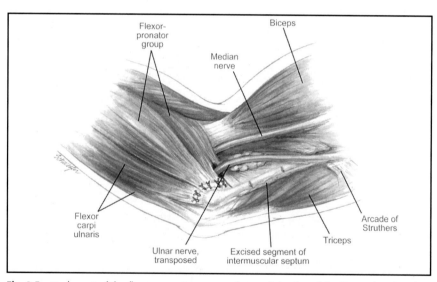

Fig. 8 Reattachment of the flexor-pronator mass to the medial epicondyle. (Reproduced with permission from Boatwright JR, D'Alessandro DF: Nerve entrapment syndromes at the elbow, in Jobe FW (ed): *Operative Techniques in Upper Extremity Sports Injuries*. St. Louis, MO, CV Mosby, 1996, pp 518–537.)

transposition of the ulnar nerve.[36] Under tourniquet control, a medial curvilinear incision is centered just posterior to the medial epicondyle extending both proximally and distally 3 to 5 cm. Identification and careful mobilization of the branches of the medial antebrachial cutaneous nerve are carried out. The ulnar nerve is then identified in the distal upper arm posterior to the medial intermuscular septum and is freed proximally for 8 cm to the arcade of Struthers. The arcade is released at this site in order to prevent any later tethering with transposition of the nerve. The cubital tunnel is then released by dividing the arcuate ligament and the nerve is isolated with a penrose drain. The articular branches of the ulnar nerve are sacrificed in order to transpose the nerve. The nerve is then followed distally between the 2 heads of the flexor carpi ulnaris and the aponeurotic band of the flexor digitorum sublimis origin is then released. Special care is taken to preserve the motor branches to these muscles. A 1- by 5-cm segment of the medial intermuscular septum of the upper arm is then excised in order to prevent kinking of the ulnar nerve along its edge. The flexor pronator muscle mass is then transversely incised from the medial epicondyle, leaving 1 cm of proximal tendon for reattachment. The flexor pronator mass is then reflected distally, revealing the underlying medial collateral ligament of the elbow. The integrity of the medial collateral ligament may be evaluated at this time. An arthrotomy can be made via a longitudinal incision along the fibers of the medial collateral ligament. The joint may be evaluated for loose bodies or spurs and valgus testing may be carried out to assess the integrity of the medial collateral ligament. The nerve is then transposed anteriorly and carefully placed atop the medial collateral ligament (Fig. 7). The flexor pronator mass is then reattached to the medial epicondylar cuff of tissue with nonabsorbable sutures (Fig. 8). The elbow is then taken through a full ROM in order to assess the flexor pronator muscle repair as well as to confirm that there are no sites of ulnar nerve entrapment or tethering. The tourniquet is then released and hemostasis is assured with electrocautery. A routine subcutaneous and skin closure are carried out, and a well-padded posterior splint is applied with the elbow at 90° of flexion and the forearm in neutral rotation.

Postoperative Rehabilitation

The postoperative rehabilitation program begins approximately 10 to 14 days after surgery, when the splint is removed. A passive ROM program is initiated, followed by active ROM exercises at the third to fourth postoperative week. A progressive strengthening program begins at 6 weeks after surgery, and at 8 to 12 weeks from surgery, a well-supervised throwing program is started. Progressive increases in throwing duration and speed continue with return to full activities by 4 months postoperatively.

Summary

Athletes who participate in overhand sports may sustain a host of injuries to the medial elbow. The chronic repetitive stress caused by the high velocity nature of the overhand throwing mechanism predisposes these athletes to overuse injuries. Medial collateral ligament instability and ulnar neuritis are common disorders seen in this patient population. A thorough understanding of the anatomy of the medial elbow as well as the pathophysiology of these disorders and their nonsurgical and surgical treatments are essential to providing these athletes with optimal care and hastening their return to sports.

References

1. Andrews JR, Craven WM: Lesions of the posterior compartment of the elbow. *Clin Sports Med* 1991;10:637–652.

2. Del Pizzo W, Jobe FW, Norwood L: Ulnar nerve entrapment syndrome in baseball players. *Am J Sports Med* 1977;5:182–185.

3. Morrey BF, An KN: Functional anatomy of the ligaments of the elbow. *Clin Orthop* 1985;201:84–90.

4. Schwab GH, Bennett JB, Woods GW, Tullos HS: Biomechanics of elbow instability: The role of the medial collateral ligament. *Clin Orthop* 1980;146:42–52.

5. Regan WD, Korinek SL, Morrey BF, An KN: Biomechanical study of ligaments around the elbow joint. *Clin Orthop* 1991;271:170–179.

6. Jobe FW, Kvitne RS: Elbow instability in the athlete, in Tullos HS (ed): *Instructional Course Lectures XL.* Park Ridge, IL, American Academy of Orthopaedic Surgeons, 1991, pp 17–23.

7. Pappas AM, Zawacki RM, Sullivan TJ: Biomechanics of baseball pitching: A preliminary report. *Am J Sports Med* 1985;13:216–222.

8. Conway JE, Jobe FW, Glousman RE, Pink M: Medial instability of the elbow in throwing athletes: Treatment by repair or reconstruction of the ulnar collateral ligament. *J Bone Joint Surg* 1992;74A:67–83.

9. Kvitne RS, Jobe FW: Ligamentous and posterior compartment injuries, in Jobe FW, Pink MM, Glousman RE, Kvitne RS, Zemel NP (eds): *Operative Techniques in Upper Extremity Sports Injuries.* St. Louis, MO, Mosby-Year Book, 1996, pp 411–430.

10. Jobe FW, Stark H, Lombardo SJ: Reconstruction of the ulnar collateral ligament in athletes. *J Bone Joint Surg* 1986;68A:1158–1163.

11. Jobe FW, El Attrache NS: Treatment of ulnar collateral ligament injuries in athletes, in Morrey BF (ed): *Master Techniques in Orthopaedic Surgery: The Elbow.* New York, NY, Raven Press, 1994, pp 149–168.

12. Woods GW, Tullos HS: Elbow instability and medial epicondyle fractures. *Am J Sports Med* 1977;5:23–30.

13. Kuroda S, Sakamaki K: Ulnar collateral ligament tears of the elbow joint. *Clin Orthop* 1986;208:266–271.

14. Glousman RE: Ulnar nerve problems in the athlete's elbow. *Clin Sports Med* 1990;9:365–377.

15. Boatright JR, D'Alessandro DF: Nerve entrapment syndromes at the elbow, in Jobe FW, Pink MM, Glousman RE, Kvitne RS, Zemel NP (eds): *Operative Techniques in Upper Extremity Sports Injuries.* St. Louis, MO, Mosby-Year Book, 1996, pp 518–537.

16. Vanderpool DW, Chalmers J, Lamb DW, Whiston TB: Peripheral compression lesions of the ulnar nerve. *J Bone Joint Surg* 1968;50B:792–803.

17. Curtis BF: Traumatic ulnar neuritis: Transplantation of the nerve. *J Nerve Ment Dis* 1898;25:480.

18. Osborne GV: Abstract: The surgical treatment of tardy ulnar neuritis. *J Bone Joint Surg* 1957;39B:782.

19. Pechan J, Julis I: The pressure measurement in the ulnar nerve: A contribution to the pathophysiology of the cubital tunnel syndrome. *J Biomech* 1975;8:75–79.

20. Childress HM: Recurrent ulnar-nerve dislocation at the elbow. *J Bone Joint Surg* 1956;38A:978–984.

21. Buehler MJ, Thayer DT: The elbow flexion test: A clinical test for the cubital tunnel syndrome. *Clin Orthop* 1988;233:213–216.

22. Dimond ML, Lister GD: Abstract: Cubital tunnel syndrome treated by long-arm splintage. *J Hand Surg* 1985;10A:430.

23. Eisen A, Danon J: The mild cubital tunnel syndrome: Its natural history and indications for surgical intervention. *Neurology* 1974;24:608–613.

24. Ogata K, Manske PR, Lesker PA: The effect of surgical dissection on regional blood flow to the ulnar nerve in the cubital tunnel. *Clin Orthop* 1985;193:195–198.

25. Buzzard EF: Some varieties of traumatic and toxic ulnar neuritis. *Lancet* 1922;1:317–319.

26. Davies MA, Vonau M, Blum PW, Kwok BC, Matheson JM, Stening WA: Results of ulnar neuropathy at the elbow treated by decompression or anterior transposition. *Aust NZ J Surg* 1991;61:929–934.

27. Manske PR, Johnston R, Pruitt DL, Strecker WB: Ulnar nerve decompression at the cubital tunnel. *Clin Orthop* 1992;274:231–237.

28. Craven PR Jr, Green DP: Cubital tunnel syndrome: Treatment by medial epicondylectomy. *J Bone Joint Surg* 1980;62A:986–989.

29. Froimson AI, Anouchi YS, Seitz WH Jr, Winsberg DD: Ulnar nerve decompression with medial epicondylectomy for neuropathy at the elbow. *Clin Orthop* 1991;265:200–206.

30. Heithoff SJ, Millender LH, Nalebuff EA, Petruska AJ Jr: Medial epicondylectomy for the treatment of ulnar nerve compression at the elbow. *J Hand Surg* 1990;15A:22–29.

31. Dellon AL: Review of treatment results for ulnar nerve entrapment at the elbow. *J Hand Surg* 1989;14A:688–700.

32. Richmond JC, Southmayd WW: Superficial anterior transposition of the ulnar nerve at the elbow for ulnar neuritis. *Clin Orthop* 1982;164:42–44.

33. Eaton RG, Crowe JF, Parkes JC III: Anterior transposition of the ulnar nerve using a noncompressing fasciodermal sling. *J Bone Joint Surg* 1980;62A:820–825.

34. Kleinman WB, Bishop AT: Anterior intramuscular transposition of the ulnar nerve. *J Hand Surg* 1989;14A:972–979.

35. Leffert RD: Anterior submuscular transposition of the ulnar nerves by the Learmonth technique. *J Hand Surg* 1982;7A:147–155.

36. Learmonth JR: A technique for transplanting the ulnar nerve. *Surg Gynecol Obstet* 1942;75:792–793.

Osteochondritis Dissecans of the Elbow

Robert K. Peterson, MD

Felix H. Savoie, III, MD

Larry D. Field, MD

Introduction

Osteochondritis dissecans of the elbow has long been recognized as a disorder of the young athlete in which outcomes vary widely and treatment remains unsatisfactory. Although the disorder is often treated with benign neglect, the clinician must recognize its potential seriousness. Tivnon and associates[1] stated that "the lesion is not benign and marks the end of hard, painless throwing for the teenage athlete," and that "prognosis is poor despite the best of treatment."

Osteochondritis dissecans is a localized lesion involving the separation of a segment of articular surface containing both articular cartilage and subchondral bone. König[2] is credited with coining the term osteochondritis dissecans in 1888, describing a pathologic process producing loose bodies in the knee or hip in the absence of trauma. The term *osteochondritis* describes an inflammation of both bone and cartilage, and dissecans is derived from the Latin *dissec*, meaning to separate. The use of this term has persisted despite the absence of inflammatory cells in histologic sections of excised osteochondral fragments and the more common belief that trauma is the primary causative factor.[3,4]

Osteochondritis dissecans of the elbow refers primarily to lesions of the capitellum, although osteochondritic lesions of the trochlea, radial head, olecranon, and olecranon fossa have been reported.[5] Descriptions of this disorder in the literature appear under a confusing array of names including osteochondritis dissecans, Panner's disease, little leaguer's elbow, osteochondrosis, osteonecrosis, osteochondral fracture or fragment, accessory centers of ossification, and hereditary epiphyseal dysplasia.[4,6] The similarities and vague differentials of these disorders should caution the reader to analyze the pertinent literature with care.

The occurrence of osteochondritis dissecans in the elbow presents the physician with the same clinical dilemmas encountered in the more common locations of the knee and ankle. The physician must have a knowledge of the current clinical data to optimize individual patient care. The natural history of this disorder is poorly understood, and no treatment regimen has proved to be universally effective.

Etiology

The precise etiology of osteochondritis dissecans remains an open question, although most investigators would agree that repetitive microtrauma plays a prominent role. Investigations have focused primarily on the roles of trauma and ischemia. Genetic factors have been proposed in sporadic reports, although there is still no convincing evidence that osteochondritis dissecans is an inherited disorder.[7] Some authors have also implied that certain patients are predisposed by constitution,[8] as suggested by the not uncommon occurrence of osteochondritis dissecans bilaterally or in multiple locations.[7,9]

The ischemic theory of osteochondritis dissecans is based on the vascular anatomy of the distal humerus and the results of histopathologic studies. Haraldsson[10] demonstrated that the immature capitellar epiphysis is supplied by 1 or 2 isolated vessels that enter the epiphysis posteriorly and traverse the cartilaginous epiphysis to supply the capitellum. No contribution was detected from the metaphyseal vasculature. Thus, the capitellar vessels function as end-arteries that pass through a pliable, cartilaginous medium. This situation may create a predisposition toward osteonecrosis.

The histopathology of osteochondritis dissecans is also seen as being consistent with an ischemic event. Findings are usually consistent with osteonecrosis of the subchondral bone. Initially, articular cartilage is intact and remains viable via nutrition from the synovial fluid. The earliest changes include hyperemia and edema. Reparative changes are seen at the interface of the necrotic subarticular segment and the healthy bone. Absorption of the necrotic bone by vascular granulation tissue occurs. This coincides with a radiographic appearance of rarefaction at the periphery of the lesion. If the articular cartilage remains intact with the necrotic segment in situ, absorption and replacement with viable osseous tissue will eventually occur. If the articular cartilage is violated, or breaks down because of insufficient mechanical support, the necrotic segment may detach and form a loose body.[7] It is believed that the new, healing bone is very vulnerable and, if fractured, may represent the essential process in the detachment of articular fragments.[11]

The importance of trauma and overuse in this process has long been assumed based on the high prevalence of the disorder in males involved in throwing sports and females involved in gymnastics, in addition to the fact that most cases occur in the dominant upper extremity. A history of repetitive overuse is common to this disorder.

Several authors have commented on the relationship between this condition, baseball pitching,[1,12–15] and competitive gymnastics.[16,17] The creation of compressive and/or shearing forces in the radiocapitellar joint is believed to be the common denominator. It has been shown that the radiocapitellar joint acts as a secondary stabilizer of the elbow, in addition to accepting up to 60% of the force of compressive axial loads.[18] The valgus stress on the elbow during the cocking phase of the throwing motion creates a compressive load at the radiocapitellar joint.[15] It is this force that may be responsible for the creation of subchondral fractures or the disruption of a tenuous local blood supply.

Repetitive microtrauma may weaken the subchondral bone of the capitellum and lead to fatigue fracture. If osseous repair fails in this setting, an avascular fragment of bone may be exposed to bony resorption and become separated. Once the mechanical support of the articular cartilage is gone, this area of cartilage is exposed to shear stresses and may break down, leading to fragmentation and the production of loose bodies.[4]

Schenck and associates[19] have demonstrated significant differences in the mechanical properties and cartilage topography between the capitellum and the radial head. Their study noted that the central radial head is significantly stiffer than the lateral aspect of the capitellum. This situation creates a mechanical mismatch that may be a factor in the creation of the osteochondritis dissecans lesion of the elbow. The predominance of involvement of the surface of the capitellum as opposed to the radial head would also be explained. These data further the case for trauma as the inciting event.

Clinical Presentation

Osteochondritis dissecans of the elbow is most commonly seen in adolescents and young adults. Males are affected far more frequently than females, and the dominant arm is predominantly affected. In most cases there is a history of chronic overuse of the upper extremity, commonly involving sports that create tremendous stress on the upper extremity such as baseball, weightlifting, racquet sports, cheerleading, or gymnastics.

The insidious and progressive development of pain is the most common presentation of the condition, although pain is not always a part of the prodrome.[17] The pain tends to be activity-related and is often relieved by rest. Examination may reveal tenderness over the lateral aspect of the elbow at the level of the radiocapitellar joint; however, the pain is commonly dull and poorly localized. Limitation of motion of the elbow is also a common complaint. Loss of extension (often 150° or more) is the most common restriction, although flexion and forearm rotation are occasionally affected.[20]

Complaints of clicking, grinding, catching, and locking should alert the examiner to the possibility of loose bodies in the joint and the elbow should always be examined for crepitus. The active radiocapitellar compression test has been recommended[21] and involves asking the patient to actively pronate and supinate the forearm with the elbow in full extension. The muscle action compresses the radiocapitellar joint and may reproduce the symptoms.

A complete upper extremity examination is routinely performed to rule out any related pathology. Osteochondritis dissecans may play a role in the ill-defined disorder that is referred to as little leaguer's elbow. Although this term has little clinical significance, its use highlights the possible association of osteochondritis dissecans and concomitant pathology of the elbow, including injury to the medial epicondyle, radial head, and the medial and lateral ulnar collateral ligaments.

Diagnostic Evaluation

Radiographic changes of the capitellum in the immature elbow occur in 2 groups that should be carefully distinguished: Panner's disease (osteochondrosis of the capitellum) and osteochondritis dissecans of the elbow. The principal differences are age of onset and degree of involvement of the capitellar secondary ossification center.

Panner's disease[22] occurs in children between the ages of 4 and 8 years and causes rarefaction and fragmentation of the entire ossific nucleus of the capitellum. Children present with dull, aching elbow pain that resolves with rest, avoidance of stress, and occasionally splinting or bracing. This is a self-limiting process of degeneration followed by reossification and resolution and is rarely associated with any long-term sequelae.[7]

In contrast, osteochondritis dissecans usually occurs between the ages of 10 and 21, involves only a portion of the capitellum, and may be associated with permanent deformity of the joint surface[4] (Fig. 1). Some authors have proposed that changes in the capitellum may occur on a continuum from osteochondroses in children to chondromalacia in the adult,[7,23] although most believe there is a clear distinction between the processes.[7,20]

Standard radiographs, including anteroposterior (AP) and lateral views of the elbow, will frequently reveal the characteristic radiolucency and rarefaction of the capitellum, along with a flattening or irregularity of the articular surface (Fig. 1). The lesion often appears as a radiolucent crater with a rim of sclerotic bone on the lateral or central portion of the capitellum. If the fragment separates, 1 or more loose bodies may be seen. Supplementary views tangential to the lesion such as a 45° AP or oblique radiographs may be helpful.[6,11]

Radiographs may also be useful in following the progression or resolution of the disease process. If the fragment does not displace, the central sclerotic fragment gradually becomes less distinct, while the surrounding area of radiolucency gradually ossifies. A relatively radiolucent bone fragment may appear over the flattened, sclerotic area of bone of the capitellum, indicating new bone

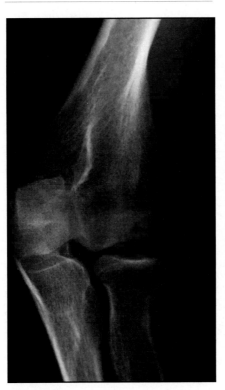

Fig. 1 Anteroposterior radiograph demonstrating radiolucency and rarefaction typical of osteochondritis dissecans of the capitellum.

formation.[11] Alternatively, if sequestration of the fragment occurs, degenerative changes of the radiocapitellar joint may be seen. Plain radiographs may also reveal compensatory changes of the radial head. This can include enlargement of the radial head, irregularity of the articular surface, and premature closure of the proximal radial physis.

In questionable cases, ancillary studies can be helpful in the detection and evaluation of osteochondritis dissecans. Conventional and computed tomography (CT) may be useful in defining the extent of the osseous lesion as well as detecting loose bodies in the joint. CT arthrography may allow for a more careful examination of the overlying cartilage.[24] Magnetic resonance imaging (MRI) has been advocated for the patient at risk,[17,25] and may be most useful in early

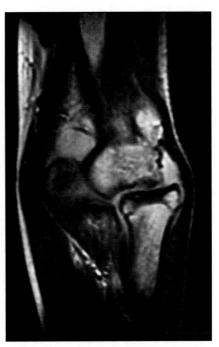

Fig. 2 Coronal magnetic resonance image of osteochondritis dissecans of the capitellum. Increased signal intensity on the T2 image indicates a detachment of the primary fragment.

detection.[11] Early in the process, T1-weighted images show low signal intensity in the superficial aspect of the capitellum, while T2 images may initially be normal.[11] Detachment of the fragment is indicated by intervening fluid seen on T2-weighted images (Fig. 2). Other studies, including bone scans and ultrasonography, may be of value, but are not in routine use.

Treatment

The treatment of osteochondritis dissecans is guided by clinical findings, radiographic appearance, status of the overlying articular cartilage, and a determination of the status of the involved segment (intact versus detached). Most authors have focused on the last factor when planning surgical care and have recognized 3 subsets: attached, partially attached, and completely detached.[7,20] Investigation of the lesion with diagnostic studies has been discussed earlier; currently, however, arthroscopy represents the most definitive method of characterizing the lesion.[5,17,20,23]

Intact capitellar lesions with no evidence of fracture of the articular cartilage are managed conservatively.[5,7,11,20] We prefer the use of a hinged elbow brace for protection and to serve as a deterrent to vigorous use. The brace may be locked for a short time if pain is the prominent complaint. Rest and protection are continued for 3 to 6 weeks until the pain is resolved. When symptoms subside, a gradual, progressive therapy program is initiated. The patient progresses in therapy through stretching, strengthening, and plyometric training to prepare for return to sport. The patient usually returns to unrestricted activity 3 to 6 months after treatment begins. Activity is monitored and adjusted for any recurrence of symptoms. Radiographic changes are followed but are not generally used as a criteria for return to play because changes may occur over several years.[7] Patients with intact lesions treated conservatively have the best prognosis, although several studies have indicated that it is prudent to counsel the patient and parents concerning the possibility of long-term sequelae.[8,16,17,26]

Indications for surgical management include persistent or worsening symptoms despite prolonged conservative care, symptomatic loose bodies, evidence of fracture of the surface of the articular cartilage, and displacement or detachment of the lesion.[5,7,20] Most of the literature concerning the surgical management of osteochondritis dissecans of the elbow discusses management with an open arthrotomy. With technologic improvements, elbow arthroscopy has become the procedure of choice in most circum-

stances and several authors have discussed the technique in excellent detail.[5,6,20,21,23]

The surgical management of osteochondritis dissecans of the elbow generally falls into 2 categories. One method involves the excision of the lesion (and removal of any loose bodies), supplemented by abrasion chondroplasty or subchondral drilling to encourage local healing and minimize future degenerative changes (Fig. 3). The other option is to attempt surgical reattachment of the fragment.

Most surgically managed osteochondritic lesions of the elbow undergo excision of the fragment followed by some type of local debridement (Fig. 3, A and B). This technique is generally performed arthroscopically, routinely inspecting both anterior and posterior compartments. Motorized shavers, burrs, suction punches, and grasping forceps are used to remove loose bodies, fragments, and debris, as well as perform an abrasion chondroplasty at the site of the lesion (Fig. 3, C). The surgeon may also opt to use the drill or microfracture technique to penetrate the subchondral bone and encourage healing by providing vascular channels (Fig. 3, D).[27]

Controversy continues concerning the role of fragment fixation in the management of osteochondritis dissecans of the elbow. Fixation can be perfomed by either open arthrotomy or arthroscopic techniques. Methods of fixation include Kirschner wires,[17,20,28] cancellous screws,[29] Herbert screws,[30] and bioabsorbable implants. A few authors[28,30] have presented satisfying results after fixation but most of the available data indicate little or no advantage to replacement or fixation of the fragment.[1,8,16,26,31,32]

Results

The longest follow-up study published in the literature to date is that

of Bauer and associates,[26] with an average of 23 years (range 11 to 35 years) of follow-up on 31 patients. Symptoms were noted in about half of the patients with impaired motion and pain on exertion being the most common complaints. Radiographic signs of degenerative joint disease were seen in over half of the group and correlated most closely with a decreased range of motion. Treatment consisted of fragment excision and removal of loose bodies. These authors do not recommend attempts at reattachment and saw no evidence to support drilling or curetting.

Woodward and Bianco[8] reported on 42 patients, all male, with an average follow-up of 12 years (range 2 to 34 years). The authors stated that "most patients thought they had normal use from their elbow." They reported that the overall prognosis was good, but some limitation of full extension (usually less than 20°) was likely to remain. They also concluded that loose bodies should be removed but that no other procedures were indicated.

Mitsunaga and associates[32] studied 66 elbows with an average follow-up period of 13.6 years. Treatment varied with the type of lesion: 42 were excised surgically, and 24 were treated nonsurgically. They concluded that loose bodies produce dysfunction, but that less than half of attached lesions progressed to detachment. These authors believe that drilling or curettage of the base of the lesion after excision was the procedure of choice.

In a marked departure from the general trend of the "conservative" approach to surgical treatment in which fragments are excised and further procedures are discouraged, Kuwahata and Inoue[30] recently reported favorable results after treating nondisplaced lesions with in situ fixation. Six patients, unresponsive to conservative care, were treated with debridement, cancellous bone grafting, replacement of the fragment in its bed, and Herbert screw fixation. The authors reported that at a minimum 12-month follow-up, all patients were pain-free and had returned to their previous sporting activities. Complete reossification of the capitellar cyst and a normally contoured joint surface were also reported.

The prognosis for return to competitive athletics varies widely in the literature. Most results suggest a guarded long-term prognosis. Tivnon and associates[1] reported that while 10 of 12 patients believed that treatment improved the function of their elbow, only 1 was able to throw at his previous level without pain. The authors stated that "the best result that one can expect is a reduction in elbow pain with a gain in extension." Only 1 of 7 elite gymnasts in the study by Jackson and associates[17] was able to return to competition. In contrast, McManama and associates[31] found that 12 of 14 patients were able to return to competitive athletics, and Singer and Roy[16] studied 5 gymnasts (2 treated conservatively) who were all able to return to competition at 3-year follow-up.

Several authors have recognized that early diagnosis and treatment greatly increase the chances for a favorable outcome.[8,11,16,17,31] A recent study[11] documented early detection of osteochondritis dissecans of the capitellum with MRI and ultrasound screening in volunteers from youth baseball teams. Three cases of osteochondritis dissecans were detected from a group of 44 players examined. Two players were withheld from play and clinical and radiographic resolution of the lesion was documented. The third patient continued to pitch against medical advice and developed

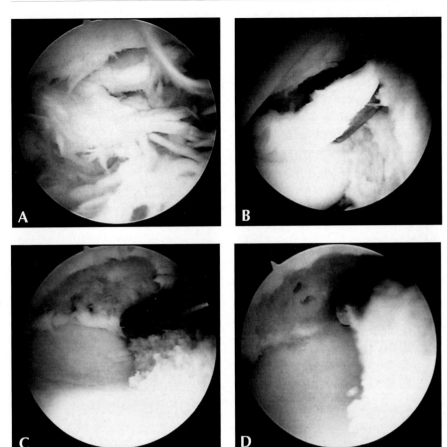

Fig. 3 Arthroscopic view using 70° arthroscope in the posterolateral portal of osteochondritis dissecans of the capitellum. **A,** Typical osteochondritis dissecans of the capitellum (capitellum is superior) with separation of the osteochondral fragment. **B,** Arthroscopic grasper introduced through the soft spot portal to remove loose bodies. **C,** Capitellum after complete debridement. **D,** Drill holes have been placed into the capitellum at the base of the lesion.

typical osteochondritis dissecans. These findings suggest the potential for spontaneous healing.

Summary

Osteochondritis dissecans of the elbow remains one of the leading causes of permanent elbow disability in adolescents and young adults engaged in throwing sports or gymnastics.[1,4] The insidious onset of lateral elbow pain and restriction of full extension should alert the physician and prompt further investigation. Early recognition and appropriate treatment may allow for the prevention of long-term sequelae.

Conservative care following early detection provides the best opportunity for a complete recovery. Surgical management at this point consists primarily of excision or removal of the osteochondral fragment with drilling or burring of the base of the lesion. Prognosis is fair with approximately half of all patients experiencing chronic pain or limitation of motion in the elbow.

Research efforts are currently focusing on the treatment of established articular surface defects. Newer procedures such as the transplantation of osteochondral, perichondral, and periosteal tissues, chondrocyte transplantation, and the biochemical manipulation of the chondrocyte environment may provide us with exciting new approaches to an old problem.[27]

Osteochondritis dissecans of the elbow continues to present a difficult challenge to the treating physician. The current literature provides very little guidance for the clinician but active and innovative investigations into the treatment of articular cartilage defects may soon provide the answers.

References

1. Tivnon MC, Anzel SH, Waugh TR: Surgical management of osteochondritis dissecans of the capitellum. *Am J Sports Med* 1976;4: 121–128.

2. König F: Ueber freie Körper in den Gelenken. *Deutsche Zeitschr Chir* 1887;27:90–109.

3. Nagura S: The so-called osteochondritis dissecans of König. *Clin Orthop* 1960;18:100–122.

4. Schenck RC Jr, Goodnight JM: Osteochondritis dissecans. *J Bone Joint Surg* 1996;78A: 439–456.

5. Chess D: Osteochondritis, in Savoie FH III, Field LD (eds): *Arthroscopy of the Elbow*. New York, NY, Churchill-Livingstone, 1996, pp 77–86.

6. Poehling GG: Osteochondritis dissecans of the elbow, in Norris TR (ed): *Orthopaedic Knowledge Update: Shoulder and Elbow*. Rosemont, IL, American Academy of Orthopaedic Surgeons, 1997, pp 363–367.

7. Shaughnessy WJ, Bianco AJ: Osteochondritis dissecans, in Morrey BF (ed): *The Elbow and Its Disorders*, ed 2. Philadelphia, PA, WB Saunders, 1993, pp 282–287.

8. Woodward AH, Bianco AJ Jr: Osteochondritis dissecans of the elbow. *Clin Orthop* 1975;110: 35–41.

9. Pappas AM: Elbow problems associated with baseball during childhood and adolescence. *Clin Orthop* 1982;164:30–41.

10. Haraldsson S: On osteochondrosis deformans juvenilis capituli humeri including investigation of intra-osseous vasculature in distal humerus. *Acta Orthop Scand* 1959;38(suppl): 1–232.

11. Takahara M, Shundo M, Kondo M, Suzuki K, Nambu T, Ogino T: Early detection of osteochondritis dissecans of the capitellum in young baseball players: Report of three cases. *J Bone Joint Surg* 1998;80A:892–897.

12. Adams JE: Injury to the throwing arm: A study of traumatic changes in the elbow joints of boy baseball players. *Calif Med* 1965;102:127–132.

13. Albright JA, Jokl P, Shaw R, Albright JP: Clinical study of baseball pitchers: Correlation of injury to the throwing arm with method of delivery. *Am J Sports Med* 1978;6:15–21.

14. Brown R, Blazina ME, Kerlan RK, Carter VS, Jobe FW, Carlson GJ: Osteochondritis of the capitellum. *J Sports Med* 1974;2:27–46.

15. Tullos HS, King JW: Lesions of the pitching arm in adolescents. *JAMA* 1972;220:264–271.

16. Singer KM, Roy SP: Osteochondrosis of the humeral capitellum. *Am J Sports Med* 1984;12: 351–360.

17. Jackson DW, Silvino N, Reiman P: Osteochondritis in the female gymnast's elbow. *Arthroscopy* 1989;5:129–136.

18. An KN, Morrey BF: Biomechanics of the elbow, in Morrey BF (ed): *The Elbow and Its Disorders*, ed 2. Philadelphia, PA, WB Saunders, 1993, pp 53–72.

19. Schenck RC Jr, Athanasiou KA, Constantinides G, Gomez E: A biomechanical analysis of articular cartilage of the human elbow and a potential relationship to osteochondritis dissecans. *Clin Orthop* 1994;299:305–312.

20. Bradley JP: Upper extremity: Elbow injuries in children and adolescents, in Stanitski CL, DeLee JC, Drez D Jr (eds): *Pediatric and Adolescent Sports Medicine*. Philadelphia, PA, WB Saunders, 1994, pp 242–261.

21. Baumgarten TE: Osteochondritis dissecans of the capitellum. *Sports Med Arthr Rev* 1995;3: 219–223.

22. Panner HJ: A peculiar affection of the capitulum humeri, resembling Calve-Perthes' disease of the hip. *Acta Radiol* 1929;10:234–242.

23. Ruch DS, Poehling GG: Arthroscopic treatment of Panner's disease. *Clin Sports Med* 1991; 10:629–636.

24. Holland P, Davies AM, Cassar-Pullicino VN: Computed tomographic arthrography in the assessment of osteochondritis dissecans of the elbow. *Clin Radiol* 1994;49:231–235.

25. Murphy BJ: MR imaging of the elbow. *Radiology* 1992;184:525–529.

26. Bauer M, Jonsson K, Josefsson PO, Linden B: Osteochondritis dissecans of the elbow: A long-term follow-up study. *Clin Orthop* 1992; 284:156–160.

27. Menche DS, Vangsness CT Jr, Pitman M, Gross AE, Peterson L: The treatment of isolated articular cartilage lesions in the young individual, in Cannon WD Jr (ed): *Instructional Course Lectures 47*. Rosemont, IL, American Academy of Orthopaedic Surgeons, 1998, pp 505–515.

28. Indelicato PA, Jobe FW, Kerlan RK, Carter VS, Shields CL, Lombardo SJ: Correctable elbow lesions in professional baseball players: A review of 25 cases. *Am J Sports Med* 1979;7: 72–75.

29. Johnson LL (ed): *Arthroscopic Surgery: Principles and Practice*, ed 3. St. Louis, MO, CV Mosby, 1986, vol 2, pp 1446–1477.

30. Kuwahata Y, Inoue G: Osteochondritis dissecans of the elbow managed by Herbert screw fixation. *Orthopedics* 1998;21:449–451.

31. McManama GB Jr, Micheli LJ, Berry MV, Sohn RS: The surgical treatment of osteochondritis of the capitellum. *Am J Sports Med* 1985; 13:11–21.

32. Mitsunaga MM, Adishian DA, Bianco AJ Jr: Osteochondritis dissecans of the capitellum. *J Trauma* 1982;22:53–55.

Arthroscopic Treatment of Posterior Elbow Impingement

Michael J. Moskal, MD
Felix H. Savoie III, MD
Larry D. Field, MD

Introduction

Posterior elbow impingement refers to a mechanical abutment of bony and soft tissues in the posterior compartment of the elbow that produces pain, stiffness, and/or locking. The clinical presentation is characterized by pain at the limits of elbow extension, with varying degrees of extension loss. In general, there are 3 broad categories of posterior elbow impingement. Posterior elbow impingement can be seen (1) as part of a primary osteoarthritic process; (2) abutment posteriorly with an intact ulnar collateral ligament, seen in athletes with hyperextension forces, and (3) bony abutment of the olecranon and the humerus, seen in overhand athletes with ulnar collateral ligamentous insufficiency. Although these categories are useful for diagnostic and treatment considerations, there is considerable overlap of the pathoanatomy encountered.

Posterior Elbow Impingement

Posterior elbow impingement in athletes occurs in 2 forms. Repetitive hyperextension of the elbow may produce posterior impingement. The pathologic entities are centrally located on the tip of the olecranon, and they usually will have reactive thickening of the bone bridge between the coronoid and olecranon fossae (Fig. 1). These lesions are seen in football linemen, gymnasts, rodeo participants, competitive weight lifters, and fast pitch softball pitchers. Radiographs in these patients are similar to those seen in patients who have primary osteoarthritis. There is usually no instability of the ligaments of the elbow, but these patients may have a mild capsular contracture anteriororly.

Instability may produce secondary posterior impingement between the outer edge of the olecranon and the inner edge of the olecranon fossae. Valgus instability produces changes on the medial side of the olecranon and the lateral aspect of the medial wall of the olecranon fossa. Varus and posterolateral instability produces lesions on the lateral aspect of the olecranon and the medial aspect of the lateral wall of the olecranon fossa (Fig. 2). Radiographs reveal eccentric changes in these areas, with no demonstrable thickening of the bone bridge between the olecranon and coronoid fossae of the distal humerus.

A significant number of competitive overhand throwers have more subtle forms of ulnar collateral ligament insufficiency. In a retrospective review of elbow surgery in professional baseball players, Andrews and Timmerman[1] noted that posterior extension injury was the most com-

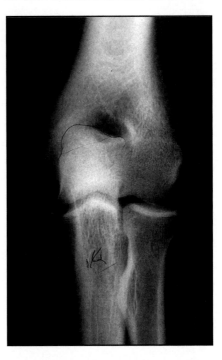

Fig. 1 Radiograph demonstrates the central spurring of the tip of the olecranon in a patient with posterior impingement.

mon diagnosis. However, ulnar collateral ligament injuries were underestimated and, of patients who required a second surgery, 25% required an ulnar collateral ligament reconstruction. They surmised that ulnar collateral ligament pathology would have been recognized more often with the arthroscopic valgus stress test[2] and recognition of undersurface tears.[3] Attenuation of the

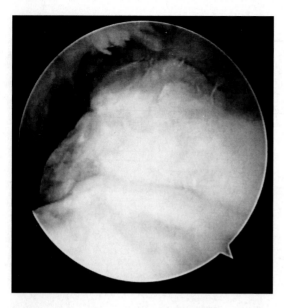

Fig. 2 Instability may produce eccentric spurring of the medial (valgus instability) or lateral (varus or posterolateral instability) olecranon.

medial stabilizing structures of the elbow allow increased valgus subluxation of the elbow during overhand throwing. Chronically, traction osteophytes along the medial aspect of the semilunar notch[4] and midsubstance calcifications of the ulnar collateral ligament[5] may develop. Increased compressive forces across the radiocapitellar joint from valgus instability can lead to chondromalacia and capitellar osteochondral lesions, in addition to posterior compartment lesions and loose bodies. In a throwing athlete, the presence of posterior impingement should focus the surgeon on instability. The arthroscopic stress test before and after spur resection should decrease the need for reoperation.

Posterior elbow impingement is also commonly encountered in degenerative and post-traumatic arthritis. Primary osteoarthritis may proceed with a predominately posterior involvement.[6] Patients are almost exclusively male and commonly present in the fourth to sixth decade of life. Mechanical abutment pain and diminished range of motion are caused by olecranon and coranoid

osteophytes, decreased volume of the olecranon fossa, and loose bodies, which may or may not be imbedded in scar tissue. Crepitance and loss of elbow extension are common. Pain loss is typically more common at the extremes of extension than at flexion. Midrange pain is more common with advanced stages.

Arthroscopic treatment for posterior impingement has evolved from open techniques. Arthroscopic assessment and treatment allows the surgeon to evaluate and treat intra-articular pathology and offers significant advantages over open procedures, including limited soft-tissue dissection and increased visualization of both the anterior and posterior compartments. In our experience, as well as in that of others,[1] arthroscopic techniques in posterior compartment surgery have proven superior to open surgery. The essentials of treatment are removal of loose bodies, olecranon tip and coronoid process osteophyte excision, deepening[7] or fenestration[8] of the distal humerus, and excision of soft-tissue lesions, such as posterolateral plicae,[9] synovitis, and/or fat pad hypertrophy. Patient

selection, technical expertise, and familiarity with both open and arthroscopic elbow surgery are all essential to success.

In addition, arthroscopic treatment for posterior impingement in throwers should also carefully assess posteromedial olecranon osteophytes with corresponding distal humeral lesions and overall humeral hypertrophy,[4] radiocapitellar degeneration,[10] posterolateral plicas,[9] and, most importantly, ulnar collateral ligament insufficiency.[11] The arthroscopic valgus stress test[2,12] before and after debridement is helpful to assess the integrity of the ulnar collateral ligament (Fig. 3).

Patient Evaluation
Information about the patient's age; occupational, athletic, and vocational activities; symptom onset; and its relation to these activities should be obtained. Patients with primary osteoarthritis are typically older, whereas patients with posterior impingement due to ulnar collateral insufficiency tend to be younger. Overhand athletes typically complain of increasing fatigue, numbness, and medial elbow pain during throwing. Overhand athletes may also complain of activity related pain in the posterolateral aspect of the radiocapitellar articulation.[13] Articular effusions are seen best posterolaterally in this radiocapitellar area. Range of motion may or may not be normal. Flexion contractures are common but are not uniformly present in patients with posterior elbow impingement.

Provocative testing is useful in the evaluation of posterior elbow impingement unrelated to primary osteoarthritis. In terminal extension, a valgus stress may be painful as the olecranon abuts against the humerus medially. Valgus stress testing can be performed with the patient sitting or

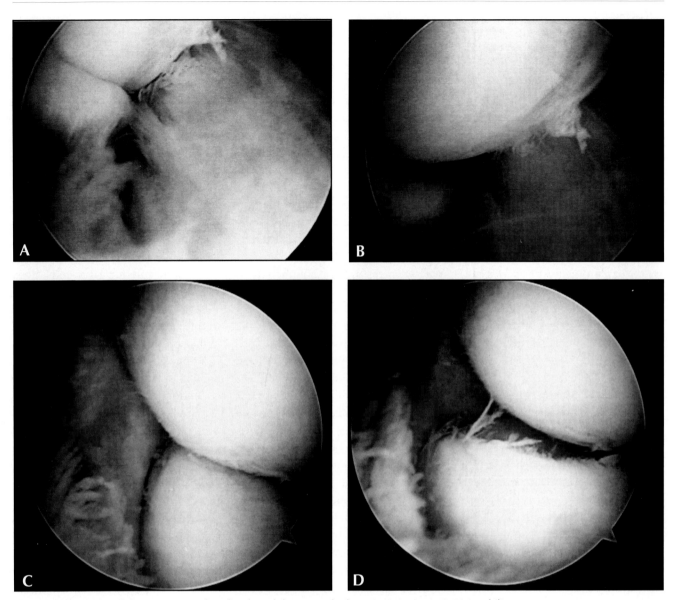

Fig. 3 Arthroscopy instability test may confirm the clinical diagnosis of valgus (**A, B**) or varus (**C, D**) instability.

lying prone. The examiner uses one hand to apply a valgus load while the other stabilizes the arm against the examining table and palpates the medial epicondyle, ulnar collateral ligament, ulnar groove, flexor-pronator origin, and the medial ulnohumeral joint. Valgus instability testing can be fairly subtle; complete anterior bundle sectioning may only increase valgus rotation by 3°.[14] Stability should be tested throughout the entire arc of motion, assessing for crepitance of the medial ulnohumeral and radiocapitellar joints as the olecranon seats into the olecranon fossa. Not all patients with posterior elbow pain have posterior impingement; for example, posterior pain can be caused by triceps tendinitis or olecranon stress fractures.[15]

Routinely, we obtain anteroposterior (AP) and lateral radiographs of the elbow; oblique and stress views are occasionally added to further assess the elbow. Loose bodies, medial epicondylar avulsion fractures, traction osteophytes of the medial semilunar notch, bony hypertrophy between the olecranon and coranoid fossae, coranoid and olecranon osteophytes are all common. Normal radiographs do not preclude symptomatic pathoanatomy, such as loose bodies and chrondral lesions. In fact, radiographs routinely underestimate the presence or numbers of loose bodies.[16,17] Computed tomography (CT) scans and magnetic resonance imaging (MRI) are occasionally helpful to further refine clinical diagnoses however, they are rarely indicated for osteoarthritic or degenerative conditions.[18]

Nonsurgical Management

The goal of treatment is the restoration of comfort and function. Patient education and nonsurgical treatment for posterior elbow impingement varies according to the primary etiology of the posterior elbow impingement and the functional requirements of the patient. The rehabilitation process for patients who have osteoarthritis as the primary etiology of posterior impingement is a gentle stretching and strengthening program. The gentle stretching program is designed to make modest gains. Patients and therapists are advised that aggressive stretching exacerbates symptoms and usually does not achieve any significant gains in motion or comfort. In general, to increase comfort after an acute injury, we recommend relative rest, cryotherapy, and, in some instances, a short term of nonsteroidal anti-inflammatory medications (NSAIDs).

After an acute injury, rest for a short period of time, to allow bleeding and swelling to subside, is beneficial. Gentle range of motion and stretching exercises, within mild pain limits are begun early. Cryotherapy diminishes pain[19] and may reduce bleeding and swelling[20] after an acute injury. The duration of ice application is limited by its potential harmful effects, such as thermal injury to subcutaneous nerves or rebound hyperemia after the cooling elements are removed.[21] NSAIDs seem to help diminish pain, but may not have a protective effect after injury.[22] We use NSAIDs for a limited time, carefully weighing their benefits against possible drug interactions and systemic side effects.

For overhand athletes, our nonsurgical and secondary postoperative rehabilitative program has evolved from the work of Wilson and associates[23] and Glousman and associates.[24] After an initial period of rest, with flexor and extensor muscle stretching, the athlete begins strengthening with low weight, high repetition isotonic exercises to build increase endurance. Isometric and isokinetic programs with gripping exercises are instituted to further increase conditioning and strengthening, advancing into plyometrics. Plyometric exercises induce a rapid transition from initial eccentric muscle contraction to concentric muscle contraction. In theory, muscle reeducation is enhanced as stretch reflexes cause the muscles to fire without conscious thought. Timing, proprioception, and muscle strength are improved. As rehabilitation continues, the rotator cuff and periscapular musculature are strengthened. As strength improves, the athlete returns to throwing using an interval throwing program.[25]

If nonsurgical therapy fails to restore comfort and function, surgical intervention is offered. The following arthroscopic surgical technique is a general approach to patients with limited motion and mechanical impingement associated with soft-tissue and bony lesions.

Surgical Technique

In all patients with a primary diagnosis of posterior elbow impingement, anterior compartment arthroscopy is performed as part of a complete arthroscopic exam. The patient is placed prone and the elbow is positioned as described by Poehling and associates.[26] Landmarks, including the medial and lateral epicondyles, olecranon tip, radiocapitellar joint and ulnar nerve, are outlined with a surgical marker. Preoperatively, we palpate the ulnar nerve to assess its stability within the cubital tunnel. We distend the elbow by injecting the joint with lactated ringers through the direct lateral (soft spot)[27] or posterocentral portal. If stiffness is significant, the average volume capacity and capsular compliance may be reduced, diminishing displacement of neurovascular structures.[28] During initial anterior portal placement, the elbow is flexed at 90° to maximize the displacement of neurovascular structures from the joint capsule. A proximal anteromedial portal is used for diagnostic evaluation of the anterior compartment (Fig. 3). Testing for varus and valgus instability is part of the initial assessment. The intra-articular pathology determines the placement of the lateral portal and the need for a transradiocapitellar inflow via the posterior soft spot.

To develop a proximal anterolateral portal an outside-in technique is the preferred method. This portal, which is placed just superior to the capitellum, is used for synovectomy, radiocapitellar joint debridement, coronoid osteophyte excision, and deepening the coronoid fossa. Viewing from the lateral portal, the proximal anteromedial portal is used as a surgical portal to excise trochlea spurs to complete the debridement. If indicated, radial head excision and/or anterior capsular release may be performed.

After anterior compartment arthroscopic surgery, the posterior compartment is evaluated using posterolateral and posterocentral portals. Inflow can be from a previous anterior portal, a posterior portal, or the viewing cannula. While viewing through the posterolateral portal, a full radius shaver is inserted through the posterocentral portal. The intervening adhesions and redundant posterior superior capsular scarring are debrided with the shaver from the posterior superior portion of the elbow and between the posterior humerus and triceps muscle. While an assistant flexes the elbow, the tip of the olecranon can be removed with mediolateral sweeps of a burr (Fig. 4). Care should be taken to avoid injury to the triceps insertion.

The medial and lateral gutters are evaluated next. The arthroscope is placed in the posterocentral portal and the shaver in the posterolateral portal. Excision of the adhesions in the lateral gutter is initiated proximally and continues distally. Occasionally, a straight lateral portal is needed to adequately debride the posterior radiocapitellar and radioulnar joints as well as a posterolateral plica, if present. The medial gutter is approached with the arthroscope in the posterolateral portal and operating from the posterocentral portal. A fully hooded shaver is used to protect the ulnar nerve during debridement. Extreme caution should be exercised, as the ulnar nerve is in close proximity normally.[29] Also, it can be displaced by scarring.

The olecranon fossa, which is frequently narrowed by bony hypertrophy, loose bodies, and scar tissue, is debrided using a combination of a shaver and burr. An ulnohumeral arthroplasty (fenestration) is initiated. A full-thickness pilot hole is made into the center of the olecranon fossa to the coranoid fossa with a 5-mm drill through the posterocentral portal, and viewing is done through the posterolateral portal. The initial pilot hole is enlarged with a burr through the posterocentral portal taking care to maintain the integrity of the medial and lateral humeral columns (Fig. 5). Adequate clearance of the coranoid and olecranon should be ensured.

In athletes who throw, increased bony clearance after posterior debridement can theoretically increase ulno-

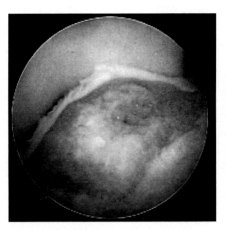

Fig. 4 Arthroscopic view of the olecranon after spur excision.

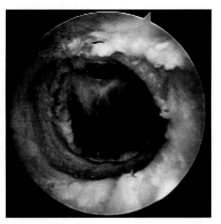

Fig. 5 Arthroscopic view of the olecranon fossa after fenestration for posterior impingement.

humeral opening, leading to valgus stress. According to Field and Altcheck,[12] medial ulnohumeral opening of 1 to 2 cm suggests complete anterior bundle insufficiency, whereas opening greater then 4-mm suggests complete medial collateral ligament insufficiency. In overhand athletes, we perform an arthroscopic valgus stress test after bony posterior debridement. We also specifically assess the trochlear notch in overhand athletes with posterolateral symptoms.[13]

Postoperative Rehabilitation

Drains may be placed in the proximal anteromedial and the posterocentral or posterolateral portals. The straight lateral portal should be routinely sutured closed, because of the lack of soft-tissue layers between the skin and joint capsule. The other portals are left open. After application of sterile dressings, the elbow is splinted in extension and supination. Early motion is instituted, with or without continuous passive motion (CPM). Patients are monitored in the hospital for 1 to 3 days, depending on the extent of surgery and the severity of disease.

Specific therapy depends on the

etiology of posterior impingement, functional requirements of the patient and secondary procedures performed. Static splinting or CPM is used at night usually for at least 3 weeks after surgery if motion gain is a significant postoperative goal. Organized therapy sessions may or may not be needed, and, again, these depend on the patient's progress and particular problem. Overhead throwers are started on a return-to-throw program that is similar to the secondary therapy described in the nonsurgical treatment section.

Results

Ogilvie-Harris and associates[30] reviewed 21 patients at an average of 35 months after arthroscopic surgery for posterior impingement due to degenerative arthritis. Anterior debridement and loose body removal was performed first, followed by posterior surgery, which consisted of removal of posterior loose bodies, removal of olecranon osteophytes, and debridement of the olecranon fossa to the point of fenestration. Significant reduction in pain, with increases in motion, strength and function, were noted. Results from arthroscopic surgery for osteoarthritis are generally good.[7,8] However, loose body removal alone does not typically improve patient's results; osteophyte excision is as important as loose body removal.[16,31]

In high-demand overhand athletes with posterior elbow impingement, reoperation rates may be high.[1] This high reoperation rate may be caused by the frequent high loads placed across the elbow, inadequate initial debridement, osteophyte reformation, unrecognized ulnar collateral insufficiency, and/or unrelated ligamentous attenuation postoperatively.

The senior author has reviewed his results of 53 arthroscopic debridements for arthrofibrosis of the elbow in 53 patients. On average, extension increased 41° (preoperative flexion contractures were reduced from 46° to 5° postoperatively) and flexion increased from 96° to 138°. Pronation increased on average 7° (75° to 82°) and supination increased 39° (47° to 86°). However, 1 patient ultimately underwent a successful elbow arthroplasty and 2 patients required a repeat arthroscopic debridement and release to maintain motion.

Conclusion

In properly selected patients, an arthroscopic approach to posterior impingement allows the surgeon to address both anterior and posterior intra-articular pathology. Arthroscopic evaluation and treatment of elbow pathology is particularly valuable because it increases visualization and diminishes soft-tissue trauma. Arthroscopic treatment of arthritic elbows is technically demanding. General techniques, as well as the sequence of procedures, should be dictated by pathology encountered during surgery and should not follow a rigid preoperative plan. Conversion to an open procedure does not represent failure.

References

1. Andrews JR, Timmerman LA: Outcome of elbow surgery in professional baseball players. *Am J Sports Med* 1995;23:407–413.

2. Timmerman LA, Andrews JR: Histology and arthroscopic anatomy of the ulnar collateral ligament of the elbow. *Am J Sports Med* 1994;22:667–673.

3. Timmerman LA, Andrews JR: Undersurface tears of the ulnar collateral ligament in baseball players: A newly recognized lesion. *Am J Sports Med* 1994;22:33–36.

4. King J, Brelsford HJ, Tullos HS: Analysis of the pitching arm of the professional baseball pitcher. *Clin Orthop* 1969;67:116–123.

5. Jobe FW, Stark H, Lombardo SJ: Reconstruction of the ulnar collateral ligament in athletes. *J Bone Joint Surg* 1986;68A:1158–1163.

6. Morrey BF: Primary degenerative arthritis of the elbow: Treatment by ulnohumeral arthroplasty. *J Bone Joint Surg* 1992;74A:410–413.

7. Ward WG, Anderson TE: Elbow arthroscopy in a mostly athletic population. *J Hand Surg* 1993;18A:220–224.

8. Redden JF, Stanley D: Arthroscopic fenestration of the olecranon fossa in the treatment of osteoarthritis of the elbow. *Arthroscopy* 1993;9:14–16.

9. Clarke RP: Symptomatic, lateral synovial fringe (plica) of the elbow joint. *Arthroscopy* 1988;4:112–116.

10. DeHaven KE, Evarts CM: Throwing injuries of the elbow in athletes. *Orthop Clin North Am* 1973;4:801–808.

11. Morrey BF, Tanaka S, An KN: Valgus stability of the elbow: A definition of primary and secondary constraints. *Clin Orthop* 1991;265:187–195.

12. Field LD, Altchek DW: Evaluation of the arthroscopic valgus instability test of the elbow. *Am J Sports Med* 1996;24:177–181.

13. Robla J, Hechtman KS, Uribe JW, Phillipon MS: Chondromalacia of the trochlear notch in athletes who throw. *J Shoulder Elbow Surg* 1996;5:69–72.

14. Callaway GH, Field LD, Deng XH, et al: Biomechanical evaluation of the medial collateral ligament of the elbow. *J Bone Joint Surg* 1997;79A:1223–1231.

15. Nuber GW, Diment MT: Olecranon stress fractures in throwers: A report of two cases and a review of the literature. *Clin Orthop* 1992;278:58–61.

16. Ogilvie-Harris DJ, Schemitsch E: Arthroscopy of the elbow for removal of loose bodies. *Arthroscopy* 1993;9:5–8.

17. Ward WG, Belhobek GH, Anderson TE: Arthroscopic elbow findings: Correlation with preoperative radiographic studies. *Arthroscopy* 1992;8:498–502.

18. Ward WG, Anderson TE: Elbow arthroscopy in a mostly athletic population. *J Hand Surg* 1993;18:220–224.

19. Speer KP, Warren RF, Horowitz L: The efficacy of cryotherapy in the postoperative shoulder. *J Shoulder Elbow Surg* 1996;5:62–68.

20. Ho SS, Coel MN, Kagawa R, Richardson AB: The effects of ice on blood flow and bone metabolism in knees. *Am J Sports Med* 1994;22:537–540.

21. Matsen FA III, Questad K, Matsen AL: The effect of local cooling on postfracture swelling: A controlled study. *Clin Orthop* 1975;109:201–206.

22. Mishra DK, Friden J, Schmitz MC, Lieber RL: Anti-inflammatory medication after muscle injury: A treatment resulting in short-term improvement but subsequent loss of muscle function. *J Bone Joint Surg* 1995;77A:1510–1519.

23. Wilson FD, Andrews JR, Blackburn TA, McCluskey G: Valgus extension overload in the pitching elbow. *Am J Sports Med* 1983;11:83–88.

24. Glousman RE, Barron J, Jobe FW, Perry J, Pink M: An electromyographic analysis of the elbow in normal and injured pitchers with medial collateral ligament insufficiency. *Am J Sports Med* 1992;20:311–317.

25. Wilk KE, Arrigo C, Andrews JR: Rehabilitation of the elbow in the throwing athlete. *J Orthop Sports Phys Ther* 1993;17:305–317.

26. Poehling GG, Whipple TL, Sisco L, Goldman B: Elbow arthroscopy: A new technique. *Arthroscopy* 1989;5:222–224.

27. Morrey BF: Arthroscopy of the elbow, in Anderson LD (ed): American Academy of Orthopaedic Surgeons *Instructional Course Lectures XXXV*. St. Louis, MO, CV Mosby, 1986, pp 102–107.

28. Gallay SH, Richards RR, O'Driscoll SW: Intraarticular capacity and compliance of stiff and normal elbows. *Arthroscopy* 1993;9:9–13.

29. Marshall PD, Fairclough JA, Johnson SR, Evans EJ: Avoiding nerve damage during elbow arthroscopy. *J Bone Joint Surg* 1993;75B:29–131.

30. Ogilvie-Harris DJ, Gordon R, MacKay M: Arthroscopic treatment for posterior impingement in degenerative arthritis of the elbow. *Arthroscopy* 1995;11:437–443.

31. O'Driscoll SW: Elbow arthroscopy for loose bodies. *Orthopedics* 1992;15:855–859.

Biceps Tendon Injury

Bernard F. Morrey, MD

Other than epicondylitis, isolated injury to the muscles or tendons about the elbow is rather uncommon.[1–5] Distal biceps tendon injury, most commonly avulsion from the radial tuberosity, although rare, is the most common tendinous injury in this region. The biceps muscle-tendon complex may be injured at the musculotendinous junction by an in-continuity tear of the tendon, and by a complete or partial tear or avulsion from the radial tuberosity.

A tear of the musculotendinous junction or an in-continuity tear of the tendon are very rare. These conditions have been seen in weightlifters and in association with anabolic steroid use. Surgical treatment is not predictable, but I have used a ligament augmentation device (LAD)™ to assist in the repair/reconstruction. Recovery is slow and incomplete. Simple plication of the stretched tendon is not reliable.

By far the most common injury is tendon avulsion, and complete avulsion is much more common than partial rupture. Even so, until recently this has been considered a rather uncommon injury.

Incidence

The rarity of the condition is exemplified by the fact that of the 355 surgeons responding to a questionnaire by Dobbie in 1941, only 51 cases were reported.[6] By 1956, there were 152 reported cases in the literature.[7] Currently the injury is well known,

and either its incidence is increasing or it is becoming recognized.[8–15]

Over 80% of the reported cases have involved the right dominant upper extremity, usually in a well developed man,[16,17] who has an average age of about 50 years,[6,18,19] ranging between 21 and 70 years.[6,17]

Mechanism of Injury

In virtually every reported case,[6,19] the mechanism of injury is a single traumatic event, often involving 40 kg or more of extension force with the elbow in about 90° of flexion. This mechanism and the tendency for anabolic steroid abuse in well conditioned, healthy, competitive weightlifters accounts for the surprisingly common occurrence of injury in this group. Preexisting degenerative changes in the tendon make rupture more likely.[20]

Etiology

The etiology of the injury has been discussed by several authors.[20,21] During pronation and supination, inflammation and degeneration of the biceps tendon are initiated by irritation from the irregularity of the radial tuberosity. Spurring of the radial tuberosity is common and is consistent with the degenerative nature of this injury. An interesting recent study on the etiology has also implicated a hypovascular zone of tendon near its attachment as a cause or contributing factor to the injury.[21] Acute pain, as in the antecubital fossa, is

noted immediately. Rarely, a patient complains of a second episode of acute pain several days later. Such a history suggests the possibility of an initial partial rupture or of secondary failure of the lacertus fibrosus.[10,22] Forearm pain has been reported but is not considered common.

Presentation
Subjective Complaints
The common symptom of distal biceps tendon rupture is a sudden, sharp, tearing pain followed by discomfort in the antecubital fossa or in the lower anterior aspect of the brachium. Activity is possible, but difficult, immediately after the injury. If the injury is not repaired with surgery, however, chronic pain with activity is common in the antecubital fossa and proximal forearm.[23] Flexion weakness of about 15% is inevitable, but it tends to decrease with time.[24] Loss of supination strength (about 40%) has been reported and is the source of considerable dysfunction. Diminution of grip strength also has been reported.[8,19]

Objective Findings
Ecchymosis is present in the antecubital fossa[6] and occasionally over the proximal ulnar aspect of the elbow joint.[25] Extensive bleeding is uncommon. With elbow flexion, the muscle contracts proximally, and a visible, palpable defect of the distal biceps muscle is obvious (Fig. 1). Local tenderness is present in the antecubital

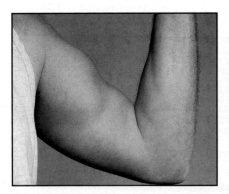

Fig. 1 Proximal migration, when present, allows the diagnosis to be readily made. (Reproduced with permission from the Mayo Foundation, Rochester, MN.)

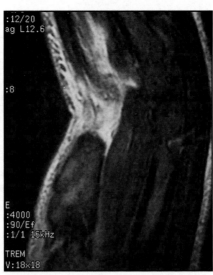

Fig. 2 Magnetic resonance imaging scan of the arm 4 days after injury. This study was of value in demonstrating retraction of the tendon and absence of tendon in the cubital fossa. (Reproduced with permission from the Mayo Foundation, Rochester, MN.)

fossa. The defect may be palpable; if not, and symptoms are otherwise consistent with the diagnosis, a partial rupture may have occurred. With partial rupture, crepitus or grinding is noted with forearm rotation.[10] Motion is not altered except possibly as a result of pain at the extremes of flexion, extension, and supination. Flexion weakness is usually and supination weakness invariably detectable by routine clinical examination.

Radiographic Changes
The routine use of the MRI has been recommended to make or confirm the diagnosis.[13] Although helpful occasionally, routine MRI is not necessary (Fig. 2).

Surgical Findings
The tendon will have recoiled into the muscle or be found to lie loosely curled in the antecubital fossa. Invariably, there is clean separation from the radial tuberosity.[6,16,19,24] The lacertus fibrosus may be attenuated, but is usually not completely torn. After several months, the tendon has retracted into the substance of the biceps muscle, making retrieval and reattachment impossible. In this instance, the lacertus fibrosus is usu-

ally torn and retracted.

Treatment
The functional superiority of surgical treatment is obvious when the results of cases treated with and without surgical intervention are reviewed.[19] The recent literature offers overwhelming documentation of the excellent results with early repair.[8,9,14,26] With a partial rupture, there is less functional loss or the tear may heal; hence, surgical management may not always be necessary.

Suture Anchor
Reattachment of the tendon to the radius by any one of several techniques[15,16,18,27] is clearly the treatment of choice. The difficulty of the anterior exposure needed to avoid radial nerve injury has prompted the development of a second incision placed over the dorsal aspect of the forearm.[25] It is of paramount importance to understand that the original 2-incision Boyd/Anderson technique has

been modified at the Mayo Clinic to lessen the likelihood of the development of ectopic bone between the radius and ulna.[27]

Because of concern over the development of ectopic bone associated with the 2-incision technique and with the advent of suture anchors, the anterior exposure using these anchors is gaining in popularity. If the procedure is done promptly, the tract of the biceps tendon is still present and is easily identified. If performed late (more than 2 weeks after injury), this tract may be obliterated, making the exposure more difficult.

I have no personal experience with these devices for distal biceps tendon rupture. The specific technique varies according to 3 variables: exposure, type of anchor used, and method of reattachment. The exposure is usually via a limited anterior approach. Two or 3 suture anchors are most often used directly into the unprepared tuberosity. Both the screw and barb designs have been described for use at the medial tuberosity (Fig. 3).

Two-Incision Technique (Mayo Clinic)
With the patient in the supine position, the extremity is prepared and draped in the usual fashion using an elbow table. A tourniquet is applied to the arm. A limited 3-cm transverse incision is performed in the cubital crease (Fig. 4). The arm is grasped and milked distally to deliver the biceps tendon. Most of the time, the tendon is readily retrieved with this maneuver. The tendon is inspected and is invariably found to have avulsed cleanly from the radial tuberosity. The distal 5 to 7 mm of degenerative tendon is resected, and two No. 5 nonabsorbable Bunnell or whip stitch (Krackow) sutures are placed in the torn tendon (Fig. 4).

The tuberosity is palpated with the index finger and a blunt, curved hemostat is carefully inserted into the space previously occupied by the biceps tendon. The instrument slips past the tuberosity and is advanced below the radius and ulna so that the tip of the instrument may be palpated on the dorsal aspect of the proximal forearm. A second incision is made over the instrument. The tuberosity is exposed by a *muscle-splitting* incision with the forearm maximally pronated. The ulna is never exposed.[28] A high-speed burr is used to evacuate a 1.5-cm wide and 1-cm deep defect in the radial tuberosity. The tendon is carefully introduced into the excavation formed in the tuberosity, and with the forearm in the neutral position the sutures are pulled tight and secured. The wounds are closed in layers, with a suction drain inserted both anteriorly and posteriorly in the depths of the wound. The elbow is placed in 90° of flexion with forearm rotation between neutral and supination. A compressive dressing is applied.

Postoperative Care The splint and surgical dressing are removed in 4 or 5 days and passive motion begun. Passive forearm rotation is encouraged as tolerated. Active flexion and extension and forearm rotation are begun at 7 to 10 days. Full active motion is attained by 3 to 4 weeks. Light weights, for example, 0.5 to 1 kg, are allowed at 4 to 6 weeks with progression as tolerated. Dynamic splints or prolonged protection are no longer used. Full activity is allowed after the third month as tolerated.

Results Strength restoration approached normal in flexion and supination. Nontreated distal biceps rupture results in a loss of about 20% flexion and 40% supination

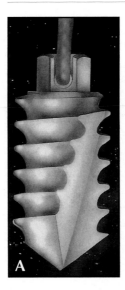
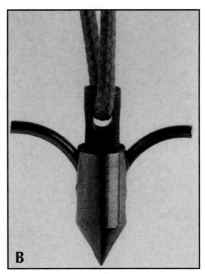

Fig. 3 Both the screw (**A**) and barbed tip (**B**) suture anchor designs had been used for biceps tendon attachment. (Reproduced with permission from the Mayo Foundation, Rochester, MN.)

strength.[19] On the other hand, restoration of normal strength has been reported,[19] and reaffirmed by Agins and associates[8] using Cybex testing for both strength and endurance. However, these authors and others[12] have observed restoration of normal strength only to the dominant extremity and a residual 20% to 30% weakness if the nondominant side was involved.

Complications To my knowledge, there are no individual reports specifically dealing with the complications of surgical treatment for distal biceps tendon rupture in the English literature. Transient radial nerve palsy with reattachment to the tuberosity has been and continues to be occasionally noted.[6,14,26,29] A delayed posterior interosseous palsy has also been reported after repair.[30] As mentioned, the use of suture anchors has become of interest to prevent injury to the nerve. Strauch and associates[15] reports 3 instances of successful treatment using a limited anterior approach and suture anchors.

Reattachment of the tendon through an anterior approach with a pullout suture to avoid ectopic bone also has received recent support.[26] In

2 recent series with 24 combined cases, this approach resulted in excellent restoration of function. There was, however, 1 musculocutaneous nerve injury and 2 temporary radial nerve palsies, which have been well documented to be associated with an anterior surgical approach for this condition.

The possibility of ectopic bone formation after the 2-incision approach is well known. We have not had a complete bridge in our practice. The possibility of this complication is lessened but continues to exist, even with suture anchors (Fig. 5). If the 2-incision technique is used, it must be emphasized that the tuberosity is exposed by a muscle-splitting approach and the ulna is never visualized (Fig. 6).

If an osseous bridge does develop, successful resection can be undertaken about 8 to 9 months after the initial surgery.[31] Some cases of extensive involvement of the interosseous space as well as site of attachment pose rather significant challenges of treatment. In some instances the biceps repair may be intimately associated with the ectopic bone. Removing the osseous bar resulted in detachment of

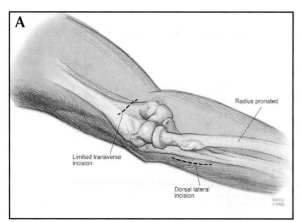

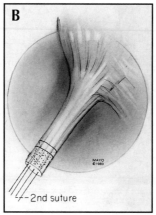

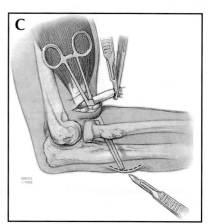

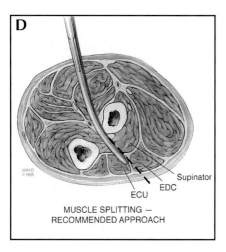

MUSCLE SPLITTING —
RECOMMENDED APPROACH

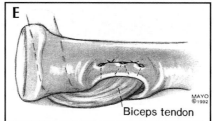

Biceps tendon

Fig. 4 A, A 3- to 4-cm transverse incision is made in the cubital space. **B,** Two heavy, nonabsorbable Bunnel sutures are placed in the end of the tendon. **C,** A blunt instrument is introduced in the tract of the biceps tendon, and the skin is indented on the volar aspect of the proximal forearm. An incision is made over this instrument. **D,** The common extensor and supinator muscles are then split to expose the radial tuberosity. The ulna is not exposed. Full pronation of the forearm brings the tuberosity into the field. **E,** The radial tuberosity is excavated using a high-speed bur and the biceps tendon is brought through its previous tract and reinserted into the radial tuberosity with the 2 nonasorbable sutures. (Reproduced with permission from the Mayo Foundation, Rochester, MN.)

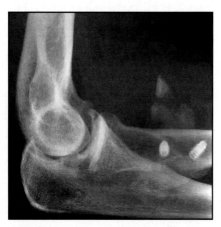

Fig. 5 Ectopic ossification associated with use of suture anchors.(Reproduced with permission from the Mayo Foundation, Rochester, MN.)

the biceps tendon, which then required reattachment into the tuberosity (Fig. 7). A good result may be anticipated but the rehabilitation must begin anew. If a bridge is excised, irradiation with 700 cGy may be administered but my experience shows that there is little tendency for recurrence of the ectopic bone.

Recurrence of the avulsion is rarely reported. There is 1 such case in a paralytic man using his arms for transfer and local motion less than 2 months after repair.

Once again, the development of proximal radioulnar synostosis is thought to be associated with exposing the periosteum of the lateral ulna, and can be avoided or at least mini-

mized with a muscle-splitting incision.[28] There is no attempt to expose the ulna. This approach allows adequate exploration of the tuberosity, reliable reattachment of the tendon, and no significant limitation of motion; it continues to be the treatment of choice.[28]

Because of the emergence of the popular suture anchor technique through an anterior approach, over 70 cases treated at the Mayo Clinic have been reviewed. Of these, 70% were treated as described above, with 2 incisions. Only 4 had a minimal amount of ectopic bone or calcification localized in the tendon and not limiting motion. Of the 9 treated with an anterior exposure and secured to the tuberosity, 2 had transient paresthesias of the radial nerve and 1 developed a small amount of ectopic bone with no consequences on motion.

Author's Preferred Treatment Method

If the diagnosis of disruption of the distal biceps tendon is made within the first 7 to 10 days after injury, reattachment to the radial tuberosity using the 2-incision technique is recommended. I have reservations about the initial strength of the suture anchors that would permit early motion.

Late Reconstruction

The individual needs of the patient and the goals of any late surgical procedure must be carefully balanced. If the patient's occupation and residual strength do not require improvement of supination strength, simple reinsertion into the brachialis muscle is performed. Although rarely indicated, this surgical procedure is easy, improves flexion strength, and is essentially free of complications. Postoperative rehabilitation is similar to that previously described except that no limitation is placed on pronation and supination in the early postoperative course.

If, after careful discussion with the patient, improved supination strength is found to be required, several reconstruction methods have been reported. A fascia lata graft has been described by Hovelius and Josefsson.[32] Others have used a free autogenous semitendinous tendon. If the tendon is retracted and shortened, which is typical, some form of breech augmentation is required. Although results were favorable, the LAD™ has been abandoned in favor of an autologous Achilles tendon graft; this tissue is ideally suited for this reconstruction. The fleck of cal-

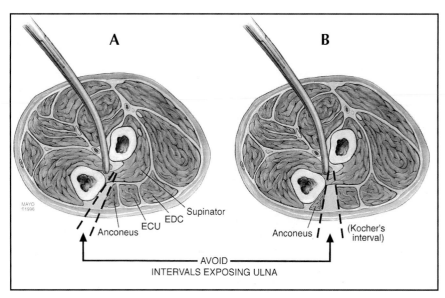

Fig. 6 The curved hemostat passes close to the radius and past the tuberosity, avoiding the ulna (**A**). Curving the instrument toward the ulna is to be avoided (**B**). (Reproduced with permission from the Mayo Foundation, Rochester, MN.)

caneus bone is trimmed and embedded into excavated radial tuberosity. Then with the elbow flexed 45° to 60°, the Achilles fascia is draped over the biceps muscle and the bone tendon stump is sewn into the muscle. This method offers a very gratifying reconstruction and allows a more aggressive rehabilitation program.

Partial (Incomplete) Distal Biceps Rupture

Partial rupture of the distal biceps tendon has been reported since the first volume of this book and has been increasingly recognized since then. Nielsen[33] documented a case in which the lacertus fibrosus was thought to have initially ruptured with a secondary elongation of the biceps tendon. Chevallier[22] reported a biceps tendon rupture with secondary stretch of the lacertus fibrosus. My experience suggests that first, a partial rupture of the biceps tendon occurs and the second episode of pain completes the rupture (Fig. 8). A secondary stretch or disruption of

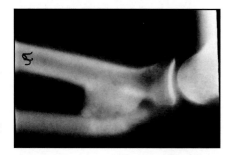

Fig. 7 Ectopic bone resulted from reattachment of an avulsed right biceps tendon to the radial tuberosity using the 2-incision technique of Boyd and Anderson, during which the ulna was exposed. (Reproduced with permission from the Mayo Foundation, Rochester, MN.)

the lacertus fibrosis may occur later.

Diagnosis of partial or impending rupture of the biceps tendon is not easy. The history of forced eccentric contracture is typical and overuse may have preceded this event. Pain subsides, but not completely. Weakness and fatigue are prominent and crepitus with forearm rotation is common. Distinction from bicipital tubercle bursitis may be difficult, especially because the 2 conditions

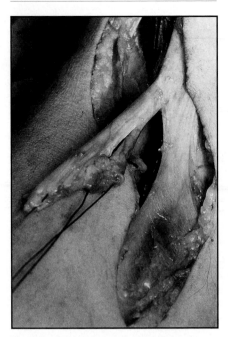

Fig. 8 Surgical photograph showing some fibers of the biceps tendon detached and retracted (lax suture), while others had remained in continuity (taut surface). Note that the lacertus fibrosus is stretched. (Reproduced with permission from the Mayo Foundation, Rochester, MN.)

may coexist. One of the 2 patients with cubital bursitis reported by Karanjia and Stiles[34] was a woman who was noted at surgery to have a distal biceps tendon degeneration in association with the bursitis. It is possible that the cubital bursitis was a reaction to the partial rupture. I have observed this finding in 1 patient in whom the initial exploration through a Henry approach revealed extensive "bursitis;" only after a careful inspection of the biceps tendon was it noted that a 50% disruption had occurred.[10]

The treatment of the partial tendon rupture may best be understood by considering the pathology of a degenerative tendon. Reimplantation of the remaining portion of the tendon to the radial tuberosity does not reliably relieve pain.[3] Complete removal of the remaining fibers, converting the

problem to a complete tear, trimming of the distal tendon, and then reattachment as if this were an acute event is the treatment of choice.

References

1. Anzel SH, Covey KW, Weiner AD, Lipscomb PR: Disruption of muscles and tendons: An analysis of 1,014 cases. *Surgery* 1959;45:406–414.

2. Brickner WM, Milch H: Ruptures of muscles and tendons. *Int Clin* 1928;2:94–107.

3. Conwell HE, Alldredge RH: Ruptures and tears of muscles and tendons. *Am J Surg* 1937;35:22–33.

4. Haldeman KO, Soto-Hall R: Injuries to muscles and tendons. *JAMA* 1935;104:2319–2324.

5. Waugh RL, Hathcock TA, Elliott JL: Ruptures of muscles and tendons: With particular reference to rupture (or elongation of long tendon) of biceps brachii with report of fifty cases. *Surgery* 1949;25:370–392.

6. Dobbie RP: Avulsion of the lower biceps brachii tendon: Analysis of fifty-one previously unreported cases. *Am J Surg* 1941;51:662–683.

7. Giugiaro A, Proscia N: Rupture of the distal tendon and of the short head of brachial biceps. *Minerva Orthop* 1957;8:57–65.

8. Agins HJ, Chess JL, Hoekstra DV, Teitge RA: Rupture of the distal insertion of the biceps brachii tendon. *Clin Orthop* 1988;234:34–38.

9. Baker BE, Bierwagen D: Rupture of the distal tendon of the biceps brachii: Operative versus non-operative treatment. *J Bone Joint Surg* 1985;67A:414–417.

10. Bourne MH, Morrey BF: Partial rupture of the distal biceps tendon. *Clin Orthop* 1991;271:143–148.

11. Hang DW, Bach BR Jr, Bojchuk J: Repair of chronic distal biceps brachii tendon rupture using free autogenous semitendinosus tendon. *Clin Orthop* 1996;323:188–191.

12. Leighton MM, Bush-Joseph CA, Bach BR Jr: Distal biceps brachii repair: Results in dominant and nondominant extremities. *Clin Orthop* 1995;317:114–121.

13. Le Huec JC, Moinard M, Liquois F, Zipoli B, Chauveaux D, Le Rebeller A: Distal rupture of the tendon of biceps brachii: Evaluation by MRI and the results of repair. *J Bone Joint Surg* 1996;78B:767–770.

14. Louis DS, Hankin FM, Eckenrode JF, Smith PA, Wojtys EM: Distal biceps brachii tendon avulsion: A simplified method of operative repair. *Am J Sports Med* 1986;14:234–236.

15. Strauch RJ, Michelson H, Rosenwasser MP: Repair of rupture of the distal tendon of the biceps brachii: Review of the literature and report of three cases treated with a single anterior incision and suture anchors. *Am J Orthop* 1997;26:151–156.

16. Bauman GI: Rupture of the biceps tendon. *J Bone Joint Surg* 1934;16:966–967.

17. Postacchini F, Puddu G: Subcutaneous rupture of the distal biceps brachii tendon: A report on seven cases. *J Sports Med Phys Fitness* 1975;15:81–90.

18. Baker BE: Operative vs. non-operative treatment of disruption of the distal tendon of biceps. *Orthop Rev* 1982;11:71.

19. Morrey BF, Askew LJ, An KN, Dobyns JH: Rupture of the distal tendon of the biceps brachii: A biomechanical study. *J Bone Joint Surg* 1985;67A:418–421.

20. Davis WM, Yassine Z: An etiological factor in tear of the distal tendon of the biceps brachii: Report of two cases. *J Bone Joint Surg* 1956;38A:1365–1368.

21. Seiler JG III, Parker LM, Chamberland PD, Sherbourne GM, Carpenter WA: The distal biceps tendon: Two potential mechanisms involved in its rupture. Arterial supply and mechanical impingement. *J Shoulder Elbow Surg* 1995;4:149–156.

22. Chevallier CH: Sur un cas de desinsertion du tendon bicipital inferieur. *Mem Acad Chir* 1953;79:137–139.

23. Jaslow IA, May VR: Avulsion of the distal tendon of the biceps brachii muscle. *Guthrie Clin Bull* 1946;15:124.

24. Lee HG: Traumatic avulsion of tendon of insertion of biceps brachii. *Am J Surg* 1951;82:290–292.

25. Boyd HB, Anderson LD: A method for reinsertion of the distal biceps brachii tendon. *J Bone Joint Surg* 1961;43A:1041–1043.

26. Norman WH: Repair of avulsion of insertion of biceps brachii tendon. *Clin Orthop* 1985;193:189–194.

27. Tendon injuries about the elbow, in Morrey BF (ed): *The Elbow and Its Disorders*, ed 2. Philadelphia, PA, WB Saunders, 1993, pp 492–504.

28. Failla JM, Amadio PC, Morrey BF, Beckenbaugh RD: Proximal radioulnar synostosis after repair of distal biceps brachii rupture by the two-incision technique: Report of four cases. *Clin Orthop* 1990;253:133–136.

29. Meherin JM, Kilgore ES Jr: The treatment of ruptures of the distal biceps brachii tendon. *Am J Surg* 1960;99:636–640.

30. Katzman BM, Caligiuri DA, Klein DM, Gorup JM: Delayed onset of posterior interosseous nerve palsy after distal biceps tendon repair. *J Shoulder Elbow Surg* 1997;6:393–395.

31. Failla JM, Amadio PC, Morrey BF: Post-traumatic proximal radio-ulnar synostosis: Results of surgical treatment. *J Bone Joint Surg* 1989;71A:1208–1213.

32. Hovelius L, Josefsson G: Rupture of the distal biceps tendon. *Acta Orthop Scand* 1997;48:280–285.

33. Nielsen K: Partial rupture of the distal biceps brachii tendon: A case report. *Acta Orthop Scand* 1987;58:287–288.

34. Karanjia ND, Stiles PJ: Cubital bursitis. *J Bone Joint Surg* 1988;70B:832–837.

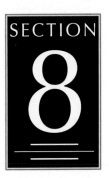

SECTION 8

Spine

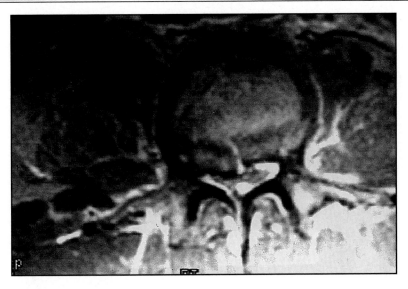

Nonsurgical Treatment of Thoracic and Lumbar Fractures

Glenn R. Rechtine, MD

Introduction

The treatment of thoracic and lumbar fractures remains as controversial as it has been over the past 50 years. Surgical and nonsurgical treatment have had their advocates with successful series in both.[1–9] There are advantages and disadvantages with each. The assumption has been that nonsurgical treatment is plagued with problems, such as pneumonia, pulmonary problems, venostasis, pulmonary emboli, late deformity, late neurologic compromise, and other complications, related to the prolonged immobilization. Over the past 25 years, with the development of more sophisticated spinal instrumentation, surgical techniques have become much more prevalent. The hypothesis is that anatomic restoration of spinal alignment and spinal canal reconstruction would result in a better functional outcome for the patient. The actual results from these techniques have not been nearly as conclusive as the initial hypothesis.

The initial treatment of any spinal injury is adequate immobilization. Once a spinal injury is suspected the patient should be immobilized. In the field, this should be done initially with extraction equipment and a spine board. On the patient's arrival at the treatment facility, the patient's hemodynamic stability and other injuries need to be evaluated and addressed. There is a high incidence of multiple

level injuries; the identification of one is the key to look for others. In a study by Henderson and associates[10] of 508 patients with spinal injuries, 15% of patients had multiple noncontiguous spinal injuries. Once the spinal injury has been identified on plain radiograph, it is prudent to follow this up with a computed tomography (CT) scan to also determine the extent of the spinal injury. A plain radiograph is not necessarily accurate in determining whether the fracture involves the middle column or creates an instability.[11] Some injuries are much more common and certain spinal injuries carry a high incidence of associated injuries. Chance-type fractures have a high association with intra-abdominal injuries. Low lumbar burst fractures are associated with high-energy injuries and are usually associated with multiple trauma as well. There is also a high association between spinal injuries and sacral and pelvic fractures. Twenty-six percent of sacral fractures will have an associated spinal fracture and almost 8% of pelvic fractures will have an associated spinal fracture.[12] When a sacral or pelvic fracture is identified, attention should be directed toward the spine, to look for an injury there as well.

The complicated biomechanics and pathophysiology of spine trauma and spinal cord injury contribute to the difficulty in being able to draw conclusions as to the most effective

treatment for these injuries. Panjabi and associates[13] pointed out in an in vitro study that the injury itself is a dynamic situation. The maximum canal compromise was 85% greater than the residual at the time the patient would have arrived for treatment at the hospital.[13] This information helps to explain papers that have reported no association between spinal canal narrowing and neurologic deficits or decompressions with neurologic recovery.[14,15] At the time of the injury, the spinal canal is markedly compromised and may already be relatively decompressed. The spinal cord injury occurred at the time of the impact.

One argument for surgical treatment is that the spinal canal must be decompressed in patients with marked canal compromise even if they are neurologically intact. The concern is that these patients will develop spinal stenosis symptoms in the future; however, they do not do so in reality. There are only rare reports of spinal stenosis symptoms developing in the future, probably because spinal canal compromise remodels spontaneously over time through an expression of Wolfe's Law.[8,16,17]

Methods of Treatment
Bracing

Bracing is one of the oldest treatment methods available. Biomechanical in vitro testing shows that an orthosis will accommodate for approximately 50% loss of stiffness at 1 level and 25% at 2 levels.[7] Cantor and associates[1] reported excellent results in a series of 33 patients who had no ligamentous injury and no neurologic deficit and were treated with bracing. Most patients were discharged within a week to 10 days after their injury.[1]

Nonsurgical Treatment of Patients Without Neurologic Deficit

There are several series in which bed rest and nonsurgical treatment were used for patients with spinal injuries. Weinstein and associates[9] presented a series of 42 patients with no neurologic deficits; at a 20-year follow-up, 2 of these patients had subsequent late surgery. In a series of 34 patients with spinal cord injuries treated nonsurgically, Davies and associates[2] reported complications of 2 pulmonary emboli and no deaths. There was no discussion as to deep venous thrombosis prophylaxis. In another report, Chan and associates[18] showed excellent results in patients treated with a combination of casts and bed rest.

Bone Remodeling

In a series of 41 neurologically intact patients, two thirds of the retropulsed bone resorbed at long-term follow-up. These data again are a reflection of bone stress and stress shielding; once the bone is no longer loaded it is resorbed.[6]

Nonsurgical Treatment of Patients With Neurologic Defects

Sandor and Barabas[8] showed that a patient with as much as 93% canal compromise resorbed the spinal canal over time with nonsurgical treatment. In a series of 63 patients with neurologic deficits, Dendrinos and associates[3] showed that there was no correlation of the neurologic deficit with canal compromise or resolution of

the deficit with decompression. In Kinoshita and associates'[5] study of 23 patients, 13 of whom had neurologic deficits, there was only 1 late surgery for progressive kyphosis. In my series of 32 patients, 12 had neurologic deficits: 3 complete and 9 incomplete. The incomplete neurologic deficits all improved at least 1 Frankel grade. The complications were 1 heel ulcer and 1 deep venous thrombosis. These did not prolong the hospitalization.

In determining which patients are candidates for nonsurgical treatment, an accurate assessment of the injury is critical. Ligamentous injuries are not candidates for nonsurgical treatment because there is a low likelihood that the ligamentous injury will heal over time. The greater the bony injury, the more likely the patient will do well with nonsurgical treatment. Multiple level injuries, particularly noncontiguous injuries, are a very good indication for nonsurgical treatment. Surgical stabilization would require immobilization of large portions of the patient's spinal column. This is particularly important when dealing with lumbar fractures where residual motion is more important.

Types of Injuries

Spinal injuries can be divided into 3 different groups because they have different characteristics both biomechanically and neurologically. Upper thoracic fractures occurring from T1 to T9-10 have the stability of the ribs, and the blood supply to the spinal cord is poor. These 2 factors combined mean that the patient is usually neurologically intact or has sustained complete neurologic injury because the stability has been overcome and the thoracic spinal cord has not withstood the high-energy injury that took place. Patients who are intact or have complete injuries are excellent candidates for nonsurgical treatment.

The thoracolumbar junction (T10 to L2) is the most common level for trauma. This is a reflection biomechanically of the junction between the stiff thoracic spine and the mobile lumbar spine. This area has the potential for any combination of neurologic injury. The neurologic injury is a combined upper motor neuron lesion and lower motor neuron lesion with injury to the conus and the cauda equina. These patients may be candidates for nonsurgical treatment because stabilization at this area, involving short-segment fixation, has a significant failure rate as a result of the high stresses involved, and using longer segment fixation will reduce significant amounts of lumbar motion.

Low lumbar fractures from L3 to L5 tend to be different both biomechanically and physiologically. These tend to be high-energy injuries, and the neurologic injury is a cauda equina injury or a lower motor neuron injury. Mick and associates[19] point out that patients with neurologic deficits and L5 fractures have more predictable results with surgery, but this is such a small series this conclusion may not be valid.

Ligamentous lumbosacral dislocations are relatively uncommon. There is a case report of 1 being reduced and treated nonsurgically, but the consensus is that this injury is best reduced open and stabilized surgically.[20] The comminuted bony injury can be treated nonsurgically.

Plan of Treatment

The protocol for nonsurgical treatment that I have used over the past 10 years includes the use of a kinetic bed with the patient rotating 40° each direction continuously. The patient must be rotating at least 6 of every 8 hours. Deep venous thrombosis prophylaxis is carried out with compression stockings and sequential compression devices. The patient is started on an active exercise program using rubber bands and weights as soon as the medical condition will allow. If the patient had other fractures and other injuries, he or she may be placed on a continuous passive motion device while on the kinetic bed. Each hatch on the kinetic bed is opened each nursing shift and the skin is inspected and massaged.

Using this protocol, the experience in Tampa now extends over 10 years. One hundred fifty patients have been treated with long-term bed rest on the kinetic bed. I also have reviewed 120 patients who were treated surgically within the same time period. The groups are comparable in age, with the average age of 32 to 33 years. There is a 70% male population, as is common with trauma. The fracture patterns are similar with slightly more burst fractures in the surgical group. There were 21% multiple-level spinal injuries with 9% noncontiguous spinal injuries. There were more complete spinal cord injuries in the nonsurgical group and more incomplete injuries in the surgically treated group. The multiple system trauma was comparable. Complications totaled 32% in the surgical group and 22% in the nonsurgical group. The difference was the 9% infection rate. Mortality was 3.3% in the surgical group and 2% in the nonsurgical group. One of the 2 fatalities in the nonsurgical group was a patient who was actually scheduled for surgery on several occasions but never stabilized medically from the time of his initial hospitalization to be a candidate for surgical treatment. The other fatality was due to a pulmonary embolus in a paraplegic patient that occurred 2 ½ weeks into his hospitalization. It is also of note that the patient had a negative color Doppler within 48 hours

prior to his fatal pulmonary embolus. Decubiti are associated with prolonged immobilization on a back board. The length of stay was longer in the nonsurgical group (41 versus 25 days) as would be expected, but in a previous study we were able to demonstrate that the overall cost was not significantly different. Without costs for surgeries and anesthesiologists, complications, and rehospitalization, the cost difference in billings is $13,000.

The key to nonsurgical treatment is an aggressive treatment plan. This is not as simple as placing the patient in a bed and ignoring him or her for 6 weeks. Some sort of kinetic bed must be used for effective immobilization. The nursing staff must be familiar with the bed and familiar with the treatment plan in order to be able to maximize the patient's eventual outcome. The patient should be exercising as early as the first injury day if possible. I am trying to avoid not only the complications of venostasis and pulmonary emboli, but also to eliminate the decreased muscle tone and muscle loss from prolonged immobilization. The patient should also have deep venous thrombosis prophylaxis with sequential compression devices and thromboembolic disease stockings, and each individual institution can decide about future prophylaxis with anticoagulation. In the initial postinjury period, anticoagulation is contraindicated for fear of creating an epidural hemaotoma.

Conclusion

The main indication for surgical treatment in a patient with a thoracic or lumbar spine injury would be to mobilize the patient sooner. This mobilization saves the patient approximately 2 weeks in acute hospitalization. The patient with a spinal cord injury will start rehabilitation

sooner. The price paid is increased mortality and morbidity, the most significant of which is an infection rate that in various series can vary anywhere from 7% to 15%. In my particular setting this rate has been approximately 9%. In my experience, which is also consistent with that of the literature, several myths associated with thoracic and lumbar trauma have evolved over time.

Myth Number 1

Any patient with a neurologic deficit requires surgical treatment. As I have already pointed out, complete injuries may be mobilized sooner but with the cost of higher complications and infection. Incomplete neurologic injuries tend to improve even with nonsurgical treatment, and if they do not improve with nonsurgical treatment, surgical treatment can be carried out at a later date with the ability to obtain similar end results.

Myth Number 2

Greater than a 50% compression of the vertebral height requires surgical restoration. To my knowledge, there has never been a study to substantiate this. Patients with multiple-level compression fractures, as long as they have been adequately immobilized and treated nonsurgically, do as well or better than those surgically treated.

Myth Number 3

Forty percent canal compromise requires surgery. This again cannot be justified in and of itself. Spinal canal compromise will resolve spontaneously over time and if the patient is asymptomatic, it is very difficult to improve that situation.

Myth Number 4

Multiple spinal fractures require surgery. Just the opposite is true. The more injuries there are, the most likely the patient should be treated nonsurgically and that the surgical stabilization would take away too much spinal motion because of the long levels of fusion required.

Myth Number 5

Nonsurgical treatment should not be used because of the increased incidence of deep venous thrombosis and pulmonary emboli. In actuality, as long as the nonsurgical treatment is done aggressively with prophylaxis, I found either the same or lower incidence in the group treated nonsurgically as in the group treated surgically.

Myth Number 6

Nonsurgical treatment should not be used because of the higher complication rates. In actuality, I have found that the complication rates and particularly significant morbidity and mortality are much lower with nonsurgical treatment.

Myth Number 7

There was less pain long term if the spine was surgically stabilized. We found this to be just the opposite. In fact, there was more pain in the groups that had fusions. There were also more patients who required late surgery in the group initially treated with surgery than in the group initially treated nonsurgically. Most of the instrumentation was removed either by protocol or rod-long and fuse short techniques.

Myth Number 8

There is better neurologic recovery with surgery. This was not substantiated in our series or in other series.[4]

Myth Number 9

Canal compromise correlates with neurologic deficits. Again, this is not true as evidenced by several studies already discussed.

Myth Number 10

Neurologic recovery correlates with spinal canal decompression. This again has been shown in several studies not to be the case. As was pointed out, it is probably biomechanically related to the fact that a great deal of the neurologic picture is determined at the time of the injury, both by the maximum canal compromise that takes place at the time of impact and by the speed of loading and the energy applied. Patients with incomplete injuries that have been stabilized can be decompressed electively.

Summary

The treatment of thoracolumbar trauma remains controversial. As more and more data are collected, there appears to be information that substantiates both surgical and nonsurgical treatment. Orthopaedic surgeons must all be cognizant of the fact that we draw our conclusions from data and not subjective prejudicial opinions. Nonsurgical treatment is still a viable and effective treatment for thoracic and lumbar fractures and should be part of the armamentarium available to all practitioners involved in the treatment of these patients.

References

1. Cantor JB, Lebwohl NH, Garvey T, Eismont FJ: Nonoperative management of stable thoracolumbar burst fractures with early ambulation and bracing. *Spine* 1993;18:971–976.

2. Davies WE, Morris JH, Hill V: An analysis of conservative (non-surgical) management of thoracolumbar fractures and fracture-dislocations with neural damage. *J Bone Joint Surg* 1980;62A:1324–1328.

3. Dendrinos GK, Halikias JG, Krallis PN, Asimakopoulos A: Factors influencing neurological recovery in burst thoracolumbar fractures. *Acta Orthop Belg* 1995;61:226–234.

4. Hartman MB, Chrin AM, Rechtine GR: Nonoperative treatment of thoracolumbar fractures. *Paraplegia* 1995;33:73–76.

5. Kinoshita H, Nagata Y, Ueda H, Kishi K: Conservative treatment of burst fractures of the thoracolumbar and lumbar spine. *Paraplegia* 1993;31:58–67.

6. Mumford J, Weinstein JN, Spratt KF, Goel VK: Thoracolumbar burst fractures: The clinical efficacy and outcome of nonoperative management. *Spine* 1993;18:955–970.

7. Patwardhan AG, Li SP, Gavin T, Lorenz M, Meade KP, Zindrick M: Orthotic stabilization of thoracolumbar injuries: A biomechanical analysis of the Jewett hyperextension orthosis. *Spine* 1990;15:654–661.

8. Sandor L, Barabas D: Spontaneous "regeneration" of the spinal canal in traumatic bone fragments after fractures of the thoraco-lumbar transition and the lumbar spine. *Unfallchirurg* 1994;97:89–91.

9. Weinstein JN, Collalto P, Lehmann TR: Thoracolumbar "burst" fractures treated conservatively: A long-term follow-up. *Spine* 1988;13:33–38.

10. Henderson RL, Reid DC, Saboe LA: Multiple noncontiguous spine fractures. *Spine* 1991;16:128–131.

11. Ballock RT, Mackersie R, Abitbol JJ, Cervilla V, Resnick D, Garfin SR: Can burst fractures be predicted from plain radiographs? *J Bone Joint Surg* 1992;74B:147–150.

12. Albert TJ, Levine MJ, An HS, Cotler JM, Balderston RA: Concomitant noncontiguous thoracolumbar and sacral fractures. *Spine* 1993;18:1285–1291.

13. Panjabi MM, Kifune M, Wen L, et al: Dynamic canal encroachment during thoracolumbar burst fractures. *J Spinal Disord* 1995;8:39–48.

14. Lemons VR, Wagner FC Jr, Montesano PX: Management of thoracolumbar fractures with accompanying neurological injury. *Neurosurgery* 1992;30:667–671.

15. Shuman WP, Rogers JV, Sickler ME, et al: Thoracolumbar burst fractures: CT dimensions of the spinal canal relative to postsurgical improvement. *Am J Neuroradiol* 1985;6:337–341.

16. Chakera TM, Bedbrook G, Bradley CM: Spontaneous resolution of spinal canal deformity after burst-dispersion fracture. *Am J Neuroradiol* 1988;9:779–785.

17. Yazici M, Atilla B, Tepe S, Calisir A: Spinal canal remodeling in burst fractures of the thoracolumbar spine: A computerized tomographic comparison between operative and nonoperative treatment. *J Spinal Disord* 1996;9:409–413.

18. Chan DP, Seng NK, Kaan KT: Nonoperative treatment in burst fractures of the lumbar spine (L2–L5) without neurologic deficits. *Spine* 1993;18:320–325.

19. Mick CA, Carl A, Sachs B, Hresko MT, Pfeifer BA: Burst fractures of the fifth lumbar vertebra. *Spine* 1993;18:1878–1884.

20. Boyd MC, Yu WY: Closed reduction of lumbosacral fracture dislocations. *Surg Neurol* 1985;23:295–298.

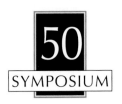

50

SYMPOSIUM

Measuring Outcomes in Cervical Myelopathy and Radiculopathy

Steven C. Ludwig, MD
Todd J. Albert, MD

Introduction

Patient-based outcome assessment for cervical myelopathy and radiculopathy has not been extensively used or reported. Currently, due to the prevalence of cervical disease and the amount of today's health-care resources used to evaluate and treat degenerative spinal disorders, the importance of outcome analysis becomes apparent.

It is intuitive that quality of life is important to patients. The influence of surgical procedures on quality of life are now being measured in patients undergoing total hip arthroplasty, coronary artery bypass, and prostate surgery, and orthopaedic spine surgeons have begun to approach patients with cervical spine disorders with similar outcome tools.[1] With regard to other spinal procedures, Albert and associates[2,3] have already demonstrated the value of applying outcome analysis to lumbar laminectomy and adult scoliosis surgery.

Currently, orthopaedic and spinal surgeons debate the correct surgical options for the treatment of cervical radiculopathy and/or myelopathy. For example, in a patient with a symptomatic cervical soft-disk herniation, a review of the literature indicates that a variety of different surgical techniques have shown similar successful results. Henderson and associates[4] reported a 96% resolution of radicular symptoms with a 91.5% good/excellent result when performing a posterior laminoforaminotomy. Similarly, Rothman and Simeone[5] reported a 96% success rate in 50 patients undergoing a posterior laminoforaminotomy. On the other hand, other authors have reported good/excellent results in 74% to 90% of patients undergoing anterior cervical decompression and fusion.[5-7] What becomes apparent after reviewing the literature is that controversy remains regarding the best treatment approach for patients with cervical radiculopathy and myelopathy, yet none of these series measures the patients' outcome as they (the patients) perceive it. Furthermore, most authors have used diverse measurements based on the surgeon's judgment.

BenDebba and associates[8] evaluated the relationship between physician-expected treatment outcome and actual outcome in patients with neck pain. Patients completed initial evaluation forms containing questions concerning pain severity, work-related activities, social/recreational activities, and treatment history. The treating physician then completed a questionnaire regarding patient clinical presentation, radiographic findings, and prescribed treatment in addition to predicting how the patients' pain, work-related activities, and social/recreational activities would change in 6 months. At 6 months the patients were contacted by telephone. Out of 503 patients, 195 presented with axial neck pain, 246 with radiculopathy, and 62 with myelopathy. Physicians prescribed conservative management for 69%, surgical intervention for 25%, and no treatment for 6%. Physicians predicted substantial improvement in pain for the majority of patients for whom they prescribed surgery, moderate improvement for the majority of patients for whom they prescribed conservative treatments, and no change for the majority of patients for whom they prescribed no treatment. Expectations for work-related activities were essentially the same but were less optimistic, while the expectations for social and recreational activities were even more conservative. No relationship was found between physician-expected outcomes and actual patient reported outcomes for pain, work-related activities, and social/recreational activities. The authors concluded that physicians were unable to predict outcome for individual patients.[8] In the past, emphasis was placed by the orthopaedist on objective criteria in order to judge the success of a surgical intervention. In addition, subjective data have been felt by many surgeons to be inadequate for research evaluations. Presently, in order to determine the success of a surgical intervention, outcome analyses that are reproducible and scientifically valid are required.

In light of the emerging changes in our health-care system, analysis of surgical outcomes may serve as a basis for future health-care policy and resource management.[9,10] Thus, with all of these considerations, the impetus for the initiation of patient-oriented outcome research becomes apparent.

What is Health Outcome Measurement?

In 1947, the World Health Organization introduced a broadened definition of health as "a state of complete physical, mental, and social well-being and not merely the absence of a disease."[11] Despite the lack of conceptual agreement, quality of life variables in outcome analysis have assumed ever increasing importance in 20th century medicine, especially in the assessment of patients with chronic disease. Outcomes research has defined outcomes in terms of patient function, well-being, satisfaction, and clinical changes resulting from medical and or surgical interventions.

Quality of life is a multidimensional concept with a variety of approaches to its measurement. It is generally agreed that health-related quality of life should assess function, including physical, psychological, social, and occupational functioning.

Quality of life following surgery is just beginning to receive attention in the orthopaedic literature.[2,3,9,12] Traditionally, quality of life issues were considered to be of secondary importance in comparison to such factors as mortality, morbidity, and bone healing and other radiographic variables. Recent interest in quality of life most likely stems from a changing pattern in the understanding of surgical diseases, the evolution of state-of-the-art surgical procedures, and the change in our health-care economy.

Why Should We Measure Health Status?

The current view of outcome assessment in orthopaedic surgery addresses a myriad of different areas. These include: assessing the quality of life, the comparison of different treatment options, monitoring and improving the quality of care, aiding in the selection of surgical candidates, aiding in policy decision-making and resource allocation, and describing the functional and psychological problems faced by the orthopaedic patient.

Recognition of changes in the pattern of surgical diseases and the subsequent development of newer techniques have necessitated the rigorous analysis of surgical outcomes. Measuring disease-specific outcomes may be important in demonstrating the efficacy of a particular procedure and may assist both patients and health-care providers in deciding between different treatment options. However, if the measurements used are only relevant for a specific disease, they are not generalizable to other populations or disease entities. It is therefore crucial to use patient-based outcome measurement to scrutinize the evolution of a new surgical technique developed for the purpose of improving the quality of life. Moreover, performing outcomes analysis may serve as a basis for the selection of the proper surgical candidate in addition to improving the timing of a therapeutic intervention. Last, these outcomes can be compared to outcomes of other disease interventions and procedures if generic metrics are used.

Why is Outcome Measurement So Important Now?

The answer to this question is multifactorial. Currently, the government and third-party payors are beginning to realize our lack of consensus regarding specific surgical interventions and their results. There is also a competitiveness of organized health care and the need for payers of health care to get the best value for their money from a medical treatment. In addition, some surgical techniques may lack a scientific basis and therefore need to be justified. What is also important to realize is that specific surgical outcomes should be individually measured. For instance, because each patient's experiences, ambitions, and plans are unique, some elements of outcome will be more important for some patients following surgical intervention than for others.[13]

If appropriately used, outcomes research should help answer questions of appropriateness of care in order to give patients the best treatment available and give them the best outcome regardless of cost. Outcomes research can also aid in allocating health-care resources in the most effective manner and in decreasing geographic variability in treatment rates and practice habits.

Health Status Instruments: Generic Versus Disease-Specific Instruments

Outcomes research was pioneered by the medical community. Outcome measures have evolved from generic health measurements that can be applied to multiple disease states or therapeutic interventions. Information that can be gathered includes demographic information, health risks, comorbidities, functional status, well-being, and satisfaction with provider services.[14] Numerous well-validated generic health profiles currently exist. In recent years, the Sickness Impact Profile (SIP),[14] the Nottingham Health Profile (NHP),[15] and the Short Form-36 item health survey (SF-36)[16,17] have been used as generic outcome measurement tools.

Disease-specific measures of outcome theoretically are more sensitive toward a particular disease entity. They may improve the sensitivity in detecting subtle changes in outcome due to intervention for a particular disease state. On the downside, disease-specific measures also prevent comparison of specific outcome measures between different disease states. Examples of disease-specific outcome measures include: the Neck Disability Index (neck pain),[18] the Oswestry Disability Index (low back pain),[19] and the Roland Disability Questionnaire (low back pain).[20]

Currently, there are a wide variety of conditions for which disease-specific instruments have not been developed. Moreover, it is thought that the generic health status instruments lack the ability to measure subtle changes related to a specific disease state. The "ceiling and floor" effects should encourage orthopaedic surgeons to develop disease-specific outcome measurement tools in order to determine whether a particular generic outcome instrument is appropriate for a disease state. The "ceiling effect" of a generic-based outcome study can be illustrated by an otherwise healthy young athlete, who, despite having a specific problem (ie, ACL tear) with a poor clinical outcome as based on a disease-specific outcome tool, may be shown by a generic health assessment instrument to have an inflated (ceiling effect) outcome score because of the lack of any significant comorbidities. As a corollary, the floor effect of a generic outcome tool can be illustrated in a patient who has multiple comorbidities, including severe degenerative joint disease of the hip requiring a total hip arthroplasty. Now despite a successful total hip replacement, which would be revealed on a disease-specific outcome measurement, the result of a generic health profile of this patient's outcome may be poor.

How Do We Judge/Select Outcome Instruments?

The surgical outcome instruments currently used must be assessed in order to determine their validity and sensitivity in detecting a patient's outcome following a specific therapeutic intervention. What is important to determine is if the outcome instrument truly measures what it is supposed to measure in specific disease states. Thus, a good outcome questionnaire should be reproducible. This is defined as the ability of the respondent to provide the same answers to the survey today and a week later, assuming there are no functional changes. Overall, the criteria surgeons should use in choosing the ideal outcomes instrument includes validity, reliability, sensitivity, practicality, cost effectiveness, and applicability to the presenting problem, along with consideration of patient comorbidities.

Is the instrument valid? Does the outcome instrument truly measure what we claim it measures? More importantly, does the health outcome tool make sense to informed observers, including both patient and physician?

Is the instrument reliable? In order for the instrument to maintain reliability, health-care outcome instruments must control for error. For example, the clinician should obtain consistent results on multiple readministrations of the instrument.

Is the instrument sensitive? In order for the health-care assessment to maintain sensitivity, it should retain the ability to detect changes in health within a group over time or with a surgical intervention.

Is the instrument practical (feasible)? How difficult is it for office personnel to administer to patients and to process? The form should not be too complex. The data should be devoid of errors as well as missed data (unanswered questions). Most importantly, standards should be derived from the normal population, so that assessments and comparisons to the disease state can be made.

Outcomes Instruments for Cervical Disorders

Disease-specific outcome instruments for cervical disorders include the Neck Disability Index (NDI), which is a modification of the Oswestry Low Back Disability Index. The NDI is a self-reporting instrument that assesses the impact of neck pain on activities of daily living.[18] This outcome assessment instrument is divided into 10 sections. It produces a 0 to 50 point score (0 = no disability; 50 = total disability). Alternatively, scores may be multiplied by 2, reporting life-style changes as percentage disability (0 to 100%).

Specific surgeon-driven measures of outcome for cervical disorders include the Odom criteria, which relate radicular pain and disability on a scale of excellent to poor.[21] Odom applied this criteria postoperatively to 175 patients who had surgery for symptomatic unilateral radiculopathy. The group with excellent results were those patients who had no complaints referable to cervical disease, and who were able to carry on their daily occupations without impairment. A good result included those patients who had intermittent discomfort that was related to cervical disease but that did not significantly interfere with their work. A satisfactory result included those who had subjective improvement but whose physical activities were significantly limited. Last, a poor result included those who did not improve or were worse as compared with their condition before their surgery.

The Nurick Criteria measures disability in patients who are myelopathic.[22] It grades disability on a scale of 0 to 5. Grade 0 is a patient with signs or symptoms of root involvement but with no evidence of spinal cord disease. Grade 1 patients have evidence of spinal cord disease but no difficulty in walking. Grade 2 is a patient who has slight difficulty in walking that does not prevent full-time employment or the ability to do daily tasks such as housework and is not severe enough to require help walking. Grade 3 patients have difficulty in walking that prevents full-time employment or the ability to do all housework, but that is not so severe as to require someone else's help to walk. Grade 4 patients can walk only with help or with a walker. Grade 5 patients have severe quadriparesis and are chairbound or bedridden.

The Japanese Orthopaedic Association Score for myelopathy measures function in activities of daily living.[23] This score, which has 17 total points, allots 3 points to subjective complaints related to bladder function and 8 points to motor function and sensation in the lower extremities and trunk. There are 4 separate categories based on upper extremity, lower extremity, sensory, and bladder function. Each category is allocated points based on severity of the myelopathic dysfunction.

For our patients with cervical radiculopathy and/or myelopathy, we are currently using the SF-36, which is a generic, self-administered health assessment instrument. It is separated into 9 domains[11] (Outline 1). The categories of the SF-36 provide an overall evaluation of health and an assessment of functional status and well-being. These domains include social and emotional aspects related to quality of life that are difficult to measure in clinical terms. Currently, it is accepted by the American Academy of Orthopaedic Surgeons as a valid outcome tool. Fortunately, the validity of all the categories of the SF-36 has already been reported.[24–27] Moreover, because the SF-36 has been applied to various diseases, it is therefore useful for comparative purposes. Data that exist comparing the results of the SF-36 tests with ratings for normal individuals of different age and sex groups allow us to compare patients with cervical radiculopathy/myelopathy with healthy individuals. Each domain of the SF-36 is scored on a scale of 0 to 100, with higher scores indicating a higher perception of quality of life within that domain.

The specific domains of the SF-36 are grouped within 3 areas of focus, including general health, functional status, and well-being. The one domain that reports on general health has scores (from low to high) indicating a range of perception from disabled/sickly to able/healthy. A low score indicates a perception of little likelihood of improvement from a poor health state; a high score indicates either a good-to-excellent health state or the anticipation of improvement. Functional status is measured by 4 domains that assess physical and social functioning and role performance. The 10 items in the physical functioning domain pro-

| Outline 1 |
| **Domains of the SF-36** |
| Physical function |
| Social function |
| Role function/physical |
| Role function/emotional |
| Mental health |
| Energy/fatigue |
| Pain |
| Health perception |
| Health change |

vide a score ranging from severe limitations in physical activities and activities of daily living to few limitations and the ability to function physically. Two items measure social functioning. This domain is assessed through social activities as limited by physical functioning. Physical role limitations and emotional and psychological role limitations measure perception of performance of work or role. The emotional and psychological aspects are included, in that functioning is related to emotional states and can be missed if not specifically measured. Well-being is a general reflection of the psychological and emotional state related to quality of life. In the mental health domain, anxiety and depressive symptoms are assessed. In addition, an overall life satisfaction question is included. The Likert scale used has been shown to be highly compatible with mental health when respondents are asked to state a feeling. Thus, the respondent is granted the opportunity to answer on a spectrum ranging from weak to strong feelings with respect to their degree of anxiety and depression in addition to their emotional control and attitude. The energy and fatigue domain are sensitive to the impact of disease and treatment on the mental health of the patient as reflected by a perception of energy. The Likert scale is also used for a range of responses to this feeling state. Lower scores reflect a diminished level of energy and possible sleep disturbances, resulting in fatigue. Bodily pain is another factor that contributes to limited functioning, but it is specific to the phenomena of pain, which has both physical and psychological components. Responses range on a 6-point scale, from no pain to very severe pain. The total score in this domain has a reverse interpretation from the other domains, in that the higher score means greater relief from bodily pain.

The SF-36 survey takes approximately 10 minutes to complete. Currently, we collect our SF-36 scores on all outpatients with cervical radiculopathy/myelopathy in the clinical office prior to their visit with a physician. In the future, newer methods of data collection through a computer-based network will be developed in order to facilitate, expedite, and improve data collection and analysis.

Conclusion

The need to assess surgical procedures in terms of their impact on overall outcome is of paramount importance. As the lay public's knowledge and interest in medicine continues to emerge, patients are beginning to participate more in surgical decision-making. Currently, when deciding about surgical intervention in patients with cervical radiculopathy/myelopathy, quality of life issues and long-term outcome may be of equal or even more importance than surgical complication rate or other surgeon-based outcome measures (ie, fusion). Therefore, application of a validated and reliable quality of life measure can produce dramatic evidence of the value of a surgical intervention in order to establish its societal value and role through its impact on patients' lives. It becomes apparent that in order to

appropriately select a health outcome instrument, we must determine its validity, reliability, sensitivity, and practicality. Moreover, it is imperative that the future reliability and validity testing of both generic and disease-specific health outcome assessments be undertaken with respect to cervical myelopathy and radiculopathy in order to determine their efficacy and utility. Last, with the current economic changes in our complex health-care system, assessing the "value for money" of a particular surgical procedure will depend on performing accurate outcome measures.

References

1. O'Boyle CA, McGee H, Hickey A, O'Malley K, Joyce CR: Individual quality of life in patients undergoing hip replacement. *Lancet* 1992;339:1088–1091.

2. Albert TJ, Purtill J, Mesa J, McIntosh T, Balderston RA: Health outcome assessment before and after adult deformity surgery: A prospective study. *Spine* 1995;20:2002–2004.

3. Albert TJ, Mesa JJ, Eng K, McIntosh TC, Balderston RA: Health outcome assessment before and after lumbar laminectomy for radiculopathy. *Spine* 1996;21:960–962.

4. Henderson CM, Hennessy RG, Shuey HM, Shackelford EG: Posterior/lateral foraminotomy as an exclusive operative technique for cervical radiculopathy: A review of 846 consecutively operated cases. *Neurosurgery* 1983;13:504.

5. Rothman RH, Simeone FA (eds): *The Spine*, ed 3. Philadelphia, PA, WB Saunders, 1992, p 608.

6. The Cervical Spine Research Society Editorial Committee (eds): Degenerative disorders, in *The Cervical Spine*, ed 2. Philadelphia, PA, JB Lippincott, 1989, pp 599–692.

7. Simpson JM, An HS (eds): *Surgery of Cervical Spine*. Baltimore, MD, Williams & Wilkins, 1994, pp 181–212.

8. BenDebba M, Long DL, Ducker T, Torgerson W: Physician-expected treatment outcome and actual outcome in patients treated for neck pain. *Orthop Trans* 1996;20:446–447.

9. Fossel AH, Roberts WN, Sledge CB: Cost-effectiveness of total joint arthroplasty in osteoarthritis. *Arthritis Rheum* 1986;29:937–943.

10. O'Boyle CA: Assessment of quality of life in surgery. *Br J Surg* 1992;79:395–398.

11. World Health Organization Constitution. *WHO Chronicle* 1947;1:29.

12. Kantz ME, Harris WJ, Levitsky K, Ware JE Jr, Davies AR: Methods for assessing condition-specific and generic functional status outcomes after total knee replacement. *Med Care* 1992;30(suppl):MS240–MS252.

13. Cohen C: On the quality of life: Some philosophical reflections. *Circulation* 1982;66:III29–III33.

14. Bergner M, Bobbitt RA, Carter WB, Gilson BS: The Sickness Impact Profile: Development and final revision of a health status measure. *Med Care* 1981;19:787–805.

15. Hunt SM, McEwen J, McKenna SP: The Nottingham health profile: User's manual, in Hunt SM, McEwen J, McKenna SP (eds): *Measuring Health Status*. London, England, Croom Helm, 1986, pp 246–283.

16. Stewart AL, Hays RD, Ware JE Jr: The MOS short-form general health survey: Reliability and validity in a patient population. *Med Care* 1988;26:724–735.

17. Ware JE Jr, Sherbourne CD: The MOS 36-item short-form health survey (SF-36): I. Conceptual framework and item selection. *Med Care* 1992;30:473–483.

18. Vernon H, Mior S: The Neck Disability Index: A study of reliability and validity. *J Manipulative Physiol Ther* 1991;14:409–415.

19. Fairbank JC, Couper J, Davies JB, O'Brien JP: The Oswestry low back pain disability questionnaire. *Physiotherapy* 1980;66:271–273.

20. Roland M, Morris R: A study of the natural history of back pain: Part I. Development of a reliable and sensitive measure of disability in low-back pain. *Spine* 1983;8:141–144.

21. Odom GL, Finney W, Woodhall B: Cervical disk lesions. *JAMA* 1958;166:23–28.

22. Nurick S: The pathogenesis of the spinal cord disorder associated with cervical spondylosis. *Brain* 1972;95:87–100.

23. Journal of the Japanese Association: Criteria on the evaluation of the treatment of cervical myelopathy. *J Jpn Orthop Assoc* 1976;50:5.

24. Brazier JE, Harper R, Jones NM, et al: Validating the SF-36 health survey questionnaire: New outcome measure for primary care. *BMJ* 1992;305:160–164.

25. Campbell A, Converse PE, Rodgers WL (eds): *The Quality of American Life: Perceptions, Evaluations and Satisfactions*. New York, NY, Russell Sage Foundation, 1976.

26. Diener E: Subjective well-being. *Psychol Bull* 1984;95:542–575.

27. Ellwood PM: Shattuck lecture: Outcomes management. A technology of patient experience. *N Engl J Med* 1988;318:1549–1556.

Surgical Management of Cervical Myelopathy

Sanford E. Emery, MD

The underlying cause of cervical myelopathy is spinal cord compression, usually resulting from herniated disks or cervical spondylosis. Other causes include ossification of the posterior longitudinal ligament, cervical kyphosis, and compensatory subluxation. Any of these factors can result in narrowing of the spinal canal and, in the case of kyphosis, draping of the spinal cord over the posterior aspect of the vertebrae and disks. The goals of surgical management of myelopathy are basically 3-fold: (1) to decompress the spinal cord, (2) to provide or maintain stability, and (3) to correct or maintain satisfactory alignment. The first goal is paramount, but the others play an important role, short term and long term, regarding neurologic and functional outcome.

Patients with symptoms and signs of cervical myelopathy should be fully evaluated with neuroradiologic studies to confirm the diagnosis and identify the exact pathology. Patients with mild myelopathy, ie, minimal gait or hand dysfunction and no significant neurologic deficits on examination, can be carefully observed over time. Some of these patients will remain stable, but in many the myelopathy will progress slowly, often in a stepwise fashion.[1,2] If functional or neurologic deterioration is noted and the patient's neuroradiologic studies show

definite cord compression, then surgical treatment is indicated. The choice of surgical procedure depends on the patient's pathoanatomy, as well as the surgeon's experience, taking into account the three goals of treatment outlined above.

Anterior Approach

Because cervical spondylosis or ossification of the posterior longitudinal ligament (OPLL) usually occurs at multiple levels, most patients with cervical myelopathy will have several levels of spinal cord compression. Appropriate surgical management necessitates removal of compression at all tight levels. If the compression is localized to the disk itself or the very edge of the end plate, then a Robinson-type anterior cervical diskectomy and fusion with tricortical iliac crest horseshoe-shaped grafts can be performed. Several millimeters of the end plate above or below the disk level can be removed (called a partial or hemicorpectomy) and a slightly larger Robinson-type graft used to provide satisfactory decompression and arthrodesis. With larger osteophytes, kyphosis, and particularly with OPLL, there is cord compression behind the vertebral bodies. This precludes decompression through the disk space alone. In order to adequately and safely decompress the spinal canal, corpec-

tomies are needed in these cases[3–6] (Fig. 1).

The technique of vertebral corpectomies involves the anterior approach, as in diskectomy and fusion procedures. The interval is between the trachea and esophagus, which are drawn medially, and the sternocleidomastoid and carotid sheath, which are drawn laterally. After carefully dissecting through the appropriate surgical planes, the anterior aspect of the vertebral bodies can be exposed in a straightforward manner. Release of the deep cervical fascia superiorly and inferiorly allows for retraction over multiple levels so that transverse incisions can be used for 3- or even 4-level corpectomy procedures. Hand-held retractors are recommended to avoid excessive and constant pressure on the soft tissues.

First, the disks are removed back to the posterior longitudinal ligament at the levels to be decompressed. Identifying the uncovertebral joints is very important to help maintain midline orientation. Distraction of the disk space will facilitate visualization of the posterior aspect of the disk, but any distraction should be done with care or avoided entirely in patients who have severe cord compression at that level. A rongeur can then be used to remove some of the anterior aspect of the vertebral body. A carbide-tip burr is used next, to channel out the middle

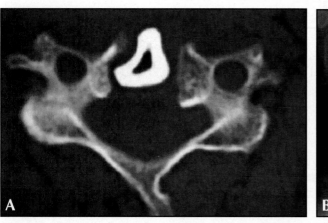
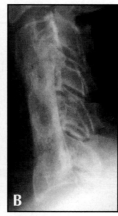

Fig. 1 A, A postoperative CT image following a 2-level corpectomy and fibular strut in a patient with cervical spondylotic myelopathy. The mid portion of the vertebra has been surgically removed, along with any disk material or OPLL that is compressing the spinal cord. The fibula strut graft is shown in cross section. **B,** A lateral radiograph of the same patient 2 years postoperatively. The graft has fully incorporated and bony remodeling is evident.

portion of the selected vertebrae. This channel is typically 16- to 18-mm wide. Any lateral deviation can endanger the vertebral artery.[7] When the posterior cortex is reached, a diamond buff is used to further thin the posterior shell and burr through the lateral gutters to the soft posterior longitudinal ligament or, in some cases, the dura. This rectangle of posterior shell then is carefully elevated off of the posterior longitudinal ligament (or off of the dura, if OPPL is present). This delicate procedure should be done using magnification and with continuous spinal cord monitoring. These steps are performed for every vertebral body to be included in the decompression. After the cord has been decompressed, intraoperative traction may be increased to help correct cervical kyphosis if present. **(CD-51.1)**

Following corpectomies, a strut graft is used for arthrodesis (Fig. 1). The superior and inferior end plates serve as docking sites for the graft. Each end plate must be prepared with a burr to flatten the surface, expose bleeding subchondral bone, and sculpt posterior and anterior lips of

bone. The graft can then be placed into the center portion of the vertebrae above and below. This placement, which provides the best distribution of stress, as well as maximum surface area for healing, is preferred over the notched graft technique which contacts only the anterior aspect of the vertebrae.[8] Traction is then released to lock the graft into place. The anterior and posterior bony lips on the docking sites discourage any graft migration. I prefer to use autogenous iliac crest bone graft as a strut following 1-level corpectomy procedures. Ilium can also be used for 2-level procedures, but I prefer to use fibula strut grafts for corpectomies of 2 or more levels. Autogenous fibula grafts have a high union rate, are exceedingly strong, and morbidity from the donor site is low.[5] Graft placement requires significant attention to detail, because the most common complications with this procedure are graft-related. If a long strut graft dislodges, it is usually associated with fracturing of the inferior vertebra and anterior displacement of the graft, which requires revision surgery in

many cases. Nonunion can occur with strut grafts, but is more problematic with multilevel diskectomy and fusion type grafts.

The use of internal fixation following anterior cervical procedures is increasing and evolving. Data exist to support the use of anterior plating with 3-level diskectomy and fusion procedures.[9] Internal fixation following corpectomy procedures for myelopathy is more controversial. I favor anterior plating following 1-level corpectomies with iliac strut grafts for the increased stability and less rigid bracing requirements. Some surgeons use long anterior plates following multilevel corpectomy and strut grafting procedures,[10] although others have reported substantial failure rates with loosening of the instrumentation or unintentionally maintained distraction.[11] A small T-shaped plate (anti-kick plate), which is secured only to the inferior vertebrae and extends upward to buttress the inferior docking site, has also been used to discourage dislodgment of the graft at the inferior pole, but its effectiveness has not been documented.

Postoperative immobilization is required after anterior decompression and fusion procedures. A soft cervical collar is recommended for 6 weeks after 1-level diskectomy and fusion procedures, or if multilevel diskectomies and fusions are done with plating. Patients having a 1-level corpectomy and strut fusion with anterior plating can also be treated safely in a soft collar. For multilevel corpectomy and strut patients, I use a rigid 2-poster type brace with underarm straps (a head-cervical-thoracic orthosis) for the vast majority of cases, for a duration of 8 weeks. If patients have preexisting instability, such as from prior laminectomies, then a halo vest is used for postoperative immobilization. At times, a 1-stage or second-stage posterior instrumentation and fusion is indicated for corpectomy and strut graft patients with severe instability, osteoporotic bone, or kyphosis.

Posterior Approach
Laminectomy
Multilevel laminectomy in the treatment of cervical myelopathy has decreased in popularity as alternative procedures, such as laminoplasty and anterior corpectomy with fusion, have evolved. Nevertheless, it is very much an appropriate tool in the spine surgeon's armamentarium for the properly selected patient. Laminectomy is a dorsal decompression technique which may be most useful if posterolateral compression from large facet joint osteophytes is present. Postlaminectomy kyphosis remains a potential complication, however, and although the exact incidence is unclear, this problem is a difficult one for the patient and the spine surgeon.[12,13] Evidence of preoperative instability, based on flexion and extension plain films, would discourage the choice of laminectomy unless it was combined with a posterior fusion technique. Typically, the pathoanatomy causing spinal cord compression is anterior to the cord; any posterior decompression technique is an indirect method. This means that relatively normal cervical lordosis is needed for the spinal cord to be able to "float away" from any anterior compressive pathology following surgical treatment from the posterior approach.

Laminoplasty
Laminoplasty was developed in Japan as an alternative posterior decompression method. There are many different techniques of laminoplasty, but they all seek to expand the spinal canal by opening the lamina in a unilateral or bilateral trap door fashion. This,

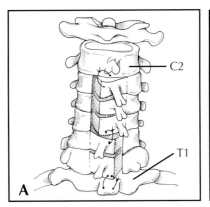
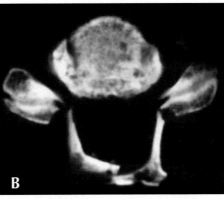

Fig. 2 A, Schematic drawing of an alternate trap-door laminoplasty technique from Chiba University, Japan. Laminae C3–C5 are opened one way and C6–C7 opened the opposite way. Three tethering sutures are used to prevent reclosure of the laminae postoperatively. **B,** A postoperative CT scan through the C5-C6 level demonstrates the opened alternate trap doors. Note the enlargement of the spinal canal.

Table 1
Anterior and posterior approaches: Advantages and disadvantages

Advantages	Disadvantages
Anterior Approach—Decompression and Fusion	
1. Direct removal compressive pathology	1. Technically demanding
2. Stabilization with arthrodesis	2. Graft complications
3. Corrects deformity	3. Postoperative bracing
4. Good axial pain relief	
Posterior Approach—Laminoplasty	
1. Less loss of motion	1. Indirect decompression
2. Not as technically demanding	2. Kyphosis limitations
3. Less bracing	3. Less axial pain relief

too, is an indirect method of decompression and relies on the cord moving posteriorly in the canal, which is promoted by normal lordosis. The theoretical advantage of laminoplasty over laminectomy includes maintaining the posterior ligament structures and allowing the paraspinal muscles to heal to the preserved bony lamina postoperatively, both of which should discourage postoperative kyphosis. Initially laminoplasty was developed for patients with OPLL over many segments,[14,15] but it has been well described for patients with cervical spondylotic myelopathy also.[16–19] With appropriate patient selection, the results of neurologic improvement

have been satisfactory, and late deformity has not been a problem although no fusion is performed, postlaminoplasty patients do lose motion.[17] Perhaps more importantly, it has been less successful than arthrodesis procedures for the relief of axial neck pain.[20]

The technique for a laminoplasty involves a standard midline posterior approach, with bilateral exposure of the lamina and facet joints. For a unilateral trapdoor-type procedure, a burr is used to make a gutter completely through the lamina on one side only, located at the junction of the lamina and facet joint. On the opposite side, a similar gutter is burred, but care is taken not to go completely through the deeper lamina cortex. After removing the interspinous ligament and ligamentum flavum at the appropriate levels, the lamina can be elevated or "swung open" using the partially buffed gutter as a hinge. In the Chiba University method, which I prefer, C3, C4, and C5 are swung open in one direction, and C6 and C7 in the other (Fig. 2). Three tethering sutures through bone keep the lamina from closing down following wound closure. Bone chips are placed in the hinge gutter to promote healing in the open position. Other methods involve midline splitting of the spinous process or use of internal fixation.[19]

Choosing an Approach

Deciding on which approach to use in the surgical treatment of cervical myelopathy depends on several patient and surgeon factors.[21] An understanding of the pathoanatomy of the canal stenosis through high-quality imaging studies is critical to sound decision making. Patients with a congenitally narrow canal and diffuse stenosis over multiple levels having normal lordosis and only mild neck pain are excellent candidates for a laminoplasty. Those patients with substantial anterior deformation of the cord, kyphosis, or preoperative instability can expect excellent results from anterior decompression and fusion techniques. Some patients are candidates for either type of approach, and the relative advantages and disadvantages for the individual patient must be considered (Table 1). As important as patient factors is the training and experience of the spine surgeon performing these high-risk surgical procedures.

References

1. Clarke E, Robinson PK: Cervical myelopathy: A complication of cervical spondylosis. *Brain* 1956;79:483–510.

2. Lees F, Turner JWA: Natural history and prognosis of cervical spondylosis. *Br Med J* 1963;2:1607–1610.

3. Bernard TN Jr, Whitecloud TS III: Cervical spondylotic myelopathy and myeloradiculopathy: Anterior decompression and stabilization with autogenous fibula strut graft. *Clin Orthop* 1987;221:149–160.

4. Okada K, Shirasaki N, Hayashi H, Oka S, Hosoya T: Treatment of cervical spondylotic myelopathy by enlargement of the spinal canal anteriorly, followed by arthrodesis. *J Bone Joint Surg* 1991;73A:352–364.

5. Emery SE, Bohlman HH, Bolesta MJ, Jones PK: Anterior cervical decompression and arthrodesis for the treatment of cervical spondylotic myelopathy: Two to seventeen-year follow-up. *J Bone Joint Surg* 1998;80:941–951.

6. Saunders RL, Bernini PM, Shirreffs TG Jr, Reeves AG: Central corpectomy for cervical spondylotic myelopathy: A consecutive series with long-term follow-up evaluation. *J Neurosurg* 1991;74:163–170.

7. Smith MD, Emery SE, Dudley A, Murray KJ, Leventhal M: Vertebral artery injury during anterior decompression of the cervical spine: A retrospective review of ten patients. *J Bone Joint Surg* 1993;75B:410–415.

8. Fernyhough JC, White JI, LaRocca H: Fusion rates in multilevel cervical spondylosis comparing allograft fibula with autograft fibula in 126 patients. *Spine* 1991;16(suppl 10):S561–S564.

9. Emery SE, Fisher JR, Bohlman HH: Three-level anterior cervical diskectomy and fusion: Radiographic and clinical results. *Spine* 1997;22:2622–2624.

10. Herman JM, Sonntag VK: Cervical corpectomy and plate fixation for postlaminectomy kyphosis. *J Neurosurg* 1994;80:963–970.

11. Paramore CG, Dickman CA, Sonntag VK: Radiographic and clinical follow-up review of Caspar plates in 49 patients. *J Neurosurg* 1996;84:957–961.

12. Mikawa Y, Shikata J, Yamarnuro T: Spinal deformity and instability after multilevel cervical laminectomy. *Spine* 1987;12:6–11.

13. Gregorius FK, Estrin T, Crandall PH: Cervical spondylotic radiculopathy and myelopathy: A long-term follow-up study. *Arch Neurol* 1976;33:618–625.

14. Hirabayashi K: Expansive open-door laminoplasty for cervical spondylotic myelopathy. (Jpn), *Shujutsu* 1978;32:1159–1163.

15. Hirabayashi K, Satomi K: Operative procedure and results of expansive open-door laminoplasty. *Spine* 1988;13:870–876.

16. Hirabayashi K, Watanabe K, Wakano K, Suzuki N, Satomi K, Ishii Y: Expansive open-door laminoplasty for cervical spinal stenotic myelopathy. *Spine* 1983;8:693–699.

17. Kimura I, Shingu H, Nasu Y: Long-term follow-up of cervical spondylotic myelopathy treated by canal-expansive laminoplasty. *J Bone Joint Surg* 1995;77B:956–961.

18. Hase H, Watanabe T, Hirasawa Y, et al: Bilateral open laminoplasty using ceramic laminas for cervical myelopathy. *Spine* 1991;16:1269–1276.

19. O'Brien MF, Peterson D, Casey AT, Crockard HA: A novel technique for laminoplasty augmentation of spinal canal area using titanium miniplate stabilization: A computerized morphometric analysis. *Spine* 1996;21:474–483.

20. Hosono N, Yonenobu K, Ono K: Neck and shoulder pain after laminoplasty: A noticeable complication. *Spine* 1996;21:1969–1973.

21. Yonenobu K, Fuji T, Ono K, Okada K, Yamamoto T, Harada N: Choice of surgical treatment for multisegmental cervical spondylotic myelopathy. *Spine* 1985;10:710–716. ·

Reference to Video

Boden S, Emery S: *Anterior Diskectomy, Corpectomy, Fusions, and Plating.* Rosemont, IL, American Academy of Orthopaedic Surgeons, Annual Meeting, 1997.

Introduction to Thoracolumbar Fractures

Jerome M. Cotler, MD

Injuries to the thoracolumbar spine are frequently encountered by orthopaedic surgeons. The incidence of such injuries that are associated with some type of neurologic deficit is approximately 1 per 20,000 per year. As with most injuries of the spine, the majority of thoracolumbar injuries occur in males, generally males between the ages of 15 and 29 years. In a multicenter review of more than 1,000 patients by the Scoliosis Research Society, 16% of injuries occurred between T1 and T10, 52% between T11 and L1, and 32% between L1 and L5.[1] The T2 to T10 area has the smallest ratio of canal size to cord diameter in the spine, which is why this area has the least tolerance to injury and a higher risk of loss of neural function. In addition, the cord area between T2 and T10 is a circulatory watershed area. The artery of Adamkiewicz provides the spinal blood supply at approximately T9 and below, and the blood supply for the area above comes from the upper thoracic area. Injuries in this area with severe thoracic fractures usually have a 6 to 1 ratio of complete to incomplete neural deficits.

The T11 to L1 area is the junction between the thoracic spine and the lumbar spine. The relative immobility of the thoracic spine and the mobility of the lumbar spine make this transition area much more vulnerable to injury, which accounts for the fact that 52% of injuries occur here. The neural elements in this area, particularly at the junction, are a commingling of cord, conus, and cauda equina, and for this reason, it is difficult to ascertain which of these elements is injured and what the ultimate outcome is likely to be. Injury to the cauda equina carries a far better prognosis, because it is a peripheral nerve and has regenerative powers not normally seen in the cord or conus. Although the lumbar spine has more sagittally oriented facets, making it more mobile in the flexion/extension mode, it nonetheless has a far better prognosis because of its increased ratio of canal area to neural tissue. Also, most of the neural tissue here is peripheral nerve tissue and is less susceptible to permanent neural damage.

Treating physicians must not lose sight of the responsibility imparted to them when seeing patients with thoracolumbar injuries. The determination must be made rapidly whether the patient is neurally intact or has an incomplete or a complete neural deficit. These baseline assessments of neural function are important, and so are early baseline assessments of the presence of bony lesions. In addition, the earliest medical status must be ascertained and recorded, and care taken not to allow any further harm or loss of function to come to the patient if at all possible. Thus, the physician must protect the neural elements and accomplish the earliest possible decompression either surgically or through closed reduction and stabilization, with the hope of obtaining some return of neural function. The physician must also determine if the patient's injury is solely in the spine or if other systems must be considered. Depending on the type of fracture, associated injuries occur in up to 50% of patients.[2-6] Half of the associated injuries result from a distraction force and involve an intra-abdominal injury, such as a rupture of a visceral organ.[7] Pulmonary injuries also occur in approximately 20% of these patients, while intra-abdominal bleeding secondary to liver and splenic injury occurs in about 10%.[8] In addition, contiguous and noncontiguous spine injuries are present in between 6% and 15%. Because the mortality rate in the first year for thoracic level paraplegia is approximately 7%,[9] the primary goal is to protect the neural elements and to maximize neural return by whatever means possible, using the pharmacologic agents available today. It also is necessary to attempt to reduce the bony deformity, whether it is a fracture-subluxation or a dislocation. Frequently, this can be done by using a traction apparatus, thus avoiding early surgery, while the patient is being stabilized and evaluated. The ultimate goal is that stabilization of the fracture will enable the patient to once again have a pain-free, stable spine and to return to the work force as a productive member of society.

Injuries at the thoracolumbar area can also lead to slow progressive deformity and vertebral body collapse (HS An, MD, personal communication). Some underlying processes that may be involved include tumors, metabolic bone disease, osteomyelitis, or osteoporosis. Of course, these latter patient groups are usually the elderly and, unfortunately, elderly females, because of their propensity to osteoporosis. Some of the issues to be addressed in subsequent chapters include thorny ones that truly require clarification, such as those in the surgical area. What are the indications for surgery, when should these types of procedures be carried out, and which is the best approach for decompression or fusion? It is also necessary to decide whether the approach should be posterior, anterior, or combined.

References

1. Gertzbein SD: Scoliosis Research Society: Multicenter spine fracture study. *Spine* 1992; 17:528–540.

2. Cotler JM, Vernace JV, Michalski JA: The use of Harrington rods in thoracolumbar fractures. *Orthop Clin North Am* 1986;17:87–103.

3. Gertzbein SD, Court-Brown CM: Flexion-distraction injuries of the lumbar spine: Mechanism of injury and classification. *Clin Orthop* 1988;227:52–60.

4. Gumley G, Taylor TK, Ryan MD: Distraction fractures of the lumbar spine. *J Bone Joint Surg* 1982;64B:520–525.

5. Saboe LA, Reid DC, Davis LA, Warren SA, Grace MG: Spine trauma and associated injuries. *J Trauma* 1991;31:43–48.

6. Weinstein JN, Collalto P, Lehmann R: Thoracolumbar "burst" fractures treated conservatively: A long-term follow-up. *Spine* 1988;13: 33–38.

7. Levine AM, Bosse M, Edwards CC: Bilateral facet dislocations in the thoracolumbar spine. *Spine* 1988;13:630–640.

8. Ducker TB, Russo GL, Bellegarrique R, Lucas JT: Complete sensorimotor paralysis after cord injury: Mortality, recovery, and therapeutic implications. *J Trauma* 1979;19:837–840.

9. Shikata J, Yamamuro T, Iida H, Shimizu K, Yoshikawa J: Surgical treatment for paraplegia resulting from vertebral fractures in senile osteoporosis. *Spine* 1990;15:485–489.

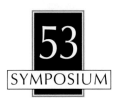

Thoracolumbar Trauma Imaging Overview

Adam E. Flanders, MD

Some of the most essential tools in the evaluation of thoracolumbar trauma are the various types of diagnostic imaging. Today, imaging of the spine and spinal axis can be performed using numerous techniques. These include plain radiographs, multiplanar tomography, myelography, computed tomography (CT) and magnetic resonance imaging (MRI). The use of these techniques is guided by the clinical assessment of the individual patient and by diagnostic algorithms.

In general, isolated thoracic spine fractures are less common than isolated cervical or lumbar fractures. The structural stability of the thoracic cage offers to the thoracic spine some protection against injury.[1] Higher forces are required to induce an injury. As a result, one half of all thoracic injuries produce a neurologic deficit.[2,3] This is attributed to the relatively smaller spinal cord diameter to spinal canal diameter ratio and the higher energies expended during injury.[2,3] Because there is relative resistance to rotation, most thoracic injuries occur in flexion and axial loading; therefore, fracture dislocations are more common than compression/burst fractures.[2]

Nondisplaced fractures of the thoracic spine may be difficult to identify on plain radiographs. Regardless, plain radiography remains the initial imaging study of choice for evaluation of thoracolumbar trauma. Standard anterior-posterior (AP) and lateral radiographs are necessary for initial evaluation because more than half of fractures are undetectable on the AP view alone.[4,5]

Lumbar level fractures are more common than thoracic injuries because of the increased mobility of the lumbar spine. The thoracolumbar junction is especially prone to injury. Anatomic differences that predispose the lumbar spine to fracture compared to the thoracic spine include the absence of ribs, the different orientation of the facet joints, and the transition from a kyphotic to a lordotic curvature.[6–8] Most lumbar fractures are classified using a variation of the Denis or McAfee schema.[9–11] The mechanisms of injury are based on the 2- and 3-column models of spinal injury proposed by Holdsworth and Denis respectively. The major difference between the 2 classification systems is the distinction between stable and unstable burst fractures in the McAfee system. The fracture subtypes include the simple compression fracture, the burst fracture, the seat belt type injury (including Chance fractures), the flexion-distraction injury, and the translational injury.[9–12]

Standard chest films are inadequate for evaluation of the spine; the radiographs must be exposed properly to optimize visualization of the spine. In the setting of acute trauma, it may be technically difficult to obtain diagnostic quality radiographs. On lateral radiographs, the upper thoracic spine is often obscured by the shoulders, and patient motion and respiration can blur bony details. A swimmer's view can prove helpful in improving the visibility of the cervicothoracic junction. In addition, cross table lateral films that are deliberately blurred by breathing artifact can improve the visibility of the spine. CT is usually reserved for imaging areas of the spine that are inadequately demonstrated on conventional radiographs. Indirect signs of thoracic fracture include a paraspinal mass, mediastinal widening, fracture of the sternum, fractures of the posterolateral or posteromedial ribs, identification of 2 spinous processes at 1 level on a frontal radiograph, and a hemothorax on a chest radiograph.[5,6]

The radiographic and clinical findings of thoracic spine fracture and traumatic aortic dissection have many similarities. Widening of the mediastinum, pleural effusions, paravertebral hematomas, and neurologic symptoms can be identified with both entities. Important distinguishing features of aortic injury on radiographs include depression of the main stem bronchus, displacement of a nasogastric tube to the right, and indistinct margins of the aortic knob.[7] Dynamic contrast CT or conventional aortography may be necessary for confirmation.

Although conventional tomography has been largely supplanted by CT in the evaluation of the spine, it is still used at many centers to delineate complex fractures. It is technically more difficult to perform than CT and requires more patient cooperation. The best application of conventional tomography is in the postoperative spine with instrumentation, because the artifacts produced by hardware degrade CT or MRI images.

CT yields significantly more diagnostic information regarding the extent of bony injury than plain radiographs. It remains the study of choice for depicting the extent of injury, as modern CT equipment with bone reconstruction algorithms provides the highest sensitivity for detecting subtle cortical abnormalities. CT has the additional advantage of computer reformatting 2-dimensional or cross-sectional information into other 2-dimensional (sagittal or coronal) or 3-dimensional views in an infinite number of potential orientations. The biggest disadvantage of CT is its limited capability for depicting soft-tissue injuries (disk herniation, epidural hematoma, ligamentous disruption, or spinal cord injury). Modern CT scanners can acquire all of the image dataset in one helical acquisition. This technique allows rapid acquisition of the clinical data with a minimum of patient cooperation. The data can then be post-processed into additional projections off-line. The quality of reconstructed images is indirectly proportional to the in-plane resolution or slice thickness.

MRI has emerged as the definitive diagnostic modality in the evaluation of spinal and spinal cord injury. The primary reason is MRI's unequaled capacity to demonstrate the soft-tissue component of spinal injury.

Formerly, soft-tissue injuries such as ligament and disk damage were inferred by the extent and type of osseous injury.[13,14] Moreover, MRI has completely supplanted myelography in the evaluation of spinal cord injury. The majority of spinal injured patients can be safely imaged with MRI during the acute period, prior to or following closed reduction of the injury. MRI-compatible monitoring and life-support equipment is also available for medically unstable patients. Absolute contraindications to MR imaging include certain biomedical implants, such as cardiac pacemakers and aneurysm clips.

While it is acknowledged that MRI is less sensitive to fractures than CT, compressive injuries to the vertebral body usually induce changes in the marrow elements, which are readily detectable with MRI. Fractures of the posterior elements, as well as nondisplaced fractures of the anterior and middle columns, are difficult to resolve on MRI. Despite these shortcomings, MRI is capable of revealing the majority of clinically significant fractures and can be used to tailor detailed imaging with CT at specific levels in question.[15] MRI also reliably demonstrates vertebral alignment and integrity.

MRI is particularly well suited for demonstrating the spectrum of soft-tissue injuries associated with spinal and spinal cord injury. The fracture classification schemes commonly in use today are based on the appearance of an injury on plain radiographs. These classification systems are useful because they attempt to predict the degree of instability and associated ligamentous damage based on the appearance on standard radiographs. The primary benefit that MRI offers over standard radiographs is direct visualization of the injured ligamentous complexes.[16]

Using MRI, spinal injury can be subdivided into 5 general injury categories: (1) vertebral fractures, subluxations, and compressive injury, (2) disk injury and herniation, (3) ligamentous disruption, (4) epidural and paravertebral hematoma, and (5) spinal cord edema and hemorrhage.

It is difficult to produce an imaging algorithm or protocol that effectively manages appropriate use of diagnostic imaging in thoracolumbar trauma. Standard, high-quality radiographs of the thoracolumbar spine should be obtained initially in any patient with a clinical examination or historical information suggestive of thoracolumbar injury. CT should be obtained through any areas of fracture and of areas that have been incompletely evaluated on the radiographs. MRI should be obtained on any patient with a neurologic deficit, regardless of the existence of a concomitant bony injury. If there is compelling evidence for a traumatic aortic injury (eg, paraspinal mass, indistinct aortic knob on chest radiograph, high speed deceleration mechanism, etc), emergent arteriography may be necessary.

References

1. Andriacchi T, Schultz A, Belytschko T, Galante J: A model for studies of mechanical interactions between the human spine and rib cage. *J Biomech* 1974;7:497–507.

2. Hanley EN Jr, Eskay ML: Thoracic spine fractures. *Orthopedics* 1989;12:689–696.

3. Meyer S: Thoracic spine trauma. *Semin Roentgenol* 1992;27:254–261.

4. Dennis LN, Rogers LF: Superior mediastinal widening from spine fractures mimicking aortic rupture on chest radiographs *Am J Roentgenol* 1989;152:27–30.

5. el-Khoury GY, Moore TE, Kathol MH: Radiology of the thoracic spine. *Clin Neurosurg* 1992;38:261–295.

6. el-Khoury GY, Whitten CG: Trauma to the upper thoracic spine: Anatomy, biomechanics, and unique imaging features. *Am J Roentgenol* 1993;160:95–102.

7. Kram HB, Appel PL, Wohlmuth DA, Shoemaker WC: Diagnosis of traumatic thoracic aortic rupture: A 10-year retrospective analysis. *Ann Thorac Surg* 1989;47:282–286.

8. Kaye JJ, Nance EP Jr: Thoracic and lumbar spine trauma. *Radiol Clin North Am* 1990; 28:361–377.

9. Denis F: Spinal instability as defined by the three-column spine concept in acute spinal trauma. *Clin Orthop* 1984;189:65–76.

10. Denis F: The three column spine and its significance in the classification of acute thoracolumbar spinal injuries. *Spine* 1983;8:817–831.

11. McAfee PC, Yuan HA, Fredrickson BE, Lubicky JP: The value of computed tomography in thoracolumbar fractures: An analysis of one hundred consecutive cases and a new classification. *J Bone Joint Surg* 1983;65A:461–473.

12. Holdsworth FW: Fractures, dislocations, and fracture-dislocations of the spine. *J Bone Joint Surg* 1963;45B:6–20.

13. Schaefer DM, Flanders AE, Osterholm JL, Northrup BE: Prognostic significance of magnetic resonance imaging in the acute phase of cervical spine injury. *J Neurosurg* 1992;76: 218–223.

14. Flanders AE, Spettell CM, Tartaglino LM, Friedman DP, Herbison GJ: Forecasting motor recovery after cervical spinal cord injury: Value of MR imaging. *Radiology* 1996;201:649–655.

15. Silberstein M, Tress BM, Hennessy O: Prediction of neurologic outcome in acute spinal cord injury: The role of CT and MR. *Am J Neuroradiol* 1992;13:1597–1608.

16. Yamashita Y, Takahashi M, Matsuno Y, et al: Chronic injuries of the spinal cord: Assessment with MR imaging. *Radiology* 1990;175:849–854.

Nonsurgical Treatment of Cervical Degenerative Disease

Glenn R. Rechtine, MD, FACS

Introduction

All of us will experience neck pain at one time or another. The severity will vary with the individual and the particular episode. Anyone who has experienced this personally can understand how the expression "pain in the neck" was born.

Surgery should not be an initial consideration, because the pain associated with most cervical disorders can be relieved by nonsurgical treatment. Although the literature is full of articles with strong opinions about the proper care of cervical disorders, unfortunately, these strong opinions have little objective data to support them. One such paper was an anecdotal report of a single case with a recommendation for chiropractic manipulation.[1] Because the natural history is benign in most cases, caretakers can be deceived into thinking that the clinical interventions used were effective.

Our goal is to return the patient to a normal work and home life as soon as possible, with the least cost to the patient, his job, his insurance company, and society in general. Ideally, the treatment would begin before the onset of symptoms, if that were possible, because preventive treatment would make further treatment unnecessary.

Patients must be educated about the disease process. Even with a severe radiculopathy, the likelihood of resolution without surgery should be explained to the patient and family. This is a difficult concept for the surgeon as well. Long-term results with nonsurgical treatment have been comparable to those with surgery.[2–5]

It is also necessary for patients to understand their role in the recovery process. They must be willing to modify any parts of their lifestyle that have contributed to the development of the problem.

Evaluation and Diagnosis

An accurate history and a careful physical examination are necessary prior to beginning any treatment program. A history that includes some form of trauma is significant for several reasons: (1) radiographs will be obtained earlier in the course; (2) flexion/extension radiographs may be necessary; and (3) it may be necessary to avoid the use of traction for fear of aggravating a ligamentous injury. Any history suggestive of tumor or infection will necessitate a thorough evaluation as well. On physical examination, an abnormality on the neurologic examination may change the initial recommendation. Any deficit must not only be identified but also recorded, so that future examinations can be compared. Indications of myelopathy will change the initial recommendation. Lung cancer, shoulder pathology, and other problems may initially present with neck and/or arm pain and must be considered in the differential diagnosis.

Radiographs

For the typical neck pain patient, radiographs may not be required for the first few weeks. If the symptoms are not responding or if there is any possibility of tumor, infection, or fracture, then radiographs or magnetic resonance imaging (MRI) may be indicated sooner. In trauma, if the standard radiographs are negative, flexion-extension views may be obtained to eliminate the possibility of ligamentous instability. The flexion and extension should be done actively by the patient and only to the extent that is comfortable. These views should be obtained only with patients who are awake, alert, sober, and cooperative, and who have a reasonably normal range of motion. These requirements are rarely met in the emergency room. If there is any suggestion of an injury, the patient is immobilized until further evaluation can be undertaken.

Routine radiographs will not help to delineate the cause of severity of the pain.[6] Disk degeneration is a chronic degenerative disease and is not associated with previous trauma.[7] If needed, cervical radiographs involve less radiation exposure than the usual lumbar films do. Exposures are less than 1.0 mR per radiograph.[8]

Acute Symptom Reduction

Patients in severe pain must initially be made more comfortable. Patients with an acute cervical radiculopathy often experience intense discomfort.

The initial recommendation is for patients to do whatever makes them feel better. They commonly present with one arm resting on the top of the head, because this helps to relieve the radicular pain. A collar can be used empirically if this helps as well. Nonsteroidal anti-inflammatory drugs (NSAIDs) can also be effective. The patient will have to experiment to find the most comfortable position for sleeping. Some will find sleeping in a recliner to be more comfortable than lying flat. Traction may be used as long as there is no reason to suspect tumor, infection, fracture, or ligamentous injury.

These simple methods will cause most patients' symptoms to start to subside within a few days. As the symptoms resolve, more vigorous daily activities can be resumed gradually. In addition, a program of regular exercise can be initiated.

Medications
Analgesics

The vast majority of patients will require nothing more than acetaminophen for pain. Care should be taken not to exceed the recommended daily dose. Liver toxicity can be severe at high doses and can even re-

sult in death. This must be explained to the patients, because they do not understand the risks of acetaminophen overdose. A great many physicians are also unaware of this risk. When a physician orders 2 tablets to be administered every 4 hours of any of the usual acetaminophen and oxycodone, codeine, or hydrocodone preparations, this constitutes an overdose of acetaminophen. Medication should be titrated as necessary for pain relief. Narcotics should be used in as small a dose and for as short a period of time as possible.

Nonsteroidal Anti-inflammatory Drugs

The pain-relieving dose of NSAIDs is less than the effective anti-inflammatory dose, but because the anti-inflammatory effect is desired, the higher doses are maintained. The anti-inflammatory effect may take 7 to 10 days. Liver and renal functions should be monitored, and routine blood counts should be taken. There is a relative contraindication in patients with a history of ulcer disease or gastrointestinal bleeding.

Steroids

Corticosteroid use has been advocated, but with very little scientific basis. Both oral and epidural steroids have been used with anecdotal success. Even with the epidural route there is a systemic steroid effect, lowering serum cortisol levels for 2 weeks.[2] Unlike lumbar epidural steroids, a single treatment is all that is used.[4] With the oral route dose-pak or short course of oral steroids, the possibility of idiosyncratic hip osteonecrosis is a possibility, even though the disease that is being treated is self-limited.

Antidepressants

Relatively small doses of the tricyclic

antidepressants can be helpful. These are usually given at bedtime, because one of the side effects of the medication is somnolence, an effect that can be helpful if the patient is having trouble sleeping.

Muscle Relaxants

Muscle relaxants have a central action and are effective in helping patients reduce their activity level. Because addiction can occur, these drugs should be for short term use only.

Modalities

Heat and ice can be used to help treat symptoms. This treatment can be done by the patient at home, and their use is predicated on the patient's response. The patient must be educated to prevent burns and frostbite from too vigorous application of thermal treatment.

Ultrasound and electrical stimulation have little if any scientific evidence to support their use. From my personal experience, what little symptomatic relief they provide is gone by the time the patient returns home.

Traction

Traction can be immediately effective for some patients, and it can be done at home in a very cost-effective manner. For these patients, the symptomatic relief, which can be demonstrated with EMG studies,[9] may be of value. If the symptoms are not relieved, there is no reason to continue the traction treatments.

Traction should not be used for patients with instability or potential instability, fracture, tumor, or infection. For this reason, traction should not be prescribed until after radiographs have been evaluated.

Trigger Point Injection

Another commonly used treatment is that of trigger point injection.

There are no controlled studies to document their effectiveness, but their use involves very little risk. If effective, they can be repeated weekly if necessary.

Transcutaneous Electrical Nerve Stimulation (TENS)

TENS units remain controversial because their effectiveness varies. TENS equipment should be tried prior to purchase, to determine if the patient is going to respond and to avoid unnecessary costs.

Exercise

Exercise is one of the mainstays of prevention and treatment of neck and arm pain.[9–14] During the acute phase of the pain, activity is decreased to reduce the patient's symptoms. As the pain decreases, the patient should begin an exercise program. In the beginning, walking on a daily basis will help prevent disuse. As the symptoms subside, the patient can begin a strengthening program as well as some form of aerobic conditioning. Flexibility and range-of-motion exercises are less helpful, and ballistic or bouncing exercises should also be avoided.

Lifestyle

The patient's home and work life should be explored for any causative activities or circumstances. Instruction in ergonomics and proper body mechanics may identify factors that could be aggravating the patient's symptoms. Factors at work can contribute to a patient's symptoms.[15,16] Something as simple as changing a computer monitor's height or keyboard level may be all that is needed to cure some patients. Eliminating a heavy briefcase or pocketbook may be helpful as well. Smoking must be discouraged.

The psychology of injury and disease must be addressed with the pa-

tient, because the better educated the patient is about the disease process, the better he or she will respond to treatment. There are no cures for degenerative conditions. Our treatments are meant to help modify the symptoms. While the prognosis is good for resolution of a current episode, it is also likely that there will be recurrences in the future.

Summary

A regular exercise program, even something as simple as a daily walk, can help to keep the ongoing degenerative process at bay. Such efforts at prevention can help with the patient's general health and should be encouraged by the spine physician. The vast majority of patients with degenerative cervical disease that is manifesting itself as neck and arm pain will respond to nonsurgical treatment. However, a very small percentage of patients who have cervical radiculopathy will require surgical treatment.[4] Each practitioner must develop his or her own protocol based on personal experience, using a combination of the methods we have just discussed.[4,17,18]

An accurate diagnosis is necessary to avoid treating the wrong problem (ie, lung cancer, shoulder impingement, etc). Patients should be knowledgeable about their disease. They should be empowered to participate in their care and encouraged to work with the physician and/or therapist to accomplish the goal of returning to a reasonable lifestyle at work as well as at home. An ongoing exercise program and an ergonomic evaluation at home and work can be helpful in reducing recurrences.

References

1. Brouillette DL, Gurske DT: Chiropractic treatment of cervical radiculopathy caused by a herniated cervical disc. *J Manipulative Physiol Ther* 1994;17:119–123.

2. Burn JM, Langdon L: Duration of action of epidural methyl prednisolone: A study in patients with the lumbo-sciatic syndrome. *Am J Phys Med* 1974;53:29–34.

3. McCormack BM, Weinstein PR: Cervical spondylosis: An update. *West J Med* 1996; 165:43–51.

4. Saal JS, Saal JA, Yurth EF: Nonoperative management of herniated cervical intervertebral disc with radiculopathy. *Spine* 1996;21: 1877–1883.

5. Wysowski S: Traction and kinesitherapy in the management of painful syndromes of the cervical spine. *Neurol Neurochir Pol* 1976;10:709–713.

6. Johnson MJ, Lucas GL: Value of cervical spine radiographs as a screening tool. *Clin Orthop* 1997;340:102–108.

7. Marchiori DM, Henderson CN: A cross-sectional study correlating cervical radiographic degenerative findings to pain and disability. *Spine* 1996;21:2747–2751.

8. Ingegno M, Nahabedian M, Tominaga GT, Scannell G, Waxman K: Radiation exposure from cervical spine radiographs. *Am J Emerg Med* 1994;12:15–16.

9. Gogia PP, Sabbahi MA: Electromyographic analysis of neck muscle fatigue in patients with osteoarthritis of the cervical spine. *Spine* 1994;19:502–506.

10. Fitz-Ritson D: Phasic exercises for cervical rehabilitation after "whiplash" trauma. *J Manipulative Physiol Ther* 1995;18:21–24.

11. Fitz-Ritson D: Therapeutic traction: A review of neurological principles and clinical applications. *J Manipulative Physiol Ther* 1984;7:39–49.

12. Highland TR, Dreisinger TE, Vie LL, Russell GS: Changes in isometric strength and range of motion of the isolated cervical spine after eight weeks of clinical rehabilitation. *Spine* 1992; 17(suppl 6):S77–S82.

13. Jordan A, Ostergaard K: Implementation of neck/shoulder rehabilitation in primary health care clinics. *J Manipulative Physiol Ther* 1996; 19:36–40.

14. Polienko EP, Galkina MG, Kochetkov IuT, Piliaev VG, Golubeva OI: Results of the complex conservative ambulatory treatment of cervical osteochondrosis including acupuncture-reflexotherapy. *Ortop Travmatol Protez* 1989;1: 36–38.

15. Alund M, Larsson SE, Lewin T: Work-related persistent neck impairment: A study on former steelworks grinders. *Ergonomics* 1994;37: 1253–1260.

16. Anderson R: The back pain of bus drivers: Prevalence in an urban area of California. *Spine* 1992;17:1481–1488.

17. Boden SD, Wiesel SW: Nonoperative management of cervical disc disease, in Camins MB, O'Leary PF (eds): *Disorders of the Cervical Spine*. Baltimore, MD, Williams & Wilkins, 1992, pp 157–160.

18. Christian CL: Medical management of cervical spine disease, in Camins MB, O'Leary PF (eds): *Disorders of the Cervical Spine*. Baltimore, MD, Williams & Wilkins, 1992, pp 147–155.

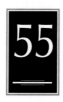

55

Classification of Thoracolumbar Fractures and Posterior Instrumentation for Treatment of Thoracolumbar Fractures

Daniel A. Capen, MD

Neurologic and Structural Classifications

In treating an injury to the thoracolumbar spine, several factors must be considered before treatment can be implemented. Outcome is governed as much by the decision-making process as by surgical or nonsurgical care. Several classification systems are available that provide the practitioner with the information needed to plan successful treatment of the injury. Any classification system must provide a guide for the clinician to permit an understanding of the injury and to allow correct treatment choice.

Injuries to the thoracolumbar spine can result from many types of trauma. Anatomic proximity to abdominal structures and intrathoracic structures often creates life-threatening injury that requires emergent attention. Head injury can also accompany spine injury, especially when high-energy trauma has occurred, such as vehicular injury or fall from heights. Once multisystem assessment is complete and life-threatening problems are cleared, the spinal surgeon can safely treat the patient's spinal injury.

The planning of treatment begins, however, with initial patient contact. A checklist can be used to glean important bits of information that will lead to appropriate treatment planning. (1) Is the injury high energy or low energy? Low-velocity gunshot wounds rarely destabilize the spine, and injuries that result from insignificant traumas, especially in older patients, must lead the practitioner to seek metabolic, metastatic, or infectious causes of the fracture. (2) Is the spinal column acutely unstable? High-energy trauma often creates an acutely unstable spine that requires emergent spine precautions. Care of life-threatening injury may delay spine surgery but must not delay spine supervision and appropriate precautions to prevent neurologic injury. If the spine is unstable acutely, does the patient need stabilization or orthotic treatment? (3) Is the neural column safe, threatened, or damaged? Imaging information may be important, but the neurologic examination is critical for appropriate decision making. Serial neurologic evaluation and appropriate grading will produce a treatment plan for successful outcome. (4) Is surgery required urgently? If canal compromise and neural deficit are documented and deterioration occurs, emergent surgery can help. If instability threatens further neurologic injury, emergent surgery can help. (5) Is surgery required for stability, neural recovery, or both?

These decisions require an understanding of the complete clinical picture. Radiographs taken of the spine at initial evaluation can often be used to diagnose spinal column injury. Computed tomography (CT) and magnetic resonance imaging (MRI) in the thoracolumbar region further clarify the picture of the spinal canal and can reveal posterior column injury, but most information regarding acute and chronic instability is present on plain radiographs. An understanding of Denis's classification of the 3-column spine will permit treatment planning for stabilization.[1] In addition to restoring spinal alignment, protecting neural elements, and preventing further injury, it is also important to avoid unneeded surgery. Even if well-performed, surgery for the wrong reason or without regard for the area of instability is subject to risk and may require revision. If appropriately applied, the Denis classification will assist the practitioner in planning the required procedure.

A mechanistic approach to thoracolumbar injury is well described by Ferguson and Allen.[2] This approach enhances the understanding of the forces applied to the spinal column at injury and helps the clinician to direct the treatment to the unstable

Table 1
Recommended treatment for various types of injury

Injury	Stability	Treatment
Vertical compression fracture	Stable	Orthosis
Missile injury	Stable	Orthosis
Distraction extension	Acutely	Surgical stabilization
Distraction flexion	Unstable	Rod-hook Screw-hooks
Translational injuries	Unstable	Reduction Rod-hooks Screw-hooks

area. From experience with the Allen classification of cervical trauma,[3] there is also some predictive information to allow nonsurgical treatment for fractures that are stable long-term. Flexion, distraction, compression, and rotational forces all produce radiographic pictures that are described in this classification.

The McAfee classification,[4] which describes 6 injury types that require CT for evaluation, also provides information regarding the forces applied at injury. This system also helps the clinician direct treatment to the area of spinal column failure. Wedge-compression, stable burst, unstable burst, Chance, flexion-distraction, and translational injuries are described, and pathology to the anterior, middle, and posterior columns associated with these injuries is described. I rely on the Allen classification because it is truly a total spine classification. However, the crucial factor is to use and become familiar with a system that will assist in understanding the pathoanatomy and enable the surgeon to plan appropriate treatment. Table 1 reflects injury type and recommended treatment.

The next factor for consideration in thoracolumbar trauma is the patient's neurologic status. Without this information, the clinician cannot plan appropriate care. Frankel grading, the standard system for many decades,[5] is generally too generic. At present, the American Spinal Injury Association (ASIA) Scoring System[6] is widely used as the standard for determining status. Waters and associates[7–9] at Rancho Los Amigos, have followed large numbers of neurologic injuries by ASIA scores to determine anticipated outcomes. The surgeon is encouraged to use this information before completing the treatment plan.

The International Standards for Neurological and Functional Classification of Spinal Cord Injury[6] defines tetraplegia as loss or impairment of motor and/or sensory function in the cervical cord. Paraplegia is loss of motor and/or sensory function in the thoracic, lumbar, or sacral cord, including caudal and conus injuries. The neurologic level is the most caudal level of bilaterally normal motor and sensory function. Incomplete injury is defined by partial motor and/or sensory function below the neurologic level. Complete injury is defined as absence of sensory and motor function in the lowest sacral segment.

The ASIA scoring system for sensory function rates dermatomes as absent = 0, impaired = 1, and normal = 2. Motor scoring is done by testing 5 muscles in the upper and 5 in the lower extremities. All tests are scored 0 to 5, and all testing is done supine. Deltoid or biceps, wrist extensors, triceps, flexor profundus, and hand intrinsics are tested for upper extremity scores. Iliopsoas, quadriceps, ankle dorsiflexors, extensor hallucis longus, and the gastrocnemius-soleus complex are scored in the lower extremities, to make a possible total of 100 points. Repeat examinations permit accurate tracking of improvement or deterioration, and pre- and postsurgical scoring is objectified.

Timing of Surgery

Complete injury is defined as the absence of motor and sensory function below the level of injury following emergence from spinal shock. Return of spinal bulbocavernosus reflex heralds emergence from spinal shock. After documentation of this, the likelihood of further neural recovery of significance is extremely small.[6] There is no current scientific justification for emergent surgery for decompression for the purpose of cord recovery in these patients. Focus must be turned to surgical or nonsurgical stabilization for enhancement of rehabilitation.[10] Needless surgery and postsurgical complications can be avoided if this is borne in mind. Some authors cite the zone of partial preservation as the target for decompression of complete injury. Some support for this viewpoint has been presented at the North American Spine Society 10th Annual Meeting by Rabinowitz (personal communication, 1995) in an animal study in which methylprednisolone was combined with decompression to produce better neural recovery, but the surgery must have reasonable likelihood of improving functional outcome.

The other group of patients with thoracolumbar trauma for whom treatment is clearly defined is the group with a perfect ASIA score, that is, normal neurologic function. This group includes patients with stable compression and burst type injuries and a few with unstable or potentially unstable injuries. It is generally agreed that, in these cases, improvement on normal neural function is impossible, while iatrogenic injury is possible.

Regardless of imaging studies, there is no justification for prophylactic decompression. In a tertiary center, such as Rancho Los Amigos Medical Center, however, it has been my experience that not all clinicians follow that caveat. The group of patients with incomplete cord injury syndromes presents the area of greatest variation in opinion and approach as to the timing and extent of surgery. The cord syndromes most frequently encountered are central, anterior, Brown-Sequard, conus, and cauda equina. Ditunno, in the ASIA standards, eloquently describes all these lesions.[6] Waters and associates[11] also describe anticipated outcomes in nonsurgical treatment for all these injuries. Before emergency intervention, the clinical status must be identified. Literature regarding cord recovery in animals by Bohlman and associates[12] and Delamarter and associates[13] has been cited most often to support emergency decompression.

The clear information is that within 6 hours after injury, the removal of compressing bone, disk, and deformity has some benefit. After 6 hours, no scientific evidence supports time as a factor in performance of decompression. I wish to stress that the time is 6 hours from time of injury, which reduces the number of patients eligible. Consideration of this factor should reduce needless high-risk surgery at midnight hours by ill-prepared surgical teams. Documented loss of neurologic function remains the 1 true indication for emergency surgery. Increased deformity, accumulation of hematoma, and cord

edema remain the most frequent causes. After adequate study, efforts should focus on both decompression and stabilization to minimize revision surgery. Laminectomy alone is to be avoided, because it serves only to further destabilize the thoracolumbar spine and often fails to adequately decompress anterior bone and disk.

In addition to maximum attention to skeletal and neurologic classification, and optimal performance of surgery, 2 other factors must be stressed. First, in most high-energy thoracolumbar patients, early surgery is likely to be adversely impacted by increased blood loss, pulmonary complications, and the sequelae of multisystem injury. Second is the incidence of neurologic complication as a result of early intervention. Marshall and associates[14] described a 2.9% complication rate in 134 cases of surgery within 48 hours. Compromised hemodynamics will compromise cord environment and injury edema also adversely affects canal manipulation.

Spine traumas that produce ligamentous and bony instability, such as Chance-type fractures, distractive flexion injuries, and translational injuries, are the most unstable of injuries to the thoracolumbar region. The preferred treatment is to stabilize the spine initially with a combination of rods, with distraction-compression type hooks above the injury and, in the very lower thoracic and lumbar spine, to use intrapedicular bone screws. Cross-links are used. In many of these fractures, especially in the L1-2 area, a posterolateral decompression can be done as well. If it is also necessary to perform anterior decompression, this can be done once the spine is reduced and stabilized. Posterior instrumentation does permit contouring of rods to preserve lumbar lordosis and thoracic kypho-

sis. Sagittal spinal balance is important for ambulation and wheelchair sitting. Unless secure fixation can be obtained with short segment fixation, at least 2 levels above and 2 levels below the injury must be incorporated. Newer FDA-approved combination rods, with pedicular hooks, transverse process hooks, and laminar hooks, provide sufficient stabilization to prevent later deformity.

As with all injuries, overdistraction or excessive compression across the traumatized area can result in neurologic worsening, because of the risk of retropulsion of bone and disk into the canal. This risk must be evaluated at the time of surgery to avoid iatrogenic neurologic injury. Understanding the mechanism of trauma and the classification of injury, together with intraoperative evaluation by radiographs, are the best methods for assurance of avoiding this complication.

In preoperative planning, if any of the posterior rod, hook, and screw combinations are going to be used, it is essential to ascertain the continuity of the planned bony structures for fixation. Ruling out occult lamina fracture, transverse process fracture, and pedicular fracture is essential. Noncontiguous spinal injury can occur, and appropriate imaging, whenever practical, can help to avoid the necessity for intraoperative change in plan. [15,16]

I prefer spinal-cord monitoring during the performance of decompression and fixation posteriorly for thoracolumbar fractures in any patient other than those with a complete neurologic injury. Even with anterior cord syndrome, monitoring impulses should be kept stable, and any manipulation of the spine must be documented. These precautions will help avoid iatrogenic neurologic worsening.

Table 2
Recommended methods for dealing with various thoracolumbar fractures

Spine Structure	Neurologic	Treatment
Stable	Normal	Nonsurgical
Stable	Complete	Nonsurgical
Stable	Incomplete	Decompression and stabilization
		Anterior or posterolateral
Unstable	Complete	Posterior stabilization
Unstable	Incomplete	Decompression and arthrodesis
		Anterior with plates
		Posterior or 360°

Posterior Instrumentation for Treatment of Thoracolumbar Fractures
Indications

The clinician must use the information contained in the classification of thoracolumbar injuries together with information regarding the patient's neurologic status in planning surgery. If the skeletal injury, the neurologic status, and the patient's multisystem health permits surgery, selection of a device for surgical fixation is the next important choice the surgeon must make.

Since the introduction of Harrington rod fixation,[17-23] there has been progressive development of instrumentation for spinal fracture fixation. Recognizing that each era had surgeons who were convinced that the "current technique" was optimal, we now have at our disposal fixation rod, hook, and cross-link systems that have been biomechanically tested. These devices are documented to provide secure fixation. The health-care industry has seen a remarkable proliferation of manufacturers of equipment, and, as a result, the surgeon can now select from multiple products.

The goals of posterior surgical treatment remain threefold. Realignment of the spine, restoration of canal anatomy, and protection against late deformity and instability are the 3 purposes for surgical intervention. The instrumentation available for treatment of thoracolumbar spine fractures permits the surgeon to create a construct that spans the area of instability and is fixed to the areas above and below the instability.

While Luque rod and wire stabilization has been shown to stabilize most fractures, the undesirable aspect of placing wires in the spinal canal adjacent to neural elements was a major drawback. Also, no distraction was possible. Current constructs, such as the Sofamor-Danek Horizon system and Acromed systems, have screw fixation systems for the pedicles below the thoracolumbar injury, and these screws are connected by a rod system to sublaminar claw and pedicular hook devices placed above the area of injury to actually grasp the spinal posterior elements. Some transverse process hooks are also available to maximize fixation above the thoracolumbar injury and to minimize the need for intracanal instrumentation. All constructs currently available emphasize the option for rods that are contoured to the spine to maintain normal or near normal sagittal balance. Numerous studies have stressed the importance of avoiding fixation in excessive kyphosis or lordosis.

The surgeon is encouraged to become familiar with a particular system and to practice working with that one instrument system until the entire operating team is aware of all the nuances of the particular device. These devices allow fixation of the minimal number of segments with maximum strength. I prefer the Horizon system by Sofamor-Danek, but this by no means indicates that other systems will not work as well. It merely reflects my familiarity with that particular device.

The success of posterior surgical treatment of thoracolumbar injuries depends on surgical judgment and appropriate indications, health of the patient at the time of the surgery, and appropriate uncomplicated application of the device at the time of the spinal surgery. Extensive operating time, staff unfamiliar with the device, and incomplete equipment can lead to substantial complications. The timing of surgery can also create hazards for the patient and intolerance of the surgical procedure. Successful outcome requires understanding and applying information from fracture classification and neurologic classification to provide appropriate treatment. Table 2 indicates the methods I prefer to use in dealing with various thoracolumbar fractures. This suggested guideline incorporates skeletal injury, neurologic status, and selected techniques for surgical intervention.

As shown in Table 2, there are several situations in which surgical intervention is not recommended. There remain indications for anterior surgery that are addressed in the anterior approaches to the thoracolumbar spine. The posterior surgical indications remain foremost with the completed neurologic injury, the unstable spine, and the desire to provide the patient with optimal early rehabilitation. As an ancillary, when anterior decompression has been performed, surgical posterior stabilization can permit full brace-free activity and rehabilitation when combined in a 360° approach.

The information provided in the 1980s by Edwards and Levine[24] remains effective in early stages to allow ligamentotaxis to decompress bony and disk elements via distraction. Although this procedure remains a viable option, the surgeon is cautioned to maintain awareness that 24- to 48-hour surgery with multisystem trauma is still beset with high incidences of complications, and a small number of spinal fractures with neurologic injury are in this category.

Summary

In treating thoracolumbar injuries, an accurate diagnosis of the structural injury to the spine is critical. I recommend the Allen classification,[2,3] but all classifications assist in obtaining an accurate understanding of the spine dynamics resulting from the injury. It is essential to remember that the majority of thoracolumbar injuries result from high-energy trauma. It is incumbent upon the spinal surgeon to ensure that multisystem trauma and life-threatening injuries, with the exception of a deteriorating neurologic injury, are cared for before embarking on spinal surgery. Even treatment of these injuries may have to be delayed if cardiovascular or abdominal hemorrhagic injuries take precedence.

A critically important piece of information is the neurologic diagnosis. I recommend the ASIA Motor Index[6] as the gold standard for diagnosing injuries and prognosticating outcome. Accurate neurologic diagnosis must be obtained prior to surgery. Finally, I recommend a firm understanding and a good working relationship with the device system used for fixation. Other instructional course authors agree that whether the anterior or the posterior approach is used, familiarity with the device nuances, by not only the surgeon but also the operating team, is very helpful in achieving a successful uncomplicated implantation. If all of the above recommendations are followed, successful outcome and optimal patient recovery can be anticipated in most cases.

References

1. Denis F: The three column spine and its significance in the classification of acute thoracolumbar spinal injuries. *Spine* 1983;8:817–831.

2. Ferguson RL, Allen BL Jr: A mechanistic classification of thoracolumbar spine fractures. *Clin Orthop* 1984;189:77–88.

3. Allen BL Jr, Ferguson RL, Lehmann TR, O'Brien RP: A mechanistic classification of closed, indirect fractures and dislocations of the lower cervical spine. *Spine* 1982;7:1–27.

4. McAfee PC, Yuan HA, Fredrickson BE, Lubicky JP: The value of computed tomography in thoracolumbar fractures: An analysis of one hundred consecutive cases and a new classification. *J Bone Joint Surg* 1983;65A:461–473.

5. Frankel HL, Hancock DO, Hyslop G, et al: The value of postural reduction in the initial management of closed injuries of the spine with paraplegia and tetraplegia: I. *Paraplegia* 1969;7:179–192.

6. American Spinal Cord Injury Association: *Standards for Neurological and Functional Classification of Spinal Cord Injury,* Revised. Chicago, IL, American Spinal Cord Injury Association, 1992.

7. Waters RL, Yakura JS, Adkins RH, Sie I: Recovery following complete paraplegia. *Arch Phys Med Rehabil* 1992;73:784–789.

8. Waters RL, Adkins RH, Yakura JS, Sie I: Motor and sensory recovery following incomplete paraplegia. *Arch Phys Med Rehabil* 1994;75:67–72.

9. Waters RL, Adkins RH, Yakura JS, Sie I: Motor and sensory recovery following complete tetraplegia. *Arch Phys Med Rehabil* 1993;74:242–247.

10. Rimoldi RL, Zigler JE, Capen DA, Hu SS: The effect of surgical intervention on rehabilitation time in patients with thoracolumbar and lumbar spinal cord injuries. *Spine* 1992;17:1443–1449.

11. Waters RL, Adkins RH, Yakura JS, Sie I: Effect of surgery on motor recovery following traumatic spinal cord injury. *Spinal Cord* 1996;34:188–192.

12. Bohlman HH, Bahniuk E, Raskulinecz G, Field G: Mechanical factors affecting recovery from incomplete cervical spinal cord injury: A preliminary report. *Johns Hopkins Med J* 1979;145:115–125.

13. Delamarter RB, Sherman J, Carr JB: Pathophysiology of spinal cord injury: Recovery after immediate and delayed decompression. *J Bone Joint Surg* 1995;77A:1042–1049.

14. Marshall LF, Knowlton S, Garfin S, et al: Deterioration following spinal cord injury: A multicenter study. *J Neurosurg* 1987;66:400–404.

15. Keenen TL, Antony J, Benson DR: Non-contiguous spinal fractures. *J Trauma* 1990;30:489–491.

16. McLain RF, Sparling E, Benson DR: Early failure of short-segment pedicle instrumentation for thoracolumbar fractures: A preliminary report. *J Bone Joint Surg* 1993;75A:162–167.

17. Davis LA, Warren SA, Reid DC, Oberle K, Saboe LA, Grace MG: Incomplete neural deficits in thoracolumbar and lumbar spine fractures: Reliability of Frankel and Sunnybrook scales. *Spine* 1993;18:257–263.

18. Stambough JL: Cotrel-Dubousset instrumentation and thoracolumbar spine trauma: A review of 55 cases. *J Spinal Disord* 1994;7:461–469.

19. Akbarnia BA, Fogarty JP, Tayob AA: Contoured Harrington instrumentation in the treatment of unstable spinal fractures: The effect of supplementary sublaminar wires. *Clin Orthop* 1984;189:186–194.

20. Keene JS, Wackwitz DL, Drummond DS, Breed AL: Compression-distraction instrumentation of unstable thoracolumbar fractures: Anatomic results obtained with each type of injury and method of instrumentation. *Spine* 1986;11:895–902.

21. Cotler JM, Vernace JV, Michalski JA: The use of Harrington rods in thoracolumbar fractures. *Orthop Clin North Am* 1986;17:87–103.

22. Dickson JH, Harrington PR, Erwin WD: Results of reduction and stabilization of the severely fractured thoracic and lumbar spine. *J Bone Joint Surg* 1978;60A:799–805.

23. Jacobs RR, Asher MA, Snider RK: Thoracolumbar spinal injuries: A comparative study of recumbent and operative treatment in 100 patients. *Spine* 1980;5:463–477.

24. Edwards CC, Levine AM: Early rod-sleeve stabilization of the injured thoracic and lumbar spine. *Orthop Clin North Am* 1986;17:121–145.

Combined Anterior and Posterior Surgery for Fractures of the Thoracolumbar Spine

Alexander R. Vaccaro, MD

Introduction

The incidence of traumatic spinal injury has increased over the last several decades, with the majority of patients being males between the ages of 15 and 29 years.[1,2] In a multicenter review of more than 1,000 patients with thoracolumbar fractures, 16% of injuries occurred between the T1 and T10 levels, 52% between the T11 and L1 levels, and 32% between the L1 and L5 levels.[3] Nearly half of the injuries in this study were the result of motor vehicle accidents, with the remainder due to falls, sporting involvement, violence, and other miscellaneous causes.[2]

Significant 3-column injuries, including fracture-dislocations, make up approximately 50% of thoracolumbar fractures, with approximately 75% of these injuries resulting in a complete neurologic deficit.[4] Spinal injuries presenting with circumferential instability usually result from a combination of significant vector forces including, but not limited to, compression, extension, rotation, and shear. In most of these unstable injuries, surgical treatment is necessary to stabilize the spinal elements and allow early mobilization; moreover there is a frequent need to decompress the neural elements. The surgeon can gain access to the anteri-or and posterior spinal elements through a variety of approaches, depending on the anatomic level.

Occasionally, because of the degree of instability, the quality of the bony and ligamentous structures, and the location of neural impingement, a circumferential surgical approach may be necessary to accomplish the goals of surgical treatment. The sequence of surgical approaches, anterior then posterior, posterior then anterior, or simultaneous, is patient- and fracture-specific and should be determined on a patient-to-patient basis. Regardless of approach, the basic goals of surgical treatment remain the same: to maintain or improve the patient's neurologic status, to realign the spine, to relieve pain, and to allow early mobilization and rehabilitation.

Anterior Followed by Posterior Approach

An anterior followed by a posterior approach is often useful in an unstable 3-column injury of the upper thoracic or lower lumbar spine in the setting of canal occlusion and an incomplete neurologic deficit. An anterior decompression followed by bone grafting is then stabilized with a posterior compression or neutralization construct. In these locations, the use of anterior instrumentation is often contraindicated because of the close proximity of the great vessels (Figs. 1–3). An anterior followed by a posterior approach may be necessary in situations where anterior instrumentation may not sufficiently stabilize the involved levels, such as in the setting of an unstable burst or shear injury that reduces adequately in the sagittal plane with recumbency (Fig. 4). In this situation, an adjunctive posterior procedure is beneficial. Shiba and associates[5] presented a series of patients who were treated surgically with an anterior decompression and bone grafting followed by posterior transpedicular fixation for unstable thoracolumbar injuries, primarily of the burst type. The authors noted a 98% rate of fusion, with 65% of patients improving by at least one Frankel grade. No patients experienced worsening of their neurologic symptoms.

A combined anterior followed by a posterior procedure is also indicated when an anterior decompression and reconstruction is needed, but anterior instrumentation is contraindicated because of the presence of significant osteoporosis. This situation often occurs in elderly patients or in patients with metabolic bone disease and poor bone quality in whom

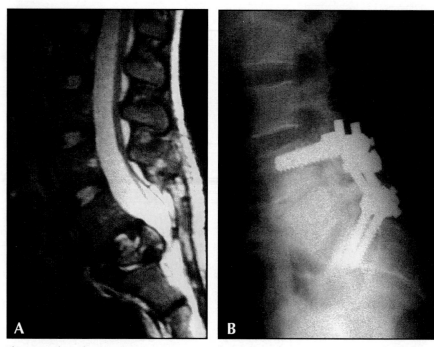

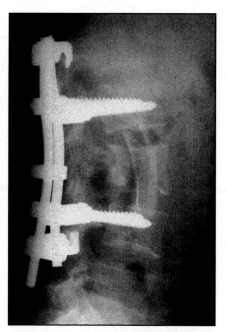

Fig. 1 A, A lateral magnetic resonance image of an L5 burst fracture in a patient with a unilateral L5 and S1 nerve root deficit. **B,** The patient underwent a posterolateral transpedicular decompression of the left L5 and S1 nerve roots and thecal sac followed by short segment posterior pedicular stabilization.

Fig. 2 A lateral plain radiograph following an anterior L3 corpectomy and strut grafting and posterior L1 to L4 hook and pedicular stabilization procedure. Anterior plate stabilization was not used because of the close proximity of the great vessels.

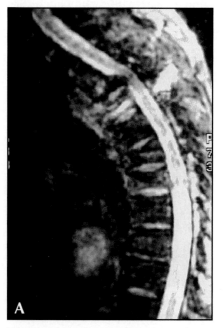

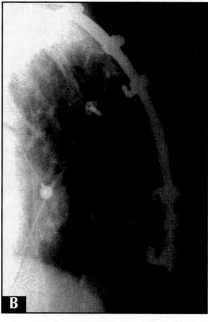

Fig. 3 A, A sagittal magnetic resonance image revealing a T3 burst fracture as well as T6 and T7 anterior compression fractures in a patient with an incomplete neurologic injury. **B,** A lateral plain radiograph following an anterior T3 carpectomy and fibula strut graft fusion with interference screw and a posterior rod hook compression and neutralization procedure. Anterior plate fixation could not be placed safely at the T2 to T4 level without risk of contact to the surrounding vasculature.

placement of anterior instrumentation carries the potential risk of screw, rod, or plate migration (Fig. 5).

Posterior Followed by Anterior Approach

A posterior followed by an anterior approach is often necessary in a significantly displaced fracture-dislocation of the thoracolumbar spine in a patient with an incomplete neurologic deficit. Adequate coronal and sagittal plane realignment is obtained through an initial posterior approach before decompressing the neural elements. Following this, the degree of canal occlusion may be assessed by intraoperative myelography, sonography, intracanal exploration, or postoperative imaging with computed tomography, myelogram, or magnetic resonance imaging. In a study by Edwards and Levine,[6] 4% of patients with an incomplete neurologic deficit who had been treated by a posterior indirect reduction had sufficient focal neurologic impingement remaining to warrant an immediate posterolateral or subsequent anterior decompression.

Occasionally, in a patient with a complete neurologic deficit, a posterior realignment procedure may result in significant loss of anterior column support and therefore not be adequately stabilized by a single-staged posterior procedure (Fig. 6). Sasso and Cotler[7] evaluated the efficacy of 3 different posterior internal fixation systems (Harrington rods and hooks, Luque rods with sublaminar wires, and AO dynamic compression plates with pedicle screws) used alone in the treatment of unstable fractures and fracture-dislocations of the thoracic and lumbar spine. At 12 months of follow-up, all 3 systems were found to be inadequate in maintaining sagittal balance, thereby illustrating the potential benefit of anterior column reconstruction and support.

Patients with ankylosing spondylitis or diffuse idiopathic skeletal hyperostosis who incur a traumatic distraction-extension injury may occasionally require a circumferential stabilization procedure (posterior, then anterior) to adequately stabilize the spine. Often, following posterior stabilization, a significant "fish mouth" anterior column defect is present, which may result in long-term instability if it is not reconstructed (Fig. 7). Also, in the setting of an open, unstable thoracolumbar injury, an initial posterior debridement followed by an anterior decompression and instrumentation fusion, if technically applicable, is recommended. Posterior instrumentation should not be used in this setting to avoid the risk of deep infection. Last, in a patient with an incomplete neurologic deficit an ante-

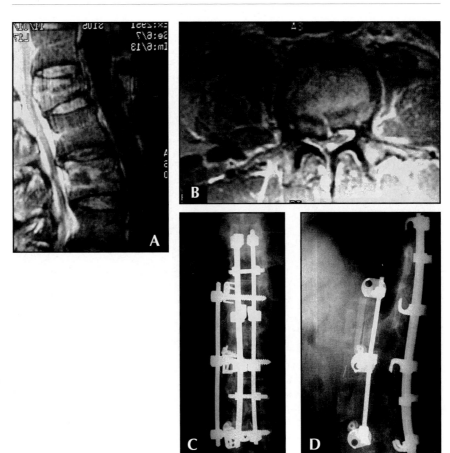

Fig. 4 A, A sagittal magnetic resonance image (MRI) of a 23-year-old man with an L1 and L3 burst fracture and an incomplete neurologic deficit. **B,** A transaxial MRI revealing the degree of canal encroachment at the L3 level. **C** and **D,** An anterior L1 and L3 corpectomy and strut graft fusion with instrumentation was followed by a neutralization and posterior stabilization because of the degree of instability. Note the single, not dual, rod application anteriorly because of the close proximity of the iliac vessels.

rior approach following an attempted posterior indirect reduction is occasionally necessary if sufficient canal clearance is not obtained during the posterior procedure. Several authors have advocated an additional anterior decompression procedure in this patient population if canal occlusion of 20% or greater is demonstrated by postoperative computed tomography scanning.[8]

Surgical Approach
In North America, a surgical team comprising of the spinal surgeon, anesthesiologist, electrophysiologist, general or thoracic surgeon, and nursing staff work in a coordinated fashion to accomplish the aforementioned surgical goals with the least potential morbidity to the trauma patient. The possibility for intraoperative adverse events, such as loss of neurologic function with positioning or fracture reduction, great vessel injury, excessive blood loss due to the length of surgery, or instrumentation malpositioning, is increased with procedures that require circumferential stabilization because of the inherent instability of these procedures.

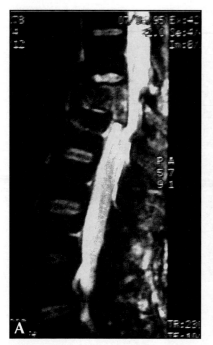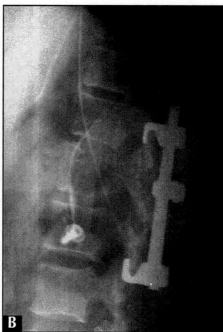

Fig. 5 A, A sagittal magnetic resonance image revealing an L1 flexion-compression burst fracture in a 68-year-old woman with significant osteoporosis. **B,** Because of the degree of osteoporosis and the potential for screw migration, an anterior plate was not applied following the corpectomy and bone grafting. A posterior compression hook and rod stabilization procedure followed the anterior procedure.

An experienced electrophysiologist using contemporary neurologic monitoring techniques greatly assists the surgeon in detecting the early onset of neurologic dysfunction. Additionally, an operating table that is equipped to rotate the patient's body axially without the need for repositioning further decreases the potential for any complications from patient movement. Most importantly, an experienced general or vascular surgeon is often of great use in anterior exposures that require exposure of the upper thoracic spine (transsternal or modified cervicothoracic approach) or lumbosacral region. Several useful posterior surgical approaches are available by which the spinal surgeon can gain access to the anterior spinal elements when a separate anterior approach is not desired. These include the posterior

transpedicular approach and lateral extracavitary approach.

Lateral Extracavitary Approach

The lateral extracavitary approach[9] allows the spinal surgeon to access the anterior thecal sac and anterolateral vertebral elements throughout the thoracic and lumbar spine. However, this approach may be difficult above the level of T2 because of the presence of the scapula, and below the level of L4 because of the presence of the iliac crest (although this can be removed during the procedure and used for bone grafting). The approach consists of a "curved hockey stick" incision beginning in the midline approximately 3 vertebral levels above to 3 levels below the lesion. The incision is extended laterally with an abrupt curve toward the side of the approach for approxi-

mately 12 to 14 cm. The subcutaneous tissue and thoracodorsal fascia are then incised along the line of the skin incision and elevated from the midline laterally off the underlying musculature. If instrumentation is to be used, subperiosteal dissection is performed to expose the posterior vertebral elements.

Exposure of the thoracic and upper lumbar spine requires the removal of ribs for adequate visualization, and resection of a portion of the posterior iliac crest is necessary for visualization of the lumbar spine. During the exposure of the thoracic spine, a surgical plane is developed along the lateral aspect of the erectae spinae muscles in order to elevate them from the ribs and retract them medially. The laterally situated muscles—the latissimus dorsi, trapezius, and serratus groups—are retracted laterally. The intercostal muscles are then dissected away from the ribs, taking care not to injure the underlying neurovascular bundles that run along their inferior surface. The intercostal artery is routinely ligated, and the nerve may be divided or left intact at the discretion of the surgeon. The band of hypesthesia that results from sacrificing the intercostal nerve is rarely problematic and generally resolves over time. Following the proximal portion of the intercostal nerve allows identification of the neural foramen. The ribs that are to be removed (the rib at the level of the lesion and usually the adjacent caudal rib) are transected 7 to 10 cm lateral to the costovertebral junction, and they are then carefully disarticulated from their costovertebral and costochondral articulations. The transverse processes are also removed at these levels.

In lower lumbar lesions, the posterior, superior, and medial portion of the iliac crest is removed following dissection of surrounding mus-

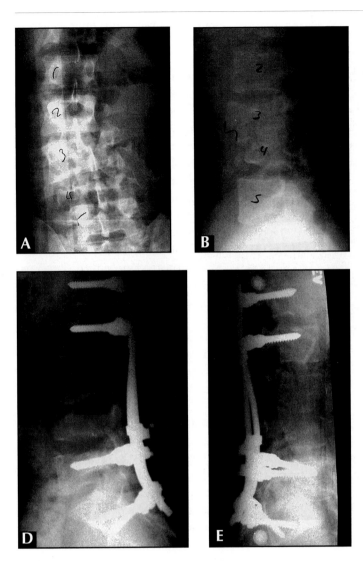

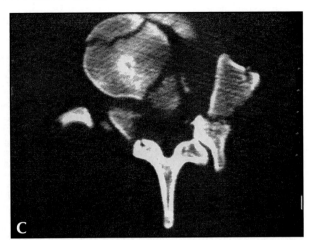

Fig. 6 **A,** anteroposterior and **B,** lateral plain radiographs of a severe rotational fracture-dislocation in a patient with a complete neurologic injury. **C,** A transaxial computed tomography scan revealed the presence of lateral vertebral subluxation as well as significant canal compromise. **D,** A lateral plain radiograph following an open posterior realignment and stabilization. **E,** Due to the degree of loss of anterior column support, an anterior L3 and L4 corpectomy and iliac crest graft reconstruction was performed.

culature and periosteum. The transverse process at the level of the lesion and the one caudal to it are dissected free of all contiguous soft-tissue structures and are removed to expose the exiting nerve roots. The nerve roots are subsequently mobilized and retracted laterally with nerve tapes and are again used to identify the neural foramen.

Subsequent to the soft-tissue exposure of the involved vertebrae, the vertebral periosteum is bluntly dissected off the ventrolateral aspect of the vertebral body and pedicle in preparation for spinal canal decompression.

Posterolateral Transpedicular Approach

The transpedicular approach may be selected in certain thoracolumbar injuries in which there is significantly lateralized or asymmetric anterior canal occlusion in a patient with symptomatic neural compression. This technique is most useful in lower lumbar injuries, in which anterior reconstructive procedures are often technically challenging and difficult to stabilize with instrumentation because of the close proximity of the great vessels. In the vast majority of cases with significant neural compression, the anterior approach provides optimal access to the anterior neural elements for decompression and reconstruction.

After posterior exposure of the involved vertebral level, the cephalad portion of the lamina, spinous process, supra-adjacent ligamentum flavum, and inferior lamina of the superior vertebrae are removed to expose clearly the medial and inferior boundaries of the pedicle to be decompressed. A burr is then used to remove the central portion of the pedicle into the fractured vertebral body. Using care to protect the transversing and exiting nerve roots, a rongeur or curette may be used to

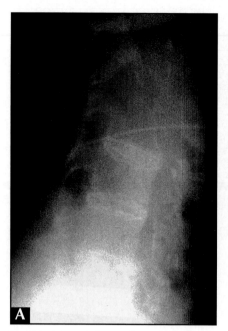
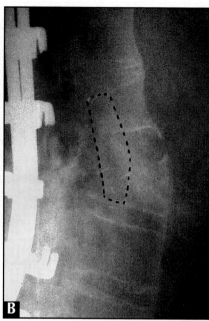

Fig. 7 A, A lateral plain radiograph of a distraction extension injury at the L1, L2 level in a patient with ankylosing spondylitis. **B,** Following a posterior stabilization procedure, an anterior column reconstruction was performed because of the presence of a large anterior "fish mouth" bony deficiency.

remove the medial cortex of the involved pedicle. A trough is then cut into the posterior portion of the vertebral body anterior to the medial pedicular wall decompression. Reverse-angled curettes are used to displace bony fragments out of the canal into the region of this trough. Large bony fragments may be removed posteriorly with gentle thecal sac retraction in the lower lumbar spine below the conus of the spinal cord.

Spinal Fixation

Spinal instrumentation allows the surgeon to manipulate the spinal elements efficiently in order to obtain proper alignment, to assist in indirectly decompressing the spinal elements, and to afford stability to allow for early mobilization. Commonly used spinal implants include hooks, screws, and wires attached to rods or plates posteriorly and screws attached to plates or rods as well as metallic interbody spacers (cages) anteriorly. The choice of implant is determined by the nature, degree, or biomechanics of the existing instability, the quality of the spinal elements in terms of bone density or osteoporosis, and the medical condition of the patient. Hooks and rods are frequently used in posterior spinal applications for thoracolumbar injuries. Converging hook patterns allow the surgeon to apply compressing forces; diverging hook patterns allow distraction. A combination of hook patterns, such as the use of claw configurations with or without supplemental sublaminar wires, allows multisegmental rigid spinal fixation, especially when a long level arm is needed for spinal manipulation. Sublaminar wires are useful in the neurologically complete patient when multiple level segmental fixation is necessary. Pedicle screw fixation is useful in lower lumbar and sacral injuries where short segment fixation is desirable as long as there is adequate anterior column support. The anatomic constraints of the pedicle in the mid and upper thoracic spine render pedicle screw applications less useful in these regions.

Techniques for anterior fixation usually involve plate and screw instrumentation. This form of fixation is generally chosen when a single approach (ie, anterior) is acceptable for neural decompression and stabilization. Circumferential procedures often use a single anterior rod and screw construct for added spinal and bone graft stability in addition to supplemental posterior instrumentation. Anterior spinal instrumentation, especially of the plating type, is generally not used in the lower lumbar and sacral region because of the close proximity of the great vessels.

Postoperative Care

Aggressive postoperative pulmonary and nutritional care is vital to the successful recovery of a patient undergoing a circumferential reconstructive procedure for an unstable thoracolumbar injury. The primary objective of such an involved procedure is to allow early patient mobilization so as to avoid the morbidity associated with recumbency. Nutritional supplementation assists in wound healing and provides the energy necessary for early patient rehabilitation.

If medically stable, patients who undergo a circumferential stabilization procedure may be mobilized in a chair on the first postoperative day. Increased mobility, either via a wheelchair or through ambulation, usually commences on approximately postoperative day 2 or at the time of chest tube removal. A standard thoracolumbosacral orthosis (TLSO) with a cervical extension is applied to fracture patterns cephalad to the T7 level. The cervical extension is used for approximately 6 weeks. Below T6, a standard TLSO is used. For fractures involving the L4, L5, or sacral levels, an additional thigh cuff attachment is used for approximately 6 weeks. The duration of brace wear ranges from 3 to 6 months, depending on the fracture type and degree of stability.

Routine upper and lower extremity range of motion and strengthening begin in the early postoperative period and are patient specific depending on the neurologic status. Following brace removal, truncal strengthening and range of motion are begun.

Outcomes

The literature is sparse on the outcomes of circumferential stabilization procedures for fracture-dislocations of the thoracolumbar spine. The obvious benefits of this procedure are the ability to decompress the anterior neural elements, provide anterior column support, and recreate or maintain sagittal balance with a variety of posterior instrumentation techniuqes. As anesthetic techniques improve and surgeons become more

experienced with circumferential stabilization techniques for thoracolumbar spinal injuries, the morbidity in terms of surgical time and blood loss will certainly be overshadowed by the satisfactory long-term outcomes of these procedures.

*At the time of this writing, bone screws placed posteriorly into vertebral elements have been cleared for use in this specific manner by the Food and Drug Administration (FDA) to provide immobilization and stabilization as an adjunct to fusion in the treatment of the following acute and chronic instability or deformities of the thoracic, lumbar and sacral spine; degenerative spondylolisthesis with objective evidence of neurological impairment; fracture; dislocation; scoliosis; kyphosis; spine tumor and failed previous fusion (pseudoarthrosis). In addition, anterior vertebral body screws (cervical, thoracic, and lumbar) are Class II devices and can be used as labeled in vertebral bodies.

References

1. Kraus JF, Franti CE, Riggins RS, Richards D, Borhani NO: Incidence of traumatic spinal cord lesions. *J Chronic Dis* 1975;28:471–492.

2. Price C, Makintubee S, Herndon W, Istre GR: Epidemiology of traumatic spinal cord injury and acute hospitalization and rehabilitation charges for spinal cord injuries in Oklahoma, 1988-1990. *Am J Epidemiol* 1994;139:37–47.

3. Gertzbein SD: Scoliosis Research Society: Multicenter spine fracture study. *Spine* 1992;17:528–540.

4. Bohlman HH: Treatment of fractures and dislocations of the thoracic and lumbar spine. *J Bone Joint Surg* 1985;67A:165–169.

5. Shiba K, Katsuki M, Ueta T, et al: Transpedicular fixation with Zielke instrumentation in the treatment of thoracolumbar and lumbar injuries. *Spine* 1994;19:1940–1949.

6. Edwards CC, Levine AM: Early rod-sleeve stabilization of the injured thoracic and lumbar spine. *Orthop Clin North Am* 1986;17:121–145.

7. Sasso RC, Cotler HB: Posterior instrumentation and fusion for unstable fractures and fracture-dislocations of the thoracic and lumbar spine: A comparative study of three fixation devices in 70 patients. *Spine* 1993;18:450–460.

8. Danisa OA, Shaffrey CI, Jane JA, et al: Surgical approaches for the correction of unstable thoracolumbar burst fractures: A retrospective analysis of treatment outcomes. *J Neurosurg* 1995;83:977–983.

9. Maiman DJ, Larson SJ: Lateral extracavitary approach to the thoracic and lumbar spine, in Rengachary SS, Wilkins RH (eds): *Neurosurgical Operative Atlas.* Park Ridge, IL, American Association of Neurological Surgeons (AANS), 1991, pp 153–161.

Evaluation of the Spine Utilizing the AMA *Guides to the Evaluation of Permanent Impairment,* 4th Edition

Robert H. Haralson III, MD

The Fourth Edition

The American Medical Association's *Guides to the Evaluation of Permanent Impairment* (AMA Guides) is now in its 4th edition.[1] In the 3rd edition and 3rd edition, revised, the only option for evaluation of the spine was to use the range-of-motion model. The difference in the 3rd edition, revised, is that in that volume the use of an inclinometer for measurement of range of motion was required, whereas the 3rd edition provided the option of using a goniometer. For a variety of reasons, it became obvious that the goniometer did not accurately measure motion in the spine, and therefore its use was abandoned.

In the 4th edition, the authors added a second method of evaluating the spine, the diagnosis-related estimates (DRE). The DRE, or injury model, has several advantages over the range-of-motion method. Despite ways to check the validity of the range-of-motion method, it is still not absolutely reliable. In addition, the range-of-motion method does not take into account the effects of aging on the spine and resulting loss of motion. Weisel reported a series of 100 patients without back pain in which he did range-of-motion studies and found up to 35% impairment based on the range-of-motion model.[2]

The range-of-motion method pe-

nalizes those patients who rehabilitate properly after injuries and/or surgery, thus regaining their motion, and it rewards those patients who do not. Use of an inclinometer measures motion of the spinal area, but it does not measure motion of the individual spinal segment, the measurement in which we are really interested. As a matter of fact, if a patient rehabilitates and regains motion of a spinal area at the expense of segments above and below a stiff segment, then, at least theoretically, the patient is worse off, because the more mobile segments have been placed at risk.

A few advantages of the range-of-motion method are certainly apparent. The range-of-motion method is fairly simple to perform. A good history and physical, along with accurate measurements using the inclinometer, gives a rather easy method of evaluating impairment. In addition, despite the fact that many spine physicians feel that range of motion has very little bearing on loss of function or impairment, it may turn out to be a good marker for impairment. Further research is necessary to prove this point. The range-of-motion method is also a good way to do an "administrative evaluation," in which a patient who is about to retire undergoes evaluation, not because of a particular injury, but in order to

determine the impairment of the patient at a certain time in his or her life.

Differentiators

The AMA Guides provide a number of differentiators to help the physician categorize patients. Differentiators are objective findings and include muscle spasm or guarding, loss of reflex, decreased circumference above and below the elbow or knee, electromyographic (EMG) diagnosis, lateral motion radiographs, loss of structural integrity, loss of bowel or bladder control, and bladder studies. The ultimate differentiator is the range-of-motion model. Determination of the loss of structural integrity is shown in Figures 1 and 2.[3]

Structural Inclusions

In addition, there are some structural inclusions that automatically place a patient in one of the categories. These are posterior element fractures, undisplaced or displaced posterior element fractures that disrupt the geometry of the spinal canal, and compression fractures, which are subdivided into less than 25%, 25% to 50%, and greater than 50%. If a patient qualifies for a particular category by way of a structural inclusion, it is not necessary to use the other criteria (differentiators).

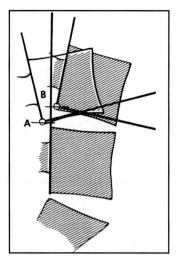

Fig. 1 Loss of motion segment integrity: translation. (Reproduced with permission from Posner I, White AA III, Edwards WT, Hayes WC: A biomechanical analysis of the clinical stability of the lumbar and lumbosacral spine. *Spine* 1982;7:374–389.)

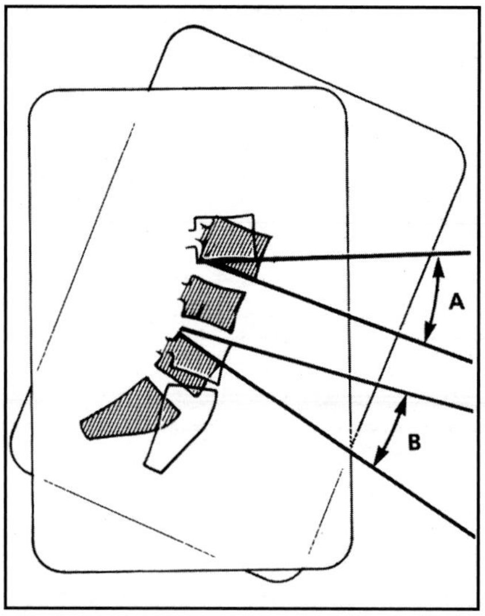

Fig. 2 Loss of motion segment integrity: angular motion. (Reproduced with permission from Posner I, White AA III, Edwards WT, Hayes WC: A biomechanical analysis of the clinical stability of the lumbar and lumbosacral spine. *Spine* 1982;7:374–389.)

Philosophy of the 4th Edition

It was the intent of the authors to make the DRE method the primary method for evaluating the spine. The range-of-motion method was to be secondary and was to be used only to assist a physician in categorizing a patient. Unfortunately, the language in the instructions was not direct enough, which has led to some confusion. The instructions, however, are fairly specific. They are that a physician is to use the DRE model as long as the patient is described by the information in Figure 3. This basically covers every situation. Further, the AMA Guides indicate that if the physician cannot decide into which DRE category to place the patient by using the differentiators, the physician then may refer to and use the range-of-motion model described in section 3.3J, for assistance in categorizing the patient. The AMA Guides further state that, using the procedures of the range-of-motion model, the physician combines an impair-

ment based on the patient's spine motion impairment with an impairment based on the patient's diagnosis (Fig. 4), and a percent based on neurologic impairment (Fig. 5), if present. The physician uses the estimate determined by the range-of-motion model to decide placement within one of the DRE categories. The proper DRE category is the one having the impairment closest to the impairment determined by the range-of-motion model.

As an example, consider a patient who has a compression fracture of the lumbar spine (LS). In the DRE model, the instructions are to determine the percentage of compression, and, as we all know, it sometimes is very difficult to determine the exact percentage of compression of a vertebral body. Many of the fractures are wedge-shaped, the adjacent vertebra may or may not be exactly the same size, and changes in radiographic techniques make the calculation difficult. In a fracture that is close to

50%, it is sometimes difficult to determine if it is 49% (LS category III), or 51% (LS category IV). However, that 2% difference might result in a 10% variance in impairment rating. In this situation, the surgeon might refer to the range-of-motion model. If the range-of-motion model indicates impairment greater than 20%, the patient would be placed in DRE category IV and given a resultant 20% impairment. If the range-of-motion model indicates impairment less than 10%, the patient should be categorized in lumbosacral category III and given a rating of 10%. If the range-of-motion model indicates impairment between 10% and 20%, the patient should be assigned to the DRE category closest to the range-of-motion impairment calculation.

The change from the 3rd edition, revised, and from the philosophy in the upper and lower extremity even in the 4th edition is that the rating for the spine should rate the result of the injury, not the treatment. Accordingly, if the patient ever has objective findings throughout his or her course, an assignment to category II is appropriate. Similarly, if a patient has significant radiculopathy anywhere in his or her course, then assignment to category III is appropriate even though the patient's symptoms may or may not improve with or without surgery. Instructions for performing evaluations are that the physician should review all of the records available, including imaging studies, and then do a complete history and physical examination. If the physician finds objective findings during the examination or evidence of objective findings in the record, assignment to the appropriate category even though the patient's symptoms may have increased or decreased with treatment (including surgery) is mandated.

Patient's condition	Category					Category *		
	I	II	III	IV	V	VI	VII	VIII
Complaints or symptoms	I							
Vertebral body compression, less than 25%		II						
Posterior element fracture, healed, stable, no dislocation or radiculopathy		II						
Transverse or spinous process fracture with dislocation of fragment, healed, stable		II						
Vertebral body compression fracture 25%–50%			III					
Posterior element fracture with spinal canal displacement or radiculopathy, healed, stable			III					
Radiculopathy			III					
Loss of motion segment integrity				IV				
Vertebral body compression, greater than 50%				IV	V			
Multilevel structural compromise				IV	V			
Cauda equina syndrome *without* bowel or bladder impairment						VI		
Cauda equina syndrome *with* bowel or bladder impairment							VII	
Paraplegia								VIII
Spondylolysis *without* loss of motion segment integrity or radiculopathy	I	II						
Spondylolysis *with* loss of motion segment integrity or radiculopathy			III	IV	V			
Spondylolisthesis *without* loss of motion segment integrity or radiculopathy	I	II						
Spondylolisthesis *with* loss of motion segment integrity or radiculopathy			III	IV	V			
Spondylolisthesis *with* cauda equina syndrome						VI	VII	VIII
Vertebral body fracture *without* loss of motion segment integrity or radiculopathy		II	III	IV				
Vertebral body fracture *with* loss of motion segment integrity or radiculopathy			III	IV	V			
Vertebral body fracture *with* cauda equina syndrome						VI	VII	VIII
Vertebral body dislocation *without* loss of motion segment integrity or radiculopathy		II	III	IV				
Vertebral body dislocation *with* loss of motion segment integrity or radiculopathy			III	IV	V			
Vertebral body dislocation *with* cauda equina syndrome						VI	VII	VIII
Previous spine operation *without* loss of motion segment integrity or radiculopathy		II	III	IV				
Previous spine operation *with* loss of motion segment integrity or radiculopathy			III	IV	V			
Previous spine operation *with* cauda equina syndrome						VI	VII	VIII
Stenosis, or facet arthrosis or disease, or disk arthrosis	I	II						

*Long-tract categories VI, VII, and VIII for long-tract signs may be combined (Combined Values Chart, p. 322) with impairment percents of cervicothoracic categories II–V or thoracolumbar categories II–IV (see Tables 73 and 74, pp. 110 and 111).

Fig. 3 Spine impairment categories for cervicothoracic, thoracolumbar, and lumbosacral regions. (Reproduced with permission from *Guides to the Evaluation of Permanent Impairment*, ed 4. Chicago, IL, American Medical Association, 1993, pp 94–138.)

The question arises as to appropriate categorization of a patient who has undergone a fusion in association with a diskectomy. If the patient's surgeon believed that a fusion after diskectomy was indicated, but the indications for the operation were radiculopathy and not loss of motion segment integrity, then the patient would still be placed in category III rather than category IV (loss of motion segment integrity), because the rating must reflect the results of the injury, not the treatment. The result of the injury was radiculopathy, not loss of motion segment integrity. A second question is whether a patient with previous surgery for radiculopathy should be awarded increased impairment after a second diskectomy. The answer, according to the 4th

Disorder	% Impairment of the whole person		
	Cervical	**Thoracic**	**Lumbar**
I. Fractures:			
A. Compression of one vertebral body			
0%-25%	4	2	5
26%-50%	6	3	7
>50%	10	5	12
B. Fracture of posterior element (pedicle, lamina, articular process, transverse process)	4	2	5
Note: An impairment due to compression of a vertebra and one due to fracture of a posterior element are *combined* using the Combined Values Chart (p. 322). Fractures or compressions of several vertebrae are *combined* using the Combined Values Chart.			
C. Reduced dislocation of one vertebra.	5	3	6
If two or more vertebrae are dislocated and reduced, *combine* the estimates using the Combined Values Chart (p. 322). An unreduced dislocation causes impairment until it is reduced; the physician should then evaluate the impairment on the basis of the subject's condition with the dislocation reduced. If no reduction is possible, the physician should evaluate the impairment on the basis of the range of motion and the neurologic findings according to criteria in this chapter and the nervous system chapter.			
II. Intervertebral disk or other soft-tissue lesion			
A. Unoperated on, with no residual signs or symptoms	0	0	0
B. Unoperated on, stable, with medically documented injury, pain, and rigidity† associated with *none to minimal* degenerative changes on structural tests, such as those involving roentgenography or magnetic resonance imaging.	4	2	5
C. Unoperated on, stable, with medically documented injury, pain, and rigidity† associated with *moderate to severe* degenerative changes on structural tests; includes unoperated on herniated nucleus pulposus with or without radiculopathy	6	3	7
D. Surgically treated disk lesion without residual signs or symptoms; includes disk injection	7	4	8
E. Surgically treated disk lesion with residual, medically documented pain and rigidity	9	5	10
F. Multiple levels, with or without operations and with or without residual signs or symptoms	Add 1% per level		
G. Multiple operations *with* or without residual symptoms:			
1. Second operation	Add 2%		
2. Third or subsequent operation	Add 1% per operation		
III. Spondylolysis and spondylolisthesis, not operated on			
A. Spondylolysis or grade I (1%-25% slippage); or grade II (26%-50% slippage) spondylolisthesis, accompanied by medically documented injury that is stable, and medically documented pain and rigidity with or without muscle spasm	6	3	7
B. Grade III (51%-75% slippage) or grade IV (76%-100% slippage) spondylolisthesis, accompanied by medically documented injury that is stable and medically documented pain and rigidity with or without muscle spasm	8	4	9
IV. Spinal stenosis, segmental instability, spondylolisthesis, fracture, or dislocation, operated on			
A. Single-level decompression *without* spinal fusion and *without* residual signs or symptoms	7	4	8
B. Single-level decompression *with* residual signs or symptoms	9	5	10
C. Single-level spinal fusion with or without decompression *without* residual signs or symptoms	8	4	9
D. Single-level spinal fusion with or without decompression *with* residual signs or symptoms	10	5	12
E. Multiple levels, operated on, with residual, medically documented pain and rigidity with or without muscle spasm	Add 1% per level		
1. Second operation	Add 2%		
2. Third or subsequent operation	Add 1% per operation		

*Instructions: 1. Identify the most significant impairment of the primarily involved region. 2. The diagnosis-based impairment estimates and percents shown above should be combined with range-of-motion impairment estimates and with whole-person impairment estimates involving sensation, weakness, and conditions of the musculoskeletal, nervous, or other organ systems. 3. List the diagnosis-based, range-of-motion, and other whole-person impairment estimates on the Spine Impairment Summary Form.

†The words "with medically documented injury, pain, and rigidity" imply not only that an injury or illness has occurred, but also that the condition is stable, as shown by the evaluator's history, examination, and other data, and that a permanent impairment exists, which is at least partly due to the condition being evaluated and not only due to preexisting disease.

Fig. 4 Whole-person impairment percents due to specific spine disorders. (Reproduced with permission from *Guides to the Evaluation of Permanent Impairment*, ed 4. Chicago, IL, American Medical Association, 1993, pp 94–138.)

edition, is that that is not appropriate. The 4th edition allows apportionment. The impairment for radiculopathy is 10%, and the 4th edition has no provision to determine the quantity of radiculopathy and, therefore, no way to increase the impairment for a second diskectomy. The argument for support of this philosophy is that the patient may have sustained more pain with the second episode, may have missed more work, and may be due an award for pain and suffering, but anatomically, is no worse off after the second operation than after the first. The problem is further complicated when the patient has a successful initial diskectomy followed by a second diskectomy that does not relieve the pain. This is even further complicated if the first surgery did not involve workers' compensation but the second one did, which is not unusual. The musculoskeletal chapter is quite specific in its direction that pain is not a consideration. Therefore, because the only difference between successful back surgery and unsuccessful back surgery is the absence of pain, and pain is not taken into account, the AMA Guides do not provide for directly awarding a patient increased impairment because of residual pain following diskectomy. The reader is reminded, however, that the AMA volume is only a guide, and that if a physician feels that it does not adequately describe the patient, then the rater is not necessarily required to follow it. Deviation does require a good explanation in the report and the addition of a reasonable award. For instance, a patient in one of the situations outlined above may be awarded an extra 5%.

Categories

There are 3 regions of the spine. The authors have renamed the areas lumbosacral, cervicothoracic and thora-

Nerve root impaired	Maximum % loss of function due to sensory deficit or pain	Maximum % loss of function due to strength deficit	Range of lower extremity impairment (%)
L3	5	20	0-24
L4	5	34	0-37
L5	5	37	0-40
S1	5	20	0-24

Fig. 5 Unilateral spinal nerve root impairment affecting the lower extremity. (Reproduced with permission from *Guides to the Evaluation of Permanent Impairment*, ed 4. Chicago, IL, American Medical Association, 1993, pp 94–138.)

columbar, new designations that better describe the function of the areas. Injuries at the lumbosacral junction act more like thoracic injuries, because the cord is involved. The lumbosacral plexus is made up of both lumbar and sacral nerve roots, and the cervical plexus is made up of both cervical and thoracic nerve roots. There are 8 categories in each of the 3 spinal areas.

Lumbosacral Area

Patients assigned to lumbosacral DRE category I have minor complaints but no objective findings of either significant injury or radiculopathy. These patients are given a rating of 0%.

In lumbosacral category II, objective findings, such as muscle spasm, dysmetria, or nonverifiable radicular pain are present, but without evidence of significant radiculopathy. Nonverifiable radicular pain is defined as pain in the distribution of a nerve root that is not verifiable by objective neurologic changes. Impairment for this category is 5%.

Lumbosacral category III is radiculopathy. Radiculopathy is diagnosed by the presence of such neurologic findings as anatomic numbness, anatomic weakness, loss of a reflex, or atrophy greater than 2 cm. A positive straight leg raising test may assist the physician in making a diagnosis of radiculopathy, but the straight leg raising test must be performed and interpreted properly. The reader is

referred to the section on straight leg raising in the AMA Guides. The impairment is 10%.

The majority of patients evaluated for spine impairments fall within the first 3 categories of the lumbosacral spine. Therefore, in most instances, the rater need make only 2 decisions. Did the patient have a significant injury, and is radiculopathy present? Most patients can be rated using these 2 decisions. The findings in the higher categories are rare in industrial settings and are not very common in automobile accidents.

One of the objective findings that allows a physician to make the diagnosis of radiculopathy are the changes in an electromyogram (EMG) as defined by the AMA Guides. These changes are unequivocal electrodiagnostic evidence of acute nerve root compromise, such as multiple positive sharp waves or fibrillation potentials; H wave absence or delay greater than 3 mm per second; or chronic changes, such as polyphasic waves in peripheral muscles. The presence of these specific EMG changes makes the diagnosis of neuropathy. However, because EMG changes are not necessary to make the diagnosis, an EMG is not appropriate in every patient.

Lumbosacral category IV is loss of structural integrity. Loss of structural integrity in the lumbosacral spine is defined as translation of 1 vertebra on another of 5 mm or more on lateral flexion and extension radiographs.

Two procedures for using this method to determine loss of structural integrity are shown in Figures 1 and 2. The impairment is 20%.

Flexion and extension radiographs are not necessary in every patient. Loss of structural integrity is rarely present in the face of normal supine anteroposterior and lateral radiographs. Therefore, unless there is a suggestion of loss of structural integrity on routine radiographs, or unless there is some other reason to feel that loss of structural integrity may exist, it is not necessary to obtain flexion and extension laterals.

Lumbosacral category V is the combination of categories III and IV, that is, radiculopathy and loss of structural integrity, and the impairment is 25%. Lumbosacral category VI is cauda equina syndrome without bowel or bladder involvement and is rated at 40%. There should be bilateral loss of lower extremity function.

Lumbosacral category VII is the same as category VI, but with the presence of bowel or bladder involvement. The history and physical examination can determine bowel and bladder involvement. Cystometrograms may confirm the diagnosis but are not necessary. The rating is 60%. Category VIII is paraplegia, defined as total or near total loss of function in the lower extremities. The impairment is 75%.

Cervicothoracic Area

The ratings for the cervicothoracic and thoracolumbar spines are very similar to those of the lumbar spine except for one major difference. In the cervicothoracic and thoracolumbar spine, an injury to the cord can produce long track signs. In such a case, it is necessary to take into account both local injury and lower extremities involvement. Therefore the impairment figures from categories VI, VII, and VIII in the cervicothoracic and thoracolumbar spine must be combined with a rating from one of the lower categories.

Cervicothoracic category I again is minor complaints with no findings and a resultant 0% impairment. Category II is the presence of objective findings and is awarded 5%. Cervicothoracic category III is radiculopathy, and in the cervical spine radiculopathy is equal to 15% impairment.

Category IV is loss of motion segment integrity or multilevel neurologic compromise, with a resultant 25% impairment. In these patients, there is significant radiculopathy in both upper extremities or radiculopathy in one extremity at more than one level. In the cervicothoracic spine, loss of motion segment integrity is defined as translation of 3.5 mm, or more. Category V is severe upper extremity neurologic compromise, requiring the use of upper extremity external functional or adaptive devices. Again, there may be total neurologic loss at a single level or severe multilevel neurologic loss.

Cervicothoracic category VII, cauda equina-like syndrome without bowel or bladder involvement, results in an impairment rating of 40%. This is not true cauda equina syndrome, which of course produces lower motor neuron symptoms, but is cauda equina-like syndrome, which causes long tract signs in both lower extremities. Long tract signs result in numbness, weakness, spasticity and hyperactive reflexes. The 40% for category VI must be combined with ratings from appropriate cervicothoracic categories II through V.

Cervicothoracic category VII is cauda equina-like syndrome with bowel and bladder involvement, and category VIII is quadriplegia. Again, the 60% from category VII or 75% from category VIII must be combined with a rating from categories II through V.

Thoracolumbar Area

Thoracolumbar categories are very similar to those in the cervicothoracic area. In thoracolumbar category I there are minor complaints but no impairment rating. Thoracolumbar category II has objective findings without radiculopathy and a resultant 5% impairment. Thoracolumbar category III, radiculopathy, again is equal to 15% impairment. Thoracolumbar category IV, loss of motion segment integrity or multilevel neurologic compromise, results in an impairment of 20%. Loss of motion segment integrity in the thoracolumbar area is translation of 5 mm or more. Thoracolumbar category IV, radiculopathy and loss of motion segment integrity (a combination of categories III and IV), results in impairment of 25%.

Thoracolumbar category VI is cauda equina-like syndrome without bowel or bladder involvement and is awarded 35% impairment. Thoracolumbar category VII is cauda equina-like syndrome with bowel and bladder involvement, 55%, and thoracolumbar category VIII is paraplegia, 70%. Again, thoracolumbar categories VI, VII, and VIII must be combined with a rating from categories II, III, or IV. In the thoracolumbar spine, the rating should not be combined with category V, because this would lead to excess impairment rating.

If the patient has the unusual circumstance in which there is involvement of the cervicothoracic or thoracolumbar spine resulting in upper extremity or truncal involvement, and bladder and/or bowel involvement without long track signs, then he or she should be given a rating from categories II through V. The bowel and bladder involvement is then rated using the chapter on the urinary and reproductive systems and the digestive system.

The Range-of-Motion Model

The instructions given by the AMA are that if a physician is having difficulty categorizing a patient in the DRE model or if two physicians disagree into which category the patient belongs, the range-of-motion method can be used as the ultimate differentiator. In addition, because some jurisdictions still use the range-of-motion model as the primary method of evaluation, knowledge of this secondary model is essential.

In the 4th edition of the AMA Guides, to assess range-of-motion in the spine, it is necessary to use an inclinometer. Several kinds of inclinometers are available. The flat-based inclinometer has a disadvantage in that the flat base rocks on the spine in many individuals. The bipedal inclinometer is more efficient. A number of computerized inclinometers are available, but these are very expensive. Although they may give extremely accurate measurements, I feel that they are merely a very expensive way to obtain a very accurate measurement of range of motion when that measurement in its most accurate state is worth very little. Certainly, hand-held inclinometers are quite adequate.

To determine range of motion in the lumbar spine, the examiner places a mark on the spinous processes of T12 and S1 with the patient in the standing position. The inclinometers are aligned with the marks and zeroed. The patient is then asked to bend forward as far as possible. The patient may place his or her hands on the knees if doing so makes the patient more comfortable. The measurement from both inclinometers is then recorded, the reading from the sacral inclinometer is subtracted from the reading of the T12 inclinometer, and the resultant figure represents true lumbar flexion. The patient is then asked to return to the standing position and to bend backwards as far as possible. Again the measurement from the lower inclinometer is subtracted from the reading from the upper inclinometer to give true lumbar extension. This procedure is repeated 3 times. It is important to record the average of each of the 3 measurements and to record the flexion and extension of the sacral inclinometer for use in the validity checks discussed later. Use of the forms shown in Figures 6, 7, and 8 provides a convenient way to record and calculate impairment.

The inclinometers are then placed flat against the lumbar spine at T12 and S1. After the inclinometers are zeroed, the patient is asked to bend to the right maximally and to the left. By performing the same calculations discussed in the flexion and extension series, it is possible to determine true right lateral bending and true left lateral bending.

There are 2 ways to check the validity of the range-of-motion measurements. The first is to perform the measurements 3 times, as mentioned above. The measurements are averaged, and all 3 measurements should be within 5° or 10% of the mean. It is important to realize that the highest of the 3 measurements is used for reporting. If any of the 3 measurements are not within 5° or 10% of the mean, the instructions are to repeat the measurements up to 6 times total in an effort to obtain 3 consecutive measurements that are within 5° or 10% of the mean. If 3 consecutive valid measurements have not been obtained after 6 attempts, that portion of the examination is invalidated or the patient is asked to return at a later date for reexamination.

The second validity check is the use of straight leg raising. The physician places the inclinometer on the crest of the tibia with the patient in the supine position and zeroes the inclinometer. The leg is then raised as far as the patient will allow, and the reading on the inclinometer is recorded. This is done for each leg and is repeated 3 times. As in the range-of-motion validity check, the examiner is attempting to gain 3 consecutive measurements that are within 5° or 10% of the mean. The lowest measurement is then compared to the sum of the sacral flexion and extension measurements. Sacral motion is really hip motion. If the lowest straight leg raising angle exceeds the sum of sacral flexion and extension angle by more than 15°, the lumbosacral flexion test is invalidated. This validity test should not be used if the total sacral (hip) motion (flexion plus extension) exceeds 55° for men or 65° for women.

The reasoning behind the first validity test is that if the measurements are not consistent, it is implied that the patient is not giving full effort. In regard to the second validity test, because sacral (hip) motion is dependent on hamstring tightness or nerve tension, if a patient allows significant straight leg raising but will not flex the sacrum, the inference again is that the patient is not giving his or her best effort.

Once these measurements have been obtained and validated, one then refers to Figures 9 and 10 to obtain impairment based on loss of motion. It should be noted that in Figure 9 (flexion and extension) increased loss in sacral (hip) flexion angle results in higher impairments for loss of true lumbar flexion. This is because it is felt that a patient with a stiff hip (as measured by sacral flexion angle) has a greater impairment

| Name _____ | Soc. Sec. No. _____ | Date _____ |

Movement	Description	Range					
Cervical Flexion	Occipital ROM						
	T1 ROM						
	Cervical flexion angle						
	±10% or 5°?	Yes	No				
	Maximum cervical flexion angle	_____					
	% Impairment	_____					
Cervical Extension	Occipital ROM						
	T1 ROM						
	Cervical extension angle						
	±10% or 5°?	Yes	No				
	Maximum cervical extension angle	_____					
	% Impairment	_____					
Cervical Ankylosis in Flexion/Extension	Position	_____	(Excludes any impairment for abnormal flexion or extension motion)				
	% Impairment						
Cervical Right Lateral Flexion	Occipital ROM						
	T1 ROM						
	Cervical right lat flexion angle						
	±10% or 5°?	Yes	No				
	Maximum cervical right lat flexion angle	_____					
	% Impairment	_____					
Cervical Left Lateral Flexion	Occipital ROM						
	T1 ROM						
	Cervical left lat flexion angle						
	±10% or 5°?	Yes	No				
	Maximum cervical left lat flexion angle	_____					
	% Impairment	_____					
Cervical Ankylosis in Lateral Flexion and Extension	Position	_____	(Excludes any impairment for abnormal lateral flexion or extension motion)				
	% Impairment						
Cervical Right Rotation	Cervical right rotation angle						
	±10% or 5°?	Yes	No				
	Maximum cervical right rotation angle	_____					
	% Impairment	_____					
Cervical Left Rotation	Cervical left rotation angle						
	±10% or 5°?	Yes	No				
	Maximum cervical left rotation angle	_____					
	% Impairment	_____					
Cervical Ankylosis in Rotation	Position	_____	(Excludes any impairment for abnormal rotation)				
	% Impairment						

Total cervical range of motion and ankylosis* impairment _____ %

*If ankylosis is present, combine the ankylosis impairment with the range-of-motion impairment (Combined Values Chart). If ankyloses in several planes are present, combine the estimates (Combined Values Chart), then combine the result with the range-of-motion impairment.

Fig. 6 Cervical range of motion. (Reproduced with permission from *Guides to the Evaluation of Permanent Impairment*, ed 4. Chicago, IL, American Medical Association, 1993, pp 94–138.)

Name _____   Soc. Sec. No. _____   Date _____

Movement	Description	Range						
Lumbar Flexion	T12 ROM							
	Sacral ROM							
	True lumbar flexion angle							
	±10% or 5°?	Yes	No					
	Maximum true lumbar flexion angle							
	% Impairment							
Lumbar Extension	T12 ROM							
	Sacral ROM							
	True lumbar extension angle							
	±10% or 5°?	Yes	No					
	Maximum true lumbar extension angle		(Add sacral flexion and extension ROM and compare to tightest straight-leg-raising angle)					
	% Impairment							
Straight Leg Raising (SLR), Right	Right SLR							
	±10% or 5°?	Yes	No	(If tightest SLR ROM exceeds sum of sacral flexion and extension by more than 15°, lumbar ROM test is invalid)				
	Maximum SLR right							
Straight Leg Raising, Left	Left SLR							
	±10% or 5°?	Yes	No	(If tightest SLR ROM exceeds sum of sacral flexion and extension by more than 15°, lumbar ROM test is invalid)				
	Maximum SLR Left							
Lumbar Right Lateral Flexion	T12 ROM							
	Sacral ROM							
	Lumbar right lateral flexion angle							
	±10% or 5°?	Yes	No					
	Maximum lumbar right lateral flexion angle							
	% Impairment							
Lumbar Left Lateral Flexion	T12 ROM							
	Sacral ROM							
	Lumbar left lateral flexion angle							
	±10% or 5°?	Yes	No					
	Maximum lumbar left lateral flexion angle							
	% Impairment							
Lumbar Ankylosis in Lateral Flexion	Position		(Excludes any impairment for abnormal flexion or extension motion)					
	% Impairment							

Total lumbar range of motion and ankylosis* impairment _____ %

*If ankylosis is present, combine the ankylosis impairment with the range-of-motion impairment (Combined Values Chart). If ankyloses in several planes are present, combine the estimates (Combined Values Chart), then combine the result with the range-of-motion impairment.

Fig. 7 Thoracic range of motion. (Reproduced with permission from *Guides to the Evaluation of Permanent Impairment*, ed 4. Chicago, IL, American Medical Association, 1993, pp 94–138.)

as a result of loss of motion in the lumbar spine.

Measurement of the cervicothoracic and thoracolumbar spines and resultant impairment calculations are similar to those used in the lumbosacral spine. These are discussed in great detail in the AMA Guides but will not be covered in this chapter.

Once the determination of impairment secondary to loss of motion is determined, the rater refers to Figure 4 to determine the possibility of any impairment secondary to the conditions listed in that table. In addition, if there is neurologic involvement, the rater refers to Figure 5. Impairment ratings from the range-of-motion study and

Name _____		Soc. Sec. No. _____		Date _____			

Movement	Description	Range						
Angle of Minimum Kyphosis (Thoracic Ankylosis in Extension)	T1 reading		XXXX	XXXX	XXXX	XXXX	XXXX	
	T12 reading		XXXX	XXXX	XXXX	XXXX	XXXX	
	Angle of minimum kyphosis		XXXX	XXXX	XXXX	XXXX	XXXX	
	% Impairment due to thoracic ankylosis	(Use larger of either ankylosis or flexion impairment)						
Thoracic Flexion	T1 ROM							
	T12 ROM							
	Thoracic flexion angle							
	± 10% or 5°?	Yes	No					
	Maximum thoracic flexion angle							
	% Impairment							
Thoracic Right Rotation	T1 ROM							
	T12 ROM							
	Thoracic right rotation angle							
	± 10% or 5°?	Yes	No					
	Maximum thoracic right rotation angle							
	% Impairment							
Thoracic Left Rotation	T1 ROM							
	T12 ROM							
	Thoracic left rotation angle							
	± 10% or 5°?	Yes	No					
	Maximum thoracic left rotation angle							
	% Impairment							
Thoracic Ankylosis in Rotation	Position	(Excludes any impairment for abnormal flexion or extension motion)						
	% Impairment							
Total thoracic range of motion and ankylosis* impairment _____ %								

*If ankylosis is present, combine the ankylosis impairment with the range-of-motion impairment (Combined Values Chart). If ankyloses in several planes are present, combine the estimates (Combined Values Chart), then combine the result with the range-of-motion impairment.

Fig. 8 Lumbar range of motion. (Reproduced with permission from *Guides to the Evaluation of Permanent Impairment*, ed 4. Chicago, IL, American Medical Association, 1993, pp 94–138.)

the 2 tables are then combined to determine the final impairment rating for that area of the spine. If more than 1 area of the spine is involved, the rater is instructed to determine the impairment in the area of the spine that has the greater involvement and then repeat the procedure in the other area or areas. Affected areas are then combined to determine the rating for the entire spine.

Again, it should be pointed out that the final rating should never come from the range-of-motion method. Instructions in the AMA Guides are that the range-of-motion method is to be used only to determine into which DRE category to place the patient.

In summary, this has been a description of the use of the *Guides to the Evaluation of Permanent Impairment* to determine impairment in the spine. The diagnosis-related estimate method is the preferred method with the range-of-motion model being used to serve as the ultimate differentiator and allow a difficult patient to be properly categorized. Once again, it is very important that the rater use all information that is available. If the patient's injury is remote and past records are not available, the rater is obligated to point out the fact that the records have not been reviewed, for it is the philosophy of the spine section of the 4th edition of the AMA Guides that if a patient has objective findings anywhere in his or her course, then that patient is deserving

The proportion of flexion and extension of total lumbosacral motion is 75%.		
Sacral (hip) flexion angle	**True lumbar spine flexion angle (°)**	**% Impairment of the whole person**
45°+	60°+	0
	45°	2
	30°	4
	15°	7
	0°	10
30 - 45	40+	4
	20	7
	0	10
0 - 29	30+	5
	15	8
	0	11

True lumbar spine extension from neutral position (0°) to:	Degrees of lumbosacral spine motion		
	Lost	Retained	
0°	25	0	7
10°	15	10	5
15°	10	15	3
20°	5	20	2
25°	0	25	0

*Use this table only if the sum of sacral (hip) flexion and sacral (hip) extension is within 15° of the straight-leg raising test on the tighter side.

Fig. 9 Impairment due to abnormal motion of the lumbosacral region: flexion and extension. (Reproduced with permission from *Guides to the Evaluation of Permanent Impairment*, ed 4. Chicago, IL, American Medical Association, 1993, pp 94–138.)

Abnormal Motion Average range of lateral flexion is 50°; the proportion of total lumbosacral motion is 40%.			
a.	**Right lateral flexion** from neutral position (°) to:	Degrees of lumbosacral motion	% Impairment of the whole person
		Lost	Retained	
	0°	25	0	5
	10°	15	10	3
	15°	10	15	2
	20°	5	20	1
	25°	0	25	0
b.	**Left lateral flexion** from neutral position (0°) to:		
	0°	25	0	5
	10°	15	10	3
	15°	10	15	2
	20°	5	20	1
	25°	0	25	0
c.	**Ankylosis** Region ankylosed at:		
	0° (neutral position)		10
	30°		20
	45°		30
	60°		40
	75° (full flexion)		50

Fig. 10 Impairment due to abnormal motion and ankylosis of the lumbosacral region: lateral flexion. (Reproduced with permission from *Guides to the Evaluation of Permanent Impairment*, ed 4. Chicago, IL, American Medical Association, 1993, pp 94–138.)

of a rating. It is not necessary that those findings be present at the time of the final examination. We are rating the results of the injury, not the results of the treatment.

References

1. Doege C, Houston TP (eds): *Guides to the Evaluation of Permanent Impairment*, ed 4. Chicago, IL, American Medical Association, 1993.

2. Lowery WD Jr, Horn TJ, Boden SD, Wiesel SW: Impairment evaluation based on spinal range of motion in normal subjects. *J Spinal Discord* 1992;5:398–402.

3. Posner I, White AA III, Edwards WT, Hayes WC: A biomechanical analysis of the clinical stability of the lumbar and lumbosacral spine. *Spine* 1982;7:374–389.

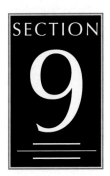
Fractures and Dislocations

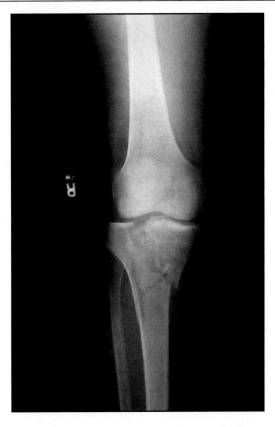

Intra-Articular Fractures of the Distal Aspect of the Radius

Thomas E. Trumble, MD
Randall W. Culp, MD
Douglas P. Hanel, MD
William B. Geissler, MD
Richard A. Berger, MD

High-energy injuries frequently cause shear and impacted fractures of the articular surface of the distal radius with displacement of the fracture fragments. Even fractures with a small amount of displacement can result in degeneration of the joint, causing pain and stiffness of the wrist. The fracture pattern, degree of displacement of the fracture fragments, and stability of the fracture determine whether surgical treatment rather than immobilization with a cast is needed. The options for surgical treatment include open reduction and internal fixation, to realign the articular surface of the radius; external fixation, for fractures with comminution of the metaphysis of the radius, to maintain the length of the radius; and bone grafting, to provide support for the articular surface of impacted fractures.

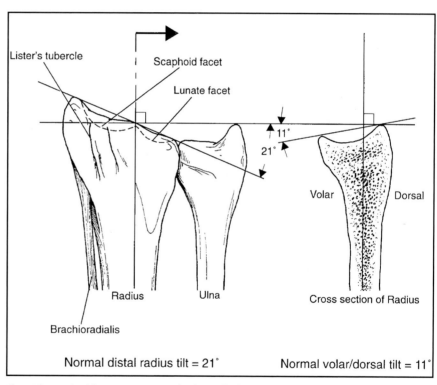

Fig. 1 The method for measurement of palmar tilt, distal radial tilt, and ulnar variance on posteroanterior and lateral radiographs of the distal radius and ulna.

Anatomy of the Articular Interface Between the Distal Radius and Ulna and the Carpus

The articular surface of the distal radius tilts 21° in the anteroposterior plane and 5° to 11° in the lateral plane (Fig. 1). The dorsal cortical surface of the radius thickens to form the Lister tubercle as well as osseous promi-

nences that support the extensors of the wrist in the second dorsal compartment. A central ridge divides the articular surface of the radius into a scaphoid facet and a lunate facet (Fig. 2). The triangular fibrocartilage extends from the rim of the sigmoid

notch of the radius to the ulnar styloid process. These areas of thickening of the metaphyseal cortex provide segments of bone that reliably resist fracture and can support internal fixation when indicated. Only the brachioradialis tendon inserts onto the distal

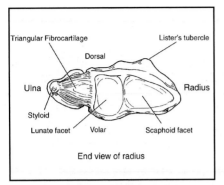

Fig. 2 The distal articular surface of the radius, which is divided into the lunate and scaphoid facets.

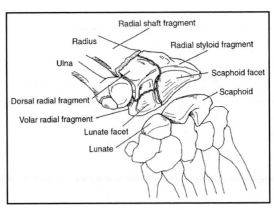

Fig. 3 Fracture lines frequently propagate between the scaphoid and lunate facets and extend dorsally adjacent to, but not through, the thicker bone that forms the Lister tubercle.

aspect of the radius; the other tendons of the wrist pass across the distal aspect of the radius to insert onto the carpal bones or the bases of the metacarpals. In addition to the extrinsic ligaments of the wrist, the scapholunate interosseous and lunotriquetral interosseous ligaments maintain the scaphoid, lunate, and triquetrum in a smooth articular unit that comes into contact with the distal aspect of the radius and the triangular fibrocartilage complex. Because of the different areas of bone thickness and density, the fracture patterns tend to propagate between the scaphoid and lunate facets of the distal aspect of the radius (Fig. 3). The degree, direction, and extent of the applied load may cause coronal or sagittal splits within the lunate or scaphoid facet.[1–3]

Effect of Intra-Articular Fracture Healing on Articular Congruity

Knirk and Jupiter[4] reported that 2.0 mm or more of displacement of the distal radial articular fragments resulted in traumatic osteoarthrosis; however, other investigators[5–7] found that displacement of even 1.0 mm resulted in pain and stiffness of the wrist. In animal models of articular fractures, the cartilage remodeled to provide a congruent articular surface when dis-

placement of the articular surface was less than 1.0 mm, whereas a step-off of 1.0 mm or more did not cause appreciable remodeling.[8,9] In one of these animal models—an articular fracture of the tibial plateau in sheep, in which the dimensions of the cartilage and bone are similar to those of the human wrist—the cartilage on the depressed segment of the tibial plateau expanded over time, whereas the cartilage on the nondepressed segment of the fracture (the so-called high side of the tibial plateau) became compressed with resultant bending of the unloaded collagen fibers[9] (Fig. 4). The cartilage on the high side of the fracture formed a shelf, which overlapped with the low side.

The ability of the cartilage to remodel may depend on its thickness. For example, the knee has a much thicker layer of cartilage than does the distal aspect of the radius, and patients appear to tolerate a much greater amount of displacement when an intra-articular fracture is in the knee than when it is in the wrist.[10–14]

Radiographic Studies

The initial standard posteroanterior, lateral, and oblique radiographs of the distal radial injury are very important because they show the extent and direction of the initial displacement. Traction radiographs assist the

surgeon in determining whether the fracture is intra-articular or extra-articular. Repeat radiographs should be made after the reduction in order to help identify the residual deformity and the degree of comminution.

Plain and computed tomographic (CT) scans, made in the sagittal and coronal planes oriented along lines parallel to the shaft of the radius, are extremely useful in helping to determine if surgery is needed when the amount of displacement is unclear or when the fracture pattern is difficult to visualize on plain radiographs (Figs. 5 and 6). CT is strongly recommended to help define the intra-articular fracture pattern, especially in association with die-punch fractures (those with a central depression of the articular surface), volar rim fractures, and fractures involving the scaphoid facet, which can be more difficult to visualize. CT also is helpful in determining the surgical approach; fractures of the lunate facet and the radial styloid process may have volar or dorsal displacement that is not evident on plain radiographs, especially if the wrist is in a cast. Radiographs made at the time of the initial injury are important in helping to determine the direction of displacement of the fracture. Traction radiographs are useful in determining the accuracy of reduction. Final displacement is mea-

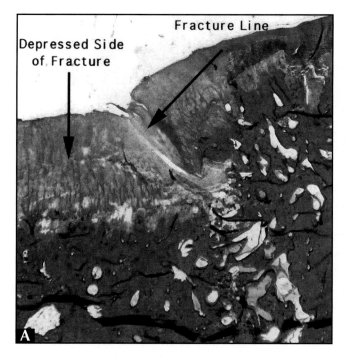

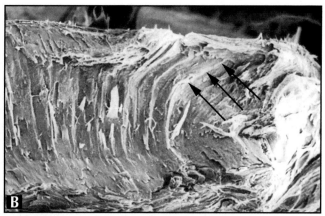

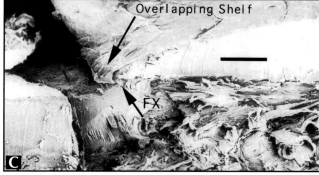

Fig. 4 Undecalcified specimen obtained from a sheep 12 weeks after a tibial osteotomy. **A,** The fracture is still evident, with ongoing bone remodeling. The low side (the depressed segment of the fracture), which has been unloaded by the osteotomy, demonstrates chondrocyte hypertrophy and expansion of the cartilage surface. Compared with sites distant to the osteotomy, the cartilage on the high side (the nondepressed segment of the fracture) is reduced in overall thickness by approximately 20% (Masson trichrome, × 200). **B,** High-power scanning electron micrograph showing the collagen fibrils on the high side of the tibial osteotomy. The arrows highlight the bending of the collagen fibrils. Bar = 100 μm. **C,** Low-power scanning electron micrograph showing an overview of the cartilage flap produced by the response of the articular surface to the osteotomy. The lower arrow demonstrates the fracture line (FX). Bar = 1 mm.

sured on radiographs or CT scans made after the reduction.

Classification of Intra-Articular Distal Radius Fractures

A number of authors have proposed systems for the classification of distal radius fractures. Many of these systems combine intra-articular and extra-articular fractures;[1,15–25] however, studies have not revealed substantial interobserver agreement among fracture types determined with use of the Frykman,[18] Mayo,[15–17] Melone,[1–3] or AO[21,23,24] classification systems.

Significant agreement ($p < 0.05$) among physicians' classifications with use of the AO system, based on reviews of the radiographs, was achieved only after the classification was reduced from 27 detailed descriptions of fractures to 3 major fracture types (extra-articular, intra-articular with part of the metaphysis intact, and intra-articular fractures with complete disruption of the metaphysis); this simplification of the system limited its usefulness.[21,26] Interobserver agreement for the other classification systems was poor.[26]

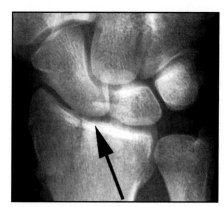

Fig. 5 A die-punch fracture (arrow) of the scaphoid facet is barely visible on this posteroanterior radiograph.

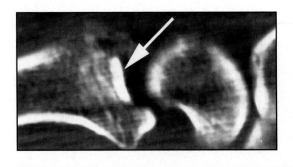

Fig. 6 Computed tomographic scan, made in the sagittal plane, clearly showing the die-punch fracture (arrow) of the scaphoid facet with 3 mm of depression that would have been easy to overlook on plain radiographs.

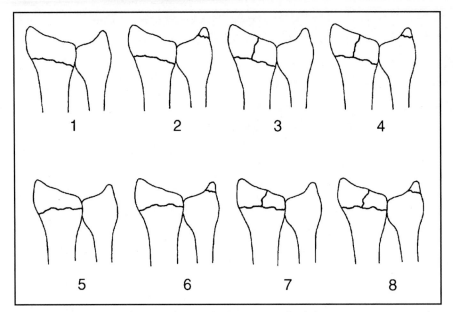

Fig. 7 The Frykman classification system.[18] The fractures are divided into 8 categories according to whether they extend into the articular surface and whether there is an associated fracture of the distal ulna.

Frykman Classification[18]

This classification focuses on the intra-articular extension of the fracture and the involvement of the ulnar styloid process, implying that the involvement of these structures contributes to the seriousness of the fracture (Fig. 7). However, it appears to be particularly difficult to determine exactly what fracture line extends where. Many fracture lines extend near the corner of a joint surface, and the decision regarding whether such a line involves the joint is often arbitrary. As one of the earliest systems for the classification of fractures of the distal aspect of the radius, this sys-

tem drew attention to the distal radioulnar joint. Because displaced and nondisplaced fractures are considered equally important, this system cannot be used to predict outcome as accurately as other systems.

Mayo Classification[15-17]

This classification system resembles that of Frykman in that the emphasis is on the extent of articular involvement (Fig. 8), but it introduces an additional variable: that of distinguishing the extension of the fracture into either the radioscaphoid or the radiolunate joint. The expected increase in variability that this might

cause is offset by the fewer general categories, as the ulnar styloid process is ignored in the Mayo system.

Melone Classification[3]

This classification system is based on the belief that the condition of the medial portion of the articular column of the distal aspect of the radius is important for determining the prognosis and the options for treatment (Fig. 9). This system was one of the first to provide an accurate description of the way in which most fractures propagate through the articular surface of the radius. By definition, this classification is relevant only to intra-articular fractures. The difficulty involved with the use of this system lies in the fact that observers often disagree about whether or not the fracture extends into the radiocarpal joint. The importance of the medial articular facet in this system resulted in 44 (88%) of 50 fractures in one study[26] being placed into class I or II; fractures that extended into the scaphoid facet were impossible to classify.

Jupiter and Fernandez Classification[20]

This classification system, a modification of the AO system, emphasizes the mechanism of injury, including bending, shear, compression, and avulsion (traction). It also includes complex fractures that result from a combination of at least two of these mechanisms of injury. Jupiter and Fernandez expanded the AO classification to include avulsion fractures caused by radiocarpal dislocation and high-velocity combined injuries. This is an excellent system that includes information on fracture displacement and the number of fracture fragments. On the basis of the main fracture type and the direction of displacement, the classification consists of approximately 25 subtypes. Because this is a newer system, scant data are available for comparing the ease and accuracy of its use with those of other classification systems.

AO Classification[21,23,24]

The AO classification system, which comprises 27 categories, is the most detailed. It also is the most inclusive, making it useful for broad anatomic categorization of large numbers of fractures for trauma registries even though it is cumbersome and lacks sufficient focus for use in clinical decision making. Andersen and associates[26] found significant ($p < 0.05$) agreement between reviewers when this system was reduced to 3 classifications: extra-articular, partial intra-articular, and complex articular. We surveyed a group of 6 orthopaedic surgeons and residents with regard to their ability to categorize only intra-articular fractures of the distal aspect of the radius with use of a slightly modified version of the AO classification. Type B1 comprised fractures of the radial styloid process; type B2, fractures of the dorsal rim; type B3, fractures of the volar rim; type B4, die-punch fractures; and type C, complex fractures as a combined group. We added type B4 as there was no convenient way, using the original AO system, to classify die-punch fractures (Fig. 10). Because fractures with at least 3 fragments that involve the entire articular surface necessitate such individualized treatment, we included these fractures together as a class, separated only into those with predominantly dorsal displacement and those with predominantly volar displacement as seen on the initial radiographs. We considered only displaced intra-articular fractures because nondisplaced fractures generally remain as a unit, similar to extra-articular fractures. With the

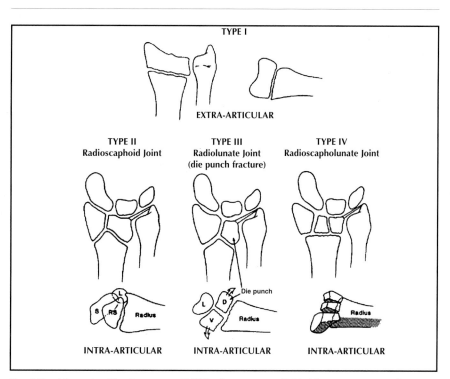

Fig. 8 The Mayo classification system.[15–17] The fractures are divided into groups according to whether they are extra-articular or intra-articular. Intra-articular fractures are divided further according to the extent of fragmentation. S = scaphoid, L = lunate, RS = radial styloid fragment, D = dorsal, and V = volar. (Adapted with permission from Missakian ML, Cooney WP, Amadio PC, Glidewell HL: Open reduction and internal fixation for distal radius fractures. *J Hand Surg* 1992;17A:745–755.)

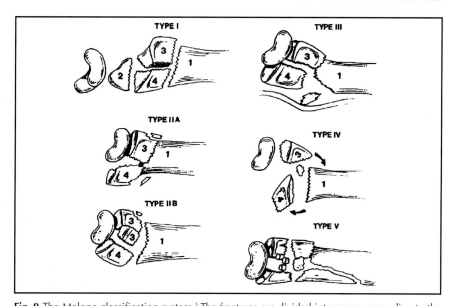

Fig. 9 The Melone classification system.[3] The fractures are divided into groups according to the amount of displacement, the pattern of the fracture, the degree of volar metaphyseal comminution, and the extension of the fracture into the diaphysis. 1 = radial shaft, 2 = radial styloid fragment, 3 = volar ulnar fragment, and 4 = dorsal ulnar fragment. (Reproduced with permission from Melone CP Jr: Distal radius fractures: Patterns of articular fragmentation. *Orthop Clin North Am* 1993;24:241.)

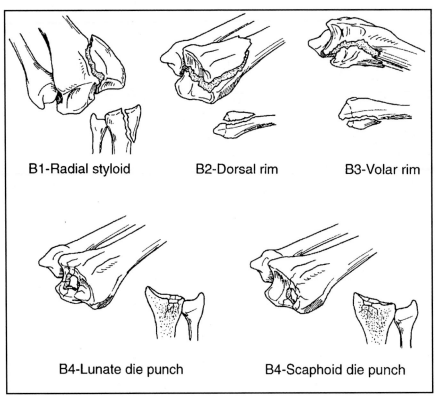

B1-Radial styloid   B2-Dorsal rim   B3-Volar rim

B4-Lunate die punch   B4-Scaphoid die punch

Fig. 10 Modification of the AO classification of partial articular fractures of the distal radius to include die-punch fracture of the scaphoid and lunate facets (subtype B4). With these fractures, a portion of the articular surface remains in continuity with the metaphysis, providing some stability even if there is loss of congruity.

Table 1
Surgical approach for open reduction and internal fixation of partial intra-articular fractures

Type of Fracture	Operative Approach
Type B1: fractures of radial styloid process	Dorsal or volar, depending on computed tomographic scans
Type B2: fractures of dorsal rim	Dorsal with buttress plate
Type B3: fractures of volar rim including those of volar ulnar corner of sigmoid notch	Volar radial (Henry) or volar ulnar with buttress plate
Type B4: die-punch fractures of scaphoid or lunate facet including those of dorsal ulnar corner of sigmoid notch	Arthroscopic or limited open reduction through dorsal approach and bone grafting with or without buttress plate

addition of CT scans and the instruction that only fractures with displacement of 1.0 mm or more should be included, the 6 physicians accurately classified 18 of 20 intra-articular fractures of the distal aspect of the radius.

Partial Intra-Articular Fractures (AO Type B) Shear injuries cause fractures of the volar and dorsal rims, fractures of the radial styloid process, and medial corner fractures, whereas impaction injuries cause die-punch fractures (Fig. 10). These injuries may include additional, smaller fractures or nondisplaced fractures that do not necessitate separate treatment, but the feature that is common to all is sparing of a portion of the articular surface that remains in continuity with the metaphysis; this adds greatly to the stability of the fracture. This simplified classification system, shown in Table 1, provides the surgeon with guidelines for treatment.

Complex Articular Fractures These injuries, which generally are higher-energy fractures than type-B fractures, often involve a combination of shear and impaction (Fig. 11). None of the articular surface remains in continuity with the metaphysis. The fractures can be classified simply as those with a dorsal pattern, those with a volar pattern, or direct impaction fractures with or without comminution. Although the fracture pattern can involve the so-called T- or Y-split of the articular surface in primarily the sagittal or coronal plane, most of these complex fractures involve a component of both (Table 2).

Marked comminution of the distal radial metaphysis is defined as involvement of more than 50% of the diameter of the metaphysis as seen on any radiograph, comminution of at least two cortices of the metaphysis, or more than 2.0 mm of shortening of the radius. The degree of comminution may not be obvious until the time of the surgery; therefore, the surgeon should always be prepared to add bone graft or bone substitute as part of the open or arthroscopic reduction and internal fixation. The injury can occur in different combinations, and a combination of tactics will be needed to treat all of the variables. For example, a 3-part fracture that includes a volar rim fracture and a die-punch fracture of the lunate facet probably will need to be treated with internal fixation with use of a buttress plate, through a volar approach (to stabilize the volar rim fracture) as well as through a dorsal or arthroscopic approach (to address the die-punch fracture).

Limits of Classification Systems

Some orthopaedists, especially those in training programs, have expressed concern that more time is spent in trying to memorize classification systems than in attempting to truly understand the fracture mechanics or the factors that have a major bearing on prognosis and treatment. A classification system, like any tool, has limitations. These systems are important when the diagnosis and treatment alternatives are being considered. A system will be sustained if it can be used to communicate the relative severity of the fracture and to describe the corresponding treatment options.

In fairness to the authors of the classification systems, it should be noted that the original systems were developed and the subsequent comparisons between them were performed without the use of CT, which has become particularly important for the diagnosis of intra-articular fractures. None of these authors expected their systems to provide answers to all of the questions regarding treatment and prognosis, and each system has added to our knowledge of these troublesome injuries. Most of the systems focus on the mechanism of injury or the geometry of the fracture. Unfortunately, most of the classifications do not correspond directly to the fracture stability.[27]

Surgical Approaches

Although there are many different surgical approaches to the distal radius, often based on the different intervals between the tendons, more than 90% of the time we have relied on 3 main approaches for open reduc-

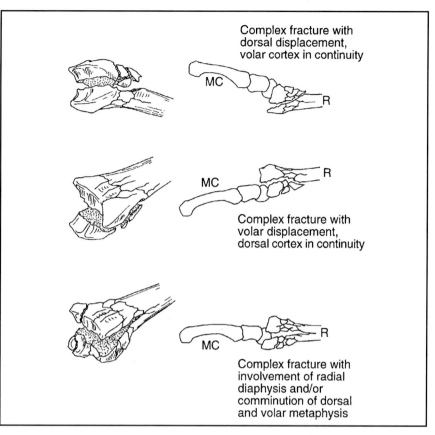

Fig. 11 Complex (type-C) fractures, described in the AO classification, have been combined into a single group. The notations indicate whether the displacement was dorsal or volar or whether the fracture was severely impacted from an axial load that caused comminution of both the dorsal and volar portions of the metaphysis or diaphysis, or both. All of these fractures involve complete separation of the metaphysis from the articular surface, making them highly unstable. MC = metacarpal, R = radius.

Table 2
Surgical approach according to the direction of displacement and the presence or absence of comminution

Direction of Displacement	Comminution	Surgical Approach	External Fixation
Dorsal	No	Dorsal	No
Dorsal	Yes	Dorsal	Yes
Volar	No	Volar	No
Volar	Yes	Volar	Yes
Direct impaction with T- or Y-split, with or without diaphyseal involvement	Yes	Dorsal and volar	Yes

tion and internal fixation of a fracture of the distal aspect of the radius.

Dorsal Approach

A longitudinal midline incision over the dorsum of the wrist provides a useful and practical exposure of the dorsum of the radius[7] (Fig. 12). The extensor pollicis longus is identified distally and traced to the third dorsal compartment. This compartment usually is distended with fracture

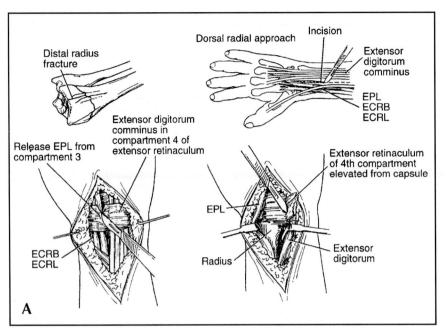

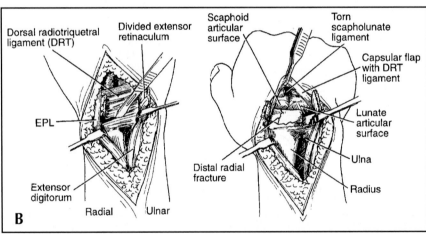

Fig. 12 The dorsal midline approach. EPL = extensor pollicis longus, ECRB = extensor carpi radialis brevis, and ECRL = extensor carpi radialis longus. **A,** The third dorsal compartment is released, and the fourth dorsal compartment is elevated off of the wrist capsule. **B,** The capsule, including the dorsal radiotriquetral ligament (DRT), is incised near its insertion onto the dorsal rim of the radius and then is reflected distally to expose the radiocarpal joint.

The joint capsule is incised obliquely and closed later at its insertion onto the dorsal rim of the radius. With this technique, it can be reflected distally to expose the articular surface of the distal aspect of the radius. Placement of traction on the fingers with use of finger-traps provides distraction to the joint and improves the exposure. Dental probes or small Freer elevators can be used to help align the articular fragments and reconstruct the articular surface. It is best to work from the deeper palmar portions of the joint to the more superficial ones. Small 0.035- or 0.045-in (0.889- or 1.143-mm) Kirschner wires (K-wires), driven just beneath the subchondral bone, provide support for the reconstructed articular surface.

After bone grafting and placement of the K-wires, the reduction is confirmed with fluoroscopy. The K-wires are cut flush with the metaphyseal surface to avoid irritating the extensor tendons. The capsule is sutured carefully to avoid any tightening that might decrease flexion of the wrist. The second and fourth extensor compartments are loosely reapproximated, but the extensor pollicis longus is left out of its compartment. The oblique course of the extensor pollicis longus prevents it from bowstringing even though the sheath of the third compartment is not repaired. **(CD–58.1)**

Limited Dorsal Approach (Without Arthrotomy)

The limited approach does not involve an arthrotomy and requires a skin incision of 3 cm or less. This approach is practical for patients who have an isolated die-punch fracture and for those in whom the articular fracture can be completely reduced in a closed manner or with manipulation with use of K-wires or small

hematoma, as most fractures that split the scaphoid and lunate facets extend into the floor of the third compartment, avoiding the stronger and thicker Lister tubercle. The third and fourth compartments are sharply elevated off the dorsal aspect of the capsule, with both the tendon compartments and the dorsal capsular ligaments, including the dorsal radiotriquetral ligament, kept intact. This avoids the need to repair the extensor retinaculum and related compartments later, which can be difficult in the presence of swelling of the tendons and the joint capsule. If the dorsal retinaculum is divided and not repaired, the tendons of the fingers and wrist will bowstring with extension of the wrist.

elevators as joysticks to impale or lever the fracture fragments into position.[28] The decision to perform a limited open reduction rather than an open reduction with an arthrotomy is based on the surgeon's evaluation of the reduction under fluoroscopy. Because the approach can easily be extended and an arthrotomy can subsequently be performed, little is lost by choosing the limited approach initially.

The radial styloid process is stabilized to the distal part of the diaphysis with 0.045-in (1.143-mm) smooth K-wires, placed percutaneously through the dorsal aspect of the radial styloid process through a soft-tissue protector sleeve that minimizes injury to the branches of the radial sensory nerve as well as the radial artery. The radial styloid fragment becomes the landmark for the subsequent realignment of the remaining displaced articular fragments. Under fluoroscopy, impacted fragments can be elevated using Freer elevators, dental probes, or K-wires as joysticks. After the fragment has been restored to its anatomic position, it can be secured with 0.035-in (0.889-mm) or 0.045-in (1.143-mm) smooth K-wires that have been introduced through the radial styloid process horizontally and dorsally, directly entering the subchondral bone of the fragment of the lunate facet. Similarly, depressed segments of the scaphoid facet can be stabilized after reduction with use of smooth K-wires, placed from the dorsal medial corner of the radius into the subchondral bone of the distal fragment.

This approach allows for the placement of a small (2.7- or 3.5-mm) buttress plate to provide support to the reconstructed dorsal rim. Supplemental cancellous bone grafting is added when a metaphyseal defect is present.

Volar Radial Approach

The most commonly used volar approach is between the radial artery and the flexor carpi radialis (Fig. 13). By extending the incision distally along the border of the thenar eminence, the flexor carpi radialis can be exposed distal to the flexion crease of the distal aspect of the wrist. The flexor carpi radialis is released from its attachments to the trapezium; this allows it to be retracted, along with all of the flexor tendons to the digits, to expose the entire volar rim, the sigmoid notch, and the distal radioulnar joint. Elevation of the pronator quadratus from the distal aspect of the radius provides the necessary exposure for the placement of a buttress plate. Large volar rim fragments can be stabilized with a buttress plate, but smaller fragments must be stabilized separately with small K-wires before application of the buttress plate (Fig. 13).

Because the articular surface cannot be visualized through the volar approach, it is important to align the fracture surfaces accurately with use of biplanar radiographs or fluoroscopy. Some authors have used arthroscopy to confirm the reduction of the volar rim fracture.[29–32] After the reduction has been confirmed with radiographs, the K-wires are cut flush with the bone and the pronator quadratus muscle is sutured to the periosteum along the radial border of the radius.

Volar Ulnar Approach for Fractures of the Volar Ulnar Corner

A longitudinal incision along the radial border of the flexor carpi ulnaris is an excellent approach for fractures of the volar ulnar corner of the distal aspect of the radius (Fig. 14). The incision can be extended distally with a release of the carpal tunnel. The ulnar nerve and artery are identified deep to the flexor carpi ulnaris tendon. The flexor tendons can be retracted radially to expose the volar rim of the distal radius and the distal radioulnar joint. The origin of the pronator quadratus on the ulna is incised and is reflected radially to expose the displaced fracture of the rim. The fragment is reduced with use of the fracture interdigitations to correct alignment, because neither the radial nor the ulnar surgical approach to the volar aspect of the radius allows visualization of the articular surface. A small 2.7-mm buttress plate frequently provides adequate stabilization.

We recommend this approach only when the ulnar segment of the volar rim is displaced. For extensive fractures of the volar rim, we advise that the radial exposure of the volar aspect of the wrist be extended by releasing the attachments of the flexor carpi radialis to the trapezium.

Combined Volar and Dorsal Approach

The combined approach is used for only approximately 10% of high-energy complex intra-articular fractures; for example, for a displaced fracture of the volar rim combined with a dorsal die-punch injury and an impacted scaphoid or lunate facet. We recommend that the volar rim be stabilized first, as described earlier, followed by use of a dorsal open or arthroscopic approach to elevate the depressed fragments. Bone grafting and internal fixation with K-wires or a dorsal buttress plate are added to stabilize articular fractures that have been elevated. These high-energy injuries often are associated with extensive swelling, and the surgery should be performed after the swelling has decreased, several days after the initial injury. Closure of the volar inci-

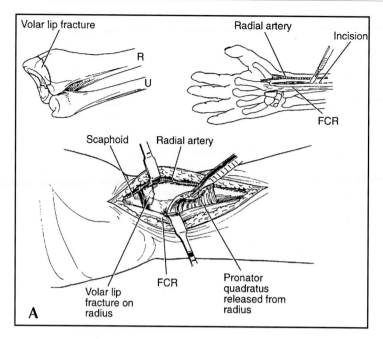

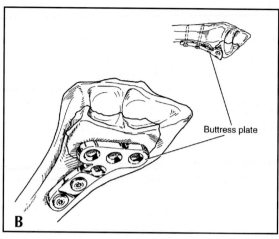

Fig. 13 The volar radial approach. **A,** The approach is through the interval between the flexor carpi radialis (FCR) and the radial artery. R = radius, U = ulna. **B,** Fractures of the volar rim can be stabilized with a contoured buttress plate.

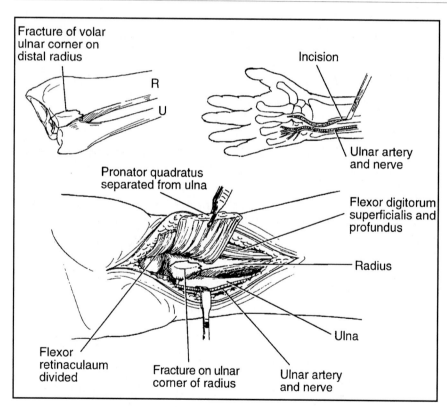

Fig. 14 The volar ulnar approach, which is through the interval between the flexor tendons to the fingers and the ulnar nerve and artery. R = radius, U = ulna.

sion before the incision for the dorsal approach is made helps to minimize the tissue swelling and wound separation that render wound closure without excessive tension difficult.

Arthroscopically Guided Reduction

In order to minimize bleeding from the fracture sites, which obscures the arthroscopic field, the surgery is performed at least 3 days after the injury. A compressive elastic bandage is wrapped around the forearm to retard extravasation of fluid into the muscle compartments during arthroscopy. The wrist is suspended in a traction tower, and 10 lb (4.5 kg) of traction is applied to the index and long fingers through finger-traps. An inflow cannula is inserted through a portal located ulnar to the extensor carpi ulnaris tendon (the 6U portal), and the joint is distended. A 20-gauge needle is inserted between the extensor pollicis longus tendon and the extensor digitorum communis tendons (the dorsal 3,4 portal). The needle should pass easily into the joint without impinging on either the carpal bones or the distal end of the radius, to ensure that the arthroscopic cannula will not be inserted into a fracture plane or an intercarpal joint, such as the scapholunate or lunotriquetral joint. The skin then is incised over the dorsal 3,4 portal by pulling it against the tip of a #11 scalpel blade, and a blunt arthroscopic cannula is inserted to prevent injury of the cutaneous nerves and dorsal veins. A small-joint arthroscope, 2.7 mm in diameter, is inserted through the cannula into the dorsal 3,4 portal (Fig. 15).

An additional portal is made between the extensor digitorum communis tendons and the extensor digiti minimi tendon (the dorsal 4,5 portal) for insertion of a small-joint shaver (2.9 mm). The shaver is used to help clear the remaining hematoma in order to provide a good view of the fracture site. Loose fragments of bone are removed with a mini-grasper. Extravasation of fluid through the fracture and capsular rents can cause troublesome soft-tissue swelling, which can be minimized by allowing the irrigation fluid to exit through the arthroscopic cannula or a separate outflow portal.

The fracture is reduced in a manner similar to the limited open approach. Smooth K-wires are inserted percutaneously through the radial styloid process into the distal diaphysis to provide the stable framework necessary for securing the remaining articular fragments. A small fragment can be elevated by means of a blunt trocar beneath the fracture fragment with use of the dorsal 4,5 portal or by means of a large (0.11-in [2.79-mm]) K-wire placed percutaneously into the metaphyseal bone proximal to the articular surface of the fragment. The K-wire can be used as a joystick to elevate and reduce the fracture fragment under arthroscopic control. Volar or dorsal rim fractures initially are stabilized with a limited approach with use of a buttress plate. Without visualization of the joint surface, the fracture is reduced with use of only the osseous land-

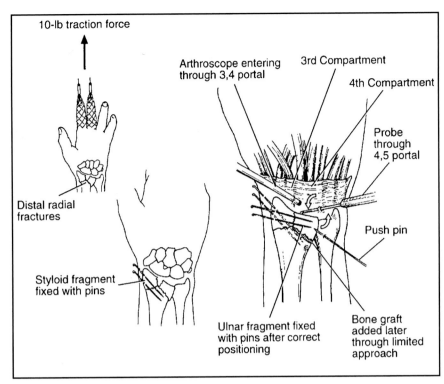

Fig. 15 The method for an arthroscopically guided reduction. The arthroscope is placed in the dorsal 3,4 portal, and a probe is inserted in the dorsal 4,5 portal. The radial styloid fragment is stabilized with percutaneous Kirschner wires.

marks of the interdigitating fracture lines. The accuracy of the reduction is confirmed with arthroscopy and is adjusted as necessary.

Associated Fractures of the Ulnar Styloid Process

Small avulsion fractures of the ulnar styloid process (type 2A[33]) do not necessitate additional treatment. The AO classification system includes 6 different types of fractures of the ulnar styloid process that are associated with fractures of the distal aspect of the radius (Fig. 16). Fractures near the base of the ulnar styloid process (type 2B[33]) include the entire insertion of the ulnar border of the triangular fibrocartilage complex; these fractures may cause instability of the distal radioulnar joint, necessitating some form of reduction and internal fixation. Injuries involving the trian-

gular fibrocartilage (type 1[33]) and complex fractures of the ulnar diaphysis or the distal articular surface of the ulna (types 3, 4, and 5[33]) are beyond the scope of this chapter. Displaced fractures near the base of the ulnar styloid process (type 2B[33]) and fractures involving the entire distal articular surface of the ulna (type 5[33]) cause displacement and deformity of the triangular fibrocartilage complex. Arthroscopy has demonstrated a high rate of involvement of the triangular fibrocartilage complex in association with intra-articular fractures of the distal aspect of the radius.[34]

The approach for stabilizing the ulnar styloid process depends on whether or not a satisfactory closed reduction can be performed. If the ulnar styloid process can be reduced, closed percutaneous fixation with

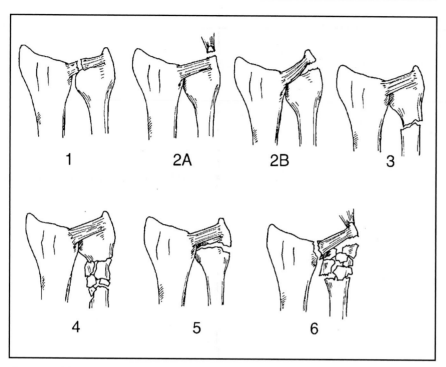

Fig. 16 Modification of the AO classification of fractures of the distal aspect of the ulna. Type-2 fractures are divided into small avulsion fractures (type 2A) and fractures near the base of the ulnar styloid process (type 2B) that cause instability of the triangular fibrocartilage complex and, consequently, the distal radioulnar joint.

use of smooth 0.035-in (0.889-mm) K-wires or a cannulated screw such as the Herbert-Whipple screw (Zimmer, Warsaw, IN) can be performed (Fig. 17). If closed reduction is not possible, an open reduction with use of an incision between the flexor carpi ulnaris and the extensor carpi ulnaris allows visualization of the avulsed ulnar styloid process.

The ulnar styloid process also can be stabilized with a tension-band-wire technique, with use of 1 or 2 smooth 0.035-in (0.889-mm) K-wires (Fig. 17). A 24-gauge stainless-steel cerclage wire then is passed through the soft tissues just distal to the ulnar styloid fragment medial to the ends of the wires, crossed, and passed through the distal aspect of the ulna. A 14-gauge needle from an intravenous catheter provides an ideal cannula for passing the cerclage wire through the ulna. The needle is drilled through the ulna with use of a power drill. The cerclage wire can be placed into the hollow needle, which then is withdrawn, bringing the wire through the ulna. The wire then is tightened to secure the fracture, and the K-wires are bent and cut short.

Associated Injuries of the Intercarpal Ligaments or the Triangular Fibrocartilage Complex

Recent advances in arthroscopically assisted reduction of intra-articular fractures have made it possible to categorize soft-tissue injuries of the wrist joint that are associated with these fractures.[12,30,31,35] In previous studies, 41 (68%) of 60 patients had soft-tissue injuries that included the triangular fibrocartilage complex in 26, the scapholunate interosseous ligament in 19, and the lunotriquetral interosseous ligament in 9.[29,30,34] (Thirteen patients had 2 injuries each.) Intercarpal injuries were identified most frequently in association with fractures involving the lunate facet of the distal articular surface of the radius.

Tears of the intercarpal ligaments were classified by Geissler and associates.[30,34] Grade-I tears involve attenuation or hemorrhage of an interosseous ligament as seen from the radiocarpal space, with no incongruency of the carpal alignment in the midcarpal space. Grade-II tears involve attenuation or hemorrhage of an interosseous ligament as seen from the radiocarpal space, with incongruency or step-off between the scaphoid and the lunate as seen from the midcarpal space. There may be a slight gap, less than the width of a probe, between the carpal bones. Grade-III tears are associated with incongruency or step-off of the carpal alignment as seen from both the radiocarpal and the midcarpal space. A probe can be placed through a gap between the carpal bones. Grade-IV tears are associated with incongruency or step-off of the carpal alignment as seen from both the radiocarpal and the midcarpal space as well as with gross instability on manipulation. A 2.7-mm arthroscope can be passed through the gap between the carpal bones.

Of the 19 patients who had an injury of the scapholunate ligament in the series of Geissler and associates,[34] 10 had a grade-II injury; 7, a grade-III injury; and 2, a grade-IV injury. Twenty-five patients had a fracture of the ulnar styloid process. Sixteen of them had a lesion of the triangular fibrocartilage complex; the lesion was ulnar type B or radial type D in 14.[34,36]

External Fixation Devices

External fixation devices are the only practical means of overcoming the force of the muscles of the forearm that pull comminuted distal radial fractures into a collapsed, shortened position. Because the loss of radial length is associated with a poorer functional outcome, an external fixation device can often be an important part of the treatment of intra-articular fractures of the distal aspect of the radius.[6,7] In many instances of severe comminution of the metaphysis, the surgeon can reconstruct the articular surface but cannot stabilize it to the shaft of the radius. An external fixation device can allow alignment of the articular surface with the shaft without reliance on support from the metaphysis.

A large variety of devices are available for external fixation of fractures of the distal aspect of the radius. All involve distraction across the wrist joint with placement of pins in the radius and the metacarpals (Fig. 18). The proximal pins are placed into the junction of the distal and middle thirds of the radius, near the insertion of the pronator teres muscle. Small incisions are made along the radial border of the forearm. The drill guide is placed between the extensor carpi radialis longus and the extensor carpi radialis brevis so that the sensory branch of the radial nerve will be protected as it exits between the extensor carpi radialis longus and the brachioradialis. The partially threaded pins can be inserted perpendicular to the shaft of the radius, unlike the smooth pins used with older external fixation devices, which had to be placed at oblique angles to one another. Placement of the pins at right angles to the radius and the metacarpals decreases skin tension and irritation. Predrilling of the pin sites (with use of a 2.0-mm drill-bit

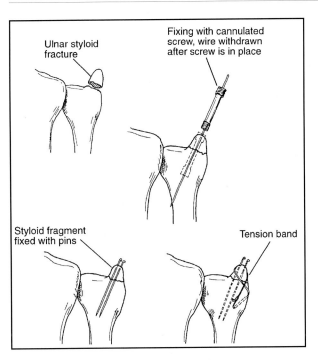

Fig. 17 The screw-fixation and tension-band-wire techniques can be used to stabilize fractures of the ulnar styloid process.

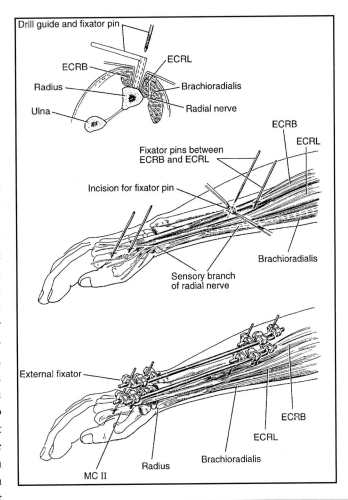

Fig. 18 The partially threaded pins for the external fixation device are inserted in the interval between the extensor carpi radialis longus (ECRL) and the extensor carpi radialis brevis (ECRB) in order to protect the sensory branch of the radial nerve. MC II = second metacarpal.

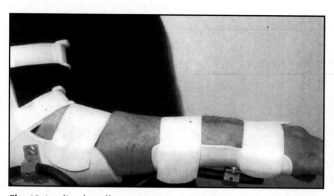

Fig. 19 A splint that allows pronation-supination to improve rotation of the forearm when 120° of combined motion has not been regained within 8 to 10 weeks after the fracture.

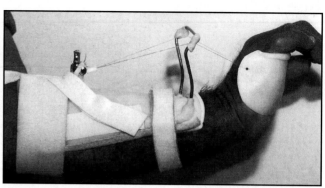

Fig. 20 A static progressive splint, used for patients who do not regain 100° of flexion and extension of the wrist within 8 to 10 weeks after the fracture.

for a 2.5-mm pin, for example) facilitates placement of the pins in hard cortical bone. The metacarpal pins also are inserted at right angles to the bone after the soft tissues have been spread to avoid injury to the smaller branches of the radial sensory nerve and the first dorsal interosseous muscle. The first pin is placed at the junction of the base and shaft of the index metacarpal. The second pin is placed near the middle or distal metaphyseal flare of the index metacarpal.

Because an external fixation device is no stronger than its weakest link, we suggest that pins of the same size be used for both the radius and the metacarpals, although other devices feature a smaller (2.5-mm) pin in the metacarpals and a larger (3.5-mm) pin in the distal aspect of the radius. The device should be placed with the wrist in neutral flexion and extension and with no more than 10 lb (4.5 kg) of distraction, demonstrated by 1.0 to 2.0 mm of distraction of the radiocarpal joint under fluoroscopy. The fingers should be able to be flexed easily into the palm with passive motion during surgery. Excessive flexion or ulnar deviation must be avoided, as either position increases the risk of compression of the median nerve, reflex

sympathetic dystrophy, and extrinsic tightness, causing stiffness of the fingers.

Advantages and Disadvantages of Open Reduction, Arthroscopically Aided Reduction, and Limited Open Reduction

Internal fixation accompanied by arthroscopically aided reduction and limited open reduction has the advantage of minimizing capsular scarring, thereby reducing stiffness of the wrist after fracture healing. To our knowledge, there are no data, retrospective or prospective, demonstrating that arthroscopically assisted reduction improves patient outcome. Arthroscopy does offer better visualization of soft-tissue injuries and the potential for treatment with repair or debridement of the triangular fibrocartilage complex. However, arthroscopic repair of the interosseous ligaments is limited to percutaneous pinning to stabilize the carpal bones, whereas an open approach provides an opportunity to suture detached ligaments to the carpal bones. In a prospective trial of 240 patients who were randomized to treatment with either limited or standard open reduction and internal fixation, limited open reduction re-

sulted in an average of 20° (15%) more motion (HL Kreder, DP Hanel, M McKee, J Jupiter, TE Trumble, unpublished data, 1998). However, in 20% of the 120 patients who had limited open reduction, the procedure failed to restore a congruent articular surface and the surgeon had to perform an open reduction. Although limited open reduction does not provide an opportunity to assess soft-tissue injury within the wrist because the reduction is guided by fluoroscopy, the data suggest that limited open reduction and internal fixation, when used successfully, improves patient outcome.

Rehabilitation After Intra-Articular Fractures of the Distal Aspect of the Radius

Distal radial fractures can be categorized as stable, as AO type B (those with a portion of the articular surface in continuity), as AO type C (those with minimum comminution), or as unstable AO type C (those with comminution necessitating an external fixation device to maintain distraction).

Patients who have a stable fracture, which may be treated without an external fixation device, must wear a splint for 4 to 6 weeks until the edema has resolved. They can begin an active range-of-motion program, with a removable splint, during the first 2 to 4 weeks, assuming that no displacement occurs. It is essential that radiographs be made during this time period. During the first 2 weeks, the patients also start an active and passive program for motion of the digits and rotation of the forearm. They then progress to a passive range-of-motion program, including exercises for the wrist (which was initially in a splint), for another 2 weeks, followed by resistive exercises for strengthening.

The goal for patients who do not have painful rotation is to regain a total of 120° of pronation and supination. If this goal is not met within 8 to 10 weeks, a program of dynamic supination and pronation splinting is begun (Fig. 19). Patients who fail to regain 100° of flexion and extension of the wrist are managed with a program of static progressive splinting (Fig. 20).

Patients who have an unstable fracture, necessitating treatment with an external fixation device, start range-of-motion exercises for the digits and rotation of the forearm immediately after surgery, in the same manner as patients who have a stable fracture not necessitating treatment with an external fixation device. The external fixation device is removed 5 to 7 weeks after surgery, depending on the surgeon's evaluation of the postoperative radiographs. After the device has been removed, active exercises for motion of the wrist are performed for the first 2 weeks, followed by passive exercises. Dynamic and static progressive devices are used after 2 weeks of passive exercise if the goals of 120° of pronation and supination of the forearm and 100° of flexion and extension of the wrist have not been achieved.

Results of Treatment

Part of the problem in comparing the clinical outcomes of different types of treatment of fractures of the distal aspect of the radius results from the use of multiple classification and evaluation systems. Even when investigators have used the same system, it is difficult to determine if fractures with similar degrees of displacement and fragmentation have been included.[4-7,15-17,33,37-39] A marked decrease in function was noted in association with fractures with more than 1.0 mm of displacement and more than 5 fragments.[6,7] Patients who had additional soft-tissue injuries and carpal fractures had a worse functional result. In one study,[7] severe AO type-C2 and C3 fractures had been treated with open reduction and internal fixation and the patients regained an average of 31 (69%) of 45 kg of grip strength, 120° of combined flexion and extension of the wrist, 41° of combined radial and ulnar deviation, and 140° of combined pronation and supination. The 301° combined motion of the wrist and rotation of the forearm corresponded to 75% of that on the contralateral side.

Other than a comprehensive study of volar rim fractures,[40] there are no reports, to our knowledge, describing the results of treatment of 2-part fractures. In that study, the combined motion of the wrist averaged 90% of that on the contralateral side and only 9 of 49 patients had osteoarthrosis at an average of 51 months after treatment. Forty-seven of the 49 patients had a grip strength that was within 10% of that on the contralateral side. The most important factors associated with a poor or fair result were osteoarthrosis as seen on the early postoperative radiographs and the reversal of normal volar tilt.

Summary

Intra-articular distal radius fractures are a heterogeneous group of injuries with different fracture patterns. The existing classification systems are helpful for describing the fractures but not for assessing their stability or for deciding which surgical approach to use. Patients who have a fracture with at least 1.0 mm of displacement of the articular surface may benefit from open surgical treatment. Improved diagnostic imaging with CT is helpful for fracture classification and surgical planning. The options for surgical treatment include limited open reduction and internal fixation, arthroscopically assisted internal fixation, and open reduction and internal fixation. The surgical approach is determined on the basis of the initial displacement of the fracture. Patients who have a displaced fracture of the volar rim may benefit from a volar approach; those who have a dorsally displaced fracture, from a dorsal approach; and those who have an impacted fracture such as a die-punch fracture, from a dorsal approach that provides better visualization of the articular surface.

The long-term functional outcome is determined in part by the severity of the fracture as defined by the amount of comminution, the initial severity of displacement, and the number of fracture fragments. The accuracy of the reconstruction of the articular surface, with the goal of establishing congruency to within 1.0 mm, is also important in order to minimize the risk of late osteoarthrosis. Of all of the extra-articular parameters, restoration of the length of the radius is the most important for enhancing recovery of motion and grip strength and for preventing problems involving the distal radioulnar joint—the so-called forgotten joint in distal radial fractures.

References

1. Melone CP Jr: Articular fractures of the distal radius. *Orthop Clin North Am* 1984; 15:217–236.

2. Melone CP Jr: Open treatment for displaced articular fractures of the distal radius. *Clin Orthop* 1986;202:103–111.

3. Melone CP Jr: Distal radius fractures: Patterns of articular fragmentation. *Orthop Clin North Am* 1993;24:239–253.

4. Knirk JL, Jupiter JB: Intra-articular fractures of the distal end of the radius in young adults. *J Bone Joint Surg* 1986;68A: 647–659.

5. Fernandez DL, Geissler WB: Treatment of displaced articular fractures of the radius. *J Hand Surg* 1991;16A:375–384.

6. Trumble TE, Schmitt SR, Vedder NB: Internal fixation of pilon fractures of the distal radius. *Yale J Biol Med* 1993;66: 179–191.

7. Trumble TE, Schmitt SR, Vedder NB: Factors affecting functional outcome of displaced intra-articular distal radius fractures. *J Hand Surg* 1994;19A:325–340.

8. Llinas A, McKellop HA, Marshall GJ, Sharpe F, Kirchen M, Sarmiento A: Healing and remodeling of articular incongruities in a rabbit fracture model. *J Bone Joint Surg* 1993;75A:1508–1523.

9. Trumble TE, Miyano J, Clark JM, et al: Intra-articular fracture: A sheep fracture model with weight bearing after internal fixation. *J Orthop Trauma*, in press.

10. Anglen JO, Healy WL: Tibial plateau fractures. *Orthopedics* 1988;11:1527–1534.

11. Lansinger O, Bergman B, Korner L, Andersson GB: Tibial condylar fractures. A twenty-year follow-up. *J Bone Joint Surg* 1986;68A:13–19.

12. Levy HJ, Glickel SZ: Arthroscopic assisted internal fixation of volar intraarticular wrist fractures. *Arthroscopy* 1993;9:122–124.

13. Rasmussen PS: Tibial condylar fractures as a cause of degenerative arthritis. *Acta Orthop Scand* 1972;43:566–575.

14. Waddell JP, Johnston DW, Neidre A: Fractures of the tibial plateau: A review of ninety-five patients and comparison of treatment methods. *J Trauma* 1981;21: 376–381.

15. Bradway JK, Amadio PC, Cooney WP: Open reduction and internal fixation of displaced, comminuted intra-articular fractures of the distal end of the radius. *J Bone Joint Surg* 1989;71A:839–847.

16. Cooney WP: Fractures of the distal radius: A modern treatment-based classification. *Orthop Clin North Am* 1993;24:211–216.

17. Cooney WP, Berger RA: Treatment of complex fractures of the distal radius: Combined use of internal and external fixation and arthroscopic reduction. *Hand Clin* 1993;9:603–612.

18. Frykman G: Fracture of the distal radius including sequelae: Shoulder-hand-finger syndrome, disturbances in the distal radioulnar joint and impairment of nerve function. A clinical and experimental study. *Acta Orthop Scand* 1967;108(suppl):3–153.

19. Graff S, Jupiter J: Fracture of the distal radius: Classification of treatment and indications for external fixation. *Injury* 1994;25(suppl 4):SD14–SD25.

20. Jupiter JB, Fernandez DL: Comparative classification for fractures of the distal end of the radius. *J Hand Surg* 1997;22A: 563–571.

21. Lichtenhahn P, Fernandez DL, Schatzker J: Analysis of the "user friendliness" of the AO classification of fractures [German]. *Helv Chir Acta* 1992;58:919–924.

22. Mehara AK, Rastogi S, Bhan S, Dave PK: Classification and treatment of volar Barton fractures. *Injury* 1993;24:55–59.

23. Müller ME, Allgöwer M, Schneider R, Willenegger H (eds): *Manual of Internal Fixation*, ed 3. New York, NY, Springer-Verlag, 1991.

24. Newey ML, Ricketts D, Roberts L: The AO classification of long bone fractures: An early study of its use in clinical practice. *Injury* 1993;24:309–312.

25. Tajima T, Saito H: A new classification of distal radius fractures and corresponding treatment methods [German]. *Handchir Mikrochir Plast Chir* 1991;23:227–235.

26. Andersen DJ, Blair WF, Steyers CM Jr, Adams BD, el Khouri GY, Brandser EA: Classification of distal radius fractures: An analysis of interobserver reliability and intraobserver reproducibility. *J Hand Surg* 1996;21A:574–582.

27. Waters PM, Mintzer CM, Hipp JA, Snyder BD: Noninvasive measurement of distal radius instability. *J Hand Surg* 1997;22A:572–579.

28. Geissler WB, Fernandez DL: Percutaneous and limited open reduction of the articular surface of the distal radius. *J Orthop Trauma* 1991;5:255–264.

29. Geissler WB: Arthroscopically assisted reduction of intra-articular fractures of the distal radius. *Hand Clin* 1995;11:19–29.

30. Geissler WB, Freeland AE: Arthroscopically assisted reduction of intraarticular distal radial fractures. *Clin Orthop* 1996; 327:125–134.

31. Whipple TL: The role of arthroscopy in the treatment of intra-articular wrist fractures. *Hand Clin* 1995;11:13–18.

32. Whipple TL, Geissler WB: Arthroscopic management of wrist triangular fibrocartilage complex injuries in the athlete. *Orthopedics* 1993;16:1061–1067.

33. Jupiter JB: Fractures of the distal end of the radius. *J Bone Joint Surg* 1991;73A: 461–469.

34. Geissler WB, Freeland AE, Savoie FH, McIntyre LW, Whipple TL: Intracarpal soft-tissue lesions associated with an intra-articular fracture of the distal end of the radius. *J Bone Joint Surg* 1996;78A:357–365.

35. Wolfe SW, Easterling KJ, Yoo HH: Arthroscopic-assisted reduction of distal radius fractures. *Arthroscopy* 1995;11: 706–714.

36. Palmer AK: Triangular fibrocartilage complex lesions: A classification. *J Hand Surg* 1989;14A:594–606.

37. Axelrod TS, McMurtry RY: Open reduction and internal fixation of comminuted, intraarticular fractures of the distal radius. *J Hand Surg* 1990;15A:1–11.

38. Edwards GS Jr: Intra-articular fractures of the distal part of the radius treated with the small AO external fixator. *J Bone Joint Surg* 1991;73A:1241–1250.

39. Fernandez DL: Fractures of the distal radius: Operative treatment, in Heckman JD (ed): *Instructional Course Lectures 42*. Rosemont, IL, American Academy of Orthopaedic Surgeons, 1993, pp 73–88.

40. Jupiter JB, Fernandez DL, Toh CL, Fellman T, Ring D: Operative treatment of volar intra-articular fractures of the distal end of the radius. *J Bone Joint Surg* 1996;78A:1817–1828.

Reference to Video

Culp R: *Isolated Sheer Fractures Limited to ORIF Volar and Distal Approaches*. Rosemont, IL, American Academy of Orthopaedic Surgeons, Annual Meeting, 1998.

Surgical Treatment of Acetabular Fractures

David C. Templeman, MD
Steven Olson, MD
Berton R. Moed, MD
Paul Duwelius, MD
Joel M. Matta, MD

Introduction

An Instructional Course Lecture published in 1986, entitled *The Surgical Treatment of Fractures of the Acetabulum*, by Matta, Letournel, and Browner, reviewed the classification of acetabular fractures, described the surgical approaches, detailed the techniques for the reduction of individual fracture types, and presented the results of Professor Emile Letournel's series of 350 cases.[1] The purpose of this chapter is to present progress made in the treatment of fractures of the acetabulum.

There has been recent widespread interest in the surgical treatment of fractures of the acetabulum, resulting in the publication of more than 100 papers between 1990 and 1997.[2] During this period, it has become evident that the protocols developed by Letournel enable the surgeon to consistently achieve accurate reductions of acetabular fractures. Letournel's protocols include the classification of the fracture, the selection of the surgical approach, and the techniques of surgical treatment.[3] Despite this knowledge, the treatment of fractures of the acetabulum remains technically demanding, and complications can result in significant disability.

Patient Assessment

Most acetabular fractures are the result of high-energy accidents. Associated injuries are common. The occurrence of aortic ruptures in combination with pelvic fractures has recently been documented.[4] Regrettably, the most common types of acetabular fractures, posterior wall fractures and the associated transverse and posterior wall fractures, are frequently associated with the failure to wear seat belts.

The initial assessment must include a detailed neurologic examination of the involved extremity. The examination is based on a thorough documentation of the 0 to 5 motor grading of the dorsiflexors and plantarflexors. The incidence of neurologic injury for all acetabular fractures ranges between 10% and 13%.[5] Letournel and associates[3,6] reported a 75% incidence of traumatic palsy of the sciatic nerve in the subset of posterior dislocations. Injuries of the peroneal nerve have a variable prognosis. When the injury to the peroneal nerve is incomplete, the prognosis for functional recovery is favorable. However, when the initial injury is severe, the prognosis for functional recovery of dorsiflexion is

poor. Patients with sciatic nerve palsy have satisfactory recovery of tibial nerve function, but they are unlikely to regain peroneal nerve function. It is difficult to predict the functional outcome for a given patient, and electromyography has not helped to predict neurologic recovery.[7]

Significant soft-tissue injuries occur in association with acetabular fractures. The Morel-Lavelle's lesion is a closed degloving injury, in which shearing forces separate the skin and subcutaneous tissue from the underlying fascia. This damages the skin, which is perfused by a vascular plexus of blood vessels that originate from deep muscles, penetrate fascial planes, and enter the subcutaneous tissue. As a result of the crushing nature of the injury and damage to the vascular plexus, necrosis of the of the skin is possible. Hypermobile skin, fluctuant swelling, and loss of local sensation are diagnostic clues.[8]

The Morel-Lavelle's lesion can occur at any site about the trunk, buttocks, or thighs. The presence of vascular compromise and necrotic fat has profound implications for the open reduction and internal fixation of adjacent fractures. This requires careful timing and planning of all skin incisions. A successful protocol for the treatment of this lesion is to perform irrigation and debridement of the entire area of degloving, proceed with open reduction and internal fixation, and then pack the wound open. Broad spectrum intravenous antibiotics and sterile wound packing are continued postoperatively. Most of these injuries are left open and are encouraged to heal by secondary intention. A few lesions are amenable to delayed primary closure, although this increases the possibility of a late infection. Despite prompt and aggressive treatment, there is a 12% incidence of infection.[8]

Dislocation or subluxation of the femoral head requires emergent reduction. The associated fracture patterns may include posterior wall fractures, which result in posterior subluxation or dislocation of the femoral head.[9] Careful study of the initial films is needed to ensure that the femoral head is not dislocated either anteriorly or posteriorly from the acetabulum. Evaluation of the obturator oblique view usually confirms whether or not the femoral head is adequately reduced. It is preferable to perform the reduction with a general anesthetic in order to avoid injury to the articular surfaces. In unusual circumstances, incarceration of large bony fragments or impingement of the femoral head against the fracture may prevent a concentric reduction. When an emergent open reduction of the dislocation is contemplated, the surgeon should be confident that open reduction and internal fixation of the acetabular fracture can be achieved at the same time. Skeletal traction is used for unstable reductions of the femoral head or when the femoral head is impacted against fracture surfaces.

Open reduction and internal fixation are rarely indicated on an emer-gent basis. A short delay ensures that the patient is adequately resuscitated, the proper imaging studies are completed, and the appropriate personnel and equipment are assembled. This delay promotes hemostasis of the fractured innominate bone, which, when coupled with hypotensive anesthesia, reduces bleeding at the time of surgery and improves visualization of the fracture.

Radiography of Acetabular Fractures

Judet and Letournel recognized the difficulty in visualizing the 3-dimensional anatomy and displacements associated with acetabular fractures as viewed with standard radiographic films. Detailed studies correlating the anatomy of the innominate bone with radiographic imaging have been performed by Letournel and associates[6,10] and Judet and associates.[11] Three radiographic projections of the pelvis are used to evaluate fractures of the acetabulum: the anterior-posterior (AP) view of the pelvis, and two oblique pelvic views known as the iliac-oblique view and the obturator-oblique view. Accurate interpretation of the plain films is based on the understanding of the correlation of the normal anatomy of the innominate bone with the pertinent radiographic landmarks of each view of the pelvis. Computed tomography (CT) can also be beneficial in evaluating acetabular fractures. However, CT does not replace the standard radiographic evaluation. Rather, it complements the information on the plain films and allows the surgeon to evaluate specific details of the fracture pattern.[3]

Anterior-Posterior View (Fig. 1)

The iliopectineal line is the major landmark of the anterior column. The inferior three fourths of the

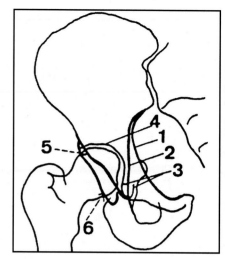

Fig. 1 There are 6 basic landmarks on the anteroposterior view: (1) iliopectineal line, (2) ilioischial line, (3) radiographic "U" or teardrop, (4) roof of the acetabulum, (5) anterior rim, and (6) posterior rim of the acetabulum.[3]

iliopectineal line correlate directly with the pelvic brim on the innominate bone. However, the superior quarter of the iliopectineal line is formed by the tangency of the X-ray beam to the superior quadrilateral surface and the posterior-superior aspect of the greater sciatic notch.[3] The ilioischial line extends from the posterior-superior greater sciatic notch to the ischial tuberosity. This radiographic landmark is formed by the tangency of the X-ray beam to the posterior portion of the quadrilateral surface of the innominate bone.[3] The ilioischial line is generally considered a radiographic landmark of the posterior column. The radiographic U, or teardrop, consists of a medial and lateral limb. The lateral limb represents the inferior aspect of the anterior wall of the acetabulum, and the medial limb is formed by the obturator canal and the anterior-inferior portion of the quadrilateral surface. The teardrop and ilioischial lines are always superimposed on the AP view

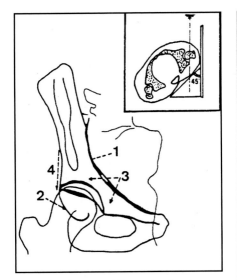

Fig. 2 The obturator oblique view is taken with the patient rotated so that the injured hip is angulated 45° toward the X-ray beam. This view projects the obturator foramen, hence its name.

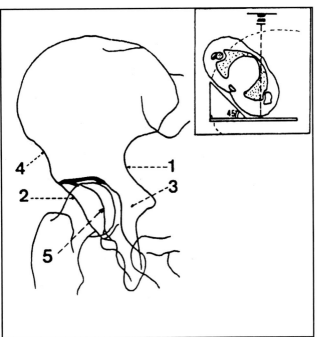

Fig. 3 The iliac oblique view is taken with the patient rotated so that the injured hip is tilted away from the X-ray beam by 45°. This view profiles the iliac wing, and projects the anterior border of the iliac wing and anterior wall of the acetabulum, as well as the greater and lesser sciatic notches of the innominate bone.

of the pelvis, because both of these landmarks are from different parts of the quadrilateral plate.[3] This means that dissociation of the teardrop with the ilioischial line suggests that either the innominate bone is rotated, or that there has been disruption and displacement of the quadrilateral surface. The dense line of the superior articular surface of the acetabulum on the AP view is known as the roof. This radiographic landmark results from the tangency of the X-ray beam to the subchondral bone in the superior acetabulum. The anterior rim and posterior rim of the acetabulum represent the peripheral contours of the anterior and posterior walls of the acetabulum, respectively.

Obturator Oblique View (Fig. 2)

The iliopectineal line can also be seen in the obturator oblique view, with the anterior column viewed in profile. Fractures of the superior and inferior pubic rami are often best detected with this obturator oblique

view. The posterior rim of the acetabulum is best visualized in this view, as are displaced fractures of the posterior wall and subtle amounts of femoral head subluxation.

Iliac Oblique View (Fig. 3)

Acetabular fractures extending into the ilium are often best visualized with the iliac oblique view. Involvement of the posterior column with disruption of the greater or lesser sciatic notch can also be best detected on this view. The anterior wall is seen in profile on the iliac oblique view, and disruption of the anterior wall can be determined by comparison with the opposite, normal hip.

Computed Tomography

The primary use of CT is to add additional information to that obtained from the plain radiographic films. After studying the plain films, the surgeon can use CT to address specific questions about the fracture pattern that may have remained unanswered.

Several aspects of acetabular fractures are better visualized with use of CT: (1) injuries to the posterior pelvic ring, (2) free intra-articular osteochondral fractures, (3) fractures of the femoral head, (4) marginal impaction of the articular surface of the acetabulum, (5) the size, rotation, comminution and displacement of anterior and posterior wall fractures, (6) rotation of fracture fragments, (7) extension of fracture lines through the quadrilateral surface, and (8) involvement of the superior acetabular articular surface, particularly with coronal plane fracture lines, such as with an anterior column fracture.[12]

Biomechanics of the Acetabulum

The hip joint functions as a ball-and-socket articulation. Recent biomechanical investigations have demonstrated that the normal acetabulum deforms small amounts under physiologic loads. Mechanical investigations of fractures of the acetabulum have demonstrated that the posterior wall component, transverse component and coronal plane components (ie, the anterior column or posterior column) of fractures result in alteration of the normal load transmission across the hip joint, with an increase in the load and contact area in the superior acetabulum.[13] This biomechanical information, combined with the general observations of Rowe and Lowell,[14] as well as those of Letournel, suggest that the maintenance of an anatomically reduced superior acetabular articular surface, and the congruent relationship of the femoral head in the acetabulum, are important factors in maintaining normal hip function.[3,13–15]

Clinical Applications

The dense radiographic line representing the roof of the acetabulum can be visualized on all 3 plain views of the pelvis. While this landmark represents the tangency of the X-ray beam to the subchondral bone of the superior acetabulum in all 3 of these views, the portion of superior acetabulum that gives rise to this landmark is different on the AP and oblique views, because the pelvis is rotated differently in each view. This observation allows the surgeon to gain insight into the location of the displaced fracture lines traversing the superior acetabulum by using roof arc measurements.[15] Matta and associates[16] developed the concept of roof arc measurements (Fig. 4) to allow the surgeon to roughly define the amount of superior acetabular articular surface that is left intact following an acetabular fracture.

A preliminary study, recently reported, used roof arc angles of 45° or greater on all 3 views, along with maintenance of a congruent relationship of the femoral head and acetabulum in the absence of posterior wall fractures, as criteria for nonsurgical

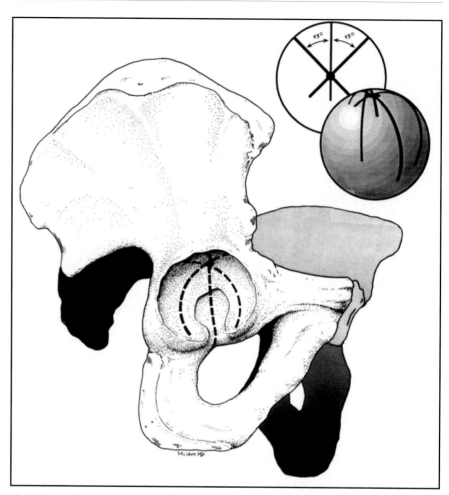

Fig. 4 The roof arc measurement is determined by finding the point representing the radiographic center of the acetabulum of the involved hip on each of the three views of the pelvis. A line is extended from this point superiorly, perpendicular to the horizontal plane. A second line is extended from the center of the acetabulum to the point along the contour of the articular surface where the fracture has disrupted the acetabulum. The angle formed by these two lines is referred to as the roof arc angle.[16,17]

treatment of the acetabulum (Fig. 5). This study documented a good-to-excellent clinical outcome in 9 of 11 patients who met these criteria for nonsurgical treatment. Seven of 12 patients who did not meet these criteria but were treated nonsurgically went on to develop a fair or poor clinical outcome.[15]

CT can be used to evaluate the superior acetabulum as well. With CT, the superior acetabulum is visualized as a series of concentric rings of dense subchondral bone. The extent of the intact acetabular surface that is necessary for a good or excellent clinical outcome, with or without surgical repair, remains unknown.[15] However, the maintenance of an anatomic reduction in the superior aspect of the acetabulum is an important factor in the long-term prognosis of the hip joint.

Postoperative CT has been shown to be unnecessary in the determination of the presence or absence of intra-articular screws in the majority of cases. However, correlation be-

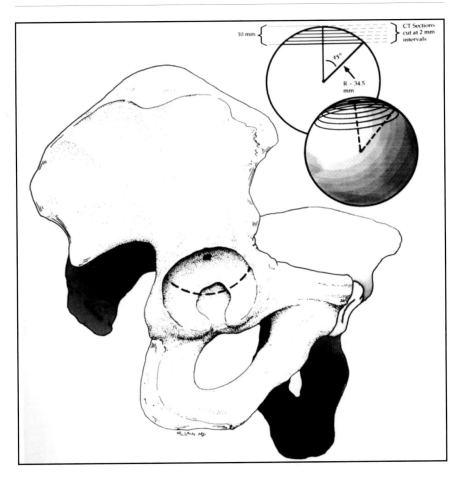

Fig. 5 The scans taken though the superior 10 mm of the acetabulum image the area equivalent to the 45° roof arc measurements on the 3 plain films.

tween postoperative reduction as evaluated with CT and long-term outcome has not been reported. It has yet to be determined whether the anatomic restoration of the subchondral arc of the superior acetabulum on post-repair CT has implications for long-term outcome.

Nonsurgical Treatment

Nonsurgical treatment for acetabular fractures is appropriate when the femoral head remains congruent with the acetabulum, and the fracture displacement occurs outside of the roof arcs and CT subchondral arc. Fractures that involve the superior acetabulum that have up to 2 mm of displacement are also appropriately

treated by nonsurgical methods. Traction should be used if there is concern that further displacement will occur; a period of 4 to 8 weeks is usually sufficient. When traction is not used, weekly radiographs are required to ensure that further displacement does not occur.[17,18]

Contraindications to Surgical Treatment

Surgical treatment is contraindicated when the above criteria for nonsurgical treatment are met. Other contraindications include the presence of local infection and the medical condition of the patient.

Severe osteoporosis associated with fractures in elderly patients is a

contraindication to surgery if the degree of osteoporosis prevents stable fracture fixation. Despite this concern, many elderly patients benefit from open reduction and internal fixation. Most fractures in this age group are secondary to falls, and result in either associated anterior column-posterior hemitransverse fractures or both column fractures. Many of these injuries in the elderly are reconstructed using the ilioinguinal approach. Helfet and associates[19] reported Harris hip scores of greater than 90 points in 16 of 17 elderly patients followed for at least 2 years after surgery.

Strategies for Open Reduction and Internal Fixation of Specific Fracture Types
Use of the Fracture Table

The protocols developed by Letournel call for strict adherence to patient positioning and the use of a fracture table.[3,6] It is our opinion that the importance of these points cannot be overemphasized. The combination of patient positioning and traction assist the surgeon in reducing the fractured acetabulum (Figs. 6 and 7).

The reduction of the fracture is the most difficult element of the surgical procedure. The use of intraoperative traction, which reduces the deforming force of the femoral head, permits a precise reduction of the fracture with the use of special clamps. Obtaining anatomic reduction is critical to achieving consistently good clinical results.

The Kocher-Langenbech approach is used for fractures of the posterior wall and posterior column and for most transverse fractures. The patient is placed in the prone position.[3] The prone position, in contrast to the lateral decubitus position, reduces the deforming force of the femoral head on the acetabulum and facilitates the reduction.

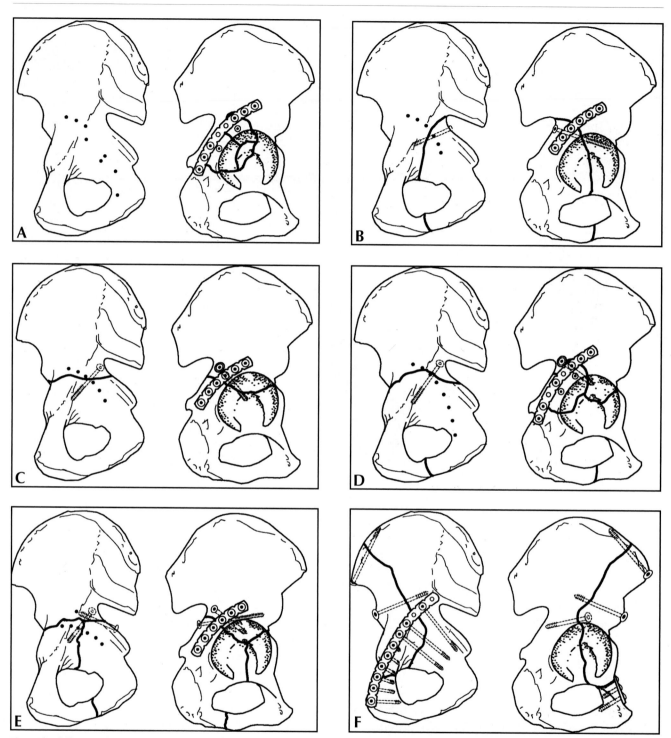

Fig. 6 The following diagrams represent 6 of the different types of acetabular fractures (3 additional types are shown in Figure 7). Standard methods of internal fixation are outlined. Careful study of the diagrams indicates that the fracture plane is frequently not perpendicular to the innominate bone and, therefore, the fracture lines are different on the outer and inner surfaces of the innominate bone. A careful study of the fracture plane is necessary to ensure that adequate fixation is achieved. Careful study of the fixation constructs as diagramed will indicate appropriate positioning of screws and plates to achieve the best fixation (often with interfragmentary screws) for the different fracture types. **A,** Multifragmented posterior wall fracture with intraarticular comminution. **B,** Posterior column fracture with a lag screw reaching the anterior column. **C,** Transverse fracture with a lag screw reaching the anterior column. **D,** Associated transverse and posterior wall fracture. **E,** Associated T-type acetabular fracture. Lag screws inserted into both the anterior and posterior columns. **F,** Anterior column fracture. Several lag screws are placed between the inner and outer tables of the innominate bone.

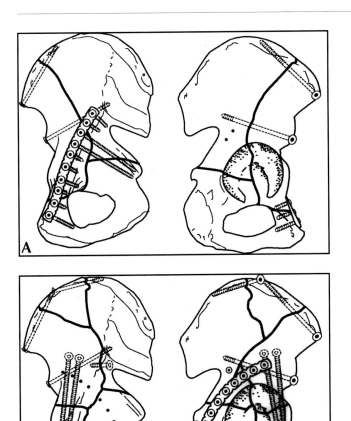

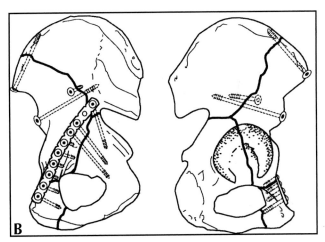

Fig. 7 Additional types of acetabular fractures. **A,** Associated anterior column and posterior hemitransverse fracture. Screws inserted from the pelvic brim must reach distal to the fracture line and engage in the posterior column. **B,** Both column fracture operated on through the ilioinguinal approach. Screws inserted from the pelvic brim reach the posterior column. **C,** Both column fracture. Internal fixation performed through the extended iliofemoral approach. Two very long screws are inserted into the anterior column and reach the superior pubic ramus.

The ilioinguinal approach is made with the patient in the supine position.[3] The supine position enhances visualization of the quadrilateral plate and reduces the deforming force of the femoral head. In selected cases, the intraoperative insertion of a trochanteric pin will assist the reduction.

The extended iliofemoral approach is made with the patient in the lateral decubitus position,[3] which allows simultaneous exposure of the external surface of the iliac wing and the retroacetabular surface. When necessary, a capsulotomy provides excellent exposure of the intra-articular surface of the acetabulum. Depending on the fracture pattern, the internal surface of the iliac wing can be exposed, but this is avoided if

a fracture of the anterior column will become devascularized.

Posterior Wall Fractures

Of the 10 fracture types, fractures of the posterior wall are the most common. Recent reports suggest, however, that despite their frequency, these fractures have a poor prognosis. The common dashboard mechanism of injury requires clinical and radiographic examination of the knee to detect associated injuries, such as patella fracture and posterior cruciate injury. Prompt and gentle reduction of the dislocated femoral head is mandatory. The incidence of osteonecrosis (ON) after a posterior fracture-dislocation of the hip is not as high as previous-

ly quoted. Recent studies indicate that ON occurs in only 5% of these cases.[3,20] Although poor results are often attributed to ON or chondral injury, most poor results are probably due to malreductions or insufficient stability of the fixation. Comminuted posterior wall fragments are particularly challenging to accurately reduce and secure with stable fixation.[21]

The patient can be placed in either the lateral decubitus or the prone position. The prone position allows better intraoperative imaging with the use of a radiolucent table. The knee must be flexed to 70° to 90° to reduce tension on the sciatic nerve. The Kocher-Langenbech approach is used. The Kocher-Langenbech approach differs significantly from the postero-lateral approach used for total hip arthroplasty. The obturator internus tendon is critical to the exposure of the retroacetabular surface. The obturator internus retracts the sciatic nerve and exposes the lesser sciatic notch for placement of a retractor.

During exposure of the posterior wall fragment, the dislocation cavity is entered. This is an area of fracture hematoma and soft-tissue disruption caused by the fracture-dislocation. Dissection in this area is often complicated by adherence of the soft tissues when the surgery is delayed. Exposure of the posterior wall fragment is a critical step in the procedure. Complete soft-tissue stripping of the wall fragment(s) must be avoided in order not to devitalize the fragment. The vascularity of the posterior wall is improved by preserving the attachment of the labrum. The hematoma is cleared from the fragment, and a gentle reduction is achieved and held with a ball spike. Lag screw fixation is used to hold the reduction. Screws are inserted oblique to the retroacetabular surface, and must be directed away from the joint.

Mechanical studies have demonstrated that when used alone, lag screws provide insufficient fixation, whereas buttress plating provides adequate fixation.[22] A curved plate that parallels the acetabulum extends from the ischium to the inferior aspect of the iliac wing. The plate is slightly undercontoured to achieve a buttress effect as screws are inserted. Dissection and the placement of plates superior to the greater sciatic notch are avoided because of potential injury to the superior gluteal nerve with subsequent abductor weakness.

Marginal impaction is present in 21% of posterior wall fractures.[3,23] Marginal impaction occurs when the femoral head depresses a segment of the articular surface at the time of the dislocation. Impaction is easy to diagnose with the preoperative CT scan. Posterior wall fractures with marginal impaction are inherently unstable and require open reduction.[3,23] The depressed segment of articular surface that is not in contact with the femoral head is elevated and reduced against the femoral head, which serves as a template for the reduction. As the impacted segment is elevated, it is important to maintain as much cancellous bone beneath the articular surface as possible. The defect beneath the articular surface is grafted with cancellous bone from the greater trochanter.[3]

Posterior Column Fractures

The patient is placed in the prone position on the fracture table and a Kocher-Langenbeck approach is made. The fracture hematoma is debrided. Reduction is usually achieved with either a pelvic manipulation clamp or a Farabeuf forceps secured to screws placed proximal and distal to the fracture. The placement of the screws for the Farabeuf procedure is critical to the force vector to reduce the fracture. The rotational displacement of the posterior column is corrected by placing a Schanz screw in the ischial tuberosity, and then using the screw as a rotational lever as the forceps compresses the fracture.

The reduction is assessed by visualization of the retroacetabular surface and palpation of the quadrilateral plate. A lag screw is inserted from posterior to anterior, and a curved plate is placed on the retroacetabular surface.

Anterior Wall Fractures

The patient is placed supine on the fracture table, and an ilioinguinal incision is made. Reduction is usually achieved through the middle window of the ilioinguinal incision, and is obtained with distraction of the femoral head and a ball spike. A curved plate extending from the superior pubic ramus to the internal iliac fossa is placed along the pelvic brim. To avoid intra-articular penetration from screws placed along the pelvic brim, the plate must be meticulously contoured, and only short screws of 12 to 14 mm in length are inserted in the area of the pectineal eminence.

Anterior Column Fractures

The ilioinguinal approach is used, with the patient in the supine position on the fracture table. The iliac wing is usually externally rotated, and maximal displacement is observed at the pelvic brim. When the iliac wing portion of the fracture line has not extended to the crest, it is sometimes necessary to complete the fracture in order to achieve the reduction. Comminution adjacent to the sacroiliac joint must be reduced prior to fixation of the anterior column.

The reduction· is assessed by inspecting the course of the fracture line across the iliac fossa, pelvic brim, and quadrilateral plate. Fixation is accomplished with interfragmentary screws along the iliac crest, and a plate placed along the pelvic brim.

Transverse Fractures

The posterior column is the site of greatest displacement in most transverse fractures. Because of this, the Kocher-Langenbeck approach is frequently used. The extended iliofemoral approach is often used for transrectal transverse fractures to ensure a perfect reduction of the acetabular roof. Reduction requires the simultaneous control of fracture displacement, and the rotation of the ischiopubic segment. Either a pelvic reduction clamp (Jungbluth) or

Farabeuf clamp is secured across the fracture to reduce the displacement. A Schanz pin is secured near the ischial tuberosity to control the rotation. The reduction is verified by palpation of the quadrilateral surface through the sciatic notch. A lag screw is directed from the retroacetabular surface, across the fracture, toward the anterior column. A plate is placed on the retroacetabular surface to complete the reduction.

Associated Posterior Column and Posterior Wall Fractures The Kocher-Langenbech approach is used with the patient in the prone position. The posterior column is first reduced. This reduction is facilitated by retracting the posterior wall fragment so that the joint can be inspected. After provisional fixation of the posterior column fracture, the posterior wall is addressed as previously described.

Associated Transverse and Posterior Wall Fractures The presence of a posterior wall fracture requires posterior exposure of the acetabulum. Most of these fractures are approached through the Kocher-Langenbech incision with the patient in the prone position. The extended iliofemoral approach is used when there is comminution of the sciatic notch, when the transverse component is transectal, or when the surgeon does not feel an anatomic reduction can be obtained through the Kocher-Langenbech approach. The transverse fracture is first reduced with the use of a pelvic reduction clamp or a Farebuef clamp, both of which are secured proximal and distal to the transverse fracture. Fracture reduction is facilitated by longitudinal traction via the fracture table. The posterior wall fracture is retracted to allow visualization of the acetabulum. A finger is inserted through the greater sciatic notch to palpate the intrapelvic surface of the quadrilateral plate in order to confirm that the rotation is correctly reduced. Fixation is achieved by placing a lag screw across the anterior column, then plating the posterior column, and finally reducing and securing the posterior wall fracture.

Associated Both-Column Fractures Most both-column fractures can be reduced through the ilioinguinal approach. Common indications for the use of the extended iliofemoral approach include presence of a posterior wall fracture, comminution of the posterior column, and involvement of the sacroiliac joint. The anterior column is first reduced at the level of the iliac crest. This reduction must be perfect; any malreduction will be propagated in subsequent steps, and the malreduction will be amplified when reducing the articular surface. The fracture of the anterior column is then reduced at the level of the pelvic brim. Typically, the "king tong" pelvic clamp is used, and the reduction is provisionally held with a lag screw directed from the fractured portion of the iliac wing into the remaining intact segment. A long reconstruction plate is fashioned to fit along the pelvic brim. It is usually necessary to contour the plate several times to achieve an accurate fit. An exact fit of the plate along the brim is required so that screws can be accurately inserted from the pelvic brim into the posterior column. Next, the posterior column is reduced using an asymmetrical pelvic reduction clamp, usually through the middle window of the ilioinguinal incision. Screws are then inserted from the brim into the posterior column using the lag screw technique.

Associated Anterior Column and Posterior Hemitransverse Fractures The ilioinguinal approach is used. The anterior column is reduced at the level of the iliac crest, and then at the pelvic brim, analogous to the both-column fracture. A plate is placed on the pelvic brim prior to reduction of the posterior hemitransverse element. Since many anterior column posterior-hemitransverse fractures occur in patients with osteoporosis, care in the reduction of the hemitransverse element is necessary to avoid additional comminution.

T-Type Fractures T-type fractures are difficult to treat, and the choice of a surgical approach is not always clear. However, most of these fractures can be reduced and stabilized through the Kocher-Langenbech approach. The anterior column fracture is exposed, with retraction of the posterior column and femoral head. The anterior column is reduced with either a bone hook or clamp, and is secured with lag screws directed from anterior to posterior. The posterior column is then reduced. If this strategy does not allow reduction of the anterior column, the posterior column is reduced and stabilized, and the patient is repositioned for a second stage ilioinguinal approach. If a second stage is needed, the screw inserted to fix the posterior column must not block the subsequent reduction of the anterior column. Depending on the configuration of the fracture pattern, the extended iliofemoral approach is occasionally chosen.

Results of Surgical Treatment

The objective of surgery is to restore the painless, durable function of the hip. It is well documented that successful clinical results are dependent on the quality of the reduction of the fracture.[3,20,24-26] The surgeon must attempt to achieve an anatomic reduction. Once committed to achieving an anatomic reduction, the surgeon must select a well-defined treatment proto-

Table 1
Literature summary

Reference	Number of Cases	Surgeons Involved	Excellent & Good Results %	Outcome Measure
Wright et al[21]	87	13	45	Harris Hip Score
Kaempffe et al[27]	50	9	62	d'Aubigné and Postel[88*]
Oransky and Sanguinetti[89]	50	1	76	d'Aubigné and Postel[88*]
Reusch et al[26]	53/89	1	81	Independent[†]
Mayo[25]	163	1	75	d'Aubigné and Postel[88*]
Matta[20]	62/494	1	76	d'Aubigné and Postel[88*]
Letournel[10]	569	1	80	d'Aubigné and Postel[88*]

*Clinical results assessed for pain, range of motion, and gait according to the method of d'Aubigne and Postel[88] with modifications for scoring the range of motion
†Clinical rating based on ability to walk, activity level, pain level and range of motion

col that will consistently result in an accurate reduction. The protocol must include the indications for surgery, the different surgical approaches (and when they are used), patient positioning, reduction techniques, and postoperative care.

However, it is often difficult to compare the results of different protocols due to variations in a number of variables present in the different series. Important differences include varying proportions of different fracture types, individual preference for surgical approaches, performance bias between surgeons, and the outcome measures used to assess clinical results.

Several trends are evident on review of the results of surgical treatment. The best results are obtained when a single surgeon or small number of surgeons have operated on a large number of patients[3,20,27] (Table 1). Given the complexities of the injury and the presence of 10 different fracture types, the acquisition of experience is critical and elusive. This reflects the well-described learning curve required for surgical proficiency.

Of the different factors that have been statistically correlated with poor results, only the quality of reduction is within the surgeon's control. Age of the patient, damage to the femoral head, and complexity of the fracture are established at the time of the injury.

Matta has reported good to excellent clinical results for 76% of 262 patients with displaced acetabular fractures that were operated on within 3 weeks of their injury.[20] The indication for surgery was displacement of 5 mm or more or a noncongruent position of the femoral head. The treatment of these patients followed a well-defined protocol. A single surgical approach was used in combination with a fracture table (see surgical technique section). Anatomic reductions were obtained in 71% of the patients in this series. Clinical results were closely related to the radiographic results. Patients with anatomic reductions had 83% good to excellent clinical results, whereas the patients with imperfect reductions had 68% good to excellent results; those with poor reductions had only 50% good to excellent

results. In this series, the following factors were prognostic of poor results: damage to the femoral head, increasing patient age, and problems with the precision of the surgical reduction.[20] It is important to note that the surgeon has control only of the surgical reduction.

The results of Matta's series provide a means to assess and describe the quality of the surgical reduction. Anatomic reductions, or those without discernible displacement, are defined as "perfect." Reductions with 1 to 3 mm of residual displacement are categorized as "imperfect." The term "acceptable" is no longer used, because reductions with residual displacement have now been statistically correlated with a poorer clinical result, and therefore should not be called acceptable. Poor reductions are those with displacements of more than 3 mm.[20]

The surgical treatment of acetabular fractures is undertaken to restore the function and longevity of the hip. The primary complication of acetabular fractures is the development of post-traumatic arthrosis. Malreductions of the articular surface alter the normal contact and pressure distribution during weightbearing. The strong relationship between the quality of the reduction and the clinical result requires that surgeons who treat these injuries must strive for perfect reductions.[20]

Complications

Judet, Judet, and Letournel delineated many of the possible complications of surgical intervention.[3,6,11] Of the multitude of potential problems associated with acetabular fracture surgery, heterotopic ossification and iatrogenic sciatic nerve injury are of specific interest (as evidenced by a rising number of reports regarding possible prophylactic intervention) due to their relatively high postoperative rate of occurrence and direct impact on limb function.

Heterotopic Ossification

Heterotopic ossification (HO) is common after acetabular fracture surgery. It has been noted in only 5% of conservatively treated patients,[28] but has been reported as occurring in as many as 90% of patients after surgical management (range, 18% to 90%), with severe involvement, as high as 50% in some patient groups.[3,29-33]

Although the specific cause of HO is obscure, numerous risk factors are implicated.[34-36] The most notable risk factor is stripping of the gluteal muscles from the external ilium.[3,20,28,29,37-39] Specifically, the use of the extended iliofemoral, Maryland, and triradiate approaches are proven to be significant risk factors for the development of HO.[20,29,30,37,40] The ilioinguinal approach is associated with an extremely low rate of ectopic bone formation.[3,20,41] A relationship between the severity of heterotopic bone formation and functional loss has been documented.[30,42,43]

Classification The term "severe heterotopic ossification" is often used to describe the amount of heterotopic ossification that is necessary to impair function. Greater than 20% loss of motion defines severe HO. However, many prior reports have defined heterotopic ossification using a single AP radiograph and the Brooker classification. Moed[28] has indicated that this method overestimates the severity of HO.

The extent of HO should be determined from the standard AP and Judet oblique views of the pelvis. This evaluation defines the location and the extent of HO better than a single AP view. Adding a review of the standard Judet oblique views (which would routinely be obtained

in the course of the patient's postoperative evaluation) to the AP view and reading them in a logical, specified sequence appears to indicate reliably the restriction of motion that can be attributed to heterotopic ossification.[43]

Incidence The extent of ectopic bone formation is evident at about 3 months after surgery. Although large numbers have been reported regarding the overall incidence of heterotopic ossification (upwards of 90% of all patients) and of "severe heterotopic ossification" (upwards of 50% of all patients), these numbers reflect series with a preponderance of extended surgical approaches and the use of the Brooker classification.[44] It is instructive to review the numbers reported by Letournel (Table 2). Using the definition of significant heterotopic bone formation as that which limits motion by greater than 20%, the overall incidence was reported to be approximately 7%.[20] In a recent series of patients not given any prophylactic treatment, Matta[20] reported a 20% reduction of motion specific to the surgical approach: Kocher-Langenbeck–9/112 (8%), extended iliofemoral–12/59 (20%), ilioinguinal–2/87 (2%).

Prophylaxis Several prophylactic treatments have been recommended. Ethyl hydroxydiphosphonate is thought to prevent osteoid mineralization, but not osteoid production.[45,46] Theoretically, discontinuation of this therapy would allow calcification of ectopic nonmineralized matrix, and produce HO.[45,47] Not surprisingly, diphosphonates have been shown to be ineffective in experimental animal studies[48] and in patients after hip surgery.[47]

The nonsteroidal anti-inflammatory drug, indomethacin, has been shown to decrease the incidence of HO after total hip arthroplasty,[38,39,49,50] after surgery for acetabular fracture,[35,42,51] and in experimental animals.[36,52-54] Indomethacin is prescribed at 25 mg 3 times per day for a 6-week postoperative course, and can be instituted per rectum at the conclusion of surgery. The drug is administered by mouth as soon as the patient has resumed a normal diet. It is well-tolerated with few reported complications, although failures have also been reported.[30,35,42,55-57] Matta and Siebenrock[34] recently reported a randomized prospective trial indicating that indomethacin was not effective.

Table 2								
Heterotopic ossification (HO)								
Incidence of HO In Patients Treated Without Prophylaxis[88]								
Time From Injury to Operation	**Surgical Approach**	**Number of Fractures**	**HO Class*** **% of Patients with HO**					
			0	**I**	**II**	**III**	**IV**	
Less than 3 weeks	Kocher-Langenbeck	281	72	4	13	9	2	
	Extended iliofemoral	26	31	4	12	19	23	
3 weeks to 4 months	Kocher-Langenbeck	81	74	1	14	5	6	
	Extended iliofemoral	37	59	3	14	16	8	
More than 4 months	Kocher-Langenbeck	62	96	0	2	2	0	
	Extended iliofemoral	21	67	9	19	5	0	

*Radiographic classification of heterotopic ossification[29]—class 0, no heterotopic bone; class I, island of bone within the soft tissue about the hip; class II, bone spurs from the pelvis or proximal end of the femur, leaving at least 1 cm between opposing bone surfaces; class III, bone spurs from the pelvis or proximal end of the femur, reducing the space between opposing bone surfaces to less than 1 cm; class IV, apparent bony ankylosis of the hip

Experimental animal studies have also shown that indomethacin will decrease the formation of new bone,[45,54,58,59] impair fracture healing,[59-61] and inhibit the remodeling of Haversian bone.[62] In the rabbit, indomethacin decreased the torsional strength of healing bone,[63] which is the most reliable method of testing long bones.[64] Clinical correlation is scarce,[59] and problems with fracture healing have not been noted in any reported series.[35,42,51,65-67]

Radiation therapy has been advocated for both total hip arthroplasty[68] and surgery for acetabular fracture.[29] Bosse and associates[29] reported a 50% incidence of HO in patients who received 1,000 cGy of radiation therapy, delivered in 200 cGy increments over a 5-day period after surgery for acetabular fracture, as compared to a 90% incidence in those who did not receive such treatment. There was also a significant difference in the incidence (10% versus 50%) of "severe" HO (class III and class IV), with and without radiation therapy, respectively. Treatment failures were attributed to a delay of more than 3 weeks before surgery and also to a delay in starting radiation. Daum and associates[69] also noted treatment failure associated with delay of radiation therapy more than 48 hours after surgery. The relationship of HO to the inflammatory process is the probable reason that prophylactic treatments, in general, appear to work only when given before or at the time of the initiation of the inductive process. A single low dose of 700 cGy has been successful in preventing HO after total hip arthroplasty,[66] and there are some preliminary data to indicate that a single dose of 800 cGY is as effective as multiple fraction therapy.[65] Radiation therapy has many risks, including induced malignant disease, sterility, and genetic alter-

ations in offspring. However, these risks are dose-related. Malignant change after low-dose radiation has not been reported.[70,71] It is expensive and time consuming, and the potential for long-term problems in young patients must be considered. A recent comparison between indomethacin and single 800 cGy dose irradiation demonstrated that they were equally effective. Noncompliance was the main problem with indomethacin. However, radiation was strikingly more expensive.

A combination of single-dose irradiation (700 cGy) and indomethacin (25 mg tid for 4 weeks) has also been advocated.[67] Irradiation acts by altering DNA transcription; this affects rapidly dividing cells and prevents osteoblastic precursor cells from multiplying and forming active osteoblasts.[29,58,72] Indomethacin and other nonsteroidal agents act through an inhibitory action on prostaglandin synthesis.[54,73,74] This theory has been challenged,[55] but experimental evidence does indicate that radiation therapy and indomethacin decrease HO by different mechanisms.[48] Thus, there is a theoretical basis for the use of combination therapy. Use of this regimen essentially eliminated postoperative heterotopic ossification in the series reported by Moed and Letournel,[67] and there was no progression of HO, even when early ossification was observed on preoperative radiographs.

Treatment Delayed excision following maturation of functionally significant heterotopic ossification remains a viable option both for treatment after failed prophylactic therapy and as an alternative to HO prophylaxis. Functional improvement can be expected in patients with congruent joint surfaces. Results with this treatment have been good, with an expected return to greater than 80% of nor-

mal motion.[17,30,75] Prophylaxis to prevent recurrent ossification is indicated in these cases. Indomethacin and radiation therapy both have been proven effective.[7,53] Accepting Matta's definition and data, it appears that even without prophylactic therapy, overall, only a small percentage of patients will require this procedure. How-ever, as discussed above, certain patient groups, notably those treated using an extended surgical approach, are at increased risk for the development of significant heterotopic ossification, and the number of these patients requiring treatment for HO will be higher.

Iatrogenic Sciatic Nerve Injury

Damage to the sciatic nerve, whether it occurs at the time of the fracture or later during the course of the patient's treatment, is one of the major complications encountered in acetabular fracture management. In 1981, Letournel and associates[6] reported an overall 11% incidence of postoperative iatrogenic nerve injury, but noted that more than a third of these patients had not undergone an adequate preoperative physical examination, leaving the actual cause of nerve injury in doubt. He stressed the need for a complete preoperative neurologic evaluation. The sciatic nerve consists of divisions which function quite independently.[76] Mixed, partial, or incomplete deficits are common[6,77,78] and are easily missed. Clinical series describing the use of a detailed preoperative neurologic evaluation report a 26% to 38% incidence of post-traumatic, preoperative nerve injury.[24,77-79] These numbers are higher than those of most other published reports,[6,17,28,80] probably indicating an increase in detection rather than an actual increase in occurrence.

Aside from obvious medicolegal implications, preoperative diagnosis of nerve injury has additional clinical importance because the previously injured nerve appears to be at greater risk for iatrogenic intraoperative injury.[75,78] Additionally, exploration of the injured nerve has been recommended for those cases allowing fracture fixation through the posterior surgical approach.[28,81] Though unpredictable, results of nerve exploration can be rewarding. Progressive or postreduction nerve deficits mandate surgical exploration.[28,81]

Patients with posterior wall or column displacement are at the greatest risk for iatrogenic, as well as posttraumatic sciatic nerve injury.[28,79,81] Iatrogenic nerve injuries are most commonly associated with the posterior and extended lateral surgical approaches,[6,78] which involve direct exposure and retraction of the sciatic nerve. However, injury can also occur at the time of indirect reduction of posterior column displacement through an anterior surgical approach.[6,79]

Nerve Monitoring Intraoperative somatosensory evoked potential (SSEP) monitoring of the sciatic nerve has been advocated as a method to decrease the incidence of intraoperative sciatic nerve injury.[77–79] SSEP monitoring requires exacting standards of technique, and the mechanical and electrical background interference, along with the practical complexities of intraoperative monitoring, can make this a frustrating and time-consuming experience.[82] The peroneal and tibial divisions of the sciatic nerve must be individually monitored to allow detection of incomplete lesions, and individually stimulated to avoid a masking effect of simultaneous stimulation.[76] Significant SSEP waveform changes do predate sciatic nerve injury that will result in a postoperative nerve deficit. However, prevention of a clinically apparent post-operative deficit requires a rapid response with removal of the offending agent, assuming that the offending agent has merely exerted pressure or traction, and has not lacerated or crushed the nerve.[76,78] This requires not only the diligence of the operating surgeon, but also the availability and attentiveness of the neurophysiologist reading the SSEP recordings.[78] In addition, SSEP monitoring is a sensory-based system and sometimes fails to provide information applicable to the motor side of the nervous system.[82,83] Preliminary results indicate that spontaneous motor potential monitoring may eventually prove to be more effective in this regard.[84]

The incidence of postoperative iatrogenic sciatic nerve injury appears to be inversely related to the experience level of the operating surgeon. Matta reported a 9% incidence in his retrospective series,[17] a 5% incidence in the subsequent prospective series,[16] and finally, 2% incidence without the aid of SSEP monitoring. These numbers compare favorably with those of series using SSEP monitoring systems, which reported a 2% to 7% incidence.[77–79,85] The question is whether SSEP monitoring, while feasible, is of real clinical value. From the total joint literature, Black and associates[86] have reported a similar 2% incidence of sciatic nerve palsy, whether or not intraoperative SSEP monitoring was employed. They concluded that routine intraoperative monitoring was not recommended because of the increased expense and expertise required. Intraoperative SSEP changes in their series were recognized, but for technical reasons they were unable to respond appropriately. However, this situation does not necessarily apply to acetabular fracture fixation, where traction and nerve retraction can be quickly altered. Therefore, specific recommendations must await a randomized prospective trial in acetabular fracture patients.

Presently, there is no substitute for attention to detail in the operating room, with careful patient positioning, maintenance of knee flexion during posterior approaches to relax the sciatic nerve, cautious placement of retractors, and limited traction on the nerve during fracture reduction. SSEP monitoring appears to be of some benefit, especially during indirect reduction of fractures with posterior displacement, but its limitations preclude absolute reliance on the intraoperative data.

Prognosis and Treatment Recovery of tibial division function can be expected despite severe initial damage. Prognosis for peroneal division recovery is more dependent on the severity of the initial injury.[5] Fassler and associates[5] reported that only one third of their patients with a severe peroneal division injury experienced a satisfactory functional return, while those with a mild injury all had a satisfactory recovery. Electromyography is helpful in defining the extent and severity of injury, but not as a prognostic indicator.[5] Return of nerve function occurs over a variable time interval with recovery noted as late as three years after surgery.[6]

Management of sciatic nerve injury consists of the use of an ankle-foot orthosis, observation and physical therapy. Medical treatment, such as carbamazepine, may be required to control pain of neurogenic origin.[5]

Infection

The prevention of infection begins with the preoperative examination. A specific search is made for degloving injuries, which are treated as previously outlined. Associated injuries, such as bladder ruptures and open fractures, must be treated to prevent systemic sepsis. Potential sites of infection from urinary catheters and intravenous lines are evaluated before surgery.

Intravenous antibiotics are given prior to making an incision. Meticulous prepping of the patient ensures a sterile surgical field. The use of a fracture table reduces movement of the patient and disruption of the surgical drapes.

Meticulous hemostasis and the use of multiple suction drains help to prevent wound hematomas. Postoperative infections are often associated with hematoma formation within the large incisions required for the internal fixation of acetabular fractures.

Clear or yellowish drainage is often observed for as long as 10 days after internal fixation. This is commonly associated with the Kocher-Langenbech approach. The presence of continued bloody drainage is considered to be evidence of an infection or a hematoma. The patient is returned to the operating room for exploration, wound cultures, and irrigation of the wound. Early treatment (first 3 weeks) usually allows primary wound closure with closed suction drainage. Late infections may require open packing of the wound. All efforts are made to diagnose and treat postoperative infections prior to abscess formation.

Matta[87] and Letournel and Judet[3] report a 5% and a 4.2% incidence of infection in two large series. In general, an intra-articular infection usually portends a poor prognosis. The clinical result after an extra-articular infection is better; however, patients who suffer an infection have a poorer clinical result than those who do not have an infection.

Total Hip Replacement After Fractures of the Acetabulum

Not all acetabular fractures will have a successful outcome. The long-term

results of Letournel and Judet[3] and Matta[20] suggest that with excellent reductions a minority of patients will require future surgery. Either fusion or total hip replacement is indicated for posttraumatic arthritis and disabling pain. What is attributed to arthritis, osteonecrosis, or chondrolysis is often the inability to achieve an anatomic reduction.

The results of total hip arthroplasty for posttraumatic arthritis after acetabular fractures are inferior to the results of primary total hip replacement performed for degenerative arthritis. Reported revision rates range from 13.5% to 50.7%. Most of these revisions were performed for aseptic loosening of the acetabular component.[72]

A number of factors are likely to compromise the longevity of the total hip.[88,89] These include prior surgical incisions, traumatic and surgical soft-tissue injuries, and the presence of heterotopic ossification. Nonunion of the acetabular fracture has also been found at the time of total hip replacement, a factor that complicates secure fixation of the acetabular component. These technical challenges have led to prosthetic dislocation and infection rates that are higher than those reported for primary total hip arthroplasty.

These reported high complication and revision rates indicate that the philosophy of performing an open reduction to restore bone stock for total hip arthroplasty has not proven to be successful. Total hip arthroplasty as a primary treatment of acetabular fractures is not recommended.

References

1. Matta JM, Letournel E, Browner BD: Surgical management of acetabular fractures, in Anderson LD (ed): American Academy of Orthopaedic Surgeons Instructional Course Lectures XXXV. St. Louis, MO, CV Mosby, 1986, pp 382–397.

2. Orthopedic Medline on CD-ROM. Rosemont, IL, American Academy of Orthopaedic Surgeons, July, 1997.

3. Letournel E, Judet R (eds): Fractures of the Acetabulum, ed 2. Berlin, Germany, Springer-Verlag, 1993.

4. Katyal D, McLellan BA, Brenneman FD, Boulanger BR, Sharkey PW, Waddell JP: Lateral impact motor vehicle collisions: Significant cause of blunt traumatic rupture of the thoracic aorta. J Trauma 1997;42:769–772.

5. Fassler PR, Swiontkowski MF, Kilroy AW, Routt ML Jr: Injury of the sciatic nerve associated with acetabular fracture. J Bone Joint Surg 1993;75A:1157–1166.

6. Letournel E, Judet R, Elson RA (eds): Fractures of the Acetabulum. Berlin, Germany, Springer-Verlag, 1981.

7. Garland DE: A clinical perspective on common forms of acquired heterotopic ossification. Clin Orthop 1991;263:13–29.

8. Hak DJ, Olson SA, Matta JM: Diagnosis and management of closed internal degloving injuries associated with pelvic and acetabular fractures: The Morel-Lavallee lesion. J Trauma 1997;42:1046–1051.

9. Roffi RP, Matta JM: Unrecognized posterior dislocation of the hip associated with transverse and T-type fractures of the acetabulum. J Orthop Trauma 1993;7:23–27.

10. Letournel E: Acetabulum fractures: Classification and management. Clin Orthop 1980;151:81–106.

11. Judet R, Judet J, Letournel E: Fractures of the acetabulum: Classification and surgical approaches for open reduction: Preliminary report. J Bone Joint Surg 1964;46A:1615–1646.

12. Olson SA, Matta JM: Surgical treatment of acetabulum fractures, in Browner BD, Jupiter JB, Levine AM, Trafton PG (eds): Skeletal Trauma: Fractures, Dislocations, Ligamentous Injuries, ed 2. Philadelphia, PA, WB Saunders, 1998, pp 1181–1222.

13. Olson SA, Bay BK, Hamel A: Biomechanics of the hip joint and the effects of fracture of the acetabulum. Clin Orthop 1997;339:92–104.

14. Rowe CR, Lowell JD: Prognosis of fractures of the acetabulum. J Bone Joint Surg 1961;43A:30–59,92.

15. Olson SA, Matta JM: The computerized tomography subchondral arc: A new method of assessing the acetabular articular continuity after fracture: A preliminary report. J Orthop Trauma 1993;7:402–413.

16. Matta JM, Mehne DK, Roffi R: Fractures of the acetabulum: Early results of a prospective study. Clin Orthop 1986;205:241–250.

17. Matta JM, Anderson LM, Epstein HC, Hendricks P: Fractures of the acetabulum: A retrospective analysis. Clin Orthop 1986;205:230–240.

18. Heeg M, Oostvogel HJ, Klasen HJ: Conservative treatment of acetabular fractures: The role of the weight-bearing dome and anatomic reduction in the ultimate results. J Trauma 1987;27:555–559.

19. Helfet DL, Borrelli J Jr, DiPasquale T, Sanders R: Stabilization of acetabular fractures in elderly patients. *J Bone Joint Surg* 1992;74A:753–765.

20. Matta JM: Fractures of the acetabulum: Accuracy of reduction and clinical results in patients managed operatively within three weeks after the injury. *J Bone Joint Surg* 1996; 78A:1632–1645.

21. Wright R, Barrett K, Christie MJ, Johnson KD: Acetabular fractures: Long-term follow-up of open reduction and internal fixation. *J Orthop Trauma* 1994;8:397–403.

22. Goulet JA, Rouleau JP, Mason DJ, Goldstein SA: Comminuted fractures of the posterior wall of the acetabulum: A biomechanical evaluation of fixation methods. *J Bone Joint Surg* 1994;76A:1457–1463.

23. Brumback RJ, Holt ES, McBride MS, Poka A, Bathon GH, Burgess AR: Acetabular depression fracture accompanying posterior fracture dislocation of the hip. *J Orthop Trauma* 1990; 4:42–48.

24. Helfet DL, Schmeling GJ: Management of complex acetabular fractures through single nonextensile exposures. *Clin Orthop* 1994;305: 58–68.

25. Mayo KA: Open reduction and internal fixation of fractures of the acetabulum: Results in 163 fractures. *Clin Orthop* 1994;305:31–37.

26. Ruesch PD, Holdener H, Ciaramitaro M, Mast JW: A prospective study of surgically treated acetabular fractures. *Clin Orthop* 1994;305: 38–46.

27. Kaempffe FA, Bone LB, Border JR: Open reduction and internal fixation of acetabular fractures: Heterotopic ossification and other complications of treatment. *J Orthop Trauma* 1991;5:439–445.

28. Moed BR: Complications of acetabular fracture surgery: Prevention and management. *Int J Orthop Trauma* 1992;2:68–81.

29. Bosse MJ, Poka A, Reinert CM, Ellwanger F, Slawson R, McDevitt ER: Heterotopic ossification as a complication of acetabular fracture: Prophylaxis with low-dose irradiation. *J Bone Joint Surg* 1988;70A:1231–1237.

30. Mears DC, Rubash HE (eds): *Pelvic and Acetabular Fractures*. Thorofare, NJ, Slack, 1986.

31. Tile M: Fractures of the acetabulum, in Schatzker J, Tile M (eds): *The Rationale of Operative Fracture Care*, ed 2. Berlin, Germany, Springer-Verlag, 1996, pp 271–324.

32. Helfet DL, Schmeling GJ: Complications, in Tile M (ed): *Fractures of the Pelvis and Acetabulum*, ed 2. Baltimore, MD, Williams & Wilkins, 1995, pp 451–467.

33. Pennal GF, Davidson J, Garside H, Plewes J: Results of treatment of acetabular fractures. *Clin Orthop* 1980;151:115–123.

34. Matta JM, Siebenrock KA: Does indomethacin reduce heterotopic bone formation after operations for acetabular fractures? A prospective randomised study. *J Bone Joint Surg* 1997;79B: 959–963.

35. Moed BR, Maxey JW: The effect of indomethacin on heterotopic ossification following acetabular fracture surgery. *J Orthop Trauma* 1993;7:33–38.

36. Moed BR, Resnick RB, Fakhouri AJ, Nallamothu B, Wagner RA: Effect of two nonsteroidal antiinflammatory drugs on heterotopic bone formation in a rabbit model. *J Arthroplasty* 1994;9:81–87.

37. Ghalambor N, Matta JM, Bernstein L: Heterotopic ossification following operative treatment of acetabular fracture: An analysis of risk factors. *Clin Orthop* 1994;305:96–105.

38. Ritter MA, Sieber JM: Prophylactic indomethacin for the prevention of heterotopic bone formation following total hip arthroplasty. *Clin Orthop* 1985;196:217–225.

39. Steenmeyer AV, Slooff TJ, Kuypers W: The effect of indomethacin on para-articular ossification following total hip replacement. *Acta Orthop Belg* 1986;52:305–307.

40. Alonso JE, Davila R, Bradley E: Extended iliofemoral versus triradiate approaches in management of associated acetabular fractures. *Clin Orthop* 1994;305:81–87.

41. Mayo KA: Efficacy and complication rates for the ilioinguinal approach to fractures of the acetabulum. *Orthop Trans* 1991;15:834.

42. Moed BR, Karges DE: Prophylactic indomethacin for the prevention of heterotopic ossification after acetabular fracture surgery in high-risk patients. *J Orthop Trauma* 1994;8:34–39.

43. Moed BR, Smith ST: Three-view radiographic assessment of heterotopic ossification after acetabular fracture surgery: Correlation with hip motion in 100 cases. *J Orthop Trauma* 1996;10:93–98.

44. Brooker AF, Bowerman JW, Robinson RA, Riley LH Jr: Ectopic ossification following total hip replacement: Incidence and a method of classification. *J Bone Joint Surg* 1973;55A: 1629–1632.

45. Plasmans CM, Kuypers W, Slooff TJ: The effect of ethane-1-hydroxy-1,1-diphosphonic acid (EHDP) on matrix induced ectopic bone formation. *Clin Orthop* 1978;132:233–243.

46. Russell RG, Smith R: Diphosphonates: Experimental and clinical aspects. *J Bone Joint Surg* 1973;55B:66–86.

47. Thomas BJ, Amstutz HC: Results of the administration of diphosphonate for the prevention of heterotopic ossification after total hip arthroplasty. *J Bone Joint Surg* 1985;67A: 400–403.

48. Ahrengart L, Lindgren U, Reinholt FP: Comparative study of the effects of radiation, indomethacin, prednisolone, and ethane-1-hydroxy-1,1-diphosphonate (EHDP) in the prevention of ectopic bone formation. *Clin Orthop* 1988;229:265–273.

49. Ritter MA, Gioe TJ: The effect of indomethacin on para-articular ectopic ossification following total hip arthroplasty. *Clin Orthop* 1982;167:113–117.

50. Schmidt SA, Kjaersgaard-Andersen P: Indomethacin inhibits the recurrence of excised ectopic ossification after hip arthroplasty: A 3-4 year follow-up of 8 cases. *Acta Orthop Scand* 1988;59:593.

51. McLaren AC: Prophylaxis with indomethacin for heterotopic bone: After open reduction of fractures of the acetabulum. *J Bone Joint Surg* 1990;72A:245–247.

52. Nilsson OS, Bauer HC, Brosjo O, Tornkvist H: Influence of indomethacin on induced heterotopic bone formation in rats: Importance of length of treatment and of age. *Clin Orthop* 1986;207:239–245.

53. Scott AC, Wong S, Ang K, Traina JF: The relative effects of indomethacin, diphosphonates and low dose radiation for the prevention of heterotopic ossification. *Trans Orthop Res Soc* 1987;12:309.

54. Tornkvist H, Bauer FC, Nilsson OS: Influence of indomethacin on experimental bone metabolism in rats. *Clin Orthop* 1985;193:264–270.

55. Russell LJ: NSAIDs and bone metabolism. *Hosp Pract (Off Ed)* 1991;26(suppl 1):13–17.

56. Saggioro A, Alvisi V, Blasi A, Dobrilla G, Fioravanti A, Marcolongo R: Misoprostol prevents NSAID-induced gastroduodenal lesions in patients with osteoarthritis and rheumatoid arthritis. *Ital J Gastroenterol* 1991;23:119–123.

57. Bardhan KD, Bjarnason I, Scott DL, et al: The prevention and healing of acute non-steroidal anti-inflammatory drug-associated gastroduodenal mucosal damage by misoprostol. *Br J Rheumatol* 1993;32:990–995.

58. Pittenger DE: Heterotopic ossification. *Orthop Rev* 1991;20:33–39.

59. Sudmann E, Hagen T: Indomethacin-induced delayed fracture healing. *Arch Orthop Unfallchir* 1976;85:151–154.

60. Graham DY, White RH, Moreland LW, et al: Duodenal and gastric ulcer prevention with misoprostol in arthritis patients taking NSAIDs: Misoprostol Study Group. *Ann Intern Med* 1993;119:257–262.

61. Bo J, Sudmann E, Marton PF: Effect of indomethacin on fracture healing in rats. *Acta Orthop Scand* 1976;47:588–599.

62. Sudmann E, Bang G: Indomethacin-induced inhibition of Haversian remodelling in rabbits. *Acta Orthop Scand* 1979;50:621–627.

63. Tornkvist H, Lindholm TS, Netz P, Stromberg L, Lindholm TC: Effect of ibuprofen and indomethacin on bone metabolism reflected in bone strength. *Clin Orthop* 1984;187:255–259.

64. Burstein AH, Frankel VH: A standard test for laboratory animal bone. *J Biomech* 1971;4: 155–158.

65. Anglen JO, Moore KD: Prevention of heterotopic bone formation after acetabular fracture fixation by single-dose radiation therapy: A

preliminary report. *J Orthop Trauma* 1996;10: 258–263.

66. Lo TC, Healy WL, Covall DJ, et al: Heterotopic bone formation after hip surgery: Prevention with single-dose postoperative hip irradiation. *Radiology* 1988;168:851–854.

67. Moed BR, Letournel E: Low-dose irradiation and indomethacin prevent heterotopic ossification after acetabular fracture surgery. *J Bone Joint Surg* 1994;76B:895–900.

68. Coventry MB, Scanlon PW: The use of radiation to discourage ectopic bone: A nine-year study in surgery about the hip. *J Bone Joint Surg* 1981;63A:201–208.

69. Daum WJ, Scarborough MT, Gordon W Jr, Uchida T: Heterotopic ossification and other perioperative complications of acetabular fractures. *J Orthop Trauma* 1992;6:427–432.

70. Brady LW: Radiation-induced sarcomas of bone. *Skeletal Radiol* 1979;4:72–78.

71. Kim JH, Chu FC, Woodard HQ, Melamed MR, Huvos A, Cantin J: Radiation-induced soft-tissue and bone sarcoma. *Radiology* 1978;129:501–508.

72. Romness DW, Lewallen DG: Total hip arthroplasty after fracture of the acetabulum: Long-term results. *J Bone Joint Surg* 1990;72B: 761–764.

73. Allen HL, Wase A, Bear WT: Indomethacin and aspirin: Effect of nonsteroidal anti-inflammato-ry agents on the rate of fracture repair in the rat. *Acta Orthop Scand* 1980;51:595–600.

74. Vane JR: Inhibition of prostaglandin synthesis as a mechanism of action for aspirin-like drugs. *Nat New Biol* 1971;231:232–235.

75. Webb LX, Bosse MJ, Mayo KA, Lange RH, Miller ME, Swiontkowski MF: Results in patients with craniocerebral trauma and an operatively managed acetabular fracture. *J Orthop Trauma* 1990;4:376–382.

76. Moed BR, Maxey JW, Minster GJ: Intraoperative somatosensory evoked potential monitoring of the sciatic nerve: An animal model. *J Orthop Trauma* 1992;6:59–65.

77. Helfet DL, Hissa EA, Sergay S, Mast JW: Somatosensory evoked potential monitoring in the surgical management of acute acetabular fractures. *J Orthop Trauma* 1991;5:161–166.

78. Vrahas M, Gordon RG, Mears DC, Krieger D, Sclabassi RJ: Intra-operative somatosensory evoked potential monitoring of pelvic and acetabular fractures. *J Orthop Trauma* 1992;6:50–58.

79. Helfet DL, Schmeling GJ: Somatosensory evoked potential monitoring in the surgical treatment of acute, displaced acetabular fractures: Results of a prospective study. *Clin Orthop* 1994;301:213–220.

80. Tile M: Fractures of the acetabulum, in Schatzker J, Tile M (eds): *The Rationale of Operative Fracture Care*. Berlin, Germany, Springer-Verlag, 1987, pp 173–213.

81. Tile M: Management, in Tile M (ed): *Fractures of the Pelvis and Acetabulum*, ed 2. Baltimore, MD, Williams & Wilkins, 1995, pp 321–354.

82. Ben-David B: Spinal cord monitoring. *Orthop Clin North Am* 1988;19:427–448.

83. Nash CL Jr, Brown RH: Spinal cord monitoring. *J Bone Joint Surg* 1989;71A:627–630.

84. Helfet DL, Anand N, Malkani AL, et al: Intraoperative monitoring of motor pathways during operative fixation of acute acetabular fractures. *J Orthop Trauma* 1997;11:2–6.

85. Baumgaertner MR, Wegner D, Booke J: SSEP monitoring during pelvic and acetabular fracture surgery. *J Orthop Trauma* 1994;8:127–133.

86. Black DL, Reckling FW, Porter SS: Somatosensory-evoked potential monitored during total hip arthroplasty. *Clin Orthop* 1991;262:170–177.

87. Matta JM: Operative treatment of acetabulum fractures, in Chapman MW, Madison M (eds): *Operative Orthopaedics*. Philadelphia, PA, JB Lippincott, 1988, pp 329–340.

88. Merle d'Aubigne R, Postel M: Functional results of hip arthroplasty with acrylic prosthesis. *J Bone Joint Surg* 1954;36A:451–475.

89. Oransky M, Sanguinetti C: Surgical treatment of displaced acetabular fractures: Results of 50 consecutive cases. *J Orthop Trauma* 1993;7: 28–32.

Fractures of the Proximal Tibia

Clayton R. Perry, MD

Robert E. Hunter, MD

Robert F. Ostrum, MD

Robert C. Schenck, Jr, MD

Fractures of the Tibial Plateau: Classification and Techniques of Management

Fractures of the tibial plateau are usually caused by one or both of the femoral condyles impacting the articular surface of the proximal tibia under varying degrees of varus or valgus force applied across the knee. Occasionally, tibial plateau fractures are caused by a direct impact to the proximal tibia (eg, a "bumper fracture"). Such fractures are a result of higher-energy trauma and generally have more complications and a worse prognosis than fractures caused by the femoral condyles.

Classification

Tibial plateau fractures are best classified based on a system described by Schatzker and associates[1] in 1979. According to this classification system, there are 6 types of tibial plateau fractures: type I, split or cleavage fracture of the lateral plateau; type II, split depressed fracture of the lateral or medial plateau; type III, central depression fracture of the lateral or medial plateau; type IV, high-energy fracture of the medial plateau; type V, bicondylar fracture, and type VI, fracture of the plateau with metaphyseal dissociation. A key point of this classification is the distinction between low- and high-energy fractures. Low-energy fractures are split, split depressed, or central depression fractures. High-energy fractures are high-energy medial condyle, bicondylar, or fractures with metaphyseal dissociation. High-energy fractures have a worse prognosis and a higher incidence of complications and associated injuries.[2] Despite the usefulness of this system, there are some atypical fractures that do not fit into the classification.

Type I, Split Fractures The split, or cleavage, fracture of the lateral plateau that occurs in young adults is best seen on the anteroposterior radiograph. The fracture line is vertical and is seldom displaced more than 3 mm. Split fractures can usually be managed with closed reduction and stabilization with percutaneous screws. Reduction is monitored fluoroscopically and is performed by applying a varus stress across the knee and manipulating the split fragment with a tenaculum through the skin. One or 2 cannulated 4.5-mm or 7.0-mm screws placed beneath the subchondral bone, with an additional screw and washer inserted distally, provide adequate stability. If a satisfactory reduction cannot be achieved, the knee is opened or examined arthroscopically to determine the block to reduction. Frequently, the lateral meniscus is found to be torn peripherally and displaced into the fracture site, blocking reduction.

Type II, Split Depressed Fractures Split depressed fractures are the most common type of tibial plateau fracture. The lateral plateau is fractured by a combination of valgus and axial stress. The lateral femoral condyle impacts the tibial plateau, splitting the lateral portion of the plateau from the proximal tibia. The injury continues as the femoral condyle impacts the articular surface of the proximal tibia, driving a segment of articular cartilage and subchondral bone into the metaphysis. The depressed articular segment is always on the medial side of the fracture, not on the split fragment. Management of these fractures is usually surgical, with elevation of the

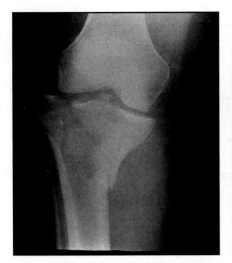

Fig. 1 A high-energy medial plateau fracture. The lateral femoral condyle has impacted the tibial spines shearing the medial condyle from the metaphysis. The lateral collateral ligament is also ruptured.

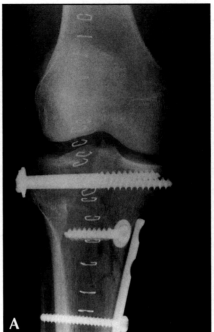
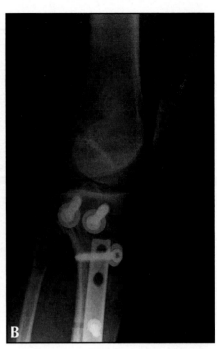

Fig. 2 A and **B,** The fracture has been reduced and stabilized with interfragmentary compression screws and a buttress plate.

depressed articular segment, bone grafting of the subchondral defect, and reduction of the split component. Stabilization is achieved with screws and plates or with cannulated screws alone.

Type III, Depressed Fractures of the Lateral or Medial Plateau. Depressed fractures of the lateral or medial plateau are low-energy fractures that occur in osteopenic patients. The mechanism of injury is a varus or valgus stress applied across the knee. As the stress is applied, the femoral condyle sinks into and depresses the articular surface without fracturing the cortical bone of the metaphysis. Because these fractures are low-energy injuries, the incidence of associated injuries is also low. One of the key factors in deciding whether management should be conservative or surgical is a functional evaluation, namely, knee stability in full extension. In cases in which medial and lateral stresses, applied while the knee is extended, do not result in an increase in varus or val-

gus angulation, conservative management will be successful. If varus or valgus angulation is greater than 10°, surgical management is indicated. The rationale is that in the stance, or weightbearing, phase of gait, angulation will occur with instability and result in deformity and chronic instability.[3] Conservative management is often indicated in elderly patients. Surgical management consists of elevating the plateau via a metaphyseal window and packing the resulting subchondral defect with bone graft.

Type IV, Medial Plateau Fractures (High Energy) These fractures are caused by an axial and valgus stress. The lateral condyle of the femur is driven into the tibial spines, shearing the medial condyle of the tibia from the proximal tibia. The fracture fragment is made up of the medial condyle, the tibial spines, and a small portion of the lateral plateau (Fig. 1). The lateral collateral liga-

ment is always ruptured or avulsed. There is a significant incidence of vascular and neurologic injuries associated with medial plateau fractures. Management consists of either wide surgical exposure, reduction, and internal fixation (Fig. 2); or limited open reduction and stabilization with an external fixator. Late collapse or fracture displacement can result unless stable fixation is achieved.

Type V, Bicondylar Fractures Bicondylar fractures involve both the medial and the lateral condyle. They are the result of high energy and are frequently associated with neurovascular and ligamentous injuries. The fracture pattern is variable, but usually the lateral condyle of the tibia is more displaced than is the medial. Management is either wide midline surgical exposure, with reduction and internal fixation, or limited open reduction and stabilization with an external fixator and cannulated screws.

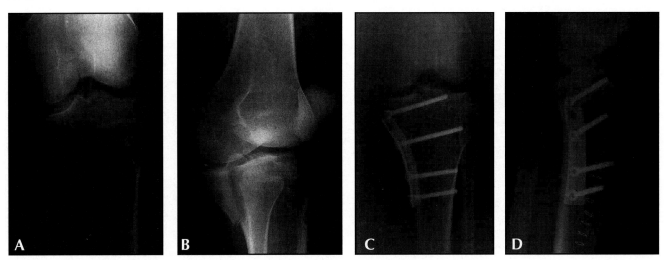

Fig. 3 A and **B,** An atypical fracture of the posterior third of the medial condyle. The degree of displacement is indicated by the oblique radiograph. Fluoroscopic examination of atypical fractures is often helpful in determining the degree of displacement. **C** and **D,** The fracture was reduced and stabilized with a posterior medial buttress plate and interfragmentary screw.

Type VI, Tibial Plateau Fractures With Metaphyseal Dissociation This type of fracture is always the result of high energy and often caused by a direct impact to the proximal tibia. As with bicondylar fractures, there may be associated neurovascular injuries. Management of these fractures is frequently complicated by nonunion and postoperative infection. In cases in which the articular surface is minimally displaced, limited open reduction and stabilization of the articular segment to the distal tibia with an external fixator is an excellent method of management. Joint reduction followed by cannulated screw stabilization allows placement of external fixation.

Atypical Fractures On occasion, fractures of the tibial plateau are encountered that do not fit into the classification system. An example is a fracture that involves only the anterior or posterior portion of the medial or lateral condyle (Fig. 3). Computed axial tomography (CT) and fluoroscopy are helpful in precisely defining the fracture pattern. The goal of management is reduction of the fracture

and early motion of the knee. The surgical exposure and technique of fixation must be tailored for each fracture (Fig. 3).

Diagnosis and Initial Management
History and Physical Examination There is a history of a varus or valgus stress or a direct impact to the knee. The knee is painful and swollen. Obvious deformity may not be present and an index of suspicion for a fracture in a swollen knee is recommended. Aspiration of the knee reveals the presence of a lipohemarthrosis.

Radiographic Examination Anteroposterior (AP), lateral, and oblique radiographs centered on the knee are obtained. On the AP radiograph, the beam is tilted 10° caudally to profile the surface of the tibial plateau. CT scans or magnetic resonance images are not indicated in all cases. They are obtained to determine the fracture pattern in high-energy fractures and to determine the amount of intra-articular displacement. Such studies are useful in planning surgical approach (incision) and sequence of fixation in cases in which the fracture

will be managed with limited open reduction.

Associated Injuries Injuries frequently associated with tibial plateau fractures are ruptures of the collateral ligaments, occlusion of the popliteal artery or the trifurcation, compartment syndrome, disruption of the extensor mechanism, and stretching of the common peroneal or posterior tibial nerve.

The collateral ligament opposite the fractured plateau is likely to be injured. Apparent ligamentous laxity with varus or valgus stressing may, in fact, be paradoxical motion through the fracture site. In questionable cases, the knee should be stressed under fluoroscopy.

Injury of the popliteal artery or the trifurcation is more likely to occur in association with high-energy fractures. Absent pulses distal to the fracture mandate an immediate arteriogram and vascular repair.

Compartment syndrome is heralded by tense swelling, an inordinate amount of pain at rest, pain with passive stretch of the muscles in the compartment, and dysesthesia

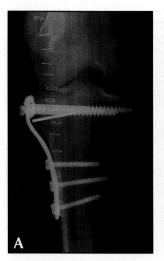 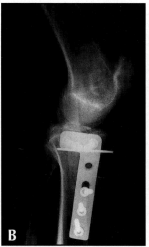 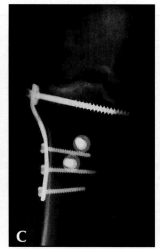 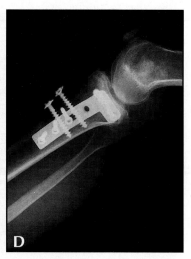

Fig. 4 A and **B,** Two weeks after fixation of a split depressed fracture in a patient with multisystem trauma, it was noted clinically that the patella was dislocated laterally. The anteroposterior radiograph is consistent with lateral subluxation. The lateral radiograph is consistent with patella alta, and, in addition, the patella is tilted. **C** and **D,** Following medial transfer of the tibial tubercle and reefing of the medial retinaculum, the patella is properly located.

or anesthesia of the skin supplied by the nerves that traverse the compartment. The 1 objective sign of compartment syndrome is an elevated compartment pressure. We use 30 mm Hg as our threshold indication for fasciotomy. Management is surgical release of the compartment.

Disruption of the extensor mechanism occasionally occurs in association with fractures of the tibial plateau. Undisplaced fracture of the patella, dislocation of the patella, and rupture of the quadriceps tendon are easily overlooked preoperatively (Fig. 4). Avulsion of the tibial tubercle and rupture of the patellar tendon are more obvious.

Injury of the common peroneal nerve is more common than injury of the posterior tibial nerve. Injury of the common peroneal nerve is indicated by loss of sensation in the first web space and inability to extend the first toe. Injury of the posterior tibial nerve is indicated by loss of sensation on the plantar aspect of the foot and inability to flex the first toe. The injury is usually due to stretching of

the nerve, and, in most cases, loss of function is temporary. However, it is necessary to rule out compartment syndrome as the cause of the neurologic loss.

Techniques of Management

Techniques of fracture management include closed treatment with casting or external fixation, wide surgical exposure and fixation with plates and screws, limited open reduction and cannulated screw fixation, limited open reduction with a bridging external fixator, and limited open reduction with external fixation using a small wire circular frame or large pin cantilever frame.

Closed Management Closed management is indicated in 3 situations: when the fracture is minimally displaced; when the fracture cannot be reduced and stabilized because of the condition of the overlying skin or because of comminution or osteopenia; and when it is necessary to delay definitive management.[4] When the fracture is nondisplaced, a hinged knee brace locked at 20° of flexion is

better tolerated than a long leg cast. Nonweightbearing is maintained for 4 to 6 weeks. At 4 weeks, range of motion exercises are initiated. When reduction and stabilization of a displaced fracture is not possible because of the condition of soft tissue or comminution/osteopenia of the fracture fragments, an external fixator can be used to stabilize the leg, allowing mobilization of the patient. A simple anterior frame is applied with 2 pins in the tibia and 2 in the femur. The pins are placed outside of the zone of injury, the knee is distracted, and the tibia is aligned with the femur in AP and lateral planes. This technique is also useful when it is necessary to delay fixation of the fracture because of the patient's overall condition or other injuries. Definitive reconstruction is carried out when the patient's local and systemic condition permits.

Wide Surgical Exposure and Fixation With Plates and Screws Wide surgical exposure with reduction and stabilization with plates and screws is the standard against which other methods of management are compared.[5,6] This method is particularly applicable to split and split depressed fractures. Its use in the management of these low-energy fractures enables the surgeon to accurately reduce and stabilize the fracture with a minimal risk of wound complications. Use of wide exposure and stabilization with plates and screws in the management of high-energy fractures (ie, high-energy medial plateau fractures, bicondylar fractures, and fractures with metaphyseal dissociation) is more controversial and is associated with a high incidence of postoperative wound complications.[7,8] Maneuvers to increase exposure of the fracture include the following: (1) incision of the coronary ligament and elevation of the meniscus; (2) incision of the anterior horn of one or both menisci and "booking" underlying split fragments open; (3) osteotomy of the tibial tubercle and retraction of the extensor mechanism proximally; and (4) use of an external fixator or femoral distractor intraoperatively to distract the knee. A number of plate and screw configurations have been described for fracture fixation. In general, the trend has been away from the use of large plates or of plates on both sides of the tibia (ie, "bone sandwich") and toward the use of smaller diameter screws.

Limited Open Reduction and Internal Fixation This method is designed to minimize the trauma of surgery.[9] It is applicable to relatively simple, minimally displaced fractures. In this technique, exposure is minimized by the use of limited incisions that are placed to provide access to a specific component of the fracture. Fragments are manipulated with a bone tamp or clamp, Kirschner wire (K-wire), or periosteal elevator. This method is applicable to simple fracture patterns, assessing reduction with fluoroscopy or arthroscopy. In

most cases, attempted reduction of complex, comminuted, or displaced fractures through 1 or 2 small incisions is futile.

Limited Open Reduction With a Bridging External Fixator This method is designed to decrease the incidence of postoperative wound complications associated with a wide surgical exposure. It is particularly applicable in the management of plateau fractures with metaphyseal dissociation when the articular surface is not particularly displaced or comminuted. Preoperative CT is useful to precisely determine the location of key fragments. Small incisions are placed to access these key fragments. The key fragments are manipulated with an elevator or a K-wire "joy stick" or through a metaphyseal window. Reduction is confirmed with the aid of fluoroscopy, and the fragments are held in place with percutaneous screws or K-wires. Because the stability of fixation is limited, an external fixator is used to bridge the knee, thus isolating the fixation from extrinsic stresses. The fixator is removed at 4 to 6 weeks. The trade-off for the decreased incidence of postoperative wound complications is that the bridging external fixator makes early motion impossible. The most commonly occurring error of technique is a failure to reduce the articular surface.

Limited Open Reduction With External Fixation Using a Small Wire Circular Frame or Large Pin Cantilever Frame This method is designed to minimize the incidence of postoperative wound complications and to allow postoperative motion.[8,10,11] A major disadvantage of this method is that the fixator pins have the potential of serving as a conduit by which bacteria reach the fracture and knee joint. Pin tract infections and osteomyelitis frequently

complicate this method of management. The limited open reduction is performed with the aid of preoperative CT and intraoperative fluoroscopy. Following reduction and stabilization of the articular segment, 1 of 3 types of external fixator are used to stabilize it to the distal tibia: a small wire circular frame, a large pin cantilever frame, or a hybrid frame in which the distal fixation is by large pins and proximal fixation is by small wires attached to a circular frame. If the articular fracture is comminuted, large pins may not provide adequate fixation, and their insertion may result in loss of reduction. In these cases, a frame with a proximal ring, either a hybrid or a small wire circular frame, is used. The 2 most commonly occurring errors of technique are failure to achieve anatomic reduction of the joint surface and failure to achieve adequate stability between the articular segment and distal tibia. In cases in which adequate stability is not achieved, stability can be increased by adding a bridging frame across the knee. This topic will be discussed in greater detail below.

Complications
The complications of tibial plateau fractures are osteoarthritis, nonunion, and infection. Osteoarthritis can occur following any type of tibial plateau fracture. It occurs more commonly following high-energy tibial plateau fractures and fractures that have not been reduced anatomically. Conservative management consists of nonsteroidal anti-inflammatory medication or intra-articular steroid injections. Surgical management consists of varus or valgus osteotomy, arthrodesis, or arthroplasty.

Nonunion occasionally complicates tibial plateau fractures with metaphyseal dissociation, and the metaphyseal component of these fractures is usually the part that fails to heal. Management consists of stable fixation and autogenous bone grafting.

Infection is the complication of tibial plateau fractures that is most difficult to manage. Management consists of debridement, dead space management, systemic antibiotics, and soft-tissue coverage. Infection frequently is associated with osteoarthritis or nonunion, adding to the difficulty of managing these complications. A history of infection should tip the scales in favor of more conservative management of osteoarthritis. If conservative management fails, an arthrodesis is less likely to activate a latent infection than is an arthroplasty.

Arthroscopic Management

The arthroscopic approach to tibial plateau fractures has become a more recognized component of the fracture surgeon's armamentarium in dealing with this complex fracture problem. However, it is critical that the surgeon have a complete understanding of fracture patterns and associated soft-tissue pathology as part of the preoperative assessment, in order that only appropriate fractures are approached using arthroscopic technology. This chapter will review preoperative assessment of tibial plateau fracture, discuss the arthroscopic option, and review surgical technique.

Preoperative Assessment

The classic history for plateau injury is one of a fall or impact causing a valgus compression to the joint and resulting in acute knee pain and a tense effusion. Of the possible sources of hemarthrosis, intra-articular fracture results in the most aggressive bleeding response and, therefore, the fastest and most tense effusion. Associated with the effu-

sion is lateral joint line pain or, more specifically, pain over the lateral tibial plateau. In this setting, stability testing is difficult, both because of guarding associated with pain and because loss of bony contour results in a false perception of laxity where no ligament damage exists.

Routine radiographic assessment includes AP and lateral radiographs of the knee and, when warranted, oblique views. However, interpreting radiographic findings requires caution. Kearns and associates[12] reviewed their experience with AP and lateral radiographs of tibial plateau fractures created in a cadaveric model. They performed 1,280 observations and came to the conclusion that a 3-mm articular defect was detected only 50% of the time, while a 5-mm defect was detected in 85% of cases. For all fractures observed, the average underestimation of displacement equaled 2.5 mm. When they added oblique views and repeated the study, 3-mm defects were detected 80% of the time, and 5-mm defects 90% of the time. With a reverse plateau view (angled 10° from the AP to account for the slope of the tibial plateau), 3-mm defects were found 90% of the time, and 100% of 5-mm displacements were identified. Given the underestimation of fractures using standard radiographs and a disturbingly low sensitivity of detection, other imaging strategies have been investigated. Barrow and associates[13] compared the use of magnetic resonance imaging (MRI) with tomography in 31 cases of plateau fracture. Joint depression was calculated equally well with either approach. Comminution, however, was better visualized on MRI. In addition, only the MRI yielded information about soft-tissue pathology. In their population, this included 32% with medial meniscus tears,

55% with lateral meniscus tears, 23% with anterior cruciate ligament (ACL) rupture, and 10% with medial collateral ligament (MCL) tears, either partial or complete.

Kode and associates[14] compared MRI with CT scan in 22 cases. They found that fracture configuration was visualized equally in 64% of cases, with MRI performing better in 23% and CT scanning superior in 13%. The soft-tissue pathology identified on MRI included complete ligament tears in 12 cases, partial tears in 15 cases, and meniscal pathology in 12 cases. They concluded that the MRI was the preferable technology. Kohut and Leyvranz[15] evaluated the importance of soft-tissue pathology on the prognosis for tibial plateau fractures. They determined that ligament, meniscus, and cartilage damage had a direct impact on the functional score as well as on osteoarthritis. Therefore, it appears that MRI adds valuable data, not only for acute management but also for prognostic purposes.

Hunter and associates evaluated the impact of MRI on fracture classification and surgical management in 53 consecutive patients meeting inclusion criteria for the study. Using the Schatzker classification, they found that the MRI changed the preoperative classification in 29% of cases that had been classified using plain radiographs and similarly changed fracture management in 29% of the population (RE Hunter, MD, T Pevny, MD, DS Aldrich, MD, MG Creighton, MD, unpublished data, 1997). Comparing the accuracy of MRI classification with the classification based on radiographs, MRI data increased the accuracy of the classification by 7%, using arthroscopic or open findings to confirm imaging studies. The MRI data were reviewed to see what additional information was gleaned regarding soft-tissue pathology. In this population, the incidence of lateral meniscus tear was 45%; MCL sprains, either partial or complete, constituted 19%; medial meniscus tears, 9%; and ACL ruptures, 8%. From these data, the authors concluded that MRI was a very valuable tool in preoperative diagnosis and surgical planning. Preoperative data are particularly important when arthroscopy is being entertained as a possible surgical approach.

Treatment

The first treatment decision to consider when faced with a plateau fracture is whether the fracture will be treated surgically or conservatively. We prefer conservative treatment for fractures that are stable on ligamentous examination and that have 2 mm or less of articular displacement. Surgical management is recommended for fractures with 2.5 mm or more of displacement, fractures that demonstrate a displaced split, or fractures that are associated with functional or ligamentous instability. This approach to surgical management is based in part on the study of Brown and associates,[16] who studied the impact of fracture displacement on lateral joint stress. In a cadaveric model, they noted stress aberrations in the lateral joint when depression was greater than 1.5 mm and a substantial change when displacement was greater than 2.5 mm. Under those loading conditions, there was a 75% increase in peak local pressures. Therefore, to avoid loads which, in the long run, could result in accelerated deterioration in the lateral compartment, surgical reduction to within 1.5 to 2 mm is recommended.

Arthroscopic Management

Bennett and Browner[2] evaluated the effectiveness of the arthroscope as a

diagnostic tool in plateau fractures. They used the arthroscope for fractures that had depression of more than 5 mm, displacement of more than 5 mm, or angular deformity in excess of 5°. In that setting, they found a 56% incidence of soft-tissue injury, including a 20% incidence of MCL rupture, 20% incidence of meniscal pathology, and 10% incidence of ACL tear. They recommended that the arthroscope be used to examine all nondisplaced fractures before conservative treatment and in conjunction with all percutaneous fixation fractures. We agree with the thorough assessment of these fractures but have found that MRI can sometimes replace the need for the arthroscope in those fractures that look to be minimally displaced or nondisplaced. A special word of caution is appropriate for those fractures that appear to be a pure split on radiographic analysis. These fractures have a high incidence of entrapped lateral meniscus, which, if untreated, will result in inadequate reduction and chronic displacement on the lateral meniscus in a bucket-handle pattern (Fig. 5).

Jennings[17] was one of the early pioneers to examine the role of arthroscopy in the management of tibial plateau fractures. With his use of an arthroscopic approach, the average hospital stay in his population was 4 days, with good results noted in 85%. Only 5% of the population had any residual decrease in range of motion.

Holzach and associates[9] reviewed their experience with 14 cases followed up for more than 1 year after being treated arthroscopically. They included both lateral depression and split depression fractures with displacement of greater than or equal to 2 mm. Excellent results were obtained in 93% and fair results in

7%. Fracture reduction was noted to be anatomic in 80% of cases. Patients expressed satisfaction in all cases and were able to resume normal activities.

Fowble and associates[18] compared arthroscopic reduction and percutaneous fixation with open reduction and internal fixation in 23 cases of split or split depression fractures, which were matched for degree of pathology. They found that the arthroscopic reduction gave an anatomic restoration in 100% of cases, compared to 55% for the open group. Hospital stay in the arthroscopic group was 5 days compared to 10 days in the open group. Range of motion was statistically better in the arthroscopic group, and complications were fewer. From this study, they concluded that the arthroscopic approach was preferable in selected fracture patterns.

Regardless of the surgical approach, the goals remain the same: anatomic reduction, rigid internal fixation, repair of associated soft-tissue injury, and early range of motion. We have found that the arthroscopic approach allows the attainment of these goals most effectively in those fractures that are either a pure depression of the lateral plateau or a split depression of the lateral compartment where the split component is easily closed and reduced (Schatzker I, II, and III).

Surgical Technique

After a thorough examination under anesthesia, a diagnostic arthroscopy is performed to evaluate the patellofemoral joint as well as the medial and lateral compartments and the intercondylar notch areas. We routinely use a leg holder to control the thigh and drop the end of the table (Fig. 6, A). This allows easy access to the lateral joint by placing the knee in flexion and varus (Fig. 6, B). Ex-

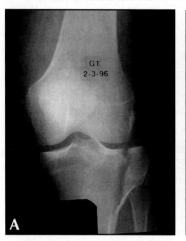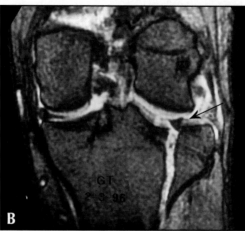

Fig. 5 A, Radiograph showing a split fracture of the lateral plateau. **B,** Magnetic resonance imaging of the fracture demonstrates a displaced lateral meniscus which is locked in the split component of the fracture (arrow).

tending the knee following reduction allows the fluoroscopy unit to be placed beneath the knee for screw fixation (Fig. 6, C). When it is confirmed that the fracture pattern lends itself to an arthroscopic approach, the anterior synovium of the knee is debrided with the arthroscope placed in the anteromedial portal and a mechanical resector in the anterolateral portal. We recommend debriding the ligamentum mucosum and whatever anterior fat pad is necessary in order to gain complete visualization of the lateral compartment in the anterolateral aspect of the knee (Fig. 7, A). In fracture patterns that involve the anterior portion of the lateral plateau, an accessory lateral portal can be very helpful to pull the anterior horn of the lateral meniscus away from the plateau, allowing for more effective visualization. This portal is 1.5 to 2 cm lateral to the standard anterolateral portal. Either a blunt probe or a blunt hook can be used to retract the meniscus without interfering with the anterolateral aspect of the knee joint (Fig. 7, B).

Using a standard drill guide (we use the ACL drill guide from our reconstruction tray), a guide wire is passed through the anterolateral skin and into the lateral joint, centered in the middle of the depressed fracture in the coronal plane and at the junction (Fig. 8, A) of the posterior and middle thirds in a sagittal plane. When placing the pin, it is important to start distal enough on the tibia that the pin enters good cortical bone below the depressed articular surface. In this way, when the anterolateral tibial cortex is drilled, it is possible to elevate the fracture without damaging the articular cartilage. This generally means that the pin enters the bone below the flare of the attachment for the anterior compartment musculature (Fig. 8, B). Once the pin is passed, a longitudinal skin incision is made from the pin proximal for 2 cm. The anterolateral cortex of the tibia is penetrated using a 9- or 10-mm cannulated reamer or a coring reamer passed over the guide wire. An angled cannulated tamp is introduced over the guide wire, and the articular surface is gently tapped up into a reduced

position. The reduction is carried out in the central aspect of the fracture, and then, using the same angled tamp with the guide wire removed, the margins of the fracture can be gently elevated in order that the entire plateau is restored to an anatomic position in contact with the undersurface of the lateral meniscus at all points (Fig. 9, A).

When reduction is obtained, the fracture is gently probed through the anterolateral portal to be certain that the fracture is elevated in all areas but not overreduced. Bone graft is used to maintain the reduction and can be easily introduced through the drill hole in the anterolateral cortex. Autogenous bone from the anteromedial tibial metaphysis or allograft croutons soaked in saline have been used effectively. Bone graft is packed gently into the lateral defect until the whole cavity is completely filled as demonstrated by digital palpation.

Using image intensification, guide wires and cannulated screws are passed from the lateral tibia beneath the plateau to exit on the medial side (Fig. 9, B). Washers are used in most cases to avoid penetrating the lateral tibial cortex with the head of the screw. A minimum of 2 and a maximum of 4 screws are used for fracture stabilization.

In those cases in which complete disruption of the MCL is demonstrated, either on examination or by MRI, we favor repairing the MCL through a small longitudinal incision on the medial side of the tibia (Fig. 10). If disrupted proximally, the repair is performed with suture anchors. Distal rupture is stabilized with 1 or 2 low profile staples. Delamarter and associates[19] reviewed the results of 39 cases followed up for greater than 1 year, comparing those cases in which all soft-tissue injuries were repaired with those in which

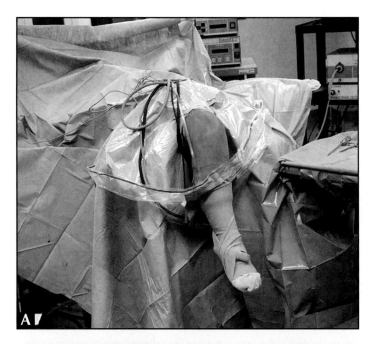

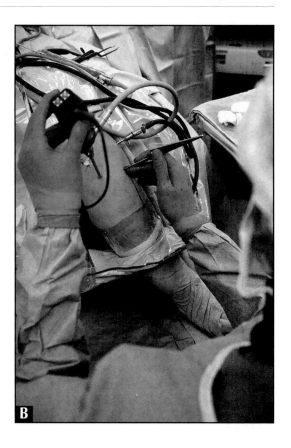

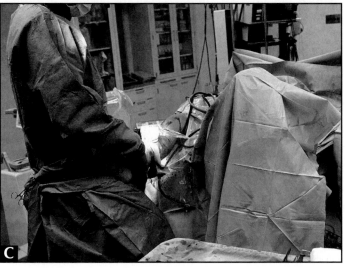

Fig. 6 A, The limb is placed in a leg holder at the end of the operating table drop allowing the operating surgeon to sit in front of the knee for maximum visualization and ease of instrumentation. **B,** By placing the foot across the lap, a varus stress can be applied to the knee allowing the lateral compartment to be both visualized and accessed without difficulty. **C,** After reduction and bone grafting, the knee is extended and the image intensifier is passed beneath the leg allowing for percutaneous insertion of cannulated screws. Slight varus stress is applied to the knee joint in order to avoid compressive loads to the lateral compartment.

only bony pathology was addressed. In the soft-tissue repair group, results were judged better or equal to good in 63% versus 50% good or better results in the fracture management only group. By contrast, poor results were noted in only 16% when ligament injuries were addressed versus 40% when only fracture reduction was undertaken.

The arthroscope has been shown to be a very effective and important tool in the management of selected tibial plateau fractures. In cases of split or split depression patterns treated arthroscopically, reduction is more effectively obtained, fixation is adequately achieved, motion is more quickly restored, and hospitalization time can be dramatically reduced. However, the arthroscope does not substitute for standard open reduction and internal fixation for more complex fractures. Thus, before embarking on an arthroscopic approach, the surgeon must do a careful preoperative assessment in order to select those cases in which arthroscopic reduction and percutaneous fixation can yield good results.

Hybrid Frame Fixation of Tibial Plateau Fractures
High-energy fractures of the proximal tibia present a challenge to the surgeon. The small proximal metaphyseal segment, often with intraarticular and cortical comminution, is difficult to reduce and hold until

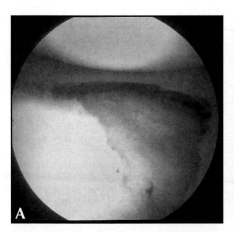 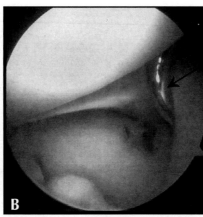

Fig. 7 A, Excellent visualization of this left lateral plateau fracture is obtained after debridement of the anterior fat pad. **B,** An ancillary lateral portal can be very helpful for introducing a blunt probe which is used to retract the lateral meniscus anterior and lateral in order to completely visualize the fracture (arrow).

union. The soft tissues are often compromised and therefore limit the possibilities for fixation. One treatment option that does not compromise soft tissues and can maintain the reduction and allow knee motion is the hybrid frame.

Hybrid frames refer to tensioned small diameter transfixation wires in the metaphyseal segment attached to partially threaded half pins in the diaphysis. The proximal ring is usually five eighths or three fourths of an inch in diameter, and the opening in the popliteal fossa allows for knee flexion. The major indication for this type of fixation is a fracture with a small extra-articular proximal tibial fragment or, more commonly, a bicondylar fracture of the tibial plateau. Although medial and lateral plate fixation can be performed, it may result in disastrous soft-tissue complications when attempted through a single midline incision. Using 2 incisions allows for less soft-tissue stripping and better soft-tissue healing, but due to comminution of both condyles, screw fixation from both sides may not provide sufficient stability to allow early motion.[1] The worst scenario

exists when open reduction of both condyles is performed, followed by postoperative immobilization. Schatzker's results demonstrated a severe decrease in range of motion in such treatment approaches.[1] The usual anterolateral approach to the lateral condyle with a second posteromedial incision for an antiglide plate allows for a sufficient soft-tissue bridge and less stripping of the bony fragments.[20]

Another option that has led to poor results is fixation of the lateral condyle alone. This ultimately results in a varus deformity and often a malunion of the posterior medial tibial condyle. Ganz has recommended lateral plate fixation with an additional external fixator for the medial plateau. If these metaphyseal half pins do not loosen or become infected, this method has yielded good results.[21]

The use of a hybrid frame offers many advantages over the previously discussed options for bicondylar tibial plateau fractures (Schatzker V and VI, AO type C).[1] If the lateral plateau is merely split and not depressed, cannulated screws can be placed subchondrally through a percutaneous incision. This allows for the insertion

of tensioned wires just below the screws, even with a small proximal juxta-articular metaphyseal fragment. When the lateral joint is severely displaced, as is often the case in fractures with diaphyseal extension, a limited anterolateral approach, with open reduction and screw fixation, is necessary. Plates are not necessary because the transfixation wires will maintain alignment of both condyles with reference to the diaphysis. This hybrid frame fixation is stable enough to permit early range of motion and partial weightbearing. The thin wires allow for some loading of the fracture fragments; however, advancement of weightbearing depends on the extent of comminution. The early results in several series demonstrated good maintenance of alignment, acceptable knee motion, a low infection rate, and rates of arthritis consistent with the extent of articular damage.[10,22–24]

Mechanical Characteristics
Several authors have looked at the stability of small diameter tensioned transfixation wires and their attachment to circular frames.[25–27] The wires are 1.5, 1.8, or 2.0 mm in diameter and can have a 4-mm olive attached on the wire which, when buttressed against the cortex, leads to increased stability by preventing translation. The most important factors in stability of a small wire circular frame include wire tension, angle between wires, number of wires, use of olive wires, proximity to the fracture site, and size of the ring[26] (Outline 1).

The wires on a full ring are tensioned to 130 kg, which makes the small diameter wire comparable in strength to a 4-mm half pin. The weakest point in the system is the slippage between the wire and the cannulated or slotted bolt. On a three

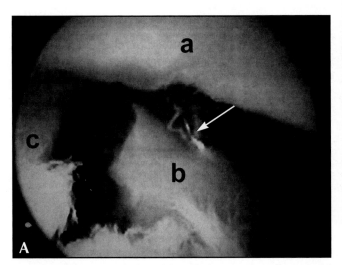
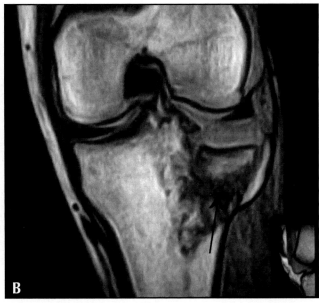

Fig. 8 A, The guide wire is passed through the anterolateral cortex of the tibia entering the fracture in the posterior third midway between the medial and lateral extent of the fracture fragment (arrow) (a: lateral femoral condyle, b: displaced lateral tibial plateau fracture, c: intact portion of lateral plateau). **B,** The guide wire must enter the anterolateral cortex of the tibia low enough that the cortical window which is drilled remains below the depressed articular fragment avoiding damage to the articular surface and allowing for elevation of the fragment with associated subchondral bone (the arrow demonstrates the point of entry of the guide wire in anterolateral hole).

quarter ring, the wires are usually tensioned to 100 kg because further tensioning leads to deformation and possible fatigue failure of the ring.

The stiffest configuration of wires is 90° to each other.[26] Unfortunately, anatomic structures about the knee do not make this possible. Studies have shown that maintenance of at least 60° between wires, which is obtainable, leads to improved fixation and stiffness.[25,26] A knowledge of the safe zones for the proximal tibia is extremely important and must be understood prior to the application of the wires.[28] Ideally, the best stability is achieved with 3 transfixation wires with a maximum spread of at least 60°. Two wires and an additional half pin directed obliquely from anterior to posterior may also be used. The most commonly used configuration consists of olive wires placed from posterolateral and posteromedial and a smooth wire between these 2. It is

important to avoid the gastrocnemius muscle and the pes anserine tendons on the medial side and to stay no further than 2 cm distal from the tip of the fibular head laterally to avoid the peroneal nerve.[29] Recently, an MRI study has shown that wires within 14 mm of the joint surface could be intra-articular, especially on the lateral side (JS Reid, MD, M Vanslyke, MD, unpublished data, 1995). These intracapsular wires, if infected, can lead to a septic joint. Although this complication is rare, it has been reported in the literature.[22,24] One possible solution to this dilemma is to place the cannulated screws in the subchondral bone where they will get the best purchase and prevent depression. The placement of wires below these screws usually prevents intracapsular placement but still allows for fixation of the proximal fragment. Placement of small diameter wires through the barrel of the cannulated

screws is discouraged, as an infected wire can lead to screw infection and possible septic arthritis.

Implications and Indications

A thorough understanding of the mechanism of injury and the amount of energy transferred in these comminuted fractures is imperative. In the multiply injured patient, an initial assessment of the patient's airway and circulation takes immediate precedence over attention to the

> **Outline 1**
> **Factors influencing stability of hybrid frames**
>
> Wire tension
> Angle between wires
> Number of wires
> Use of olive wires
> Wire proximity to the fracture site (closer leads to increased stability)
> Size of the ring (smaller diameter rings are more stable)

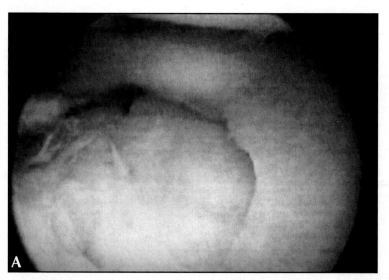

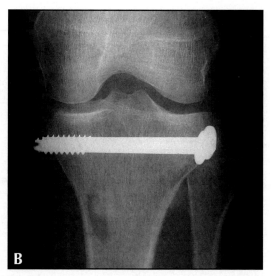

Fig. 9 A, After complete reduction, the lateral plateau should contact the undersurface of the lateral meniscus throughout its entire periphery and the articular surfaces should be level with the adjoining intact articular cartilage. **B,** Small lateral puncture wounds are used to insert the cannulated screws which buttress the elevated lateral plateau (also shown is a small anteromedial metaphyseal window used to obtain autogenous bone graft).

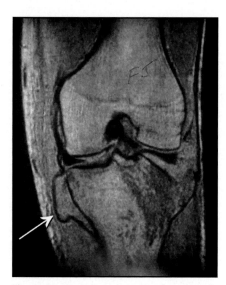

Fig. 10 Magnetic resonance imaging of a split depressed lateral plateau fracture showing associated grade 3 laxity of the medial collateral ligament with disruption distally (arrow).

injured extremity. This should not preclude examining the patient and developing treatment options during the resuscitation phase.

The initial limb assessment should focus on the neurologic and vascular status of the extremity. There should be a high index of suspicion in order to rule out compartment syndrome. Complicating factors can include an open injury and coexisting peripheral nerve injuries along with compartment syndrome. Once the patient has been sufficiently evaluated and stabilized, the treatment plan for the limb can be formulated.

Even when radiographs have been obtained in the emergency room, it is often extremely helpful to get anteroposterior and lateral traction radiographs of the limb once the patient has been anesthetized (Fig. 11). Hybrid fixation may be the definitive treatment of choice but often is impractical in the emergency setting. A bridging external fixator across the knee is the simplest and fastest way to manage the traumatized limb. If the condition of the soft tissues is acceptable and the fracture is minimally displaced, then percutaneous screw fixation can be done during the initial setting. For more comminuted, dis-

placed, and depressed fractures, it is often advantageous to perform ligamentotaxis with a bridging external fixator and get a postoperative computed tomography (CT) scan prior to joint stabilization.

Hybrid frames are indicated for small proximal extra-articular fractures (AO type A). These fractures have a tendency to go into procurvatum and valgus with intramedullary nailing. The major indication is bicondylar tibial plateau fractures with and without diaphyseal extension (Schatzker V and VI, AO type C). If the joint surface is displaced or depressed, a limited, CT-informed arthrotomy is performed with cannulated screw fixation followed by a hybrid frame. The use of a hybrid frame does not preclude a good open reduction of the joint, and after skin closure the frame acts as a buttress and neutralization plate in all planes.

A useful indication for the hybrid frame is the injury with compromised soft tissues that would not

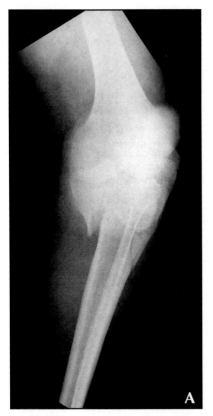
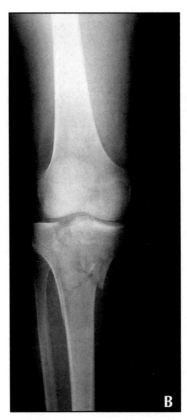
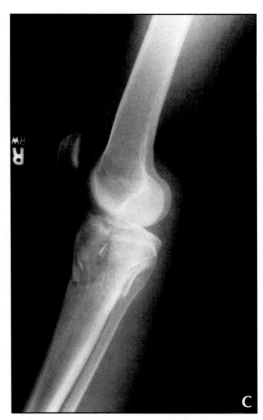

Fig. 11 A, Emergency room radiograph of proximal tibia fracture-dislocation. **B** and **C,** anteroposterior and lateral traction radiographs performed in the operating room after general anesthetic reveals the morphology and extent of the fracture allowing better preoperative planning. Lateral diaphyseal extension and anterior comminution are now evident.

otherwise allow metaphyseal fixation. This is especially true for fractures with metaphyseal diaphyseal dissociation. Small diameter wires do not damage traumatized soft tissues but do allow stable fixation, early motion, and partial weightbearing with good maintenance of alignment. The use of previously described surgical exposures for internal fixation is to be avoided when there is recognized or even anticipated soft-tissue injury.

Surgical Technique

The entire limb, up to the groin, is sterilely prepped and draped. The foot is left exposed so that pulses can be evaluated by palpation or sterile Doppler. The patient is placed on a radiolucent table and biplanar fluo-

roscopy is available. Folded sheets are placed under the knee to allow slight flexion. If the joint is minimally displaced or there is a simple split type fracture, percutaneous reduction and compression with a tenaculum can be attempted. The articular surface is then checked under fluoroscopy with the knee slightly flexed and fully extended. When the reduction is judged to be acceptable, a small lateral incision is made just below the joint line. Two large diameter (7.0 or 7.3 mm) cannulated, cancellous screws with washers are placed parallel to the knee joint in the subchondral bone. The anterior screw is directed in a posteromedial direction and the posterior screw is placed in an almost straight medial direction. Again, these screws and

the joint surface must be checked under fluoroscopy. If deemed to be satisfactory, the skin is closed prior to wire placement.

In the event that the lateral joint cannot be reduced in a closed fashion, a limited open reduction is necessary, usually through an anterolateral or midlateral vertical incision starting proximal to the joint and extending about 7 cm below the joint line. After elevation and retraction of the meniscus, the articular surface is reduced and grafted as is standard technique for displaced tibial plateau fractures. Two cancellous screws are placed as previously described. The meniscus is repaired to the capsule, and the capsule and skin are closed. The use of a hybrid frame does not preclude a good open reduction of the joint. *Note that reduction of the articular surface is the most important step in treatment of all articular fractures and is independent of the method of stabilization chosen.*

Following joint reduction, the small diameter wires can be inserted. The first wire is inserted, under image intensification, from the tip of the fibular head and directed in a posterolateral to anteromedial direction. This wire should be parallel to the joint just below the previously inserted screws. Placing the wires within 15 mm of the joint runs the risk of an intracapsular wire with the possibility of septic arthritis.[22,24] Subchondral screw placement with wire placement just below should allow for good articular compression and avoid intracapsular wire placement (Fig. 12). The proximal five-eighths ring is then attached to the wire, which is tensioned to 100 kg. Using the ring as a guide, the second wire is inserted parallel to the joint in a posteromedial to anterolateral direction. The use of olive wires for these first 2 wires is encouraged to increase the stability of the fixation and to prevent translation.[26] The angle between these 2 wires should be close to 60° to achieve maximum stability. After connecting and tensioning this wire to the frame, a third smooth wire is placed parallel to floor and bisecting the 2 previously placed wires. Another option to the third wire is a half pin in the proximal fragment either posteromedial or posterolateral. This half pin should not be directed posteriorly towards the popliteal vessels but rather in an oblique fashion. Use of 3 wires or 2 wires plus a half pin is necessary for stable proximal fixation. Placement of these wires must be checked with the knee in 30° of flexion and extension to ensure that these wires are not intracapsular.

Following the application of the proximal small diameter tensioned wires and the partial ring to the metaphyseal segment, a gross reduction is attempted by manual traction under fluoroscopic examination. Two or 3 5-mm half pins are inserted through the anterior or anteromedial face of the tibia diaphysis. These half pins are then attached to a bar or ring that is connected to the proximal ring. After alignment has been obtained with traction, the joints connecting the diaphyseal segment, with half pins, to the ring are then tightened. At this point, it is necessary to check alignment in both the anteroposterior and the lateral planes. It is often helpful to obtain plain radiographs in both planes in the operating room to better determine axial alignment. Assessment of the joint surface may be difficult, especially on the lateral radiograph, because of the presence of the frame and bolts. Oblique views in several planes will often allow visualization of the joint surface. If a bony defect is present in the metaphysis or the fracture is open, then autologous bone grafting at 4 to 6 weeks is recommended through an anterolateral approach once the soft tissues have healed.

The pins are then wrapped with sterile bandages to soak up any serous drainage and to prevent crusting of eschars around the pins and possible infection. Some authors recommend dilute hydrogen peroxide, antibiotic ointment, sterile saline, or manufactured sponges for the pin sites. Although each of these is possible, simple pin wrapping can be used if that is the surgeon's preference. Intravenous antibiotics are administered for 48 hours postoperatively. A foot plate with a thick rubber band extension can be added to prevent equinus contracture and allow ankle exercises. In severely compromised

distal soft tissues or patients with head injuries, a half pin can be placed into the first metatarsal and incorporated into the frame. This pin is usually removed at 4 to 6 weeks. The patient can be allowed to ambulate with toe touch to 30% partial weight-bearing following frame application. Weightbearing can be advanced as tolerated, depending on the extent of comminution, until the patient can bear full weight with crutches in a 4-point gait prior to frame removal. Early passive motion of the knee with heel cord stretching is imperative in the early postoperative phase. Unfortunately, passive motion and continuous passive motion (CPM) machines promote atrophy and should be used in conjunction with active motion. With most frames, the patient can achieve 90° of flexion while the circular frame is in place. The proximal thin wires may become inflamed or even infected with knee motion due to the skin moving. If pin infection does ensue, resolution within a few days is usually seen with the administration of an oral first generation cephalosporin. Should drainage and infection continue, cultures may be appropriate, along with intravenous antibiotics, release of tight inflamed skin edges, or even wire removal.

Progressive weightbearing can be initiated over time; however, radiographs rarely show any substantial callus in the metaphyseal fracture location. The average time until frame removal is between 10 and 18 weeks.[10,22–24] Dynamization of the frame or loosening of the frame in the office with a clinical examination may be useful prior to frame removal. The hazards of early frame removal include malunion, mostly drifting into varus, and nonunion. Application of a patellar weightbearing cast for 1 or 2 months postoperatively can prevent malunion and enhance bony contact and union. Frame removal is most commonly performed in the operating room because of the pain associated with removal of the intraosseous transfixation wires. At that time, an examination under anesthesia, knee manipulation, and cast application can be done.

Results

There are few published reports with long-term follow-up in the orthopaedic literature.[10,22–24] The results at present are extremely encouraging, and the soft-tissue complication rate is very low. Pin tract infection, when extra-articular, responded readily to oral antibiotics.

Stamer and associates[10] reported 3 deep wound infections, which responded to debridement and intravenous antibiotics. They had only 1 pin tract infection, 1 deep venous thrombosis, and one 5° varus malunion. Their knee score results revealed that 16 patients (70%) had good or excellent results, and the 3 failures were all in patients with deep infection.[10]

In a study of 48 patients with 50 fractures, Weiner and associates[24] demonstrated that the average overall knee score was 90; however, the intra-articular fractures had a lower average score of 84. Poor results were not seen in the 6 patients with an anterior cruciate ligament (ACL) avulsion or in 6 patients with varus/valgus ligamentous laxity. Two patients, with proximally placed intracapsular wires, developed septic knee joints. Good and excellent results were seen clinically in 98% of patients and radiographically in 82% of fracture reductions.[24]

Of 5 patients in the series by Murphy and associates,[22] 1 patient with a proximally placed wire developed a septic joint but still had a good

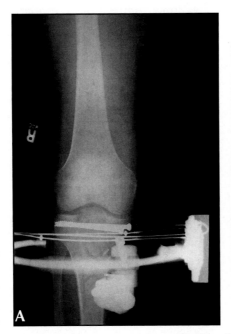
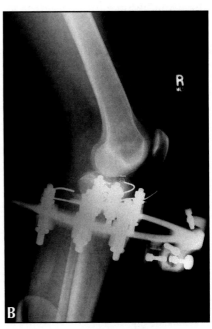

Fig. 12 A and **B,** Anteroposterior and lateral radiographs of recommended construct. Compression screws are placed subchondral and transfixation wires are just below avoiding intracapsular insertion. Note the difficulty in assessing the joint on the lateral radiograph due to the presence of hardware.

result. In 31 Schatzker VI high-energy fractures, Watson[23] reported an average Hospital for Special Surgery knee score of 82. Despite 1 infection in a grade IIIC fracture, which resulted in an amputation, there was only 1 nonunion, which healed with bone grafting and no serious pin tract problems. In this study, the frames were used on average for 15 weeks, resulting in an average knee range of motion of 106°.[23]

Hybrid frame fixation appears to be a reasonable and viable option in the treatment of severe proximal tibia fractures, especially those with soft-tissue compromise. The percentage of good and excellent results is consistent with other series on open reduction and internal fixation of these higher energy fractures.[1,20,30]

The 2 most important factors in the treatment of comminuted intra-articular tibial plateau fractures are accurate joint reduction and preserva-

tion of traumatized soft tissues. Hybrid frame fixation, with a limited open reduction of the joint when necessary, is an excellent treatment alternative. The thin wires afford excellent fixation of the small proximal periarticular fracture fragment, and ligamentotaxis of the metaphyseal-diaphyseal extension leads to good alignment of the mechanical axis and bony union without violating intact soft tissues. Careful attention to the cross-sectional anatomy and maintenance of 15 mm from the joint surface will avoid any serious complications. For the more difficult open fractures or for those associated with compartment syndromes or compromised soft tissues, the hybrid frame should be considered the treatment of choice.

Tibial Plateau Fractures: Postoperative Treatment

Suction drainage of the knee joint as well as intravenous antibiotics is usually continued for 48 hours postoperatively. A small compression dressing with early motion is appropriate for stable fracture fixation constructs. Those fractures with associated knee ligamentous injuries or with less rigid fixation can be treated with adjunctive cast bracing. As previously mentioned, immobilization of the knee joint following open reduction with internal fixation leads to extremely poor knee motion.[1] It is advantageous to achieve complete extension and least 90° of flexion within the first few weeks after surgery.

There are 2 basic premises in the postoperative care of the patient with a surgically treated tibial plateau fracture: early range of motion and delayed weightbearing. This regimen, however, must be individualized to each patient and fracture.

For the simple noncomminuted split fracture, early range of motion and strengthening can be started immediately postoperatively. At 6 to 8 weeks, partial weightbearing can be initiated, with full weight on the extremity by 10 to 12 weeks. For fractures with more depressed articular fragments and for those with metaphyseal comminution, weightbearing should be delayed for 12 to 15 weeks. Continuous passive motion (CPM) machines are beneficial in the immediate postoperative period but must be used in conjunction with active motion and muscle strengthening.

When a hybrid frame is used, partial weightbearing can be initiated early if the metaphyseal comminution is not extensive. Full weightbearing by 3 weeks, with frame removal by 12 to 15 weeks is a useful guideline for most patients. CPM machines can be used in conjunction with hybrid frames.

Multiply injured patients, especially those with head injuries, should be given special consideration. The tendency for these patients to develop heterotopic bone and knee flexion contractures is extremely high. Early passive stretching to the muscle's limit and CPM machines are useful in the early postoperative period. The major emphasis should be placed on maintaining good passive knee motion and avoiding equinus contractures of the ankle. When the patient is able to cooperate with therapy, the standard rehabilitation protocol can commence. One of the problems with internal fixation in osteoporotic bone is not in obtaining fracture reduction but rather maintaining that reduction. Schatzker's group demonstrated the loss of initial alignment and fixation in patients with poor bone quality.[1] These patients may need an adjunctive cast brace to maintain alignment. Weightbearing in these patients must be delayed at least 12 to 15 weeks, and the patient must have full extension and good quadriceps strength prior to walking.

Although the principles in postoperative management are simple, each fracture must have its own individualized postoperative regimen. Articular displacement, metaphyseal comminution, rigidity of fixation, ligamentous injuries, and the patient's overall condition are all important factors that must be considered in the rehabilitation phase. It is important to remember that the final outcome depends not only on the surgical treatment of these fractures but also on appropriate care during the postoperative management period as well.

References

1. Schatzker J, McBroom R, Bruce D: The tibial plateau fracture: The Toronto experience 1968–1975. Clin Orthop 1979;138:94–104.

2. Bennett WF, Browner B: Tibial plateau fractures: A study of associated soft tissue injuries. J Orthop Trauma 1994;8:183–188.

3. Rasmussen PS: Tibial condylar fractures: Impairment of knee joint stability as an indication for surgical treatment. J Bone Joint Surg 1973;55A:1331–1350.

4. Duwelius PJ, Connolly JF: Closed reduction of tibial plateau fractures: A comparison of functional and roentgenographic end results. Clin Orthop 1988;230:116–126.

5. Perry CR, Evans LG, Rice S, Fogarty J, Burdge RE: A new surgical approach to fractures of the lateral tibial plateau. J Bone Joint Surg 1984;66A: 1236–1240.

6. Fernandez DL: Anterior approach to the knee with osteotomy of the tibial tubercle for bicondylar tibial fractures. J Bone Joint Surg 1988;70A:208–219.

7. Benirschke SK, Agnew SG, Mayo KA, Santoro VM, Henley MB: Immediate internal fixation of open, complex tibial plateau fractures: Treatment by a standard protocol. J Orthop Trauma 1992;6:78–86.

8. Mallik AR, Covall DJ, Whitelaw GP: Internal versus external fixation of bicondylar tibial plateau fractures. Orthop Rev 1992;21: 1433–1436.

9. Holzach P, Matter P, Minter J: Arthroscopically assisted treatment of lateral tibial plateau fractures in skiers: Use of a cannulated reduction system. J Orthop Trauma 1994;8:273–281.

10. Stamer DT, Schenk R, Staggers B, Aurori K, Aurori B, Behrens FF: Bicondylar tibial plateau fractures treated with a hybrid ring external fixator: A preliminary study. J Orthop Trauma 1994;8:455–461.

11. Ries MD, Meinhard BP: Medial external fixation with lateral plate internal fixation in metaphyseal tibia fractures: A report of eight cases associated with severe soft-tissue injury. Clin Orthop 1990;256:215–223.

12. Kearns RJ, Mendelow M, Soltes G, Gartsman GM, Tullos HS: Abstract: Radiographic view and quality in the assessment of the tibial plateau fracture: Are we missing something? J Orthop Trauma 1989;3:167.

13. Barrow BA, Fajman WA, Parker LM, Albert MJ, Drvaric DM, Hudson M: Tibial plateau fractures: Evaluation with MR imaging. Radiographics 1994;14:553–559.

14. Kode L, Lieberman JM, Motta AO, Wilber JH, Vasen A, Yagan R: Evaluation of tibial plateau fractures: Efficacy of MR imaging compared with CT. Am J Roentgenol 1994;163:141–147.

15. Kohut M, Leyvranz PF: Cartilaginous, meniscal and ligamentous lesions in the prognosis of tibial plateau fractures. Acta Orthop Belg 1994; 60:81–88.

16. Brown TD, Anderson DD, Nepola JV, Singerman RJ, Pedersen DR, Brand RA: Contact stress aberrations following imprecise reduction of simple tibial plateau fractures. J Orthop Res 1988;6:851–862.

17. Jennings JE: Arthroscopic management of tibial plateau fractures. *Arthroscopy* 1985;1:160–168.

18. Fowble CD, Zimmer JW, Schepsis AA: The role of arthroscopy in the assessment and treatment of tibial plateau fractures. *Arthroscopy* 1993;9:584–590.

19. Delamarter RB, Hohl AM, Hopp E Jr: Ligament injuries associated with tibial plateau fractures. *Clin Orthop* 1990;250:226–233.

20. Georgiadis GM: Combined anterior and posterior approaches for complex tibial plateau fractures. *J Bone Joint Surg* 1994;76B:285–289.

21. Mast J, Jakob R, Ganz R: *Planning and Reduction Technique in Fracture Surgery*. Heidelberg, Germany, Springer-Verlag, 1989, pp 168–178.

22. Murphy CP, D'Ambrosia R, Dabezies EJ: The small pin circular fixator for proximal tibial

fractures with soft tissue compromise. *Orthopedics* 1991;14:273–280.

23. Watson JT: High-energy fractures of the tibial plateau. *Orthop Clin North Am* 1994;25:723–752.

24. Weiner LS, Kelley M, Yang E, et al: The use of combination internal fixation and hybrid frame external fixation in severe proximal tibia fractures. *J Orthop Trauma* 1995;9:244–250.

25. Orbay GL, Frankel VH, Kummer FJ: The effect of wire configuration on the stability of the Ilizarov external fixator. *Clin Orthop* 1992;279:299–302.

26. Kummer FJ: Biomechanics of the Ilizarov external fixator. *Clin Orthop* 1992;280:11–14.

27. Calhoun JH, Li F, Bauford WL, Lehman T, Ledbetter BR, Lower R: Rigidity of half-pins for the Ilizarov external fixator. *Bull Hosp Joint Dis* 1992;52:21–26.

28. Freye E: *Transfixation: Atlas of Anatomical Sections for the External Fixation of Limbs*. Heidelberg, Germany, Springer-Verlag, 1987.

29. Stitgen SH, Cairns ER, Ebraheim NA, Neimann JM, Jackson WT: Anatomic considerations of the pin placement in the proximal tibia and its relationship to the peroneal nerve. *Clin Orthop* 1992;278:134–137.

30. Lansinger O, Bergman B, Korner L, Andersson GB: Tibial condylar fractures: A twenty-year follow-up. *J Bone Joint Surg* 1986;68A:13–19.

Knee Dislocations

Robert C. Schenck, Jr, MD
Robert E. Hunter, MD
Robert F. Ostrum, MD
Clayton R. Perry, MD

Knee dislocations present with a wide spectrum of severity and associated injuries. They are most commonly a result of high-energy trauma (typically a motor vehicle accident), but they can also result from contact sporting injuries.[1-4] Furthermore, knee dislocations can present either as isolated injuries or as one injury in a multiply injured patient. In the latter situation, the difficulty of proper management, including the eventual plan for the ligament surgery, involves prioritization of the other orthopaedic injuries. As will be outlined, the risk of arterial injury is present with any type of knee dislocation. However, once arterial damage is ruled out, the ligamentous management can be delayed after immediate stabilization and reduction of the knee is performed and other more pressing fractures and injuries are treated.

Any injury to the knee joint with significant displacement (dislocation or fracture-dislocation) requires evaluation for possible vascular injury, including frank tearing of the popliteal artery or compartment syndrome of the leg. The well-established risk of arterial injury remains, but many authors have questioned the need for arteriography in all dislocated knees.[4-7] Clinical examination, in conjunction with noninvasive vascular studies, has been increasingly used to follow patients with a normal initial examination (pulses, capillary refill).[5,6] Regardless, the need for a careful vascular examination remains, and a high index of suspicion for arterial injury is essential. Frequently, this requires arteriography to rule out arterial injury (Fig. 1, A).

Once limb-threatening vascular injuries are carefully excluded, a well-conceived plan is necessary to treat the various combinations of ligamentous, articular, and musculotendinous injuries to the knee. Functional restoration of knee stability with a full range of motion can be challenging in light of the complexity of multiple ligament injuries and gross instability.[7-10] The risk of stiffness in the pursuit of knee stability is commonly the underlying issue in the outcome of a knee dislocation.

General Concepts

The diagnosis, pathology, and treatment of knee dislocations have been historically reviewed in detail.[7] In this chapter, we will discuss pertinent historical areas and will also include current concepts.

Kendall[11] published a classic paper on the dislocated knee in 1963. In his paper he combined clinical experience with a cadaveric study of dislocation mechanisms. Furthermore, he defined the classification of the knee dislocations based on position, and outlined the risk of arterial injury with dislocations. Clinically, he noted remarkably good results with closed treatment but recommended surgical management. Many of his clinical cases were referrals and descriptions from other clinicians in Canada. His cadaveric studies are very useful in describing the sequence of injury during hyperextension with a resultant anterior knee dislocation: the anterior cruciate ligament (ACL) tears first, the posterior cruciate ligament (PCL) and capsule tear at 30° hyperextension, and the popliteal artery tears at 50°. The author was unable to reproducibly create a posterior knee dislocation, most commonly creating a fracture of the knee itself.

The classification of knee dislocations has been commonly based on position, energy, or, more recently, anatomic involvement (Fig. 1, B). Spontaneous reduction of knee dislocations occurs, and the position of a knee dislocation (even if known) does not reproducibly determine which ligaments are involved or the surgical approach to be used. Position classification is useful for reduction maneuver (Fig. 2) and for alerting the clinician to a complex dislocation, as

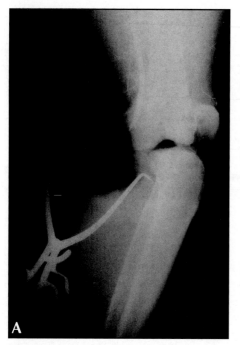
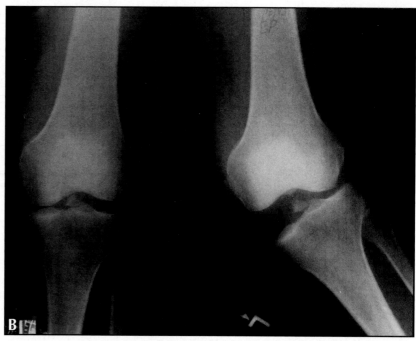

Fig. 1 A, Intraoperative knee radiograph showing a dislocated knee with torn popliteal artery (note arteriogram) from an open high-energy knee injury. Because of complete tibial and peroneal nerve injury with an insensate foot, the patient required an above knee amputation. **B,** Initial anteroposterior radiograph of a spontaneously reduced knee dislocation after injury while playing softball (hyperextension) and anteroposterior stress radiograph of the same knee in full extension (classified as KDIIIM). The patient underwent multiple ligament reconstruction and currently has returned to functional activities.

in a posterolateral injury. Low-energy dislocations, as in sporting activities, may have a lower incidence of arterial injury, as shown in the study by Shelbourne and associates.[4] The classification of knee dislocations by the structure(s) torn is useful for surgical planning as well as for comparison of like injuries. Comparing a PCL-intact knee dislocation and an injury in which all 4 ligaments are torn is like comparing an ACL injury to an injury to both cruciates. The classification involves the use of 4 classes with 5 basic injury patterns (Table 1).

Further definition is on the basis of associated injuries (vascular, neural, tendinous, or ligament-midsubstance or ligament-avulsion); for example, KDIIIL-CN is an ACL/PCL/lateral corner dislocation with vascular and neural injuries.[7,10,12,13] The system is useful in determining the appropriate surgical approach, in classifying injuries for comparison, and as a tool for communication.

Physical Examination

Once a dislocation is diagnosed or suspected, the tendency is to evaluate the ligamentous injury. However, the appropriate step is to focus immediately on the vascular examination, followed by a careful evaluation of the neurologic/motor examination of the lower extremity. Palpation of pulses, capillary refill, and skin color should be assessed carefully in both legs. Any abnormality should make the clinician suspicious of an arterial injury. If ischemia is present despite appropriate joint reduction maneuvers, immediate intraoperative arterial evaluation and repair is required. If arterial repair is delayed more than 6 to 8 hours, limb loss will be imminent.[14]

Historically, the presence of a knee dislocation mandated an arteriogram, with an accepted incidence of arterial tears in 33% of knee dislocations.[15-17] One trend in treatment of dislocations with a normal vascular examination involves serial clinical examinations with adjunctive use of noninvasive vascular studies (sonography and pulse pressures or ankle-arm indices).[1,4-6] Despite the possible complications of arteriography, the onus is on the clinician to rule out or treat arterial injury promptly in the dislocated knee. Arteriograms are still very useful and should be performed, following surgeon and institution preference, in the multitrauma patient. Any equivocal clinical examination requires an arteriogram. Furthermore, vascular observation should be performed in the presence of a vascular specialist or under a specific protocol.

Neurologic examination is important and, commonly, will find evidence of a peroneal nerve palsy, especially with lateral sided injuries. The finding of tibial nerve involvement is rarer, and should direct one to an additional diagnosis of vascular injury, compartment syndrome, and severe displacement with the dislocation (ie, KDIV pattern). Findings of diffuse stocking-glove paresthesias should make one suspicious of a compartment syndrome.

Ligamentous examination of the knee can frequently be difficult at the time of injury because of pain. Use of the Lachman and stabilized Lachman for evaluation of both posterior and anterior translation may be the only cruciate examination possible immediately after injury, due to difficulty flexing the knee to 90°. Varus or valgus opening with the knee positioned in full extension implies tears of a collateral/posterior capsule and both cruciate ligaments. Gross knee swelling in spite of a "normal" radiograph should wake the clinician's suspicions of a bicruciate injury or a dislocated but spontaneously reduced bicruciate injury.[12] Frequently, examination under anesthesia (EUA) is necessary to perform a complete evaluation. This is especially important in those patients with a PCL-intact dislocation (KDI), in which there is magnetic resonance imaging (MRI) evidence of a partial PCL tear and the functional integrity of the PCL is in question.

Radiographic Evaluation

Plain radiographs, anteroposterior (AP) and lateral, are necessary for evaluation of displacement and joint position, and for verification of reduction maneuvers. Careful inspection for bony avulsion injuries is helpful and can help guide the surgeon in the ultimate ligamentous diagnosis and

Table 1
Classification of knee dislocations

Class	Injury*
KDI	PCL-intact knee dislocation, usually ACL and LCL torn, also includes ACL-intact knee dislocation with complete PCL tear
KDII	ACL and PCL torn, collaterals intact
KDIII	
IIIM	ACL, PCL, and MCL-corner torn, lateral side intact
IIIL	ACL, PCL, and LCL-corner torn, medial side intact
KDIV	All 4 ligaments torn

*PCL, posterior cruciate ligament; ACL, anterior cruciate ligament; LCL, lateral collateral ligament; MCL, medial collateral ligament.

treatment. Frequently, the only evidence of injury is slight tibiofemoral joint distraction on AP view, as over 20% of knee dislocations reduce spontaneously at the time of injury.[10]

Because of the difficulty of ligamentous examination, due to pain, a useful adjunct is MRI. It allows accurate evaluation of ligamentous injury and type (avulsion, midsubstance tears) and of evidence of bone bruises and meniscal injuries (Fig. 3). MRI can be useful in planning surgical approaches and in anticipating cruciate graft needs and autologous tendon availability (for example, in the presence of a patellar tendon injury).[7,18,19]

Treatment

Taylor and associates,[20] in 1972, reported a series of knee dislocations with good results with closed treatment. In their series, knee dislocations were treated closed if simple (normal artery, reducible, closed) and open only if requiring immediate management (open injuries, arterial injuries). The authors noted better results with closed treatment but related the results to the severity of injury, rather than the mode of treatment. The authors, however, noted very useful information with respect to the length of immobilization when treating a knee dislocation closed, recommending a period of 4 to 6

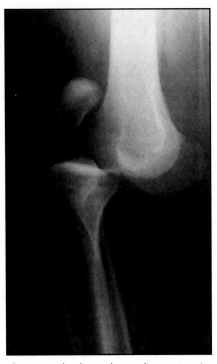

Fig. 2 Lateral radiograph revealing an anterior dislocation which reduced with axial traction. The injury was eventually diagnosed as a posterior cruciate ligament intact knee dislocation (KDI). Note the proximity of the tibia and femur, as well as the position of the patella. In a complete bicruciate ligament injury, the patella will parallel the femur.

weeks. In their study, knees immobilized less than 4 weeks had no evidence of motion loss but had unacceptable knee joint laxity, whereas knees immobilized longer than 6 weeks had very stable knees, but

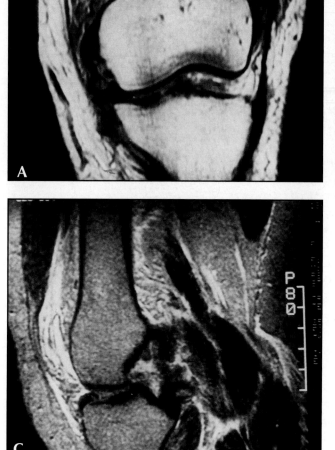

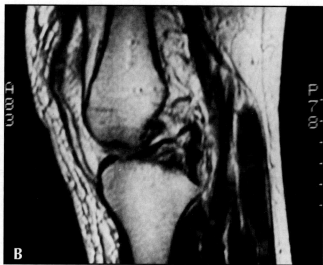

Fig. 3 A, Magnetic resonance (MR) image revealing a tibial avulsion of the medial collateral ligament in a knee dislocation. **B,** MR image of a reduced knee dislocation revealing a femoral avulsion of the posterior cruciate ligament (PCL). The ligamentous injury is that of stripping from the medial femoral condyle without a bony fragment, also referred to as a "peel-off" injury. **C,** MR imaging of the notch revealing midsubstance tears of both the anterior and posterior cruciate ligaments.

unacceptable stiffness or arthrofibrosis. Closed treatment for 4 to 6 weeks is useful in treating a combined arterial injury/knee dislocation when external fixation is used and no ligamentous repair can be performed (Fig. 4). However, the associated complications of immobilization and the advancements in knee ligament surgery make surgical management a more viable approach when indicated. Closed treatment for 6 weeks, to be definitive, probably requires manipulation and arthroscopy, at a minimum, followed by extensive rehabilitation.

Surgical ligamentous management

of simple knee dislocations has been recommended by many authors, and initially by Meyers and Harvey,[8] who showed poorer results (unacceptable laxity) with those patients treated closed. In their follow-up study, these authors noted the possibility of a PCL-intact knee dislocation and continued poor results with closed management. Sisto and Warren[9] also noted improved results with surgical intervention, but warned the clinician of the risk of stiffness and arthritis with the surgical approach. Shelbourne and associates[4] noted the use of staged surgery with low veloc-

ity dislocations: initial surgery treated the PCL and corner, followed by ACL reconstruction once range of motion (ROM) was regained. Fanelli and associates[21] have discussed delayed simultaneous ACL/PCL treatment using allograft tissues after establishing ROM and have reported good results. No studies have compared open versus closed treatment or immediate versus staged reconstructions in similar types of knee dislocations.

The decision for open or closed management depends on the severity of injury, arterial involvement, and other injuries present. Closed treatment (ie, external fixation) may be the most appropriate management in the multitrauma patient, despite the desire to treat the ligamentous involvement surgically. Surgical management of ligamentous injuries requires vascularity, skin coverage, and the ability to perform rehabilitation. The decision for immediate versus delayed reconstruction depends on many factors, including the ligaments involved. For this reason, initial closed treatment (early ROM) with delayed ACL reconstruction can be used successfully for a PCL-intact knee dislocation. Because knee dislocations present with a wide severity of injury and involvement, the treatment plan depends on the individual patient situation.

Surgical Management

The dislocated knee is a complicated reconstructive challenge for the orthopaedic surgeon and requires preoperative planning and experience with open and arthroscopic ligament reconstruction procedures about the knee. Treatment of both cruciate and collateral injuries is necessary and options for both are necessary. Arthroscopy within the first 10 to 14 days after injury (complete capsular tears) carries significant risk of fluid extravasation and even compartment syndrome. Depending on the surgeon's preference and experience, arthroscopic reconstructive procedures after reestablishment of ROM can be useful in patients with delayed presentation of knee dislocation and in the PCL-intact knee dislocation (KDI). Early (within 5 days of injury) surgical open reconstruction or repair is recommended, but it can still be complicated by arthrofibrosis, arthritis, and decreased function. Need for reconstruction or repair depends on the ligament injury present. As noted earlier,

knee dislocations present in a range of severity from ACL/LCL (lateral collateral ligament) injuries (PCL-intact knee dislocation) to severe injuries with all 4 ligaments torn. Unlike combined injuries of the ACL/MCL (medial collateral ligament), the collateral associated with dislocated or bicruciate knee injuries is usually more severe, with involvement of the ligamentous corner of the knee. Thus, it is usually recommended to reestablish the PCL and associated collateral(s) initially, with ACL reconstruction either immediate or delayed. When performing simultaneous PCL and ACL surgery, tensioning of the PCL should be performed before tensioning of the ACL. Tensioning the ACL first can potentially cause posterior tibiofemoral subluxation.[4] Reconstruction of midsubstance cruciate tears, reattachment of cruciate avulsions, and repair of collateral tears are recommended approaches.[4,7,9] Simultaneous ACL/PCL reconstructions with allograft tissues can be successful, but require great care in the creation of tibial and femoral tunnels.[21]

The exposure of the bicruciate-injured knee should be performed with future surgical needs in mind as well as access to the PCL and collateral(s). Placement of the incision over the involved collateral allows exposure of the corner and can be supplemented with a more anteriorly placed incision to inspect the notch and its contents[1,4,22] (Fig. 5).

The approach to the PCL requires knowledge of posterior knee anatomy. The straight posterior approach requires prone positioning with a need to turn the patient to approach the anterior aspect of the knee. We have used the posteromedial and, in specific situations (KDIIIL, complete tears of the ACL, PCL, and posterolateral corner), the posterolateral approach to access the tibial side of

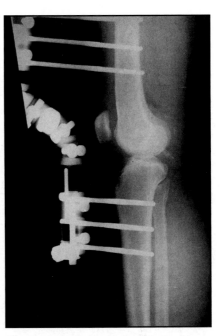

Fig. 4 Lateral radiograph of a dislocated knee after placement of anterior external fixation. Notice the bony posterior cruciate ligament avulsion from the tibia.

the PCL (Fig. 6). Approach to the posteromedial corner and PCL can be made through the same incision medially, using the approach recommended by Burks and Schaffer.[23] When approaching a KDIIIM injury, we find it useful to modify this approach by making the incision from the back edge of the tibia to the femoral epicondyle. This allows repair of the collateral as well as the tibial approach to the PCL by going above the pes and anterior to the gastrocnemius. Approach to the lateral side of the knee requires great care with initial release of the peroneal nerve. Depending on the degree of displacement at the time of injury, varying degrees of ligamentous and tendinous injuries will be seen. Injury to the iliotibial band, biceps tendon, fibular collateral ligament (FCL), arcuate ligament, popliteus tendon, and popliteofibular ligament can occur. In general, if both cruci-

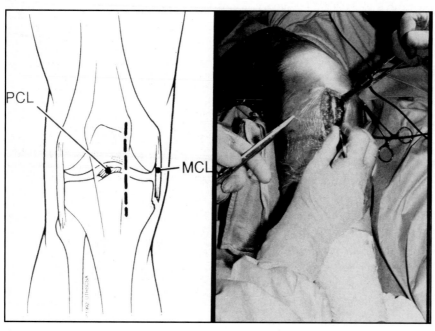

Fig. 5 Paramedian approach to allow access to anterior knee and ligament repair. If magnetic resonance imaging reveals a midsubstance posterior cruciate ligament (PCL) tear, the incision can be placed posteriorly over the collateral edge to access the posterior tibia for placement of a bony trough for PCL reconstruction.

ates and the posterolateral corner are torn completely (KDIIIL), the tibial side of the PCL can be approached through a lateral incision. Although it is difficult to create a tibial trough from the lateral side secondary to the overlying popliteus muscle, an endoscopic cannulated tibial tunnel from the posterior (and lateral) side can be made without great difficulty in such situations. It should be emphasized that such an approach, however, requires complete tears of the ACL, PCL, and posterolateral corner. Regardless, establishing the PCL in its proper position in the presence of its tibial insertion ledge is of primary importance.

Repair or reattachment is performed with braided nonabsorbable sutures (ie, No. 5 Ethibond) and is useful for collateral injuries and stripping of the PCL. PCL reattachment requires much less surgery

than reconstruction and can be a simple procedure when indicated. The knee dislocation, when secondary to hyperextension (anterior), frequently occurs with stripping of the PCL off the femoral origin (also referred to as a "peel-off" injury),[24] and in such injuries the stripped PCL can be successfully reattached with heavy sutures in a Krackow fashion.[25,26] Collateral ligament reattachments can use both suture and washer/screw techniques. A locking whipstitch, as described by Krackow, works very well and can be used to repair midsubstance or avulsion type collateral tears.[25,26] The Krackow (a locking whip) stitch is especially useful when repairing gracile ligaments or tendons where the locks can be taken into the normal substance of the ligament or tendon. In a midsubstance repair of a collateral structure, careful placement of the first lock is

important as that will determine the length of the ligament when sutures are tightened.

Graft selection is controversial and includes consideration of an allograft. PCL midsubstance tears are best reconstructed with an allograft Achilles/patellar tendon or autograft patellar tendon/quadriceps tendon. Presence of extensor or hamstring rupture may preclude the use of autograft. We prefer to use autograft in the surgical plan for ligamentous treatment in knee dislocations when possible. Again, degree of injury, surgeon preference and experience, patient education, geographic preferences, and risks/benefits determine the graft selection. Simultaneous ACL/PCL reconstructions are best performed with allograft, because reestablishment of motion with harvested autograft tissues for simultaneous ACL/PCL reconstruction is difficult.

Tightening of collateral repairs and the PCL reconstruction or reattachment deserves comment. Use of the intact collateral (if present) with the knee flexed can provide protection against overtensioning and tibiofemoral subluxation. With a medial-sided injury and repair (ie, KDIIIM), the leg should be externally rotated to put the knee in a figure 4 position. The PCL should be tightened and fixed initially, checking the resistance to posterior subluxation at 90° of knee flexion and insuring that the knee will fully extend as well. Once satisfied with proper position and PCL function, tighten (tie) the medial repair at 25° knee flexion again with the leg externally rotated. This position allows the MCL to be properly tensioned against the grossly intact LCL. Any reconstructions require intraoperative radiographs to assure proper tibiofemoral alignment. Presence of multiple ligament

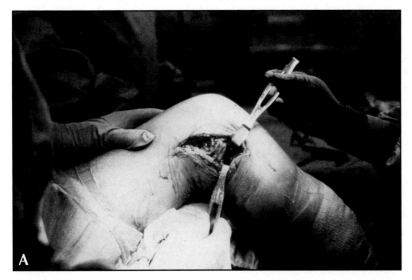
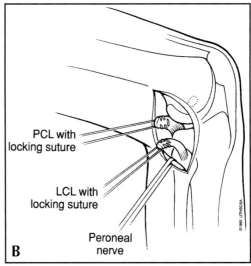

Fig. 6 A, Posterolateral approach with initial release of nerve allowing access to posterolateral corner and knee contents. An anteriorly placed short paramedian approach is frequently helpful to allow full notch inspection and ligament (anterior cruciate/posterior cruciate repair). **B,** Drawing of the posterolateral exposure, including initial exposure of the peroneal nerve. (Reproduced with permission from Schenck RC Jr: The dislocated knee, in Schaefer M (ed): *Instructional Course Lectures 43*. Rosemont, IL, American Academy of Orthopaedic Surgeons, 1994, pp 127–136.)

injuries can lead to overtensioning and partial knee subluxation during a reconstruction, which must be corrected before leaving the operating room.[22]

Managing Combined Arterial and Ligamentous Injuries

Combined arterial injuries and knee dislocations are difficult problems and can be complicated by a concomitant open knee injury. External fixation with an anterior frame is an excellent option to provide immediate stabilization to allow arterial reconstruction. Ligamentous repair should be considered secondary to limb salvage and, if necessary, soft-tissue coverage. The severity of the soft-tissue injury and added insult of ischemia creates an environment for poor ligament healing, possibility of infection, and arthritic change. Such injuries require management of many problems, including fasciotomy, initial immobilization, and final decision for possibility of ligament

repair. Because of associated problems such as these noted, ligament surgery is frequently not possible and the knee is immobilized to allow ligament healing. In our experience, despite immobilization, symptomatic laxity can still occur, which frequently requires bracing. As noted initially, the severity of the knee dislocation must be considered in deciding treatment options.

Conclusion

The dislocated knee can be a significant limb-threatening injury, and the range of severity of a dislocation is an important consideration in deciding appropriate treatment. Evaluation and immediate treatment of vascular insufficiency is primary, but, once this is ruled out, ligament injury becomes the most challenging and common concern. Treating the knee, based on the ligaments involved, with early anatomic repair/reconstruction is the recommended approach.

References

1. Bunt TJ, Malone JM, Moody M, Davidson J, Karpman R: Frequency of vascular injury with blunt trauma-induced extremity injury. *Am J Surg* 1990;160:226–228.

2. Cooper DE, Speer KP, Wickiewicz TL, Warren RF: Complete knee dislocation without posterior cruciate ligament disruption: A report of four cases and review of the literature. *Clin Orthop* 1992;284:228–233.

3. Hughston JC, Bowden JA, Andrews JR, Norwood LA: Acute tears of the posterior cruciate ligament: Results of operative treatment. *J Bone Joint Surg* 1980;62A:438–450.

4. Shelbourne KD, Porter DA, Clingman JA, McCarroll JR, Rettig AC: Low-velocity knee dislocation. *Orthop Rev* 1991;20:995–1004.

5. Dennis JW, Jagger C, Butcher JL, Menawat SS, Neel M, Frykberg ER: Reassessing the role of arteriograms in the management of posterior knee dislocations. *J Trauma* 1993;35:692–697.

6. Kendall RW, Taylor DC, Salvian AJ, O'Brien PJ: The role of arteriography in assessing vascular injuries associated with dislocations of the knee. *J Trauma* 1993;35:875–878.

7. Schenck RC Jr: The dislocated knee, in Schaefer M (ed): *Instructional Course Lectures 43*. Rosemont, IL, American Academy of Orthopaedic Surgeons, 1994, pp 127–136.

8. Meyers MH, Harvey JP Jr: Traumatic dislocation of the knee joint: A study of eighteen cases. *J Bone Joint Surg* 1971;53A:16–29.

9. Sisto DJ, Warren RF: Complete knee dislocation: A follow-up study of operative treatment. *Clin Orthop* 1985;198:94–101.

10. Walker DN, Hardison R, Schenck RC: A baker's dozen of knee dislocations. *Am J Knee Surg* 1994;7:117–124.

11. Kendall JC: Complete dislocation of the knee joint. *J Bone Joint Surg* 1963;45A:889–904.

12. Nonweiler DL, Schenck RC Jr, DeLee JC: The incomplete bicruciate knee injury: A report of two cases. *Orthop Rev* 1993;22:1249–1252.

13. Schenck RC, Burke R, Walker D: The dislocated knee: A new classification system. *South Med J* 1992;85:3S–61.

14. DeBakey ME, Simeone FA: Battle injuries of the arteries in World War II: An analysis of 2,461 cases. *Ann Surg* 1946;123:534–579.

15. Walker DN, Rogers W, Schenck RC Jr: Immediate vascular and ligamentous repair in a closed knee dislocation: Case report. *J Trauma* 1994;36:898–900.

16. Green NE, Allen BL: Vascular injuries associated with dislocation of the knee. *J Bone Joint Surg* 1977;59A:236–239.

17. Muscat JO, Rogers W, Cruz AB, Schenck RC Jr: Arterial injuries in orthopaedics: The posteromedial approach for vascular control about the knee. *J Orthop Trauma* 1996;10:476–480.

18. Schenck RC Jr, McGanity PLJ: Reattachment of avulsed cruciate ligaments: Report of a technique. *Orthop Trans* 1992;16:77.

19. Reddy PK, Posteraro RH, Schenck RC Jr: The role of MRI in evaluation of the cruciate ligaments in knee dislocations. *Orthopedics* 1996;19:166–170.

20. Taylor AR, Arden GP, Rainey HA: Traumatic dislocation of the knee: A report of forty-three cases with special reference to conservative treatment. *J Bone Joint Surg* 1972;54B:96–102.

21. Fanelli GC, Giannotti BF, Edson CJ: Arthroscopically assisted combined anterior and posterior cruciate ligament reconstruction. *Arthroscopy* 1996;12:5–14.

22. Schenck RC: Management of PCL injuries in knee dislocations. *Oper Tech Sportsmed* 1993;1:143–147.

23. Burks RT, Schaffer JJ: A simplified approach to the tibial attachment of the posterior cruciate ligament. *Clin Orthop* 1990;254:216–219.

24. Horner CD, Hoher J: Evaluation and treatment of posterior cruciate ligament injuries. *Am J Sports Med* 1998;26:471–482.

25. Mandelbaum BR, Myerson MS, Forster R: Achilles tendon ruptures: A new method of repair, early range of motion, and functional rehabilitation. *Am J Sports Med* 1995;23:392–395.

26. Krackow KA, Thomas SC, Jones LC: A new stitch for ligament-tendon fixation: Brief note. *J Bone Joint Surg* 1986;68A:764–766.

Pediatric Orthopaedics

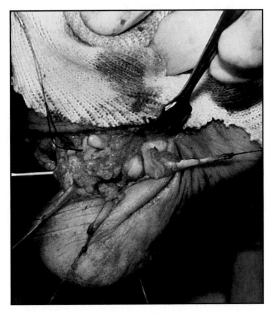

Back Pain in Childhood and Adolescence

B. Stephens Richards, MD
Richard E. McCarthy, MD
Behrooz A. Akbarnia, MD

Introduction

During childhood and adolescence back pain is less common than during adulthood, a period when reportedly 60% to 80% of adults experience episodes of discomfort.[1] In fact, the number of children with complaints of back pain who are seen in pediatric orthopaedic practice has been reported to account for less than 2% of referrals.[2] Unlike the adult, underlying pathology is often detectable in young children, particularly through the use of various imaging studies.

The incidence of back pain in the young, presumably normal population has not been clearly defined. Three commonly mentioned studies reported prevalence of 11.5%, 26%, and 33%, with pain most commonly seen in the age range of 13-15 years, and an equal distribution between sexes.[3-5] A recent study reported that the annual incidence of low back pain rose from 12% at age 12 years to 22% by age 15 years.[6] Lifetime prevalence of low back pain rose from 12% at age 11 years to 50% by age 15 years. Recurrent pain was common, but few children required treatment. Another recent study reported a very low prevalence of low back pain in 7 year olds (1%) and 10 year olds (6%), a higher prevalence in 14- to 16-year-old adolescents (18%), and, as above,

found no differences between genders.[7] From this information, then, approximately 10% to 30% of the normal young population can be expected to experience back pain, particularly low back pain, by their teenage years.

A variety of disorders can lead to back pain in children (Outline 1). If a careful evaluation is made, the etiology often can be determined. The orthopaedic literature reports a 52% to 84% likelihood of identifying the cause, with the more common diagnoses being spondylolisthesis and Scheuermann's kyphosis.[2,8,9] However, a recent report that used single photon emission computed tomography (SPECT) as an adjunctive study successfully identified a pathologic condition in only 22% of 226 children.[10] In all of the studies mentioned, plain radiographs were found to be the best screening test.

Medical Evaluation

History

A detailed history should be obtained from the patient and parents. General questions, with emphasis on the initial onset and duration of symptoms, history of trauma or infection, location of the pain, and frequency and intensity of the discomfort, will often provide the orthopaedist with the

---

Outline 1
Back pain in childhood and adolescence

Differential Diagnoses
    Developmental
        Scheuermann's kyphosis
        Painful scoliosis
    Infection-"infectious spondylitis"
        Diskitis
        Vertebral osteomyelitis
        Tuberculous spondylitis
    Traumatic
        Spondylolysis and spondylolisthesis
        Herniated disk
        Slipped vertebral apophysis
        Fractures
        Muscle strain
    Neoplasms
        Benign
        Posterior
            Osteoid osteoma, osteoblastoma, aneurysmal bone cyst
        Anterior
            Histiocystosis
        Malignant
        Leukemia, lymphoma, sarcoma
    Visceral
        Awareness of abdominal neoplasms, pyelonephritis, appendicitis, retro peritoneal abscess

(Reproduced with permission from Richards BS: Clinical assessment of back pain in children. *J Musculoskel Med* 1998;15:31–40.)

---

information necessary to formulate a provisional differential diagnosis.[11-14] For example, mild pain that has been present for a short duration following intense athletic training may represent muscle strain or overuse.

Further workup would not be necessary and symptoms may resolve with rest. On the other hand, pain that persists for weeks or months following active athletic training, particularly in football, gymnastics, or dance may represent an underlying lumbar spondylolysis or spondylolisthesis.

Location of the pain is important to note. It may localize to a small area of the back, as seen with spondylolysis or tumors, or it may be generalized, as seen following overuse activities or inflammatory disorders. Generalized thoracic discomfort in the adolescent is commonly seen in Scheuermann's disorder. Radiation of pain into the buttock or lower extremity with or without numbness, weakness, or tingling may be a reflection of disk herniation, an uncommon problem in children. Constant, progressive night pain, particularly if it is unrelated to physical activity and does not improve with rest, may be representative of a neoplasm involving the spine or spinal cord.

The age of the child may help in differentiating between disorders. Young children are unlikely to exaggerate symptoms. In those under age 4, the differential diagnosis should always include infection (particularly diskitis) or tumor. In general, adolescents are more likely to have less worrisome disorders, such as spondylolysis or Scheuermann's kyphosis.

Neurologic status, including continence of bowel and bladder, should always be investigated. Worsening of balance, coordination, or gait may be a reflection of spinal cord pathology.

Finally, changes in the general medical condition should alert the orthopaedist to the possibility of an underlying systemic disorder. Fever, chills, lethargy, pallor, bruising, bleeding, or weight loss may indicate a malignant or infectious etiology. Six percent of children with acute lymphocytic leukemia present with complaints of back pain.[15]

Physical Examination

A general screening examination (which includes assessment of the head, neck, upper and lower extremities, and gait) should be performed initially. By doing this, any associated abnormalities may quickly become apparent. The spinal examination includes an assessment of posture, alignment, and skin condition (particularly midline defects such as sinuses, hemangiomas, or hair patches). Scoliosis, trunk decompensation, and muscle spasm may be readily apparent. The forward bending test assesses for thoracic and lumbar asymmetry and spinal flexibility. When stiffness in the lumbar spine is present during this examination, there should be suspicion of associated underlying pathology. Midline skin defects may communicate with underlying neural structures and should be thoroughly investigated.

A careful neurologic examination consisting of motor and sensory testing, reflex testing, and gait evaluation should be routinely performed. The presence of clonus or an abnormal Babinski reflex may be indicative of a central abnormality. Asymmetry in abdominal reflexes is often found in those with spinal cord abnormalities (ie, syringomyelia).

Imaging Studies

Plain radiographs, technetium bone scans, single photon emission computed tomography (SPECT), CT scans, and MRI scans are all valuable studies. Rarely would all be needed together.

Plain radiographs consistently are found to be the most helpful imaging study. In most instances, anteroposterior and lateral radiographs of the spine should be obtained during the initial evaluation. This is especially true for children who are 4 years of age or younger, have had back pain longer than 2 months, have pain that awakens them from sleep, or have associated constitutional symptoms. Disk space narrowing, vertebral endplate irregularities, vertebral scalloping, destructive radiolucent or radiodense lesions, fractures, pars defects, and scoliosis are several of many abnormalities that can be detected. Often additional oblique radiographs will provide further detail of bony pathology in the area of concern, ie, spondylolysis. Adequate visualization of the pelvis is required, as some pathologic conditions that involve the pelvis can lead to complaints of back pain.

When plain radiographs are normal and the patient's neurologic examination is normal, a technetium bone scan should be the next imaging study obtained. This study should be limited to the entire spine and pelvis. The bone scan is quite sensitive, though not specific, in detecting abnormalities such as infection, benign and malignant neoplasms, and occult fractures. Single photon emission computed tomography (SPECT) may be useful when the plain bone scan is negative or equivocal and is usually obtained at the radiologist's recommendation. SPECT's superiority is recognized in detecting spondylolysis and for more precise localization of lesions within the spine.

If the child's neurologic examination is abnormal, imaging of the spinal cord and spinal canal is necessary and should be obtained prior to bone scan. Magnetic resonance imaging (MRI) is the optimal study for assessing the neural axis and is invaluable in diagnosing spinal cord tumors, syringomyelia, bone tumors, diskitis, and herniated disks (Fig. 1). Caution must be exercised to avoid overreading

MRI scans as positive for disk pathology in the adolescent and thereby assuming the back pain is a result of this abnormality. However, a recent prospective MRI study of 15-year-olds with and without back pain found that adolescents with early disk degenerative changes or disk protrusions were indeed at greater risk for having low back pain or developing it in the near future when compared to those without disk abnormalities.[1]

Bone tumors or stress fractures can also be seen on MRI, but surrounding soft tissue edema may lead to some difficulty in interpretation of the bone abnormalities. When a bone lesion is identified on plain radiographs or bone scan, a CT scan remains the best imaging study to clarify the extent of the pathology. CT myelography may still provide additional useful information in the evaluation of disk herniation.

Laboratory Evaluation

A complete blood count (CBC) with differential and an erythrocyte sedimentation rate (ESR) are the most useful screening tests and should be obtained early in young children, those complaining of night pain, and those with constitutional symptoms in which infection, lymphoma, or leukemia may be suspected. Testing for rheumatoid factor, antinuclear antibody, and HLA B27 may be helpful if a rheumatologic disorder is suspected.

Scheuermann's Disorder

Scheuermann's disorder is the most common cause of thoracic back pain and structural kyphosis in adolescents. The pain is described as dull, aching, and nonradiating, is generally localized to the midscapular area, and may be aggravated by standing, sitting, and physical activity. Often, poor posture is the presenting complaint,

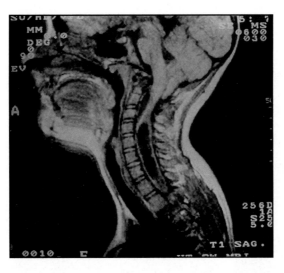

Fig. 1 MRI is currently the optimal study for assessing the neural axis. A large cervical syringomyelia is seen well on this MRI scan of the head and neck. (Reproduced with permission from Richards BS: Clinical assessment of back pain in children. *J Musculoskel Med* 1998; 15:31–40.)

with pain being present but not severe.[14,16] The physical examination demonstrates an increased, inflexible thoracic kyphosis (Fig. 2). Compensatory lumbar hyperlordosis may be present. The neurologic examination is usually normal.

The diagnosis is confirmed radiographically. Kyphosis exceeds 45° (normal range 20° to 45°) and is accompanied by wedging of at least 5° in 3 adjacent vertebra, vertebral end plate irregularities, narrowing of disk height, and occasional protrusion of disk material into the vertebral body (Schmorl's nodes). The apex of the deformity is usually located in the T7-T8 region (Fig. 3). Structural stiffness is often apparent when a lateral radiograph is taken with the patient lying supine over a bolster in an effort to hyperextend the spine. Further imaging studies are unnecessary.

The etiology of Scheuermann's disorder remains unknown. Theories include familial predisposition, hormonal abnormalities, collagen defects, juvenile osteoporosis, excessive manual labor, athletic injuries, and vitamin deficiencies. Ultrastructural studies have demonstrated thinning or absence of vertebral endplates and

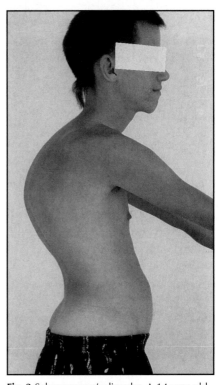

Fig. 2 Scheuermann's disorder. A 14-year-old boy with inflexible thoracic hyperkyphosis.

physes, disorganized chondrocytes, altered proteoglycan content, reduced amounts of collagen fibrils, and abnormal ossification.

Significant kyphosis or pain in adolescence is often cited as evidence of impending adult disability and, therefore, is a reason to initiate treat-

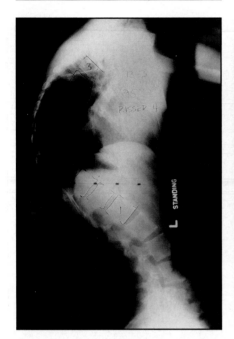

Fig. 3 A lateral radiograph of the patient in Figure 2 demonstrates the hyperkyphosis in the thoracic spine. Vertebral wedging and narrowed disk spaces are present.

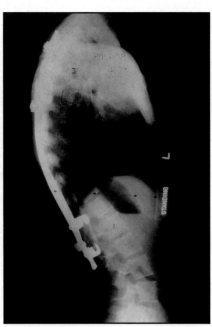

Fig. 4 A postoperative lateral radiograph of the patient in Figure 2 demonstrates the improved sagittal alignment in the thoracic spine.

ment. However, a recent natural history and long-term follow-up study found that those with Scheuermann's kyphosis adapted well to their condition and had few limitations.[17] When compared to controls, they had more intense back pain, jobs that tended to have lower requirements for activity, less motion in extension of the trunk, and different localization of pain. However, they did not differ from controls with respect to education, work absence because of low-back pain, self-esteem, medication use for back pain, or level of recreational activities. Pulmonary function was normal in those whose kyphosis was less than 100°. Mild scoliosis was noted but spondylolisthesis was not.

The majority of patients are treated nonsurgically. Brace treatment can improve the kyphosis during the time of spine growth.[18] The most effective brace is the Milwaukee brace, which applies a three-point force, anteriorly on the pubis and

sternum and posteriorly at the apex of deformity. Lower profile braces have not been shown to be effective. Factors suggestive of brace success include moderate deformity (< 70°), lower apex (T9 or below), flexibility, diffuse kyphosis instead of severe focal deformity, meaningful growth potential (> 2 years), and genuine interest in the deformity on the part of the child. If the kyphosis is rigid, serial casting may be needed before bracing. Exercises to stretch the hamstrings and lumbodorsal region and to strengthen abdominal muscles may improve symptoms of pain but will not change the deformity.

If surgical intervention is under consideration, acceptable indications for surgery include large deformities (> 70°), progressive deformity, pain, and genuine concern regarding appearance. Successful outcomes have been reported either by combining anterior release with posterior fusion/instrumentation or by posterior proce-

dure alone.[19,20] The role of anterior release remains controversial and its best indication appears to be in large, stiff deformities with focal kyphosis. Dual rod, multiple hook, segmental fixation systems are the preferred posterior instrumentation (Fig. 4). The complication of progressive short segment kyphosis immediately above or below the fusion is caused by failing to include every vertebra in the kyphotic segment.[21] Excessive deformity correction (more than 50%) increases the risk of proximal kyphosis. Failure to include the first lordotic disk space and non-wedged vertebrae inferiorly increases the risk of short segment kyphosis below the fusion.

Lumbar Scheuermann's disorder consists of the classic type, with 3 or more consecutive wedged vertebrae, or the atypical type, with only 1 or 2 affected vertebral bodies, Schmorl's nodes located anteriorly, and disk space narrowing.[22] In general, symptoms of back pain are found in the atypical form. Conservative management is recommended.

Painful Scoliosis

Generally, children and adolescents with scoliosis (idiopathic being the most frequently encountered) present for evaluation because of cosmetic concerns rather than back discomfort. However, in a recent study of 2,442 adolescent idiopathic scoliosis patients, some back pain was present in 23% of patients at the time of presentation and in an additional 9% during the course of follow-up.[23] Of patients with discomfort, only 9% were found to have an identifiable pathologic condition. When discomfort is present in this group of children, it usually is mild, nonspecific, intermittent, nonradiating, resolves with rest, and does not limit normal activities. Further investigation of the discomfort is usually not necessary.

However, when persistent severe back pain is the prominent complaint and a scoliotic deformity is noted secondarily, a thorough investigation into the source of pain is needed. Painful scoliosis is not a specific diagnosis, but it is a physical finding that may be associated with many of the disorders seen in Outline 1.

The physical examination may demonstrate stiffness in the lumbar spine due to muscle spasm. The position of the head, which is normally centered over the pelvis in children with idiopathic scoliosis, may be noticeably shifted out of balance (Fig. 5). Movement onto the examination table may be awkward as might the patient's gait. If the neurologic examination is abnormal, pathology involving the spinal cord is likely. It is, however, uncommon for patients with syringomyelia and scoliosis to present with back pain.

The initial investigation requires plain AP and lateral radiographs of the entire spine. Further views focusing on the more painful regions of the spine (or pelvis) may be needed. The radiographs should be carefully scrutinized for congenital abnormalities, disk space narrowing, lucencies or increased densities, pars defects, and bone erosions or expansions. An abnormality may be evident in the apical region of the curve.

If the patient's plain radiographs are unremarkable, and the neurologic examination is normal, then CBC, ESR, and technetium bone scan should be obtained next. Infection, neoplasms of the bone, and stress fractures of the pars can usually be localized with these tests. If the patient's neurologic examination is abnormal, an MRI of the spine should precede the technetium bone scan. Syringomyelia, spinal cord tumors, and disk herniation can readily be appreciated by

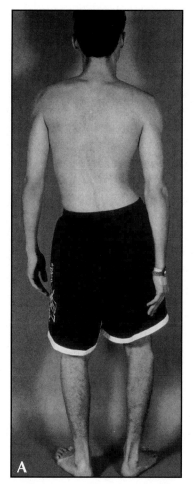

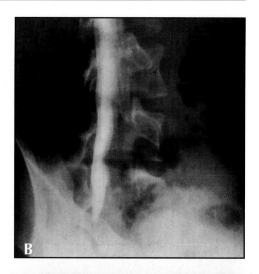

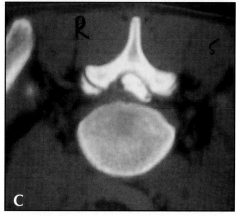

Fig. 5 A 16-year-old boy with a herniation of the L5-S1 disk. Clinical appearance demonstrates the out-of-balance convex left scoliosis (**A**). Radiograph and CT myelography clearly show the nerve root compression secondary to the L5-S1 disk herniation (**B, C**).

MRI. CT myelography may provide additional useful information when evaluating disk herniations. Once identified, the pathologic condition should be treated by the appropriate methods.

Infection
Infectious Spondylitis
Infectious causes must be considered in the differential diagnosis of back pain in children. Infectious spondylitis includes pyogenic infections of the vertebra-disk unit, including diskitis, vertebral osteomyelitis, non-specific spondylitis, and benign osteomyelitis of the spine.[24–26] Ring and associ-

ates[24,27] and Wenger and associates[28] have offered us the insight into some of the mechanisms for the propagation of infection in the child (Fig. 6). It is thought to spread from hematogenous sources initiated by bacteremia of multiple potential causes (URI, otitis, etc). Some have made theoretical association between trauma (frequently seen in youngsters) and bacteremia causing osteomyelitis.[29–31] Low-grade infection originating in the vertebral end plate can spread to the adjacent disk space through small vascular channels. Reaction in the adjacent vertebral marrow, if there is a delay in treat-

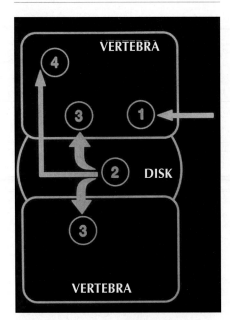

Fig. 6 The mechanism for propagation of infectious spondylitis is best understood using the disk-vertebra-disk model. Hematogenous bacteria settle in the apophysis (1), spread to both sides of the disk (2), affecting the adjacent vertebrae (3), and if there is a delay in treatment osteomyelitis can establish in the vertebra (4).

ment, can develop into vertebral osteomyelitis with late presentation.[32–35]

The apoplyses have end arteriolarvenous channels with sluggish blood flow, diminishing the clearance of bacteria by white cells with development of micro abscesses.[30,36] Disks are more vascular in children with direct vascular channels which close by 20 years of age when end plate ossification occurs. This difference in blood supply accounts for the rarity of true vertebral osteomyelitis in children and the predominance of osteomyelitis in adults and diskitis in children.[36,37]

Diskitis

Diskitis is the earliest phase in the spectrum of infectious spondylitis. Its diagnosis is based on clinical symptoms in the child, marked by limp, abdominal pain, hamstring spasm, or back pain. There is generally an elevation in the sedimentation rate (ESR) and radiographically a narrowed disk space can be noted. Diskitis affects children most commonly between 1 and 17 years of age. Symptoms will depend on the age of the child.[5] Those children less than 3 years of age will present with loss of ability to walk or to stand, not wanting to be moved very much. Not uncommonly there is fever and malaise. In the slightly older age group, between 3 and 8 years of age, abdominal pain is the primary symptom with a mild fever and elevation in the white blood cell count. The diskitis is generally in the low thoracic region. The older age group, between the ages of 8 and 17, will be characterized by back pain and may stand with an abnormal posture. This can be one of the causes of what is referred to as "painful scoliosis". A delay in diagnosis is common in this age group.

Physical examination begins with initial observation of the child in whatever position is most comfortable. Watching the child play with toys sitting on the floor, one might note a painful cry when he is coaxed to stand or held in a standing position.[29] Small children will cry and resist when their spine is flexed with the knees flexed and then pushed against the abdomen. This produces an increased pressure in the disk and elicits a painful response in the infected child. The hip examination will be negative. Children with diskitis may be able to crawl, but they generally do so without any lumbar lordosis and with a great deal of paraspinal muscle spasm. In the slightly older age group, between 3 and 8 years of age, there is a vague description of back or abdominal pain.[29] There are no localizing signs of peritonitis or specific areas of tenderness. There may be poorly localized areas of tenderness to percussion in the back. Children in this age group may be able to walk, but bending forward is difficult for them due to the increased pressure produced in the disk space. The 8- to 17-year group is generally able to verbalize sufficiently to localize the site of their pain. They generally have tenderness in their back with a clinical loss of lumbar lordosis with lack of reversal of the spinous processes on forward bending. They may maintain a normal posture except with flexion.

The workup includes a careful history including any antecedent infection, the chronicity of the complaints, and the onset of the symptoms. Previous otitis media is very common in the smaller children, with bouts of bacteremia. The history of how the patient has progressed over the previous few days prior to the examination can allow the physician some insight into how rapidly this has progressed as the parents tell the story of how much limitation there has been in play activity and how much time there has been simply holding the child for reassurance. The physical examination should start with uninvolved areas and progress to the more painful tests last. A neurologic examination is important to complete in the child. Plain radiographs, including AP and lateral views of the spine, should be done in the position of function, ie, standing or sitting. It should be remembered that plain radiographs may be normal early on, with disk space narrowing seen later in the course. The CBC may not be especially high, but the sedimentation rate is generally in the range of 50.[28,34] Other studies, including bone scan and MRI, may be necessary for the diagnosis and if there is an elevation in the sedimentation rate or there is strong suspicion, a bone scan offers the advantage of being less expensive and allowing for localization of the problem (Fig. 7). The MRI is very specific and diagnostic in infants and young children and will be necessary in the setting of any neurologic symptoms to visualize the spinal canal or in settings where the surrounding soft tissues need to be better analyzed.[26,27,38-40] The needle biopsy is only necessary when the child has not responded to the normal course of therapy.[28]

The most common organism that has been identified in children is *Staphylococcus aureus*.[24,28,29,31-35,41-43] The treatment is designed to treat this organism and most commonly first generation cephalosporins are administered intravenously until the signs and symptoms decrease markedly.[24,44] Some practitioners wait until the sedimentation rate begins to drop and then the child is switched to antibiotics by mouth for another 3 or 4 weeks. In the past, some authors have recommended benign neglect as a form of treatment for this disorder; however, with better understanding, it seems quite conclusive that the withholding of antibiotics is a mistake in these children.[24,28,31,32,42] Rest and immobilization certainly help in the healing process and occasionally this may include a corset brace, TLSO, or a body cast to enforce the rest. The chronicity of the symptoms will determine the need for immobilization.

Rarely, surgery for debridement of an abscess will be necessary and this should always be considered if the child is not responding appropriately to antibiotic therapy. A needle biopsy may be helpful to better direct antibiotics, especially if there is suspicion of tuberculosis.[28] If surgery is necessary, drainage alone is usually sufficient.[34] If debridement is extensive, anterior bone grafting with the use of rib or allograft fibula may be necessary for stability.

Vertebral Osteomyelitis

Later in the phase of infectious spondylitis, vertebral osteomyelitis develops. It can present with an acute or chronic presentation with systemic symptoms frequently seen including fever, back pain, and increased sedimentation rate.[24,28,32,35,43] Vertebral osteomyelitis occurs when bacteria spread from the disk area to the vertebral body, where they become established; this entity represents only 1% of pyogenic osteomyelitis.[32,35] Vertebral osteomyelitis generally occurs between 2 weeks and 8 years of age, the majority in the perinatal period. Correa and associates[32] reported on a series of 48 patient whose symptoms were fever (54%), back pain (43%), neck pain (14%), chest pain (8%), abdominal pain (14%), or flank pain (8%). Neurologic deficit occurred in 19% of patients, 1 with permanent sequelae. Gait abnormality, noted as a limp, occurred in 14% and it was associated with other areas of osteomyelitis in 10% of patients. A history of trauma is common.[28,32]

Vertebral osteomyelitis generally occurs in the lumbar spine but can also be seen in the thoracic, cervical, or lumbosacral areas.[32-35,41] Physical examination is similar to that for diskitis, but children are generally systemically ill with an elevated temperature, a great deal of tenderness, and stiffness on examination.[32]

The sedimentation rate will be elevated, with the mean ESR 58 (range 34–125).[32,43] Because of the more involved nature of this disorder, the white count is more commonly elevated, above 15,000. In patients who are younger than 3 months of age, the white count can be in the range of 24,000 to 59,000.[32] Bone scans are helpful for localization of infection

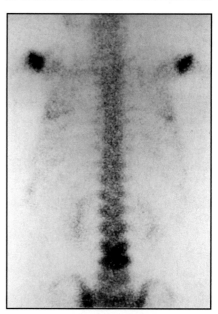

Fig. 7 Bone scan with increased uptake of technetium dye in adjacent vertebra of lumbar spine in a child with diskitis.

and then, if necessary, an MRI will better define the extent of the destruction in the surrounding tissues.[45]

Diagnostically, the onset from symptoms to actual diagnosis is often delayed by an average of 5 weeks.[24,32-35,41] Blood cultures or aspirate of the bone are positive 80% of the time and the organism is most commonly *Staphylococcus aureus* or Salmonella.[32] Treatment is directed at the specific bacteria. Radiographic changes in the spine appear 2 to 6 weeks from the onset of symptoms. The bone scan may be abnormal within 7 days of onset of symptoms, leaving a window during which the bone scan could be falsely negative. The MRI offers a specific localization of the infection. One might think of the bone scan as an aerial photograph to establish the diagnosis and localize the area. MRI is a cone-down view to more specifically outline surrounding tissue involvement, including the epidural space and the psoas muscle where abscesses tend to form.[24,35]

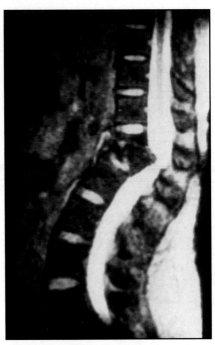

Fig. 8 Fifteen-year-old on chronic steroids with T12 vertebral osteomyelitis and collapsing kyphosis secondary to atypical mycobacterium.

The treatment takes longer than for diskitis, generally 6 weeks.[32,43]

Tuberculous Spondylitis

Spinal osteomyelitis secondary to *Mycobacterium tubercolosis* is common in children of developing countries and is a diagnostic problem in industrial countries because of its rarity.[46,47] The incidence of tuberculosis in North America is presently rising especially in immigrant populations, North American Indians, and in immunosuppressed individuals.[34,46,48] In these patients, the spine is a secondary area for infection, the primary being the pulmonary or genitourinary systems. A search for a primary site should be part of the evaluation. Infection in the spine occurs through lymphatic or hematogenous spread.[36]

The most common organism causing this infection is *Mycobacterium tuberculosis*, but atypical forms exist.

The vertebral body is affected, with collapse of the body producing vertebra plana. Frequently, more than a single level is involved in the infectious process leading to collapse, most commonly at the thoracolumbar junction with kyphosis[43] (Fig. 8). Neurologic signs may be present due to encroachment of the spinal canal by debris from the infectious process or by collapse producing kyphotic angulation and tension on the spinal cord itself.[46] Presentation depends on the stage of illness of the child; symptoms are frequently present for more than a year with symptoms consistent with chronic illness, that is, weight loss, malaise, anorexia, night sweats, and pain about the spine. The age at presentation is less than 5 years of age in 76% of patients.[49] These patients generally have a positive purified protein derivative (PPD) test with sputum and/or urine cultures positive for the primary. Paraplegia is seen in 50% of pediatric patients, but this is lower than seen with adults.[49] The white blood cell count and ESR are elevated; however the C-reactive protein is within normal limits.[30] MRI is especially helpful in detecting and defining an abscess, which can commonly occur.[48] Because of the high incidence of paraplegia, an MRI is necessary to visualize the spinal canal.

Treatment with antituberculous drugs, including streptomycin, rifampin, and Isoniazid, is started 1 to 2 weeks prior to debridement unless an emergency decompression is necessary for paraplegia, which has a good chance for recovery.[43] Surgery is almost always necessary, with anterior debridement of the diseased tissue and insertion of a strut for stability.

Spondylolysis and Spondylolisthesis

Spondylolysis appears as a stress fracture of the pars interarticularis in the lumbar spine, most commonly at L5. It occurs at the junction between the relative stability of the sacrum and the mobility of the lumbar segments. Spondylolysis can occur unilaterally or bilaterally and occurs more commonly in the setting of spina bifida occulta, where there is deficiency of the posterior sacral elements. It affects 4% to 6% of the population, but the exact incidence of low back pain in this population is unknown.[50,51] It usually appears beyond walking age and not at birth, implying man's upright bipedal position as a component in this disorder.[52–54] Spondylolisthesis is the forward slippage of the vertebral body away from the posterior elements. This can progress between ages 5 and 20, that is, during the growth period.[52]

The disorder is produced by an increased degree of lumbar lordosis over normal producing stress on the pars area leading to fracture with repetitive loading activities. Those activities that tend to load the pars area in young people are gymnastics, weight lifting, and other sports that require a hyperlordotic lumbar position.[51,55–57] A genetic predisposition appears likely, because it is frequently seen in other members of the same family.[51,53,57]

These patients frequently present in early adolescence with mid-line low lumbar pain, with or without sciatica, only occasionally will there be complaints of postural deformity.[55,58] Historically, the pain is initiated either during activity or afterwards. The pain is activity related and relieved by rest. Without treatment, it frequently progresses to the point of voluntary cessation of the activities that cause the pain.

On physical examination, the pain can be reproduced by hyperextension of the spine. In the area of the pars fracture, deep palpation over the midline or slightly off midline can reproduce the pain, and in the setting of spondylolisthesis, a palpable step off between the area of the unaffected lumbar spine and the loose posterior elements at the affected area can be noted. Hamstring tightness occurs in 80% of symptomatic patients.[52] With retroversion of the pelvis, in advanced stages of spondylolisthesis, a shortened torso may be seen. Uncommonly an abnormal gait may be noted with a pelvic waddle.[52]

Diagnosis may be difficult in the prefracture state. Clinical suspicion is necessary in order to make this diagnosis in patients whose oblique radiographs are normal. An increased amount of sclerosis in the area of the pars may be the only initial sign.[58] Upright AP and lateral radiographs (Fig. 9) of the lumbar spine and supine obliques are usually diagnostic in this condition. The upright lateral spot of the L5-S1 area is the most helpful radiograph for follow-up, observing for progression of the spondylolisthesis during the adolescent growth spurt. Bone scan with spectrometry has a high positive correlation with active disease.[59,60] A positive bone scan implies a state of activity that is amenable to treatment; a cold scan implies that the body's attempts at healing have ceased.[60] Spectrometry has added a higher level of diagnostic ability by identifying the disorder in its early phases before the appearance of a pars fracture radiographically or on a regular scan.[59] Occasionally, a CT scan (Fig. 10) with sagittal reconstruction may be necessary to better define the disorder, and MRI may be useful in the early diagnosis of spondylolysis. MRI is most useful for evaluation of the nerve roots.

Spondylolisthesis is best evaluated radiographically with the lateral view of the low lumbar spine and hips. Taillard described the percentage of

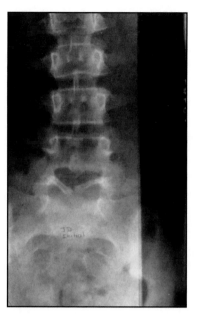 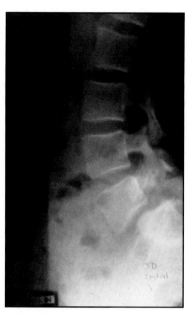

Fig. 9 AP and lateral erect views of lumbar spine in an 11-year-old with grade II spondylolisthesis and spina bifida occulta.

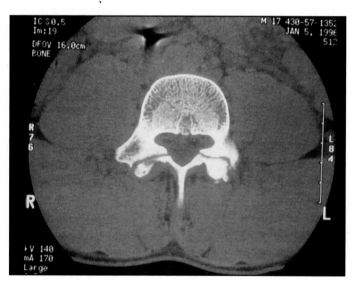

Fig. 10 CT scan of 16-year-old weight lifter with spondylolysis at L4.

slippage of L5 off of the top of S1 similar to Meyerding's classification, which divides the upper sacrum into quadrants. A grade I is less than 25% slip, grade II between 25% and 50% slip, grade III 50% to 75% slip, grade IV 75% to 100% slip, and a grade V greater than 100% slip, referred to as spondyloptosis.[28] Other measurements have been described that reflect the secondary rounding in the

upper sacrum or lower aspect of L5. The slip angle describes the forward rotation of L5 with slippage beyond 50%. As the sagittal rotation increases, the slip angle increases (Fig. 11). This is a poor prognostic sign and indicates a greater likelihood for further progression and a poor outcome from surgery.[61]

Wiltse has given us a classification system in which type I, congenital,

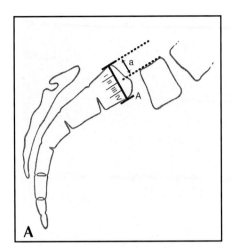
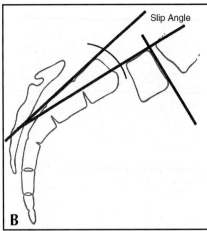

Fig. 11 A, The percentage slip of L5 on S1 is a/A and the grade of slippage is I to IV. B, The slip angle reflects sagittal rotation of L5, measured by intersection of lines from the posterior edge of L5 (perpendicular to the top of vertebra) and the posterior sacral line.

includes a dysplastic, elongated pars interarticularis with facets that subluxate at the L5-S1 level. It is important to recognize this classification in children because these patients are more prone to recurrent symptoms and deformity.[62,63] Type 2, isthmic, is characterized by a fracture of the pars interarticularis; subtype B is characterized by an elongation of the pars with a fracture, healing, and recurrent fracture pattern. Type 3, degenerative, type 4, traumatic, and type 5, pathologic, complete the major portion of the classification system. Of importance when considering back pain in children is a more recently noted type 6 secondary to surgical changes after laminectomy,[50] which has importance in spastic pediatric or adolescent patients having undergone rhizotomy. A 20% incidence of type 6 spondylolisthesis after rhizotomy has been reported.[64]

Nonsurgical Treatment

Nonsurgical treatment includes thoughtful counseling of the patient and the family regarding how the spinal disorder impacts on their present and future goals. Not uncommonly, spondylolysis occurs in aggressive young athletes who had hoped to achieve careers in professional sports. In this setting, there is a great deal of anxiety over potential scholarships and careers. Time taken discussing these anxieties in a realistic sense is time well spent. Bracing as an option for nonsurgical treatment has been promoted by some. In one study, a full-time brace program over 6 months produced healing of the pars in a third of patients. The healing of the pars is more likely to occur when the defect is unilateral and positive on bone scan.[59,61] Bracing produces a resolution of symptoms in the vast majority of patients even when healing is not effected.[55,65–67] It also allows patients to return to participation in their desired sport in the brace. The bone scan can be used to determine if the brace should be worn for the 6-month regimen with healing as the goal.

Physical therapy is helpful for abdominal and back strengthening and for education regarding the avoidance of risky activities such as barbell weights on the shoulders or overhead.[50,55,60] Activities that tend to load the lower lumbar spine in aggressive weightbearing and hyperextension activities can retard the healing process and worsen the symptoms.[28] Follow-up radiographs using the L5 spot lateral are important to watch for progression during the growth years. Generally nonsteroidal anti-inflammatory drugs are avoided because they can slow ossification and healing of the pars.

Surgical Treatment

Posterior intrasegmental fixation has been advocated by some for direct repair of the spondylolytic defect.[68,69] It is generally reserved for older adolescents with minimal slippage (< 7 mm) and a competent disk at the level of the pars defect.[57]

A posterolateral fusion has been the mainstay of surgical management for adolescents and young adults with persistently symptomatic spondylolysis or grade I and grade II spondylolisthesis.[52,62,69–74] The persistence of symptoms in spite of bracing and the absence of any other findings on further workup are prerequisites. Patients at greatest risk for surgery are those with acute spondylolisthesis, very tight hamstrings, females, and dysplastic types.[52,56] Some controversy exists regarding who qualifies for fusion, at what age, and at what degree of slippage.[61] Grade III or more in young adolescents, especially those with a worsening slip angle are at a high risk for progression and warrant surgery.[50,75–82] Grade II patients are at risk for further progression and should be considered as potential candidates for fusion.[52,76,82] Occasionally grade I older adolescents who have persistent symptoms will require fusion.

The mainstay of surgery is posterolateral intertransverse fusion, avoiding the Gill procedure unless decompression is felt to be necessary.[50,52,62,69,70–73,76–81,83] Symptomatic relief of leg pain is accomplished in the majority of young people undergoing in situ fusion alone.[61] The grade III, IV, and V immature patients pose a dilemma. There is some disagreement in the literature regarding the proper way to approach these patients surgically. Wiltse has promoted the use of in situ fusion alone, including L4 in the fusion mass if the superior boarder of the L5 is greater than 55° with reference to the horizontal on a standing film.[84] Others have noted nonunion and bending of the fusion mass with progression in high grade slips.[52,72,76] Rare cases of cauda equina have been reported after in situ fusion and require late decompression with sacroplasty (removal of prominent bone of posterosuperior corner of S1).[61,85,86] Because of this controversy, instrumentation techniques have been proposed to prevent further slippage of higher grade spondylolisthesis in young people. The use of pedicle screws, Luque wires, and supplemental casts as well as additional bone graft techniques have been recommended, although pedicle screws have not yet been approved for use in children.[78,81,83] With reduction maneuvers, root injuries can occur with any of these techniques.[77,81] It must be kept in mind that these procedures are technically difficult and in any reduction maneuver the emphasis should be on safe correction of the sagittal rotation. Translatory displacement is only corrected secondarily.

Additional procedures to enhance fusion have included the use of a fibular strut placed across the L5-S1 junction for interbody stabilization[87] (Fig. 12). Gaines has used an L5 vertebrectomy for older individuals with the placement of L4 on the sacrum in situations of spondyloptosis.[88] Post-

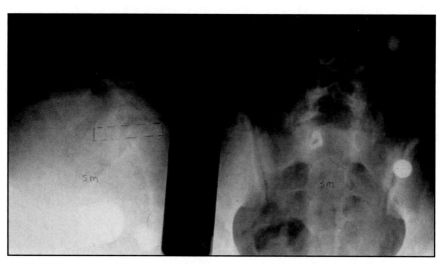

Fig. 12 Postoperative radiograph of a 15-year-old with in situ L5-S1 fusion supplemented with autogenous fibula placed posteriorly from S1 to L5.

operative immobilization in a pantaloon cast or braces incorporating thigh cuffs has also been helpful to enhance the L5-S1 fusion.[52] When considering additional supplemental procedures, it is important to remember that excellent results have been reported in most children undergoing an in situ fusion alone.[76] Supplemental intraoperative maneuvers and hardware offer additional risk and should be carefully considered prior to their utilization.

Herniated Disk and Slipped Vertebral Apophysis

The incidence of disk herniation in children with back pain has been reported to be from 0.8% to 3.2%. Children and adolescents account for approximately 1% of surgically treated patients. It is diagnosed equally in males and females but females predominate in the younger age group and males in older children (between 16 to 18 years of age). The diagnosis of herniated disk is difficult to establish as the symptoms are intermittent. The children tend to have a paucity of neurologic findings. Disk herniation is most commonly diagnosed at L4-

L5 and L5-S1 levels. A history of trauma is given as a precipitating factor in 37% to 50% of patients. There are often associated congenital abnormalities, such as transitional vertebra, congenital spinal stenosis, and spina bifida occulta.[89] Occasionally there is a positive family history of disk herniation.[7,90–92]

The most common symptoms are back pain presenting as "stiffness" and leg pain. The symptoms may be aggravated by prolonged sitting and standing and by coughing and sneezing. True motor weakness and bowel and bladder symptoms are rare.[93] The symptoms are often long standing (from several months to a year). On physical examination, there is back stiffness and limitation of range of motion in the lumbar spine, especially during flexion. There is tenderness in the lower lumbar spine and loss of normal lumbar lordosis. Scoliosis is seen in some patients, often with an exaggerated trunk shift. The most common finding, that of positive straight leg raising test, is noted in almost all patients. There are subtle sensory, motor or reflex changes in about 50% of patients. It is often difficult to localize the level of disk herniation based on clinical examination.

Plain radiographs may show a sagittal or a coronal deformity due to spasticity in the paraspinal musculature. Occasionally there is narrowing of the disk space. The most helpful imaging study is MRI. CT-myelogram is occasionally used and often confirms the diagnosis.

Although the treatment for herniated disks in children often needs to be aggressive, the patients should be offered a course of nonsurgical treatment if there is no neurologic deficit. This treatment includes a short period of complete bed rest and medications, including analgesic muscle relaxants and anti-inflammatories. Once the symptoms have subsided, a period of stretching and physical therapy may be helpful. Occasionally an epidural steroid injection may be helpful, but this has not been studied in children and the long-term effects are not known.

There are few long-term studies of conservative treatment of disk herniation in children.[94] Approximately 50% of patients show improvement after this type of treatment. The indications for surgical treatment include failed nonsurgical treatment or presence of significant neurologic deficit. It is very important to determine if the ring apophysis is fractured. If there is a ring fracture, a simple laminectomy may not be adequate and a formal decompression for spinal stenosis is needed to prevent possible neurologic deficit. If there is only disk herniation, a laminectomy, microdiskectomy, or chemonucleolysis is done. There are reports that the chemonucleolysis with surgery as a backup procedure has a good long-term success.[95] The minimally invasive techniques used in the adult population have not been widely used in the pediatric age group.

Spine Fractures

Children with spine fractures usually have a history of a major traumatic episode to explain their symptoms. The incidence of thoracic and lumbar fractures in children is not known, but spinal fractures in children are reported to account for 2% to 3% of all injuries in children. The incidence of pediatric spine injuries peaks in 2 age groups, children 5 years old or younger and children older than 10. Twenty percent of patients have associated neurologic deficit.[96,97]

Spinal injuries unique to children include slipped vertebral apophysis, spinal cord injury without radiographic abnormalities (SCIWORA) and injuries in child abuse.

SCIWORA

Traction, cord rupture, traumatic infarction, blunt abdominal trauma, interference of the vascular supply, and soft-tissue enfolding are all possible etiologic factors in SCIWORA. This injury accounts for 16% to 90% of spinal cord injuries in children. Kewalramani and associates[98] reviewed several series of SCIWORA in the infant to 16-year age group and found that 23 of 33 patients (70%) had paraplegia from spinal cord injuries below T1. Although most of the injuries were from motor vehicle accidents, other causes, such a fall and electrocution, were found. Although myelography has been used to diagnose this problem, MRI seems to be a more accurate diagnostic tool.

Slipped Vertebral Apophysis

Slipped vertebral apophysis is an injury characterized by avulsion of bony fragment from the posterior rim of the vertebral body associated with the central disk herniation. It is often the result of repetitive trauma, which separates the apophyseal ring from the vertebral body through its weak osteocartilaginous junction. It is more common in males than females and in the inferior border of L4 and the superior border of S1. Children often present acutely following trauma, and the mechanism of injury is usually flexion and rotation. Takata and associates[99] divided these fractures into 3 types and Epstein and Epstein[100] introduced a type IV to this classification as follows. Type I fractures are pure avulsions of posterior cortical margins without attendant osseous defect (pure cartilage injuries). Type II fractures are larger central fractures that include portions of cancellous and cortical bony rim. Type III fractures are more localized and lateral as tear drop fractures. Type IV fractures span the entire length and breadth of the posterior vertebral body.

These injuries may present clinically with findings similar to a herniated disk. This injury is often missed or the diagnosis may be delayed for weeks (Fig. 13). In a series reported by Epstein from 27 patients, stiffness and spasm were seen in 27, numbness and weakness in 23, neurologic claudication in 24, and cauda equina in 2. The imaging studies included plain radiograph, which was positive in 5, and MRI, positive in 6 (Fig. 13). All 27 CT-myelogram studies were diagnostic.

Fractures Resulting from Child Abuse

The incidence of spinal fractures in child abuse is from 0% to 3% and it is important to have a high index of suspicion for this injury.[96,101,102] Many times young children show no evidence of spine deformity despite significant spinal injury. A lateral spine radiograph should be included in all skeletal surveys to detect subtle compression fractures of the vertebral

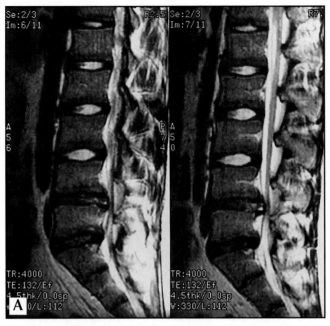
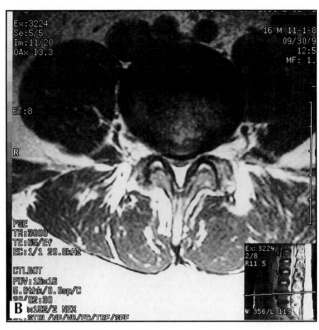

Fig. 13 A 17-year-old boy with a 16-month history of back pain. He sustained an injury playing basketball and continued to be symptomatic off and on and presented with stiffness and inability to move his lumbar spine. He had no neurologic deficit. **A** and **B**, Magnetic resonance imaging showing narrow spinal canal as well as degenerative changes at L4-L5 and L5-S1 and disk herniation at L4-L5 with end plate fracture. Note the compression of the dural sac.

body, disk narrowing, or true subluxation or dislocation. Spinal injuries in children may go unrecognized and only present with a vague history of back pain (Fig. 14). Plain radiographs are the primary method of detection. However, MRI and other more accurate imaging studies may demonstrate a more detailed picture. Radiographically, these injuries most commonly affect vertebral bodies, with anterior compression and notching near the superior end plates. There may be narrowing of the disk space, mimicking diskitis, or a true fracture dislocation may be seen. These changes must be differentiated from normal developmental changes that occur in the growing vertebral bodies.

Neoplasms

Spinal tumors can cause back pain and spinal deformity in children. The child usually has a tight back and tends to deviate to the side while bending forward. There may be local tenderness in the area of the tumor. The pain may present day or night and is not fully relieved by bed rest.

Benign Tumors

These tumors are relatively rare and because of structural complexity of the spine, frequently cause problems in diagnosis and treatment.[103,104]

Osteoid Osteoma and Osteoblastoma Osteoid osteoma accounts for approximately 1% of all spinal tumors and 11% of all primary benign tumors.[105–108] Ten percent of osteoid osteomas are seen in the spine. The age range is from 10 to 25 years and the male to female ratio is 2:1. These tumors have a strong predilection for the posterior vertebral elements, with the lamina and pedicle being the most frequent sites. Scoliosis develops because of the asymmetric involvement of the vertebra and subsequent muscle spasm (Fig. 15). Tumors usually are located around the apex of the curve on the concave side. Bone scan

is the most sensitive method of localizing an osteoid osteoma. In 80% of patients the diagnosis is made within 2 years of onset.

Osteoblastoma accounts for 1% of all primary benign tumors, and more than 40% are located in the spine. The size of the tumor is larger than an osteoma and usually more than 2 cm in diameter. The location of the tumors is similar to that of osteoid osteoma, with the lamina and pedicle being the most frequent sites. In this lesion, nonsteroidal anti-inflammatory medications are usually ineffective. Spinal deformity with neurologic deficit is often observed. In some instances, lesions may mimic other conditions such as aneurysmal bone cyst.[109]

In their retrospective study of 44 museum cases of spinal osteoid osteoma or osteoblastoma, and using a meta analysis of 421 additional cases from the literature, Saifuddin and associates[110] found that, overall, 63%

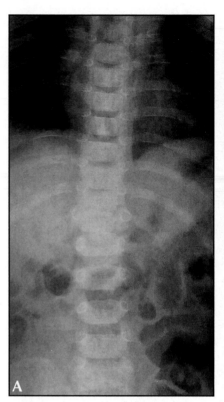
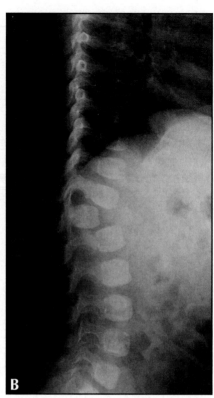
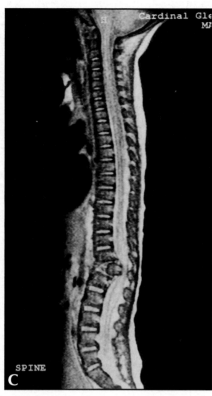

Fig. 14 A 10-month-old boy with a 5-day history of irritability and unwillingness to move his neck. He was taken to the pediatrician's office because of stiffness and inability to stand. He was admitted to the hospital with a tentative diagnosis of aseptic meningitis and a workup revealed T12 fracture-dislocation. **A** and **B,** AP and lateral views of the spine showing the fracture-dislocation. **C,** MRI sagittal reconstruction and the dislocation of T12 posteriorly. At surgery it was noted that the cartilaginous end plate had split in the coronal plane and the anterior half of the superior end plate had remained with the T11-T12 disk. The posterior half of the superior end plate had moved posteriorly into the canal along with the vertebral body. The entire inferior end plate remained with the T12-L1 disk and had not extruded posteriorly.

of subjects had scoliosis. All the lesions except 3 were typically present on the concave aspect of the curve.[110] They found that the scoliosis was significantly more common in cases of osteoid osteoma than in cases of osteoblastoma. Lesions were more common in the thoracic and lumbar levels than cervical levels. Age, gender, and duration of symptoms were not significant. They concluded that the findings support the concept that scoliosis is secondary to asymmetric muscle spasm in these patients.

The treatment may include nonsteroidal anti-inflammatories in cases of osteoid osteoma, but surgical excision is the treatment of choice in both tumors. Using different imaging techniques, such as bone scan and MRI, the lesion should be precisely localized before surgery. If scoliosis is present for a long time (more than 15 months), and especially in osteoblastoma, it is more likely to become structural and less likely to improve after surgery. Following excision, the margins of the tumor with the host should be carefully labeled to rule out any possibility of incomplete excision. Incomplete excision may lead to a 10% recurrence rate. Radiation therapy remains controversial and has been reported by some investigators to be ineffective.

Aneurysmal Bone Cyst The etiology of aneurysmal bone cysts is unclear, and they may arise from bones with preexisting lesions. Twenty percent are located in the spine, more commonly in the lumbar spine. Sixty percent of cases are located in the posterior elements and 20% to 40% of cases involve more than a single vertebra.[111] Clinical presentation includes back pain, loss of lumbar range of motion, scoliosis, swelling around the vertebral column, local tenderness, and neurologic deficit.

The treatment is usually surgical, with curettage and excision being the treatment of choice. Embolization may be indicated to prevent excessive bleeding. Radiation is rarely indicated, as it may lead to myelitis and malignant transformation.[112]

Eosinophilic Granuloma (Histiocytosis) Eosinophilic granuloma usually is seen in children younger than 10 years of age, and it is very common in the spine. The pain may or may not be a predominant feature and neurologic deficit is rare. In younger children, rapid collapse causes vertebra plana; in older children, wedge-shaped deformity is present. Once the other causes of vertebral collapse are ruled out, observation is usually all that is needed.

Malignant Tumors

Leukemia is the most common cancer in children, and patients can present with a history of back pain. The symptoms are nonspecific and the diagnosis is difficult to make unless there is a high index of suspicion. Usually a bone scan is not helpful and blood tests lead to the diagnosis. Other malignant tumors include Ewing's sarcoma and osteosarcoma. Metastatic tumors have unique characteristics and should be considered on rare occasions.[113-115]

Summary

A variety of disorders can account for back pain in the child or adolescent (Outline 1). Some of these can result in significant morbidity if not properly diagnosed and treated. Fortunately, nearly all can be correctly diagnosed by taking a thorough medical history, performing a complete physical examination, and obtaining appropriate imaging and laboratory studies. Although back pain in children and adolescents may result from overuse or minor trauma and will respond to rest and anti-inflammatories, this review should enable the orthopaedist to systematically recognize those back disorders in need of more aggressive medical intervention.

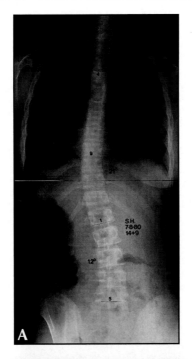
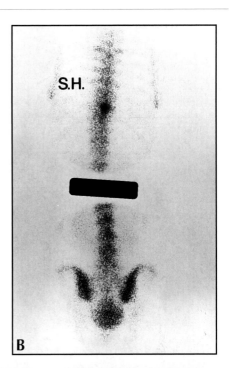
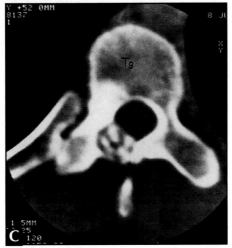
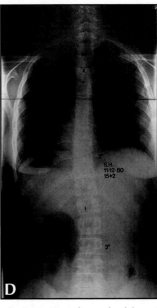

Fig. 15 14-year-old-girl with a history of back pain and scoliosis. **A,** PA radiograph of the spine showing a left thoracic scoliosis with the apex at T9. **B,** A bone scan was positive. **C,** CT scan shows precise location of osteoid osteoma in the right lamina. **D,** Following excision of the tumor the spinal deformity and pain completely resolved.

References

1. Salminen JJ, Erkintalo M, Laine M, Pentti J: Low back pain in the young: A prospective three-year follow-up study of subjects with and without low back pain. *Spine* 1995;20:2 101–2107.

2. Turner PG, Green JH, Galasko CS: Back pain in childhood. *Spine* 1989;14:812–814.

3. Fairbank JC, Pynsent PB, Van Poortvliet JA, Phillips H: Influence of anthropometric factors and joint laxity in the incidence of adolescent back pain. *Spine* 1984;9:461–464.

4. Grantham VA: Backache in boys: A new problem? *Practitioner* 1977;218:226–229.

5. Balague F, Dutoit G, Waldburger M: Low back pain in school children: An epidemiological study. *Scand J Rehabil Med* 1988;20:175–179.

6. Burton AK, Clarke RD, McClune TD, Tillotson KM: The natural history of low back pain in adolescents. *Spine* 1996;21:2323–2328.

7. Taimela S, Kujala UM, Salminen JJ, Vijanen T: The prevalence of low back pain among children and adolescents: A nationwide, cohort-based questionnaire survey in Finland. *Spine* 1997;22:1132–1136.

8. Hensinger RN: Back pain in children, in Bradford DS, Hensinger RN (eds): *The Pediatric Spine*. New York, NY, Thieme, 1985, pp 41–60.

9. King HA, Tufel D: Prospective study of back pain in children *Orthop Trans* 1986;10:9–10.

10. Feldman DS, Wright JG, Hedden DM: Back pain in children and adolescents. *Orthop Trans* 1995;19:350.

11. Davids JR, Wenger DR: Back pain in children and adolescents: An algorithmic approach. *J Musculoskel Med* 1994;11:19–32.

12. Karol L: Evaluation of back pain, in Richards BS (ed): *Orthopaedic Knowledge Update: Pediatrics*. Rosemont, IL, American Academy of Orthopaedic Surgeons, 1996, pp 11–18.

13. King H: Back pain in children, in Weinstein SL (ed): *The Pediatric Spine: Principles and Practice*. New York, NY, Raven Press, 1994, pp 173–183.

14. Thompson GH: Back pain in children. *J Bone Joint Surg* 1993;75A:928–938.

15. Rogalsky RJ, Black GB, Reed MH: Orthopaedic manifestations of leukemia in children. *J Bone Joint Surg* 1986;68A:494–501.

16. Koop S: Scheuermann's disorder, in Richards BS (ed): *Orthopaedic Knowledge Update: Pediatrics*. Rosemont, IL, American Academy of Orthopaedic Surgeons, 1996, pp 125–127.

17. Murray PM, Weinstein SL, Spratt KF: The natural history and long-term follow-up of Scheuermann kyphosis. *J Bone Joint Surg* 1993;75A:236–248.

18. Sachs B, Bradford D, Winter R, Lonstein J, Moe J, Willison S: Scheuermann kyphosis: Follow-up of Milwaukee-brace treatment. *J Bone Joint Surg* 1987;69A:50–57.

19. Lowe TG, Kasten MD: An analysis of sagittal curves and balance after Cotrel-Dubousset instrumentation for kyphosis secondary to Scheuermann's disease: A review of 32 patients. *Spine* 1994;19:1680–1685.

20. Sturm PF, Dobson JC, Armstrong GW: The surgical management of Scheuermann's disease. *Spine* 1993;18:685–691.

21. Reinhardt P, Bassett GS: Short segmental kyphosis following fusion for Scheuermann's disease. *J Spinal Disord* 1990;3:162–168.

22. Blumenthal SL, Roach J, Herring JA: Lumbar Scheuermann's: A clinical series and classification. *Spine* 1987;12:929–932.

23. Ramirez N, Johnston CE, Browne RH: The prevalence of back pain in children who have idiopathic scoliosis. *J Bone Joint Surg* 1997;79A:364–368.

24. Ring D, Johnston CE II, Wenger DR: Pyogenic infectious spondylitis in children: The convergence of discitis and vertebral osteomyelitis. *J Pediatr Orthop* 1995;15:652–660.

25. Crawford AH, Kucharzyk DW, Ruda R, Smitherman HC Jr: Diskitis in children. *Clin Orthop* 1991;266:70–79.

26. Szalay EA, Green NE, Heller RM, Horev G, Kirchner SG: Magnetic resonance imaging in the diagnosis of childhood discitis. *J Pediatr Orthop* 1987;7:164–167.

27. Ring D, Wenger DR: Magnetic resonance-imaging scans in discitis: Sequential studies in a child who needed operative drainage. A case report. *J Bone Joint Surg* 1994;76A:596–601.

28. Wenger DR, Bobechko WP, Gilday DL: The spectrum of intervertebral disc-space infection in children. *J Bone Joint Surg* 1978;60A:100–108.

29. Freeman BL: Disc space infections, in Wood GW (ed): *Spinal Infections*. Philadelphia, PA, Hanley & Belfus, 1989, pp 453–459.

30. Whalen JL, Fitzgerald RH Jr, Morrissy RT: A histological study of acute hematogenous osteomyelitis following physeal injuries in rabbits. *J Bone Joint Surg* 1988;70A:1383–1392.

31. Spiegel PG, Kengla KW, Isaacson AS, Wilson JC Jr: Intervertebral disk-space inflammation in children. *J Bone Joint Surg* 1972;54A:284–296.

32. Correa AG, Edwards MS, Baker CJ: Vertebral osteomyelitis in children. *Pediatr Infect Dis J* 1993;12:228–233.

33. Eismont FJ, Bohlman HH, Soni PL, Goldberg VM, Freehafer AA: Vertebral osteomyelitis in infants. *J Bone Joint Surg* 1982;64B:32–35.

34. Joughin E, McDougall C, Parfitt C, Yong-Hing K, Kirkaldy-Willis WH: Causes and clinical management of vertebral osteomyelitis in Saskatchewan. *Spine* 1991;16:261–264.

35. Schwartz ST, Spiegel M, Ho G Jr: Bacterial vertebral osteomyelitis and epidural abscess. *Semin Spine Surg* 1990;2:95–105.

36. Whalen JL, Parke WW, Mazur JM, Stauffer ES: The intrinsic vasculature of developing vertebral end plates and its nutritive significance to the intervertebral discs. *J Pediatr Orthop* 1985;5:403–410.

37. Coventry MB, Ghormley RK, Kernohan JW: The intervertebral disk: Its microscopic anatomy and pathology. I: Anatomy, development, and physiology. *J Bone Joint Surg* 1945;27A:105–112.

38. du Lac P, Panuel M, Devred P, Bollini G, Padovani J: MRI of disc space infection in infants and children: Report of 12 cases. *Pediatr Radiol* 1990;20:175–178.

39. Forster A, Pothmann R, Winter K, Baumann-Rath CA: Magnetic resonance imaging in non-specific discitis. *Pediatr Radiol* 1987;17:162–163.

40. Gabriel KR, Crawford AH: Magnetic resonance imaging in a child who had clinical signs of discitis: Report of a case. *J Bone Joint Surg* 1988;70A:938–941.

41. Eismont FJ, Bohlman HH, Soni PL, Goldberg VM, Freehafer AA: Pyogenic and fungal vertebral osteomyelitis with paralysis. *J Bone Joint Surg* 1983;65A:19–29.

42. Scoles PV, Quinn TP: Intervertebral discitis in children and adolescents. *Clin Orthop* 1982;162:31–36.

43. Wenger DR, Davids JR, Ring D: Discitis and osteomyelitis, in Weinstein SL (ed): *The Pediatric Spine: Principles and Practice*. New York, NY, Raven Press, 1994, pp 813–835.

44. Nelson JD, Bucholz RW, Kusmiesz H, Shelton S: Benefits and risks of sequential parenteral-oral cephalosporin therapy for suppurative bone and joint infections. *J Pediatr Orthop* 1982;2:255–262.

45. Modic MT, Feiglin DH, Piraino DW, et al: Vertebral osteomyelitis: Assessment using MR. *Radiology* 1985;157:157–166.

46. Upadhyay SS, Sell P, Sajim J, Sell B, Yau AC, Leong JC: Seventeen year prospective study of surgical management of spinal tuberculosis in children: Hong Kong operation compared with debridement surgery for short- and long-term outcome of deformity. *Spine* 1993;18:1704–1711.

47. Medical Research Council Working Party on Tuberculous of the Spine: A 10-year assessment of a controlled trial comparing debridement and anterior spinal fusion in the management of tuberculosis of the spine in patients on standard chemotherapy in Hong Kong. *J Bone Joint Surg* 1982;64B:393–398.

48. Desai SS: Early diagnosis of spinal tuberculosis by MRI. *J Bone Joint Surg* 1994;76B:863–869.

49. Bailey HL, Gabriel M, Hodgson AR, Shin JS: Tuberculosis of the spine in children: Operative findings and results in one hundred consecutive patients treated by removal of the lesion and anterior grafting. *J Bone Joint Surg* 1972;54A:1633–1657.

50. Pizzutillo PD, Hummer CD III: Nonoperative treatment for painful adolescent spondylolysis or spondylolisthesis. *J Pediatr Orthop* 1989;9:538–540.

51. Stinson JT: Spondylolysis and spondylolisthesis in the athlete. *Clin Sports Med* 1993;12:517–528.

52. Hensinger RN: Spondylolysis and spondylolisthesis in children and adolescents. *J Bone Joint Surg* 1989;71A:1098–1107.

53. Turner RH, Bianco AJ Jr: Spondylolysis and spondylolisthesis in children and teen-agers. *J Bone Joint Surg* 1971;53A:1298–1306.

54. Lucey SD, Gross R: Painful spondylolisthesis in a two-year-old child. *J Pediatr Orthop* 1995;15:199–201.

55. Blanda J, Bethem D, Moats W, Lew M: Defects of pars interarticularis in athletes: A protocol for nonoperative treatment. *J Spinal Disord* 1993;6:406–411.

56. Jackson DW, Wiltse LL, Cirincione RJ: Spondylolysis in the female gymnast. *Clin Orthop* 1976;117:68–73.

57. Schlenzka D, Poussa M, Seitsalo S, Osterman K: Intervertebral disc changes in adolescents with isthmic spondylolisthesis. *J Spinal Disord* 1991;4:344–352.

58. Halperin N, Copeliovitch L, Schachner E: Radiating leg pain and positive straight leg rais-

ing in spondylolysis in children. *J Pediatr Orthop* 1983;3:486–490.

59. Collier BD, Johnson RP, Carrera GF, et al: Painful spondylolysis or spondylolisthesis studied by radiography and single-photon emission computed tomography. *Radiology* 1985;154:207–211.

60. Jackson DW, Wiltse LL, Dingeman RD, Hayes M: Stress reactions involving the pars interarticularis in young athletes. *Am J Sports Med* 1981;9:304–312.

61. Newton PO, Johnston CE II: Analysis and treatment of poor outcomes following in situ arthrodesis in adolescent spondylolisthesis. *J Pediatr Orthop* 1997;17:754–761.

62. Seitsalo S, Osterman K, Poussa M, Laurent LE: Spondylolisthesis in children under 12 years of age: Long-term results of 56 patients treated conservatively or operatively. *J Pediatr Orthop* 1988;8:516–521.

63. Papageloupoulos PJ, Peterson HA, Ebersold MJ, Emmanuel PR, Choudhury SN, Quast LM: Spinal column deformity and instability after lumbar or thoracolumbar laminectomy for intraspinal tumors in children and young adults. *Spine* 1997;22:442–451.

64. Peter JC, Hoffman EB, Arens LJ: Spondylolysis and spondylolisthesis after five-level lumbosacral laminectomy for selective posterior rhizotomy in cerebral palsy. *Childs Nerv Syst* 1993;9:285–287.

65. Steiner ME, Micheli LJ: Treatment of symptomatic spondylolysis and spondylolisthesis with the modified Boston brace. *Spine* 1985;10:937–943.

66. Bell DF, Ehrlich MG, Zaleske DJ: Brace treatment for symptomatic spondylolisthesis. *Clin Orthop* 1988;236:192–198.

67. Morita T, Ikata T, Katoh S, Miyake R: Lumbar spondylolysis in children and adolescents. *J Bone Joint Surg* 1995;77B:620–625.

68. Nicol RO, Scott JH: Lytic spondylolysis: Repair by wiring. *Spine* 1986;11:1027–1030.

69. Buck JE: Direct repair of the defect in spondylolisthesis: Preliminary report. *J Bone Joint Surg* 1970;52B:432–437.

70. Burkus J, Lonstein J, Winter RB, Denis F: Long-term evaluation of adolescents treated operatively for spondylolisthesis: A comparison of in situ arthrodesis only with in situ arthrodesis and reduction followed by immobilization in a cast. *J Bone Joint Surg* 1992;74A:693–704.

71. Lenke LG, Bridwell KH, Bullis D, Betz RR, Baldus C, Schoenecker PL: Results of in situ fusion for isthmic spondylolisthesis. *J Spinal Disord* 1992;5:433–442.

72. Sherman FC, Rosenthal RK, Hall JE: Spine fusion for spondylolysis and spondylolisthesis in children. *Spine* 1979;4:59–66.

73. Stanton RP, Meehan P, Lovell WW: Surgical fusion in childhood spondylolisthesis. *J Pediatr Orthop* 1985;5:411–415.

74. Velikas EP, Blackburne JS: Surgical treatment of spondylolisthesis in children and adolescents. *J Bone Joint Surg* 1981;63B:67–70.

75. Hilibrand AS, Urquhart AG, Graziano GP, Hensinger RN: Acute spondylolytic spondylolisthesis: Risk of progression and neurological complications. *J Bone Joint Surg* 1995;77A:190–196.

76. Boxall D, Bradford DS, Winter RB, Moe JH: Management of severe spondylolisthesis in children and adolescents. *J Bone Joint Surg* 1979;61A:479–495.

77. Bradford DS: Closed reduction of spondylolisthesis: An experience in 22 patients. *Spine* 1988;13:580–587.

78. Fabris DA, Constantini S, Nena U: Surgical treatment of severe L5-S1 spondylolisthesis in children and adolescents: Results of intraoperative reduction, posterior interbody fusion, and segmental pedicle fixation. *Spine* 1996;21:728–733.

79. Freeman BL III, Donati NL: Spinal arthrodesis for severe spondylolisthesis in children and adolescents: A long-term follow-up study. *J Bone Joint Surg* 1989;71A:594–598.

80. Johnson JR, Kirwan EO: The long-term results of fusion in situ for severe spondylolisthesis. *J Bone Joint Surg* 1983;65B:43–46.

81. Schwend RM, Waters PM, Hey LA, Hall JE, Emans JB: Treatment of severe spondylolisthesis in children by reduction and L4-S4 posterior segmental hyperextension fixation. *J Pediatr Orthop* 1992;12:703–711.

82. Harris IE, Weinstein SL: Long-term follow-up of patients with grade-III and IV spondylolisthesis: Treatment with and without posterior fusion. *J Bone Joint Surg* 1987;69A:960–969.

83. Boos N, Marchesi D, Aebi M: Treatment of spondylolysis and spondylolisthesis with Cotrel-Dubousset instrumentation: A preliminary report. *J Spinal Disord* 1991;4:472–479.

84. Wiltse LL, Winter RB: Terminology and measurement of spondylolisthesis. *J Bone Joint Surg* 1983;65A:768–772.

85. Maurice HD, Morley TR: Cauda equina lesions following fusion in situ and decompressive laminectomy for severe spondylolisthesis: Four case reports. *Spine* 1989;14:214–216.

86. Schoenecker PL, Cole HO, Herring JA, Capelli AM, Bradford DS: Cauda equina syndrome after in situ arthrodesis for severe spondylolisthesis at the lumbosacral junction. *J Bone Joint Surg* 1990;72A:369–377.

87. Smith MD, Bohlman HH: Spondylolisthesis treated by a single-stage operation combining decompression with in situ posterolateral and anterior fusion: An analysis of eleven patients who had long-term follow-up. *J Bone Joint Surg* 1990;72A:415–421.

88. Lehmer SM, Steffee AD, Gaines RW Jr: Treatment of L5-S1 spondyloptosis by staged L5 resection with reduction and fusion of L4 onto S1 (Gaines procedure). *Spine* 1994;19:1916–1925.

89. Epstein JA, Epstein NE, Marc J, Rosenthal AD, Lavine LS: Lumbar intervertebral disk herniation in teenage children: Recognition and management of associated anomalies. *Spine* 1984;9:427–432.

90. Garrido E: Lumbar disc herniation in the pediatric patient. *Neurosurg Clin N Am* 1993;4:149–152.

91. Kling T: Herniated nucleus pulposus and slipped vertebral apophysis, in Weinstein SL (ed): *The Pediatric Spine: Principles and Practice.* New York, NY, Raven Press, 1994.

92. Silvers HR, Lewis PJ, Clabeaux DE, Asch HL: Lumbar disc excisions in patients under the age of 21 years. *Spine* 1994;19:2387–2391.

93. Martinez-Lage JF, Martinez Robledo A, Lopez F, Poza M: Disc protrusion in the child: Particular features and comparison with neoplasms. *Childs Nerv Syst* 1997;13:201–207.

94. DeLuca PF, Mason DE, Weiand R, Howard R, Bassett GS: Excision of herniated nucleus pulposus in children and adolescents. *J Pediatr Orthop* 1994;14:318–322.

95. Bradbury N, Wilson LF, Mulholland RC: Adolescent disc protrusions: A long-term follow-up of surgery compared to chymopapain. *Spine* 1996;21:372–377.

96. Chambers HG, Akbarnia BA: Thoracic lumbar and sacral spine fractures and dislocations, in Weinstein S (ed): *The Pediatric Spine: Principles and Practice.* New York, NY, Raven Press, 1994.

97. Ferguson RL: Thoracic and lumbar spinal trauma of the immature spine, in Rothman RH, Simeone FA (eds): *The Spine.* Philadelphia, PA, WB Saunders, 1992, pp 501–512.

98. Kewalramani LS, Tori JA: Spinal cord trauma in children: Neurologic patterns, radiologic features, and pathomechanics of injury. *Spine* 1980;5:11–18.

99. Takata K, Inoue S, Takahashi K, Ohtsuka Y: Fracture of the posterior margin of a lumbar vertebral body. *J Bone Joint Surg* 1998;70A:589–594.

100. Epstein NE, Epstein JA: Limbus lumbar vertebral fractures in 27 adolescents and adults. *Spine* 1991;16:962–966.

101. Akbarnia BA: The role of the orthopaedic surgeon in child abuse, in Morrissy RT, Weinstein SL (eds): *Lovell aned Winter's Pediatric Orthopaedics,* ed 4. Philadelphia, PA, JB Lippincott, 1996, pp 1315–1331.

102. Akbarnia BA, Torg, JS, Kirkpatrick RT, et al: Manifestations of the battered-child syndrome. *J Bone Joint Surg* 1974;456:1159.

103. Beer SJ, Menezes AH: Primary tumors of the spine in children: Natural history, management, and long-term follow-up. *Spine* 1997;22:649–658.

104. Weinstein JN: Differential diagnosis and surgical treatment of primary benign neoplasms, in Frymoyer JW (ed): *The Adult Spine: Principles and Practice.* New York, NY, Raven Press, 1994, pp 830–850.

105. Akbarnia BA, Bradford DS, Winter RB: Osteoid osteoma of the spine. *Orthop Trans* 1982;6:373.

106. Azouz EM, Kozlowski K, Marton D, Sprague P, Zerhouni A, Asselah F: Osteoid osteoma and osteoblastoma of the spine in children: Report

of 22 cases with brief literature review. *Pediatr Radiol* 1986;16:25–31.

107. Marsh BW, Bonfiglio M, Brady LP, Enneking WF: Benign osteoblastoma: Range of manifestations. *J Bone Joint Surg* 1975;57A:1–9.

108. Pettine KA, Klassen RA: Osteoid-osteoma and osteoblastoma of the spine. *J Bone Joint Surg* 1986;68A:354–361.

109. Akbarnia BA, Rooholamini SA: Scoliosis caused by benign osteoblastoma of the thoracic or lumbar spine. *J Bone Joint Surg* 1981;63A: 1146–1155.

110. Saifuddin A, White J, Sherazi Z, Shaikh MI, Natali C, Ransford AO: Osteoid osteoma and osteoblastoma of the spine: Factors associated with the presence of scoliosis. *Spine* 1998;23: 47–53.

111. Tillman BP, Dahlin DC, Lipscomb PR, Stewart JR: Aneurysmal bone cyst: An analysis of ninety-five cases. *Mayo Clin Proc* 1968;43:478–495.

112. Akbarnia BA, Ganjavian MS: Aneurysmal bone cysts of the spine. *Orthop Trans* 1987;11:41.

113. Gupta P, Lenke LG, Bridwell KH: Incidence of neural axis abnormalities in infantile and juvenile patients with spinal deformity: Is a magnetic resonance image screening necessary? *Spine* 1998;23:206–210.

114. Mottl H, Koutecky J: Treatment of spinal cord tumors in children. *Med Pediatr Oncol* 1997;29: 293–295.

115. Weinstein JN: Spine neoplasms, in Weinstein SL (ed): *The Pediatric Spine: Principles and Practice.* New York, NY, Raven Press, 1994.

Current Concepts in Myelomeningocele

James C. Drennan, MD

Myelomeningocele Foot Deformities

Foot deformities, the most common orthopaedic problem in the spina bifida population, generally result from muscle imbalance. The lower lumbar and sacral nerve roots supply the extrinsic and intrinsic muscles to the foot, and these are the levels most commonly affected in these patients.[1]

The articular cartilage of the hind and midfoot bones serve both as the articular joint surface and also as growth cartilage. These bones are particularly vulnerable to in utero deformation caused by muscle imbalance (Hueter-Volkmann law) (Fig. 1). In addition, patients with a high level of neurologic loss may also develop foot deformities because of the unopposed adverse effects of gravity.

Rehabilitation goals include a braceable plantigrade foot that retains its correction and permits upright activities at an appropriate age for desired motor development. Several general principles must be observed in the management of these insensate foot deformities: (1) The skin and neurovascular structures are frequently contracted, which may limit the degree of surgical correction. Infant management by gentle manipulation and serial casting generally allows skin closure at the time of surgery. (2) Complete surgical correction of the hindfoot and midfoot deformity must be accomplished or

recurrence can be expected. (3) Any muscle imbalance should be addressed at the time of correction of the bony architecture. A single tendon that is active can be neutralized by transfer to the midline, eg, tibialis anterior to the heel during correction of a calcaneovarus deformity. (4) Tenotomy or tendon resection may be necessary. The major exception to this rule is the tibialis posterior muscle, which can be lengthened but should never be sacrificed. Loss of hindfoot inversion can lead to iatrogenic hindfoot valgus, which is difficult to manage orthotically.

The age of the child determines the type of surgical correction. Children younger than 4 years of age should have surgery limited to soft-tissue structures. Older children may benefit from the addition of osteotomies. Arthrodeses are not recommended because they may unnecessarily shorten the foot and may produce rotational overload on adjacent joints, which could lead to either arthritic or neuropathic joint changes.

Management of Specific Foot Deformities

Equinovarus Deformity

This rigid form of clubfoot is generally associated with retained activity or contracture of the tibialis anterior and tibialis posterior muscles, particularly in patients with L-4 level myelomeningocele. Serial gentle manipula-

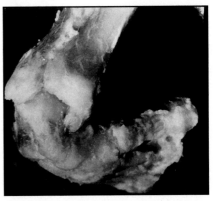

Fig. 1 The ankle joint protects the talar body. The talar neck and head as well as the other bones of the hindfoot and midfoot are deformed by the muscle imbalance.

tions and casting during the first 6 months mobilize the soft tissues and permit primary closure of the skin at the time of surgery. A comprehensive clubfoot release, performed through a Cincinnati incision, includes lengthening of the tibialis posterior and the Achilles tendon as well as transfer of active tibialis muscle to the dorsal midfoot. Thickened capsular structures may make dissection tedious. Correction of the subtalar rotational deformity is essential. Kirschner wire fixation of the talocalcaneal and talonavicular joints is followed by 4 months of long leg casting. The patient is then transferred into an ankle-foot orthosis.

Equinovarus has the highest incidence of recurrence of any type of

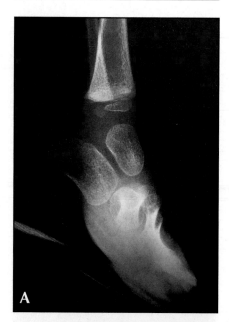

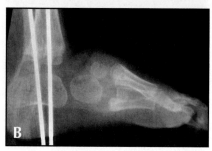

Fig. 2 A, Preoperative lateral maximum dorsiflexion radiograph demonstrates severe equinovarus deformity. **B,** Following talectomy and heelcord lengthening, the foot achieves a plantigrade position.

foot deformity. Children younger than 4 years of age benefit from repeat comprehensive release. A talectomy through an anterolateral approach may be more appropriate when there is scarification and loss of mobility of the medial heel soft tissue[2] (Fig. 2). Residual hindfoot varus can be managed by a lateral closing wedge calcaneal osteotomy or a lateral displacement horizontal calcaneal osteotomy. Residual forefoot adduction in children older than 5 years of age can be effectively corrected by metatarsal osteotomies. When the deformity occurs in the midfoot,

shortening of the lateral column of the foot through the os calcis or cuboid may be combined with an opening medial cuneiform osteotomy. Hindfoot arthrodeses should be avoided because of the risk of the development of neuropathic changes in the neighboring joints.

Tarsal medulostomy offers an additional method of managing a rigid equinocavovarus deformity. This procedure has the advantage of not requiring general anesthesia because the foot is insensate. Enucleation of the calcaneus and cuboid is followed by manual correction of the deformity. This procedure is most commonly indicated to allow the introduction of ankle-foot orthoses and shoes. Proper foot placement on the wheelchair foot rest improves the patients sitting stability and weight distribution.

A variety of opening and closing wedge osteotomies can be used. The lateral column can be lengthened or shortened through the calcaneal neck as well as through the cuboid. Medial cuneiform lengthening is effective in correcting forefoot adduction.

Vertical Talus

The congenital vertical talus combines rigid hindfoot equinus with forefoot dorsiflexion and eversion (Fig. 3). The dorsal dislocation of the navicular onto the anterior talar head and neck is the hallmark of the rigid medial longitudinal column deformity. The more severe form includes a dorsal subluxation or dislocation of the calcaneocuboid joint, which indicates that the lateral longitudinal column is also involved. Paresis of the tibialis posterior has been implicated in this severe form of a flatfoot.[3] The rigid hindfoot is plantarflexed beneath the tibia. The dislocation of the transverse tarsal articulation occurs in line with the anterior border of the tibia.

Preliminary soft-tissue serial cast-

ing begins in the newborn period with surgical correction through a Cincinnati incision undertaken at the age of 9 months. The one-stage open reduction includes lengthening of all extrinsic muscles to the foot except the tibialis posterior muscle which is shortened (Fig. 4). Muscle imbalance to the hindfoot and forefoot is corrected by transferring the tibialis anterior to the talar neck and the peroneus longus to the navicular with its distal segment reattached to the peroneus brevis. Extensive capsular releases include the calcaneocuboid joint when the lateral column is involved. After 4 months of plaster immobilization, the patient is fitted with an ankle-foot orthosis. When surgery is delayed until 5 years of age, it may be necessary to excise the navicular to shorten the medial longitudinal column.

Hindfoot Valgus

Hindfoot valgus can develop at the subtalar or ankle joints or a combination of both joints. Accurate radiographic documentation is important to locate the level and plan correction.

Subtalar Valgus

The presence or absence of subtalar motion determines the type of surgical approach. A medial displacement calcaneal osteotomy performed through a lateral heel exposure is recommended when the subtalar joint has restricted motion, eg, as a result of previous surgery.[4,5] The lateral column is shortened in the flexible pes planovalgus foot. This permits the unsupported talar head to plantarflex into a weight-bearing position and results in potential skin embarrassment. Mobile subtalar and transverse tarsal articulation joints permit use of a calcaneal lengthening osteotomy.[6] Dilwyn Evans[7] stated that the normal foot is composed of 2 longitudinal columns, which should be equal in length. The lateral column is lengthened through an opening wedge osteotomy of the calcaneal neck, which repositions the distal calcaneus beneath the talar head. Equalization of the length of the columns also restores the medial longitudinal arch.

Ankle Valgus

These patients demonstrate a weight-bearing radiologic triad, which includes shortening of the fibula, lateral wedging of the distal tibial epiphysis, and lateral tilt of the talus.[8]

Ankle valgus greater than 7° may require surgical management to avoid medial malleolar skin embarrassment. Tenodesis of the Achilles tendon to the distal fibular diaphysis has been effective in patients younger than 8 years of age.[9] Placement of multiple small staples over the distal medial tibial epiphysis is the preferred technique for patients between the ages of 8 and 12 years, with the goal being correction to at least neutral alignment of the ankle mortise[10] (Fig. 5). Older patients gain correction by a closing wedge supramalleolar osteotomy. Choosing this approach in younger patients may result in progressive distal tibial diaphyseal deformity secondary to the continued growth of the distal tibia. Supramalleolar derotational osteotomy can be used in patients as young as 4 years of age for isolated rotational correction.

Equinus Deformity

This deformity results from failure to protect the flail foot from the effects of gravity or, occasionally, from retained reflex sacral activity in the triceps surae and long toe flexors. Proper use of prophylactic orthotics that extend to the toes can prevent this deformity. Fixed paralytic equinus that exceeds 20° of fixed contracture requires a posterior release.

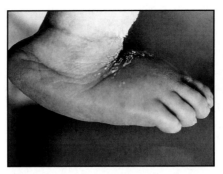

Fig. 3 Congenital convex pes valgus foot deformity shows the rocker-bottom contour as well as a hollow sulcus anterior to the lateral malleolus.

Equinus secondary to reflex activity has a propensity to recur. It is most appropriately managed by radical resection of the offending tendons, which alternatively may be transferred into the distal tibia.

Cavus

Pes cavus refers to forefoot equinus and generally results from a loss of intrinsic musculature. The addition of terms such as equinus and calcaneus describe the position of the hindfoot, which is critical in determining the method for correction. Weightbearing radiographs are necessary to understand the location of the deformity.

Cavus deformities in myelomeningocele patients present most frequently during adolescence and may be associated with cock-up toe deformity secondary to intrinsic loss. Isolated cavus can be addressed by combining metatarsal osteotomies with soft-tissue correction of the toe deformity, including lengthening of the long toe extensors, dorsal metatarsophalangeal capsulotomies, and tenodesis of the long toe flexor to their first phalanx. Kirschner wire fixation for 6 weeks is recommended.

Equinocavus deformity requires a

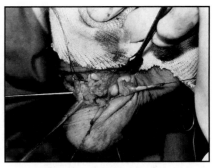

Fig. 4 A Kirschner wire introduced into the talar body gives control to the surgeon and permits the bone to be dorsiflexed. The midfoot is plantarflexed to reduce the talonavicular joint which is fixed under direct vision.

2-stage approach. The cavus correction is achieved by soft-tissue plantar release, with the forefoot being dorsiflexed against the fixed hindfoot. A staged second procedure can then correct the plantarflexed hindfoot deformity.

Calcaneocavus deformity can progress rapidly because of unopposed retained activity of the dorsal musculature, combined with the progressive dorsal calcaneal rotation. Soft-tissue procedures include the early transfer of the conjoined tendon of the tibialis anterior and hypertrophied peroneus tertius through the interosseous membrane to the os tuber, with additional selective lengthening of the other dorsiflexors. Older children may benefit from a posterior displacement calcaneal osteotomy combined with metatarsal osteotomies.[11]

Brinker and associates[12] recently reported that long-term review of sacral level myelomeningocele patients demonstrated a significant adult loss of their previous independent ambulation. One third of the patients, who initially were community ambulators, had lost this skill when examined at age 30 years. Progressive loss of plantar sensation coupled with the loss of plantarflex-

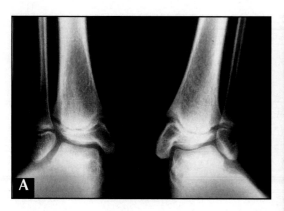

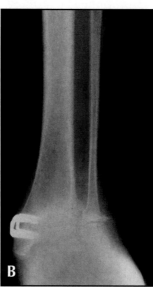

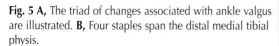

Fig. 5 A, The triad of changes associated with ankle valgus are illustrated. **B,** Four staples span the distal medial tibial physis.

ion muscle power was believed to be responsible. Plantar ulceration developed secondary to excessive localized skin pressure particularly beneath the os calcis and metatarsal heads. Five of his 29 patients eventually required below-knee amputation.

Orthotics

Lower extremity orthoses provide functional advantages to the spina bifida population. The brace can stabilize a weightbearing joint that lacks adequate muscle control, thereby promoting upright function. Bracing may facilitate daytime activities by providing stability at the expense of limiting joint motion. The physician must balance the functional need for joint motion with the need for stabilization of that joint. Orthotics cannot correct a fixed deformity but can control the corrected limb following surgery and maintain a plantigrade position of the foot. Orthotics may permit wearing shoes both for ambulation and protective coverage. Well-padded night-time orthotics can passively control position to prevent unnecessary or recurrent contracture.

Patients who retain antigravity strength in their quadriceps and medial hamstring muscles can be expected to be functional adult ambulators. Upright activities provide both physiologic and psychologic benefits to the patient. Braces may allow the patient to achieve appropriate motor milestones at an age comparable to their uninvolved peers. Orthotics may free the upper extremities to permit development of bimanual skills. My personal philosophy favors bracing high to ensure that the patient succeeds at mastering a specific upright activity. This achievement increases the patient's physical performance and self confidence. The level of bracing can be decreased as the patient's motor skills and social maturation improve, which is accomplished by an increased comprehension of the goals of the therapist and family. The absence of sensation in the lower extremity denies the patient distal proprioceptive feedback. This problem may also necessitate an initial high level of bracing for transference of sensation and perception

of motion to more proximal sensate joints.

Orthotics for the Lower Extremities
Ankle-Foot Orthoses (AFOs)

Orthotic stabilization of the ankle joint, a keystone to upright activity, can be accomplished by the use of an AFO, which replaces the weak or absent triceps surae muscle. Most unbraced myelomeningocele patients have excessive ankle dorsiflexion during stance, which compels the more proximal knee and hip joints to adapt to a flexion posture and makes ambulation very cumbersome. The AFO also acts to protect the insensate and uncontrolled ankle joint from excessive degenerative stress or risk of neuropathic changes. Proper positioning of the feet on the wheelchair foot plate aids balance and reduces pressure on the buttocks and thighs.

Plastic AFOs are constructed from high temperature thermoplastic materials, such as polypropylene, polyethylene, or copolymer, which is a combination of the two. The positive mold permits modifications for relief, and the orthotics are vacuum formed for accurate fit. The most utilitarian is the solid ankle AFO, which includes a posterior shell with anterior calf-strap. The orthotic foot plate is extended to the tips of the toes to protect the insensate phalanges.

A floor-reaction AFO stabilizes the ankle joint and uses plantarflexion of a few degrees in the foot component to transfer its reactive force to assist in knee extension. Patients who lack antigravity quadriceps may find that the floor reaction AFO will increase their functional quadriceps strength by one-half grade. A prerequisite for successful use is the ability to fully extend the knee joint. Flexion contractures of greater than 10° cause the reactive force to dissi-

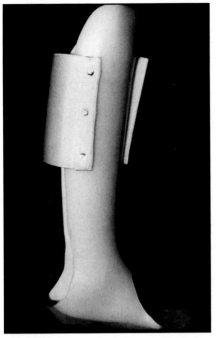
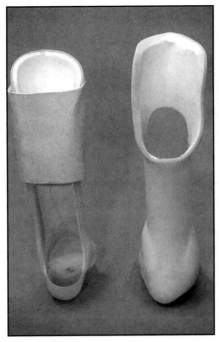
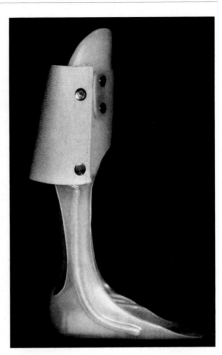

Fig. 6 The differences between the posterior entry and anterior entry floor-reaction ankle-foot orthosis braces are shown.

pate anterior to the axis of motion of the knee. Currently, floor reaction AFOs are commonly used for patients with midlumbar motor levels. This form of orthosis can also be incorporated as a component in a more extensive bracing system. Both front entry and rear entry single-unit, floor-reaction AFOs can be used (Fig. 6). The posterior entry has the potential advantage of offering rigid, circumferential orthotic extension over the dorsum of the ankle joint. This enables the patient to stand upright with the ankle locked in a neutral alignment. The posterior entry form has a potential disadvantage, because its distal dorsal edge may irritate and eventually ulcerate the insensate skin. Frequent inspection is necessary, and care must be taken to respond to any skin irritation, particularly in patients whose feet are prone to dependent swelling. The posterior heel lip may also irritate the insensate fat pad and necessitate reverting to the more traditional

anterior entry form, which does not stabilize the ankle joint as rigidly.

Patients with short, stubby feet may benefit from a metal double upright AFO with a 90° ankle stop. All dorsiflexion is blocked to stabilize the ankle. The uprights are attached to a steel shank in the shoe and use a proximal leather cuff. Leather T-straps may be added for control of ankle varus or valgus and act to pull the leg over the foot. The soft leather is more forgiving than the rigid plastic material and the shoe can comfortably adapt to the individual foot shape. Extra depth shoes may be needed. Metal braces are heavier, and shoe styles are limited, which can pose social problems for adolescents.

The introduction of a varus or valgus window to an AFO is the plastic equivalent of the leather T-strap.[13,14] The concept is again to take advantage of the more durable skin and subcutaneous fat of the calf to draw the leg over the foot and spare skin

embarrassment over the vulnerable malleoli (Fig. 7).

Knee-Ankle-Foot Orthoses (KAFOs)

Most forms of KAFOs use double uprights and knee hinges to join the thigh cuff to the AFO. Knee flexion contractures of greater than 20° may prevent adequate bracing, and these can be corrected by prone-lying with the patient taking advantage of gravitational forces on the unsupported leg. Occasionally a surgical correction is required.

A variety of hinges can be used, with the traditional droplock the most commonly employed. There is the occasional need for posterior offset hinges or bail locks. A ratchet type of knee joint can be used to gain the final few degrees of necessary extension. A KAFO with a free knee joint may be used to control a patient who has adequate motor strength to ambulate with below knee bracing, but whose gait pattern results in a valgus and external rota-

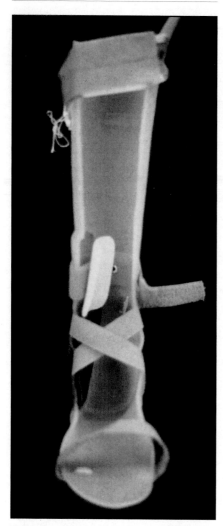

Fig. 7 The addition of a valgus-producing window assists in the control of hindfoot varus.

tional force at the knee joint. A varus producing strap or knee cage are additional options.

Hip-Knee-Ankle-Foot Orthoses (HKAFOs)

Thoracic level patients require orthotic control of all lower extremity joints. Their prescription includes hip and knee joints equipped with droplocks. A unilateral hip abduction hinge permits the patient to perform self catheterization. A molded pelvic girdle or a pelvic band may be used. These patients generally develop a swing-to or swing-through type of gait, because they cannot actively initiate hip flexion. Children in HKAFOs have a significantly higher energy consumption rate than children in reciprocal gait orthoses. Children with a swing-through pattern in HKAFOs had significantly faster velocity.[15]

Reciprocal-Gait Orthoses (RGOs)

Reciprocal-gait orthoses can be used by patients who have either a thoracic or high lumbar motor level and who cannot expend sufficient energy to walk with traditional HKAFOs.[15] The system supplies a flexion assist and requires a pelvic band. The gear type RGO combines flexion of one hip with obligatory extension of the opposite hip. The flexion power of one hip is used to extend the contralateral hip. Hip flexion can be controlled by adding gluteal extenders or a posterior lumbosacral shell in lieu of the pelvic band.

Standing-Frame Orthoses

Standing-frame orthotics offer a similar level of support to the HKAFO but are mounted on a base plate. This design allows hands-free, crutchless standing and limited mobility by a swiveling technique. These are most commonly used in children between the ages of 1 and 2 years with a thoracic or high level lumbar lesion. The parapodium, Orthotic Research and Locomotor Assessment Unit (ORLAU) swivel walker and the A-frame designs are examples of this level of bracing. Adults with myelomeningocele using the ORLAU ParaWalker had the same rate of compliance as patients who became paraplegic following an adult traumatic spinal injury.[16]

Latex Allergy

The diagnosis and management of latex allergies has become a major concern to physicians caring for myelomeningocele. The initial case of contact dermatitis due to latex surgical gloves was reported in 1979.[17] Anaphylactic reactions to latex products have become increasingly common, because these products are ubiquitous in today's health care industry. Current literature suggests that 6% of all medical personnel and 18% to 40% of spina bifida patients develop latex sensitivity.[18] Patients with major congenital urologic anomalies are another high-risk group. Persons allergic to bananas, water chestnuts, kiwi, passion fruit, and avocados are also considered high-risk individuals. Latex sensitivity occurs in only one of 3,000 persons in the general population.

The initial exposure for most spina bifida patients occurs at the time of newborn closure of the myelomeningocele. Repeated urologic self-catheterization has also been identified as a major contributor to the problem in susceptible individuals. All spina bifida patients should be screened for latex allergy prior to admission or before any ambulatory procedure. It is very important to obtain a detailed history of previous latex exposure and possible allergic reactions.

Types of Reaction

Type I Type I is a rare immediate response, which can be life threatening. These patients develop an IgE antibody to a latex sap antigen that remains as a residual free protein material after the rubber vulcanization process.[19] The anaphylactic reaction is triggered by a sudden release of histamine from mast cells and basophiles. The term 'anaphylaxis' describes an exaggerated allergic immunologic reaction to a foreign protein and includes a blood pressure drop of greater than 30 ml, stridor, wheezing, rash, angioedema, and bronchospasm. Clinically, the anesthetized patient rapidly develops tachycardia, precipitous hypotension, bronchospasm, and upper body flushing. These cutaneous, respiratory, and circulatory events are the result of peripheral vasodilation due to increased vascular permeability and decreased intravascular volume. The conscious patient may initially note perioral tingling and a feeling of warmth. The patient may experience difficulty swallowing, become apprehensive, and develop physical findings similar to those of an anesthetized patient.

Exposure can occur by skin, inhalation, mucous membranes, or intravenous means, and the patient may become sensitized to the latex antigen. Major mucosal or pleuroperitoneal exposure, eg, during an anterior spinal fusion, make the patient susceptible to the rapid entrance of antigenic substances into the bloodstream.[18] Powder on rubber products such as gloves or catheters may act as the vehicle for transmission of the protein allergen, which can easily be eluded from the surfaces of the latex products.[20] This type of anaphylactic reaction occurs between 40 to 300 minutes after anesthetic induction. In contrast, reactions to anesthetic agents generally occur within 5 minutes after the initiation of anesthesia.

Type IV Type IV reaction, the most common form of latex allergy, represents a delayed hypersensitivity whose response is mediated by T-lymphocytes. The response may not be seen until 2 days following the antigenic exposure. The skin reacts to the released histamine by developing a contact urticaria, eg, swollen lips after balloon contact. Pulmonary problems include bronchospasm and laryngeal edema. Rhinoconjunctivitis is also common. Treatment of type IV

reactions is limited to the use of antihistamine medications.

Preoperative Management
Preoperative protocols for latex allergy prophylaxis have been developed for myelomeningocele patients who have been identified as having a risk for, or are known to have an allergy to latex. This approach reduces their exposure to a systemic reaction to latex. The specific protocol varies with the documented type of previous allergic reaction. Patients requiring intravenous (IV) prophylaxis need to be admitted with sufficient time allowed for the administration of medications. Patients needing oral prophylaxis have to be scheduled to accommodate their specific medication regimen. Preoperative planning should include the use of stopcocks for drug injection, nonlatex gloves and tourniquets, as well as appropriate medications with the individual drug dose calculated per weight.

Preoperative Latex Allergy Prophylaxis
Type I Reaction Patients are admitted 24 hours before the procedure and an IV is started on admission to the unit. Prophylactic medications are administered intravenously prior to surgery and continued for 24 hours postoperatively. Medications for these patients are: (1) diphenhydramine, 1 mg/kg every 6 hours (minimum 3 doses preoperatively; maximum 50 mg/dose); (2) methylprednisolone, 1 mg/kg every 6 hours (minimum 3 doses preoperatively; maximum 40 mg/dose); (3) cimetidine, 1 mg/kg every 6 hours (minimum 3 doses preoperatively; maximum 300 mg/dose) or ranitidine, 1 to 2 mg/kg every 8 hours (minimum 3 doses preoperatively, maximum 150 mg/dose), which should be substituted in patients receiving medications such as

anticonvulsants, theophylline, or oral contraceptives, or for patients with hepatic disease whose metabolism may be affected by cimetidine; (4) albuterol administered every 6 hours for patients with reactive airway disease (asthma); (5) aerosol (inhaler), 1 to 2 metered inhalations (when each delivers 90 mcg); (6) nebulization, 0.5 ml of 0.5% solution in 2.5 normal saline (0.25 ml dose for children 2 years of age in 2.5 normal saline).

Preoperative Latex Allergy Prophylaxis for Type IV Reaction An anesthetist will administer IV prophylaxis 1 hour prior to surgery. Alternatively, oral prophylaxis is administered 24 hours prior to surgery. Medications for these patients are: (1) diphenhydramine, 3 doses preoperatively; maximum 50 mg/dose); (2) prednisone, 2 mg/kg every 6 hours (minimum 3 doses preoperatively; maximum 60 mg/dose); (3) cimetidine, 1 mg/kg every 6 hours (minimum 3 doses preoperatively; maximum 300 mg/dose).

Additionally, patients in a high-risk group with the diagnosis of spina bifida or congenital urologic anomalies who have not demonstrated a latex allergy but who have been exposed to latex are treated with the following oral prophylactic regimen given 12 hours prior to surgery: (1) diphenhydramine, 1 mg/kg every 6 hours (minimum 3 doses preoperatively; maximum 50 mg/dose); (2) prednisone, 1 mg/kg every 6 hours (minimum 3 doses preoperatively; maximum 60 mg/dose); (3) cimetidine, 1 mg/kg every 6 hours (minimum 3 doses preoperatively; maximum 300 mg/dose).

Patients who must undergo an emergency or urgent procedure, who have had or who are at risk for latex allergy, should be treated as type I patients and receive intravenous prophylaxis as soon as feasible. Cimetidine and ranitidine should be excluded from these regimens for patients who have a significant history of asthma in addition to latex allergy susceptibility.

Intraoperative Protocol These patients should be scheduled as the first cast of the day, irrespective of their age, to decrease their exposure to airborne latex. It is imperative that latex exposure be avoided during surgery. This can be accomplished by using nonlatex equipment, eg, silicone or plastic catheters, syringes, and drapes; the use of plastic anesthesia circuits, including endotracheal tubes, oxygen masks, and neoprene anesthesia bags; rinsing the nonlatex gloves; and protecting the blood pressure cuff from skin contact by cotton padding. Postoperatively, the patient should avoid latex during the entire hospitalization, have latex-free products at the bedside, and warning signs on the door and bed so that visitors are made aware of the medical problem.

General Precautions These patients should wear a Medic Alert bracelet. Patients with type I response should carry autoinjectable epinephrine. A radioallergosorbent test (RAST) is helpful but not diagnostic and currently lacks the sensitivity and specificity to be recommended as a routine screening test.

References

1. Sharrard WJ, Grosfield I: The management of deformity and paralysis of the foot in myelomeningocele. *J Bone Joint Surg* 1968;50B:456–465.

2. Menelaus MB: Talectomy for equinovarus deformity in arthrogryposis and spina bifida. *J Bone Joint Surg* 1971;53B:468–473.

3. Drennan JC, Sharrard WJ: The pathological anatomy of convex pes valgus. *J Bone Joint Surg* 1971;53B:455–461.

4. Koutsogiannis E: Treatment of mobile flat foot by displacement osteotomy of the calcaneus. *J Bone Joint Surg* 1971;53B:96–100.

5. Trieshmann H, Millis M, Hall J, Watts H: Sliding calcaneal osteotomy for treatment of hindfoot deformity. *Orthop Trans* 1980;4:305.

6. Mosca VS: Calcaneal lengthening for valgus deformity of the hindfoot: Results in children who had severe, symptomatic flatfoot and skewfoot. *J Bone Joint Surg* 1995;77A:500–512.

7. Evans D: Calcaneo-valgus deformity. *J Bone Joint Surg* 1975;57B:270–278.

8. Malhotra D, Puri R, Owen R: Valgus deformity of the ankle in children with spina bifida aperta. *J Bone Joint Surg* 1984;66B:381–385.

9. Stevens PM, Toomey E: Fibular-Achilles tenodesis for paralytic ankle valgus. *J Pediatr Orthop* 1988;8:169–175.

10. Burkus JK, Moore DW, Raycroft JF: Valgus deformity of the ankle in myelodysplastic patients: Correction of stapling of the medial part of the distal tibial physis. *J Bone Joint Surg* 1983;65A:1157–1162.

11. Mitchell GP: Posterior displacement osteotomy of the calcaneus. *J Bone Joint Surg* 1977;59B:233–235.

12. Brinker MR, Rosenfeld SR, Feiwell E, Granger SP, Mitchell DC, Rice JC: Myelomeningocele at the sacral level: Long-term outcomes in adults. *J Bone Joint Surg* 1994;76A:1293–1300.

13. Lin RS: Application of the varus T-strap principle to the polypropylene Ankle Foot Orthosis. *Orthot Prosthet* 1982;36:67–70.

14. White FJ: Orthotics, in Drennan JC (ed): *The Child's Foot and Ankle*. New York, NY, Raven Press, 1992, pp 71–95.

15. Cuddeford TJ, Freeling RP, Thomas SS, et al: Energy consumption in children with myelomeningocele: A comparison between reciprocating gait orthosis and hip-knee-ankle-foot orthosis ambulators. *Dev Med Child Neurol* 1997;39:239–242.

16. Stallard J, Major RE, Patrick JH: The use of the Orthotic Research and Locomotor Assessment Unit (ORLAU) ParaWalker by adult myelomeningocele patients: A seven year retrospective study. Preliminary results. *Eur J Pediatr Surg* 1995;5(suppl 1):24–26.

17. Nutter AF: Contact urticaria to rubber. *Br J Dermatol* 1979;101:597–598.

18. Banta JV, Bonanni C, Prebluda J: Latex anaphylaxis during spinal surgery in children with myelomeningocele. *Dev Med Child Neurol* 1993;35:543–548.

19. Tosi LL, Slater JE, Shaer C, Mostello LA: Latex allergy in spina bifida patients: Prevalence and surgical implications. *J Pediatr Orthop* 1993;13:709–712.

20. D'Astous J, Drouin MA, Rhine E: Intraoperative anaphylaxis secondary to allergy to latex in children who have spina bifida: Report of two cases. *J Bone Joint Surg* 1992;74A:1084–1086.

The Treatment of Neuromuscular Scoliosis

John V. Banta, MD
Denis S. Drummond, MD
Ronnie L. Ferguson, MD

Introduction

Major advances in the treatment of pediatric neuromuscular disorders have occurred in the past 30 years, and with increased survivorship, many children and adolescents now present with major spinal deformities that were not previously recognized.[1-4] With the virtual elimination of poliomyelitis in all but regions of Africa and Asia, a wide spectrum of neurologic and neuromuscular diseases present a major treatment challenge to the orthopaedic surgeon. As an example, at the Rancho Los Amigos Hospital in 1975, Bonnet and associates[5] reported the changing prevalence of perioperative complications encountered in the surgical management of paralytic scoliosis (Table 1). Improvements in surgical technique and changes in postoperative management resulted in a reduction in the pseudarthrosis rate; curve progression was eliminated, but wound infections persisted and perioperative mortality rose as more complex deformities were treated.

The prevalence of spinal deformity varies from 20% in children with cerebral palsy to 60% in patients with myelodysplasia, and rises to 90% in males with Duchenne muscular dystrophy. With improved management of childhood traumatic paraplegia, it

is now evident that 100% of children injured when younger than 10 years of age will develop scoliosis and/or kyphosis.[6]

Outcomes Analysis

Integral to our knowledge of what may be offered to the patient and what expected result can be explained to the family is a fundamental understanding of a current outcomes analysis. Therefore, a review of current literature allows us to combine patients with similar diagnoses and treatments thereby identifying trends in surgical outcomes. Data were extracted from 30 papers written since 1972 concerning the surgical treatment of neuromuscular scoliosis in 902 patients who were followed up for a minimum of 24 months.[4,7-24]

Diagnoses and number of cases reported were: spina bifida, 362; cerebral palsy, 387; and muscular dystrophy and spinal muscular atrophy, 153. Although these diagnoses do not encompass all of the diagnostic categories, these groups had large enough numbers of patients to make their averages meaningful. Anterior instrumentations were not separated from anterior releases and fusions because instrumentation has not been shown to give significantly greater correction in neuromuscular spinal deformity. All of the patients reported had instrumentations used for their posterior arthrodeses, and all were administered prophylactic antibiotics. Specific areas of interest were correction, complications, and functional outcomes. These topics were reported in the aggregate, by

Table 1
Paralytic scoliosis: The Rancho Los Amigos experience

Complications	1954-1956 (%)	1967-1975 (%)
Deep wound infections	6	6
Pseudarthrosis	38	27
Curve progression	38	0
Curve extension	25	8
Superficial infection	19	8
Death	19	8
Stiff hips	0	14

(Reproduced with permission from Bonnett C, Brown JC, Perry J, et al: Evolution of treatment of paralytic scoliosis at Ranchos Los Amigos Hospital. *J Bone Joint Surg* 1975;57A:206–215.)

diagnosis, by instrumentation system, and by surgical approach.

Correction

Posterior fusion with instrumentation led to an average correction of 39% when all patients were combined without regard to diagnosis. If anterior and posterior spinal fusions were performed, the average correction rose to 59%. Patients with Harrington instrumentation and postoperative casting averaged 37% correction, but when this was combined with anterior fusion and postoperative casting, the average correction increased to 60%. Those patients treated with posterior segmental instrumentation systems averaged 48% correction, which increased to an average of 58% when combined with anterior arthrodesis. Pelvic obliquity was corrected an average of 31% with posterior instrumentation and fusion and 66% when anterior and posterior fusions were performed. The data suggest that the newer segmental fixation systems have more efficacy for correction when used alone but give no greater correction than Harrington instrumentation combined with anterior and posterior arthrodesis. By including an anterior release and arthrodesis with the posterior fusion, approximately 20% more correction can be obtained. Furthermore, anterior procedures yield twice as much correction of pelvic obliquity as a single posterior approach.

Complications

Complications were classified according to implant, medical, and technical problems. Implant problems consisted of pseudarthrosis and implant failure. Medical complications dealt with wound infection, skin breakdown or dehiscence, urinary tract infection, pulmonary distress, and death. Tech-

nical problems related to surgical judgment or error, including error in determining fusion level, neurologic injury, or patient selection criteria.

Pseudarthrosis occurred in 28% of patients fused posteriorly with Harrington instrumentation alone, 7% fused with posterior segmental instrumentation alone, 24% of patients with myelodysplasia, 17% of patients with cerebral palsy who were fused posteriorly alone, and only 7% of cerebral palsy patients who underwent both anterior and posterior fusion.

Instrumentation failure occurred overall in 15% of the 902 patients. Harrington instrumentation had the highest failure rate (19%), whereas the newer segmental instrumentations with better design characteristics (smooth nonnotched rods) had only a 3% incidence of rod breakage, hook dislodgement, or significant wire failure. The failure rate in the segmental spinal instrumentation (SSI) systems could increase with follow-up, because many of the newer systems do not fail until up to 4 years after implantation when an unrecognized pseudarthrosis is present. Myelodysplastic patients had the highest instrument failure rate (20%), whereas the cerebral palsy population had only a 12% failure rate.

Wound infections occurred in 8% of all cases. All of the patients included were from series in which prophylactic antibiotics were used. The myelodysplastic population had the highest infection rate of (15%); the rate in patients with cerebral palsy was only 6%. According to those papers reporting infecting organisms, 54% were mixed gram negative and gram positive organisms, whereas only 22% were *Staphylococcus aureus*. Infections were more common after staged anterior-posterior procedures than after same-day sequential ante-

rior-posterior fusions.

Urinary tract infections were reported to be prevalent in all neuromuscular patients, especially those who had a history of previous urinary sepsis. Pulmonary distress causing prolonged intubation, reintubation, or pneumonitis most often occurred in patients with a forced vital capacity (FVC) less than 50% and in conjunction with anterior surgery. These trends did not have large numbers but were reported by numerous authors.

Skin pressure lesions, especially in those patients with insensitive skin or where casting was used as an adjunct to immobilize spinal instrumentation, were common. Because SSI with or without bracing is now commonly used without casting, pressure sores have decreased. Yet 26% of the myelodysplastic patients developed gluteal pressure sores that were related to excessive flattening of the lumbar lordosis and incomplete correction of pelvic obliquity, both of which led to excessive or unequal ischial pressure in the seated position.

Deaths occurred, on average, at a rate between 1% and 2%. The 2 major causes were excessive intraoperative blood loss and pulmonary complications. Once a patient approaches a total blood volume loss, the patient's intrinsic clotting factors become so diluted that clotting mechanisms fail. This amount of blood volume loss is not uncommon, especially in those patients undergoing staged anterior-posterior spinal fusions. Replacement of these factors with fresh frozen plasma, cryoprecipitate, and platelet transfusions will help restore the homeostatic clotting mechanisms. Pulmonary complications tend to occur more often when the FVC is less than 50%. When calculating FVC, the arm span and not the truncal height must be used because spinal deformity provides falsely elevated FVC predictions.

Comparing medical complications between 16 patients undergoing same day versus 29 patients having staged spinal surgery revealed 36 major and minor complications in the staged group versus only 14 complications in the same-day surgical group. Those undergoing a staged procedure experienced longer surgical and anesthetic time, greater blood loss, decreased nutritional indices, and a longer hospital stay.[25]

Technical

Technical complications were small in number, but several trends were reported by numerous authors. Kyphosis occurred above the instrumentation, particularly if the fusion stopped at the apex of the thoracic kyphosis, leading authors to recommend extension of fusion to the T2 or T3 level. Failure to extend the fusion to the pelvis could result in residual or recurrent pelvic obliquity, particularly in those patients with prolonged longevity who had long paralytic "C" shaped curves. Severe permanent neurologic injury rates averaged 1%. Patients with athetoid cerebral palsy who did not have a combined approach appeared to have an increased pseudarthrosis rate.

Function

Postoperative improvement in function relates directly to truncal balance. Percent correction of deformity was not as important as restoration of spinal compensation. In patients with myelodysplasia, spinal surgery with fusion to the pelvis may result in loss of walking ability, noted in 25% of patients. This loss may relate to increased residual hip flexion deformity in a marginally ambulatory patient

or caused by increased pelvic flexion following instrumentation, or it may be secondary to the age at which surgery is performed, coinciding with natural progression to a wheelchair for mobility. Improved expiratory volumes have been measured in patients following correction of congenital kyphosis, and improved expiratory flow with greater endurance has been measured in spina bifida patients following correction of curves over 60°.[26]

It is evident from these studies that sequential anterior and posterior spinal fusion is preferable in the appropriate patient because the complication rate is reduced.[27] The technique of segmental spinal instrumentation provides multiple fixation sites to distribute the corrective forces over many spinal levels, which is of utmost importance in patients with disuse osteopenia. The child with a neuromuscular disorder requires a meticulous preoperative assessment to avoid or minimize the high incidence of complications so common in these diseases.[28] Careful attention to nutritional parameters, the status of the urinary tract and pulmonary function, and routine use of prophylactic antibiotics are essential to achieving optimum postoperative results.

Preoperative Assessment
Treatment Goals

The highest priority in the surgical treatment of the patient with neuromuscular scoliosis is to achieve spinal balance. Frontal and sagittal plane balance provides a comfortable seating posture, which allows increased wheelchair sitting endurance and, thereby, improved facility in the activities of daily living. A compensated spine indicates correction in the sagittal, coronal, and transverse planes and no fixed pelvic obliquity. Poor balance leads to seating problems, secondary difficulties with

head control, and increased risk for pressure sores, particularly in those patients who are insensate. In the normal person, seating pressures are distributed, with 60% of the body weight anterior beneath the fleshy thighs and only 40% posterior with equal pressures beneath the ischial tuberosities; coccygeal pressures are measured at less than 11%. Myelomeningocele patients with neuromuscular scoliosis, pelvic obliquity, and pressure sores had at least 1 of the following: 60% of pressure distributed posterior, 30% or more on 1 ischial tuberosity, or 11% or more under the coccyx.[29]

Spinal Alignment

In the frontal plane, balance is measured in relationship to the central sacral line (CSL). This is a perpendicular line from the center of S1 extending proximally at right angles to the intercristal plane, a line joining the top of the iliac crests (Fig. 1). Frontal balance is determined by measurement of the translation of the apical vertebra of the scoliosis curve from the perpendicular to the floor, or to the bottom of the radiograph. Acceptable frontal balance, by definition, requires minimal apical translation from the CSL, no fixed pelvic obliquity, and no oblique takeoff of L5 on S1.

Sagittal balance is determined by the relationship of the spine to the weight reaction line that extends from the occiput as a plumb line, passing anterior to the thoracic spine, posterior to the lumbar spine, and through the body of S1 (Fig. 2). When the weight reaction line bisects S1, the forces at the lumbosacral junction are relatively neutral. If the weight reaction line passes anterior to S1 resulting in relative lumbar kyphosis, the normal compression forces in the lumbar spine are now in

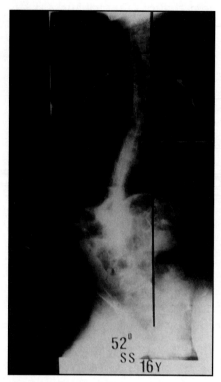

Fig. 1 The central sacral line (CSL) is shown. Balance in the frontal plane is defined by the relationship of the spine to this line.

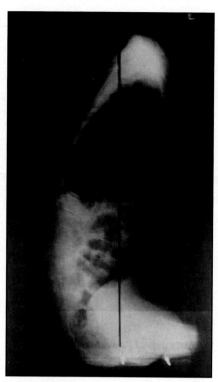

Fig. 2 The weight reaction line is shown. With sagittal balance, this line passes anterior to the thoracic spine, posterior to the lumbar spine, and through the body of S1. In this example the spinal balance is poor.

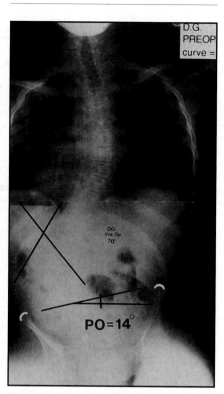

Fig. 3 Neuromuscular scoliosis with pelvic obliquity measuring 14°.

distraction, which will likely result in a lumbosacral pseudarthrosis.

Pelvic obliquity is measured as the angle formed between the intercristal plane and a line parallel to the horizontal plane (Fig. 3). Thus, any measured obliquity is a pathologic condition that causes imbalance in the frontal plane and unbalanced sitting with unequal distribution of sitting pressures, which are not tolerated by the patients with insensate skin under the buttocks. Pelvic obliquity may be a result of spinal deformity or imbalance of the hips with contracture with or without dislocation (Fig. 4). Preoperative surgical planning must include a thorough evaluation of both hips. When corrected, spinal deformity with excessive lumbar lordosis and pelvic obliquity will accentuate fixed hip contractures.

Restoration of more normal trunk height is an important goal of surgical correction, which results in improved diaphragmatic efficiency[26,30] and improved appetite, and frees the upper extremities for functional activities. However, patients with spinal muscle atrophy frequently deteriorate in upper extremity function following spinal fusion because a rigid spine removes the compensatory skills they used preoperatively to accommodate for proximal limb weakness.[12,31]

Surgical Concepts

Deformity alters normal spinal biomechanics. Bending forces are increased in direct proportion to the magnitude of the curve. Bending loads applied to the apex of the curve vary directly with curve size and the moment arm, which runs perpendicular from the central sacral line to the apical vertebra. With a 59% correction of the curve, the moment arm is similarly reduced and the resultant bending forces are reduced by half. These changes, in turn, reduce the convex tension forces at the apex, resulting in less tendency for pseudarthrosis formation (Fig. 5). The same principle applies in the sagittal plane, where a similar moment arm exists from the lumbosacral junction anteriorly to the weight reaction line (Fig. 6). The resultant tension forces associated with lumbar kyphosis explain the relatively high rate of fusion failure at the lumbosacral junction.

Corrective Forces

Modern surgical techniques employ both axial and translational forces to

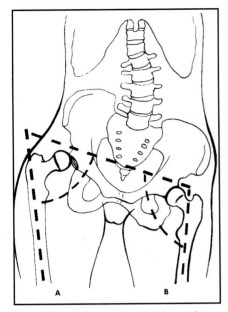

Fig. 4 Pelvic obliquity. With windswept hips, some of this deformity can be defined as femoropelvic obliquity.

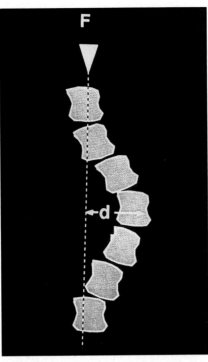

Fig. 5 Frontal plane view of a spine with scoliosis. Following surgery, bending forces directed at the spinal implants and the arthrodesis are directly proportional to the moment arm "d," which extends between the central sacral line and the apical vertebra.

achieve correction in all 3 planes. Ancillary forces include distraction and compression, which were the methods of choice with Harrington instrumentation. Distraction elongates the spine, correcting the end vertebrae to the horizontal, and approximates the apical vertebra toward the CSL in the frontal plane. However, distraction simultaneously flattens the sagittal contours, producing thoracic hypokyphosis and lumbar flat back. The former causes a reduction in pulmonary volumes and the latter leads to unbalanced sitting. Translational corrective forces are horizontally applied in either tension, as with progressive tightening of sublaminar wires, or through forces imparted by the cantilever maneuver of the contoured rod pressed against the apex of the deformity. The major advantage of segmental spinal fixation is the ability to apply powerful corrective forces in all planes without producing loss of normal sagittal contours.[22] In addition, the use of multi-

ple purchase sites not only increases the stability of the construct but also allows for the application of gradual progressive correction with wide distribution of forces to each vertebra, thus reducing the risk for failure at the bone-implant interface.[7,32] This concept is particularly important with neuromuscular deformities, which are often large and rigid with osteopenic bone.

Anterior release and arthrodesis are essential to achieve maximum safe correction and, more importantly, to restore anatomic spinopelvic alignment. Indications for anterior release and fusion include rigid deformity, which prevents reduction of the scoliosis to at least 50° on stress radiographs, an inadequate fusion area caused by deficient posterior ele-

ments as seen in spina bifida or following laminectomy, and structural kyphosis. Typically, a transthoracic, posterior retroperitoneal or combined thoracoabdominal approach is used. Anterior release in the thoracic spine can be accomplished by a video-assisted thoracoscopy technique; however, many neuromuscular curve patterns require a combined thoracoabdominal approach. The anterior approach allows for a complete release of the anterior longitudinal ligament, annulectomy, and diskectomy, which mobilizes the vertebra for both angular and rotational mobility as well as providing an excellent fusion area in the excised disk spaces.

Many patients with neuromuscular scoliosis in addition to disuse osteopenia secondary to their sedentary wheelchair existence have a relative decrease in pelvic bone mass, thereby reducing the availability of a source of autogenous bone graft. Allogeneic bone has been successfully used for many years and has been proven effective even though it provides only osteoconductive properties.[33]

Fusion Levels

Most nonambulatory patients with neuromuscular spinal deformity require fusion and instrumentation to the pelvis. The main exception is for those few patients who retain walking skills and need preservation of lower lumbar motion. In such patients, to fuse short of the sacrum there must be neither fixed pelvic obliquity nor an oblique takeoff of L5 on the S1 vertebra so that the lowest instrumented level remains horizontal. Another group in whom the fusion is not extended to the pelvis consists of select patients with Duchenne muscular dystrophy who have smaller curves without associated pelvic obliquity.[34–36]

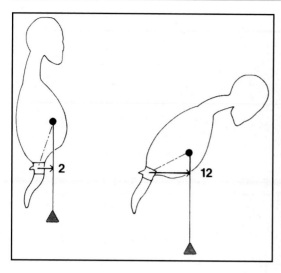

Fig. 6 Biomechanical forces that lead to failure of an arthrodesis at the L5-S1 junction are related to a moment arm extending from the lumbosacral junction and the weight reaction line. The diagram shows how these forces are magnified by forward flexion. Similarly, sagittal plane imbalance with lumbar kyphosis increases these forces.

Instrumentation

There has been a proliferation of implant systems to provide segmental spinal fixation. However, not infrequently, there is a conflict between achieving certain stability while providing a smaller construct with a so-called "low profile." The technique most commonly used in North America today is the Luque-Galveston technique, which provides the advantages of segmental spinal fixation: versatility, cost, and an implant of minimum bulk that can be contoured to achieve an optimum profile.[14,21,37–41] The construct is made up of 2 contoured rods, one on either side of the midline fixed intimately to each laminar surface with sublaminar wires. With the introduction of rigid cross-linking devices, a strong rectilinear construct provides rigid immobilization with restoration of near normal anatomic alignment in both the sagittal and coronal planes (Fig. 7).

The Galveston technique of pelvic fixation developed by Allen and Ferguson is accomplished by implanting the pelvic portion of the rods into the posterior column or transverse bar of the ilium, which contains the greatest bone mass and where the fixation is least likely to fail (Fig. 8). Although there are proponents of multiple hook and rod fixation devices to obtain fixation to the pelvis in cases of neuromuscular deformity,[18] the Galveston technique is considered superior for pelvic fixation.[42]

Subsequent to the development of the Luque-Galveston technique, there have been some refinements such as the unit rod. After this single contoured rod is inserted into the transverse iliac bar, the resultant long lever arm is used to gradually correct the spine by progressive tightening of the sublaminar wires, thus providing greater corrective forces to reduce pelvic obliquity while correcting the scoliosis.[9,38,43]

The Galveston technique has proved to be very effective because there are no connections with iliac screws, which theoretically create points of fatigue, and the multiplanar configuration of the rod provides an excellent triangulation fixation to the pelvis.[44] There are 2 theoretical disadvantages of the Luque-Galveston technique. First, the instrumentation crosses the sacroiliac joint and can potentially cause pain associated with sacroiliac joint degeneration. Second, many patients develop radiolucency around the tip of the pelvic limb of the rods. Long-term studies, however, have not shown problems of sacroiliac pain, and the radiolucency about the tip of the rod resolves as the fusion matures.[11,45]

Hybrid constructs are occasionally useful in more difficult situations. For example, the distraction forces applied with the Luque rod can be increased by selective placement of laminar and pedicle hooks applied in a distraction mode on the concave rod. Sublaminar wires, hooks, and pedicle screws can be used as a hybrid construct, and anterior instrumentation may be used to reduce a large lordotic deformity that prevents easy access to the pelvis for the posterior Galveston pelvic rod placement (Fig. 9).

In select instances, very young children with progressive scoliosis can be treated with spinal instrumentation without fusion, thereby allowing for successive distraction on rods placed in a subfascial plane. The patient must be protected by full-time orthotic support. In addition, progressive structural changes occur in the apex of the spinal deformity, which in our opinion severely limit the applicability of this procedure for cases of neuromuscular scoliosis.[46]

Specific Disease Problems
Cerebral Palsy

Cerebral palsy is one of the most common diagnoses associated with spinal deformity. The incidence is proportional to the degree of neurologic involvement, with the incidence rising to 60% to 75% in those individuals with spastic quadriplegia.[47] Orthotic treatment does not halt the progression of deformity in these patients.[48] Early reports of surgical treatment included high complication

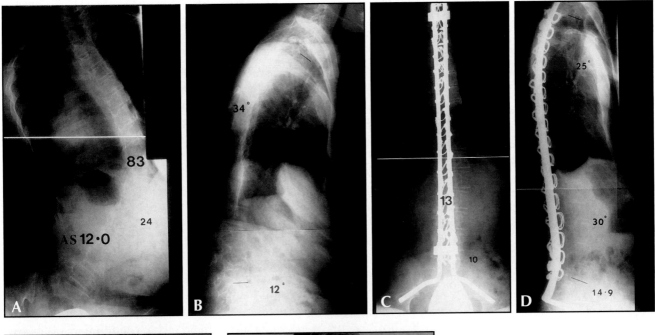

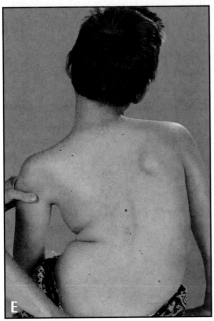

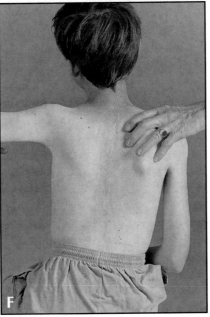

Fig. 7 A, Preoperative 83° thoracolumbar scoliosis with 24° pelvic obliquity in a 12-year-old male with Duchenne muscular dystrophy. **B,** Preoperative lateral view showing 34° thoracic kyphosis. Note the reversal of lumbar lordosis. **C** and **D,** Postoperative posteroanterior and lateral radiographs show correction of coronal, sagittal plane deformity. **E** and **F,** Pre- and postoperative clinical photographs.

rates,[37] but detailed analysis clarified 2 distinct patterns of deformity: group 1 curves, with little pelvic obliquity; and group 2 curves, in which a large lumbar or thoracolumbar curve extended into the pelvis with resultant pelvic obliquity that necessitated combined anterior and posterior fusion.[16] Recognition of the importance of preoperative nutritional supplements[49] coupled with the surgical techniques outlined above have resulted in a marked reduction in the rate of perioperative complications.[14,21,23] Recent reports have focused on the functional outcomes of surgery for the severely handicapped child and questioned the risk-benefit ratio of this major complex surgery.[50,51] For the child with increasing deformity and deterioration in function, the improvement in sitting balance, stabilization of pulmonary function, and perceived ease of management by the attendants caring for that child confirm the value of surgical treatment.[38,47]

Spina Bifida

Spina bifida occurs in approximately 0.5 to 1 per 1,000 live births, and sco-

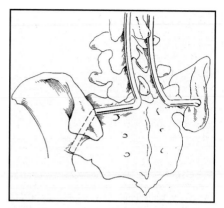

Fig. 8 Diagram shows the Galveston method of fixing the pelvic limb of the rod to the posterior column of the ilium. Because the construct extends through 2 planes, this provides triangulation, which is a biomechanically important feature contributing to stability.

liosis occurs in approximately 60% of affected children, with the highest incidence in those patients with a thoracic level paraplegia. Surgical treatment of this complex spinal disorder has been characterized by a high rate of pseudarthrosis formation, infection, and incomplete correction.[52] The concept of staged anterior interbody fusion coupled with posterior fusion and instrumentation led to dramatically improved results.[8,17,19,53] This combined circumferential fusion technique provided for correction of pelvic obliquity, more rapid postoperative mobilization,[54] and a reduction in the incidence of pressure sores.[3] Controversy now centers on whether the fusion should extend into the pelvis, because the loss of lumbar motion segments can hinder functional ambulation by restricting elevation of the hemipelvis in swing phase as well as interfere with the normal transverse plane rotation of the pelvis so necessary to paraplegic ambulation.[55] Commonly, many ambulatory patients with mid to upper lumbar level function select the wheelchair for mobility in the second decade of

life to conserve the energy costs associated with ambulating with orthoses and crutches.[56] If the scoliosis does not extend into the pelvis, the fusion may be stopped at the lowest level lumbar vertebra. However, there are no long-term studies to show if there is an increased risk of neurotrophic degeneration below the fusion. Recently, pedicle screw fixation has been used to augment posterior segmental spinal fixation with reported good results, without anterior arthrodesis.[57] Long-term follow-up is needed to confirm that either isolated posterior or anterior fusion with newer segmental fixation implants will have fusion rates equal to those of patients having anterior-posterior arthrodesis.

Kyphosis occurs in up to 20% of newborns with spina bifida and presents the complex challenge of correction of severe sagittal plane deformity with absent posterior laminar arches. The critical goal is to restore normal sagittal alignment by resection of the upper limb of the kyphotic deformity, not just the apical vertebra. Recent reports indicate that resection of the proximal limb of the kyphotic deformity in the upper lumbar region and fusion, followed by orthotic support, can allow for further spinal growth, thereby deferring a definitive long arthrodesis until the child is older.[58] Preoperative neurologic examination frequently reveals that observed lower limb motion is often reflexive or synergistic and not under voluntary cortical control. If the malformed distal cord is resected, the distal cord should not be ligated because ligation can alter intraventricular pressure, with occlusion of the central canal of the cord, which remains open in those patients with hydrocephalus.

Various techniques have been developed to provide stable fixation in the pelvis to provide a cantilever

corrective force to restore normal sagittal alignment after resection of the apical deformity.[58–62] It is important to note that the conventional Galveston technique is not good for the kyphotic spine because the iliac wings are not oriented in the normal oblique fashion from the sacral ala but are more parallel to one another, which can result in backing out of the iliac limbs of the Luque rod (Fig. 8).

Children with spina bifida, congenital genitourinary anomalies, and, more recently, children with spinal cord injury have become sensitized to Latex.[63] The allergic reaction ranges from mild urticarial reaction to life-threatening anaphylaxis.[64] The standard of care today requires treatment of such children in a latex-free environment in both the office and the operating room. Protocols have been established for prevention and, in many cases, prophylaxis prior to beginning surgical procedures.[65] Close collaboration between surgeon, anesthesiologist, and intensive-care unit physician are necessary to prevent this untoward, potentially life-threatening complication.

With the introduction of magnetic resonance imaging, it became apparent that the neural contents adhere to the site of the closure of the myelomeningocele defect. The pathophysiology of the so-called tethered cord syndrome involves progressive deterioration of the remaining neural elements in the distal cord, and this process is aggravated by traction on the neural elements.[66] Although shunt dysfunction can lead to scoliosis, which can be stabilized by correction of the shunt malfunction,[67] there is no clear evidence at this time that release of the caudal end of the cord will alter the incidence of scoliosis in this patient population. The tethered cord syndrome is based on clinical, not radiographic, findings. Recent data confirm that the neural elements frequently readhere to the site of release, and the need for further orthopaedic procedures is common.[68]

Myopathies

The introduction of segmental spinal instrumentation has changed the management philosophy and the surgical treatment of Duchenne muscular dystrophy. Approximately 95% of all males will develop scoliosis, but the important factor is that Duchenne dystrophy is accompanied by restrictive pulmonary disease, which is first evident as a decrease in vital capacity when the patient is no longer able to stand.[69] Each 10° increase in deformity corresponds to approximately a 4% further decrease in forced vital capacity (FVC).[30] The current recommendation is to perform a spinal fusion once the curve exceeds 20°. If the FVC drops below 35% of predicted value, the risk of perioperative pulmonary complications rises.[34,70] Previous authors suggested that if the FVC fell below 40% of predicted value and the patient had a nonproductive cough, preoperative tracheostomy was required.[20] More recent advances in anesthesiology and postoperative management suggest tracheostomy is less frequently required.[71,72] Patients with Duchenne dystrophy maintain a stable FVC for approximately 36 months following spinal fusion surgery and show improvement in peak expiratory flow rate. Although spinal fusion does not alter the course of cardiomyopathy, the ultimate cause of death in the third decade of life, reducing the discomfort associated with poor sitting posture greatly enhances the quality of life for these patients.[73]

Spinal muscular atrophy is an autosomal recessive disorder of unknown etiology. A functional classification

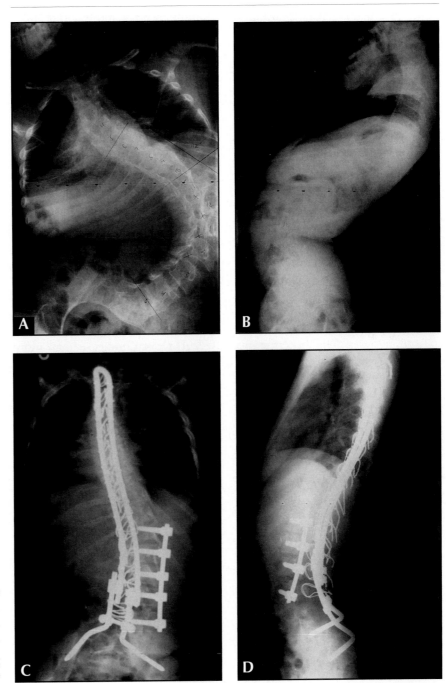

Fig. 9 A, An anteroposterior radiograph of a severe neuromuscular scoliosis in a 16-year-old boy with spastic quadriplegia. **B,** The sagittal deformity in which the extreme lumbar lordosis makes placement of Galveston pelvic fixation very difficult. Both frontal and sagittal deformities were rigid. **C,** Frontal radiograph following surgery shows a hybrid approach. Following anterior release and fusion, as well as anterior instrumentation, the sagittal deformity was improved enough to make placement of the short pelvic rods possible. The use of 4 rods and dominos, which are a type of cross links to connect rods in parallel, further expedited the Luque-Galveston technique. Note also a reverse curve was shaped into the rods proximally to help achieve spinal balance. **D,** Lateral radiograph shows that good sagittal balance has been achieved. Note that by rotating the anterior rod into kyphosis, correction of the severe lordotic deformity was accomplished.

describes prognosis in relationship to the progression of deformity. Group I never develop sitting ability, develop scoliosis at an early age, and have a short life span. Group II sit but cannot stand, group III have limited walking ability, and group IV walk, climb stairs, and have a potentially normal life span.[74] Orthotic support may provide enhanced sitting balance for the very young child, but significant chest wall deformity with loss of lung volume occurs with growth. Early surgical intervention is recommended before significant loss of pulmonary function.[4,75] Patients with myopathies have an increased risk of malignant hyperthermia, characterized by a rapid rise in temperature with muscle rigidity and hypoxia. The hyperthermia often is triggered by succinyl choline and halothane anesthetic agents. Dantrolene is the drug of choice to reverse these effects. Accurate preoperative anesthetic evaluation is necessary, including tests for creatinine phosphokinase levels.[71]

Scoliosis in patients with Friedreich's ataxia is commonly classified as neuromuscular; however, recent work by Labelle and associates[76] indicated that many curves were not progressive and showed no relationship to muscle weakness. The major factors in curve progression requiring surgery were the age at onset of the disease and the presence of deformity before the onset of puberty.[76]

Rett syndrome was first described in 1966 as a progressive neurologic disorder affecting females. Four stages of progressive deterioration have been described, which are accompanied by mental deterioration, autism, loss of ambulatory skill with ataxia, and characteristic hand wringing movements. The incidence of scoliosis increases with age. It affects nearly 80% of those patients attaining puberty, and is commonly a long "C shaped" pattern. Bracing is recommended for those curves measuring less than 40°, and fusion is recommended for those curves showing further progression.[77,78]

Neurologic Complications

The patient's loss of neurologic function is the dread of every spinal surgeon. Neurologic compromise in the child with neuromuscular spinal deformity will compound the preexisting disability. The early results of spinal cord monitoring suggested that as a result of impaired function of the motor cortex, as in cerebral palsy or abnormal spinal tracts, reliable tracings could not be attained.[79] Recent reports suggest that more accurate monitoring is possible by combining somatosensory-evoked potentials with motor-evoked potentials.[80–82] With improved techniques, real-time monitoring of cord function has greater potential than the wake up test, which is difficult to use in children with neuromuscular disabilities. Winter[83] summarized the major potential problems that must be considered to prevent neurologic compromise: careful preoperative evaluation, delicate exposure and instrumentation, avoidance of excessive distraction, accurate monitoring, awareness that hypotension reduces cord blood flow, and that all of these factors are additive.

Conclusion

With the increase in spinal instrumentation techniques for the treatment of neuromuscular spinal deformity, the 1992 editorial comment of Apley and Rowley[84] is just as relevant today, "But we do believe that it is not enough to train surgeons to be expert metal workers; they need to master all the available techniques of treatment, and then develop the wisdom to choose between them."[84]

★At the time of this writing, bone screws placed posteriorly into vertebral elements have been cleared for use in this specific manner by the Food and Drug Administration (FDA) to provide immobilization and stabilization as an adjunct to fusion in the treatment of the following acute and chronic instability or deformities of the thoracic, lumbar, and sacral spine: degenerative spondylolisthesis with objective evidence of neurological impairment; fracture; dislocation; scoliosis; kyphosis; spinal tumor and failed previous fusion (pseudoarthrosis). In addition, anterior vertebral body screws (cervical, thoracic, and lumbar) are class II devices and can be used as labeled in vertebral bodies.

References

1. Balmer GA, MacEwen GD: The incidence and treatment of scoliosis in cerebral palsy. *J Bone Joint Surg* 1970;52B:134–137.

2. Garrett AL, Perry J, Nickel VL: Stabilization of the collapsing spine. *J Bone Joint Surg* 1961;43A:474–484.

3. Harris MB, Banta JV: Cost of skin care in the myelomeningocele population. *J Pediatr Orthop* 1990;10:355–361.

4. Riddick MF, Winter RB, Lutter LD: Spinal deformities in patients with spinal muscle atrophy: A review of 36 patients. *Spine* 1982;7:476–483.

5. Bonnett C, Brown JC, Perry J, et al: Evolution of treatment of paralytic scoliosis at Rancho Los Amigos Hospital. *J Bone Joint Surg* 1975;57A:206–215.

7. Allen BL Jr, Ferguson RL: L-rod instrumentation for scoliosis in cerebral palsy. *J Pediatr Orthop* 1982;2:87–96.

8. Banta JV: Combined anterior and posterior fusion for spinal deformity in myelomeningocele. *Spine* 1990;15:946–952.

9. Bell DF, Moseley CF, Koreska J: Unit rod segmental spinal instrumentation in the management of patients with progressive neuromuscular spinal deformity. *Spine* 1989;14:1301–1307.

10. Bonnett C, Brown JC, Grow T: Thoracolumbar scoliosis in cerebral palsy: Results of surgical treatment. *J Bone Joint Surg* 1976;58A:328–336.

11. Broom MJ, Banta JV, Renshaw TS: Spinal fusion augmented by Luque-rod segmental

instrumentation for neuromuscular scoliosis. *J Bone Joint Surg* 1989;71A:32–44.

12. Brown JC, Zeller JL, Swank SM, Furumasu J, Warath SL: Surgical and functional results of spine fusion in spinal muscular atrophy. *Spine* 1989;14:763–770.

13. Ferguson RL, Allen BL Jr: Staged correction of neuromuscular scoliosis. *J Pediatr Orthop* 1983; 3:555–562.

14. Gersoff WK, Renshaw TS: The treatment of scoliosis in cerebral palsy by posterior spinal fusion with Luque-rod segmental instrumentation. *J Bone Joint Surg* 1988;70A:41–44.

15. Hensinger RN, MacEwen GD: Spinal deformity associated with heritable neurological conditions: Spinal muscular atrophy, Friedreich's ataxia, familial dysautonomia, and Charcot-Marie-Tooth disease. *J Bone Joint Surg* 1976;58A:13–24.

16. Lonstein JE, Akbarnia A: Operative treatment of spinal deformities in patients with cerebral palsy or mental retardation: An analysis of one hundred and seven cases. *J Bone Joint Surg* 1983;65A:43–55.

17. McMaster MJ: Anterior and posterior instrumentation and fusion of thoracolumbar scoliosis due to myelomeningocele. *J Bone Joint Surg* 1987;69B:20–25.

18. Neustadt JB, Shufflebarger HL, Cammisa FP: Spinal fusions to the pelvis augmented by Cotrel-Dubousset instrumentation for neuromuscular scoliosis. *J Pediatr Orthop* 1992;12: 465–469.

19. Osebold WR, Mayfield JK, Winter RB, Moe JH: Surgical treatment of paralytic scoliosis associated with myelomeningocele. *J Bone Joint Surg* 1982;64A:841–856.

20. Sakai DN, Hsu JD, Bonnett CA, Brown JC: Stabilization of the collapsing spine in Duchenne muscular dystrophy. *Clin Orthop* 1977;128:256–260.

21. Sponseller PD, Whiffen JR, Drummond DS: Interspinous process segmental spinal instrumentation for scoliosis in cerebral palsy. *J Pediatr Orthop* 1986;6:559–563.

22. Sullivan JA, Conner SB: Comparison of Harrington instrumentation and segmental spinal instrumentation in the management of neuromuscular spinal deformity. *Spine* 1982; 7:299–304.

23. Swank SM, Cohen DS, Brown JC: Spine fusion in cerebral palsy with L-rod segmental spinal instrumentation: A comparison of single and two-stage combined approach with Zielke instrumentation. *Spine* 1989;14:750–759.

24. Ward WT, Wenger DR, Roach JW: Surgical correction of myelomeningocele scoliosis: A critical appraisal of various spinal instrumentation systems. *J Pediatr Orthop* 1989;9:262–268.

25. Ferguson RL, Hansen MM, Nicholas DA, Allen BL Jr: Same-day versus staged anterior-posterior spinal surgery in a neuromuscular scoliosis population: The evaluation of medical complications. *J Pediatr Orthop* 1996;16:293–303.

26. Banta JV, Park SM: Improvement in pulmonary function in patients having combined anterior and posterior spine fusion for myelomeningocele scoliosis. *Spine* 1983;8:765–770.

27. Powell ET IV, Krengel WF III, King HA, Lagrone MO: Comparison of same-day sequential anterior and posterior spinal fusion with delayed two-stage anterior and posterior spinal fusion. *Spine* 1994;19:1256–1259.

28. Winter S: Preoperative assessment of the child with neuromuscular scoliosis. *Orthop Clin North Am* 1994;25:239–245.

29. Drummond D, Breed AL, Narechania R: Relationship of spine deformity and pelvic obliquity on sitting pressure distributions and decubitus ulceration. *J Pediatr Orthop* 1985;5: 396–402.

30. Miller F, Moseley CF, Koreska J, Levison H: Pulmonary function and scoliosis in Duchenne dystrophy. *J Pediatr Orthop* 1988;8:133–137.

31. Furumasu J, Swank SM, Brown JC, Gilgoff I, Warath S, Zeller J: Functional activities in spinal muscular atrophy patients after spinal fusion. *Spine* 1989;14:771–775.

32. Asher MA, Strippgen WE, Heinig CF, Carson WL: Isola instrumentation, in Weinstein SL (ed): *The Pediatric Spine: Principles and Practice.* New York, NY, Raven Press, 1994, vol 2, pp 1619–1658.

33. Bridwell KH, O'Brien MF, Lenke LG, Baldus C, Blanke K: Posterior spinal fusion supplemented with only allograft bone in paralytic scoliosis: Does it work? *Spine* 1994;19: 2658–2666.

34. Brook PD, Kennedy JD, Stern LM, Sutherland AD, Foster BK: Abstract: Spinal fusion in Duchenne muscular dystrophy. *J Bone Joint Surg* 1994;76B(suppl 2 and 3):105.

35. Mubarak SJ, Morin WD, Leach J: Spinal fusion in Duchenne muscular dystrophy: Fixation and fusion to the sacropelvis? *J Pediatr Orthop* 1993;13:752–757.

36. Sussman MD: Advantage of early spinal stabilization and fusion in patients with Duchenne muscular dystrophy. *J Pediatr Orthop* 1984;4: 532–537.

37. Boachie-Adjei O, Lonstein JE, Winter RB, Koop S, vanden Brink K, Denis F: Management of neuromuscular spinal deformities with Luque segmental instrumentation. *J Bone Joint Surg* 1989;71A:548–562.

38. Drummond DS, Ferguson RL, Banta JV: Advances in the treatment of neuromuscular scoliosis. *Semin Spine Surg* 1997;9:181–193.

39. Maloney WJ, Rinsky LA, Gamble JG: Simultaneous correction of pelvic obliquity, frontal plane and sagittal plane deformities in neuromuscular scoliosis using a unit rod with segmental sublaminar wires: A preliminary report. *J Pediatr Orthop* 1990;10:742–749.

40. Stevens DB, Beard C: Segmental spinal instrumentation for neuromuscular spinal deformity. *Clin Orthop* 1989;242:164–168.

41. Luque ER: The anatomic basis and development of segmental spinal instrumentation. *Spine* 1982;7:256–259.

42. Camp JF, Caudle R, Ashmun RD, Roach J: Immediate complications of Cotrel-Dubousset instrumentation to the sacro-pelvis: A clinical and biomechanical study. *Spine* 1990;15: 932–941.

43. Bulman WA, Dormans JP, Ecker ML, Drummond DS: Posterior spinal fusion for scoliosis in patients with cerebral palsy: A comparison of Luque rod and Unit Rod instrumentation. *J Pediatr Orthop* 1996;16:314–323.

44. Marchesi D, Arlet V, Stricker U, Aebi M: Modification of the original Luque technique in the treatment of Duchenne's neuromuscular scoliosis. *J Pediatr Orthop* 1997;17:743–749.

45. McKeon BP, Thomson JD, Banta JV: Long term (minimum ten year) followup of neuromuscular spinal fusion augmented by Luque-rod segmental instrumentation for neuromuscular scoliosis. *Orthop Trans* 1996;20:118.

46. Klemme WR, Denis F, Winter RB, Lonstein J, Koop SE: Spinal instrumentation without fusion for progressive scoliosis in young children. *J Pediatr Orthop* 1997;17:734–742.

47. Lonstein JE: Cerebral palsy, in Weinstein SL (ed): *The Pediatric Spine: Principles and Practice.* New York, NY, Raven Press, 1994, vol 2, pp 977–998.

48. Miller A, Temple T, Miller F: Impact of orthoses on the rate of scoliosis progression in children with cerebral palsy. *J Pediatr Orthop* 1996;16:332–335.

49. Jevsevar DS, Karlin LI: The relationship between preoperative nutritional status and complications after an operation for scoliosis in patients who have cerebral palsy. *J Bone Joint Surg* 1993;75A:880–884.

50. Askin GN, Hallett R, Hare N, Webb JK: The outcome of scoliosis surgery in the severely physically handicapped child: An objective and subjective assessment. *Spine* 1997;22:44–50.

51. Cassidy C, Craig CL, Perry A, Karlin LI, Goldberg MJ: A reassessment of spinal stabilization in severe cerebral palsy. *J Pediatr Orthop* 1994;14:731–739.

52. Sriram K, Bobechko WP, Hall JE: Surgical management of spinal deformities in spina bifida. *J Bone Joint Surg* 1972;54B:666–676.

53. Mayfield JK: Severe spine deformity in myelodysplasia and sacral agenesis: An aggressive surgical approach. *Spine* 1981;6:498–509.

54. Kahanovitz N, Duncan JW: The role of scoliosis and pelvic obliquity on functional disability in myelomeningocele. *Spine* 1981;6:494–497.

55. Mazur J, Menelaus MB, Dickens DR, Doig WG: Efficacy of surgical management for scoliosis in myelomeningocele: Correction of deformity and alteration of functional status. *J Pediatr Orthop* 1986;6:568–575.

56. Muller EB, Nordwall A, von Wendt L: Influence of surgical treatment of scoliosis in children with spina bifida on ambulation and motoric skills. *Acta Paediatr* 1992;81:173–176.

57. Rodgers WB, Williams MS, Schwend RM, Emans JB: Spinal deformity in myelodysplasia: Correction with posterior pedicle screw instrumentation. *Spine* 1997;22:2435–2443.

58. Lintner SA, Lindseth RE: Kyphotic deformity in patients who have a myelomeningocele: Operative treatment and long-term follow-up. *J Bone Joint Surg* 1994;76A:1301–1307.

59. Heydemann JS, Gillespie R: Management of myelomeningocele kyphosis in the older child by kyphectomy and segmental spinal instrumentation. *Spine* 1987;12:37–41.

60. McCarthy RE, Dunn H, McCullough FL: Luque fixation to the sacral ala using the Dunn-McCarthy modification. *Spine* 1989; 14:281–283.

61. Torode I, Godette G: Surgical correction of congenital kyphosis in myelomeningocele. *J Pediatr Orthop* 1995;15:202–205.

62. Warner WC Jr, Fackler CD: Comparison of two instrumentation techniques in treatment of lumbar kyphosis in myelodysplasia. *J Pediatr Orthop* 1993;13:704–708.

63. Vogel LC, Schrader T, Lubicky JP: Latex allergy in children and adolescents with spinal cord injuries. *J Pediatr Orthop* 1995;15:517–520.

64. Emans JB: Allergy to latex in patients who have myelodysplasia: Relevance for the orthopaedic surgeon. *J Bone Joint Surg* 1992;74A:1103–1109.

65. Dormans JP, Templeton J, Schreiner MS, Delfico AJ: Intraoperative latex anaphylaxis in children: Classification and prophylaxis of patients at risk. *J Pediatr Orthop* 1997;17: 622–625.

66. Yamada S, Zinke DE, Sanders D: Pathophysiology of "tethered cord syndrome." *J Neurosurg* 1981;54:494–503.

67. Hall P, Lindseth R, Campbell R, Kalsbeck JE, Desousa A: Scoliosis and hydrocephalus in myelocele patients: The effects of ventricular shunting. *J Neurosurg* 1979;50:174–178.

68. Archibeck MJ, Smith JT, Carroll KL, Davitt JS, Stevens PM: Surgical release of the tethered spinal cord: Survivorship analysis and orthopaedic outcome. *J Pediatr Orthop* 1997;17: 773–776.

69. Smith AD, Koreska J, Moseley CF: Progression of scoliosis in Duchenne muscular dystrophy. *J Bone Joint Surg* 1989;71A:1066–1074.

70. Miller F, Moseley CF, Koreska J: Spinal fusion in Duchenne muscular dystrophy. *Dev Med Child Neurol* 1992;34:775–786.

71. Murray DJ, Forbes RB: Anesthetic considerations, in Weinstein SL (ed): *The Pediatric Spine: Principles and Practice.* New York, NY, Raven Press, 1994, vol 2, pp 1105–1155.

72. Rawlins BA, Winter RB, Lonstein JE, et al: Reconstructive spine surgery in pediatric patients with major loss in vital capacity. *J Pediatr Orthop* 1996;16:284–292.

73. Galasko CS, Delaney C, Morris P: Spinal stabilisation in Duchenne muscular dystrophy. *J Bone Joint Surg* 1992;74B:210–214.

74. Evans GA, Drennan JC, Russman BS: Functional classification and orthopaedic management of spinal muscular atrophy. *J Bone Joint Surg* 1981;63B:516–522.

75. Phillips DP, Roye DP Jr, Farcy JP, Leet A, Shelton YA: Surgical treatment of scoliosis in a spinal muscular atrophy population. *Spine* 1990;15:942–945.

76. Labelle H, Tohme S, Duhaime M, Allard P: Natural history of scoliosis in Friedreich's ataxia. *J Bone Joint Surg* 1986;68A:564–572.

77. Lidstrom J, Stokland E, Hagberg B: Scoliosis in Rett syndrome: Clinical and biological aspects. *Spine* 1994;19:1632–1635.

78. Bassett GS, Tolo VT: The incidence and natural history of scoliosis in Rett syndrome. *Dev Med Child Neurol* 1990;32:963–966.

79. Ashkenaze D, Mudiyam R, Boachie-Adjei O, Gilbert C: Efficacy of spinal cord monitoring in neuromuscular scoliosis. *Spine* 1993;18: 1627–1633.

80. Ecker ML, Dormans JP, Schwartz DM, Drummond DS, Bulman WA: Efficacy of spinal cord monitoring in scoliosis surgery in patients with cerebral palsy. *J Spinal Disord* 1996;9:159–164.

81. Noordeen MH, Lee J, Gibbons CE, Taylor BA, Bentley G: Spinal cord monitoring in operations for neuromuscular scoliosis. *J Bone Joint Surg* 1997;79B:53–57.

82. Owen JH, Sponseller PD, Szymanski J, Hurdle M: Efficacy of multimodality spinal cord monitoring during surgery for neuromuscular scoliosis. *Spine* 1995;20:1480–1488.

83. Winter RB: Neurologic safety in spinal deformity surgery. *Spine* 1997;22:1527–1533.

84. Apley AG, Rowley DI: Editorial: Fixation is fun. *J Bone Joint Surg* 1992;74B:485–486.

Treatment of Hip and Knee Problems in Myelomeningocele

Walter B. Greene, MD

In the 1960s, effective techniques were developed for shunting hydrocephalus and for early closure of neural tube defects. As a result, orthopaedic surgeons were presented with the challenge of managing an emerging population of children who have myelomeningocele. Initially, the musculoskeletal problems in these children were treated with the modalities and expectations that had been learned from the treatment of poliomyelitis. However, it soon became apparent that the management of children who have myelomeningocele was not so simple. Additional factors include a decrease or loss of sensation affecting some or all parts of the lower extremities, associated congenital anomalies of the spine and lower extremities, and muscle imbalance that affects skeletal development over the entire period of growth. Furthermore, some patients who have myelomeningocele have a static encephalopathy that impairs coordination and results in the loss of strength of the lower and upper extremities.[1-3] Also, progressive neurologic deterioration may occur because of tethered cord syndrome or syringomyelia.[4] As a result, the evaluation and treatment of musculoskeletal problems in these patients can be quite difficult.

The purpose of this chapter is to review the natural history of myelomeningocele as well as the types of deformity that are associated with it, the treatment options that are available, and the expected results of treatment of hip and knee problems related to myelomeningocele. Although other factors must be considered, the neurologic level is the key to understanding the hip and knee deformities seen in these patients. Unless otherwise specified, a modification of the classification system described by Asher and Olson[5] will be used to define the neurological level (Table 1). This classification is based on muscle strength, is simple to use, and, in my experience, has been helpful in predicting gross motor function and potential problems.

Before any decision is made concerning the treatment of hip and knee deformities in myelomeningocele, the physician and the parents must understand the realistic goals with respect to functional walking—that is, walking independently either in the community or about the house.[6] Patients who have thoracic myelomeningocele may be able to walk during the first decade of life, but experience has shown that these patients become dependent on a wheelchair as they attain adult body mass.[6,7-12] Even

Table 1
Definition of neurological level*

Level	Function
Thoracic	No grade 3 strength in muscles of lower extremity
L1-L2	Hip flexion or adduction
L3	Knee extension
L4	Knee flexion
L5	Ankle dorsiflexion
Sacral	Ankle plantarflexion

*Based on the lowest level of antigravity (at least grade 3) strength on the patient's best side

patients who have upper lumbar (first or second lumbar) myelomeningocele seldom retain the capacity for functional walking by the time growth is complete.[8] The prognosis is certainly better for patients who have midlumbar (third or fourth lumbar) myelomeningocele or lumbosacral (fifth lumbar or first sacral) myelomeningocele; however, it must be remembered that even these patients may eventually lose the capacity for functional walking because of other factors. Indeed, it previously was thought that all patients who had sacral myelomeningocele were able to walk independently.[6] However, in 1 study of 36 such patients who were evaluated as adults, 6 had become dependent on a wheelchair as a result of neurologic deterioration, ulceration of the feet, and other problems.[13]

Problems About the Hip
Natural History

The neurologic level is a critical factor in determining the type of deformity of the hip. Patients who have thoracic myelomeningocele lack active movement of the lower extremity muscles. Therefore, the lower extremities tend to lie in abduction, external rotation, and flexion. This posture may facilitate early stabilization of the hip joint, but it also causes the progressive development of a flexion-abduction-external rotation contracture. It is important to note that the severity of the flexion contracture will not be appreciated if the hip is allowed to abduct while the Thomas test is performed (Fig. 1). Tightness of the iliotibial band also causes external tibial torsion and contributes to a flexion deformity of the knee. In addition, tethered cord syndrome, which is more common in patients who have thoracic myelomeningocele, may cause spasticity of the adductors and subluxation of the hips similar to that observed in patients who have cerebral palsy.

A contracture of the unopposed hip flexors typically develops in patients with upper lumbar myelomeningocele. A mild contracture of the unopposed hip adductors may also occur; however, the restriction of hip abduction is usually mild and is not clinically important.

Patients who have mid-lumbar myelomeningocele typically have normal strength in the hip flexors and adductors but no function of the hip extensors or abductors. Therefore, a flexion contracture of the hip and some limitation of abduction frequently develop in these patients. More importantly, this pattern of muscle imbalance predis-

poses to progressive subluxation of the hip.

The probability of subluxation or a severe flexion contracture of the hip is low in patients who have lumbosacral myelomeningocele. This is particularly true if the myelomeningocele is at the sacral level, but adequate stability and an adequate range of motion of the hip are usually maintained even in patients with fifth lumbar myelomeningocele who have only grade 2 or 3 strength of the hip abductors and absent or trace strength of the hip extensors. Apparently, this degree of activity of the hip abductors combined with activity of the hamstrings can be an effective counterbalance to hip flexors and adductors of normal strength. These patients should have periodic radiographs during early childhood to monitor the development of the hip joint.

In a multicenter study of 1,061 patients who had myelomeningocele, measurement of the flexion contractures of the hip in older children (9 to 11 years old) revealed that the greatest average value was in the patients who had thoracic or upper lumbar myelomeningocele.[14] Dislocation, defined as no area of congruity between the femoral head and the acetabulum, was most commonly observed in the patients who had thoracic myelomeningocele. Dislocation tended to occur by the age of 3 to 4 years in the patients who had mid-lumbar myelomeningocele, but those who had thoracic or upper lumbar myelomeningocele continued to have dislocation of the hip even after the age of 10 years. By the age of 9 to 11 years, there had been no dislocation or surgery on the hip in 42% of the patients who had third lumbar myelomeningocele, 67% of the patients who had fourth lumbar myelomeningocele, and 80% of the patients who had fifth lumbar myelomeningocele. A possible criticism of

this study is that the authors excluded hips that were subluxated, a factor that is particularly relevant for patients who have mid-lumbar myelomeningocele.

In a review by Fraser and associates,[15] subluxation or dislocation at the age of 1 year was observed in 25 of 29 patients who had third lumbar myelomeningocele and in 8 of 19 who had fourth lumbar myelomeningocele. Of the 15 hips that were stable at the age of 1 year, only 1 subsequently dislocated.

Treatment of Problems in Children Who Have Thoracic or Upper Lumbar Myelomeningocele

Numerous studies have demonstrated that the ability to walk is not affected by dislocation of the hip in patients who have thoracic or upper lumbar myelomeningocele.[7–11,14–17] Therefore, reconstructive procedures to correct dysplasia of the hip are rarely indicated for these patients because relocation of the hip does not provide functional gains and may cause complications, such as pathologic fracture or the more devastating complication of a stiff hip joint.

Because children who have myelomeningocele at an upper level rarely retain the ability to walk after reaching adulthood, some authors have recommended that these patients use a wheelchair when they are young.[18,19] Others have advocated an intensive program of bracing and gait-training during early childhood.[20,21] Charney and associates[20] found that, with such therapy, 45 of 87 patients (52%) who had myelomeningocele at an upper level were able to walk about the community by 5 years of age. However, deficient balance reactions and weakness of the upper extremities coupled with the extensive bracing that is needed prevent some of these children from achieving a functional walking ability.

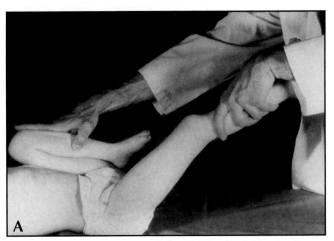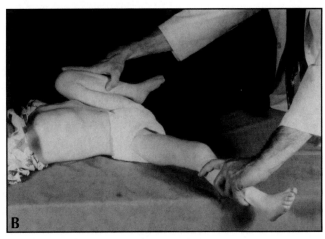

Fig. 1 A patient who had myelomeningocele at the thoracic level. **A,** Measurement of extension of the hip in the neutral plane demonstrates a 60° flexion contracture. **B,** If the extremity is positioned in abduction, the flexion contracture will be underestimated.

The potential benefits of walking by patients with myelomeningocele at an upper level include strengthening of the upper extremities, protection against obesity, better bone density, and prevention of contractures of the lower extremities. However, in my opinion, the most striking and important benefit is the tremendous sense of accomplishment that these children express when they achieve the ability to be upright and to move around a room like other children of their age. This psychological boost has also been noted in other reports on children who have myelomeningocele at an upper level.[21,22] Furthermore, in 1 study, patients with this level of myelomeningocele who were managed with bracing and early walking had fewer fractures and pressure sores and were more independent in transfers, even when they eventually switched to a wheelchair, compared with patients who had always used a wheelchair.[21] However, these children were hospitalized more often, for surgical procedures to allow bracing. Obesity, dexterity of the upper extremities, and the ability to perform other activities of daily living did not differ between the 2 groups.

My approach to the treatment of problems related to the hip in patients who have myelomeningocele begins at birth. At this age, it is not possible to identify which children are candidates for bracing and walking; therefore, all parents are taught a therapy program that targets anticipated problems. For patients who have thoracic and upper lumbar myelomeningocele, the program includes stretching exercises for the iliotibial band, the hip and knee flexors, and the ankle plantarflexors.

Patients with myelomeningocele at an upper level who have good upper-body strength and adequate balance reactions are candidates for bracing and walking. The braces for these patients must extend proximal to the hip, and walking is most easily achieved with a swing-to or swing-through gait. Because of the coordination and upper body strength that are required for such walking, gait-training should be delayed until the child is approximately 2 years old (range, 18 to 36 months). Between the age of 1 year and the initiation of gait-training, a standing frame can be helpful. This device positions the child upright and also acts to stretch flexion contractures at the hip and

knee. The wooden base of the frame is large enough to prevent falling. Parents are taught how to construct a simple table with a semicircular cutout. When the child is in the standing frame, the table is positioned around the child to allow him or her to play and do other activities in an upright position.

The brace that is initially prescribed for patients who have myelomeningocele at an upper level provides adequate support and has maximum adaptability for growth. A pelvic band is adequate for most patients who have second lumbar myelomeningocele, but patients who have thoracic myelomeningocele need a more extended plastic mold to support the lower part of the trunk. For patients who have lumbar kyphosis, the molded trunk support also minimizes skin ulceration over the spinal gibbus. Drop-lock hinges are used at the hips, but knee joints are not part of the initial orthotic. The incorporation of knee joints into a brace made for a small child markedly restricts how much the brace can be lengthened as the child grows. This brace has few disadvantages because young children can sit comfortably in most chairs without bending the knees. However, before the child goes to school, a brace that does have drop-lock knee hinges is prescribed.

A parapodium is an option for patients who have myelomeningocele at an upper level and are not candidates for independent walking. The swivel-walker type of parapodium, although more expensive, has many advantages.[23] Its heavy base prevents the child from falling, and the swivel action makes it possible for a child who has deficient balance reactions to propel himself or herself around the house, to a limited degree. The psychological boost and the additional benefits accrued from being in an upright position make the effort worthwhile.

Children with myelomeningocele at an upper level who are candidates for walking and who have flexion contractures of the hip of more than 25° to 30° must be managed surgically in order to achieve optimum bracing and walking ability. The procedure is best done when the child is ready to start gait-training. If the surgery is performed at an earlier age, the contractures will recur. Patients who have thoracic myelomeningocele do not have pain postoperatively, and the procedure usually can be done on an outpatient basis.

All components of the hip deformity should be corrected.[24] A lateral approach, centered over the greater trochanter, provides adequate exposure and minimizes problems with wound-healing and recurrent contracture. The iliotibial band, gluteus medius and minimus, tensor fasciae latae, sartorius, rectus femoris, and iliopsoas tendon are released sequentially. To protect the femoral vessels during exposure of the iliopsoas tendon, the femoral nerve should be identified first as it crosses the pelvic brim and then the femoral nerves

and vessels should be retracted medially. With severe contractures, it is also necessary to release the external rotators and the anterolateral aspect of the joint capsule.

The flexion contracture of the hip should be completely corrected by the end of the procedure. Failure to achieve full correction predisposes to early recurrence. Therefore, even when surgery is performed unilaterally, both hips are draped so that the contralateral hip can be fully flexed in order to assess the flexion contracture adequately during the procedure.

The lower extremities are immobilized postoperatively in a bilateral above-the-knee cast with a cross-bar that keeps the hips in 5° to 10° of abduction and 20° to 30° of internal rotation. This type of cast prevents the skin problems that are associated with a spica cast. Immediately after the surgery, the child is positioned with the hips in some degree of flexion. As the swelling and pain decrease, the hips are positioned to gain full extension. The child is then kept in either the supine or the prone position with the hips fully extended for at least 18 hours a day. Short periods of sitting are allowed to facilitate feeding, transportation, and other activities. The cast is worn for 4 weeks. A longer period of immobilization does not seem to lower the risk of recurrent contracture and increases the risk of pathologic fracture. To minimize the risk of recurrent contracture, it is important that bracing begin directly after the cast treatment has been discontinued.

Treatment of Problems in Children Who Have Midlumbar Myelomeningocele

Before these patients are discharged from the newborn nursery, the parents are taught a stretching program that targets the unopposed hip flexors and adductors. Radiographs of

the pelvis are made during periodic visits to the clinic. If subluxation occurs, it usually does so before the age of 3 years.

The role of surgical intervention for dysplasia of the hip in children who have myelomeningocele at the midlumbar level is controversial. Some authors have noted no association between walking ability and dislocation of the hip, whereas others have reported that dysplasia reduced the walking ability of patients who had midlumbar myelomeningocele.[5,7–10,12,16,17,25] Asher and Olson,[5] in a study that combined detailed analysis and clear separation of the patients who had third lumbar myelomeningocele from those who had fourth lumbar myelomeningocele, demonstrated a significant association between hip deformities and walking ability in both groups. In fact, deformity of the hip was the only variable that was significantly associated (< 0.05) with walking status in the group that had third lumbar myelomeningocele. Only 1 of the 8 patients who had third lumbar myelomeningocele (average age, 16 years) and a unilateral or bilateral dislocation of the hip was capable of functional walking, compared with 5 of the 12 patients who had third lumbar myelomeningocele but did not have a dislocation. Although the many variables involved make statistical analysis difficult, it has been my observation that hip dysplasia adversely affects walking ability as patients who have midlumbar myelomeningocele reach the second decade of life.

It is also true that the treatment of dysplasia of the hip in patients who have midlumbar myelomeningocele is difficult and is not universally successful. The final decision to operate must be tempered by the analysis of other factors, including the strength of the upper extremities, balance reactions, the strength of the quadriceps and medial hamstring muscles, and the severity of the acetabular and proximal femoral malalignment. Furthermore, it is important to do whatever is necessary to stabilize the hips with the first operation. The goal of treatment of hip problems in patients who have myelomeningocele is to minimize the number of operations needed and the period of immobilization in a spica cast.[26] Repeated attempts at reconstruction of the hip predisposes to pathologic fracture or, even worse, a stiff hip that affects wheelchair activities and accelerates the development of painful arthrosis.

Posterolateral transfer of the iliopsoas, as described by Sharrard,[27] is meant to correct muscle imbalance and to stabilize or correct dysplasia of the hip in patients who have myelomeningocele. The concept of the Sharrard procedure is to transfer the deforming force of the iliopsoas to a position where it can substitute for the nonfunctional hip extensors and abductors. The iliopsoas tendon and the iliacus muscle are freed up so that both can be transferred through a drill-hole made in the ilium. This requires the creation of a relatively large window. The iliopsoas tendon is inserted through the drill-hole into the posterior aspect of the greater trochanter, and the origin of the iliacus is sutured to the ilium in a position corresponding to the origin of the gluteus medius.

Initially, the Sharrard procedure was done on virtually all patients with myelomeningocele who had a dysplastic hip.[27] However, disenchantment was subsequently voiced.[8,26,28–30] The surgery was noted to be extensive and to seldom provide active antigravity extension. Furthermore, a high rate of recurrent subluxation was reported in some series.[8,26,28–30] Additional analysis, however, revealed that the latter prob-

lem was partly related to the inclusion of patients who had thoracic or upper lumbar myelomeningocele; we now understand that this procedure is inappropriate for these patients.

Posterolateral transfer of the iliopsoas should be limited to a select group of patients. In 1983, Sharrard[31] recommended that the transfer should be combined with an adductor release, should be done before osseous deformity develops (between 1 and 2 years of age), and should be limited to patients who have fourth lumbar myelomeningocele. The third guideline is perhaps too stringent as good results have been observed in patients with third lumbar myelomeningocele who have good (grade 4) strength of the quadriceps muscle.[12,17,28]

The study by Stillwell and Menelaus[12] provided useful data concerning the effectiveness of the Sharrard procedure. It should be noted that all 47 patients in that series had release of the adductors to obtain 60° of abduction. Most of the operations were performed before the patients were 3 years old. Ten years or more postoperatively, the results were relatively good: 35 patients (74%) were capable of functional walking and most of these 35 could climb stairs. Functional walking was associated with the neurologic level and at least grade 3 strength of the quadriceps. At the time of follow-up, none of the 3 patients who had second lumbar myelomeningocele, 10 of the 16 patients who had third lumbar myelomeningocele, 13 of the 15 patients who had fourth lumbar myelomeningocele, and 12 of the 13 patients who had fifth lumbar myelomeningocele were capable of functional walking. A flexion contracture of more than 20° was not observed in any patient, and only 5 of the 79 hips had a contracture of 20°. Before the surgery, 8 hips were

subluxated and 23 were dislocated. At the most recent follow-up evaluation, 2 hips were subluxated and 2 were dislocated. No patient in that study was excluded from the analysis because of loss of neurologic function.

It is now clear that posterolateral transfer of the iliopsoas does not provide active extension or abduction against gravity, and it is doubtful that this out-of-phase transfer provides any noticeable extension or abduction during the gait cycle. A recent study using 3-dimensional gait analysis revealed no improvement in abnormal pelvic obliquity in patients with fourth lumbar myelomeningocele who had been managed with iliopsoas transfer.[29] In my opinion, the primary benefit of posterolateral transfer of the iliopsoas is that it not only removes a deforming force but also provides an active restraint or tenodesis effect that greatly minimizes the risk of a recurrent flexion contracture of the hip. When there is no flexion contracture, walking mechanics are improved and, more importantly, standing is possible with little or no support. In contrast, patients with mid-lumbar myelomeningocele who have a flexion contracture of more than 20° cannot stand and rest but must expend considerable energy just to stay upright. As a result, walking is difficult. The iliopsoas transfer, combined with an adductor release and osteotomies as needed, can stabilize progressive subluxation of the hip and help to maintain functional walking (Fig. 2), but whether this approach is optimum for these patients is still debatable.

Transfer of the external oblique muscle has been advocated as an alternative to transfer of the iliopsoas for patients who have myelomeningocele at the midlumbar level as well as a dysplastic hip.[32–34] This procedure does not weaken the iliopsoas.

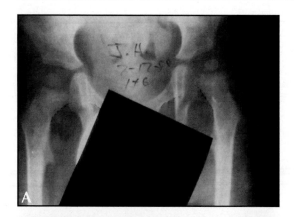

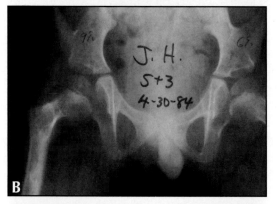

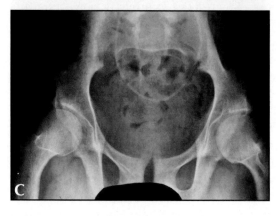

Fig. 2 Anteroposterior radiographs of a boy who had myelomeningocele at the third lumbar level. **A,** At 1 year and 6 months of age, there is early subluxation of the left hip. Bilateral dysplasia ultimately developed, and the patient had a bilateral staged adductor myotomy, transfer of the iliopsoas, and femoral osteotomy. **B,** At 5 years of age, there is adequate containment. Note the size of the iliac window necessary for a standard Sharrard transfer. **C,** At 16 years of age, the containment is satisfactory. The patient was able to walk about the community with use of a knee-ankle-foot orthosis on the left, an ankle-foot orthosis on the right, and forearm crutches.

Therefore, the power of the hip flexors and the ability to climb stairs should be maintained. Some authors[35] have stated that transfer of the external oblique muscle improves hip mechanics during midstance; however, gait-analysis studies have demonstrated that the transferred external oblique muscle mainly functions during the swing phase of gait.[35] Therefore, it is doubtful that this transferred muscle imitates the activity of the hip abductors or extensors during walking.

Phillips and Lindseth[33] described the results of transfer of the external oblique muscle in 47 patients (89 hips). With that method, the hip adductors were transferred to the ischium and the tensor fasciae latae were moved to a more lateral position. Although those authors reported functional walking by all patients, the duration of follow-up averaged

only 4.5 years, and 6 patients were excluded from the analysis because of loss of neurologic function. With the more limited follow-up and the exclusion of certain patients, it is doubtful that the results reported by Phillips and Lindseth are markedly different than those observed after transfer of the iliopsoas.

In a study of 34 children (66 hips) with third, fourth, or fifth lumbar myelomeningocele who had a femoral osteotomy combined with transfer of the external oblique and adductor muscles, Tosi and associates[34] reported the maintenance of stability of 37 of 51 hips (73%) in the 26 children who remained neurologically stable; however, only 8 of 15 hips in the 8 children who had a progressive loss of neurologic function remained stable. The poorest results were for the hips that had dislocated previously. Only 2 of the 10 hips in this group had a successful result. The transferred muscle was noted to be weak, as no patient demonstrated active abduction even in the supine position. The average duration of follow-up in that study was relatively long (10.9 years), but the wide range of follow-up (0.7 to 20.0 years) limits conclusions concerning functional status as these children reached adult body size. At the most recent evaluation, 21 of the 26 children (81%) who had not lost neurologic function were able to walk about the community.

It is difficult to compare studies of transfer of the iliopsoas with those of transfer of the external oblique muscle. Reports vary with regard to how the neurologic level and the results are defined. In addition, the definition of progressive loss of neurologic function is imprecise, and not all studies have provided a separate analysis of patients with such loss. Furthermore, it seems that, in the large series, the procedure was done on virtually all patients who had midlumbar myelomeningocele.[12,33,34] Perhaps this protocol was used because previous authors had suggested that the muscle imbalance in these patients eventually causes dysplasia of the hip and that tendon transfers should be done, if possible, before marked subluxation and osseous changes develop.[28,31] However, it is now understood that progressive dysplasia does not develop in all patients who have myelomeningocele at the midlumbar level (Fig. 3), and experienced observers, such as Broughton and associates[14] now recommend a selective approach for surgical intervention.

In my opinion, both transfers are major procedures and are indicated only for patients in whom subluxation has developed and who have at least grade 4 strength of the quadriceps. Transfer of the external oblique muscle has the advantage of maintaining the function of the iliopsoas, but the external oblique muscle is relatively small and there is a legitimate concern that patients managed with this procedure are at greater risk for recurrent dysplasia and a recurrent flexion contracture of the hip. Maintaining neutral extension of the hip and the ability to stand without the support of the upper extremities is a long-term benefit of transfer of the iliopsoas; however, moving the entire iliacus muscle to the posterior aspect of the ilium is an extensive dissection. Perhaps the results would be just as good if only the iliopsoas tendon was transferred to the greater trochanter and the iliacus muscle was left in place. Longer follow-up after transfer of the external oblique muscle as well as comparative gait analysis studies will allow a more definitive statement concerning the best approach.

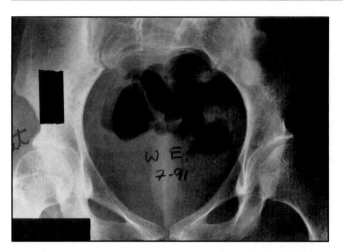

Fig. 3 Anteroposterior radiograph of a 23-year-old woman who had myelomeningocele at the fourth lumbar level. She was able to walk about the community with use of forearm crutches and an ankle-foot orthosis on each side. She did not have any surgery on the hip.

The Role of Concomitant Procedures

Whether one prefers transfer of the external oblique muscle or the iliopsoas, it is clear that either procedure must be combined with release or transfer of the adductors, to correct adduction contractures and to provide a better biomechanical environment for the transfer. This concept was corroborated by Yngve and Lindseth,[36] who documented better radiographic results when adductor and abductor procedures had been combined.

Transfer of the adductors to the ischium should provide better power of hip extension, but this concept has not been proved. Compared with adductor myotomy, transfer of the hip adductors requires more dissection and, in children who had cerebral palsy, was associated with a pullout rate of 33% (11 of 33 hips) despite an average duration of immobilization in a cast of 5.7 weeks.[37] In my opinion, this duration of immobilization is contraindicated for patients who have myelomeningocele.

Muscle transfers for the treatment of dysplasia of the hip associated with myelomeningocele are insufficient to correct severe osseous deformities. Malalignment of the proximal part of the femur or the acetabulum is par-

ticularly common after the age of 3 years, and this problem should be corrected either before or at the same time as the muscle transfers. A femoral varus rotation osteotomy corrects abnormal valgus angulation and anteversion. The type of pelvic osteotomy that best serves these patients is less clear. Acetabular deficiency in patients who have myelomeningocele is often global (anterior and posterior).[38] For that reason, a Pemberton or modified Dega procedure may be better than other pelvic osteotomies that are commonly used for the management of young children who have congenital dislocation of the hip.[39,40]

Patients who have myelomeningocele are at risk for pathological fracture, particularly after immobilization in a spica cast. Therefore, such immobilization should be limited to 4 weeks, an approach that requires adequate fixation of the sites of both the tendon transfers and the osteotomies (Fig. 4).

Dysplasia of the Hip Before the Age of One Year in Children Who Have Midlumbar Myelomeningocele

Subluxation or dislocation of the hip that develops before the age of 1 year in patients who have midlumbar

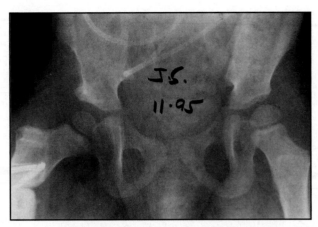

Fig. 4 Anteroposterior radiograph of a 2-year and 6-months-old girl with myelomeningocele at the fourth lumbar level in whom early subluxation of the right hip developed. She was managed with transfer of the external oblique muscle, adductor myotomy, and femoral osteotomy. Blade-plate fixation of the osteotomy site and good suture techniques for the tendon transfer made it possible for the cast to be removed after 4 weeks of immobilization.

myelomeningocele is difficult to treat. Typically, the problem is noted in the first few months of life. Use of a Pavlik harness or some other brace designed for congenital dysplasia of the hip is seldom successful over the long term for patients who have myelomeningocele. Furthermore, when the hip extensors are nonfunctional, these braces exacerbate a flexion contracture in a neonate.

Transfer of the iliopsoas or the external oblique muscle has also not been successful in this group of patients. In the study by Stillwell and Menelaus,[12] 5 of 9 patients who had had an iliopsoas transfer before they were 1 year old were not walking at the time of the most recent follow-up, at least 10 years postoperatively. Tosi and associates[34] reported redislocation of 2 of 4 hips that had had transfer of the external oblique muscle and femoral osteotomy after initial treatment with a Pavlik harness. The reason for the dislocations is unclear, but they may be explained by the timing of surgery in this unique subset of patients. In my experience, when dysplasia develops in the first year of life in patients who have midlumbar myelomeningocele, it develops by the age of 3 or 4 months. Indeed, many of these patients probably have dislocation of the hip at birth, but the treatment of other medical problems prevents its documentation. If intervention is delayed, the rapid growth during infancy coupled with an underlying muscle imbalance may result in severe dysplasia that cannot be stabilized with soft-tissue procedures.

My method of treatment for this problem is an iliopsoas recession and adductor myotomy.[41] The surgery is typically performed between the age of 2 and 4 months because, by that time, other medical problems have stabilized. The iliopsoas recession moves the psoas tendon to a position at which it cannot block a concentric reduction or compress the medial femoral circumflex artery. The hips can then be reduced and immobilized in a position of extension, abduction, and internal rotation. This position, although good for the stabilization of congenital dysplasia, was abandoned because of its association with osteonecrosis. However, after an adductor myotomy and iliopsoas recession, the risk of osteonecrosis from positioning the hips in extension is virtually eliminated.

Immobilization after the iliopsoas recession and adductor myotomy can be accomplished effectively with the application of a bilateral above-the-knee cast with cross-bars that keep the hips in abduction and internal rotation. Use of this cast eliminates the serious nursing problem that occurs when small infants who have neurogenic dysfunction of the bowel and bladder are placed in a spica cast. Extension of the hip can be adequately maintained with appropriate positioning. Immobilization typically lasts for 2 months and is followed by treatment with an abduction splint.

My experience with this method for treating myelomeningocele is limited to 3 patients, but the dislocation was corrected in all 3 (Fig. 5). If dysplasia of the hip recurs, reconstructive procedures can be performed without the surgeon having to contend with the extreme acetabular dysplasia and joint contractures that would have developed without the described treatment.

Dysplasia of the Hip in Older Children Who Have Midlumbar Myelomeningocele

Progressive subluxation of the hip in an adolescent patient presents a dilemma. Muscle imbalance coupled with complicated acetabular dysplasia leads to a substantial rate of recurrent subluxation. There is no set answer for these patients. Certainly, the evaluation should include assessment for a possible tethered cord syndrome and consideration of a computed tomography scan with reconstruction to define the extent and location of the acetabular deformity.[38,42] Treatment must be individualized, but I have most often performed a Chiari pelvic osteotomy

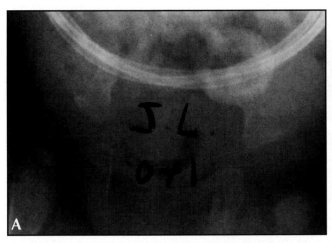
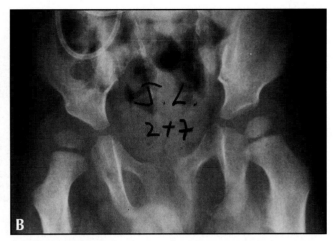

Fig. 5 Anteroposterior radiographs of a boy who had myelomeningocele at the midlumbar level. **A,** Bilateral dislocation of the hip was evident at the age of 2 months. The patient was managed with iliopsoas recession and adductor myotomy. **B,** At the age of 2 years and 7 months, the hips were located but still dysplastic. Additional procedures will most likely be necessary, but the improvement in the interval definitely made the procedure worthwhile.

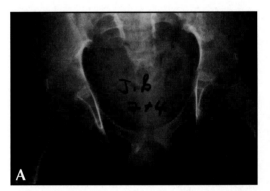
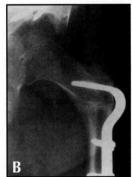
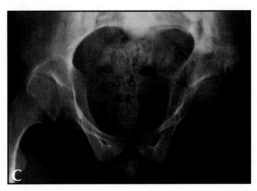

Fig. 6 A boy who had myelomeningocele at the fourth lumbar level and subluxation of the left hip. **A,** Anteroposterior radiograph made at the age of 7 years. Two years later, the subluxation had progressed and there was 52% migration. **B,** Anteroposterior radiograph made after Chiari pelvic and proximal femoral osteotomies. **C,** Anteroposterior radiograph made at the age of 16 years. There was still satisfactory coverage.

and femoral varus rotation osteotomy in this group of patients (Fig. 6). I have also recommended observation or no treatment for adolescent patients who have a history of surgery, no functional abductor muscles, and a markedly dysplastic acetabulum. In this situation, the chance of success is low and reconstructive surgery may cause the hip to become stiff and painful.

Problems About the Knee

Surgical treatment of the knee is needed considerably less often than surgery on the hip and foot in chil-dren who have myelomeningocele. However, it has recently become apparent that arthropathy of the knee may develop in relatively young adults who have myelomeningocele. In a study of adult patients who ranged in age from 23 to 39 years, Williams and associates[43] noted severe symptoms related to the knee in 17 of 72 patients (24%) who functioned as community ambulators.[6] Patients with myelomeningocele who have absent or diminished strength of the hip abductors and the ankle plan-tarflexors walk with an increased valgus-external rotation thrust applied to the knee during midstance. These forces are exacerbated when these patients walk without the use of forearm crutches, a situation that is almost universal during the adolescent years. As they reach the second decade of life, these patients should be counseled concerning the abnormal biomechanics and the fact that total joint arthroplasty is not a good option for them as young adults. Most importantly, they need to understand that the use of forearm crutches can decrease the abnormal forces acting to accelerate degenerative arthrosis of the knee joint.

Congenital hyperextension of the knee is occasionally seen in patients who have thoracic myelomeningocele. Patients who have rigid deformities should not be managed with a cast because the risk of skin ulceration or bowing of the tibia is too great. Treatment involves either a V-Y lengthening of the quadriceps tendon, a percutaneous release, or a division of the patellar ligament.[44–46] The latter is a simple procedure, and it is my preferred method for the treatment of extension deformities of the knee in patients who have thoracic myelomeningocele.

The natural history of flexion contracture of the knee associated with myelomeningocele was described by Wright and associates.[47] Patients who had thoracic myelomeningocele had the most severe deformity; the flexion contracture averaged 30° at maturity. However, the standard deviation was large for all groups except the patients who had sacral myelomeningocele. Therefore, severe deformities are less likely to occur in patients who have lumbar myelomeningocele but they may occur.

Bracing and walking are affected by flexion contractures of more than 20° to 25°. My primary reason for release of a knee flexion contracture associated with myelomeningocele is to improve or allow bracing. Unless there is a tethered cord, the severity of the flexion contracture of the knee is not markedly different when measured with the hip in flexion. This indicates that contraction of the posterior aspect of the knee capsule, as opposed to the hamstrings, is the primary pathologic finding. Therefore, a complete release of the capsule is necessary to correct the problem.

My technique for releasing a flexion contracture of the knee is

through a single midline posterior incision. Occasionally, 2 incisions, 1 posteromedial and 1 posterolateral, are used in a small child who has a severe contracture. In either case, the incision does not cross the popliteal crease. If the hamstrings have at least grade 3 strength, they are lengthened; however, if these muscles are weak, a tenotomy is done. Because the gastrocnemius is inactive in these patients, the medial and lateral heads

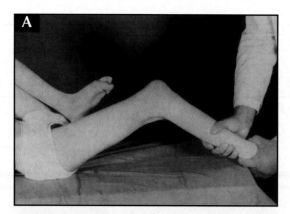

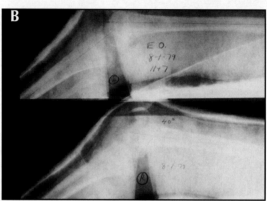

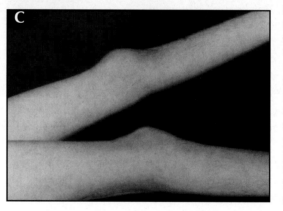

Fig. 7 A boy who had myelomeningocele at the fourth lumbar level. A, Photograph showing severe flexion contracture of the knee, which developed at the age of 11 years following a period of inactivity imposed by a burn injury to the lower extremity. The patient was managed with a radical posterior release of the contracture. B, Lateral radiographs, made after the first postoperative cast-wedging, demonstrating posterior subluxation of the tibia. A Quengle cast was used to provide anterior translation of the tibia. C, Photograph, made at the completion of treatment with the cast, showing full extension of the knee. Fourteen years after the procedure, the patient was still able to walk about the community with use of forearm crutches and a bilateral ankle-foot orthosis.

are released from the femoral condyle. The posterior aspect of the knee capsule is incised from the posterior margin of the medial collateral ligament to the posterior margin of the lateral collateral ligament. Occasionally, one or both cruciate ligaments must be released.

If full extension is not achieved, wedging of the cast is initiated on the second or third postoperative day. After a radical posterior knee release, no more than 2 or 3 wedges are required to obtain full extension. To perform the wedging, the cast is cut almost circumferentially at the level of the adductor tubercle (the instant center of knee motion). To prevent anterior translation and breakage of the cast, an anterior strip (4 to 5 cm long) is left intact. The integrity of this tongue of plaster is enhanced by 2 vertical cuts (6 cm long) at the medial and lateral margins of the strip. The child is then placed in the prone position with the feet hanging off the table. The knee is extended, and the corrected position is secured by a block of wood inserted on the posterior margin of the cast. The block is made with a lip on either end to prevent dislodgment and skin ulceration. A roll of plaster of Paris secures the block and stabilizes the cast.

Skin ulceration may develop at the heel after postoperative cast-wedging, despite appropriate precautions. This is not surprising because the heels of these patients are insensate. Frequent inspection of the cast identifies the problem before serious complications occur.

When a patient has a severe contracture, cast-wedging may cause posterior subluxation of the tibia (Fig. 7). Although this problem is uncommon in patients with myelomeningocele who have had a posterior release of the knee capsule, a lateral radiograph should be made to exclude the possibility. If posterior subluxation occurs, alternative treatment, such as the use of a Quengle cast[48] with antisubluxation hinges or 2-pin skeletal traction through the distal aspect of the femur and the proximal aspect of the tibia, is necessary to correct the subluxation and obtain full extension.

Extension osteotomy of the distal aspect of the femur is another technique that can be used to treat a flexion deformity of the knee.[49] This procedure, however, has several disadvantages that, for the most part, preclude its use in children who have myelomeningocele. The osteotomy does not correct the primary deformity but rather straightens the knee by creating a second deformity. More importantly, there is rapid recurrence of the deformity when the procedure is performed at a young age, the time when most flexion deformities in patients who have myelomeningocele are treated.

Overview

While the treatment of hip and knee deformities associated with myelomeningocele can be quite challenging, progress has been made in our understanding of these problems. A procedure to correct severe contractures of the hip and knee may be indicated for a patient with myelomeningocele at an upper level who is a candidate for bracing and walking; however, the parents must understand that the deformity will recur when walking stops. Procedures to stabilize progressive subluxation of the hip are indicated for patients with a lesion at the midlumbar level who have good strength of the quadriceps. The procedure should correct the hip flexor and adductor imbalance and should also correct severe osseous deformities. At present, it is unclear whether transfer of the iliopsoas or transfer of the external oblique muscle is the better procedure.

References

1. Mazur JM, Stillwell A, Menelaus M: The significance of spasticity in the upper and lower limbs in myelomeningocele. *J Bone Joint Surg* 1986;68B:213–217.

2. Mazur JM, Menelaus MB, Hudson I, Stillwell A: Hand function in patients with spina bifida cystica. *J Pediatr Orthop* 1986;6:442–447.

3. Turner A: Hand function in children with myelomeningocele. *J Bone Joint Surg* 1985;67B:268–272.

4. Archibeck MJ, Smith JT, Carroll KL, Davitt JS, Stevens PM: Surgical release of tethered spinal cord: Survivorship analysis and orthopedic outcome. *J Pediatr Orthop* 1997;17:773–776.

5. Asher M, Olson J: Factors affecting the ambulatory status of patients with spina bifida cystica. *J Bone Joint Surg* 1983;65A:350–356.

6. Hoffer MM, Feiwell E, Perry R, Perry J, Bonnett C: Functional ambulation in patients with myelomeningocele. *J Bone Joint Surg* 1973;55A:137–148.

7. Barden GA, Meyer LC, Stelling FH III: Myelodysplastics: Fate of those followed for twenty years or more. *J Bone Joint Surg* 1975;57A:643–647.

8. Bazih J, Gross RH: Hip surgery in the lumbar level myelomeningocele patient. *J Pediatr Orthop* 1981;1:405–411.

9. De Souza LJ, Carroll N: Ambulation of the braced myelomeningocele patient. *J Bone Joint Surg* 1976;58A:1112–1118.

10. Feiwell E: Surgery of the hip in myelomeningocele as related to adult goals. *Clin Orthop* 1980;148:87–93.

11. Samuelsson L, Skoog M: Ambulation in patients with myelomeningocele: A multivariate statistical analysis. *J Pediatr Orthop* 1988;8:569–575.

12. Stillwell A, Menelaus MB: Walking ability after transplantation of the iliopsoas: A long-term follow-up. *J Bone Joint Surg* 1984;66B:656–659.

13. Brinker MR, Rosenfeld SR, Feiwell E, Granger SP, Mitchell DC, Rice JC: Myelomeningocele at the sacral level: Long-term outcomes in adults. *J Bone Joint Surg* 1994;76A:1293–1300.

14. Broughton NS, Menelaus MB, Cole WG, Shurtleff DB: The natural history of hip deformity in myelomeningocele. *J Bone Joint Surg* 1993;75B:760–763.

15. Fraser RK, Hoffman EB, Sparks LT, Buccimazza SS: The unstable hip and midlumbar myelomeningocele. *J Bone Joint Surg* 1992;74B:143–146.

16. Keggi JM, Banta JV, Walto C: The myelodysplastic hip and scoliosis. *Dev Med Child Neurol* 1992;34:240–246.

17. Lee EH, Carroll NC: Hip stability and ambulatory status in myelomeningocele. *J Pediatr Orthop* 1985;5:522–527.

18. Butler C, Okamoto GA, McKay TM: Powered mobility for very young disabled children. *Dev Med Child Neurol* 1983;25:472–474.

19. Shurtleff DB: Mobility, in Shurtleff DB (ed): *Myelodysplasias and Exstrophies: Significance, Prevention, and Treatment.* New York, NY, Grune & Stratton, 1986, pp 313–356.

20. Charney EB, Melchionni JB, Smith DR: Community ambulation by children with myelomeningocele and high-level paralysis *J Pediatr Orthop* 1991;11:579–582.

21. Mazur JM, Shurtleff D, Menelaus M, Colliver J: Orthopaedic management of high-level spina bifida: Early walking compared with early use of a wheelchair. *J Bone Joint Surg* 1989;71A:56–61.

22. Liptak GS, Shurtleff DB, Bloss JW, Baltus-Hebert E, Manitta P: Mobility aids for children with high-level myelomeningocele: Parapodium versus wheelchair. *Dev Med Child Neurol* 1992;34:787–796.

23. Lough LK, Neilsen DH: Ambulation of children with myelomeningocele: Parapodium versus parapodium with Orlau swivel modification. *Dev Med Child Neurol* 1986;28:489–497.

24. Menelaus MB: The hip in myelomeningocele: Management directed towards a minimum number of operations and a minimum period of immobilisation. *J Bone Joint Surg* 1976;58B:448–452.

25. Feiwell E, Sakai D, Blatt T: The effect of hip reduction on function in patients with myelomeningocele: Potential gains and hazards of surgical treatment. *J Bone Joint Surg* 1978;60A:169–173.

26. Drummond DS, Moreau M, Cruess RL: The results and complications of surgery for the paralytic hip and spine in myelomeningocele. *J Bone Joint Surg* 1980;62B:49–53.

27. Sharrard WJW: Posterior iliopsoas transplantation in the treatment of paralytic dislocation of the hip. *J Bone Joint Surg* 1964;46B:426–444.

28. Carroll NC, Sharrard WJ: Long-term follow-up of posterior iliopsoas transplantation for paralytic dislocation of the hip. *J Bone Joint Surg* 1972;54A:551–560.

29. Duffy CM, Hill AE, Cosgrove AP, Corry IS, Mollan RAB, Graham HK: Three-dimensional gait analysis in spina bifida. *J Pediatr Orthop* 1996;16:786–791.

30. Sherk HH, Ames MD: Functional results of iliopsoas transfer in myelomeningocele hip dislocations. *Clin Orthop* 1978;137:181–186.

31. Sharrard WJ: Management of paralytic subluxation and dislocation of the hip in myelomenin-

gocele. *Dev Med Child Neurol* 1983;25:374–376.

32. Dias LS: Hip deformities in myelomeningocele, in Tullos HS (ed): *Instructional Course Lectures XL*. Park Ridge, IL, American Academy of Orthopaedic Surgeons, 1991, pp 281–286.

33. Phillips DP, Lindseth RE: Ambulation after transfer of adductors, external oblique, and tensor fascia lata in myelomeningocele. *J Pediatr Orthop* 1992;12:712–717.

34. Tosi LL, Buck BD, Nason SS, McKay DW: Dislocation of the hip in myelomeningocele: The McKay hip stabilization. *J Bone Joint Surg* 1996;78A:664–673.

35. Dias LS, Thomas SS, Robinson C, Porcelli R, Sarwark J: Hip dislocation in spina bifida: The external oblique transfer. *Orthop Trans* 1992;16:624–625.

36. Yngve DA, Lindseth RE: Effectiveness of muscle transfers in myelomeningocele hips measured by radiographic indices. *J Pediatr Orthop* 1982;2:121–125.

37. Loder RT, Harbuz A, Aronson DD, Lee CL: Postoperative migration of the adductor tendon after posterior adductor transfer in children with cerebral palsy. *Dev Med Child Neurol* 1992;34:49–54.

38. Buckley SL, Sponseller PD, Magid D: The acetabulum in congenital and neuromuscular hip instability. *J Pediatr Orthop* 1991;11:498–501.

39. Mubarak SJ, Valencia FG, Wenger DR: One-stage correction of the spastic dislocated hip: Use of pericapsular acetabuloplasty to improve coverage. *J Bone Joint Surg* 1992;74A:1347–1357.

40. Pemberton PA: Pericapsular osteotomy of the ilium for treatment of congenital subluxation and dislocation of the hip. *J Bone Joint Surg* 1965;47A:65–86.

41. Breed AL, Healy PM: The midlumbar myelomeningocele hip: Mechanism of dislocation and treatment. *J Pediatr Orthop* 1982;2:15–24.

42. Abel MF, Sutherland DH, Wenger DR, Mubarak SJ: Evaluation of CT scans and 3-D reformatted images for quantitative assessment of the hip. *J Pediatr Orthop* 1994;14:48–53.

43. Williams JJ, Graham GP, Dunne AB, Menelaus MB: Late knee problems in myelomeningocele. *J Pediatr Orthop* 1993;13:701–703.

44. Curtis BH, Fisher RL: Congenital hyperextension with anterior subluxation of the knee: Surgical treatment and long-term observations. *J Bone Joint Surg* 1969;51A:255–269.

45. Roy DR, Crawford AH: Percutaneous quadriceps recession: A technique for management of congenital hyperextension deformities of the knee in the neonate. *J Pediatr Orthop* 1989;9:717–719.

46. Sandhu PS, Broughton NS, Menelaus MB: Tenotomy of the ligamentum patellae in spina bifida: Management of limited flexion range at the knee. *J Bone Joint Surg* 1995;77B:832–833.

47. Wright JG, Menelaus MB, Broughton NS, Shurtleff D: Natural history of knee contractures in myelomeningocele. *J Pediatr Orthop* 1991;11:725–730.

48. Greene WB, Wilson FC: Nonoperative management of hemophilic arthropathy and muscle hemorrhage, in Murray JA (ed): American Academy of Orthopaedic Surgeons *Instructional Course Lectures XXXIII*. St. Louis, MO, CV Mosby, 1983.

49. Zimmerman MH, Smith CF, Oppenheim WL: Supracondylar femoral extension osteotomies in the treatment of fixed flexion deformity of the knee. *Clin Orthop* 1982;171:87–93.

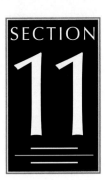

SECTION 11

Orthopaedic Oncology

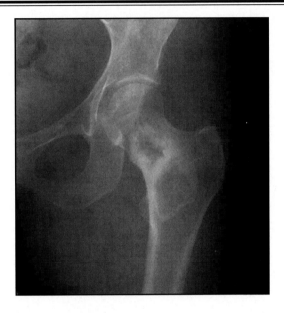

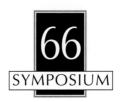

Orthopaedic Oncology for the Nononcologist Orthopaedist: Introduction and Common Errors to Avoid

William G. Ward, Sr, MD

Introduction

This update on orthopaedic oncology, based on a symposium entitled "Orthopaedic Oncology for the Nononcologist Orthopaedist" presented at the 1998 American Academy of Orthopaedic Surgeons Annual Meeting is designed to provide the practicing general orthopaedist with a practical straightforward review of current orthopaedic oncology principles and practices, without being encyclopedic in approach. The symposium was well received and the attendee feedback was quite positive. The authors and editor have now assembled this material into a series of chapters on orthopaedic oncology, reviewing the same material presented during the symposium. Mastery of the material presented should give the general orthopaedist a good overview of orthopaedic oncology and provide a practical framework for use in the evaluation, treatment, and follow-up of patients with orthopaedic tumors. The material will also educate the general orthopaedist on the common pitfalls and errors encountered in treating patients with orthopaedic tumors, hopefully allowing the practitioner to avoid repeating many of the same errors and pitfalls to which we are all prey, due to the subtle nature of many tumors, and the infrequency with which these problems are encountered in the general orthopaedist's practice.

There have been many advances in the field of orthopaedic oncology over the past 2 decades. Limb salvage surgery is now possible in the majority of patients with sarcomas. Long-term survival of 50% to 75% of patients is regularly achieved in osteosarcoma and many other orthopaedic neoplasms. These potentially good results depend heavily on prompt and proper management of the patients. In order to update the general orthopaedist on current concepts in orthopaedic oncology, this chapter will present the more common pitfalls and errors to which all orthopaedists are subject in the management of these problems. A number of actual exemplary cases will be presented to illustrate these concepts.

Index of Suspicion

General orthopaedists infrequently mismanage an orthopaedic tumor once the neoplastic process is recognized. Such patients are usually referred to an orthopaedic oncologist. However, the defensive approach of referring all tumor cases to an orthopaedic oncologist will not always keep the general orthopaedist out of trouble, because the diagnosis of neoplasia is established late in many patients with tumors. Because most patients with orthopaedic tumors are otherwise healthy, an index of suspicion for neoplasia should always be maintained whenever treating any patient, especially those with a soft-tissue mass or painful bony lesion. For example, a recently treated 18-year-old male presented to his orthopaedist complaining of knee pain. He was not asked about night pain, and a mechanical problem (meniscal tear) was diagnosed. The knee radiograph was interpreted as normal (Fig. 1, A and B). He underwent arthroscopic examination and no significant abnormalities were found. When he returned for follow-up 3.5 months later, the clinical and radiographic findings had progressed (Fig. 1, C and D). His night pain was now severe, he had a palpable mass and osteosarcoma was easily diagnosed.

Misdiagnoses usually fall into 1 of 2 categories. The first is misdiagnosis due to the lack of detection of an abnormality, such as a radiographic finding, that would suggest a neoplastic process. The second is misdiagnosis from attributing an abnormal radiographic or clinical finding to a benign etiology, such as a hematoma. Thus, in both situations, the orthopaedic surgeon fails to maintain an index of suspicion, either that a neoplastic process is present, or that an abnormality

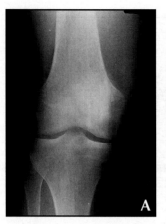
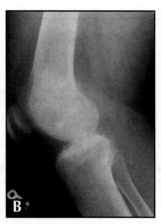
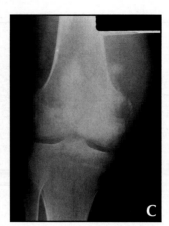
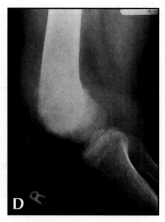

Fig. 1 Anteroposterior (AP) and lateral knee radiographs (**A** and **B**) of an 18-year-old male with knee pain. Note the subtle supracondylar sclerosis. This sclerosis was overlooked because the history of night pain was not obtained and the radiograph was not studied with an index of suspicion for neoplasia. Bone scan or MRI would demonstrate the tumor well at this stage. AP and lateral radiographs (**C** and **D**) of the same patient 2½ months later. Note the increased lysis, sclerosis, and soft-tissue extension of the osteosarcoma.

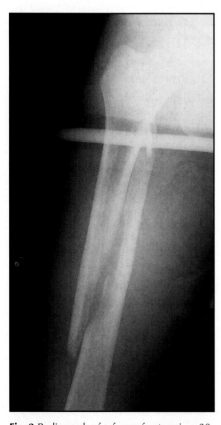

Fig. 2 Radiograph of a femur fracture in a 20-year-old male. Note the subtle permeation due to Ewing's sarcoma. The history of a nontraumatic initial fracture led the treating physicians to obtain special projections to demonstrate the anomaly.

Outline 1
Presentation of orthopaedic tumors

Mass
Pain
Pathologic fracture
Serendipitous finding

reflects a neoplastic process. By maintaining an index of suspicion, and obtaining an appropriate history, most neoplasms can be detected.

A recently treated 20-year-old male fractured his femur while hiking in the mountains. Upon further questioning by the residents in the emergency room, it was determined that he did not break his femur in a fall, but rather his femur broke during the "push off" phase of a jump while jumping from one rock to another in the mountains. His radiographic abnormality (aside from the obvious fracture) was subtle at best (Fig. 2); a small amount of a permeative abnormality of the cortex could be appreciated in 1 of the 5 radiographic projections obtained. These multiple projections were obtained purely because of the high index of suspicion for a pathologic fracture, based entirely on the history of the mechanism of injury. On one AP view, there was a hint of a permeative process in the posterior cortex. At open biopsy the cortex grossly appeared normal, as did the periosteum, surrounding hematoma, and the other soft tissues. Biopsy of these areas was normal also. Only a 1.5- to 2-inch section of marrow in the fracture site itself harbored pathologically detectable Ewing's sarcoma.

In the evaluation of patients with potential neoplasms, the physician must rely on the history, physical examination, and laboratory findings, as in the evaluation of any patient. Patients with musculoskeletal tumors generally present in 1 of the 4 manners listed in Outline 1. These presentations include the presence of a mass, pain, pathologic or impending pathologic fracture, or a serendipitous finding.

Mass

Whenever a patient presents with a new mass, it should be considered a sarcoma until proven otherwise. The lack of other symptoms, such as pain, is the rule rather than the exception with soft-tissue sarcomas. Soft-tissue sarcomas are far more common than osseous sarcomas. Few surgeons would mistake a sizeable mass as anything other than a tumor. However, smaller masses are frequently misdiagnosed as hematomas, ganglions, lipomas, or other benign processes, presumably because the physician did not consider the possibility of neoplasia.

Hematomas

Hematomas do not spontaneously occur in patients without a history of significant trauma, use of anticoagulation medication, or some other coagulopathic process. When a tumor bleeds, it bleeds into itself from central necrosis. The hematoma does not disseminate into the surrounding soft tissues due to capsular and pseudocapsular compartmentalization and containment of the tumor. Thus, subcutaneous ecchymosis will not be present in the extremity of a hemorrhagic sarcoma. There will be no observable "bruising." These blood-filled cavities tend to grow over time, presumably due to recurrent bleeding. Alternatively, when a muscle tears or a muscle-tendon unit ruptures, or if there is any other significant traumatic tissue disruption that causes a soft-tissue bleed, the blood in those situations generally will extend along fascial planes. Ecchymosis will be present in subcutaneous locations, especially in the gravitationally dependent locations. Over several weeks this ecchymosis will generally be reabsorbed. If there is no observable ecchymosis, do not diagnose a hematoma.

An 80-year-old male was referred after he had had 2 aspirations of a supposed anterior thigh muscle hematoma. The 2 aspirates reported-

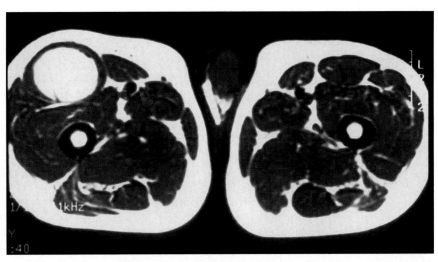

Fig. 3 Axial MRI scan demonstrating a lesion isolated to the rectus femoris. Biopsy confirmed a thin-walled malignant fibrous histiocytoma with a large central hemorrhagic cavity.

ly revealed only blood. He had no observable ecchymosis. Magnetic resonance imaging (MRI) demonstrated a process isolated to his rectus femoris muscle (Fig. 3). Radical resection of his rectus femoris revealed a thin-walled, high-grade sarcoma with a large central hematoma. He remains recurrence-free at 4-year follow-up.

A 68-year-old female fell on her porch steps and "bumped" her buttock on the steps. She developed a lump in the buttock that was thought to be a hematoma despite the absence of subcutaneous ecchymosis. The presumed hematoma was aspirated by her family physician twice. The hematoma kept recurring. The patient was then referred to a general surgeon who "drained" the hematoma cavity twice. Only when the patient developed an open infected wound, and "a nodule of tumor rolled out of the wound onto the examination table" did the surgeon consider the possibility of a hemorrhagic sarcoma. Despite subsequent chemotherapy and aggressive resection, the patient died 10 months later of metastatic disease.

Pulled Muscles

Patients do not develop pulled muscles unless they are performing a relatively vigorous activity or have some other reason for a vigorous or violent muscle contraction sufficient to cause a tissue tear or disruption. A significant pulled muscle should have associated hemorrhage and ecchymosis. A 39-year-old athletically inclined woman developed an enlarging mass in her right medial thigh and groin. Her family physician diagnosed a pulled muscle to which she replied, "If that is your diagnosis, then find me another doctor. I have been athletic all my life and I know that this is not a pulled muscle." The physician then ordered an MRI scan that demonstrated a large inhomogeneous soft-tissue mass (Fig. 4), which biopsy revealed to be an extraosseous Ewing's sarcoma.

Muscle Hypertrophy

Exercise does not produce isolated muscle hypertrophy. An athlete with long-standing exercise asymmetry may on occasion develop diffuse hypertrophy of an entire extremity

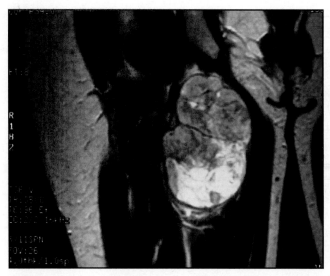

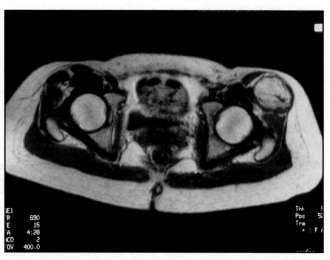

Fig. 4 Coronal MRI scan of an extraosseous soft-tissue Ewing's sarcoma that was briefly misdiagnosed as a "pulled groin muscle."

Fig. 5 MRI scan revealing an anterior groin liposarcoma. Unlike most patients with soft-tissue sarcomas, this patient's complaint was pain. Due to her mild obesity, her mass was not palpable.

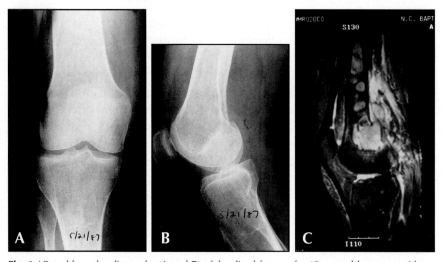

Fig. 6 AP and lateral radiographs (**A** and **B**) of the distal femur of a 45-year-old woman with leukemia and knee pain. The radiographs were remarkably unrevealing compared to the extent of disease identified on MRI scan (**C**).

the "knee sprain," the diagnosis of osteosarcoma was easily established after her follow-up radiographs more clearly demonstrated lysis, sclerosis, and periosteal reaction. Although the initial radiographic findings in this case, as in the case illustrated in Figure 1, were subtle, with proper history and clinical suspicion, a bone scan or an MRI could have been obtained and would have led to the proper diagnosis and treatment much sooner.

Persistent Pain

If a physician diagnoses arthritis or any other process that does not respond to treatment as expected, then a more sophisticated study such as a bone scan, computed tomography (CT) scan, or MRI scan may be indicated to rule out an underlying neoplastic, infectious, or other occult process. A recently treated 40-year-old female executive had seen 4 physicians for pain in her anterior groin. She was minimally overweight. None of the 4 initial physicians nor I could palpate an abnormality in her groin or thigh region. However, the

relative to the contralateral side in such sports activities as place kicking, throwing/pitching, or tennis, but asymmetry in a single muscle, or muscle group, for all practical purposes, rarely if ever occurs. Whenever a single muscle or muscle group is enlarged, suspect a soft-tissue sarcoma, and do not fall prey to the temptation to attribute it to asymmetric muscle hypertrophy from exercise.

Pain

If a patient develops rest pain, it is a tumor or infection until proven otherwise. A recently treated teenager was initially diagnosed as having a knee sprain, although her knee only hurt her at night and she denied any injury. Her initial knee radiographs revealed only subtle changes in the distal femoral metaphysis. After 2 months of conservative treatment for

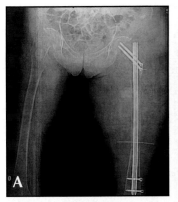
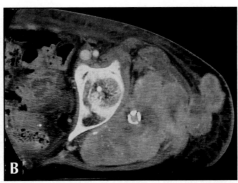
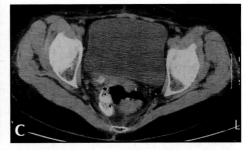

Fig. 7 CT scout radiograph (**A**) of the femur of a 56-year-old woman 3 months after intramedullary nailing of an impending pathologic fracture that was initially thought to be associated with breast cancer. It proved to be a new onset chondrosarcoma that was metastatic at presentation. The CT scout film and the CT axial cut (**B**) demonstrate the local spread of the chondrosarcoma from the intramedullary (IM) nailing procedure. Note the diffuse spread into the soft tissues, including the gluteal muscles, along the tract of the IM rod, due to the "transplantability" of chondrosarcoma. Note specifically the lack of any tumor in the gluteal region on a pelvic CT scan of the same region obtained 1 month preoperatively (**C**). I recommend tumor resection and endoprosthetic bone replacement for metastatic chondrosarcomas rather than IM rods.

fourth examining physician had obtained an MRI scan, which demonstrated a lesion subsequently proven to be a liposarcoma (Fig. 5).

Mechanical Pain

Tumors can cause pain on weightbearing. Orthopaedists are cautioned to remember that not everyone in the world with pain on weightbearing has arthritis. Impending pathologic fractures also cause mechanical pain. Although an arthritic hip will cause pain with weightbearing and activity, so will an impending pathologic hip fracture. Physicians must remember that the initial presentation of up to one fourth of all patients with metastatic carcinoma is due to the bony involvement. Most of these lesions are apparent on plain radiographs, so the physician is well advised to always take a radiograph of any extremity with bone pain or pain on weightbearing.

Pathologic and Impending Pathologic Fractures

Several common errors occur in the diagnosis and management of pa-

tients with pathologic and impending pathologic fractures. The first requirement is to recognize the diagnosis. In many patients, a pathologic or lytic lesion will not be obvious upon inspection of the fracture radiograph (Fig. 2). Thus, the surgeon must always question the mechanism of injury and maintain an index of suspicion for neoplasia in all cases of fractures that arise without significant trauma. A 40-year-old patient with history of leukemia was referred for evaluation of mechanical knee pain by her radiation oncologist. Her initial radiographs were relatively unrevealing. An MRI scan, however, demonstrated extensive disease within her marrow space (Fig. 6). Permeative cortical destruction was more apparent on subsequent radiographs obtained a week later. CT scan is generally the preferable study to quantitate the extent of bony destruction and to aid the surgeon in best estimating the risk of pathologic fracture. As demonstrated in the case illustrated in Figure 2, an index of suspicion for pathologic fracture must be maintained whenever exam-

ining any patient with a fracture. Failure to diagnose or suspect a sarcoma can lead the surgeon to perform such ill-advised surgical procedures as intramedullary nailing of a suspected metastatic carcinoma, only to find out later that sarcomatous tumor tissue has been spread throughout the bone and extremity (Fig. 7). Such tumor spread can convert a potential limb salvage sarcoma case into an extended amputation.

Adjuvant treatment should be employed postoperatively for metastatic bony lesions, or the tumor will recur and progress, even after curettage and internal fixation. Adjuvant options include chemotherapy, hormonal therapy, bisphosphonate administration, and/or radiation therapy.[1] With the recently demonstrated benefits of pamidronate and other bisphosphonates,[2–7] consultation with a hematologist/oncologist or other physician familiar with administration of bisphosphonates is indicated in the majority of patients with myeloma and metastatic carcinomas.[2–4,8,9] Such administration has been demonstrated to diminish the

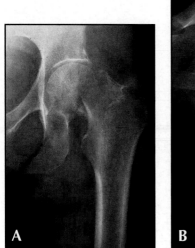
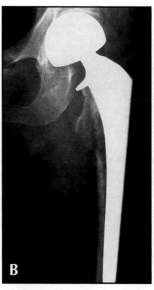
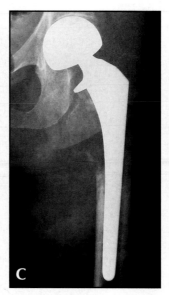
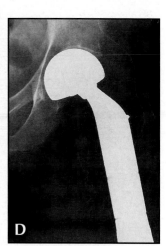

Fig. 8 A 75-year-old woman sustained a pathologic fracture of the femoral neck (**A**) that was treated with hemiarthroplasty (**B**). Three months later, during which time the patient received no radiation therapy nor any other adjuvant therapy, the tumor had progressed (**C**), requiring massive proximal femoral endoprosthetic replacement (**D**).

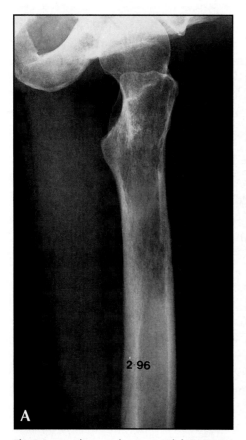
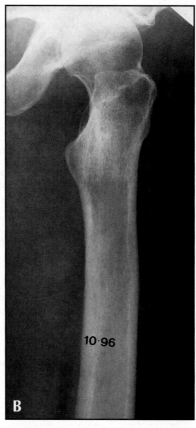

Fig. 9 A recently treated patient with breast carcinoma metastatic to her subtrochanteric area (**A**) declined surgery. She was treated with radiation and 2 months of protected weightbearing. Radiographs 8 months later confirmed excellent sustained healing (**B**).

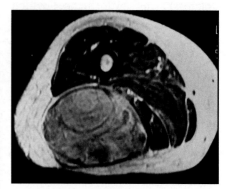

Fig. 10 An 80-year-old female patient presented with a large mass in her posterior thigh. Although it possessed distinct margins on MRI scan, it was a high grade sarcoma. Note the inhomogeneity of the signal within the lesion which is a common feature of malignant tumors.

bony destructive process and pain.[2–9]

A 75-year-old woman with squamous cell carcinoma of the esophagus presented to an orthopaedic surgeon with hip pain. A hemiarthroplasty was performed to treat a femoral neck pathologic fracture (Fig. 8, *A* and *B*). The patient was not given radiation therapy, chemotherapy, or any other antineoplastic therapy postoperatively. The tumor progressed, ultimately requiring a proximal femoral resection 3 months later (Fig. 8, *C* and *D*). Once a pathologic fracture has been stabilized, effective adjuvant therapy must be used to slow disease progression in the involved bone. Some tumors, particularly breast carcinoma metastatic to bone, respond very favorably to radiation therapy (Fig. 9).

MRI

Most orthopaedic surgeons are well aware that benign and slow-growing neoplasms appear well marginated on plain radiographs and that malignant and aggressive benign lesions appear poorly marginated, possessing permeative or moth-eaten borders. Some orthopaedists and many inexperienced radiologists mistakenly extrapolate this information to the appearance of MRI scans. Many mistakenly believe that a well-marginated lesion on MRI scan must be benign. In my experience, many soft-tissue tumors appear to be well-marginated, regardless of their etiology. Soft-tissue sarcomas push the surrounding fascia into a pseudocapsule as they grow. This pseudocapsule makes the lesions appear encapsulated on MRI scan. Naive radiologists who infrequently encounter soft-tissue MRIs may think that a sharp margin equates with a benign lesion (Fig. 10). A large, well-marginated lesion in the soft tissue with inhomogeneity of the MRI signal of the lesion itself is almost always a malignant or aggressive neoplasm. Infiltrative or indistinct borders on MRI scans do not necessarily imply malignancy either. While lymphomas, some sarcomas, and some carcinomas may appear to have indistinct borders, so do infections, stress fractures, and other reactive lesions (Fig. 11).

The value of the plain radiograph

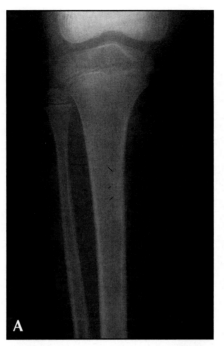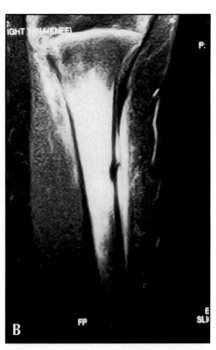

Fig. 11 Radiograph (**A**) and MRI (**B**) of a 12-year-old boy with a stress fracture of the tibia that developed while training for his school's cross country track team. Note the indistinct "permeative borders" of this benign process.

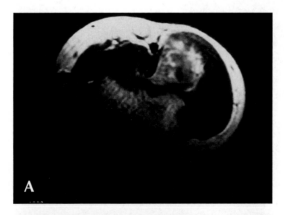

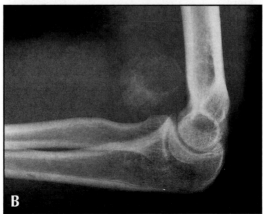

Fig. 12 A 29-year-old woman complained of a lump in her proximal forearm. An MRI (**A**) had been obtained initially, revealing an aggressive appearing inhomogeneous soft-tissue mass. Plain radiographs (**B**) revealed a typical pattern of myositis ossificans, demonstrating the value of plain radiographs.

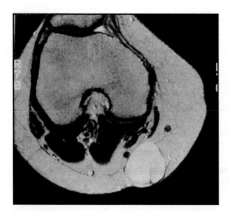

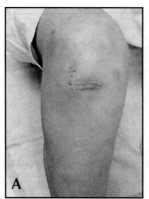

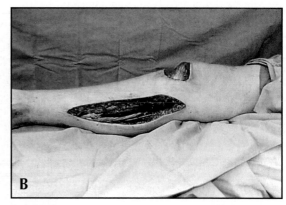

Fig. 13 The cystic mass noted in the posterior knee region depicted on this MRI appears well circumscribed and loculated. The pathology, however, revealed telangiectatic extraosseous osteosarcoma.

Fig. 14 A 67-year-old female had a meniscal "cyst" resected by her orthopaedic surgeon through a transverse incision (**A**). The pathology revealed leiomyosarcoma. This necessitated a fairly extensive resection and a medial gastrocnemius rotation flap (**B**) to remove all the contaminated tissue and provide soft-tissue coverage. Had a simple transillumination, a needle aspiration, or a fine needle aspiration biopsy of this cyst been performed prior to surgery, a lesser resection would have sufficed.

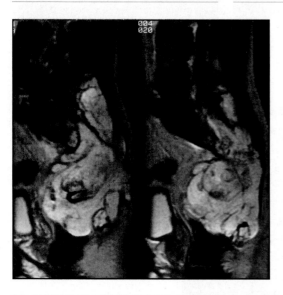

Fig. 15 MRI scan of a 37-year-old man with 3 years of low back pain. By the time the tumor was diagnosed, a curative-intent excision would have rendered the patient an L4-5 level paraplegic, a condition he was not willing to accept. Despite debulking and radiation treatment, his tumor progressed over the subsequent 4 years and he remains alive with metastatic disease at the time of this writing.

cannot be overstated. The MRI appearance of a bone or soft-tissue lesion can be quite alarming. However, the plain radiograph is usually a better indicator of the aggressiveness of the lesion (Fig. 12).

Ganglions

Many errors occur in the treatment of presumed ganglions. If what appears to be a ganglion is in an unusual location, it is probably not a ganglion (Fig. 13). It is quite simple to transillumi-

nate all ganglions with a pen light or other small focused beam of light. When the light source is touched to the skin overlying a ganglion, the entire ganglion should glow homogeneously. If transillumination cannot be performed, then a simple aspiration to verify that the lesion contains the typically clear, gelatinous, mucinous material will confirm the diagnosis and prevent the inadvertent mistreatment of a small sarcoma.

I generally perform a fine needle

aspiration biopsy in the clinic on all lesions prior to surgery, even small ones that are probably benign. This biopsy generally avoids surgical surprises (Fig. 14). It is performed with a 25-gauge needle, without anesthesia, and is well-tolerated by patients.

Unexpected Tumor Encounters

When an unexpected tumor is encountered at surgery by a nontumor surgeon, the best course of action is usually to resect only a sufficient amount of tissue for an adequate biopsy. A frozen section should be obtained and the pathologist should verify that sufficient tissue has been obtained for diagnosis. Additional samples for additional stains or studies can be obtained at that time if required. The surgeon should obtain hemostasis and avoid opening tissue planes. He should then close the wound. If a drain is required, it should be brought through the skin in line with the incision so that the drain tract can be excised along with the biopsy tract. If a subsequent wide resection

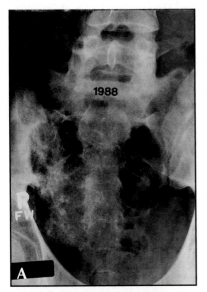

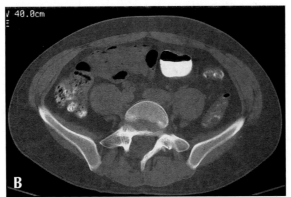

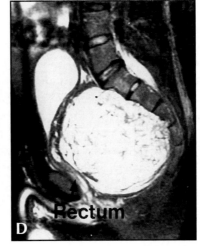

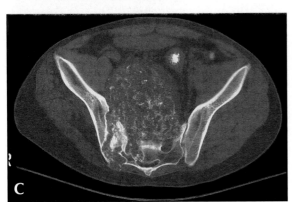

Fig. 16 A 30-year-old man underwent laminectomy in 1988 for right-sided leg pain. His pain persisted. An AP radiograph at the time of surgery suggested an intrapelvic mass (**A**), but this finding was not appreciated. He was told by his physician that there was nothing else that could be done for the pain that failed to respond to laminectomy. Six years later, he added an additional complaint that his stools had become thin and ribbon-like. He still had pain. CT scan confirmed the laminectomy defect (**B**) as well as massive chondrosarcoma filling the pelvis (**C**). MRI scan confirmed the extent of the pelvic mass (**D**).

is required, it is technically much easier to perform if there is still some tumor to palpate. Do not "debulk" the entire lesion. The only exception involves small tumors that can be safely excised with a margin of normal tissue and in which, if the margin is inadequate, a wide excision can still be accomplished without difficulty. The other exception involves bone tumors in which the bleeding cannot be controlled without resecting the tumor. In these tumors, a resection or curettage of the entire lesion with packing of the tumor cavity with polymethyl methacrylate will usually suffice.

Scheduled Unplanned Resections

Probably the most frustrating experiences for orthopaedic oncologists follow incomplete tumor resections of large neoplasms by well-intentioned, but uninformed or inexperienced surgeons. It is inappropriate for a general or orthopaedic surgeon to attempt to resect a large tumor without having obtained a preoperative MRI or CT scan to define the anatomic extent of the lesion. The surgeon, having entered the tumor and contaminated wide areas of otherwise salvageable tissue, then often turns to a radiation oncologist or a hematologist-oncologist and asks them to salvage the situation. These

surgeons do not understand the importance of proper anatomic mapping and wide resection. Such tumor contamination and incomplete excision are unacceptable. A wide re-resection or amputation is often required. In one study of osteosarcoma, every patient in whom there was a microscopic tumor-containing margin ultimately developed metastases. These recurrences occurred despite adjuvant treatment, demonstrating the importance of complete tumor excisions.[10] Resection of large masses should be undertaken only by those familiar with the management of such cases. Otherwise, many patients will develop local recurrences, with increased likelihood of death, and they will require amputations or extensive resections that would not have been required had the proper surgery been performed initially.

Low Back Pain

A rectal exam should be performed on all patients with persistent low back pain, especially if the pain is in the very low back or sacral area. Chordomas usually originate in the lower sacrum. They are easily excised and the patients are easily cured when these are detected while still small. Chordomas are usually relatively small when the lesion is restricted to the lower sacrum where they originate. These lesions can be readily palpated on a digital rectal examination. Failure to do such an examination can have disastrous consequences (Fig. 15).

Reconsider the Diagnosis

If a patient's condition or problem does not resolve as expected, consider the possibility of a misdiagnosis. By reexamining the patient, and restudying the problem, the proper diagnosis can often be determined, avoiding disastrous delays and poor results (Fig. 16).

Summary

A number of the more frequently encountered diagnostic and management errors and pitfalls have been discussed. However, if a physician will recognize his or her own limits and will always consider the diagnostic possibility of a neoplastic process, then appropriate steps can usually be taken, improving the patient's health care. The following chapters will outline the appropriate steps in the evaluation and work-up of patients with suspected tumors, as well as the currently recommended approach for biopsy, treatment, and follow-up.

References

1. Janjan NA: Radiation for bone metastases: Conventional techniques and the role of systemic radiopharmaceuticals. *Cancer* 1997;80(suppl 8):1628–1645.

2. Rogers MJ, Watts DJ, Russell RG: Overview of bisphosphonates. *Cancer* 1997;80(suppl 8): 1652–1660.

3. Adami S: Bisphosphonates in prostate carcinoma. *Cancer* 1997;80(suppl 8):1674–1679.

4. Coleman RE, Purohit OP, Vinholes JJ, Zekri J: High dose pamidronate: Clinical and biochemical effects in metastatic bone disease. *Cancer* 1997;80(suppl 8):1686–1690.

5. Kanis JA, McCloskey EV: Clodronate. *Cancer* 1997;80(suppl 8):1691–1695.

6. Burckhardt P: Ibandronate in oncology. *Cancer* 1997;80(suppl 8):1696–1698.

7. Body JJ: Clinical research update: Zoledronate. *Cancer* 1997;80(suppl 8):1699–1701.

8. Berenson JR: Bisphosphonates in multiple myeloma. *Cancer* 1997;80(suppl 8):1661–1667.

9. Lipton A: Bisphosphonates and breast carcinoma. *Cancer* 1997;80(suppl 8):1668–1673.

10. Ward WG, Mikaelian K, Dorey F, et al: Pulmonary metastases of stage IIB extremity osteosarcoma and subsequent pulmonary metastases. *J Clin Oncol* 1994;12:1848–1859.

Biopsy

Albert J. Aboulafia, MD

Stedman's Medical Dictionary defines biopsy as the "process of removing tissue from living patients for diagnostic examination."[1] Although the definition is accurate, it is incomplete as related to the biopsy of primary bone and soft-tissue sarcomas. The goals of the biopsy of musculoskeletal sarcomas include more than simply removing tissue for diagnostic examination; considerations for the ultimate management of the lesion must be taken into account. The ultimate goal of treating patients with primary bone and soft-tissue sarcomas is to obtain local and distant control of the tumor while maximizing function. Given that more than 90% of patients with extremity sarcomas can now be managed with limb-sparing surgery, it is critical that the physician who performs the biopsy be familiar with limb-sparing techniques if these goals are to be met. Complications resulting from biopsy have been well documented.[2,3] In some cases an inappropriate biopsy may provide tissue for diagnosis, but in so doing, compromise the goals of achieving local control and maximal function.

A more fitting definition of biopsy, as related to musculoskeletal tumors, includes not only removal of tissue, but also minimizing the risks to the patient while optimizing local control and function. Given this "working definition," it seems evident that "whereas biopsy frequently demands relatively few technique skills, the decisions related to the performance of the biopsy require considerable thought and experience" as suggested by Simon and Biermann.[4] The biopsy should not be performed until the workup and considerations outlined in the sections on the workup of bone and soft-tissue lesions have been completed. A more complete workup is generally expected prior to open biopsy; however, closed biopsy should not be performed without consideration of all facets of the biopsy, including such factors as biopsy site and needle tract trajectory. Most agree that the biopsy should be performed by the physician who will perform the definitive resection.

It is simply a fact that some suspected nonneoplastic conditions, such as infections, hematomas, and ganglions, and some benign neoplastic conditions, such as lipoma, treated by nononcologic orthopaedists will prove to be malignant at the time of surgery. Understanding the principles of the biopsy and approaching all lesions as if they may be malignant optimizes the subsequent management of patients with lesions that later prove to be malignant.[5]

Principles and Techniques
Various options for obtaining tissue for diagnosis exist. A biopsy may be performed as an open or closed procedure. Closed procedures are performed percutaneously and may be either fine needle aspiration or core biopsy. An open biopsy may be either incisional or excisional. Each technique has associated risks and benefits, and no one technique can be recommended for all patients. The ultimate choice of which biopsy procedure is most suited for an individual patient depends on the nature and location of the lesion as well as the experience of the institution's pathologists and surgeons. However, some general rules for all biopsies exist.

Principles
Principle Number 1 The biopsy should be performed so as not to compromise subsequent definitive resection. All open biopsy or core biopsy tracts should be located such that they can be excised en bloc at the time of definitive resection. This procedure requires that the biopsy tract be located and aligned along the surgical excision tract for the future limb-salvage resection. The fact that the surgeon must be familiar with limb-sparing techniques to properly place a biopsy has led to the dictum, "Biopsies of potentially malignant and aggressive lesions should be performed by the surgeon who will provide the definitive care." In the extremities, the incision should be oriented longitudinally; transverse

biopsy incisions are to be avoided. When the biopsy tract, including the skin, is excised, wound closure is simplified with longitudinally oriented defects compared to transverse ones. Suboptimal biopsy technique can also complicate amputation by contaminating flaps used for closure.

Surgical approaches used in general orthopaedics may be relatively contraindicated as surgical approaches for musculoskeletal biopsies. For example, an approach to the proximal humerus through the deltopectoral interval would be contraindicated because tumor cells can contaminate the deltopectoral interval muscle plane and the chest wall. Alternatively, the proximal humerus should be approached through the anterior third of the deltoid, contaminating only such tissues as can subsequently be resected en bloc with the proximal humerus at the time of limb-sparing surgery.

Principle Number 2 Meticulous hemostasis must be achieved. Following biopsy, some bleeding will occur irrespective of the technique chosen, be it fine needle, core, or open biopsy. The resultant bleeding from the tumor has the potential of seeding previously uninvolved areas, making subsequent local control difficult and at times impossible. A history of bleeding disorder, easy bruising, or use of medications that could cause bleeding should be obtained prior to biopsy and appropriate steps taken to facilitate surgical hemostasis. Whether hemostasis is achieved by biopsy obtained with or without tourniquet control depends on the surgeon's training and ability. However it is obtained, hemostasis must be achieved prior to wound closure. Bone holes generally require plugging with either polymethylmethacrylate, gel foam, bone wax, or some other suitable substance. A

drain is often indicated, and the drain tract should exit the skin in line with the biopsy incision to allow subsequent drain tract excision at the time of en bloc resection.

Principle Number 3 The biopsy should be performed such that it does not contaminate compartments that are not involved by the tumor. It may be tempting to biopsy a lesion in the distal femur through a lateral approach because this is a common approach used in orthopaedics for fracture care. However, if the soft-tissue mass extends beyond the bone to involve the medial compartment, the oncologic treatment will require a medial approach. Consequently, a limb-salvage procedure would be difficult and would require removal of more tissue than would otherwise been necessary.

Principle Number 4 Avoid iatrogenic complications such as fractures from stress risers whenever possible. To minimize the risk of pathologic fracture following biopsy of bone tumors, the surgeon should first assess whether or not the bone itself needs to be biopsied. In the majority of bone sarcomas, there is extension of tumor beyond the cortex. In such instances, the soft-tissue component of the tumor should be biopsied. If the bone needs to be biopsied, the area of maximal cortical thinning should be opened if possible. When making a cortical window, a small circular or oval hole should be created rather than a square or rectangular defect to minimize the stress riser. The cortical window should be plugged with bone cement, bone wax, or gel foam to prevent bleeding into the surrounding soft tissue, as previously mentioned.

Treatment

Open Biopsy An open biopsy is one in which an incision is made. The biopsy may be incisional, in which a

small portion of the tumor is removed, or excisional, in which the entire tumor is removed. Incisional biopsy remains the gold standard to which all other biopsy techniques should be compared. The main advantage of open biopsy compared to closed biopsy is that it yields a larger tissue sample. This helps to avoid problems associated with sampling error and may help the pathologist make a correct diagnosis. The disadvantages of open biopsy compared to closed biopsy include wound healing problems, pathologic fracture, increased potential for infection and tumor contamination of the biopsy site, and increased cost. Many of these complications can be minimized if not avoided when an incisional biopsy is performed with attention to details.

Once the decision has been made to proceed with an open biopsy, the surgeon must consider whether to perform an incisional or excisional biopsy. The advantages of excisional biopsy, when done correctly, include a single surgical procedure, minimal risk of tumor spillage, and complete tissue sampling. The disadvantages of excisional biopsy include inability to assess response to neoadjuvant therapy, more extensive surgical procedure than may be necessary if the lesion is benign, and contamination of a larger surgical field if wide margins are not achieved and the tumor is malignant or locally aggressive.

Excisional biopsy is best reserved for those tumors known to be benign and small subcutaneous lesions that can be removed widely with little or no additional morbidity than marginal excision. Bone tumors, such as osteochondromas and osteoid osteomas, and soft-tissue tumors such as lipomas can frequently be diagnosed with great accuracy based on clinical and radiographic information. Such lesions are well suited for excisional biopsy. Additionally, small subcutaneous masses, which are likely to be benign, may be removed with a cuff of normal tissue (wide margin) without additional morbidity to the patient.

Although primary excisional biopsy of suspected malignant bone and soft-tissue tumors has been described, this practice should be reserved for exceptional situations. Many bone and soft-tissue tumors treated with preoperative radiation and/or chemotherapy will dramatically decrease in size and develop a more defined pseudocapsule. This allows for limb-sparing surgeries to be performed with better local control and more functional results. Additionally, the response to preoperative chemotherapy has significant prognostic value in the case of osteosarcoma and possibly other neoplasms. When primary excision of malignant bone and soft-tissue tumors is performed, the advantages of preoperative treatment may be sacrificed.

Complications resulting from incisional biopsy include poor wound healing, infection, lack of adequate tissue sampling, tumor spillage, pathologic fracture, and contamination of uninvolved compartments. Many of these complications can be minimized by following the general principles outlined above. However, some additional considerations most germaine to performing an incisional biopsy need emphasizing. General orthopaedic surgeons are accustomed to draining abscesses through an incision centered over the area of maximum fluctuance or "the top of the mountain." The biopsy of musculoskeletal tumors should avoid this site. The area of maximum tenting of the skin is vulnerable to poor wound healing because it is under tension. Additionally, the skin over this area is fre-

quently thin and ischemic, further compromising the potential for wound healing. In cases of rapidly growing tumors, the tumor growth rate exceeds the potential for local wound healing and the tumor may grow rapidly through the slow-healing wound. The incision should be small but adequate to allow visualization of the surgical field and avoid excessive retraction of the skin. A tiny incision that does not allow for adequate visualization of the surgical field and meticulous hemostasis lends itself to complications resulting from hematoma formation.

Irrespective of whether an incisional biopsy or closed biopsy is performed, it is necessary to obtain viable tumor. The portion of the tumor to be biopsied should be chosen with an understanding of the biology of tumor growth and following interpretation of imaging studies. Because sarcomas grow in centrifugal fashion, the center of the tumor is the most mature, and the periphery the least mature. As sarcomas grow, the more mature center may undergo hemorrhagic necrosis and a biopsy from this area may yield nondiagnostic tissue. Therefore, the ideal biopsy should be performed with an attempt to obtain tissue from the periphery of the viable tumor. Intraoperative frozen sections or touch preparations should be performed prior to conclusion of the procedure to confirm that adequate viable tumor has been obtained, and not simply reactive or necrotic tissue. Frozen section or touch preparation samples also alert the pathologist to the possible need for special handling of tissue. If the biopsy reveals a small round blue cell tumor, the pathologist may separate or request additional tissue for further studies, such as flow cytometry, cytogenetics, and special stains. In cases where infection is possible, antibi-

otics should not be administered until cultures have been obtained. The dictum: "Biopsy what you culture, and culture what you biopsy" will avert an overlooked diagnosis in many cases. Osteomyelitis frequently is clinically indistinguishable from Ewing's sarcoma, histiocytosis, and lymphoma on the basis of clinical findings alone. Errors in diagnosis of these lesions are not uncommon.

Closed Biopsy There are 2 types of closed biopsies. They include fine needle aspiration biopsy (FNAB) and core needle biopsy. In both cases, the tumor sampling is performed percutaneously. Consequently, the incidence of infection and wound complications is reduced compared to open biopsy. Additionally, because there is no, or at most a tiny incision, neoadjuvant radiation and/or chemotherapy may begin immediately without the need to wait for wound healing. Moreover, percutaneous biopsy can be performed in the office under local or no anesthesia, making it expedient, convenient, and cost effective. The disadvantages of closed biopsy include a tumor sample that is smaller than that obtained with open procedures. Irrespective of the type of biopsy performed, the same general rules apply.

Fine needle aspiration involves aspirating the tumor mass with a small syringe and a 25-gauge needle. After identifying the most appropriate site for aspiration, the skin is prepped using betadine or other skin preparation solution. The skin and subcutaneous tissue may be anesthetized using local anesthetic, although this is usually unnecessary. The needle, attached to the syringe, is advanced into the tumor. Suction is applied by withdrawing the syringe plunger, and the needle is advanced and withdrawn within the tumor in a repetitive motion. The needle can be directed in various directions within the tumor to increase the probability of obtaining viable and representative tumor cells. The suction is released, the needle withdrawn, and the aspirated tissue expelled onto glass slides. The syringe and needle are rinsed with saline and the fluid centrifuged into a tissue pellet. The slides are stained and studied microscopically. Manual pressure maintained on the biopsy site for several minutes after the biopsy will generally prevent subsequent hemorrhagic tumor spread. The major disadvantage of FNAB compared with other biopsy techniques is the small amount of tumor tissue retrieved. However, by making 2 or 3 passes, tissue for immunohistochemical stains and cytogenetic analysis, and clotted tissue for standard histologic preparation and staining, can be readily obtained. Although FNAB of musculoskeletal tumors is commonly used at some centers in Europe and the United States, many clinicians and pathologists in the United States prefer core biopsy or open biopsy.[6] FNAB is especially useful for the evaluation of clinically enlarged lymph nodes and to evaluate areas of suspected local recurrence,

and to evaluate suspected metastatic carcinomas.

Core needle biopsy is performed percutaneously using local anesthesia. In most cases it can be performed in the office without radiographic assistance. Radiographic aid may be necessary when biopsying tumors involving the spine or pelvis. When a biopsy is performed in the radiology suite, either with the aid of fluoroscopy or computed tomography, the approach to the lesion should be carefully selected by the surgeon who will perform the definitive resection. For example, a periacetabular lesion approached posteriorly risks contamination of the gluteal muscles, making subsequent local control more difficult. A variety of needles are available to perform core biopsy, and the selection of which needle to use will depend on whether or not the cortex of bone is intact. The tru-cut needle (Baxter Healthcare Corporation, Deerfield, IL) is especially useful for the biopsy of soft-tissue tumors or the soft-tissue component of a bone tumor. If the cortex of the bone is intact and not significantly weakened by the

bone, a needle designed to penetrate bone is required.

Summary

Obtaining tissue for diagnosis of bone and soft-tissue tumors is one of the goals of all biopsies. The biopsy, however, must be well planned so as to avoid creating inadvertent tumor spread, thereby compromising the ability to perform limb-sparing resectional surgery.

References

1. Stedman TL: *Stedman's Medical Dictionary*, ed 2. Baltimore, MD, Williams & Wilkins, 1995.

2. Mankin HJ, Lange TA, Spanier SS: The hazards of biopsy in patients with malignant primary bone and soft-tissue tumors. *J Bone Joint Surg* 1982;64A:1121–1127.

3. Mankin HJ, Mankin CJ, Simon MA: The hazards of the biopsy, revisited: Members of the Musculoskeletal Tumor Society. *J Bone Joint Surg* 1996;78A:656–663.

4. Simon MA, Biermann JS: Biopsy of bone and soft-tissue lesions, in Schafer M (ed): *Instructional Course Lectures 43.* Rosemont, IL, American Academy of Orthopaedic Surgeons, 1994, pp 521–526.

5. Springfield DS, Rosenberg A: Biopsy: Complicated and risky. *J Bone Joint Surg* 1996;78A:639–643.

6. Kreicbergs A, Bauer HC, Brosjo O, Lindholm J, Skoog L, Soderlund V: Cytological diagnosis of bone tumours. *J Bone Joint Surg* 1996;78B:258–263.

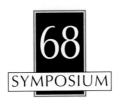

68
SYMPOSIUM

Treatment Options for Orthopaedic Oncologic Entities

Robert J. Zehr, MD

Much has been learned about the natural history and characteristics of musculoskeletal neoplasms over the past 30 years. This understanding has, in turn, led to an astonishing expansion of specialized treatment and reconstructive techniques. Limb salvage, once an oddity for malignant lesions, is now the standard of care for the orthopaedic oncologist. Additionally, very aggressive benign lesions, such as giant cell tumor, aneurysmal bone cyst, and fibromatosis, can present a debilitating threat to overall limb function and are frequently referred to an orthopaedic oncologist for definitive care.

Fortunately, far more musculoskeletal neoplasms are benign than malignant. The average practicing orthopaedic surgeon is typically capable of identifying the clinical and radiographic features that differentiate the malignant from the benign lesion. This ability has become a key issue of practice with the advent of "gatekeeper medicine." There is intense pressure and reluctance to refer simple things to a specialist outside the system.

This chapter is intended to be a brief overview of the current treatment options of the more common benign and malignant, bone and soft-tissue lesions that practicing orthopaedic surgeons are likely to encounter at some point in their career. Additional and more detailed

reviews are available of the principles and techniques presented.[1–5]

Staging

The appropriate treatment of a musculoskeletal neoplasm varies depending on the tumor's natural history, its behavior pattern, and the point in time at which treatment is begun. Staging is a process of determining at what point along the spectrum of a tumor's natural history it is presenting to the physician. Several prognostic criteria are considered when staging a tumor: grade, location, size, and metastasis. When considered collectively, these variables provide a means of separating the less worrisome benign processes from the highly aggressive malignant lesions. The histologic grade of a lesion is obtained through a biopsy, but the clinically observed growth rate is also important in providing an overall understanding of grade. Radiographic assessment of the lesion delineates size and proximity to vital structures. Bone scan and computed tomography (CT) are used to establish the current status of metastatic disease.

A system of staging neoplasms developed by Enneking[6] and accepted by the Musculoskeletal Tumor Society is currently used by most orthopaedic oncologists to assist them in providing patients a prognosis for their tumor. Malignant lesions are

either high grade (II) or low grade (I), either in a well-defined tissue compartment (A) or in 2 or more compartments or no well-defined compartment (B), and have known metastatic disease (III) or not.

Although other staging systems are used with malignant musculoskeletal neoplasms, this is the only staging system that addresses the benign neoplasms. Benign lesions are staged with the designations 1, latent; 2, active; and 3, aggressive, depending on the biologic behavior and known natural history of these lesions.

Treatment of Common Benign Bone Tumors

Most stage 1 benign bone lesions are treated by simple curettage. For most stage 2 and some stage 3 lesions, extended curettage with or without various adjuvants, or with localized resection is satisfactory. On rare occasion with advanced aggressive lesions, such as in stage 3 giant cell tumor or aneurysmal bone cyst, en bloc resection is necessary. These situations often require more involved reconstructive techniques.

Osteoid Osteoma and Osteoblastoma

Most authorities regard osteoid osteoma and osteoblastoma as separate, but related lesions. Histologically these osteoblastic lesions appear very similar, and differentiation is typically achieved based on clinical location and radiographic appearance. These are osteoblastic lesions that often invoke the production of reactive bone about a fibrovascular, variably mineralized nidus.

Osteoid osteoma is smaller, with a nidus less than 1.5 cm, and is most often found in the femur, tibia, distal humerus, and the small bones of the hand. When found in a juxta-articular location such as the femoral neck or olecranon fossa a synovitis is common, but the typical reactive bone may be absent as a result of the lack of periosteum in these areas. This common bone lesion accounts for approximately 10% of benign bone tumors and is twice as common in men as in women. The presence of persistent night pain is a very common historical finding; however, response to various antiprostaglandin medications is variable. Osteoblastoma is very rare, generally larger than 1.5 cm, and has a predilection for the spine and jaw. The nidus does not typically incite development of surrounding reactive bone, and night pain is uncommon.

Treatment options for osteoid osteoma include conservative care because spontaneous healing of the lesion is possible over many years. Medical management with an anti-inflammatory regimen is generally the first line of treatment if the patient has not already discovered this on his or her own. Problems with compliance, intolerance, and ineffectiveness often lead to abandonment of this course.

Alternatively, surgical removal is the more commonly offered treatment and is more likely to resolve the painful symptoms. Removal of the offending nidus can, however, be difficult , especially if the nidus is not well visualized. The nidus can be localized with CT scanning that includes anatomic reference landmarks that can readily be found in surgery. However, intraoperative measurements from palpable landmarks may be inaccurate, and even with fluoroscopic equipment the nidus can be elusive. The use of a technetium-99 isotope probe to preoperatively label the lesion has been described, but also presents logistic difficulties.

An en bloc resection of a wide area of bone around the nidus has been favored historically. This is most effectively done using a high-speed burr with a pencil tip to facilitate a controlled scribing of the hard, reactive bone. Intraoperatively, the removed bone is radiographed to confirm the presence of a nidus. After en bloc resection in weight-bearing long bones, the residual section defect may necessitate stabilization with an intramedullary nail or a dynamic compression plate to prevent fracture.

An alternative procedure to en bloc resection described by Ward and associates[7] involves the "burr-down" technique. The nidus must be well-localized on the periosteal cortex or in the cortical bone. The maximally raised area of reactive bone is burred in a circumscript fashion until the nidus becomes visible. The nidus is removed with a curet and sent for pathologic evaluation, and the residual cavity is extended with the burr. This technique will result in the removal of less bone and, thereby, lessen the need for additional stabilizing procedures. Percutaneous burr excision under CT guidance has been recently described, but is best considered experimental at this point because of a high incidence of recurrence.

Enchondroma

Enchondromas are common benign cartilage lesions that occur most frequently in the small bones of the hands and feet. Another typical location is in the metaphysis and diaphysis of long bones, especially the femur and humerus. This lesion composed of mature cartilage has limited growth potential, generally presenting as a stage 1 or 2 lesion. It can be identified by "stippled" or "popcorn" calcifications on plain radiographs. Usually asymptomatic, enchondromas are often discovered incidentally on radiographs taken for unrelated reasons. Bone scans typically reveal modest uptake of technetium isotope.

Enchondromas in the small bones of the hands and feet often cause endosteal erosion, which results in pathologic fracture. Pain in long-bone lesions often indicates the transition to a malignant process and dictates further investigation. Biopsy of a cartilaginous lesion is often of limited value in differentiating benign from low-grade malignant cartilage. The radiographic and clinical picture must be relied upon to determine appropriate treatment.

Most incidentally discovered lesions in the long bones should be observed and the patient educated to return if the involved area develops persistent pain. On occasion, large lesions (over 3 cm) or symptomatic lesions require surgical treatment. A biopsy that reveals low-grade cartilage indicates a lesion that can be treated with an extended curettage and the cavity filled with allograft. Low-grade cartilage malignancies treated in this manner have a small risk of local recurrence and if followed closely have a very small risk of metastasis. High-grade or dedifferentiated chondrosarcoma requires a wide resection as discussed later in this chapter.

Chondroblastoma

Chondroblastoma is a benign cartilage lesion uniquely associated with the epiphysis of adolescent long bones. This lesion is characterized histologically by the production of immature oval shaped cartilage cells with interwoven fine linear matrix that can calcify, generating the so-called "chicken wire" pattern. Osteoclast-like giant cells are typically scattered throughout the pattern. These multinucleated giant cells were responsible for this tumor once being considered a variant of giant cell tumor.

Clinically, chondroblastoma presents as a painful joint with synovial swelling and decreased motion. Radiographically, a geographic, lytic, central epiphyseal lesion circumscribed by reactive bone is often found. These tumors present as stage 2 or rarely stage 3 benign lesions. Favored locations include the epiphyses of the knee and proximal humerus, the patella, the talus, and the greater trochanteric apophysis.

Adequate treatment of this lesion is achieved with a thorough curettage and cavity extension with a high-speed burr. The defect can be filled with bone graft preferably, or polymethylmethacrylate cement if the defect is very large. Because these lesions are epiphyseal, the extra-articular approach to the lesion often involves crossing the epiphysis. It is far more important to obtain a sufficient oncologic margin than to risk recurrence through a minimalist approach through the epiphysis. Similarly, intra-articular contamination with chondroblastoma should be avoided because recurrence from the transplanted tumor is likely. On occasion, the lesion is extensive and requires resection and a complex reconstruction with an osteoarticular allograft or megaprosthesis. These lesions are generally best treated by an orthopaedic oncologist.

Osteochondroma

Osteochondroma is considered the most common benign bone lesion, accounting for approximately 40% of bone tumors.[8] It is arguably a hamartomatous lesion and not a true tumor, resulting from the growth of displaced physeal cartilage through the perichondrial ring, which gives rise to an exophyte or exostosis.[9] This outgrowth is composed of a bony stalk, either pedunculated or sessile, and is covered by a cartilaginous cap generally less than 1 cm in depth. A solitary, painless, hard mass of long duration is a typical presentation.

Radiographically, the confluence of the cancellous bone of the medullary canal with that of the stalk is characteristic of the osteochondroma. This transition zone is best seen with CT scanning, which also delineates the cartilage cap well. The cartilage cap is influenced by growth hormones and should cease growth at skeletal maturity. Continued growth or growth later in adulthood should be eyed with suspicion. Malignant degeneration of an osteochondroma is probably less than 1%. Symptoms are generally related to overlying bursae, neurovascular compromise, fractures of pedunculated stalks, or malignant degeneration.

These lesions can be treated conservatively or surgically. Because most osteochondromas are stage 1 lesions, surgical intervention is not imperative. Surgical excision is considered on occasion for cosmetic reasons, or if the lesion has become symptomatic. The recommended excisional margin in an adult is a marginal margin around the cartilage cap and intralesionally through the base of the stalk. Local recurrence is rare, and reconstruction of bone or soft tissue is almost never indicated.

If the lesion is found prior to skeletal maturity, observation through the period of skeletal growth is recommended. Local recurrence is higher when these lesions are excised in the immature patient. If no problems have arisen by early adulthood, the patient is educated to report any new onset of persistent pain or swelling and discharged.

Unicameral Bone Cyst

Solitary or unicameral bone cysts are not true neoplasms. The descriptive term, "unicameral" is misleading because many of these lesions are multilocular.[10] Most, however, are unicompartmental cystic lesions filled with serous fluid. The majority of cases present in children between ages 3 and 14 years. The proximal humerus accounts for approximately 50% of cases, with the proximal femur next most common.

The most common presentation is pain after a pathologic fracture through the weakened cortical bone surrounding the bone cyst. Most unicameral bone cysts are otherwise asymptomatic and go undiscovered unless found incidentally by radiograph or bone scan. On plain radiograph, the lesion can be characterized as a geographic, central, radiolucent lesion in the metaphysis, often extending into the diaphysis. Those lesions adjacent to the epiphysis are active; whereas, those in which the reactive boundary does not involve the physis are typically considered latent.

Unicameral bone cysts present as stage 1 or stage 2 lesions. Because most lesions will heal uneventfully after skeletal maturity, the goal of treatment is the prevention of fracture. Although contact sports should not be encouraged, further restriction of activity in an asymptomatic patient is not necessary or practical. Observation and serial radiographs at regular intervals through skeletal maturity are sensible.

Recurrent fracture or the presence in a weightbearing bone are relative indications for intervention. Open surgical procedures, however, are rarely required. Several authors have reported that single or multiple injections of methylprednisolone acetate are a safe and effective means of stimulating most cysts to heal. The most common technique used requires the placement of 2 large-bore needles (12 to 14 gauge) into the cyst under fluoroscopic guidance. Yellow, serous fluid should be aspirated, characteristic of the unicameral bone cyst. An injection of water-soluble contrast is often used to evaluate the cavity. If the contrast material fills the lesion, the injection of the steroid can follow. If gross bloody fluid is aspirated, but the lesion fills with contrast the steroid injection can be used. If bloody fluid is aspirated and the lesion does not fill with contrast, a space-occupying lesion should be suspected, and a biopsy of the lesion should be done.

Water-soluble contrast is often used to assess the nature of the chambers. Quick runoff of the contrast is suggestive of a very active cyst and short deposition time for the steroid. The dose of steroid depends on the size of the lesion. Most authors have reported the injection of 40 to 200 mg of methylprednisolone acetate. This procedure is repeated as needed based on bimonthly assessments and radiographs until ossification of the cyst occurs.

Open reduction with internal fixation is needed for pathologic fracture of the proximal femur. The cyst is thoroughly curetted, followed by grafting and fixation. Although autograft has been the standard filler material, recent advances with synthetic materials, allografts, and bone marrow aspirates show promise as useful alternatives.

Aneurysmal Bone Cyst

Aneurysmal bone cyst (ABC) is a multiloculated cystic lesion that, like unicameral bone cyst, is not considered a true neoplasm. It is thought to initiate through an injury to the bone's vascular network, resulting in an expansile destructive process propagated by the capillary pressures. The lesion is found most often in the femur and tibia, with the pelvis and spine as additional sites. The lesion often develops centrally with an eccentric expansion of the process, but subperiosteal presentation is also observed. ABCs are unusual in patients over the age of 20 years.

These locally destructive lesions present with pain, swelling, and sometimes fracture. The characteristic plain radiographic appearance is a ballooned or blowout expansion of the cortical bone with a thin rim of reactive bone containing the lesion. Magnetic resonance images or CT scans often indicate a fluid-fluid level typical of the ABC (Fig. 1).

Secondary ABCs develop in many lesions, such as giant-cell tumor, chondroblastoma, fibrous dysplasia, and giant-cell reparative granuloma. Rarely does ABC coincide with a malignant process; however, the differential diagnosis of telangiectatic osteosarcoma can be very difficult to exclude without a biopsy.

ABC presents as a stage 2 or 3 lesion that requires intervention, because it is rarely an indolent process. As a result of a high incidence of recurrence with simple curettage, surgeons have resorted to more aggressive marginal excisions in functional bones or wide excisions in expendable bones. Locally these lesions can be as destructive as high-grade malignancies and require the same complex resection and reconstruction.

Fortunately, most ABCs can be controlled with an extended curet-tage and filling of the residual defect with bone graft, especially in children. They can be filled with polymethylmethacrylate cement in skeletally mature adolescents and young adults. Hemorrhage is often brisk when curetting these lesions, and adequate exposure of the lesion prior to puncturing the reactive bony rim will facilitate the procedure by decreasing blood loss. On entering the cyst, the surgeon should expect the lesion to bleed until all of the fibrous tissue is removed. In large lesions of weightbearing bones, adequate internal fixation should be considered.

Radiation therapy for benign conditions such as aneurysmal bone cyst has a limited role. In areas, such as the spine or pelvis, in which surgery may render significant functional deficits, moderate doses have been employed.[11] Typically, these lesions are first treated with embolization before considering the use of radiation because the incidence of secondary sarcomas is a real concern.

Fibrous Dysplasia

Fibrous dysplasia is a condition occurring both as solitary (monostotic) and multifocal (polyostotic) variants, whereby the bone forming mesenchymal tissue is unable to produce mature lamellar bone. The production of bone does not advance beyond the level of woven bone. The monostotic form of the condition is more common and typically affects the femur, tibia, and ribs. The polyostotic variation is more severe, affecting the skin with café-au-lait spots and often with severe involvement of various endocrine systems as observed with Albright's syndrome.

Radiographic evaluation reveals a central geographic lesion with a classic "ground glass" appearance, often with

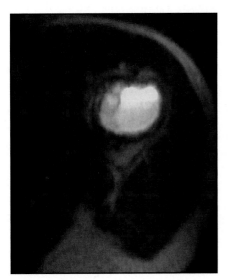

Fig. 1 Aneurysmal bone cyst of proximal humerus demonstrates bi-fluid level on T2 magnetic resonance images.

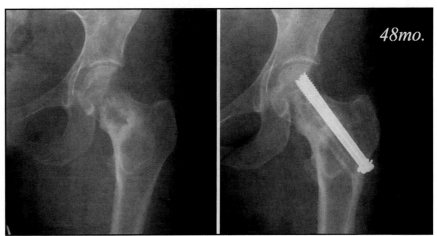

48mo.

Fig. 2 Fibrous dysplasia of the proximal femur treated with curettage, cortical fibular allograft, and cannulated screws.

a circumferential rim of reactive bone. These lesions have moderately intense uptake on bone scans even in the older age population. Rib lesions will frequently have an expansile appearance. Histologically, fibrous dysplasia is characterized by spindle cells in a whorled configuration admixed with trabeculae of immature woven bone with conspicuously absent rimming osteoblasts. Malignant transformation is exceedingly rare but has been reported coincident with radiation as a treatment.

Fibrous dysplasia is a benign condition and not a neoplasm. The lesion may progress during development, but generally halts at skeletal maturity. Asymptomatic lesions need no treatment. The weak quality of the bone may lead to fatigue fractures in weightbearing bones. Typically, surgical stabilization is indicated for persistent pain unresponsive to conservative management. In children, a simple curettage will result in recurrence of the dysplastic bone, and surgery is inadvisable before skeletal maturity. Alternatively, curettage in

the symptomatic adult with a cortical allograft filler and internal stabilization is often highly successful in relieving painful symptoms (Fig. 2). The use of autograft as a filler material should be discouraged with fibrous dysplasia because it has been shown to remodel with dysplastic bone.[12] Cortical allografts remodel very slowly and maintain structural integrity better that autograft.

Giant Cell Tumor
Giant cell tumor is an unusual and often very challenging neoplasm for both the general orthopaedic surgeon and the subspecialist. This lesion accounts for up to 10% of benign bone neoplasms in most large series in persons between 20 and 40 years of age. It most often occurs in the epiphyses of the knee, but is also found in the distal radius and proximal humerus. Although found in the sacrum, it is rare elsewhere in the spine. Presenting complaints are of localized pain in up to 30% of cases.

The characteristic radiographic appearance is that of a radiolucent, eccentric, geographic lesion abutting the articular surface of the epiphysis with extension into the metaphyseal

bone. Cortical destruction is common, and soft-tissue extension is seen with the more aggressive lesions. Intramedullary reactive bone is not typically seen with giant cell tumor. Campanacci and associates[13] are credited with a 3-grade staging system based on radiographic appearance of giant cell tumor, but the correlation with recurrence and prognosis has not been corroborated.

Grossly the tumor can be very vascular, presenting an intraoperative problem if the surgeon is ill-prepared for hemorrhage. The lesion can have a large cystic cavity similar to ABC or be quite solid and brownish in color from hemosiderin staining. Much has been written about the microscopic appearance with 2 populations of cells; the plump, spindle-shaped mononuclear background cells are interspersed with multinucleated giant cells that may have 100 nuclei or more.

Current treatment methods respect the aggressive potential of this tumor. Giant cell tumors present as stage 2 or 3 lesions that require extended curettage and adjuvant treatment or a wide resection to control the localized process. In the assessment stage, when the patient presents with a radiograph consistent with giant cell tumor, it is wise to obtain a baseline chest radiograph. Pulmonary metastasis occurs in up to 3% of patients with giant cell tumor. Although thought by most authors to be "benign" and cured with pulmonary wedge resection, reports of a more aggressive course have surfaced.

Suspected giant cell tumors are currently treated with an extended curettage after an open biopsy has confirmed the diagnosis. Rapid removal of the fleshy tumor will usually halt the occasionally intense bleeding. The curettage is extended with a high-speed burr through a cortical window that has been opened and widened to give a clear view of the entire cavity. Residual tumor will often remain on the cortical bone near an inadequate opening and will lead to unnecessary recurrence. Pulsatile lavage of the cavity is important as the burring proceeds. The area nearest the joint is particularly tedious to clean, but must be well purged of the involving tumor. The articular cartilage is typically a barrier to tumor extension into the joint and most often can be preserved.

Once it has been adequately prepared, the cavity is most commonly filled with polymethylmethacrylate bone cement (PMMA). An adjuvant effect attributed to PMMA by some authors clinically may relate to a lower recurrence rate over autograft or allograft fillers. Some authors, however, have advocated the use of a layer of autograft or allograft bone adjacent to the articular cartilage in addition to PMMA in those circumstances in which a good portion of the subchondral bone has been burred away. Local recurrence with the extended curettage and PMMA filler has been estimated to be up to

20% to 25%. If autograft is harvested from the iliac crest, it is imperative that separate, uncontaminated instruments, and gowns, gloves, and drapes not used earlier in the case be used to retrieve the graft. Otherwise, the surgeon risks implanting the tumor into the pelvis.

Some of the more advanced lesions or those that recurred multiple times will require an en bloc resection of the entire end of the bone along with a substantial soft-tissue cuff. These procedures and reconstructive problems are often handled more effectively at tertiary centers.

Treatment of Common Benign Soft-Tissue Tumors

It is well established that benign musculoskeletal soft-tissue neoplasms far outnumber their malignant counterparts. One conservative estimate is that benign lesions are 100 times more common than malignant soft-tissue sarcomas. The majority of benign soft-tissue lesions can be intralesionally or marginally excised if appropriately indicated. The challenge, however, for the general orthopaedic surgeon is to recognize those features that should raise a suspicion for a malignant process so that the case can be referred to an oncologist for biopsy and treatment.

Lipoma

This may be the most common soft-tissue tumor recognized. Most lipomas occur in the adult population and are found incidentally as asymptomatic subcutaneous lesions with a prolonged growth history. They are found commonly across the shoulders, back, and neck. Occasionally, if it recently has been traumatized or when it is pressing on an adjacent nerve, a lipoma will present as a symptomatic lesion. The less common subfascial or intramuscular

lipoma tends to be infiltrative and often attains considerable size before being discovered. Many high-grade sarcomas have been mishandled under the mistaken diagnosis of intramuscular lipoma.

Radiographic characterization by magnetic resonance imaging (MRI) or CT scan is very helpful in distinguishing between fat and other tissue. If the lesion is not completely homogeneous and of the same signal intensity as subcutaneous fat, then the lesion is not going to be a simple lipoma. The lesion should be treated as a potential malignancy and evaluated with tissue taken through a small, carefully placed open biopsy incision as outlined elsewhere in this section.

The common subcutaneous lipoma can either be observed or marginally excised if symptomatic or a cosmetic issue. The deep intramuscular lesion, once proven to be benign fat by biopsy or radiographic study can be removed with a marginal margin with an anticipated low expectation of local recurrence and minimal functional morbidity.

Atypical lipoma has been used to describe those deep extremity lesions that have the histologic appearance of a well-differentiated liposarcoma without the potential to metastasize. This lesion often presents as a very large, deforming mass with a long, asymptomatic clinical history. On MRI it is usually homogeneous with a few more low signal edema strands coursing through the lesion than in the true lipoma. Treatment of the atypical lipoma is debatable. Marginal excision has the least functional impairment but will have a high associated local recurrence. Recurrence brings with it the risk, albeit low, of a more malignant process. Wide margins will lessen the risk of recurrence but will sacrifice to a greater degree the function of the limb. Radiation is not typically used in either case.

Schwannoma (Neurilemoma)

This typically small, unifocal lesion occurs in middle-aged adults on peripheral nerves, specifically peroneal and ulnar nerves, and occasionally in spinal nerve roots, especially of the neck and sympathetic chain. Presenting complaints of tingling or numbness occur as the tumor grows. Delay in seeking medical attention is usual because this lesion typically causes few symptoms unless confined by the neural canal or tight fascial compartments.

Grossly these tumors are encapsulated by epineurium, and the involved nerve skirts around the circumference of the lesion, not through it as in the case of neurofibroma (Fig. 3). Microscopically, the hallmark features are 2 distinct cell elements: a highly ordered arrangement of spindle-shaped cells (Antoni A) with areas of palisading nuclei (Verocay bodies) and a loose collection of less densely packed myxoid cells (Antoni B). There is intense staining with S-100 protein, which is useful in differentiating schwannoma from neurofibroma.

This lesion is treated with careful marginal dissection of the tumor from the nerve, generally preserving function of the nerve. The incision through the capsule of the neurilemoma must be oriented longitudinally to prevent inadvertent transection of a significant portion of the nerve fibers splayed out over the tumor. Recurrence is rare if careful removal is performed. The incidence of malignant transformation is negligible.

Neurofibroma

Solitary neurofibroma is a lesion of young adults, 20 to 30 years of age, and is not associated with the ge-

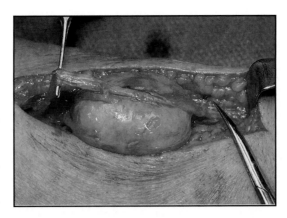

Fig. 3 Neurilemoma on superficial radial nerve demonstrates how nerve "skirts around" tumor.

netically determined condition of neurofibromatosis (NF) or von Recklinghausen's disease. The incidence of solitary neurofibroma is much more common than that of NF, but the diffuse distribution pattern is no different from the peripheral form of neurofibromatosis (NF-1). These lesions occur on any subcutaneous surface. Although often asymptomatic they can, on occasion, be associated with intense pain and are easily aggravated by touch.

Intraoperative examination of the neurofibroma will reveal a lesion intimately entwined with the involved nerve. There is no capsule as with the schwannoma, and surgical excision of the lesion is generally at the expense of the host nerve. In the case of major peripheral nerve involvement and if the lesion has shown no evidence of malignant transformation, it may be prudent to leave the lesion alone, thereby preserving function. Microscopic dissection is possible if severe pain prompts intervention on a major nerve, but removal of the lesion with an oncologically acceptable margin is not feasible if nerve preservation is the goal.

Fibromatosis (Extra-Abdominal Desmoid)

The family of benign proliferative fibrous lesions that is collectively referred to as fibromatosis is quite large. This discussion will be confined to the extra-abdominal desmoid variant. This lesion is quite common, arising over a period of months to years in young adults. Trauma or previous surgery have been associated with the site of subsequent desmoid development in a minority of patients.

Although this lesion can arise virtually anywhere, there is a strong association with the chest, shoulder, and upper arm regions, as well as the pelvic girdle. Extra-abdominal desmoid presents as a dense, often deep, poorly circumscribed lesion that grows insidiously. Pain on presentation is common, but not typical. Patients often demonstrate an unusual ability to detect recurrence by the new onset of pain before the clinical presence of the lesion is established.

The benign histologic appearance of these lesions has often lured the unwary surgeon into a false sense of nonchalance. In fact, local recurrence is frequent with this process and generally a more complex problem. Small lesions that can be excised should be excised with a wide margin because this lesion is exceedingly infiltrative through muscle and fascial planes. Therefore, locally, this lesion should be treated like a sarcoma. In

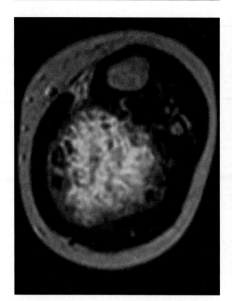

Fig. 4 Intramuscular hemangioma of the soleus muscle in a 2-year-old child demonstrated with gadolinium enhanced T1 magnetic resonance image.

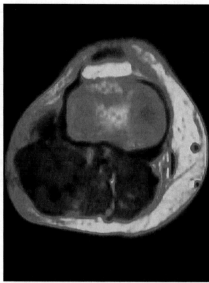

Fig. 5 Fibromatosis of the proximal leg involving the peroneal nerve and lateral compartment of the leg.

circumstances where the achievement of wide margins might entail the sacrifice of neurovascular structures, it is generally preferable to preserve these structures, accept a marginal margin, and add postoperative radiation (Fig. 4).

Alternatives to surgery have been used when ablative surgery or severe functional impairment would be the result of surgical intervention. High-dose radiation, as given for high-grade sarcomas, has halted tumor growth and given symptomatic pain improvement. Likewise, various chemotherapeutic regimens with hormonal, anti-inflammatory, or antineoplastic agents have had variable success in local control of the disease process.

Although death by local extension of uncontrolled disease occurs, fibromatosis is basically a benign process with a high rate of local recurrence, even with appropriate oncologic margins. Control of recurrent disease is often less successful than primary excision. As a consequence, this lesion

can be frustrating for a community orthopaedic surgeon not comfortable with his or her ability to achieve an adequate surgical margin, as well as for orthopaedic oncologists confronted with a recurrent lesion.

Intramuscular Hemangiomas

Cutaneous hemangiomas are quite common, are ordinarily identified in infancy or early childhood, and are not lesions of great concern to the orthopaedic surgeon. The more rare intramuscular hemangioma is a lesion of interest and can present diagnostic challenges. These lesions are generally identified in adults younger than 30 years and are frequently found in the thigh. Presenting history involves an aching or painful muscular area that worsens with exercise. The explanation for the pain is the increased blood flow expanding the thin-walled vessels. A characteristic serpiginous pattern of interwoven poorly formed vessels gives a typical MRI appearance. Occasionally plain radiographs

will reveal smooth calcifications or phleboliths.

Treatment of intramuscular hemangiomas is fraught with difficulty and disappointment. Obtaining a wide margin around small lesions will adequately control these lesions, but in larger lesions, such a margin may result in profound disability (Fig. 5). A less aggressive margin will leave residual tumor with a high rate of recurrent disease and usually worse pain. Angiographers have had variable success with sclerosing agents such as ethanol injected into painful areas of the lesion. Embolization is invasive, and the effect may be only transient with potential muscle, skin, and nerve necrosis problems to consider. This technique is useful if used preoperatively when excising large lesions to minimize surgical bleeding.

Treatment of Common Malignant Bone Tumors

The incidence of malignant primary bone tumors is low, but virtually every orthopaedic surgeon will one day encounter such a challenge. These lesions often present a profound and emotional encounter with the involved patient. The understanding, recognition, and course of action taken by the surgeon in the evaluation of these bone lesions and the malignant counterpart in soft tissues will often make the greatest impact on survival and limb salvage.

Osteosarcoma and Ewing's sarcoma found in children and young adults and chondrosarcoma in older adults are the most common bone malignancies, excluding metastatic disease and multiple myeloma, to affect the community orthopaedic surgeon. It is highly recommended that if the surgeon suspects a primary malignant bone lesion after a preliminary assessment, the case be referred to a specialist. All invasive procedures, especially the placement and technique of the biopsy will critically affect the outcome of the case. A brief overview of currently accepted surgical treatment and reconstructive techniques is presented and is not intended to be all inclusive. The reader is referred to the reference texts for an expanded review of these principles.[1–5]

Surgical Margins

No understanding of the treatment of malignant bone or soft-tissue lesions can be attempted without a thorough appreciation of the concept of oncologic surgical margins. Enneking[14] has established widely accepted terminology describing 4 possible surgical dissections based on the relationship of the lesion to the surrounding tissues. An intralesional margin describes a violation of the reactive pseudocapsule, entering into the tumor and results in a piecemeal removal of the lesion. This margin would be associated with curettage and is adequate for stage 1 and 2 benign lesions. A marginal margin describes a plane of dissection that involves the pseudocapsule of the lesion. The typical "shell-out" procedure is generally a marginal margin. This margin is acceptable for stage 2 benign bone lesions, benign infiltrating soft-tissue tumors (ie, intramuscular lipoma), and stage 3 benign bone tumors when combined with an adjuvant (PMMA, phenol, liquid N_2). A wide margin is achieved when the tumor, its pseudocapsule, and a cuff of normal tissue circumferentially about the lesion are removed en bloc. The size of the cuff is dictated more by experience of the surgeon than by any specified distance from the tumor. This is the margin most commonly sought in the removal of musculoskeletal malignancies. A radical margin is one in which the entire compartment in which the

tumor resides is removed. This margin is reserved for those instances in which the lesion is very large, taking up most of the compartment with tumor; for recurrent sarcomas; and for pathologic fractures through bone sarcomas with extensive extravasation of hematoma and/or tumor along tissue planes.

For malignant lesions of bone and soft tissue (stage IA/B or IIA/B) only wide and radical margins will give adequate control of the local disease. In the case of high grade lesions (stage IIA/B), adjuvant chemotherapy and radiation are often required to improve the chances of both patient survival and local control of the tumor. Marginal margin and intralesional margins in the treatment of skeletal malignancy are grossly inadequate and will require additional treatment in the form of reexcision and adjuvant therapies in most instances.

Limb Salvage Techniques

With the advent of modern surgical and chemotherapeutic techniques, surgeons are faced with a wonderful problem, that of the long-term cancer survivor. The problem is that the salvage of an afflicted limb requires durable, functional, and sometimes replaceable reconstructions. This remains a true frontier of development and cooperation between patient, doctor, and medical industry. The variety of limb salvage techniques and available devices is quite extensive. A few of the more common techniques will be discussed as an overview.

The four A's of limb reconstruction as they have come to be known are: Amputation, Arthrodesis, Allograft, and Arthroplasty. Each technique has many nuances as it applies to the practice of oncology. Amputation is often initially rejected by patients if alternatives exist, yet this may be the

most cost effective and lowest maintenance reconstruction to patient and society. Arthrodesis is very durable, but in the case of tall patients, knee and hip fusion makes sitting in a car or plane very difficult. Allografts have problems with infection, fracture, and nonunion in the early postoperative years, but fewer problems in subsequent years. Arthroplasty with large, oncologic megaprostheses allows immediate weightbearing in most instances, but the long-term integrity of these mechanical devices may be problematic.

Amputation Amputation has been used far less frequently in the past 20 years. However, with the improved understanding of the natural history of most lesions, it is still the treatment of choice in up to 10% of presenting musculoskeletal malignancies. In those lesions where the neurovascular bundles are intimately involved in the tumor, amputation is preferred over the high risk of recurrence that an inadequate margin of resection will create. Amputation margins must adhere to the same principles as for limb salvage. Specifically, a wide margin amputation must be obtained.

Rotationplasty is a variant amputation typically used in the very young child with many years of growth remaining. Tumors of the distal femur or proximal tibia with intraarticular extension or adherent vessels in which above-knee amputation might be considered can be resected and the reconstruction performed as a below-knee amputation. The distal leg is rotated and fixed to the femur in such a way that the foot functions as the below-knee amputation stump, the ankle as a knee joint, and the gastrocnemius muscle joined to the quadriceps performs stump extension function via ankle plantarflexion. The improved function of

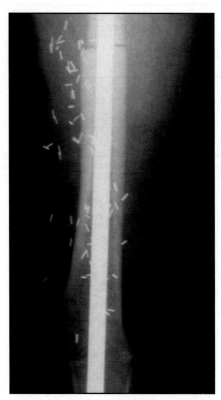

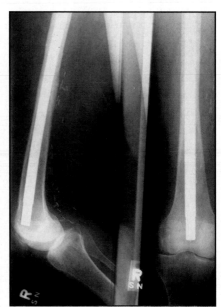

Fig. 7 Distal femoral osteoarticular allograft reconstruction of the knee with well healed host allograft junction.

Fig. 6 Intercalary allograft arthrodesis of distal femur with intramedullary nail fixation at 6 months, with distal host allograft junction healed but proximal junction with minimal evidence of union.

a below-knee amputation over an above-knee amputation and the complete lack of phantom pain problems makes this a viable alternative to above knee amputation.

Arthrodesis Arthrodeses of the knee, hip, or shoulder are typically strong, enduring reconstructions of the involved limb. Knee arthrodesis is a reasonable alternative to amputation when the extensor mechanism is involved in the tumor process and must be resected. A knee fusion after tumor resection often relies on an intercalary allograft or autograft spanning between the remaining host bone, fixed with compression plates or long intramedullary nail (Fig. 6). Arthrodesis of the hip following pelvic resection gives a stable and painless reconstruction despite a

very high pseudarthrosis rate. Fusion of the shoulder is a demanding operation, but results in the strongest, least debilitating of the reconstructive alternatives.

Allograft The use of large structural allografts to reconstruct skeletal defects has been highly successful in the field of orthopaedic oncology. Nevertheless, complications such as infection, fracture, and nonunion are problems that are of great concern and result in the overall early loss of approximately 30% of the reconstructions. Osteoarticular allografts matched to the patient's joint can provide a biologic restoration to the knee, shoulder, and distal radius where these grafts are typically used (Fig. 7). Intercalary allografts provide a means to span a large diaphyseal defect or provide bone to an arthrodesis. Another important value of the allograft is in the soft-tissue attachments. The patellar tendon of the proximal tibia, the hip abductor attachments to the greater trochanter,

and the rotator cuff tendons of the proximal humerus are valuable in providing attachment points to the allografts near joints.

Arthroplasty The use of large, modular, oncologic prosthetic devices sometimes known as megaprostheses provides a versatile and quick means of reconstructing large bone defects in and around major joints (Fig. 8). These prostheses have improved greatly over recent times, with the understanding of the biomechanics of the joint forces and fatigue properties of the prosthesis and components. Modularity has provided a means of addressing worn bearing surfaces and periprosthetic fracture. Nevertheless, instability, infection, and loosening are complicating events that result in reported 10-year revision-free endurance rates of only 60% to 80% in the knee and hip.

Soft-tissue attachment to the megaprosthesis is often unreliable and is a problem that has prompted significant investigation. The use of allograft-prosthesis composites is a means of providing a more secure soft-tissue attachment to bone through the tendinous attachments on the allograft and still achieve the reliability of the modern prosthetic bearing surfaces (Fig. 9).

In summary, the type of reconstruction selected depends on several variables, the site of resection, the amount of soft tissue removed, the wishes of the patient, and the experience and biases of the surgeon. Rarely is only 1 reconstructive technique the only possibility. Over time, as complications occur, several of the various alternatives may be used in any individual patient.

Treatment of Malignant Soft-Tissue Tumors

It has been estimated that approximately 6,500 soft-tissue sarcomas are diagnosed annually in the United States, with 50% of these occurring in the extremities. The community orthopaedic surgeon will encounter these lesions. The common soft-tissue sarcomas that present to the orthopaedic surgeon are malignant fibrous histiocytoma and liposarcoma in middle-aged to older adults, and synovial sarcoma in younger adults. These lesions generally present as painless masses, deep to the fascia, which often grow insidiously and are discovered when clothes fit poorly or an adjacent joint loses motion. The examining physician must take the approach that deep, firm masses in an adult are malignant until proven otherwise.

The innocuous presentation of soft-tissue sarcomas often leads the patient to ignore the lesion until it has attained great size. Approximately 10% of soft-tissue sarcomas present with pulmonary metastases. High-grade lesions with a presenting size greater than 5 cm have a higher risk of metastasis than the smaller lesions. In general terms for all groups collectively, the 5-year survival rate for soft-tissue sarcomas is 60% to 70% with adequate surgery and adjunctive therapies. Statistically, larger lesions do more poorly than smaller; high grade lesions do worse than low grade; and limb salvage does not put patient survival at a higher risk than would an amputation if adequate surgical margins are achieved.

The treatment of soft-tissue sarcomas has many similarities to that of primary bone malignancy. It is not the goal of this short overview to examine in depth the surgical approaches that are quite elaborately reviewed elsewhere. Rather, this section is a synopsis of the accepted principles followed in the treatment of soft-tissue sarcomas. Limb salvage is considered a reasonable alternative to amputation when an adequate

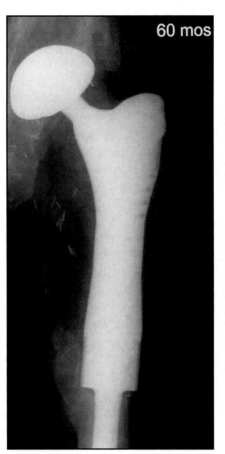

Fig. 8 Megaprosthesis reconstruction of the proximal femur at 5 years.

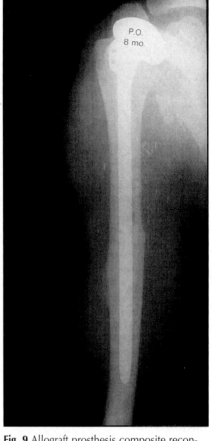

Fig. 9 Allograft prosthesis composite reconstruction of the proximal humerus.

margin can be achieved in the removal of the lesion and function of the spared limb would be better than that of an amputation.

An adequate surgical margin must be achieved to reduce the chance of local recurrence, which is associated with a decreased rate of patient survival. This may require a radical resection of the involved compartment(s) or an amputation in a large, deep tumor. More commonly a wide surgical margin is adequate to gain local control of most low-grade soft-tissue sarcomas; whereas, in high-grade lesions adjunctive treatment with the addition of pre- or postoperative radiation therapy to a wide margin is standard for local control. It is a grave assumption that poor surgery

with inadequate margins can be "fixed" with radiation. In addition, the use of chemotherapy is recommended for the patient with a large, high-grade lesion at high risk for metastatic spread.

Chemotherapy

The use of high-dose chemotherapy has revolutionized the current treatment of high-grade bone sarcomas, specifically, osteosarcoma and Ewing's sarcoma, and is generally accepted for use in high-grade soft-tissue sarcomas. Historically, local control of high-grade sarcomas did not equate to improved survival. For osteosarcoma prior to the advent of chemotherapy, amputation was the standard of treatment, yet survival rates of 15% were

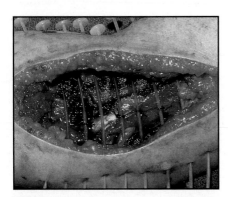

Fig. 10 Brachytherapy technique applied to the surgical bed in the antecubital fossa.

observed. The presence of micrometastases at presentation, although usually not visualized on chest CT scan has dictated the routine use of pre- and postoperative chemotherapy in high-grade lesions both for bone and soft tissue. The improved rate of survival for bone malignancies has been well documented. The unequivocal improvement in survival using chemotherapy for soft-tissue sarcomas remains to be established, but investigational protocols for these malignancies are currently being used by most large centers.

Radiation

The use of modern radiation therapy techniques has greatly improved the local control rate of soft-tissue sarcomas and has resulted in improved limb function by allowing less than radical resection margins. Radiation is delivered in several fashions, depending on the situation. Conventional external beam radiation is given preoperatively to inspire the development of a thickened pseudocapsule or rind. This seems to affect the tumor cells within the reactive zone, allowing for a closer resection margin particularly at vessels and nerves. Wound complications are generally higher with preoperative radiation. Postoperative external beam radiation typ-

ically requires higher doses of radiation over a broader area, but there are fewer wound problems with no reported differences in ultimate patient survival.

Brachytherapy is a technique that has allowed for the deliverance of radiation to the surgical bed, minimizing the effect to the surrounding soft tissues and bone. Surgery can be performed soon after diagnosis. Plastic tubes are placed intraoperatively, and radiation is given in the form of iridium seeds placed within the tubes postoperatively. The tubes are removed shortly thereafter (Fig. 10). Brachytherapy has been equally as effective as external beam radiation in controlling local recurrence rates with a much shorter treatment period. The use of preoperative external beam radiation with the addition of brachytherapy has been advocated for large high-grade lesions abutting the neurovascular structures or bone when limb salvage has been elected.

Summary

Over the past 2 decades, tremendous advancement in the understanding of tumor natural history and treatment has occurred. If the basic principles are followed, the evaluation and appropriate treatment of musculoskeletal tumors can be reproduced successfully by any conscientious surgeon. Many benign bone and soft-tissue tumors can and probably should be treated by the community orthopaedic surgeon, and this chapter is biased toward treatment of those lesions. The encounter of a malignant lesion is probably beyond the scope of practice of most practicing orthopaedic surgeons. The assessment of the patient and treatments rendered in the first meetings may well dictate the ultimate outcome of survival and limb preservation; thus, patients with such lesions

should be treated by experienced orthopaedic oncologists. With the small numbers of these lesions and the extreme consequences of mishandling them, it would be imprudent to do otherwise.

References

1. Conlon KC, Brennan MF: Soft tissue sarcomas, in Murphy GP, Lawrence W Jr, Lenhard RE Jr (eds): *American Cancer Society Textbook of Clinical Oncology*, ed 2. Atlanta, GA, American Cancer Society, 1995, pp 435–450.

2. Dorfman HD, Czerniak B (eds): *Bone Tumors*. St. Louis, MO, Mosby-Year Book, 1998.

3. Enneking WF (ed): *Musculoskeletal Tumor Surgery*. New York, NY, Churchill Livingstone, 1983.

4. Enzinger FM, Weiss SW (eds): *Soft Tissue Tumors*, ed 2. St. Louis, MO, CV Mosby, 1988.

5. Simon MA, Springfield D, Conrad EU, Eckardt JJ, Finn HA, Gebhardt MC, et al (eds): *Surgery for Bone and Soft-Tissue Tumors*. Philadelphia, PA, Lippincott-Raven, 1998.

6. Enneking WF: Staging musculoskeletal tumors, in Enneking WF (ed): *Musculoskeletal Tumor Surgery*. New York, NY, Churchill Livingstone, 1983, pp 69–88.

7. Ward WG, Eckardt JJ, Shayestehfar S, Mirra J, Grogan T, Oppenheim W: Osteoid osteoma diagnosis and management with low morbidity. *Clin Orthop* 1993;291:229–235.

8. Dahlin DC, Unni KK (eds): *Bone Tumors: General Aspects and Data on 8,542 Cases*. Springfield, IL, Charles C Thomas, 1986, pp 18–32.

9. Milgram JW: The origins of osteochondromas and enchondromas: A histopathologic study. *Clin Orthop* 1983;174:264–284.

10. Dorfman HD, Czerniak B: Cystic lesions, in Dorfman HD, Czerniak B (eds): *Bone Tumors*. St. Louis, MO, CV Mosby, 1998, pp 855–912.

11. Serber W, Dzeda MF, Hoppe RT: Radiation treatment of benign disease, in Perez CA, Brady LW (eds): *Principles and Practice of Radiation Oncology*, ed 3. Philadelphia, PA, Lippincott-Raven, 1998, pp 2167–2185.

12. Enneking WF, Gearen PF: Fibrous dysplasia of the femoral neck: Treatment by cortical bone-grafting. *J Bone Joint Surg* 1986;68A:1415–1422.

13. Campanacci M, Baldini N, Boriani S, Sudanese A: Giant-cell tumor of bone. *J Bone Joint Surg* 1987;69A:106–114.

14. Enneking WF: Surgical procedures, in Enneking WF (ed): *Musculoskeletal Tumor Surgery*. New York, NY, Churchill Livingstone, 1983, pp 89–122.

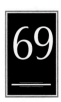

Appropriate Follow-up of Orthopaedic Oncology Patients

G. Douglas Letson, MD
William G. Ward, MD

Introduction

Follow-up of orthopaedic oncology patients is not a clearly defined subject; there are no clinical trials that define the appropriate time intervals. A wide range of follow-up intervals are presently being used throughout the United States at major institutions. Although they were not specifically reported as recommended regimens, prior publications have reported or alluded to our follow-up practices.[1,2] These range from a yearly chest radiograph for malignant neoplasms to a chest computed tomography (CT) scan for high-risk patients at 3-month intervals (WG Kraybill, MD, personal communication, 1997). A yearly chest radiograph in the early follow-up of high-grade sarcomas is probably inadequate, allowing extensive metastases to develop before discovery and treatment. Obtaining a chest CT scan every 3 months is a very sensitive approach to detect the early progression of malignant disease, but may be considered too costly by some insurers and others in today's cost containment environment. The optimum follow-up care is probably somewhere between these 2 ranges. A clinical study is currently being performed at the Roswell Park Cancer Institute to further define the follow-up practices for sarcoma patients.

Follow-up requirements must be separated into those for neoplasms without the potential to metastasize and neoplasms with the potential to metastasize. Neoplasms capable of metastasizing include such entities as chondroblastoma and giant cell tumor of bone, both "benign" lesions that can metastasize and even cause death.[3-5] Nonmetastasizing benign neoplasms need only be followed-up for local recurrence, whereas potentially metastasizing neoplasms need follow-up evaluations for both local recurrence and metastatic disease. There is no outcomes-based, data-substantiated standard regimen for the timing of follow-up of patients with musculoskeletal neoplasms. The physicians must therefore define an arbitrary schedule of follow-up evaluations based on the natural history of the disease, the risks of disease recurrence or progression, and the perceived risks of delay in the detection of disease progression. Factors to consider in planning the follow-up include the histologic diagnosis, the stage, and the extent of disease at presentation.

Many follow-up regimens, however, are well defined by the chemotherapy protocols into which most of these patients are enrolled. Ideally, the orthopaedic oncologist and the medical oncologist should collaborate on the plans for long-term follow-up. The time to detectable local recurrence or detectable metastatic disease depends on the rate of cell replication. Patients with high-grade lesions will manifest disease recurrence or progression much earlier than patients with slow-growing, low-grade lesions.[6] For example, in patients who have high-grade osteosarcoma, most metastases are detected within the first 2 postoperative years, and most deaths occur within the first 3.5 years postoperatively,[1] confirming the need for more frequent surveillance in the first 2 to 3 years. Thus, for aggressive or rapidly growing neoplasms, an initial follow-up interval of every 2 to 4 months seems reasonable. After 2 progression-free years, then 6-month intervals for the third year, yearly for the fourth and fifth years, and every other year thereafter seem reasonable. This approach has been used in the past with acceptable results;[1] however, these time intervals have not been tested in a rigorous manner and are therefore presented as unproven guidelines. As more effective salvage therapies for disease progression are developed, earlier detection will likely become even more important.

Common sense and anecdotal experience dictate that some reasonable regimen of surveillance for disease progression must be employed in all patients to avoid the unchecked progression of disease to an untreatable stage or to a stage that is more difficult to treat, as in the patient

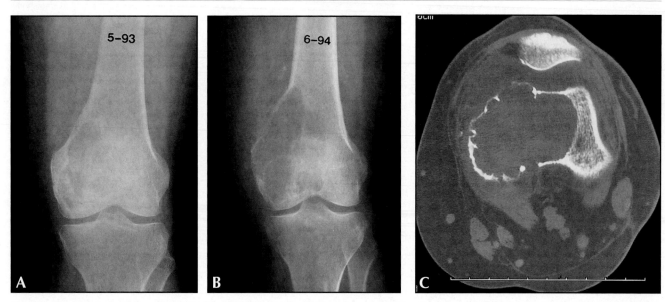

Fig. 1 A, Anteroposterior (AP) radiograph of the distal femur of a 26-year-old woman 4 years after giant cell tumor excision and bone grafting at another institution. No treatment was instituted. **B** and **C,** AP radiograph (**B**) and computed tomography (CT) scan (**C**) of the distal femur of the same extremity 13 months later, showing the extensive further destruction of the distal femur caused by the persistently recurrent giant cell tumor. She sustained a pathologic fracture through this lesion, requiring distal femoral allograft replacement, a much more complex reconstruction than the initial recurrence of giant cell tumor would have required had the tumor been treated 13 months previously.

illustrated in Figure 1. As a general overview, the follow-up guidelines we use are shown in Table 1.

Local Recurrence

Local recurrence can occur with both benign and malignant neoplasms. The signs and symptoms of local recurrence are similar to the signs and symptoms of the primary disease. In the follow-up, the history, physical examination, and imaging studies of the tumor site must be considered. Many sarcomas are symptomatically silent, thus local recurrences may be symptomatically silent.

Office physical examination is the primary evaluation for local recurrence. Because many sarcomas present as a painless mass, a local recurrence will also likely be a painless mass that may be detected strictly by palpation. Serial examinations of the surgical site facilitate the surgeon's ability to differentiate recurrent tumor from scar. Recurrent tumor is

often firm and rounded, whereas scar is often thinner and more elongated. Deep masses and subsequent deep recurrences may not be palpable, such as in the proximal thigh, pelvis, or shoulder girdle. A large periarticular tumor and, consequently, a large periarticular tumor recurrence may cause restricted limb motion, a feature that should be detected on routine follow-up examination.

Imaging studies should be obtained whenever there is any question of recurrence. Plain radiographs are easily obtained, are good for identifying bone lesions, and may show soft-tissue lesions. A magnetic resonance imaging (MRI) scan is usually the best study to evaluate for local recurrences of soft-tissue neoplasms. However, some experience is required to differentiate postoperative changes, such as edema, scar tissue, and seromas, from local recurrence on MRI scans. Most local recurrences will present as somewhat rounded discrete masses,

whereas surgical changes are usually thinner, elongated, and more diffuse abnormalities. We do not routinely obtain MRI scans of areas that can be reliably examined by manual palpation. However, for deep-seated resection beds or fibrotic postirradiation tumor beds, serial imaging studies may be required to reliably exclude the possibility of recurrent tumor. CT scans may be helpful for the evaluation of local recurrence of soft-tissue neoplasms, but MRI scans provide better information. CT scans are less expensive and are best in the evaluation for local recurrence in difficult to see bone lesions, such as around the polymethylmethacrylate cement in previously treated giant cell tumors. Technetium bone scans can be useful in the follow-up of musculoskeletal neoplasms, because most have increased activity. Following most bony surgical procedures, the bone scan should normalize within 12 to 24 months. Whenever abnormal activity

Table 1
Authors' general follow-up practices (frequency of examinations)

Location	Examination*	Year 1	Year 2	Year 3	Years 4&5	Years 6–10	After Year 10
Bone							
High-grade sarcomas†	Clinical examination	q 3 mo	q 3 mo	q 6 mo	q 12 mo	q 12-24 mo	q 24 mo
	Radiograph	q 3 mo	q 3 mo	q 6 mo	q 12 mo	q 12-24 mo	q 24 mo
	CXR	q 3 mo	q 3 mo	q 6 mo	q 12 mo	q 12-24 mo	q 24 mo
	Chest CT scan§	q 3-12 mo	q 3-12 mo	q 12 mo prn	q 12 mo prn	Rarely	–
	MRI¶	Rarely	Rarely	Rarely	Rarely	Rarely	–
Low-grade sarcomas**	Clinical examination	q 3 mo	q 6 mo	q 6-12 mo	q 12 mo	q 12 mo	q 24 mo
	Radiograph	q 3 mo	q 6 mo	q 6-12 mo	q 12 mo	q 12 mo	q 24 mo
	CXR	q 3- 6 mo	q 3-6 mo	q 6-12 mo	q 12 mo	q 12 mo	q 24 mo
	Chest CT scan§	q 12 mo	q 12 mo prn	q 12 mo prn	q 12 mo prn	Rarely	–
	MRI¶	Rarely	Rarely	Rarely	Rarely	Rarely	–
Soft Tissue							
High-grade sarcomas‡	Clinical examination	q 3 mo	q 3 mo	q 6 mo	q 12 mo	q 12 mo	q 24 mo
	Radiograph	q 3 mo prn	q 3 mo prn	q 6 mo prn	q 12 mo prn	q 12 mo prn	q 24 mo
	CXR	q 3 mo	q 3 mo	q 6 mo	q 12 mo	q 12 mo	q 24 mo
	Chest CT scan§	q 3-12 mo	q 6-12 mo	q 6-12 mo prn	q 12 mo prn	Rarely	–
	MRI***	q 6-12 mo	q 6-12 mo	q 6-12 mo prn	q 12 mo prn	Occasionally	–
Low-grade sarcomas	Clinical examination	q 3 mo	q 3 mo	q 6 mo	q 12 mo	q 12-24 mo	q 24 mo
	Radiograph	q 6-12 mo	q 6 mo prn	q 6 mo prn	q 12 mo prn	q 24 mo prn	q 24 mo
	CXR	q 6-12 mo	q 6-12 mo	q 6-12 mo	q 12 mo	q 24 mo	q 24 mo
	Chest CT scan§	q 12 mo prn	q 12 mo prn	q 12 mo prn	q 12-24 mo	Rarely	–
	MRI***	q 12 mo prn	q 12 mo prn	q 12 mo	q 12-24 mo	Occasionally	–

(Generic table derived from a compilation of our suggested 1998 follow-up practices. In our practices, many individual variations from these guidelines are present. These are merely suggested guidelines, not a data-tested, outcomes-substantiated regimen.)

*CXR = chest radiograph, CT = computed tomography, MRI = magnetic resonance imaging scan, q = every, mo = months, prn = as needed

†For example, osteosarcoma, chondrosarcoma, Ewing's sarcoma

§Obtained more frequently if patient's CXR or baseline CT is abnormal; Note: CXR and chest CT scan are obtained only in those patients at risk for pulmonary metastases

¶MRI of primary site following bony reconstruction cannot usually be performed, even if desirable, due to metallic implants or fixation hardware; need for follow-up MRI of primary tumor bed depends on physician's ability to palpate site for recurrence (ie, depth of prior lesion, scarring, radiation effect)

**For example, parosteal sarcomas

‡For example, malignant fibrous histiocytoma, liposarcoma (myxoid round cell and pleomorphic)

***Usually obtain a baseline follow-up MRI sometime 3–12 months after resection

is detected after a 12-month period, the surgeon must consider the possibility of local recurrence. Bone scans are excellent at revealing bony metastatic disease. Newer modalities, such as positron-emission tomography (PET) scans, may have increasing roles in the postoperative surveillance of patients with sarcomas, and PET scans can detect both local recurrent and metastatic disease.[7]

Metastatic Disease

Essentially all musculoskeletal neoplasms that metastasize do so most commonly to the lung.[8] The lung should therefore be the site of most intense evaluations for metastatic disease in follow-up. Periodic evaluation of the lungs should be performed in the follow-up of patients with neoplasms capable of metastasizing.

The chest radiograph and chest CT scans are the 2 most commonly performed follow-up studies. The chest radiograph is simple, relatively inexpensive, and can be done in the office setting. The disadvantage is that it cannot reliably detect lesions smaller than 2.0 cm in size. The CT scan is much more sensitive in revealing metastatic disease and can detect lesions as small as 0.5 mm in size. However, the CT scan is more expensive, time consum-

ing, and cannot be routinely obtained in the office setting. The CT scan will add about 10% to 15% additional sensitivity to the screening, but is nonspecific and may detect many more clinically irrelevant benign nodules than metastatic nodules.[9]

Lymph node metastasis is uncommon in primary musculoskeletal neoplasms, and only certain tumors show evidence of frequent metastases to the lymph node. These include synovial cell sarcomas, clear cell sarcomas, and epithelioid sarcomas. Thus, periodic regional lymph node examination (palpation) should be performed when following up patients with sarcomas, especially patients with the 3 sarcomas that frequently metastasize to lymph nodes. Whenever questions arise, the CT scan is excellent for evaluating lymph nodes, especially in the pelvic and retroperitoneal areas.

The retroperitoneal area is a common area for metastases of liposarcoma.[10] The role of routine evaluation of the retroperitoneal area in the follow-up of patients with liposarcomas is unclear, but might include periodic CT scans or MRI scans.

Sarcomas may metastasize to other bones. The phenomenon of metachronous osteosarcoma is most likely simply late bone metastases. The tumors that most commonly develop metastatic disease to other bones include Ewing's sarcoma and other marrow cell diseases. The role of routine periodic bone scans in the follow-up of patients with sarcomas is unclear and undefined at this point.

Summary

In summary, there is no gold standard of the appropriate follow-up of orthopaedic patients. Patients with musculoskeletal neoplasms should be watched closely for local recurrence. Those patients whose tumors have metastatic potential should be followed up closely for metastatic disease. The timing of the suggested follow-up intervals varies, depending on the aggressiveness and growth rate of the tumor. There is no objective, data-based study to define the optimal follow-up intervals for the various entities. In general, the earlier recurrent or progressive disease can be detected, the better the chance of disease eradication. However, there is still some question as to whether the earlier detection of metastatic disease will change the eventual outcome in these patients.

References

1. Ward WG, Mikaelian K, Dorey F, et al: Pulmonary metastases of stage IIB extremity osteosarcoma and subsequent pulmonary metastases. *J Clin Oncol* 1994;12:1849–1858.

2. Lawrence W Jr, Donegan WL, Natarajan N, Mettlin C, Beart R, Winchester D: Adult soft tissue sarcomas: A pattern of care survey of the American College of Surgeons. *Ann Surg* 1987; 205:349–359.

3. Kay RM, Eckardt JJ, Seeger LL, Mirra JM, Hak DJ: Pulmonary metastases of benign giant cell tumor of bone: Six histologically confirmed cases, including one of spontaneous regression. *Clin Orthop* 1994;302:219–230.

4. Huvos AG, Marcove RC: Chondroblastoma of bone: A critical review. *Clin Orthop* 1973;95: 300–312.

5. Green P, Whittaker RP: Benign chondroblastoma: Case report with pulmonary metastasis. *J Bone Joint Surg* 1975;57A:418–420.

6. Letson GD: Diagnosis and treatment of soft tissue sarcomas. *Cancer Control Journal* 1994; 6:566–567.

7. Lucas JD, O'Doherty MJ, Wong JC, et al: Evaluation of fluorodeoxyglucose positron emission tomography in the management of soft-tissue sarcomas. *J Bone Joint Surg* 1998; 80B:441–447.

8. Frassica FJ, Lindsey J, Heitmiller RF, Choong PFM, Sim FH: Evaluation and treatment of pulmonary metastases, in Simon MA, Springfield D, Conrad EU, et al (eds): *Surgery for Bone and Soft-Tissue Tumors*. Philadelphia, PA, Lippincott-Raven, 1998, pp 105–109.

9. Chalmers N, Best JJ: The significance of pulmonary nodules detected by CT but not by chest radiography in tumour staging. *Clin Radiol* 1991;44:410–412.

10. Cheng EY, Springfield DS, Mankin HJ: Frequent incidence of extrapulmonary sites of initial metastasis in patients with liposarcoma. *Cancer* 1995;75:1120–1127.

Presentation and Evaluation of Bone Tumors

W. Seth Bolling, MD
Christopher P. Beauchamp, MD

Introduction

Bone tumors are a relatively rare occurrence in an orthopaedic practice. They can be difficult to recognize early, and unless the possibility of a tumor is included in the differential diagnosis, it can easily be missed. Some lesions are obvious and the diagnosis can be easily made such as with an osteochondroma; others are more difficult because the clinical and radiographic presentations can mimic a wide range of pathologic entities. An example of this is the tremendous overlap in presentation of Ewing's sarcoma, eosinophilic granuloma, and osteomyelitis. Despite the rarity of these conditions, it is important for the orthopaedic surgeon to have a good knowledge base of common bone neoplasms. The surgeon must recognize when a patient needs investigation of a lesion and when a patient needs to see an oncologic surgeon. Despite efforts to educate physicians about the dangers associated with the workup, investigation, and diagnosis (biopsy) of these lesions, the care of many patients continues to be compromised simply by the surgeon not understanding the problem. Joyce and Mankin[1] illustrated this point precisely in their report of a number of patients who underwent arthroscopic knee procedures for unrecognized underlying tumors of the distal femur or proximal tibia.

Clinical Presentation

Perhaps the most common error orthopaedic surgeons commit in the evaluation of patients is the development of an incomplete or abbreviated differential diagnosis. If, after the physician arrives at a diagnosis and prescribes a treatment, the patient returns without improvement, it is necessary to evaluate the patient again and revisit the differential diagnosis. Patients with bone tumors usually present in 1 of 5 ways.[2,3]

Pain Typically, pain of tumor origin is present constantly, at rest and especially at night. It is a disturbing pain, and the history is worrisome to the physician. A detailed pain history is especially important; otherwise, the possibility of a bone tumor will be overlooked and a more common musculoskeletal diagnosis will be initially considered. Sometimes the pain is of a mechanical origin, such as with a large osteochondroma beneath the scapula, or there may be a history of trauma that unmasks an otherwise asymptomatic lesion.

Mass Patients may present with only a mass, which may or may not be painful. The mass can be a subtle enlargement that is barely noticeable or a very large lesion. The surgeon should ask several questions: When did it begin? Is it getting larger? Does it change in size? Was it the result of an injury?

Deformity Bone lesions can affect the growth, development, and structural integrity of the skeleton and may present initially as a deformity. Fibrous dysplasia and multiple hereditary exostoses are examples of lesions that can be very deforming.

Fracture Pathologic fracture is not an uncommon presentation of bone pathology. Sometimes it is not easy to recognize the underlying pathologic disorder, and a high index of suspicion may be necessary to recognize the problem.

Incidental Finding This is a fairly common method of presentation. This situation usually arises when a lesion is detected during a radiographic evaluation of an injury or a screening bone scan is done for other reasons. Incidental findings are frequently benign, nonprogressive lesions that usually can be diagnosed with plain radiographs. They sometimes mimic metastatic disease and may require further investigations, including biopsy.

Bone infarcts, bone islands, enchondromas, nonossifying fibromas, osteochondromas, fibrous dysplasia, degenerative cysts, and radiation osteitis are the most common incidental findings seen radiographically, and it is important for orthopaedic surgeons to be comfortable diagnosing lesions on plain radiographs.

The evaluation of the patient should then include a thorough review of family history, past medical and surgical history, and review of systems. Relevant family information may reveal a history of hereditary exostosis. Past history and review of systems will be particularly important in patients presenting with a potential metastatic lesion. At times the distinction between a primary and secondary malignancy of bone may be difficult both clinically for the diagnostician and for the pathologist examining the biopsy tissue. Information about a prior lung carcinoma, for example, is obviously very helpful, even if it was in the distant past, because metastatic disease can develop many years after the primary disease has been treated. Bone tumors present diagnostic challenges on all fronts, and these situations demand a thorough collection of all patient data.

Physical Examination

A detailed thorough examination should be conducted both locally and systemically. The orthopaedic surgeon may need to examine unfamiliar systems during the course of patient assessment.

Locally, the lesion should be assessed by a complete evaluation of the mass, which includes location, dimension, size, shape, surface, consistency, tenderness, inflammation, mobility, and anatomic relations.[4] Does it transilluminate? Is there a bruit? The local assessment should also include the presence or absence of atrophy, local functional limitations, and distal neurovascular status. Careful assessment of lymphadenopathy is necessary even though bone tumors seldom involve lymphatics.

The remainder of the examination is directed toward the detection of metastatic disease, a primary tumor

elsewhere, or the physical stigmata suggestive of a more widespread disorder. The presence of a breast mass, prostatic nodule, splenomegaly, or pigmented skin lesions should be carefully examined and noted. The ideal goal of the history and physical examination is to obtain a diagnosis. The ultimate examination, the biopsy, ideally should be a confirmation of the orthopaedist's clinical impression.

Laboratory Investigations

Laboratory tests complement the history, physical examination, and radiographic imaging studies. White blood cell count, sedimentation rate, and C-reactive protein are helpful tests for infection, but may be positive with widespread disease or extensive tumor necrosis. The presence or absence of anemia can provide evidence of systemic disease or myeloma. Serum calcium, phosphorus, and alkaline phosphatase can provide clues to the metabolic activity of some tumors or the systemic effect on the skeleton from widespread disease. Other blood tests may provide further evidence of specific diagnoses, such as prostate specific antigen, serum protein electrophoresis, and parathyroid hormone assays. A urinalysis may indicate renal carcinoma or multiple myeloma.

Radiographic Examination

The single, most important diagnostic test in the evaluation of a bone tumor is the plain radiograph.[5] Most of the other modalities used in the staging of bone tumors do not provide as much information regarding the diagnosis as does the plain radiograph. Radiographs should be biplanar, of good quality, and carefully examined. Subtle periosteal reactions or endosteal calcifications can be difficult to see on poor or overpenetrated films. Radiographs are sometimes

obtained after isotope scans. Occasionally, as in the case of a small, hard to find osteoid osteoma, the isotope scan is used to guide the radiographic examination.

When examining the radiograph, it must be viewed systematically. Each lesion should be viewed keeping in mind the 4 questions of Enneking.[6]

First, where is the lesion? The particular location of a tumor within a bone can provide clues to its identity. Outline 1 and Figure 1 list specific sites within bone commonly associated with tumors.[7,8] However, these lesions can occur elsewhere. Tumors sometimes occur on or near the surface of the bone. When you see juxtacortical lesions think of the tumors listed in Outline 2.[9]

Second, what is the lesion doing to the bone? Is the lesion behaving aggressively, appearing destructive and ill defined, or is it well circumscribed and localized? Malignant and aggressive benign lesions have a wide zone of transition, are permeative in nature, and the bone has little time to respond. Infections can have this appearance as well. Well-demarcated geographic lesions with a narrow zone of transition are more likely to be benign.

Third, what is the bone doing (endosteally and periosteally)? Is there any reaction to the lesion? Is there a periosteal reaction (Outline 3)? Is it smooth, suggestive of a benign process? Is there an onion-skin or sunburst reaction? Reactive bone formation provides a clue to the biologic activity of the disease process.[10]

Fourth, what is in the lesion? Is there calcification indicating a cartilaginous lesion, bone formation, or other tissue?[11]

Two further questions can be added to the list: Fifth, what is the patient's age? Age is an important factor in evaluating patients with bone tumors. The differential diagnosis changes considerably as patients grow older. Table 1 categorizes tumors by age group.[12–14]

Finally, is there more than 1 lesion? The presence of multifocal disease gives rise to a relatively short list of diagnostic possibilities. When multiple lesions are present, the orthopaedic surgeon should think of the lesions listed in Outline 4.[15,16]

In many cases, the diagnosis can be made on plain radiographs. The above questions guide the differential diagnosis. Lesions that can often be comfortably diagnosed on plain films without further investigation or biopsy are listed in Outline 5.[15,17] It is important for orthopaedic surgeons to be able to recognize these lesions and not embark on further unnecessary investigations or cause undue patient anxiety when the diagnosis can be readily made on plain radiograph unless surgical treatment is required. If there is any uncertainty regarding the diagnosis at this point, most orthopaedic oncologists are more than willing to provide assistance with a radiographic opinion. This opinion can be reassuring to the surgeon and the patient. Many times the diagnosis is obvious and a biopsy is not required, although the lesion may require periodic follow-up to confirm its inactivity and a benign clinical course. Such is the case of a typical enchondroma. If, however, the lesion does not fit a definite diagnosis or the lesion is symptomatic and requires surgical management, further investigation is necessary.

Some lesions mimic bone tumors. It is important for the orthopaedic surgeon and the radiologist to be mindful of other processes that can masquerade as bone neoplasms. Trauma, stress fractures, osteonecro-

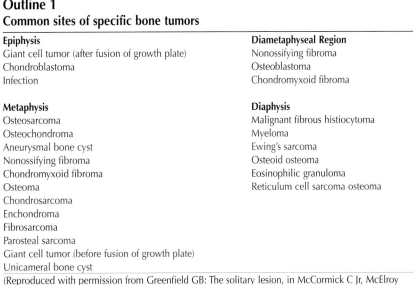

Outline 1
Common sites of specific bone tumors

Epiphysis	Diametaphyseal Region
Giant cell tumor (after fusion of growth plate)	Nonossifying fibroma
Chondroblastoma	Osteoblastoma
Infection	Chondromyxoid fibroma

Metaphysis	Diaphysis
Osteosarcoma	Malignant fibrous histiocytoma
Osteochondroma	Myeloma
Aneurysmal bone cyst	Ewing's sarcoma
Nonossifying fibroma	Osteoid osteoma
Chondromyxoid fibroma	Eosinophilic granuloma
Osteoma	Reticulum cell sarcoma osteoma
Chondrosarcoma	
Enchondroma	
Fibrosarcoma	
Parosteal sarcoma	
Giant cell tumor (before fusion of growth plate)	
Unicameral bone cyst	

(Reproduced with permission from Greenfield GB: The solitary lesion, in McCormick C Jr, McElroy MB (eds): *Radiology of Bone Diseases*, ed. 5. Philadelphia, PA, JB Lippincott, 1990, pp 579–732.)

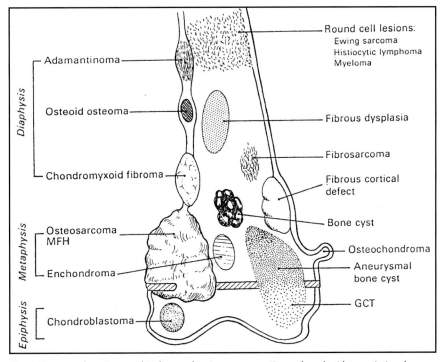

Fig. 1 Common locations within bone of various tumors. (Reproduced with permission from Madewell JE, Ragsdale BD, Sweet DE: Radiographic and pathologic analysis of solitary bone lesions: Part I. Internal margins. *Radiol Clin North Am* 1981;19:715–748.)

sis, Paget disease, hyperparathyroidism, pigmented villonodular synovitis, degenerative cysts, and infections can all present as a bone tumor.

Isotope Scans

Skeletal scintigraphy is a helpful tool in the evaluation of bone tumors. The technetium-99 bone scan is a very sensitive test in the investigation

Outline 2
Differential diagnosis of juxtacortical bone tumors[9]

Osteochondroma
Periosteal osteosarcoma
Periosteal chondroma
Periosteal chondrosarcoma
Aneurysmal bone cyst
Parosteal osteosarcoma

Outline 3
Differential diagnosis of periosteal reactions[10,11]

Solid Periosteal Reaction
Benign neoplasms (osteoid osteoma)
Eosinophilic granuloma
Infection (sclerosing osteomyelitis)
Stress fractures
Hypertrophic pulmonary osteoarthropathy

Aggressive Periosteal Reaction
Osteomyelitis
Malignant neoplasms
Osteosarcoma
Chondrosarcoma
Fibrosarcoma
Lymphoma
Leukemia
Metastasis

Benign Neoplasms
Aneurysmal bone cyst
Giant cell tumor

Table 1
Age distribution of various bone lesions[14–16]

Age	Malignant	Benign
0 to 10	Leukemia	Osteomyelitis
	Metastatic neuroblastoma	Osteofibrous dysplasia
	Metastatic rhabdomyosarcoma	
	Ewing's sarcoma (tubular bones)	
0 to 20		Simple bone cyst
10 to 20	Osteosarcoma	Chondroblastoma
	Leukemia	Osteoid osteoma
	Adamantinoma	Nonossifying fibroma
	Ewing's sarcoma	Eosinophilic granuloma
		Fibrous dysplasia
10 to 30	Ewing's sarcoma (flat bones)	Osteochondroma
		Enchondroma
		Chondromyxoid fibroma
		Osteoblastoma
		Desmoplastic fibroma
		Aneurysmal bone cyst
15 to 35		Osteoma
20 to 40	Parosteal sarcoma	Giant cell tumor
30 to 40	Fibrosarcoma	
	Hemangioendothelioma	
	Reticulum cell sarcoma (histiocytic lymphoma)	
	Lymphoma	
30 to 50	Chondrosarcoma	
	Malignant giant cell tumor	
30 to 60	Chordoma	
40 to 60	Metastatic bone disease	Hyperparathyroidism
	Myeloma	Paget disease
	Paget sarcoma	Mastocytosis
	Postradiation sarcoma	
	Chondrosarcoma	

of patients with painful disorders. There are a number of circumstances when it is useful and some when it is not.[18]

A bone scan can be helpful in evaluating a patient with a lesion not readily evident on plain radiograph. The scan can point the clinician to the area of abnormality where other diagnostic modalities can be applied. A bone scan is the most efficient method for the detection of skeletal metastasis. Not only is metastatic disease well demonstrated by bone scan, but other multifocal lesions are also well defined. A bone scan also may draw attention to other unrelated disorders. A common situation is a patient who undergoes a screening scan during staging of other malignant disorders. The bone scan may discover incidental lesions that may require further investigation or even biopsy.

There is an erroneous belief that a positive bone scan infers a more ominous diagnosis in an otherwise benign appearing lesion. Some common examples of lesions that appear warm on bone scans include enchondroma, osteoid osteoma, Paget disease, and fibrous dysplasia. A positive bone scan does not imply a more aggressive benign or malignant character. It may be important to obtain a scan in this situation, however, so that other lesions may be detected.

Some bone tumors do not yield a positive bone scan. Multiple myeloma, very aggressive metastatic carcinomas, and Langerhan's cell histiocytosis usually do not image well with technetium-99. These multifocal lesions are best viewed with a skeletal plain radiographic survey. Primary bone lesions need to be studied with a whole body bone scan to determine the presence or absence of distant bony metastasis, multifocal disease, or skip metastasis.

Computed Tomography

The computed tomography (CT) scan is quite valuable for evaluating musculoskeletal neoplasms, especially of bone. It is able to precisely localize the lesion, outline its extent, define its anatomic relations, and, in some instances, may facilitate the diagnosis with a CT-guided biopsy. The major reasons for obtaining a CT scan for a bone tumor include to detect the extent of the process, to aid in surgical planning, to judge the effect of preoperative therapy, and to provide diagnostic information related to the CT characteristics of a particular lesion.[19] A CT scan is best for evaluating lesions containing calcium, such as enchondromas, or osteoid as seen in the rim of an aneurysmal bone cyst. It is the most sensitive method to evaluate bone destruction, periosteal new bone formation, or soft-tissue mineralization. In the past it was limited to axial imaging, but with new software, sagittal reconstructions have become increasingly more useful today.

Magnetic Resonance Imaging

Whereas the CT scan is an excellent tool for evaluating bone, the magnetic resonance imaging (MRI) scan is an excellent tool for evaluating everything else. MRI is superior to CT in that it can image in multiple planes. This makes surgical planning and treatment easier in that 3-dimensional understanding of the lesion is facilitated. MRI shows soft tissues much better than CT, so it is useful in bone tumors that have soft-tissue components to them. An MRI is particularly useful in detecting the intraosseous extent of tumors because the demarcation between normal marrow and tumor is sharply displayed.[20] Most lesions have low signal intensity on T1-weighted images and high signal on T2-weighted images. The T1 images provide a high contrast at the lesion-marrow interface. The T2 images provide high contrast at the lesion and surrounding muscle. Both T1 and T2 images in 2

orthogonal planes are needed to assess tumor extent accurately. The MRI is extremely sensitive. Inflammation, edema, and reaction to prior injury/surgery sometimes make interpretation of images difficult. It is for this reason that all imaging of the lesion should be completed before biopsy.

Angiography

Once used extensively for the evaluation of bone and soft-tissue tumors, today angiography is rarely used for diagnostic purposes. MRI and magnetic resonance angiography have largely eliminated the need for angiography. Angiography still has a role in the evaluation of the degree of vascularity of the lesion and is commonly used preoperatively for embolizaton of very vascular lesions. It is extremely important to be aware of the potential of massive bleeding from metastatic bone lesions, especially thyroid and kidney carcinomas.

Conclusion

Bone tumors, while not common, are encountered in every orthopaedic surgeon's practice. The importance of understanding bone pathology is indeed reflected in the content of the

Outline 4
Differential diagnosis of multiple bone lesions[15,16]
Fibrous dysplasia
Eosinophilic granuloma
Enchondroma
Metastasis
Hyperparathyroidism (brown tumors)
Osteochondroma
Enchondroma
Myeloma
Nonossifying fibroma
Hemangiosarcoma
(Adapted with permission from Richardson ML (ed): *Approaches to Differential Diagnosis in Musculoskeletal Imaging*. Seattle, WA, University of Washington Department of Radiology, 1994, pp 1–7.)

Outline 5
Tumors that are often diagnostic by plain film alone[15,17]
Osteochondroma
Nonossifying fibroma
Unicameral bone cyst
Osteoid osteoma (classic)
Bone infarct
Bone island
Fibrous dysplasia (classic)

in-training examination and part I of the Board examinations. A sound understanding of the presentation and evaluation of bone tumors and tumor-like conditions is necessary in every practice. It is particularly important to avoid unnecessary investigations for lesions that can be readily diagnosed on plain radiography and equally important to recognize lesions that need further investigation and referral to a musculoskeletal oncologist.

References

1. Joyce MJ, Mankin HJ: Caveat arthroscopes: Extra-articular lesions of bone simulating intra-articular pathology of the knee. *J Bone Joint Surg* 1983;65A:289–292.

2. Buckwalter JA: Musculoskeletal neoplasms and disorders that resemble neoplasms, in Weinstein SL, Buckwalter JA (eds): *Turek's Orthopaedics: Principles and Their Application*, ed 5. Philadelphia, PA, JB Lippincott, 1994, pp 290–295.

3. Wheeless CR: *Atlas of Pelvic Surgery*, ed 3. Baltimore, MD, Williams and Wilkins, 1996, pp 133–135.

4. D'Ambrosia RD (ed): *Musculoskeletal Disorders: Regional Examination and Differential Diagnosis*, ed 2. Philadelphia, PA, JB Lippincott, 1986, pp 1–19.

5. Resnick D (ed): *Diagnosis of Bone and Joint Disorders*, ed 3. Philadelphia, PA, WB Saunders, 1995, vol 6, pp 3613–3627.

6. Enneking WF (ed): *Musculoskeletal Tumor Surgery*. New York, NY, Churchill Livingstone, 1983, pp 87–89.

7. Greenfield GB (ed): *Radiology of Bone Diseases*, ed 5. Philadelphia, PA, JB Lippincott, 1990, pp 579–732.

8. Madewell JE, Ragsdale BD, Sweet DE: Radiographic and pathologic analysis of solitary bone lesions: Part I. Internal margins. *Radiol Clin North Am* 1981;19:715–748.

9. Netter FA, Enneking WF, Conrad EU III: Section II: Tumors of musculoskeletal system,

in Netter FH, Dingle RV, Freyberg RH, Hensinger RN (eds): *The Ciba Collection of Medical Illustrations: Musculoskeletal System. Part II: Developmental Disorders, Tumors, Rheumatic Diseases, and Joint Replacement*. Summit, NJ, CIBA-GEIGY, 1990, vol 8, pp 117–153.

10. Ragsdale BD, Madewell JE, Sweet DE: Radiologic and pathologic analysis of solitary bone lesions: Part II. Periosteal reactions. *Radiol Clin North Am* 1981;19:749–783.

11. Richardson ML (ed): *Approaches to Differential Diagnosis in Musculoskeletal Imaging*. Seattle, WA, University of Washington Department of Radiology, 1994, pp 1–4.

12. Resnick D, Fix CF (eds): *Bone and Joint Imaging*, ed 2. Philadelphia, PA, WB Saunders, 1996, pp 979–1091.

13. Ferguson AB, D'Ambrosia RD: Roentgenogram interpretation, in D'Ambrosia RD (ed): *Musculoskeletal Disorders: Regional Examination and Differential Diagnosis*, ed 2, Philadelphia, PA, JB Lippincott, 1986, pp 21–57.

14. Frassica FJ, McCarthy EF Jr: Orthopaedic pathology, in Miller MD (ed): *Review of Orthopaedics*, ed 2. Philadelphia, PA, WB Saunders, 1996, pp 292–335.

15. Helms CA (ed): *Fundamentals of Skeletal Radiology*. Philadelphia, PA, WB Saunders, 1989, pp 10–66.

16. Richardson ML (ed): *Approaches to Differential Diagnosis in Musculoskeletal Imaging*. Seattle, WA, University of Washington Department of Radiology, 1994, pp 1–7.

17. Bogumill GP: Tumors of the musculoskeletal system, in Wiesel SW, Delahay JN, Connell MC, Bogumill GP (eds): *Essentials of Orthopaedic Surgery*. Philadelphia, PA, WB Saunders, 1993, pp 95–114.

18. Alazraki N: Radionuclide techniques, in Resnick D (ed): *Diagnosis of Bone and Joint Disorders*, ed 3. Philadelphia, PA, WB Saunders, 1995, pp 430–474.

19. Andre M, Resnick D: Computed tomography, in Resnick D (ed): *Diagnosis of Bone and Joint Disorders*, ed 3. Philadelphia, PA, WB Saunders, 1996, pp 118–169.

20. McEnery KW, Murphy WA Jr: Resonance imaging: Practical considerations, in Resnick D (ed): *Diagnosis of Bone and Joint Disorders*, ed 3. Philadelphia, PA, WB Saunders, 1996, pp 191–218.

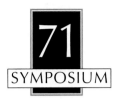

SYMPOSIUM

The Pathologist's Role in the Diagnosis of Bone Tumors: Informed Versus Uninformed

Scott E. Kilpatrick, MD
William G. Ward, Sr, MD

Introduction

It is impossible to underestimate the value of clinical and radiographic correlation in the diagnosis of musculoskeletal tumors. Although a diagnosis may be rendered on pathologic material alone in most cases, such practice is unwise and potentially dangerous. Radiographic assessment of features, such as anatomic location, lesional size and shape, pattern of bone destruction, matrix, margins, periosteal reactions, and concomitant soft-tissue abnormalities generally correlates with the aggressiveness (biologic behavior) of the lesion in question and allows for a more specific diagnosis. Knowledge of the clinical symptomatology attributable to the lesion itself (eg, pain versus asymptomatic) is also useful, especially in the differential diagnosis of cartilaginous tumors. Thus, open communication between the biopsying surgeon and the interpreting pathologist is imperative. To simply label a biopsy specimen as "bone lesion" or "soft-tissue lesion" without any additional information is an inadequate level of communication and will often lead to an inadequate and/or an inappropriate interpretation. To illustrate the importance of clinicoradiologic correlation for the diagnosis of musculoskeletal neopla-

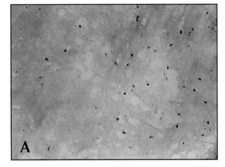 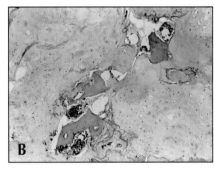

Fig. 1 A, Enchondroma characterized by hypocellular hyaline cartilage (hematoxylin & eosin × 100). **B,** Chondrosarcoma with characteristic permeation pattern and entrapment of trabecular bone. Note the similarities and overlap between the cellularity of enchondroma and that observed in low grade chondrosarcoma (hematoxylin & eosin × 40).

sia, selected examples of potentially difficult diagnoses will be analyzed and discussed.

Chondroma (Enchondroma, Soft-Tissue Chondroma, Periosteal Chondroma) Versus Chondrosarcoma

Nowhere is the correlation with clinicoradiologic findings more necessary than in establishing a diagnosis of chondroma versus chondrosarcoma. This fact should not imply, however, that specific morphologic findings do not exist for these entities. Microscopic features supporting a diagnosis of chondrosarcoma include enlarged chondrocytes with atypical nuclei, hypercellularity,

myxoid changes, and permeation (and entrapment) of medullary bone.[1] However, in most cases of chondrosarcoma, the degree of cellularity is not appreciably different from that observed with enchondroma (Fig. 1). Permeation and bone entrapment often is not obvious in small biopsy or curettage specimens. The presence of binucleated chondrocytes also may not be helpful in this distinction.[1] Complicating matters further, the degree of acceptable cellularity in chondroma depends, at least in part, on anatomic site (origin). For example, enchondromas of the phalanges and soft-tissue chondromas of the distal extremities are often significantly hypercellular,

Table 1

Clinicopathologic features of soft-tissue chondroma, periosteal chondroma, enchondroma, and chondrosarcoma

Tumor	Age Range* (years)	Anatomic Location	Clinical Symptoms	Radiologic Features	Pathologic Findings
Soft-tissue chondroma	30 to 60	Distal extremities, especially hands and feet; most common location is the fingers	Usually painless swelling or soft-tissue mass	Well-circumscribed soft-tissue mass; calcifications frequently present	Well-circumscribed, variably cellular lobulated with fibrous tissue septae containing epithelioid and multinucleated histiocytes; chondrocyte atypia is often marked
Periosteal chondroma	10 to 30	Proximal extremities, especially the femur and humerus	Painless swelling or soft-tissue mass	Juxtacortical mass, saucerization of the underlying cortex, < 3 cm, metaphyseal or disphyseal; may be calcified	Well-circumscribed and often hypercellular with atypical chondrocytes
Enchondroma	10 to 50	Small bones of the hands and feet, less commonly long bones; rare in axial skeleton	Often asymptomatic, incidental findings; pain is rare	Intramedullary, lytic, sharply marginated with punctate calcifications; metaphyseal/diaphyseal localization; cortical thinning and endosteal erosion in small bones only	Hypocellular, mature hyaline cartilage, may be encased by bone; rarely hypercellular
Chondrosarcoma	40 to 60	Most common in pelvic bones, proximal femur and humerus, ribs	Pain usually present; soft-tissue mass may also be seen	Intramedullary, bone expansion and cortical thickening, endosteal erosion	Variably cellular, myxoid changes frequent, permeation and entrapment of medullary bone

*Age range = most common age range; potentially any age may be affected

with the latter frequently displaying bizarre and atypical chondrocytes.[2] Similar findings in an intramedullary femoral lesion would require a diagnosis of chondrosarcoma. Likewise, periosteal chondromas tend to be more cellular than their classical intramedullary counterparts but, radiologically, are juxtacortical and associated with saucerization of the underlying bone.[3]

Because of the considerable overlap in the histologic findings, especially in low-grade chondrosarcomas and enchondromas, a definitive diagnosis requires analysis of other pertinent clinical features. Reliance on the clinical presence of pain favors the diagnosis of chondrosarcoma. Clin-

ically, pain is only rarely experienced by patients with enchondroma. Most enchondromas are asymptomatic, incidental findings. The pain of chondrosarcomas is most often a deep aching pain, often felt at night and unrelated to activity. With severe bone erosion, the pain may be mechanical from impending pathologic fracture. However, the surgeon must be cautious in the interpretation of pain. Pain from a coexistent process, such as rotator cuff tendinopathy or internal derangement of the knee, often leads to the radiographic study such as a plain radiograph or a magnetic resonance imaging study that detects the abnormality. The surgeon must use clinical skills to

determine whether the patient's pain is related to a nontumorous orthopaedic condition or to the neoplasm. This has important implications for the diagnosis. Because the presence of a pathologic entity (ie, enchondroma) does not necessarily account for the patient's pain, the clinician and the pathologist should not base diagnostic decisions on the presence or absence of pain alone, but, also, on the character of the pain.

The radiographic picture of bone expansion and cortical thickening in a long bone is virtually pathognomonic of chondrosarcoma. Endosteal erosion and soft-tissue extension are also frequently observed. In contrast, enchondromas tend to be sharply marginated, lack endosteal erosion, and frequently exhibit punctate and ring-like calcifications. For all practical purposes, conventional chondrosarcoma arising in soft tissues is nonexistent. The clinical, radiologic, and pathologic features of soft-tissue chondroma, periosteal chondroma, enchondroma, and chondrosarcoma are summarized in Table 1.

Giant Cell Tumor Versus Metaphyseal Fibrous Defect (Nonossifying Fibroma)

Clinically and radiologically, the distinction between giant cell tumor and metaphyseal fibrous defect is not difficult. Giant cell tumors typically arise as lytic, epiphyseal-centered lesions within the long bones of patients between the ages of 20 and 40 years. As the name implies, metaphyseal fibrous defects are probably nonneoplastic proliferations arising within the metaphyseal regions of skeletally immature patients. Radiologically, the latter are well-marginated with scalloped borders, appear predominately lytic, and are eccentrically located. In spite of the obvious clinicoradiologic differences between these 2 entities, significant histomorphologic overlap may occasionally occur, potentially confounding the diagnosis.

Microscopically, giant cell tumors are usually composed of numerous multinucleated osteoclast-type giant cells within a background of mostly uniform ovoid to spindle-shaped cells, the nuclei of which approximate, both in size and shape, the nuclei of the osteoclast-type giant cells.[4] On the other hand, metaphyseal fibrous defects are characterized by a fibroblastic, spindle cell proliferation arranged in obvious storiform patterns[5] (Fig. 2). Nevertheless, occasional examples of giant cell tumor may appear significantly

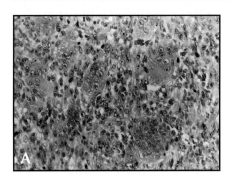
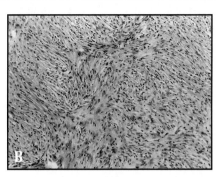

Fig. 2 A, Classic microscopic picture of giant cell tumor with numerous multinucelated osteoclast-type giant cells within an ovoid to spindle cell stroma (hematoxylin & eosin × 200). **B,** Metaphyseal fibrous defect characterized by a benign-appearing fibroblastic proliferation arranged in a classic storiform pattern (hematoxylin & eosin × 200).

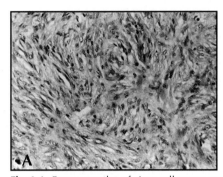
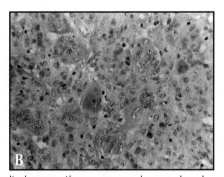

Fig. 3 A, Rare examples of giant cell tumor may display a storiform pattern and appear largely devoid of the characteristic multinucleated osteoclast-type giant cells. Such a pattern may cause diagnositic confusion with metaphyseal fibrous defect (hematoxylin & eosin × 200). **B,** Metaphyseal fibrous defect composed of numerous osteoclast-type giant cells, mimicking the microscopic appearance of giant cell tumor (hematoxylin & eosin × 200).

fibrous, displaying prominent storiform patterns, whereas metaphyseal fibrous defects may contain innumerable multinucleated osteoclast-type giant cells, mimicking the appearance of giant cell tumor (Fig. 3). Reactive bone rimmed by a single layer of osteoblasts may be seen in both lesions. Thus, without clinicoradiographic correlation, a significant pathologic misdiagnosis could occur.

Fibrous Dysplasia Versus Parosteal Osteosarcoma

The clinical and radiologic features separating fibrous dysplasia and parosteal osteosarcoma are obvious.

Fibrous dysplasia usually involves the skull/craniofacial region, femur, tibia, and ribs, arising in patients between the ages of 10 and 20 years.[6] The lesions are intramedullary, metaphyseal or diaphyseal, lytic, sharply marginated, and frequently reveal scattered ground glass-like densities. By contrast, parosteal osteosarcomas form juxtacortical lesions most commonly afflicting patients between the ages of 20 and 30 years.[7] The vast majority of cases involve the posterior distal femur. With adequate clinical and radiologic information, a pathologist will have little difficulty rendering the correct diagnosis. However, in the absence of such information, a less

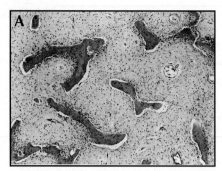 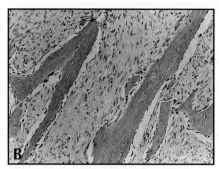

Fig. 4 A, Fibrous dysplasia with characteristic fibrous stroma and woven bony spicules (hematoxylin & eosin × 40). **B,** Parosteal osteosarcoma displaying a deceptively benign-appearing fibrous stroma and mostly mature bony trabeculae.

than accurate diagnosis may be given.

Microscopically, fibrous dysplasia is characterized by a dense fibrous tissue stroma containing a uniform population of fibroblasts with short, blunt-ended nuclei. Emanating from the fibrous stroma are bony trabeculae, often arranged in a haphazard, nonfunctional pattern. Occasional bony trabeculae exhibit a "mosaic pattern" of the so-called cement lines, mimicking Paget's disease. Like fibrous dysplasia, parosteal osteosarcoma is associated with a bland-appearing fibrous stroma accompanied by deceptively benign-appearing bony trabeculae (Fig. 4). Although the bony trabeculae tend to be longer with a lamellated appearance in parosteal osteosarcoma, spicules of bone virtually identical to those seen in fibrous dysplasia may also occur. Albeit extraordinarily rare, the intraosseous counterpart of parosteal osteosarcoma, the so-called well-differentiated intraosseous osteosarcoma, may also cause diagnostic confusion. The distinction of the latter from fibrous dysplasia requires meticulous attention to histomorphology (eg, permeation) and clinical and radiologic features.

Conclusion

The diagnosis of bone tumors is usually relatively straightforward when appropriate clinical and radiologic information is reviewed. It is important for both the pathologist and the orthopaedic surgeon involved with bone tumor diagnoses to understand the necessity of a multidisciplinary approach and interdisciplinary communication. In this manner, patient care is substantially improved and the likelihood of mistreatment is significantly reduced.

References

1. Mirra JM, Gold R, Downs J, Eckardt JJ: A new histologic approach to the differentiation of enchondroma and chondrosarcoma of the bones: A clinicopathologic analysis of 51 cases. *Clin Orthop* 1985;201:214–237.

2. Fletcher CD, Krausz T: Cartilaginous tumours of soft tissue. *Appl Pathol* 1988;6:208–220.

3. Nojima T, Unni KK, McLeod RA, Pritchard DJ: Periosteal chondroma and periosteal chondrosarcoma. *Am J Surg Pathol* 1985;9:666–677.

4. Hutter RVP, Worcester JN Jr, Francis KC, Foote FW Jr, Stewart FW: Benign and malignant giant cell tumors of bone: A clinicopathological analysis of the natural history of the disease. *Cancer* 1962;15:653–690.

5. Ritschl P, Karnel F, Hajek P: Fibrous metaphyseal defects: Determination of their origin and natural history using a radiomorphological study. *Skeletal Radiol* 1988;17:8–15.

6. Henry A: Monostotic fibrous dysplasia. *J Bone Joint Surg* 1969;51B:300–306.

7. Okada K, Frassica FJ, Sim FH, Beabout JW, Bond JR, Unni KK: Parosteal osteosarcoma: A clinicopathological study. *J Bone Joint Surg* 1994;76A:366–378.

Evaluation of Soft-Tissue Tumors

Dempsey Springfield, MD

Introduction

The good news about soft-tissue sarcomas is that they are uncommon. Fewer than 7,000 new soft-tissue sarcomas were diagnosed in 1997, and only a few more than 4,000 deaths due to soft-tissue sarcomas occurred that same year.[1] The bad news is that there are many more patients who present with a soft-tissue mass. Most of these masses are benign and need no treatment, but it is extremely difficult to know who has a benign tumor and who has a malignant one. The physician must decide which are benign and which are malignant. It is not practical or appropriate to biopsy, or even completely work up, every patient with a soft-tissue mass. However, a soft-tissue sarcoma should not be ignored and it would be inappropriate to just observe every lesion to see which proved to be a sarcoma. It is important to know when to observe, when to do an evaluation, and when to biopsy.

Systemic symptoms are not helpful. Patients who have a sarcoma generally are not sick. They have no systemic symptoms, and specifically do not complain of pain, tachypnea, fatigue, fever, night sweats, weight loss, or other systemic conditions. They are active, healthy individuals who usually simply noted a mass. There are no blood tests or specific radiographic findings that are diagnostic. The physician must ascertain the risk of a lesion being malignant, based on the initial presentation, using less than precise data.

History

As is the case with all medical evaluations, the history is important. Most of us sustain trauma to our extremities during the course of our daily activities, and patients tend to relate a mass to a specific traumatic event whether or not the 2 are related . Many patients first become aware of their mass due to trauma. The physician must be cautious in believing there is a relationship and should make the diagnosis of a residual hematoma rarely, if ever. Deep hematomas do occur, but are limited almost entirely to patients with bleeding disorders or those on anticoagulants.

A pseudoaneurysm, a mass that is related to trauma, can be confused with a neoplasm. It is caused by a lesion of the intima of an artery that results in bleeding within the wall of the vessel, producing a mass. Pseudoaneurysms are most commonly seen in the axilla where they are caused by blunt, nonpenetrating trauma. They can also be seen due to penetrating trauma at any site. The patient's history should be reviewed carefully for history of a traumatic event, and pulsatile masses must be approached carefully.

The patient should be questioned to establish the duration of any lesion and its recent behavior. If a mass has been unchanged for years, it is unlikely to be a malignancy. However, if the patient says the mass has grown over the last 1 to 2 months, the physician should be suspicious that the mass is malignant or locally aggressive. However, a word of caution must be expressed. Not infrequently, a patient's mass will appear to the physician to have been present for a long time, but the patient believes it has arisen overnight. This is probably the result of the mass not producing symptoms. When it is finally noticed, the patient cannot believe it could have been present without having been aware of it. Thus, if other data suggest a mass has been present for a longer time than the patient believes, it is better to believe the data than the patient.

Physical Examination

The physical examination of soft-tissue lesions can be extremely important. The examination is better at distinguishing nonneoplastic from neoplastic masses than it is at distinguishing between benign and malignant neoplastic masses. Neoplastic masses are usually not tender or inflamed. When a mass is particularly tender and inflamed the physician should suspect an abscess and the patient should be treated accordingly, remembering that a sarcoma is rarely inflammatory. The examination should reveal whether the mass is subcutaneous or deep. Deep is defined as deep to the superficial fascia. The size of the mass should be measured. Its movement should be noted and classified as movable, tethered, or fixed. Sarcomas and locally aggressive benign neoplasms are more commonly deep, larger than 5 cm, and tethered or fixed.

The physical findings of nonneoplastic lesions are valuable in deciding how extensive an evaluation should be done. As previously stated, abscesses are tender and inflamed. Suspected abscesses can be aspirated for diagnostic material. Aneurysms and pseudoaneurysms are pulsatile and may have a bruit. Ganglions are almost always adjacent to a joint (wrist and knee most commonly), firm, and usually can be transilluminated. If the physical findings suggest a ganglion and additional confirmation is needed, an aspiration can be done. A type of ganglion that often confuses the physician is one that arises from the proximal tibiofibular joint and extends distally in the anterior or lateral compartment of the leg. These may produce peroneal nerve dysfunction. Most schwannomas will be associated with a Tinel's sign, and this is almost always diagnostic.

Malignancies are less common in the subcutaneous tissues than in the deep tissues. When the physical examination suggests that the lesion is subcutaneous, measures less than 3 cm in diameter, and is movable, then it is reasonable to follow the patient clinically without further evaluation. If the patient wants the mass removed, it is safe to excise these lesions, but the tissue should be examined pathologically. All lesions deep to the fascia should be evaluated, because all of these should be considered malignant until proven otherwise.

Radiographic Examination

Plain radiographs are an important component of the evaluation of the patient with a deep soft-tissue mass. The density of the mass, the presence of calcifications or ossification, and any changes in the bone on the plain radiograph should be noted. Deep lipomas can usually be suspected by their low density on the plain radiograph. Calcifications seen in hemangiomas are usually small and smooth, while myositis ossificans will have peripheral ossification. Synovial sarcoma often has irregular central calcification or ossification. Benign neoplasms occasionally cause pressure changes in the adjacent bone, but bony changes usually reflect malignant or locally aggressive neoplasms.

After a plain radiograph, magnetic resonance imaging (MRI) is the single best means of further evaluating almost all soft-tissue masses. MRI provides an anatomic map of the lesion and can suggest the histologic diagnosis. The MRI characteristics of a benign lesion differ from those of most malignant lesions. A lipoma can be diagnosed from its characteristics on an MRI. It will have the identical signal characteristics of the subcutaneous tissues and be homogeneous. Ganglia will have the signal of fluid, dark on T1 and bright on T2. Hemangiomas can often be diagnosed or, at least, highly suspected with their characteristic combination of fat signal and round low density vessels. When this appearance on MRI is combined with a plain radiograph with small round calcifications, a diagnosis of hemangioma can be made. Schwannoma are usually recognized when the lesion is noted to be in continuity with a nerve. Additional tissue-specific diagnoses are unusual. Malignant lesions commonly are not well defined, have an inhomogeneous signal, and are surrounded by an inflammatory reaction. They will enhance with gadolinium. Benign lesions tend to be well defined, to have a homogenous signal, and have no or minimal associated surrounding inflammation.

An MRI scan should be done before the biopsy in order to know exactly where the lesion is located, which makes doing the biopsy easier. The biopsy will change the signal characteristics and may make defining the exact location more difficult.

Computed tomography (CT) is of less value but sometimes is used if the patient cannot tolerate the claustrophobic experience of an MRI scan. If a CT scan is done, it should be both with and without intravenous contrast. The radiologist should measure the density of the mass before and after contrast has been injected. Small amounts of calcification or ossification and subtle bone erosion are best seen on a CT scan. Technetium bone scans and gallium bone scans are of limited value and are not routinely recommended. Angiograms are done only when the vessels are not adequately seen on the MRI scan and involvement of the vessels is suspected.

When a patient is suspected of having a malignancy, a chest radiograph and whole lung CT scan should be done. A whole lung CT scan is best done prior to general anesthesia, when needed, because general anesthesia produces pulmonary changes that make the interpretation of the CT difficult, at least for several days postoperatively.

Biopsy

Biopsy is the last step of the evaluation. It should be planned and done carefully. Based on the prebiopsy evaluation, the surgeon should have a reasonably good idea of what will be found. The surgeon should discuss the biopsy with the pathologist before doing the procedure, and the surgeon doing the biopsy should be willing to manage the patient after the biopsy.

There are several alternative biopsy techniques available, including fine needle aspiration (FNA), core needle, open incisional, and open excisional. Each has its advantages and disadvantages, and the surgeon should select the technique appropriate for the patient. Fine needle aspiration is easy and convenient for the patient and surgeon. It requires only a small needle stick and can be done in the office. The material obtained is limited and only cytologic details are obtained. The pathologist must be experienced in making diagnoses from FNAs, and it may be difficult to histologically grade a tumor from an FNA. Placement of the fine needle is important but the risk of a recurrence if the needle tract is not excised is thought to be minimal.

Core needle biopsy is a little more difficult but usually can be done in the office with local anesthesia. The small cores of tissue obtained provide the pathologist with a more traditional specimen from which to make a diagnosis. The needle tract from these cores should be excised when the tumor is resected. Incisional biopsy provides the most tissue and is considered the standard means of doing a biopsy. It requires anesthesia and results in greater tissue contamination. When an incisional biopsy is done, longitudinal incisions are recommended, the dissection should be through muscle rather than between, and neurovascular bundles should not be exposed. An excisional biopsy is occasionally preferred; when done, it is recommended that the entire lesion be removed along with a surrounding cuff of normal tissue.

Summary

Soft-tissue masses present a challenge to the practicing physician. Most are of little or no concern and do not need medical attention, but the consequences of missing a sarcoma are significant. It is important to give careful consideration to each soft-tissue mass seen and decide which need further evaluation and which do not. Periodic reexamination is recommended for patients with masses not thought to need biopsy. Patients with more worrisome soft-tissue masses should have at least an MRI scan and then, usually, a biopsy.

Reference

1. Parker SL, Tong T, Bolden S, Wingo PA: Cancer statistics, 1997. *CA Cancer J Clin* 1998;47:5–27.

Cartilage and Bone

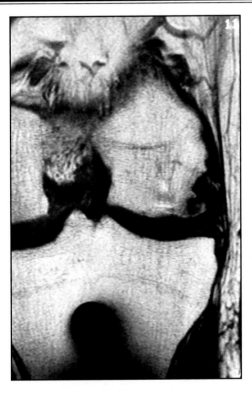

Biologic Restoration of Articular Surfaces

Victor M. Goldberg, MD
Arnold I. Caplan, PhD

Introduction

The statement by Hunter in 1743 that "ulcerated cartilage is a troublesome thing, once destroyed is not repaired" remains true today. Articular cartilage is a complex tissue that provides the diarthrodial joint with a low-friction surface. This surface comprises a low percentage of chondrocytes embedded in a 3-dimensional collagen network with an extracellular matrix of negatively charged hydrophilic proteoglycans.[1,2] Hyaline cartilage is not a uniform tissue, but has different properties depending on the location. The cells of the top layer have a flattened appearance, for example, and cells in the deeper layer are more rounded. Similarly, the extracellular matrix has different composition and properties. For example, type II collagen fibrils in the superficial layers are horizontal; in the deeper layers they are vertically oriented and appear to act as scaffolding material.

The structural differences of hyaline articular cartilage give rise to 4 distinct zones. The superficial zone is a cell-free layer known as the lamina splendens. In the transitional zone, the chondrocytes are situated parallel to the surface, and the collagen fibrils are tangential to the lamina splendens. The radial zone is characterized by chondrocytes that are larger and arranged in columns, and the collagen fibrils are radially dispersed. The deep, fourth layer is called the calci-

fied zone, and there is a visible border between the third and fourth zones that is known as the tidemark. The calcified zone is an important transition to the subchondral bone. The biomechanical properties of these distinct zones are directly dependent on the articular cartilage's biochemical and structural characteristics.[3]

Cartilage Injuries

Cartilage injuries may be characterized into 2 major types.[1] In the first type, mechanical damage is confined to loss of the matrix components without damage to the chondrocytes or collagen scaffold. Usually, the chondrocytes are able to synthesize new proteoglycans so that the cartilage can be completely restored. The second type of cartilage injury is mechanical destruction of the cells and the matrix, including the collagen scaffolding, by either blunt or penetrating trauma. It is possible for the chondrocytes to repair the damage, but their ability to do so depends on the extent of the injury as well as the location of the injured cartilage area and whether the injury extends into the vascular subchondral marrow cavity. Generally, significant trauma that does not penetrate to the subchondral bone and that significantly disrupts the collagen matrix as well as the chondrocytes has little or no capacity to heal. By contrast, full-thickness injuries that penetrate the

vascular subchondral marrow with its resident progenitor cells do have the capability to repair. However, the repair that ensues is variable and depends a great deal on the extent of the injury, the location of the cartilage injury (eg, loaded versus unloaded areas), and the age of the animal.[1,4–7]

Until recently, there has been no evidence that any treatment can result in normal articular cartilage in skeletally mature animals, and usually any repair tissue that is present will ultimately fail and will not function long-term. However, this concept has been recently challenged by a number of investigators who suggest that articular cartilage does have the potential to restore itself, and a number of procedures have been used to take advantage of this potential.[4,5,8–16] These procedures can be divided into 2 categories: those that stimulate repair and regeneration of articular cartilage, and those that use transplanted tissue or cells. Those methods that stimulate articular cartilage repair and regeneration include the drilling, resection, or abrasion of the subchondral plate; the decrease of articular surface contact loads by osteotomy; and the implantation of growth factors, with or without artificial matrices. Transplantation methods include both autografts and allografts of articular cartilage and soft-tissue grafts as well as cells, including chondrocytes and mesenchymal stem cells.[5,17–23] Although there have been a significant number of recent publications describing these approaches to the restoration of articular cartilage, there has been great difficulty in determining which procedures have the best potential to restore functional articular surfaces.

Definition of Repair

The repair of articular cartilage, which is avascular, aneural, and alymphatic, differs from the classic response to injury. Response to tissue injury is usually divided into 4 stages: necrosis, inflammation, repair, and scar remodeling. The vascular system is essential in this repair sequence. The lack of vascular response in the avascular hyaline cartilage is central to the inability of cartilage to repair itself.[24] Healing is usually defined as restoring the structural integrity and function of a damaged tissue. Repairing implies replacing the damaged or lost cells or matrix with new cells or matrix, but not necessarily restoring the tissue to its original function and structure. Regeneration implies that the damaged tissue has been replaced by the repair tissue, with new cells and matrix identical to the original tissue and with function that is biomechanically identical to that of normal hyaline cartilage. The focus of this report is on the strategies used to restore biologically (regenerate) articular cartilage to its original form with new cells and matrix.

Strategies to Biologically Restore Articular Cartilage
Osteochondral Grafts

Transplantation of osteochondral grafts has been shown to be an effective technique for replacing confined areas of damaged articular cartilage.[1,17,18,20,21,25] The graft can restore both joint contour and subchondral bone and provide a biomechanically satisfactory tissue integrated with its host.

Autografts A number of recent studies have reported the use of autogenous osteochondral grafts to treat osteochondral defects of the femoral condyles.[23] These reports indicate that the technique can restore articular surfaces and provide satisfactory clinical outcome. However, the limited availability of autografts and the difficulty in ensuring biomechanical properties identical to those of the lost tissue restrict the use of this approach to small articular surface defects in relatively nonloaded areas.

Allografts Osteochondral allografts have been used more frequently because of their greater availability and because they can be prepared in any size.[1] Clinical experience with both fresh and frozen allografts indicates that they can integrate to the host tissue and functionally restore articular surfaces.[1,17,18,20,21,25] Because of the issues of availability and transmission of diseases, preserved frozen osteochondral allografts have been used. The success of fresh osteochondral grafts has been reported as 64% in 10 years,[18] while frozen osteochondral allografts appear to produce results that compare favorably with fresh graft when used to replace localized defects in the distal femoral articular surfaces.[1] The controversial issues in regard to frozen allografts include preservation techniques, cell viability, and immune responses to the cells or matrix.

Perichondrial and Periosteal Grafts

Periosteal and perichondrial soft-tissue grafts can be used to deliver a new cell population to the cartilage defect site. Animal and clinical experiments have shown that both these grafts, when placed in articular cartilage defects, can produce new cartilage.[1,4,26–33] O'Driscoll and associates[31,32] showed that adult periosteum regenerated acceptable repair tissue in adult rabbits as well as in a small group of patients with isolated chondral and osteochondral defects. Other recent studies reporting the use of periosteal grafts to repair small osteochondral defects suggest that the outcomes may be acceptable for a short time with significant improvement of symptoms. Similar promising results have been reported with the use of perichondrium to repair partial and full-thickness cartilage defects.[26–29] However, the long-term durability of these grafts, both clinically and experimentally, still remains uncertain. Long-term studies have indicated that the graft tissue ultimately degenerates, that it integrates poorly into the host tissue, and that ultimately the surfaces become denuded down to subchondral bone. The best results of the use of these tissues have been in younger patients who have localized posttraumatic defects in the distal femoral condyles.

Growth Factors

Many growth peptides, such as fibroblastic growth factors, insulin-like growth factors, transforming growth factor betas, and bone morphogenetic proteins, affect cartilage metabolism and development.[1,4,16,34,35] Although there have been extensive studies demonstrating the effect these growth factors have on chondrocyte metabolism, there have been limited studies investigating their potential to stimulate restoration of articular surfaces.[1,4,14] Recent studies suggest, however, that local treatment of partial- and full-thickness articular cartilage defects with growth factors such as transforming growth factor beta has the potential to stimulate regeneration of an articular surface.[6,14] However, growth factor use alone may be limited because of the complexity of the interaction between growth factors and cartilage progenitor cells.

Tissue Engineering

The primary goal of tissue engineering is to restore, maintain, or improve tissue function, using the principles of engineering and life sciences. Tissue engineering merges the fields of cell biology, engineering, materials science, and surgery to synthesize new functional tissue using living cells, biomatrices, and signaling molecules. The paradigm of this technology is presently applied in the area of artificial skin, where isolated keratinocytes and dermal fibroblasts are mitotically expanded in tissue culture and combined with a biocompatible collagen vehicle to form an in vitro artificial skin. This tissue is then used to repair skin loss in, for example, burn patients. The application of this technology to articular cartilage defects requires the transplantation of viable cells. Experimental and preliminary clinical work has shown that both committed chondrocytes and undifferentiated mesenchymal cells placed in articular cartilage defects survive and produce a new cartilage matrix.[5,9,11–13,19,22,24,36–42] Committed chondrocytes isolated and grown in a culture environment can be transplanted to articular cartilage defects and produce a tissue with the characteristics of hyaline cartilage. Brittberg[4] and Brittberg and associates[9] have reported the use of autologous chondrocyte transplantation under a sutured periosteal flap to repair deep cartilage defects in the knee. The clinical results of these studies indicate that, at 2 years after surgery, approximately 80% of the patients were clinically improved. Biopsies of repaired tissue indicated that the repaired tissue had the appearance of hyaline cartilage. These results indicate that cultured autologous chon-

drocytes combined with a periosteal graft have the potential to restore articular surfaces. However, the long-term durability of this tissue remains in doubt, and additional studies are required to define the role of this tissue-engineering technique.

Wakitani and associates[41] have used osteochondral progenitor cells isolated from periosteum and bone marrow to repair large, full-thickness defects of the articular cartilage in rabbits. These adherent cells were isolated in vitro, dispersed in a type I collagen gel, and transplanted into a large, full-thickness defect in the medial femoral condyle. Within the first 4 weeks, these chondroprogenitor cells had differentiated into chondrocytes (Fig. 1). The implanted cells appeared to recapitulate the embryonic sequence. Rapidly, the implanted mesenchymal stem cells differentiated into characteristic embryonic cartilage. The chondrocytes at the surface appeared to be hyaline articular cartilage and rapidly synthesized a metachromatic matrix. The chondrocytes at the base of the defect appeared to be replaced by vascularized cancellous bone that appeared to be derived from host cells. The surface cartilage remained as articular cartilage, while the tissue at the base of the defect remodeled to become subchondral bone and resembled host bone histologically. There was satisfactory integration of the transplanted repair tissue with the host; however, the surface cartilage was roughened and thinner than the surrounding host articular surface. During the subsequent 44 weeks, the repair cartilage resembled the surrounding hyaline cartilage; however, the neocartilage became thinner and demonstrated a fibrillated and irregular surface. These findings were in sharp contrast to unrepaired defects and those repaired with a type I colla-

gen gel delivery vehicle, which remained fibrous and had few characteristics of adult hyaline cartilage. Mechanically, the repair tissue was more compliant than normal cartilage but stiffer than unrepaired defects.

Additional experimental studies have established some of the principles relevant to the clinical repair and regeneration of articular cartilage.[24] These studies have shown that an optimal number of appropriate chondroprogenitor cells delivered in a supportive vehicle provides a methodology in which regeneration of articular cartilage can be observed.[24] Further, the pretreatment of the defect with a highly dilute solution of trypsin provides a host surface more amenable to accepting a cell-based transplant. Electron microscopy has indicated that protease-treated matrix has a much less structured water content and a decreased concentration of small proteoglycans. This perhaps allows the newly synthesized matrix and the expanding repair tissue to infiltrate the host tissue.

Recent studies from this laboratory are addressing the use of unique matrices such as hyaluronic acid derivatives as biologic carriers that can be used to stabilize the cells and growth factors in the defect. These studies suggest that biomatrices may act not only as carrier material but also as a chondroconductive material. Future research will continue to address the issue of the ideal combination of cells, biomatrices, and growth factors to effectively treat both partial- and full-thickness defects of articular surfaces. Because of the complexity of the injuries seen clinically, it is unlikely that any one therapeutic strategy will be successful in biologically restoring all articular cartilage defects, and a number of different strategies will be necessary to address specific cartilage defects.

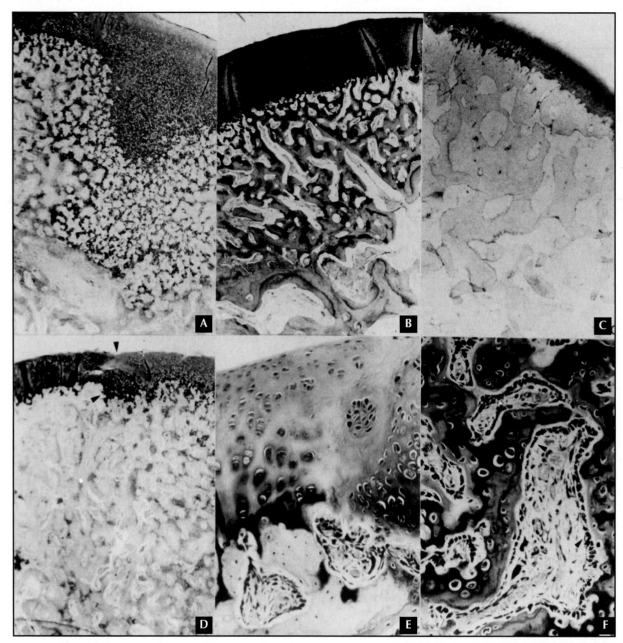

Fig. 1 Full-thickness defects in the medial femoral condyle were filled with culture-expanded autologous mesenchymal stem cells in a type I collagen gel. The rabbits were sacrificed at **(A)** 3 weeks, **(B, D, E,** and **F)** 1 month, or **(C)** 6 months, and the knees were processed routinely for histologic study. **A,** All of the cells in the defect have differentiated into embryonic-like chondrocytes that produce a rich, cartilaginous matrix. From the bony walls of the defect inward and upward, the cartilage was being replaced and endochondral bone was forming (stain, toluidine blue; magnification × 30). A higher magnification view of the lining osteoblasts fabricating this new bone is seen in **E** and **F.** One month after implantation, the endochondral bone formation produces trabecular bone of a density different from that of the host bone **(B)**; (stain, Mallory/Heidenhain; magnification × 40) comparing the bone with that in **C. C,** At 6 months after implantation, the bone density and articular cartilage were indistinguishable from host (stain, toluidine blue; magnification × 40). **D** and **E,** Various degrees of host; regenerate integration of cartilage can be observed. **D** shows a mixture of highly cellular cartilage and repair tissue at the junction of host and repair tissue [arrowhead] (stain, toluidine blue; magnification × 20) whereas **(E)** shows the relatively intact host cartilage on the left and repair cartilage on the far right. Between these two zones was an interface zone that seems to be continuous with the repair and host zones and that clearly contains host cells that are cloning, as often is seen in repairing osteoarthritis (stain, toluidine blue; magnification × 250). **(F)** Arrowheads point to sheets of bone-forming osteoblasts (stain, Mallory/Heidenhain; magnification × 250). (Reproduced with permission from Caplan AL, El Yaderani M, Mochizuki S, Goldberg VM: Principles of cartilage repair and regeneration. *Clin Orthop* 1997;342:254–269.)

References

1. Buckwalter JA, Mankin HJ: Articular cartilage: Part II. Degeneration and osteoarthrosis, repair, regeneration, and transplantation. *J Bone Joint Surg* 1997;79A:612–632.

2. Buckwalter JA, Mankin HJ: Articular cartilage: Part I. Tissue design and chondrocyte-matrix interactions. *J Bone Joint Surg* 1997;79A:600–611.

3. Mow VC, Rosenwasser M: Articular cartilage: Biomechanics, in Woo S-LY, Buckwalter JA (eds): *Injury and Repair of the Musculoskeletal Soft Tissues.* Park Ridge, IL, American Academy of Orthopaedic Surgeons, 1988, pp 427–463.

4. Brittberg M: Cartilage Repair: *On Cartilaginous Tissue Engineering With the Emphasis on Chondrocyte Transplantation.* Göteburg, Sweden, Institute of Laboratory Medicine, Vasatadens Bokbinderi, 1996. Thesis.

5. Goldberg VM, Caplan AI: Cellular repair of articular cartilage, in Kuettner KE, Goldberg VM (eds): *Osteoarthritic Disorders.* Rosemont, IL, American Academy of Orthopaedic Surgeons, 1995, pp 357–363.

6. Rosenberg L, Hunziker EB: Cartilage repair in osteoarthritis: The role of dermatan sulfate proteoglycans, in Kuettner KE, Goldberg VM (eds): *Osteoarthritic Disorders.* Rosemont, IL, American Academy of Orthopaedic Surgeons, 1995, pp 341–356.

7. Shapiro F, Koide S, Glimcher MJ: Cell origin and differentiation in the repair of full-thickness defects of articular cartilage. *J Bone Joint Surg* 1993;75A:532–553.

8. Aston JE, Bentley G: Repair of articular surfaces by allografts of articular and growth-plate cartilage. *J Bone Joint Surg* 1986;68B:29–35.

9. Brittberg M, Lindahl A, Nilsson A, Ohlsson C, Isaksson O, Peterson L: Treatment of deep cartilage defects in the knee with autologous chondrocyte transplantation. *N Engl J Med* 1994;331:889–895.

10. Brittberg M, Nilsson A, Lindahl A, Ohlsson C, Peterson L: Rabbit articular cartilage defects treated with autologous cultured chondrocytes. *Clin Orthop* 1996;326:270–283.

11. Caplan AI, Fink DJ, Goto T, et al: Mesenchymal stem cells and tissue repair, in Jackson DW, Arnoczky SP, Woo SLY, Frank CB, Simon TM (eds): *The Anterior Cruciate Ligament: Current and Future Concepts.* New York, NY, Raven Press, 1993, pp 405–417.

12. Chu CR, Coutts RD, Yoshioka M, Harwood FL, Monosov AZ, Amiel D: Articular cartilage repair using allogeneic perichondrocyte-seeded biodegradable porous polylactic acid (PLA): A tissue-engineering study. *J Biomed Mater Res* 1995;29:1147–1154.

13. Grande DA, Pitman MI, Peterson L, Menche D, Klein M: The repair of experimentally produced defects in rabbit articular cartilage by autologous chondrocyte transplantation. *J Orthop Res* 1989;7:208–218.

14. Hunziker EB, Rosenberg LC: Repair of partial-thickness defects in articular cartilage: Cell recruitment from the synovial membrane. *J Bone Joint Surg* 1996;78A:721–733.

15. Langer F, Gross AE: Immunogenicity of allograft articular cartilage. *J Bone Joint Surg* 1974;56A:297–304.

16. Reddi AH: Regulation of cartilage and bone differentiation by bone morphogenetic proteins. *Curr Opin Cell Biol* 1992;4:850–855.

17. Bayne O, Langer F, Pritzker KP, Houpt J, Gross AE: Osteochondral allografts in the treatment of osteonecrosis of the knee. *Orthop Clin North Am* 1985;16:727–740.

18. Beaver RJ, Mahomed M, Backstein D, Davis A, Zukor DJ, Gross AE: Fresh osteochondral allografts for post-traumatic defects in the knee: A survivorship analysis. *J Bone Joint Surg* 1992;74B:105–110.

19. Bentley G, Smith AU, Mukerjhee R: Isolated epiphyseal chondrocyte allografts into joints surfaces: An experimental study in rabbits. *Ann Rheum Dis* 1978;37:449–458.

20. Convery FR, Meyers MH, Akeson WH: Fresh osteochondral allografting of the femoral condyle. *Clin Orthop* 1991;273:139–145.

21. Gross AE, Beaver RJ, Mahomed MN: Fresh small fragment osteochondral allografts used for posttraumatic defects in the knee joint, in Finerman GAM, Noyes FR (eds): *Biology and Biomechanics of the Traumatized Synovial Joint: The Knee as a Model.* Rosemont, IL, American Academy of Orthopaedic Surgeons, 1992, pp 123–141.

22. Itay S, Abramovici A, Nevo Z: Use of cultured embryonal chick epiphyseal chondrocytes as grafts for defects in chick articular cartilage. *Clin Orthop* 1987;220:284–303.

23. Outerbridge HK, Outerbridge AR, Outerbridge RE: The use of a lateral patellar autologous graft for the repair of a large osteochondral defect in the knee. *J Bone Joint Surg* 1995;77A:65–72.

24. Caplan AI, Elyaderani M, Mochizuki Y, Wakitani S, Goldberg VM: Principles of cartilage repair and regeneration. *Clin Orthop* 1997;342:254–269.

25. Garrett JC: Fresh osteochondral allografts for treatment of articular defects in osteochondritis dissecans of the lateral femoral condyle in adults. *Clin Orthop* 1994;303:33–37.

26. Amiel D, Coutts RD, Abel M, Stewart W, Harwood F, Akeson WH: Rib perichondrial grafts for the repair of full-thickness articular-cartilage defects: A morphological and biochemical study in rabbits. *J Bone Joint Surg* 1985;67A:911–920.

27. Engkvist O, Ohlsén L: Reconstruction of articular cartilage with free autologous perichondrial grafts: An experimental study in rabbits. *Scand J Plast Reconstr Surg* 1979;13:269–274.

28. Engkvist O: Reconstruction of patellar articular cartilage with free autologous perichondrial grafts: An experimental study in dogs. *Scand J Plast Reconstr Surg* 1979;13:361–369.

29. Engkvist O, Johansson SH: Perichondrial arthroplasty: A clinical study in twenty-six patients. *Scand J Plast Reconstr Surg* 1980;14:71–87.

30. Korkala O, Kuokkanen H: Autogenous osteoperiosteal grafts in the reconstruction of full-thickness joint surface defects. *Int Orthop* 1991;15:233–237.

31. O'Driscoll SW, Keeley FW, Salter RB: The chondrogenic potential of free autogenous periosteal grafts for biological resurfacing of major full-thickness defects in joint surfaces under the influence of continous passive motion: An experimental investigation in the rabbit. *J Bone Joint Surg* 1986;68A:1017–1035.

32. O'Driscoll SW, Keeley FW, Salter RB: Durability of regenerated articular cartilage produced by free autogenous periosteal grafts in major full-thickness defects in joint surfaces under the influence of continuous passive motion: A follow-up report at one year. *J Bone Joint Surg* 1988;70A:595–606.

33. Rubak JM: Reconstruction of articular cartilage defects with free periosteal grafts: An experimental study. *Acta Orthop Scand* 1982;53:175–180.

34. Guenther HL, Guenther HE, Froesch ER, Fleisch H: Effect of insulin-like growth factor on collagen and glycosaminoglycan synthesis by rabbit articular chondrocytes in culture. *Experientia* 1982;38:979–981.

35. Lotz M, Blanco FJ, von Kempis J, et al: Cytokine regulation of chondrocyte functions. *J Rheumatol* 1995;43(suppl):104–108.

36. Caplan AI: Mesenchymal stem cells. *J Orthop Res* 1991;9:641–650.

37. Hendrickson DA, Nixon AJ, Grande DA, et al: Chondrocyte-fibrin matrix transplants for resurfacing extensive articular cartilage defects. *J Orthop Res* 1994;12:485–497.

38. Peterson L: Articular cartilage injuries treated with autologous chondrocyte transplantation in the human knee. *Acta Orthop Belg* 1996;62(suppl 1):196–200.

39. Robinson D, Halperin N, Nevo Z: Fate of allogeneic embryonal chick chondrocytes implanted orthotopically, as determined by the host's age. *Mech Ageing Dev* 1989;50:71–80.

40. Vacanti CA, Kim W, Schloo B, Upton J, Vacanti JP: Joint resurfacing with cartilage grown in situ from cell-polymer structures. *Am J Sports Med* 1994;22:485–488.

41. Wakitani S, Goto T, Pineda SJ, et al: Mesenchymal cell-based repair of large, full-thickness defects of articular cartilage. *J Bone Joint Surg* 1994;76A:579–592.

42. Wakitani S, Kimura T, Hirooka A, et al: Repair of rabbit articular surfaces with allograft chondrocytes embedded in collagen gel. *J Bone Joint Surg* 1989;71B:74–80.

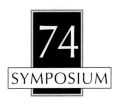

74

The Role of Cartilage Repair Techniques, Including Chondrocyte Transplantation, in Focal Chondral Knee Damage

Tom Minas, MD, FRCSC, MS

Introduction

Renewed interest in cartilage repair, as a result of new repair techniques,[1–3] has caused considerable debate among orthopaedists concerning new technologies, indications, effectiveness, and costs as compared to the role of traditional cartilage repair techniques performed arthroscopically.[4–6] The role of these techniques in the armamentarium of the treating orthopaedist has not been elucidated. To assist the orthopaedist in the decision-making process, this chapter seeks to outline the clinical results that can be expected with available cartilage repair techniques. In this way, a treatment may be selected to match the patient's needs and expectations.

Prevalence of Chondral Injuries, and the Natural History of Osteoarthritis

Full-thickness chondral injuries secondary to work-related and sporting activities are common, with an incidence of between 5% and 10% of acute hemarthrosis.[7] A retrospective review of 31,516 knee arthroscopies demonstrated an incidence of 41% Outerbridge grade III chondral lesions and 19.2% Outerbridge grade IV lesions. In those patients younger than 40 years of age, 5% had unipolar grade IV injuries to the medial femoral condyle (MFC), which were believed to be treatable by autologous chondrocyte transplantation (ACT).[8] Overall, there was a prevalence of 20% grade IV chondral lesions to the MFC, with the majority (72%), occurring in patients older than 40 years. This chapter seeks to define the patient population suitable for cartilage grafting. Possibly, new cartilage repair techniques could alter the progression of chondral disease to osteoarthritis.

Although orthopaedists note anecdotally that chondral injuries often progress to osteoarthritis, this claim has not been validated in a prospective fashion, probably largely due to the inability to accurately diagnose chondral injuries by noninvasive techniques and follow them over time. However, a recent study, which evaluated 31 patients followed up for 14 years, demonstrated at follow-up that greater than 50% of patients had radiographic evidence of joint space narrowing when a unipolar, unicompartmental injury was initially noted arthroscopically. These adolescent patients had 28 Outerbridge grade III lesions and 3 grade IV lesions, and they underwent arthroscopic assessment and localized debridement alone. Functionally, 14 years later, 21 patients were able to return to sports and 22 patients had good or excellent knee scores. However, progression of disease in this initially adolescent population was still noted radiographically.[9]

A recent Swedish cohort study evaluated the natural history and progression of osteoarthritis over 20 years. Those knees with early involvement had a variable progression, and those starting with advanced involvement had a consistent progression of disease. Specifically, patients with Ahlback stage 1 osteoarthritis (50% joint space narrowing) demonstrated progression of radiographic joint space narrowing in 61% of cases, with 39% remaining stable without further reduction in the joint

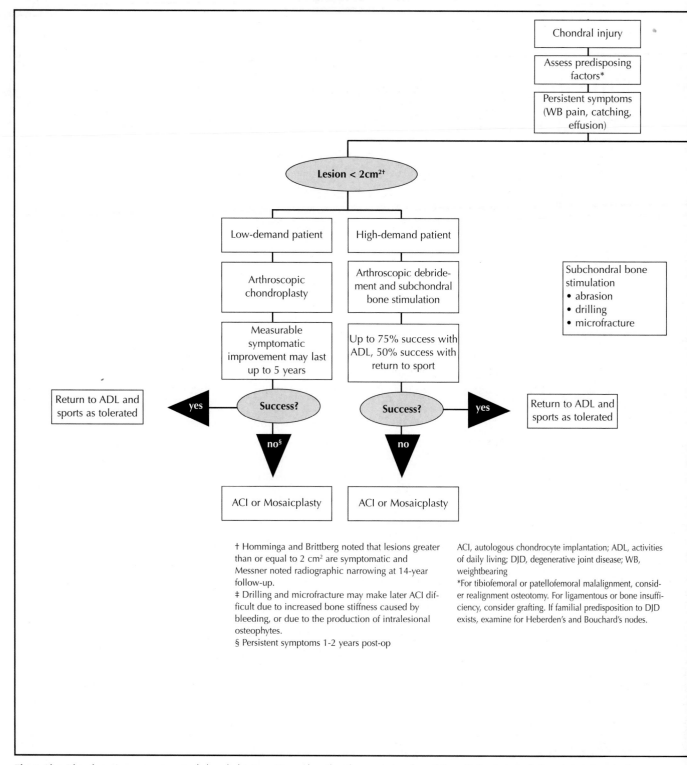

Fig. 1 Algorithm for primary treatment of chondral injury. (Reproduced with permission from Minas T: Treatment of chondral defects in the knee. *Orthop Spec Ed* 1997;3:69–74.)

space. Of patients with Ahlback stage 0 osteoarthritis (as defined by osteophyte or subchondral bone sclerosis with normal joint space), 57% would progress over time. However, all patients with Ahlback stages 2, 3, 4, and 5 osteoarthritis demonstrated progression of disease.[10]

Therefore, it would be difficult to

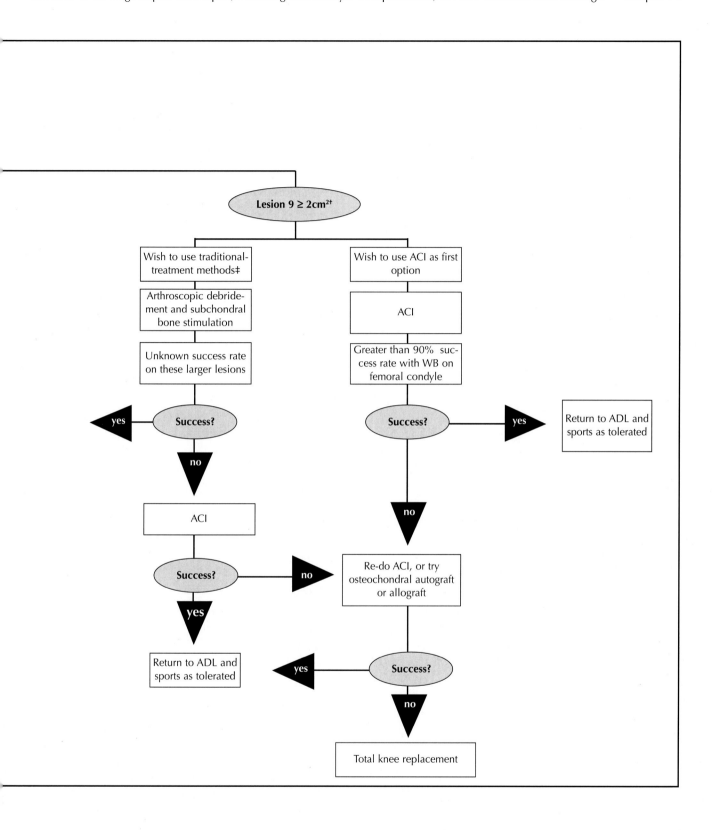

speculate on which lesions would progress, because isolated chondral injuries would be pre-Ahlback stage 0

disease radiographically. The natural course of a single or focal chondral lesion is not known. However, in

experimental studies, incongruity or step-off in joint articulation leads to degeneration of the cartilage and subchondral bone that mimics osteo-arthritis.[11]

Hence, as the natural history of an isolated chondral injury is unknown once it is discovered incidentally at the time of arthroscopy, the surgeon should be cautious prior to engaging in cartilage repair surgery. The surgeon's best judgment correlating the lesion to the presence of symptoms and disability is the best guide for intervention. A knowledge of the available treatments and success rates would allow the surgeon to make a rational treatment choice.[12] The algorithm shown in Figure 1 was developed as a practical guide, after review of the literature, as well as my own experience, in the management of a primary chondral lesion.

Chondral Lesion Site and Size

Most researchers have assumed that unrepaired full-thickness chondral injuries progress to osteoarthritis by secondary friction and overload to the opposing articular pole. However, when the subchondral bone plate is well shouldered, stimulation to that nerve-rich area may not occur, and the patient may remain asymptomatic (Figs. 2 and 3). Similarly, progression may be very slow. Although a weight-bearing site may be a key factor in progression, size may also be important. Of the lesions treated by Brittberg and associates[1] some 3 years after the onset of symptoms, with chondral injuries with an average defect size of 2 to 3 cm², opposing articular damage was not noted. Hence, lesions of this size, although symptomatic, may not progress over a short period of time. However, using an absolute surface area of 2 cm² as a cutoff to progression may not be appropriate, because it is the size of the lesion relative to the surface area of the weightbearing condyle that is important. An example of this would

be a 2-cm² lesion in the small weight-bearing condyle of a 5'1" woman versus a 6'2" man. The implications of the 2-cm² chondral defect would be much more serious in the smaller surface area of the woman's weight-bearing femoral condyle. Other factors that could contribute to a more rapid progression of the chondral injury include malalignment, obesity, family history of osteoarthritis, and impact-loading activities.[13–15]

Pain

Joint pain may have contributions from various component structures of the joint. With cartilage loss and loss of the cushioning function of the articular surface, the subchondral bone layer is exposed to pressure. Pain receptors of the periarterial nerve fibers of this layer are then stimulated. The bone undergoes eventual sclerosis, with secondary vascular stages in the condyle that include increased venous blood flow and subchondral cancellous bone congestion with further arterial nerve stimulation. These changes may account for the sensations of sharp pain and achiness in the joint. Parallel to these reactions, enzymatic metabolites from cartilage breakdown cause a painful synovitis with eventual capsular distention and further discomfort. Treatments that alter any of these mechanisms of pain production may result in symptom relief.[16]

Evaluation of Chondral Injuries

A history of symptoms, which include catching, crepitus, pain, and effusion, is typical of full-thickness chondral injuries. A magnetic resonance imaging (MRI) evaluation that does not demonstrate ligamentous or meniscal injury does not definitively exclude a chondral injury. MRI techniques, although improving steadily, may still under- or overdiagnose chondral injuries, because of their

lack of sensitivity and specificity. The literature reports values of 75% to 93%.[17] Arthroscopy remains the gold standard for evaluation of the articular surface when considering cartilage repair.

Useful screening tools for evaluating patients who may be candidates for cartilage repair techniques, specifically chondrocyte transplantation, include standing anteroposterior (AP) and 45° bent posteroanterior (PA) radiographs, which would demonstrate joint-space narrowing with bipolar disease.[18] The evidence of joint-space narrowing implies global thinning of articular surfaces and osteoarthritis, which is not optimal for patients undergoing cartilage repair procedures. In this situation, realignment osteotomy would be more appropriate. Fibrocartilage repair in the face of osteoarthritis has not been shown to improve the clinical outcome alone[19,20] or in addition to osteotomy.[21,22]

Symptom Management

Jackson[23] noted serendipitous relief of symptoms after diagnostic arthroscopy. Since then, several other authors have noted similar improvement in patient symptoms in the face of mild to severe osteoarthritis of the knee.[24,25] Arthroscopic lavage is thought to be beneficial in that it removes degenerative articular cartilage debris and the mediators of inflammation produced by the synovium of the joint. Hence, although arthroscopy may alleviate such symptoms as rest and night pain in the first year after treatment it does not affect cartilage repair, and patients do not experience a further measurable outcome improvement. When debridement is added, to remove cartilaginous flaps and to contour the condyles, the results are somewhat improved.

A randomized, controlled trial of arthroscopic surgeries versus closed needle joint lavage for patients with osteoarthritis of the knee demonstrated no significant difference between the groups of patients. After 1 year, 44% of patients undergoing arthroscopy reported improvement, as did 58% of subjects undergoing in-office joint lavage. However, this study was small and subgroups, such as those with meniscal tears, could not be adequately assessed.[26]

Similarly, arthroscopic debridement assessed in the osteoarthritic knee offered no improvement for 39% of patients, temporary improvement in 9%, and good or excellent improvement in 52% at an average of 33 months' follow-up. These were self-reported scales and when Hospital for Special Surgery (HSS) scores were employed, it was noted that, although patients claimed improvement, no improvement was noted on an outcome measurement scale.[27] Sprague[28] noted similar results.

A recent study performed by Hubbard,[29] which prospectively randomized similar disease states of unipolar Outerbridge grade III or IV medial femoral condyle injuries to either arthroscopic debridement or lavage only, noted a significant improvement in those patients treated by debridement. Over half the patients were free of pain 5 years after treatment when debridement was employed. Using a Lysholm knee score evaluation, there was continued measurable improvement at 4.5 years in the debridement group and negligible change in the lavage group.[29] This study did not suffer from a mixed population of disease states. However, the study did lack follow-up arthroscopies to evaluate whether the chondral injuries had progressed in size despite continued symptom relief. Unfortunately, defect sizes and

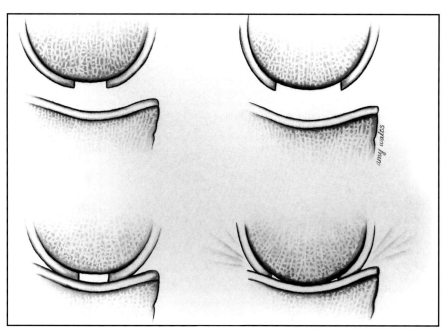

Fig. 2 Schematic representation of loading focal femoral defects. Small lesions (left) contain the defect and protect the tibial surface. Wider lesions (right) allow abrasion of the tibial articular surface resulting in mechanical symptoms and early cartilage degeneration. (Reproduced with permission from Minas T, Nehrer S: Current concepts in treatment of articular cartilage defects. *Orthopedics* 1997;20:525–538.)

follow-up weightbearing radiographs were not reported to assess whether there was progression to osteoarthritis.

When performing arthroscopic debridement in the face of osteoarthritis, factors associated with a better outcome include normal limb alignment, history of mechanical symptoms, minimal radiographic degeneration, and a short duration of symptoms. Variables associated with a poor outcome include varus or valgus malalignment, loading symptoms, severe radiographic degeneration, previous surgeries, and chronic symptoms.[30]

In summary, it would appear that in the nonarthritic knee, focal chondral injuries, when treated by debridement, maintain measurable pain relief in over 50% of patients for up to 5 years. Lavage may relieve symptoms for up to 1 year. Arthroscopy in the face of osteoarthritis, although not

demonstrating measurable outcome improvement, offers symptomatic relief for up to 3 years in approximately 60% of patients.[27,28]

Cell-Based Therapies Aimed at Cartilage Repair
Marrow Stimulation Techniques
Delivery of pluripotential marrow stem cells to the articular surface defect has been a technique used to enhance cartilage repair. These techniques originated during open surgery,[31,32] but with the advent of arthroscopy, they have become increasingly popular, and they have less morbidity than open techniques. However, despite their widespread use, well-controlled studies to evaluate outcomes are lacking. Tippett,[33] when combining arthroscopic drilling with unloading osteotomy, found that results were minimally improved over osteotomy alone, despite an

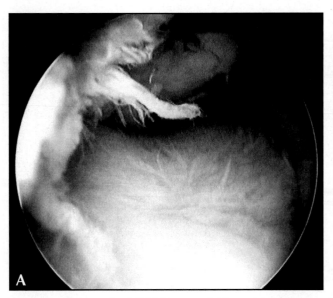 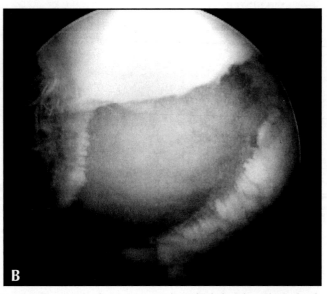

Fig. 3 A, Large, traumatic, full-thickness medial femoral condyle injury (2.5-cm wide × 1.5-cm long). Note grade II tibial chondromalacia developing early after the traumatic full-thickness femoral lesion has started to produce mechanical symptoms. **B,** The femoral lesion is effectively unshouldered due to its width; exposed bone is abrading the opposing tibial articular surface. (Reproduced with permission from Minas T, Nehrer S: Current concepts in treatment of articular cartilage defects. *Orthopedics* 1997;20:525–538.)

increase in the damaged joint space, shown radiographically, and the appearance of second-look repair tissue noted at the sites of drilling.

The results of arthroscopically performed abrasion arthroplasty have been variable. Friedman and associates[34] noted that the results were best in patients younger than 40 years of age. Overall, 60% of patients who underwent abrasion arthroplasty showed improvement. The knee remained unchanged in 44%, and was made worse in 6% (all with grade IV articular changes). In those patients younger than 40 years of age, there was a trend towards improvement in patients treated with abrasion versus debridement alone.

Bert and Maschka[19] reported on the results of arthroscopic abrasion arthroplasty versus arthroscopic debridement alone. They noted that the results were slightly better for those patients treated by arthroscopic debridement alone (in the presence of radiographic osteoarthritis).

Similarly, Akizuki and associates,[22] who prospectively evaluated the effect of abrasion arthroplasty on cartilage repair in osteoarthritic knees with eburnation when osteotomy was combined with abrasion versus osteotomy alone, noted no clinical improvement between groups. However, arthroscopic second looks at both treatment groups demonstrated that there was a significant repair of defect tissue in the group treated by abrasion arthroplasty. This was also noted by biopsy study. However, despite the presence of repair tissue, clinical results did not improve.[22] These results suggest that the biomechanical properties of the repair tissue were not sufficient to provide symptom improvement by protecting the pain-sensitive subchondral bone from mechanical stimulation.

Hence, it appears that although abrasion is not useful as an adjunctive procedure to the osteoarthritic knee to improve clinical outcome, it may have a role in the treatment of unipolar

focal chondral defects in the non-arthritic knee in patients younger than 40 years of age.

Steadman and associates[35] have popularized marrow stimulation by microfracture technique. An arthroscopic awl is used to make multiple holes or "microfractures" in the subchondral bone plate, usually 3 to 4 mm apart, but not so close as to break into one another, which would damage the subchondral bone plate between them. This microfracture is done after the defect is debrided back to healthy, intact margins and the subchondral bone plate is scraped. A tourniquet is then let down and a "super clot" is produced with the desired marrow stem cells. A protected weightbearing protocol and continuous passive motion (CPM) are used postoperatively. In young active patients, this technique provided pain relief at 3 to 5 years in 75% of patients, but 20% remained unchanged and 5% worsened. Parameters of activities of daily living and work showed improvement in 67% of patients, and no changes in 20%; the other 13% were made worse. Patients involved in strenuous sports and labor had an improvement rate of 65%.[35]

Autologous Tissue Derived Cell Therapies

Cell-based therapies derived from autologous tissue transplants include perichondrium and periosteum with or without cultured articular chondrocytes. Numerous experimental animal studies have demonstrated the ability of these tissues to produce a hyaline cartilage repair response.[36-40]

The mechanical environment of these tissues during repair may also affect the quality of the repair tissue. This has been demonstrated in the case of continuous passive motion to stimulate neochondrogenesis in the rabbit.[38] Continuous passive motion has also been shown to provide benefit in the clinical situation with regard to the quantity of repair tissue.[41]

Perichondrium

In 1990, Homminga and associates[42] reported on the use of autologous perichondrium derived from the rib in the treatment of full-thickness chondral defects in the knee. Perichondrium was noted to provide a significant clinical improvement, with an average defect size of 2 to 3 cm². An increase in HSS score from preoperative 73 to postoperative 90 at 1 and 2 years after transplantation was noted. Arthroscopic second-look assessment and biopsies in a few patients demonstrated a hyaline repair tissue. However, it was noted that calcific radiodensity occurred by 2 years in the grafts of 21 of 30 patients implanted. The significance of these findings was not known at the time of publication.

In my own personal clinical series, I have found that calcific radiodensity,

when present, resulted in failure of the transplant and clinical result by enchondral ossification within the graft substance to the surface of the repair site, eventually resulting in graft failure and recurrence of symptoms.[43] This eventual failure occurred in 7 out of 10 patients transplanted. Although clinical results were excellent in the first 2 to 3 years, by 5 years failure, by enchondral ossification or delamination, occurred.

Periosteum

The use of periosteum alone for weightbearing femoral condyles in the management of osteochondritis dissecans showed early promise;[44] however, the long-term results have been disappointing (P Angermann, MD, personal communication, 1997). A recent survey of 15 of 23 patients (age 14 to 25 years) demonstrated graft failure in 6 patients, with recurrence of symptoms. The other 9 patients remained clinically satisfactory.[45]

The early results of periosteum transplantation for the treatment of the patella appeared to be promising;[46] however, the long-term results similarly demonstrated near uniform failure (G Sandelin, MD, personal communication, 1997).

Autologous Chondrocyte Transplantation (ACT)

Swedish Series The use of in vitro cultured autologous chondrocytes for reimplantation under a periosteal patch has been reported.[1] Unipolar lesions in nonarthritic knees are treated by this technique. This pilot study demonstrated that weightbearing femoral condyles did best, with 14 of 16 patients having good and excellent results; 11 of 15 biopsies demonstrated hyaline cartilage. When the patella was treated, only 2 of 7 patients had good and excellent results, and only 1 of 7

transplants demonstrated hyaline repair tissue.

The 2- to 9-year follow-up of the first 100 patients treated in Sweden using cultured articular chondrocytes demonstrated that clinical improvement occurred in 92% of patients treated for isolated weightbearing femoral condyle lesions, in 89% of those treated for osteochondritis dissecans lesions, and in 75% when the weightbearing condyle was treated along with anterior cruciate ligament reconstruction. Overall 62% of chondral lesions treated on the patella did well, and over 60% of multifocal lesions treated had demonstrated improvement.[47]

United States Series, 1998 After approval by the human ethics committees of the hospitals I use, a prospective outcome series was undertaken in March 1995 to evaluate the efficacy of the use of autologous cultured articular chondrocytes. Demographic data; prior surgical histories; defect location, site, and size; as well as baseline quality-of-life health utility instrument data were collected by a research assistant, independent of the surgeon. These data were independently analyzed after collection at time-points of 6, 12, 18, and 24 months, and at yearly intervals thereafter (AACT-Abt Associates Clinical Trials, Cambridge, MA).

Quality-of-life health-care instruments included SF-36 (short form 36 questionnaire), WOMAC scores (Western Ontario MacMaster osteoarthritis scale), KSS (Knee Society Scores), Modified Cincinnati Knee Score, and a patient satisfaction survey. In addition to clinical outcomes, adverse events were reported. An optional 2-year MRI scan, video arthroscopy with quantitative mechanical indentation probing, and biopsy of the repair site and host ref-

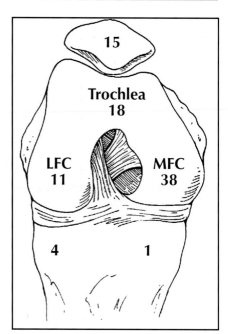

Fig. 4 Schematic representation of defect locations treated by autologous chondrocyte transplantation (ACT) in the first 44 patients (87 lesions) with greater than 6 months' follow-up. LFC = Lateral femoral condyle. MFC = Medial femoral condyle.

erence articular surfaces is underway. The biopsy repair tissue and reference tissues were then stained for histochemical and immunohistochemical markers for cartilage repair.

Demographics

To date, 70 patients (23 women and 47 men) have been treated by ACT, and 44 have passed 6-month follow-up data collection. The ages were 14 to 55 years old at the time of surgery, with an average age of 35.8 years. The average size of the defect treated was 5.5 cm² (range 1.5 to 21 cm²), with an average of 2 defects per knee. Eighty-seven percent of patients had prior surgery in the 5 years preceding ACT. Of these, 55.3% had prior cartilage repair surgery including abrasion, drilling, microfracture, or perichondrial graft transplantation that had failed. On average, the patients had

2.5 prior surgeries. This is compatible with my tertiary referral practice. FDA labeling and approval of this technique occurred on August 22, 1997 for focal defects of the femur. This study was underway.

Indications

Symptomatically disabled patients with focal chondral lesions of a traumatic or degenerative nature were treated. Based on an earlier report, isolated unipolar femoral articular lesions were felt to be ideal lesions for treatment.[1] However, lesions of the patella, trochlea, tibia, multifocal lesions, and even bipolar or "kissing" lesions were treated when the radiographic joint space was maintained and the lesions were focal in nature.

The patients were then broadly categorized into 3 treatment categories, so that outcomes could be correlated to the stage of disease at the time of treatment. Further subcategories would eventually be developed as the sample sizes for each subcategory became numerous enough to develop meaningful statistical and clinical interpretations.

The lesions for which complete data were collected are represented schematically in Figure 4. Forty-four patients with 87 chondral graftings by ACT had outcome data collected with greater than 6 months' follow-up (represented). Thirty-three were greater than 1 year and 7 at 2 years (outcome data presented in Tables 1 through 4).

Categories

A previously described classification[43] consisted of simple, complex, and salvage categories, listed as follows:

Simple This category includes those with isolated unipolar chondral lesions localized to the weightbearing femoral condyles, healthy joint, and surrounding articular chondromala-

cia < Outerbridge I–II.

Complex This category includes those patients with unipolar single or multifocal lesions, patella, trochlea, or tibia. These cases may require realignment osteotomy for tibiofemoral or patellofemoral malalignment, ligamentous reconstruction for concomitant instability, or staged bone reconstitution with bone grafting prior to articular resurfacing (in cases of deep osteochondritis dissecans lesions or bone cysts). The joint is otherwise without advanced chondromalacia as in the simple category.

Salvage This category of patients includes those with radiographic and arthroscopically defined cases of osteoarthritis (OA) at the earliest stage of disease. Radiographic criteria of OA (Altman) are defined by osteophyte formation, as well as Ahlback stage of disease: 0, osteophytes; stage I < 50% radiographic joint space narrowing on standing AP radiographs. It also includes arthroscopically determined bipolar or "kissing" lesions, or evidence of generalized Outerbridge chondromalacia ≥ grade II, even with unipolar lesions (unusual).

Presumably the lesions treated in the combined categories of simple and complex do not suffer from an inherent degenerative condition and may have different outcomes and survivorship outcomes. Long-term data, however, will be required to validate this hypothesis.

Although these categories include a broad variety of conditions treated (especially the complex category), they are useful with smaller sample sizes in statistical analyses. The first 2 groups are relatively homogeneous, in that the articular surfaces are healthy and do not have generalized degeneration (Outerbridge chondromalacia < grade II). The salvage category of patients, however, has radiographically defined osteoarthritis

Table 1
SF36

	Preop	12 Months	24 months
Physical Health			
Overall	33	41, $p = 0.014$	42, $p = 0.019$
Bodily pain	41	57, $p = 0.02$	67, $p = 0.04$
Role physical	22	53, $p = 0.01$	50, $p = 0.03$
Physical function index	40	58, $p = 0.04$	57, $p = 0.24$
Mental Health			
Overall	49	532, NS	59, NS
Vitality	52	66, $p = 0.03$	74, NS
Social functioning	57	81, $p < 0.001$	75, NS
General health	75	81, NS	89, NS
Role emotional	62	66, NS	81, NS
Mental health	67	74, NS	89, NS

n = 26 patients @ 12 months
n = 7 patients @ 24 months
paired, 2-tailed + t-test, sig $p < 0.05$

Table 2
WOMAC Scores

	Preop	12 Months	24 Months
Overall	35	23, $p = 0.014$	25, NS
Physical function	24	16, $p = 0.02$	16, NS
Pain	9	6, $p = 0.002$	6, NS
Stiffness	3	3, NS	3, NS

n = 30 patients @ 12 months
n = 8 patients @ 24 months
paired, 2-tailed +t-test, sig $p < 0.05$

(Altman) or arthroscopically proven bipolar "kissing" lesions (OA).

Results

In general, as a group, the simple and complex category patients recovered more rapidly than the salvage category of patients and had higher outcome scores. But the scores and satisfaction of the salvage category patients remain satisfactory. Failures were defined as arthroscopically demonstrated graft delamination or degeneration with a poor clinical outcome. There were 5 treatment failures in the first 70 patients treated.

The quality-of-life instruments used demonstrated significant improvements clinically and in patient well-being (Tables 1 through 4). Quality-of-life improvements, as measured by the SF-36 questionnaire, demonstrated clinically and statistically significant improvements (2-tailed paired t-test, $p < 0.05$) in physical health-overall score and each of its component scores (bodily pain, role physical, physical function index) by 12 months, which were sustained at 2 years. All patient categories (simple, complex, and salvage) were included together in the analyses.

The overall mental health component summary similarly demonstrated a trend towards improvement by 1 year, and this was sustained at 2 years. However, the subgroups of emotional well-being, consisting of vitality ($p = $ 0.03) and social functioning ($p = $ 0.001), were significantly improved by 1 year and were maintained by 2 years.

Joint-specific evaluations included the WOMAC, Knee Society (KSS), and Cincinnati scores. These evaluative tools were chosen because they were complementary, in that they assessed outcome from differing points of view. The WOMAC score assessed the impact of the joint on physical parameters usually reserved for the arthritic patient with significant impairment. KSS was developed to assess the impact of arthroplasty in the management of the arthritic knee. The Cincinnati knee score was developed to evaluate the impact of intervention in the high-level functioning athlete with instability and was modified to assess the stable knee of a high-level functioning patient.

All scales demonstrated significant improvement in the first year after surgery, with maintenance or further improvement during the second. The simple and complex categories of patients in general achieved higher scores than the salvage group, and they recovered more quickly. However the failures were not taken out of the analyses, and the 4 failures that occurred in the complex group undervalued the otherwise excellent results in this group (Table 3).

MRI, arthroscopic assessment, and biopsy specimens for histologic evaluation are now underway but are preliminary. An example is noted in Figure 5. This 27-year-old man had 4 surgeries prior to ACT repair of large chondral defects to the articular surfaces of the lateral femoral condyle, trochlea, and patella (salvage category), and is presently doing well 2 years after ACT.

Complications

In the first 70 patients there were 26 complications (37%) that required

Table 3
Knee Society Scores

		Knee Score	
	Preop	12 Months	24 Months
All patients	51	68, $p < 0.001$	70, $p = 0.005$
Simple and complex	55	69, $p = 0.008$	81, $p = 0.019$
Salvage	41	65, $p = 0.015$	52, $p = 0.003$
		Function Score	
	Preop	12 Months	24 Months
All patients	63	73 $p = 0.03$	73, NS
Simple and complex	64	73, NS (0.09)	85, NS
Salvage	62	72, NS	53, NS

n = 33 @ 12 months (23 simple and complex, 10 salvage)
n = 8 @ 24 months (5 simple and complex, 3 salvage)
paired, 2-tailed + t-test, sig $p < 0.05$

surgical intervention. These occurred in the first 8 months postoperatively. Early problems included stiffness from adhesions after femoral periosteum was used for large or multiple lesions, and these required arthroscopic lysis of adhesions, followed by manipulation. Later interventions were for catching symptoms, with pain and effusion, which developed as a result of periosteal hypertrophy. These tended to occur between 3 and 7 months postoperatively. Arthroscopic resection of prolific tissue to the level of the surrounding articular surfaces resulted in resolution of symptoms. One patient, who had also undergone osteotomy, developed an acute deep venous thrombosis day 1 postoperatively. After heparinization, a hematoma developed, which required surgical evacuation. There were no deep infections.

Failures

There were 5 failures (7%) in the first 70 patients. Three patients sustained falls early during their recovery, with traumatic partial or complete graft delamination. They were managed successfully by repeat ACT. Two patients developed adhesions to a graft in a multiply transplanted knee (1 complex and 1 salvage patient). A partial delamination resulted in 1 patient who accepted his lessened outcome after partial graft excision arthroscopically. The other patient underwent removal of graft with eventual carbon-fiber transplant with cells (in Gothenberg, Sweden) with an excellent result.

Although a correlative study to compare MRI images, arthroscopic assessment, and histology from biopsy is early, the first specimens appear promising, with correlative high clinical scores 2 years after ACT (Fig. 3).

Rehabilitation to Enhance Tissue Repair for Cell-Based Therapies

The concept of a time course of healing for cell-based therapies is useful in the postoperative management and in understanding tissue repair.[12] Animal models have demonstrated cell proliferation and fill (proliferative phase), followed by matrix macromolecular production (transitional phase) and an ongoing remodeling of the matrix framework over time (remodeling phase).[48] If the mechanical environment is protective and stimulatory to the repair process, an ongoing remodeling of the tissue will occur and the tissue will mature (stage of maturation). If the tissue undergoes mechanical overload early in the remodeling process it may degenerate (stage of degradation). Hence, early active and passive motion (including continuous passive motion) and a protected and progressive weightbearing program during the proliferative and transitional stages (0 to 12 weeks) followed by a functional use of the limb without impact loading are important in the first year after cartilage repair during matrix remodeling. This regimen would allow the optimal environment for the repair tissue to mature (Table 5).

This process of repair theoretically is similar for all cell-based cartilage repair techniques, differing only in the population and mix of cell lines and their containment at the repair site, ie, marrow stimulation techniques may include bone, cartilage, and fibrous and hematopoetic cell lines and, because they do not have a containing membrane, there may be an incomplete defect fill or a mixed tissue response. Autologous tissue implants have a contained defect (depending on the technique used) and a more likely directed and committed cell line response.

Assessing the predisposing factors for cartilage injuries is also critical to success. Tibiofemoral or patellofemoral malalignment as well as ligamentous instability, if present, must be addressed prior to, or at the time of the cartilage repair procedure.

Failure to recognize instability or malalignment may result in compressive or shear force overload to immature tissue before mechanical integration of the repair tissue, with resultant degradation or delamination and repair tissue failure.

Table 4
Modified Cincinnati Knee Score

	Clinician Evaluation				Patient Evaluation			
	Baseline	12	24	p value	Baseline	12	24	p value
Overall								
12 mos n = 26	3.38	4.96	–	< 0.001	3.77	5.31	–	0.004
24 mos n = 8	3.00	5.25	6.0	0.031 (baseline) 0.170 (1-2 yr)	3.13	5.75	5.25	0.185 0.487
Simple and Complex								
12 mos n = 19	3.53	5.32	–	0.002	3.84	5.68	–	0.006
24 mos n = 5	2.67	5.33	7.33	0.037 (baseline) 0.179 (-2 yr)	3.40	7.00	6.80	0.190 0.847
Salvage								
12 mos n = 16	3.44	5.06	–	0.005	3.88	5.44	–	0.007
24 mos n = 3	2.67	5.33	7.33	0.184 (baseline) 0.184 (1-2 yr	4.00	6.33	7.33	0.289 (baseline) < .000 (1-2 yr)

Table 5
Rehabilitation Guidelines to Enhance Tissue Repair for Cell-Based Therapies

Time	0-3 Months	3-6 Months	> 6 Months
Stage	Proliferation	Remodeling (affected by extrinsic factors)	Maturation (histologic maturation occurs 2-3 yr) or degeneration
Treatment	Correct ligamentous stability and patello-femoral and tibiofemoral alignment	Assess pain, catching, and edema	Continued follow-up
Activities	Progression to partial WB CPM: Full ROM on WB condyles, 0° - 40° ROM for trochlea/patella, 6-8 h/d x 8 wk postop	Progression to full WB Limited activity to protect repair tissue	Patients with lesions < 2 cm: Full activities after 9-12 months depending on symptoms: Patients with lesions ≥ 2 cm:Full activities after 12 months depending on symptoms

CPM, continuous passive motion
ROM, range of motion
WB, weightbearing

Osteochondral Transplantation
Multiple Osteochondral Autograft Transplantation

The first clinical autogenic osteochondral transplantation, reported in 1985, used an osteochondral block taken from the nonweightbearing position of the joint to repair osteochondritis dissecans.[49] This was followed in 1993 by a report of arthroscopically placed multiple osteochondral transplants to correct a chondral defect associated with an anterior cruciate ligament (ACL) disruption.[50] Since then, Bobic[2] and Hangody and associates[3] have also reported on the use of autogenic cylindrical osteochondral bone plugs to treat full-thickness chondral defects. Bobic reported on the treatment of chondral defects when accompanied by ACL tears, and 10 of 12 cases had good and excellent results (at 2-year follow-up). The notchplasty site was used for the osteochondral bone plugs during the ACL reconstruction. Lesions ranged from 10 to 22 mm in diameters. Donor site morbidity was not reported.[2]

Hangody and associates[51] reported on the use of this technique from 1992 to January 1996, in 168 patients from Budapest, Hungary, and Portsmouth, New Hampshire. The average age was 32.4 years, an average of 8 grafts were used (1-18), and the longest patient follow-up was 5 years. The average modified HSS score was 82.5 (65 to 100), and a donor site morbidity score (Bandi score for patellar complaints) demonstrated problems in 5 cases. No baseline data were provided in a prospective fashion to determine improvements, nor was information given on the average size of defect treated.[51]

Important considerations noted for a successful result included pro-

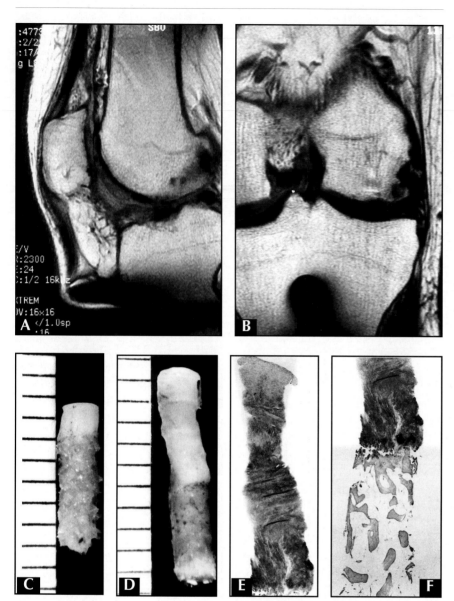

Fig. 5 A, Magnetic resonance image (MRI; sagittal image) of the knee of a patient treated by autologous chondrocyte transplantation (ACT) for lesions of the patella, trochlea, and weight-bearing lateral femoral condyle (salvage category). Note especially, the abundant repair thickness of the trochlea, but also the fill of the patella, and the lateral femoral condyle. **B,** MRI (coronal view) of the same patient with complete fill of the lateral femoral condyle. Note the edema in the subchondral plate and the void appearance in the underlying bone from a prior failed drilling procedure. **C,** Two-year biopsy of the host reference cartilage. **D,** The adjacent trochlea ACT repair site. The repair tissue thickness is 5 mm and the host, 1.5 mm. There is good integration to the underlying bone and a smooth firm surface. **E,** Safranin O histochemical staining for proteoglycans, demonstrating the superficial portion of the biopsy in *D*. **F,** The deep portion of the graft integrated to the underlying bone. Note the somewhat fibrillar nature of the deep portion integrating to the subchondral bone plate, the homogeneous staining for proteoglycans, and the fibrous nature of the surface (presumably the periosteal remnant).

tected weightbearing for 8 weeks postoperatively, to allow consolidation without collapse of the condyle.

In a canine model used to evaluate osteochondral autografts, one third of the weightbearing condyles collapsed.

It was suggested that the condylar collapse was secondary to the inability of the canine to be nonweightbearing during bony union.[3]

This technique appears promising for small chondral injuries when accompanied by ACL reconstruction, or to treat isolated defects of relatively small proportion so that donor site morbidity would not be an issue. Technical considerations for reconstituting the chondral curvature in both the sagittal and coronal planes with multiple osteochondral bone plugs are of paramount importance. Protected rehabilitation, to prevent collapse of the condyle in the postoperative period, is also mandatory.[51]

Osteochondral Allograft Transplantation (Fresh/Cryopreserved)

When damage to cartilage and bone involvement are present, the use of fresh osteochondral allografts for posttraumatic defects in the knee has been successful.[52–56] Unloading osteotomies are paramount to the success of these osteoarticular allografts, as is chondrocyte viability, gained by using fresh cadaveric allografts.

A success rate of 75% at 5 years, 64% at 10 years, and 63% at 14 years was noted. The failure rate was higher for bipolar grafts than for unipolar grafts, and for those patients older than 60 years of age. Outcome was not dependent on the sex of the patient or the compartment grafted. Unloading osteotomy with fresh cadaveric allografts and meticulous inlay were critical to the success of osteochondral defect repair.[57]

Meniscal Allograft Transplantation

Meniscal allograft transplantation is a viable treatment alternative for patients who have symptomatic compartments without advanced degenerative change or malalignment. Factors important to success include normal tibiofemoral alignment, chondromalacia no greater than Outerbridge grade II, a well-matched tibial plateau radiographically for meniscus sizing, technical placement of interior and posterior horn origins, and revascularization of the periphery.

Clinical outcomes of 23 patients at 2 to 5 years after treatment were assessed in the Netherlands. Ten patients had a good result and 10 had a fair result. Three of the patients had poor results when the allograft became detached from the capsule and was removed. Joint line discomfort and effusion or discomfort from nonabsorbable sutures developed in 5 patients.[58] Poor results were associated with malalignment, instability, or grade IV advanced chondromalacia. In Noyes' series,[59] a 58% failure rate may have been secondary to a high level of gamma irradiation (2.5 Mrads).

ACL Reconstruction with Focal Chondral Damage

Stabilization of the ACL-deficient knee in itself, when arthroscopically documented Outerbridge grade III/IV chondral lesions are present, has been noted to provide clinical benefit. When malalignment was not present, Noyes noted that significant improvements, 37 months after ACL allograft reconstruction, were found in pain, giving way, and function. Fifty-five percent had returned to light athletics (avoiding impact sports) and were asymptomatic.[59]

Conclusion

Treatment rationale for the treatment of cartilage damage in young patients depends on a thorough understanding of the predisposing factors for the chondrosis and the stage of disease. Arthroscopic lavage and debridement provide symptom relief, which may

last as long as 5 years in patients with unipolar damage and low-demand activities. However, debridement does not promote cartilage repair, and disease progression is likely. For the 50% of patients who do not experience relief with arthroscopic debridement and who desire high-level activities, cartilage repair by alternative arthroscopic or open techniques may be necessary. Arthroscopic marrow stimulation techniques must be followed by a suitable rehabilitation program, which will allow for a time course of healing for the cartilage repair tissue. When the lesions are relatively small (< 2 cm^2), these techniques can allow a return to sports in up to 65% of patients and improvement for activities of daily living in 75% of patients.

Multiple osteochondral autografts may be used when lesions are small and combined with an ACL reconstruction. This technique, however, violates subchondral bone and affects the bone-cartilage functional unit. Its theoretic advantage is rapid recovery after bone union, as the cartilaginous cap is mechanically mature and for small lesions donor site morbidity should not be an issue. Early results have been impressive; however, issues of donor site morbidity, maximal treatment size, and resulting joint incongruity are still of concern.

Transplantation of autologous cultured chondrocytes allows for resurfacing of larger defect areas with reproducibly excellent results in over 90% of patients when weightbearing femoral condyles are treated. Autologous chondrocyte transplantation (ACT) involves an open technique with the inherent disadvantages of adhesions and a more prolonged recovery. The symptomatic occurrence of graft margin overgrowth or periosteal hypertrophy requires surgical intervention for graft "chondroplasty" to allow the graft to mature

uneventfully (15% to 20%). The occurrence of adhesions in multiply transplanted knees and of periosteal hypertrophy accounts for my high complication rate (37%), defined as the need for postoperative intervention. Graft outcome was protected by these interventions in that normal repair proceeded thereafter and patient outcomes have been improved. Quality-of-life instruments used prospectively to evaluate patient outcomes undergoing ACT have demonstrated significant improvements, up to 2.5 years in the United States and 10 years in Sweden.

Allogeneic, fresh osteochondral allografts combined with unloading osteotomies have proven successful in treating injuries to both bone and articular cartilage and are especially useful for large posttraumatic deformities. Allogeneic transplantation of cryopreserved, nonirradiated meniscus is indicated in the symptomatic well-aligned knee with no greater than grade II chondromalacia. Allogeneic ACL reconstruction in the face of early arthritic damage may also provide clinical benefit in the short term.

When bipolar damage is present, standard osteotomy techniques around the knee are used, accompanied by arthroscopic debridement or supplemented with ACL reconstruction if required. These techniques may return patients to high levels of subjective satisfaction and a high level of function.[60]

The techniques of cartilage repair have varying degrees of success for differing situations of lesion size, patient age, and activity level. This challenges the surgeon to match the procedure used to patient expectations. An algorithmic approach has been offered, based on the available literature results and my experience, in order to assist in procedure selection for each situation. In order to validate such a guideline, however, prospective randomized outcome data are required to determine success and failure rates for these procedures, including survivorship data, costs, and quality-of-life improvements. In the absence of randomization, well-planned prospective outcome studies capturing the parameters of interest are still useful in comparing standardized outcome instruments for like parameters, and will aid in determining procedural efficacy and procedural cost-effectiveness. These are our tasks for the future.

References

1. Brittberg M, Lindahl A, Nilsson A, Ohlsson C, Isaksson O, Peterson L: Treatment of deep cartilage defects in the knee with autologous chondrocyte transplantation. *N Engl J Med* 1994;331:889–895.

2. Bobic V: Arthroscopic osteochondral autograft transplantation in anterior cruciate ligament reconstruction: A preliminary clinical study. *Knee Surg Sports Traumatol Arthrosc* 1996;3: 262–264.

3. Hangody L, Kish G, Karpati Z, et al: Autologous osteochondral graft technique for replacing knee cartilage defects in dogs. *Orthopedics* 1997;5:175–181.

4. Jackson DW, Simon TM: Chondroctye transplantation. *Arthroscopy* 1996;12:732–738.

5. Messner K, Gillquist J: Cartilage repair: A critical review. *Acta Orthop Scand* 1996;67:523–529.

6. Brittberg M, Lindahl A, Homminga G, Nilsson A, Isaksson O, Peterson L: A critical analysis of cartilage repair. *Acta Orthop Scand* 1997;68: 186–191.

7. Noyes FR, Bassett RW, Grood ES, Butler DL: Arthroscopy in acute traumatic hemarthrosis of the knee: Incidence of anterior cruciate tears and other injuries. *J Bone Joint Surg* 1980;62A: 687–695.

8. Curl WW, Krome J, Gordon ES, Rushing J, Smith BP, Poehling GG: Cartilage injuries: A review of 31,516 knee arthroscopies. *Arthroscopy* 1997;13:456–460.

9. Messner K, Maletius W: The long-term prognosis for severe damage to weight-bearing cartilage in the knee: A 14-year clinical and radiographic follow-up in 28 young athletes. *Acta Orthop Scand* 1996;67:165–168.

10. Sahlström A, Johnell O, Redlund-Johnell I: The natural course of arthrosis of the knee. *Clin Orthop* 1997;340:152–157.

11. Lefkoe TP, Trafton PG, Dennehy DT, Ehrlich MG, Akelman E: A new model of articular step-off for the study of post-traumatic arthritis. *Trans Orthop Res Soc* 1992;17:207.

12. Minas T: Treatment of chondral defects in the knee: *Orthop Spe Ed* Summer/Fall, 69–74, 1997.

13. Radin EL, Ehrlich MG, Chernack R, Abernethy P, Paul IL, Rose RM: Effect of repetitive impulsive loading on the knee joints of rabbits. *Clin Orthop* 1978;131:288–293.

14. Radin EL, Martin RB, Burr DB, Caterson B, Boyd RD, Goodwin C: Effects of mechanical loading on the tissues of the rabbit knee. *J Orthop Res* 1984;2:221–234.

15. Radin EL, Schaffler M, Gibson G, Tashman S: Osteoarthrosis as a result of repetitive trauma, in Kuettner KE, Goldberg VM (eds): *Osteoarthritic Disorders*. Rosemont, IL, American Academy of Orthopaedic Surgeons, 1995, pp 197–203.

16. Huber J, Gasser B, Perren SM, Bandl W: Changes in retropatellar pressure values in relation to the position of the tibial tuberosity. *Knee* 1994;1(suppl 1):S19–S43.

17. Linklater JM, Potter HG: Imaging of chondral defects. *Op Tech Orthop* 1997;7:279–288.

18. Rosenberg TD, Paulos LE, Parker RD, Coward DB, Scott SM: The forty-five-degree posteroanterior flexion weight-bearing radiograph of the knee. *J Bone Joint Surg* 1988;70A:1479–1483.

19. Bert JM, Maschka K: The arthroscopic treatment of unicompartmental gonarthrosis: A five-year follow-up study of abrasion arthroplasty plus arthroscopic debridement and arthroscopic debridement alone. *Arthroscopy* 1989;5:25–32.

20. Johnson LL: Arthroscopic abrasion arthroplasty, in McGinty JB, Caspari RB, Jackson RW, Poehling GG (eds): *Operative Arthroscopy*. New York, NY, Raven Press, 1991, pp 341–360.

21. Rand JA, Ritts GD: Abrasion arthroplasty as a salvage for failed upper tibial osteotomy. *J Arthroplasty* 1989;4:S45–S48.

22. Akizuki S, Yasukawa Y, Takizawa T: Does arthroscopic abrasion arthroplasty promote cartilage regeneration in osteoarthritic knees with eburnation? A prospective study of high tibial osteotomy with abrasion arthroplasty versus high tibial osteotomy alone. *Arthroscopy* 1997;13: 9–17.

23. Jackson RW: Arthroscopic treatment of degenerative arthritis, in McGinty JB, Caspari RB, Jackson RW, Poehling GG (eds): *Operative Arthroscopy*. New York, NY, Raven Press, 1991, pp 319–323.

24. Livesley PJ, Doherty M, Needoff M, Moulton A: Arthroscopic lavage of osteoarthritic knees. *J Bone Joint Surg* 1991;73B:922–926.

25. Gibson JN, White MD, Chapman VM, Strachan RK: Arthroscopic lavage and debridement for osteoarthritis of the knee. *J Bone Joint Surg* 1992;74B:534–537.

26. Chang RW, Falconer J, Stulberg SD, Arnold WJ, Manheim LM, Dyer AR: A randomized, controlled trial of arthroscopic surgery versus closed-needle joint lavage for patients with osteoarthritis of the knee. *Arthritis Rheum* 1993; 36:289–296.

27. Baumgaertner MR, Cannon WD Jr, Vittori JM, Schmidt ES, Maurer RC: Arthroscopic debridement of the arthritic knee. *Clin Orthop* 1990; 253:197–202.

28. Sprague NF III: Arthroscopic debridement for degenerative knee joint disease. *Clin Orthop* 1981;160:118–123.

29. Hubbard MJ: Articular debridement versus washout for degeneration of the medial femoral condyle: A five-year study. *J Bone Joint Surg* 1996;78B:217–219.

30. Novak PJ, Bach BR Jr: Selection criteria for knee arthroscopy in the osteoarthritic patient. *Orthop Rev* 1993;22:798–804.

31. Pridie KH: Abstract: A method of resurfacing osteoarthritic knee joints. *J Bone Joint Surg* 1959;41B:618–619.

32. Ficat RP, Ficat C, Gedeon P, Toussaint JB: Spongialization: A new treatment for diseased patellae. *Clin Orthop* 1979;144:74–83.

33. Tippett JW: Articular cartilage drilling and osteotomy in osteoarthritis of the knee, in McGinty JB, Caspari RB, Jackson RW, Poehling GG (eds): *Operative Arthroscopy*. New York, NY, Raven Press, 1991, pp 325–339.

34. Friedman MJ, Berasi CC, Fox JM, Del Pizzo W, Snyder SJ, Ferkel RD: Preliminary results with abrasion arthroplasty in the osteoarthritic knee. *Clin Orthop* 1984;182:200–205.

35. Steadman JR, Rodkey WG, Singleton SB, Briggs KK: Microfracture technique for full-thickness chondral defects: Technique and clinical results. *Op Tech Orthop* 1997;7:300–304.

36. Amiel D, Coutts RD, Harwood FL, Ishizue KK, Kliener JB: The chondrogenesis of rib perichondral grafts for repair of full thickness articular cartilage defects in a rabbit model: A one year postoperative assessment. *Connect Tissue Res* 1988;18:27–39.

37. Homminga GN, van der Linden TJ, Terwindt-Rouwenhorst EA, Drukker J: Repair of articular defects by perichondral grafts: Experiments in the rabbit. *Acta Orthop Scand* 1989;60:326–329.

38. O'Driscoll SW, Salter RB: The induction of neochondrogenesis in free intra-articular periosteal autografts under the influence of continuous passive motion: An experimental investigation in the rabbit. *J Bone Joint Surg* 1984; 66A:1248–1257.

39. Grande DA, Pitman MI, Peterson L, Menche D, Klein M: The repair of experimentally produced defects in rabbit articular cartilage by autologous chondrocyte transplantation. *J Othop Res* 1989;7:208–218.

40. Brittberg M, Nilsson A, Lindahl A, Ohlsson C, Peterson L: Rabbit articular cartilage defects treated with autologous cultured chondrocytes. *Clin Orthop* 1996;326:270–283.

41. Rodrigo J, Steadman JR: Improvement of full-thickness chondral defect healing in the human knee after debridement and microfracture using continuous passive motion. *Am J Knee Surg* 1994;7:109–116.

42. Homminga GN, Bulstra SK, Bouwmeester PS, van der Linden AJ: Perichondral grafting for cartilage lesions of the knee. *J Bone Joint Surg* 1990;72B:1003–1007.

43. Minas T, Nehrer S: Current concepts in the treatment of articular cartilage defects. *Orthopedics* 1997;20:525–538.

44. Angermann P, Riegels-Nielsen P, et al: Osteochondritis dissecans of the femoral condyle treated with periosteal transplantation: A preliminary study of 14 patients. *Orthopedics* 1994; 2:425–428.

45. O'Driscoll SW: Cartilage regeneration through periosteal transplantation: Basic scientific and clinic studies. Proceedings of the American Academy of Orthopaedic Surgeons 64th Annual Meeting, San Francisco, CA. Rosemont, IL, American Academy of Orthopaedic Surgeons, 1997, p 183.

46. Ritsila VA, Santavirta S, Alhopuro S, et al: Periosteal and perichondral grafting in reconstructive surgery. *Clin Orthop* 1994;302:259–265.

47. Peterson L: Current approaches and results of chondrocyte transplantation. Proceedings of the American Academy of Orthopaedic Surgeons 64th Annual Meeting, San Francisco, CA. Rosemont, IL, American Academy of Orthopaedic Surgeons, 1997, p 183.

48. Breinan H, Minas T, Barone L, et al: Histological evaluation of the course of healing of canine articular cartilage defects treated with cultured chondrocytes. *Tissue Eng* 1997;4: 101–114.

49. Yamashita F, Sakakida K, Suzu F, Takai S: The transplantation of an autogeneic osteochondral fragment for osteochondritis dissecans of the knee. *Clin Orthop* 1985;201:43–50.

50. Matsusue Y, Yamamuro T, Hama H: Arthroscopic multiple osteochondral transplantation to the chondral defect in the knee associated with anterior cruciate ligament disruption. *Arthroscopy* 1993;9:318–321.

51. Hangody L, Kish G, Karpati Z, Eberhart R: Osteochondral plugs: Autogenous osteochondral mosaicplasty for the treatment of focal chondral and osteochondral articular defects. *Op Tech Orthop* 1997;7:312–322.

52. Outerbridge HK, Outerbridge AR, Outerbridge RE: The use of a lateral patellar autologous graft for the repair of a large osteochondral defect in the knee. *J Bone Joint Surg* 1995;77A:65–72.

53. Zukor DJ, Gross AE: Osteochondral allograft reconstruction of the knee: Part 1. A review. *Am J Knee Surg* 1989;2:139–149.

54. Garrett J: Osteochondral allografts for reconstruction of articular defects of the knee, in Cannon DW Jr (ed): *Instructional Course Lectures 47*. Rosemont, IL, American Academy of Orthopaedic Surgeons, 1998, pp 517–522.

55. Convery FR, Meyers MH, Akeson WH: Fresh osteochondral allografting of the femoral condyle. *Clin Orthop* 1991;273:139–145.

56. Garrett JC: Treatment of osteochondral defects of the distal femur with fresh osteochondral allografts: A preliminary report. *Arthroscopy* 1986;2:222–226.

57. Beaver RJ, Mahomed M, Backstein D, Davis A: Zukor DJ, Gross AE: Fresh osteochondral allografts for post-traumatic defects in the knee: A survivorship analysis. *J Bone Joint Surg* 1992; 74B:105–110.

58. van Arkel ER, de Boer HH: Human meniscal transplantation: Preliminary results at 2 to 5-year follow-up. *J Bone Joint Surg* 1995;77B: 589–595.

59. Noyes FR, Barber-Westin SD: Arthroscopic-assisted allograft anterior cruciate ligament reconstruction in patients with symptomatic arthrosis. *Arthroscopy* 1997;13:24–32.

60. Boss A, Stutz G, Oursin C, Gachter A: Anterior cruciate ligament reconstruction combined with valgus tibial osteotomy (combined procedure). *Knee Surg Sports Traumatol Arthrosc* 1995;3:187–191.

The Biology of Bone Grafting

Robert M. Kerry, MB, FRCS (Orth)
Bassam A. Masri, MD, FRCSC
Donald S. Garbuz, MD, FRCSC
Andrei Czitrom, MD, FRCSC
Clive P. Duncan, MD, FRCSC

Introduction

Orthopaedic procedures continue to increase in complexity from the simple closed procedures done for the treatment of fractures in the early days of our specialty, to the major reconstructions of multiply failed joint replacements, limb-salvage reconstructions for malignant bone tumors, and complex spine reconstructions for instability, deformity, and paralysis. Regardless of the particular details of each of these procedures, there has been an increased demand for bone grafts and bone substitutes, particularly allograft bone.

Despite the increased publicity that organ transplantation has received over the past decade, bone was one of the first tissues to be transplanted, with autograft use described as early as 1820 by Phillips von Walter in Germany in order to fill skull defects after trepanotomy.[1] The first recorded use of allograft bone was the replacement of the proximal two thirds of a humerus by Macewen[2] in Scotland. The original uses of bone grafts were for the purposes of helping fractures or nonunions unite, and for allowing

diseased joints to fuse, well before the days of joint replacement.[3] In these situations, the size, shape, and quantity of graft material from the host is usually sufficient. Although these applications are as important today as they were over 50 years ago, recent procedures have demanded a more abundant source than the human body can afford. Furthermore, these new operations require structural bone, which is usually impossible to obtain from the live host, with the exception of perhaps fibular grafts. Such new applications include the reconstruction of a skeletal defect following tumor excision (Fig. 1), reconstruction of bone stock deficits after total joint arthroplasty (Fig. 2), and, to a lesser extent, reconstruction of skeletal defects after massive injuries. For these applications, allograft bone from a deceased donor is ideal. It has been estimated that in the United States the total number of procedures using allograft bone exceeds 200,000 per annum.[4]

Allograft bone is used in various ways in revision hip surgery on both the acetabular and femoral sides. On the acetabular side, allografts have

been used as morcellized chips to fill contained or containable defects[5,6] (Fig. 3) or as structural grafts to support acetabular components (Fig. 4) in uncontainable defects.[7–9] On the femoral side, allograft bone has been used to replace the proximal femur[10] (Fig. 2), as cortical struts to reinforce the femoral bone stock,[11] and, more recently, as morcellized graft with the technique of impaction grafting.[12,13] Recent studies[14] have called into question the longevity of hip reconstructions using structural allografts; however, the overall clinical experience with the use of allografts in joint revision surgery has been positive,[8–10] and the complication rate has been acceptable.[7,10] On the other hand, reconstructive oncological procedures with allografts have been plagued with a high rate of complications, including infection, fracture of the allograft, and nonunion of the graft-host junction.[15–17] Despite this high rate of complications, most patients favor limb salvage techniques to limb-ablative options.

In addition to excellent technical skills, successful bone allograft surgery requires a thorough understand-

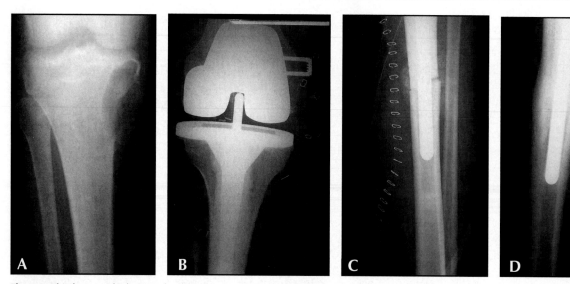

Fig. 1 A, This lesion, which proved to be an osteosarcoma of the proximal tibia, was treated using limb salvage techniques, with resection of the proximal tibia and reconstruction with not only allograft bone, but also allograft extensor mechanism, to restore the function of the quadriceps muscle. **B,** The proximal tibial allograft, with its attached extensor mechanism was used to reconstruct the proximal tibia, and was fixed to the distal tibia using a press-fit stem distally. A constrained knee replacement was performed through the allograft bone. **C,** The allograft-host junction was augmented with autograft bone. **D,** Eight months later, the allograft is well united to the host bone, the extensor mechanism is functioning well, and the patient is completely asymptomatic and free of disease. Prior to the introduction of these techniques, the only option would have been an above knee amputation.

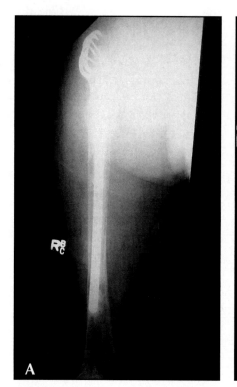
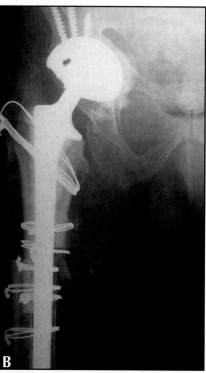

Fig. 2 A, This young man, with a history of ankylosing spondylitis, presented with a failed revision total hip arthroplasty with severe osteolysis involving the entire proximal femur. **B,** The hip replacement was revised using a structural proximal femoral allograft along with a cortical strut to augment the deficient bone stock distally.

ing of the biology, immunology, and biomechanics of allograft behavior. This chapter will summarize the current understanding of bone transplant biology and immunology.

Biologic Properties of Bone Grafts

Bone is often thought of as a structural entity that affords the body rigidity and mobility, with very little change over the years. Nothing can be further from the truth. Through the processes of osteogenesis (bone formation by osteoblasts) and osteoclastic resorption (bone breakdown), normal bone can remodel and can turn over under normal and abnormal biochemical and biomechanical conditions. These unique characteristics of bone formation and bone resorption, which under normal circumstances are carefully balanced to avoid excessive bone formation and resorption, are critical for fracture healing and repair, as well as for the incorporation of bone grafts.

Had it not been for these properties, most of the field of orthopaedic surgery would be nonexistent today.

When cancellous bone is used as bone graft, the ability to form bone is retained, but to a lesser degree than in native well-vascularized bone. This is known as the osteoinductive capacity of bone. Osteoinduction is the ability of bone graft to stimulate new bone formation by recruitment of pluripotential mesenchymal cells from the surrounding host bed. This unique property of bone is mediated by several bone matrix-derived soluble proteins, of which the best characterized group is the family of bone morphogenic proteins (BMP). The function of these proteins does not require the presence of living cells within the bone graft, and its activity is triggered by removing bone mineral.[18–20] Another property of bone grafts that allows successful bone formation is osteoconduction. This refers to the ability of bone graft to function as a scaffold for the ingrowth of capillaries and perivascular tissue, and for the orderly proliferation of osteoprogenitor cells from the host bed. This scaffold is critical to the remodeling of bone and allows gradual replacement of the bone graft over time by resorption of old bone trabeculae and formation of new bone, a process described by Phemister as creeping substitution.[21] In addition to the properties of osteoinduction and osteoconduction, autogenous bone graft contains some viable cells that contribute to the processes of osteogenesis, which is the third property of autogenous bone. In contrast, processed allograft bone only possesses the property of osteoconduction. This helps to explain why autograft heals and incorporates faster than allograft bone. From a clinical standpoint, the success of a bone graft is defined as the time when the host-graft interface

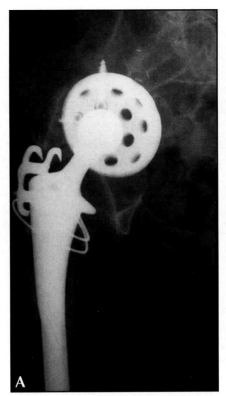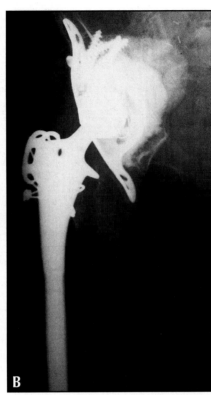

Fig. 3 A, This patient presented with an intrapelvic acetabular component following a failed revision total hip arthroplasty. The bone stock within the acetabular fossa is clearly deficient. **B,** This hip was salvaged using a reconstruction cage and morcellized cancellous allograft bone obtained femoral heads. The patient is asymptomatic 1 year following revision arthroplasty.

unites and the graft-host bone construct tolerates physiologic weight-bearing without fracture or pain.[22] Clinical success varies depending on the type of bone that is being grafted. In cancellous grafting to a defect in trabecular bone, the graft remodels and incorporates while sustaining physiologic loads. On the other hand, in cases in which a massive cortical graft is used in revision hip arthroplasty, the graft has to unite to host bone for a successful clinical result but need not, and will not, incorporate or remodel completely. Despite this lack of biologic incorporation, an allograft construct can be a clinical success when united and supported by internal fixation. Complete incorporation may appear to be the aim from a bio-

logic, and often theoretic point of view, but this may not be necessary for satisfactory clinical function, nor is it a clinical reality in the vast majority of cases. Indeed, it may be undesirable, because of the risk of bone resorption and extreme weakening while undergoing vascularization.[23–26]

Autogenous Bone Graft

Healing and incorporation of autogenous grafts is a process very much akin to the process of fracture healing. The early phase after transplantation is dominated by inflammation. Some osteoblasts and osteocytes of the graft survive and are capable of producing early new bone.[18,23,24] During this early phase, vascular invasion from the host bed occurs. Along with these new

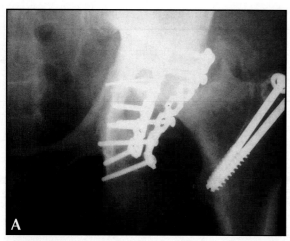 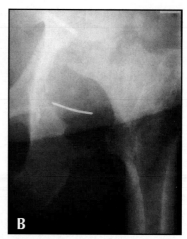 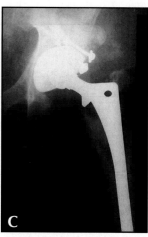

Fig. 4 A, This patient presented a few months after internal fixation of a posterior wall fracture-dislocation of the left acetabulum. Preoperative investigations revealed occult sepsis as the cause of failure of the reconstruction. **B,** A debridement was required to remove the implants and necrotic and infected bone. This left him with a substantial deficiency of the posterior wall of the acetabulum. **C,** The hip was salvaged in a staged fashion, and, after the infection was eradicated, the posterior wall was recreated using a structural femoral head allograft, which was fixed to the pelvis using two screws. This allowed the reconstruction of the hip with a cementless total hip arthroplasty.

blood vessels come pluripotential mesenchymal cells, which can differentiate into osteoblasts as part of the mechanism known as osteoinduction. These newly formed osteoblasts produce seams of osteoid around the central core of necrotic bone.[18] The new bone grows around the lattice formed by the graft bone. This process of osteoconduction continues for some time. Both the transplanted bone and its recipient bed contribute osteogenic cells.[25] The early phase following transplantation is similar for both cancellous and cortical autografts. The late phase after autogenous bone grafting differs significantly between cancellous and cortical bone. In cancellous grafting, bone formation and bone resorption occur concomitantly. Thus, osteoblasts produce seams of osteoid on the surface of necrotic bone, while osteoclasts gradually resorb the dead trabeculae. This process of creeping substitution[18,19] characterizes the late phase of autogenous cancellous bone grafting. This phase eventually results in complete replacement of the graft by host bone

and marrow. In cortical grafting, bone formation occurs only after resorption of dead lamellar bone. Dense Haversian systems have to be completely broken down by osteoclasts before any bone formation can occur. This is a very slow process reflected in the slow revascularization[23,25] of cortical autografts. Unlike cancellous grafts, resorption predominates for long periods of time in cortical grafts. Widespread graft resorption can be seen as early as 2 weeks after transplantation and can last for many months or years,[23,26] with the consequence that the graft will be weaker than normal bone. Another major difference between cancellous and cortical autografts is that cancellous grafts are completely remodeled (ie, replaced by host bone), while cortical grafts are never completely remodeled and will, to all intents and purposes, always be a combination of necrotic and living bone. The fundamental processes involved in the incorporation of cortical and cancellous bone grafts may be qualitatively similar but there are significant quantitative differences.

The knowledge of the biology of autogenous bone grafts is important for an understanding of the sequence of events associated with the healing and incorporation of allograft bone. Although autogenous bone possesses all of the unique features required for successful healing and incorporation, it has limitations in its use because of the lack of a suitable quantity for many procedures and significant donor site morbidity. These limitations have led to the increasing clinical use of allograft bone.

Allograft Bone
Allograft bone is an attractive alternative to autogenous bone. It is available in potentially almost unlimited quantities in various shapes that can be tailored to the defect encountered at surgery, and it avoids donor site morbidity. These characteristics make it an attractive biologic alternative in revision joint arthroplasty, where bone stock deficiencies are often encountered. The fundamental biologic processes involved in allograft bone healing and incorporation are

similar to those seen in autograft healing, as discussed in the preceding section, with further important quantitative differences. The main differences are the lack of viable donor cells that can contribute to healing and the potential for immunologic reaction to constituents of the donor bone. As a result, the incorporation of cancellous bone and the healing (union) of cortical allografts is generally slower and less complete than that of similar autogenous grafts.[19]

An understanding of the biology of allograft incorporation and the various mechanisms that can affect this biology is critical to the successful application of allografts in revision total joint arthroplasty. Bone loss in revision joint procedures is usually classified as cavitary or segmental.[10] The process of allograft incorporation varies with the clinical situation in which it is used. The most critical factor in allograft incorporation is the recipient host bed. For example, in an acetabular reconstruction in which there is a cavitary defect, morcellized allograft has been successfully used as filler.[5,27] From a biologic point of view, this is the ideal host environment, consisting of a well-vascularized bed. This recipient bed aids the incorporation of the allograft through a combination of revascularization, osteoconduction, and remodeling. This contrasts with cases in which a segmental femoral allograft is used to replace diaphyseal bone loss in revision total hip arthroplasty. In these cases, the junction between graft and host is cortex to cortex, and the vast majority of the allograft is in contact with soft tissue. In such situations, it has been shown that the allograft can unite to the host, but there will be very limited internal remodeling of the allograft, even after prolonged periods.[28]

Allograft incorporation has been studied extensively in animals. These findings may not be directly applicable to humans, but they do help us understand the principles of the processes involved in allograft incorporation. Fresh allografts are rejected by the host immune system. The initial response in fresh allografts is inflammation, followed by complete graft resorption or marked delay in graft incorporation.[29] Because of the immune response to fresh allografts, bone allografts used in clinical surgery are processed. The most common methods of processing are freezing, freeze drying, and irradiation. These techniques allow long-term preservation of the graft. Bone frozen at -70° C has a shelf life of 5 years.[29] These techniques have been shown to decrease or eliminate the immunogenicity of bone allografts, but they also decrease their biologic activity by killing all cells.

Allograft use in revision surgery in the form of morcellized chips to fill cavitary defects, has had good clinical success.[5,27] These grafts biologically lack osteogenic potential but do possess osteoconductive properties, and they remodel like cancellous autografts, but at a slower rate.[19] Despite their slower incorporation, cancellous allografts are widely accepted as a reconstructive alternative in well-vascularized cavitary host defects.

The use of structural allografts in revision surgery is controversial. Although early clinical results were successful, long-term results have been less consistent.[8,9,30] In addition, complications such as infection, nonunion, and fracture have been reported in approximately 25% to 35% of cases.[15,16,31] Structural grafts can be cortical, as in proximal femoral replacement, or corticocancellous, as in acetabular reconstruction. These structural grafts have limited biologic activity. The first stage in the healing of structural allografts is the inflammatory response, which brings in the pluripotential cells required for new bone formation. In most cases, union then occurs at the allograft host junction. The degree of union is highly dependent on the host. Revascularization, creeping substitution, and remodeling[25,32] occur to a very limited degree in processed bulk allografts. Many factors have been implicated as affecting structural allograft incorporation, including immune response and mechanical factors such as graft host stability.[3] Despite these multiple factors, animal experiments that have controlled for them[23,32,33] have shown that processed structural allograft bone unites to the host but lacks the ability to remodel and relies on internal fixation devices for clinical function.

Controlled animal experiments have provided insight into the basic science of allograft incorporation, but ultimately the biologic response and clinical fate of allografts in humans is of primary concern. Human retrieval studies[28,34] have provided great insight into the biologic behavior of frozen allografts in humans. Enneking's study looked at retrieval of 16 massive allografts. It was found that union occurs at the host graft junction slowly at cortical cortical junctions by formation of external callus from the host. In addition, he found that internal repair (remodeling) took place on the superficial ends of the graft and involved less than 20% of the graft. An important clinical finding was that soft tissues become firmly attached to the graft by a seam of new bone. This human retrieval study confirmed previous results from animal experiments. Frozen structural allografts only possess the osteoconductive property of bone grafts. They are relatively inert and therefore function as implants. This has important biologic and biomechanical consequences.

Once union occurs at the graft-host junction, an allograft prosthesis composite such as would be used in the reconstruction of a massive proximal femoral deficiency can be considered a clinical success. To achieve union can be difficult, because the allograft is only osteoconductive. To improve the rate of union, autograft can be placed at the graft-host junction. This autograft can be harvested from the iliac crest, or residual host femur can be wrapped around the junction as suggested by Gross.[10] This autograft possesses cells capable of osteogenesis and proteins capable of osteoinduction, 2 properties lacking in frozen allografts.

After healing of the graft-host junction, allograft composites can continue to function well clinically in spite of the fact that they are incapable of complete remodeling. This lack of ability to remodel has important clinical implications in terms of methods of fixation of allograft to host bone. It has been shown that holes in allografts and the use of plates increases the risk of fracture,[35,36] which is both a common and serious complication. Intramedullary fixation, on the other hand, decreases this risk of fracture because of the lack of screw holes and potential stress risers. When allografts are used in femoral reconstruction, the prosthesis serves as the intramedullary fixation device. The prosthesis should span the complete allograft, because any stress riser may eventually lead to fracture of this biologically inert graft. Allografts, being inert, are particularly susceptible to fatigue fracture. Irradiated allografts are more brittle than allografts that have not been irradiated, because of damage to their collagen structure, but the clinical significance of this is uncertain.[37]

Most of the knowledge of allograft biology from the clinical literature pertains to cancellous allograft used to fill cavitary defects or structural allografts used to reconstruct segmental defects. More recently there has been growing enthusiasm for the technique of impaction grafting both in revision femoral[12,13] and acetabular[6] surgery. One consideration with regard to the biology of impaction grafting is whether or not bone cement has any effect on the incorporation of cancellous allograft. Clinical studies on impaction allografting on both the femoral and acetabular sides have been encouraging. Radiographic follow-up indicates that the impacted allograft does incorporate.[13] Radiographs, however, are unreliable indicators of bone incorporation. Recent studies[38,39] have looked at biopsies of cases that previously had undergone impaction allografting. In all patients, allograft incorporation was seen on histology. The grafts were revascularized, remodeled, and underwent creeping substitution. Because these were limited biopsies, it is not certain whether or not incorporation was complete. Animal experiments support the fact that allograft used in impaction grafting does incorporate, at least partially. Schreurs and associates[40] looked at the histology of impaction grafting in goat femora. They found that by 12 weeks, the grafted area was an admixture of necrotic and live bone. This indicates partial graft incorporation that is very similar to the situation when morcellized allograft is used in cavitary defects without cement. There is no reason to suppose that the presence of cement rather than prosthesis in contact with the graft should have an adverse effect on graft incorporation. Although clinical and experimental data on the biology of allografts in impaction grafting are limited, there is no evidence that cement interferes with the incorporation process.

Allograft incorporation is a complex process that is dependent on many factors. Complete incorporation, (ie, replacement by new bone derived from the host) may not be necessary in order to achieve the goal in all clinical situations. Although complete incorporation often occurs in cancellous grafting, the goal in cortical structural grafting is union at the graft-host junction, with limited incorporation or remodeling. Clinical success ultimately depends on the bone graft providing adequate mechanical support for the skeleton and soft tissues. The potential role of the immune response in determining the ultimate fate of allograft bone has been increasingly recognized in recent years.

Immunology of Allografts

Fresh unmatched allograft bone will inevitably invoke an immune response in the host. This immune response can result in graft resorption or marked delay in graft incorporation. For this reason, techniques were developed to decrease the immunogenicity of transplanted allograft bone. The most common clinical techniques used today are deep freezing, freeze drying, and irradiation. These methods allow for long-term preservation and storage of allograft bone. Allograft processing has been shown to reduce the host immune response.[41] It was thought that, because processed allografts have no living cells, they would not elicit a strong alloreactive immune response when transplanted. With the advent of modern immunologic assay techniques, it has become apparent that fresh and processed allograft bone can invoke immune responses. In 1 study by Friedlander and associates,[42] both deep frozen and freeze-dried allograft bone elicited a humoral and cell-mediated immune response in rabbits. However, both methods of processing, particularly freeze drying, decreased this response in comparison to the response to fresh allogeneic bone. Although most authors[4,43] agree that processed allograft bone can elicit a host immune response, the exact role of immunology in its biologic incorporation is unclear. It has been suggested that this immune reaction may, in part, be responsible for the unpredictable outcome of allografts in revision surgery.[3]

The major histocompatibility complex (MHC) class I and class II antigens on specialized antigen presenting cells are responsible for the immune response of allograft bone.[22,29] Animal studies have examined the role of these antigens by studying transplants in animals matched at the MHC, those with minor mismatches, and in animals with major mismatches. Bos and associates[44] looked at the effects of histocompatibility matching on the incorporation of frozen bone transplanted in rats. This study confirmed that in rats with major histocompatibility differences frozen bone elicits a strong immune response and that in closely related donors the immune response is almost undetectable. Despite these marked differences in immune response, no significant effect was seen on the biology of graft incorporation. A further study[33] addressed the issue of freezing and histocompatibility matching on rat cortical bone graft incorporation in a weightbearing environment. Incorporation was followed sequentially over time. This study concluded that histocompatibility matching and freezing were the most important determinants of graft incorporation. Frozen grafts with a major mismatch (the most commonly used grafts in clinical practice) were unpredictable in terms of incorporation, with a trend towards lack of revascularization and failure. A further study in dogs also showed a detectable difference in immune response between matched and unmatched grafts.[45]

Studies using immunosuppressive agents have lent further support to a critical role for immunology in bone graft incorporation. In a study on transplantation in rats, cyclosporine was used in animals with a major histocompatibility mismatch.[46] When animals with a major mismatch were immunosuppressed with cyclosporine, the incorporation of allograft was similar to that of autograft. Immunosuppression, although theoretically attractive, has no defined role at present in revision surgery because of its potentially serious side effects.

Collective evidence from experimental studies indicates that processed allograft bone is definitely immunogenic. However, the importance of this immune response in determining the degree of allograft bone incorporation is not clearly defined.

A few studies have looked at the effect of human leukocyte antigen (HLA) matching in humans and the immune response to allograft bone. A recent multicenter study[47] has shown sensitization to HLA after transplantation of frozen allograft bone. Whether this immune response had any biologic or clinical effects was not ascertained. Muscolo and associates[48,49] looked at HLA matching in human allograft recipients. These studies looked at the effect of matching on radiographic incorporation of allografts. Their data showed an increased radiographic score for patients with 1 or more HLA class I antigen matches compared with the group that was totally mismatched. However this difference was not statistically significant.

From all of the data available, it is clear that immunologic events play an important role in bone graft incorporation. The exact nature of the interplay between the immune system and bone physiology has yet to be determined. It has recently been shown that bone allografts can cause sensitization that may preclude subsequent organ transplantation,[50] confirming that much remains to be understood. The ultimate aim must be to eliminate antigenicity, while preserving biologic activity and mechanical properties, even though this is not necessarily mandatory for clinical success.

Summary

Allograft bone continues to play an important role in revision hip and knee arthroplasty with well documented clinical success. A basic understanding of allograft biology and immunology is important in order to optimize outcome. The importance of the interaction of immunologic factors with the biologic processes involved in bone graft incorporation has yet to be fully understood. A better understanding may, in the future, enable an improvement in the quality and uniformity of clinical outcome.

References

1. Chase SW, Herndon CH: The fate of autogenous and homogenous bone grafts: A historical review. *J Bone Joint Surg* 1955;37A:809–841.

2. Macewen W: Observation concerning transplantation of bone. Illustrated by a case of interhuman osseous transplantation whereby over two thirds of the shaft of a humerus was restored. *Proc R Soc London* 1881;32:232–247.

3. Aro HT, Aho AJ: Clinical use of bone allografts. *Ann Med* 1993;25:403–412.

4. Friedlaender GE: Bone allografts: The biological consequences of immunological events. *J Bone Joint Surg* 1991;73A:1119–1122.

5. Berry DJ, Muller ME: Revision arthroplasty using an anti-protrusio cage for massive acetabular bone deficiency. *J Bone Joint Surg* 1992;74B:711–715.

6. Slooff TJ, Buma P, Schreurs BW, Schimmel JW, Huiskes R, Gardeniers J: Acetabular and femoral reconstruction with impacted graft and cement. *Clin Orthop* 1996;324:108–115.

7. Garbuz D, Morsi E, Gross AE: Revision of the acetabular component of a total hip arthroplasty with a massive structural allograft: Study

with a minimum five-year follow-up. *J Bone Joint Surg* 1996;78A:693–697.

8. Paprosky WG, Magnus RE: Principles of bone grafting in revision total hip arthroplasty: Acetabular technique. *Clin Orthop* 1994;298: 147–155.

9. Paprosky WG, Perona PG, Lawrence, JM: Acetabular defect classification and surgical reconstruction in revision arthroplasty: A 6-year follow-up evaluation. *J Arthroplasty* 1994; 9:33–44.

10. Gross AE: Revision arthroplasty of the hip using allograft bone, in Czitrom AA, Gross AE (eds): *Allografts in Orthopaedic Practice.* Baltimore, MD, Williams & Wilkins, 1992, pp 147–173.

11. Emerson RH Jr, Malinin TI, Cuellar AD, Head WC, Peters PC: Cortical strut allografts in the reconstruction of the femur in revision total hip arthroplasty: A basic science and clinical study. *Clin Orthop* 1992;285:35–44.

12. Gie GA, Linder L, Ling RS, Simon JP, Slooff TJ, Timperley AJ: Contained morselized allograft in revision total hip arthroplasty: Surgical technique. *Orthop Clin North Am* 1993;24: 717–725.

13. Gie GA, Linder L, Ling RS, Simon JP, Slooff TJ, Timperley AJ: Impacted cancellous allografts and cement for revision total hip arthroplasty. *J Bone Joint Surg* 1993;75B:14–21.

14. Kwong LM, Jasty M, Harris WH: High failure rate of bulk femoral head allografts in total hip acetabular reconstructions at 10 years. *J Arthroplasty* 1993;8:341–346.

15. Berrey BH Jr, Lord CF, Gebhardt MC, Mankin HJ: Fractures of allografts: Frequency, treatment, and end-results. *J Bone Joint Surg* 1990; 72A:825–833.

16. Lord CF, Gebhardt MC, Tomford WW, Mankin HJ: Infection in bone allografts: Incidence, nature, and treatment. *J Bone Joint Surg* 1988; 70A:369–376.

17. Dick HM, Strauch RJ: Infection of massive bone allografts. *Clin Orthop* 1994;306:46–53.

18. Goldberg VM, Stevenson S: Biology of bone and cartilage allografts, in Czitrom AA, Gross AE (eds): *Allografts in Orthopaedic Practice.* Baltimore, MD, Williams & Wilkins, 1992, pp 1–13.

19. Goldberg VM, Stevenson S, Shaffer JW: Biology of autografts and allografts, in Friedlaender GE, Goldberg VM (eds). *Bone and Cartilage Allografts: Biology and Clinical Applications.* Park Ridge, IL, American Academy of Orthopaedic Surgeons, 1991, pp 3–12.

20. Reddi AH, Wientroub S, Muthukumaran N: Biologic principles of bone induction. *Orthop Clin North Am* 1987;18:207–212.

21. Phemister DB: The fate of transplanted bone and regenerative power of its various constituents. *Surg Gynecol Obstet* 1914;19:303–333.

22. Stevenson S, Horowitz M: The response to bone allografts. *J Bone Joint Surg* 1992;74A: 939–950.

23. Burchardt H, Jones H, Glowczewskie F, Rudner C, Enneking WF: Freeze-dried allogeneic segmental cortical-bone grafts in dogs. *J Bone Joint Surg* 1978;60A:1082–1090.

24. Chalmers J: Transplantation immunity in bone homografting. *J Bone Joint Surg* 1959;41B: 160–179.

25. Burchardt H: Biology of bone transplantation. *Orthop Clin North Am* 1987;18:187–196.

26. Enneking WF, Burchardt H, Puhl JJ, Piotrowski G: Physical and biological aspects of repair in dog cortical-bone transplants. *J Bone Joint Surg* 1975;57A:237–252.

27. Padgett DE, Kull L, Rosenberg A, Sumner DR, Galante JO: Revision of the acetabular component without cement after total hip arthroplasty: Three to six-year follow-up. *J Bone Joint Surg* 1993;75A:663–673.

28. Enneking WF, Mindell ER: Observations on massive retrieved human allografts. *J Bone Joint Surg* 1991;73A:1123–1142.

29. Czitrom AA: Biology of bone grafting and principles of bone banking, in Weinstein SL (ed): *The Pediatric Spine: Principles and Practice.* New York, NY, Raven Press, 1994, vol 2, pp 1285–1298.

30. Oakeshott RD, Morgan DA, Zukor DJ, Rudan JF, Brooks PJ, Gross AE: Revision total hip arthroplasty with osseous allograft reconstruction: A clinical and roentgenographic analysis. *Clin Orthop* 1987;225:37–61.

31. Head WC, Berklacich FM, Malinin TI, Emerson RH Jr: Proximal femoral allografts in revision total hip arthroplasty. *Clin Orthop* 1987;225:22–36.

32. Stevenson S, Li XQ, Martin B: The fate of cancellous and cortical bone after transplantation of fresh and frozen tissue-antigen-matched and mismatched osteochondral allografts in dogs. *J Bone Joint Surg* 1991;73A:1143–1156.

33. Stevenson S, Li XQ, Davy DT, Klein L, Goldberg VM: Critical biological determinants of incorporation of nonvascularized cortical bone grafts: Quantification of a complex process and structure. *J Bone Joint Surg* 1997;79A:1–16.

34. Hooten JP Jr, Engh CA, Heekin RD, Vinh TN: Structural bulk allografts in acetabular reconstruction: Analysis of two grafts retrieved at post-mortem. *J Bone Joint Surg* 1996;78B: 270–275.

35. Thompson RC Jr, Pickvance EA, Garry D: Fractures in large-segment allografts. *J Bone Joint Surg* 1993;75A:1663–1673.

36. Vander Griend RA: The effect of internal fixation on the healing of large allografts. *J Bone Joint Surg* 1994;76A:657–663.

37. Hamer AJ, Strachan JR, Black MM, Ibbotson CJ, Stockley I, Elson RA: Biochemical properties of cortical allograft bone using a new method of bone strength measurement: A comparison of fresh, fresh-frozen and irradiated bone. *J Bone Joint Surg* 1996;78B:363–368.

38. Buma P, Lamerigts N, Schreurs BW, Gardeniers J, Versleyen D, Slooff TJ: Impacted graft incorporation after cemented acetabular revision: Histological evaluation in 8 patients. *Acta Orthop Scand* 1996;67:536–540.

39. Nelissen RG, Bauer TW, Weidenhielm LR, LeGolvan DP, Mikhail WE: Revision hip arthroplasty with the use of cement and impaction grafting: Histological analysis of four cases. *J Bone Joint Surg* 1995;77A:412–422.

40. Schreurs BW, Buma P, Huiskes R, Slagter JL, Slooff TJ: Morsellized allografts for fixation of the hip prosthesis femoral component: A mechanical and histological study in the goat. *Acta Orthop Scand* 1994;65:267–275.

41. Burwell RG: Studies in the transplantation of bone: V. The capacity of fresh and treated homografts of bone to evoke transplantation immunity. *J Bone Joint Surg* 1963;45B:386–401.

42. Friedlaender GE, Strong DM, Sell KW: Studies on the antigenicity of bone: I. Freeze-dried and deep-frozen allografts in rabbits. *J Bone Joint Surg* 1976;58A:854–858.

43. Langer F, Czitrom A, Pritzker KP, Gross AE: The immunogenicity of fresh and frozen allogeneic bone. *J Bone Joint Surg* 1975;57A:216–220.

44. Bos GD, Goldberg VM, Zika JM, Heiple KG, Powell AE: Immune responses of rats to frozen bone allografts. *J Bone Joint Surg* 1983;65A: 239–246.

45. Stevenson S, Shaffer JW, Goldberg VM: The humoral response to vascular and nonvascular allografts of bone. *Clin Orthop* 1996;326:86–95.

46. Lee WP, Pan YC, Kesmarky S, et al: Experimental orthotopic transplantation of vascularized skeletal allografts: Functional assessment and long-term survival. *Plast Reconstr Surg* 1995; 95:336–349.

47. Strong DM, Friedlaender GE, Tomford WW, et al: Immunologic responses in human recipients of osseous and osteochondral allografts. *Clin Orthop* 1996;326:107–114.

48. Muscolo DL, Ayerza MA, Calabrese ME, Redal MA, Santini Aravjo E: Human leukocyte antigen matching, radiographic score, and histologic findings in massive frozen bone allografts. *Clin Orthop* 1996;326:115–126.

49. Muscolo DL, Caletti E, Schajowicz F, Aravjo ES, Makino A: Tissue typing in human massive allografts of frozen bone. *J Bone Joint Surg* 1987; 69A:583–595.

50. Lee MY, Finn HA, Lazda VA, Thistlethwaite JR Jr, Simon MA: Bone allografts are immunogenic and may preclude subsequent organ transplants. *Clin Orthop* 1997;340:215–219.

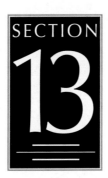
Additional Topics of Practical Interest

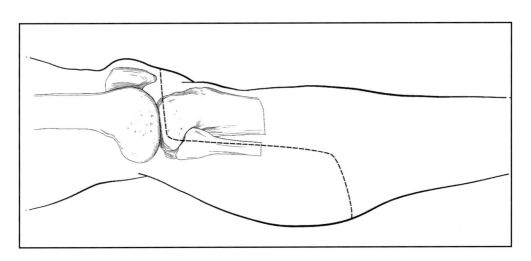

Current Options and Approaches for Blood Management in Orthopaedic Surgery

E. Michael Keating, MD

Introduction

Although the implementation of blood-screening measures has vastly reduced the risk of transmission of the human immunodeficiency virus (HIV) through transfusion of donated blood products, several factors preclude the blood supply from achieving a zero-risk status. Patients who receive perioperative allogeneic blood transfusions, for instance, have been reported to have higher rates of infection[1-3] (although this finding remains controversial[4,5]) and perioperative blood loss, longer hospital stays,[6,7] more consecutive days of fever and administration of antibiotics, and a postoperative decrease in natural killer cells.[3] Furthermore, in a retrospective quantitative analysis of transfusion-associated immunomodulation, transfusion was the most important prognostic factor for postoperative infection.[8] Finally, the risk of transmission of infectious diseases, such as those caused by hepatitis-B and -C viruses[9] and, to a lesser extent, cytomegalovirus[10] and Epstein-Barr virus,[11] as well as the risk of transfusion reactions, alloimmunization, and immunomodulation, remains substantive. Optimization of blood management is thus as important today as it was a decade ago, despite the markedly improved safety of allogeneic blood.

Cost-management pressures in the 1990s and continued public concern about the safety of the blood supply have precipitated a concerted movement among the surgical specialties to refine the existing blood-conservation measures as well as to develop new approaches.[12,13] These efforts have included development of transfusion practice standards; improvement in the techniques of surgical hemostasis; perioperative blood salvage; promotion of preoperative autologous blood donation (PAD); and, more recently, development of blood substitutes or temporary oxygen carriers (currently under investigation)[14-16] and clinical utilization of recombinant human erythropoietin (epoetin alfa) to stimulate erythropoiesis[6,7,17-22] (Table 1). These strategies and options, and their potential importance in orthopaedic surgical procedures, are reviewed.

Transfusion Practice Standards

Gidelines for blood management in orthopaedic procedures have been developed and promoted as a way to improve, in a cost-effective manner, the outcomes associated with perioperative loss of red blood cells (that is, to reduce patient exposure to allogeneic blood transfusion).[23] In general, the guidelines encourage and support good operative anesthetic and hemostatic technique, PAD, intraoperative and postoperative blood salvage, acute normovolemic hemodilution, unit-by-unit transfusion when blood is necessary, and pharmacologic intervention with epoetin alfa when indicated. Allogeneic blood transfusion should be limited on the basis of individual need. Despite the development of general blood-management guidelines related to the hemoglobin level and the hematocrit to trigger transfusion, the transfusion-triggering levels should be established for each patient on the basis of that patient's overall health.[24,25]

One of the challenges in the implementation of transfusion practice standards is to change the way that surgeons approach transfusion or to change their behavior, or both. Changes in transfusion practice—for instance, the lowering of transfusion-triggering thresholds for well-characterized physiologic indicators such as the hemoglobin level or the hematocrit—have been suggested as a way to reduce the need for transfusion. Clinical data indicate that adequate tissue oxygenation is supported at hemoglobin concentrations of less than 100 g/l, the level previously considered an indicator for transfusion,[23-30] these data provide a rationale for the tolerance of more periopera-

Table 1
Current blood management options in orthopaedic surgery

Option	Comment
Transfusion practice standards	Lower transfusion triggers: hemoglobin concentration of less than 70 to 80 g/l
Surgical technique	Emphasis on maintaining careful surgical technique. Modified surgical technique (for example, modified approach). Hypotensive anesthesia has potential
Topically or locally active agents	Thrombin, collagen, and fibrin glue. Antifibrinolytics (aprotinin, tranexamic acid, and ε-aminocaproic acid)
Blood salvage	Intraoperative and postoperative collection, processing, and transfusion of blood
Preoperative autologous blood donation	Considered a standard of care in some orthopaedic procedures. Often used in conjunction with perioperative administration of epoetin alfa
Perioperative administration of epoetin alfa	Increases reticulocyte count, red blood-cell production, hematocrit, and hemoglobin concentration. Facilitates preoperative autologous blood donation and reduces need for allogeneic blood transfusion during elective orthopaedic procedures in patients who have a hemoglobin concentration of > 100 to ≤ 130 g/l

tive blood loss without intervention with use of allogeneic blood. Thus, although a hemoglobin level of 100 g/l is a transfusion trigger in patients with impaired cardiac function and in those with cardiopulmonary disease, the trigger is 70 to 80 g/l in otherwise healthy patients having orthopaedic procedures.[28] However, surgeons generally recognize that the hemoglobin level alone is not a basis for transfusion and that multiple clinical factors should be assessed for each patient.[31]

Blood Management in the Orthopaedic Setting
Surgical Technique and Pharmacologic Intervention

Surgeons should minimize blood loss by carefully maintaining surgical hemostasis.[28] Several surgical techniques, including electrocautery, argon-beam coagulation, and use of topical agents, reduce blood loss safely and effectively.[32–34] Furthermore, many orthopaedic procedures have been modified to reduce blood loss and to minimize the need for transfusion of allogeneic blood.[35,36] The application of hypotensive anesthesia is also gaining credibil-

ity as an option for blood management in the orthopaedic setting.[37]

In addition to improvements in surgical technique, several pharmacologic options for blood management are available to orthopaedic surgeons or are under active investigation. Many topically or locally active agents, such as thrombin, collagen, and fibrin glue, may hold promise for the maintenance of perioperative hemostasis.[28,38] Another class of pharmacologic agents, the antifibrinolytics, includes promising agents such as aprotinin, tranexamic acid, ε-aminocaproic acid, and, to a lesser extent, desmopressin. The antifibrinolytics are administered intraoperatively or postoperatively, are generally safe, and are variably effective in reducing perioperative blood loss and the need for allogeneic blood transfusion. The ε-aminocaproic acid is administered as an intravenous injection of 10 g, followed by infusion of 2 g/hr for 5 hours; tranexamic acid, as an intravenous injection of 10 mg/kg of body weight, followed by infusion of 1 mg/kg of body weight per hour for 10 hours; aprotinin, as an intravenous infusion of 2 million

kallikrein inactivation units (a unit of measure referring to inhibition of kallikrein) over a 20-minute period preoperatively, followed by infusion of 500,000 kallikrein inactivation units per hour intraoperatively; and desmopressin, as an intravenous infusion of 0.3 mg/kg of body weight over a 20-minute period.

Although its mechanism of action is still unknown, aprotinin is an antifibrinolytic agent that has been approved by the Food and Drug Administration to reduce blood loss in cardiopulmonary bypass procedures, and it has recently been investigated for use in patients having major orthopaedic procedures.[39–45] In the orthopaedic setting, aprotinin has been shown to be safe[39,40,42] and effective in reducing intraoperative blood loss[40,41] postoperative blood loss[40,44] and the need for allogeneic blood transfusion.[40,42] However, Hayes and associates[39] found no effect of aprotinin on blood loss or transfusion requirements in patients having total hip replacement.

Tranexamic acid is another promising antifibrinolytic agent. This agent, which is administered intravenously near the conclusion of surgery, has been found to markedly reduce postoperative blood loss[46–50] and patient exposure to allogeneic blood.[48–50] No difference was found, in several studies, with regard to the prevalence of thrombolytic events in patients who had received tranexamic acid and those who had been given a placebo.[48–50]

A third antifibrinolytic agent, ε-aminocaproic acid, is effective in reducing blood loss when it is administered before cardiac procedures.[51–53] However, its use in the orthopaedic setting has not yet been investigated.

Several clinical studies have suggested that desmopressin is ineffective in reducing blood loss and the need for allogeneic blood transfusion in the orthopaedic setting.[54-56]

As a class of agents, the antifibrinolytics (aprotinin, tranexamic acid, and ε-aminocaproic acid) have an important role in the management of perioperative blood loss and exert no apparent adverse effect on the prevalence of thrombolytic events.

Blood Salvage

Despite numerous advances in surgical technique and intraoperative pharmacologic interventions, blood loss in orthopaedic procedures may be extensive.[57,58] Intraoperative and postoperative blood salvage is a technique that is used to return washed or unwashed autologous blood to the patient, potentially reducing the need for allogeneic blood transfusion. Blood-salvage devices currently in use or that are under active investigation include the Cell Saver (Haemonetics, Braintree, MA), the ConstaVac Blood Conservation System (Stryker, Kalamazoo, MI), and Solcotrans Plus (Smith and Nephew Richards, Memphis, TN). The lost blood is collected by aspiration or drainage and then is filtered, washed or unwashed (the Solcotrans Plus system does not wash the blood), and centrifuged before being transfused. The necessity of washing collected blood before autotransfusion has been questioned; however, filtering alone does not markedly reduce cytokine concentrations in the processed blood.[59] Intraoperative blood salvage can allow as much as 60% of the red blood cells that are lost during the surgical procedure to be recovered for subsequent autotransfusion.[60]

There also may be a large amount of blood drainage from the wound postoperatively. For example, after primary or revision joint arthroplasty, postoperative blood salvage resulted in autotransfusion of approximately

437 ml after primary total hip procedures and 883 ml after primary total knee procedures; volumes of salvaged blood were as high as 946 ml.[61,62] However, the cost-effectiveness of returning washed autologous blood to patients has been questioned because the technique requires an expensive device and technical expertise to operate it.[63] In contrast, reinfusion of unwashed filtered autologous blood has been shown to be cost-effective in decreasing the need for allogeneic blood transfusion.[64] Ideally, unwashed autologous blood should be filtered and transfused within 4 hours after collection to avoid potential febrile reactions.[65]

Both the safety and the efficacy of intraoperative and postoperative-blood salvage have been documented in the orthopaedic setting.[61,62,64,66-68] Blood salvage has reduced the need for allogeneic blood transfusion in several orthopaedic procedures, including total hip and knee arthroplasty and bilateral total knee arthroplasty.[61,66,68] Although blood salvage is safe and can provide a considerable volume of autologous blood, it does not decrease the need for allogeneic blood transfusion in many orthopaedic procedures.[68,69] Furthermore, the use of salvaged blood that is washed before autotransfusion may be too costly to be recommended as a standard practice. Blood salvage may be most effective in reducing the need for allogeneic blood transfusion when it is used in conjunction with other blood-management options, particularly PAD.[66,68,70]

Preoperative Autologous Blood Donation

PAD donation is based on the premise that the patient's own blood is the safest blood. It decreases the need for allogeneic blood transfusion in elective surgical procedures in

which a large amount of blood loss is expected,[31,71-74] and it has become a standard of care as a blood-conservation strategy in some orthopaedic procedures.[75,76] However, its usefulness may be limited in many patients because of preexisting medical conditions, such as anemia, advanced age, an unacceptable preoperative hematocrit and hemoglobin concentration, and a poor erythropoietic response to phlebotomy.

A poor erythropoietic response to phlebotomy has been observed by numerous investigators in patients who have donated autologous blood preoperatively.[77-79] Kickler and Spivak[79] noted that the degree of anemia caused by repeated phlebotomy was inadequate to increase erythropoietin production, resulting in the onset of mild anemia in most donors. A mathematical analysis used to examine the benefits and detriments of PAD showed that patients who donate blood preoperatively are more likely to need transfusion earlier and more frequently than are nondonating patients.[77] A prospective study of 72 consecutive patients who were scheduled to have an elective orthopaedic procedure demonstrated an inadequate erythropoietic response in 33 (58%) of 57 patients who had donated blood preoperatively.[78] This study and others[79,80] also demonstrated that a major portion of the donated units had red blood-cell volumes that were less than the minimum standards for blood donation. PAD alone thus may not stimulate erythropoiesis sufficiently to meet the need for blood in orthopaedic procedures.

Another limitation to the successful implementation of a PAD program is the high cost. Not only are there logistic obstacles, such as the collection, storage, and transfusion of the blood, but a high percentage of predonated autologous blood units are never used.[81-83] Two studies revealed that approximately 50% of predonated autologous blood units (no numbers were reported) are routinely wasted[82-84] and a rate of waste as high as 70% (164 of 234 units) has been reported.[83] Such waste reduces the cost-effectiveness of any PAD program.

Acute Normovolemic Hemodilution

A proposed alternative to the high cost of PAD is acute normovolemic hemodilution, a blood-management technique in which whole blood is withdrawn preoperatively or intraoperatively and is isovolumetrically replaced with colloid or crystalloid solutions.[85] Patients thus lose fewer red blood cells during procedures involving ongoing blood loss, and the collected units are held in reserve until the hemoglobin concentration or the hematocrit reaches a predetermined level or the patient demonstrates a physiological need for transfusion. Acute normovolemic hemodilution is contraindicated in patients who have coronary artery, renal, or pulmonary disease and in those who have severe hepatic disease.[86]

Acute normovolemic hemodilution (ANH) has been investigated in the orthopaedic setting, although only superficially. Of 17 patients who had a total hip arthroplasty and were managed with hemodilution, seven required autologous blood compared with 12 of 16 patients in the control group[87] The clinical safety and efficacy of ANH for reducing the need for allogeneic blood transfusion is under investigation; however, because of the short duration of many orthopaedic procedures and the precision with which the technique must be implemented, it may be impractical in many orthopaedic settings.[60] Nevertheless, there undoubtedly will be additional investigation of ANH as a strategy for blood management in orthopaedic procedures.

Pharmacologic Strategies for Blood Management

The rationale behind the use of pharmacologic strategies for blood management includes a forecasted shortage of 4 million units of red blood cells by the year 2030;[88] the high cost of acquisition, screening, storage, transport, and administration of blood; the goal of elimination of transmission of disease,[10,89,90] transfusion reactions, and suppression of normal immune function;[91] preexisting medical conditions such as anemia; and inadequate erythropoietic response to phlebotomy.[77-79] Thus, several temporary oxygen carriers and blood substitutes are now under investigation in phase III clinical trials. Furthermore, epoetin alfa, administered perioperatively, has been shown to be safe and effective for treating anemia and decreasing patient exposure to allogeneic blood transfusion.[6,7]

Oxygen Carriers

The potential for oxygen carriers to temporarily increase oxygen delivery and tissue oxygenation during procedures associated with high blood loss, as well as for the treatment of conditions such as cerebral hypoxia, is compelling. However, numerous obstacles, including a short shelf-life, difficulty of use, side effects and the low concentrations that must be used to avoid them, and a short intravascular half-life, have slowed the emergence of oxygen carriers in the surgical setting. Nevertheless, 2 classes of oxygen carriers—those that are hemoglobin-based and perfluorocarbons—have shown clinical potential (Table 2). Both classes include agents that are currently under phase II or phase III clinical development.

Hemoglobin-Based Oxygen Carriers (Red Blood-Cell Substitutes)

Research involving hemoglobin-based oxygen carriers, as a class, has necessarily evolved from the initial investigation of free hemoglobin, which is nephrotoxic,[92,93] to the study of structurally modified hemoglobin. Hemoglobin has been structurally modified in various ways, by cross-linking, polymerization, conjugation, lipid encapsulation, and genetic engineering,[94] in an attempt to prevent nephrotoxicity and to circumvent other, unexpected deleterious biological interactions. However, many of these modified hemoglobins continue to elicit unexpected adverse effects, including fever, headache, chest, and abdominal pain, and hypertension, in the clinical setting.[94] Further modification of the hemoglobin molecule may reduce many of these side effects.

Numerous hemoglobin-based oxygen carriers have been developed and have been investigated in phase I and phase II clinical trials. Much of the preliminary data indicates that many of the limitations, with regard to biologic safety, of previous hemoglobin-based oxygen-carrier formulations have been overcome.[95] However, data demonstrating that these hemoglobin-based oxygen carriers support tissue oxygenation in humans as well as transfusion does are not yet available. In the next 2 to 3 years, data on safety and efficacy should emerge from phase-III trials of several hemoglobin-based oxygen carriers.

Temporary Oxygen Carriers (Perfluorocarbons)

As a class, perfluorocarbons are inert organic compounds that have an exceptionally high solubility for gases, including oxygen and carbon dioxide. The oxygen-carrying capacity of perfluorocarbons is directly proportional to the ambient partial pressure of oxygen.[96] Unlike hemoglobin, which is saturated at oxygen partial pressures of 100 torr (13.3 kilopascals) (room air), perfluorocarbons can continue to load oxygen in a linear manner as oxygen partial pressure is increased. Thus, perfluorocarbons can carry more oxygen at a point at which hemoglobin is already fully saturated with oxygen and can provide no additional benefit[97] (Fig. 1).

Of the perfluorocarbons that are under investigation, only perfluorodecalin, a first-generation perfluorocarbon, has been approved by the Food and Drug Administration for use in humans having percutaneous transluminal coronary angioplasty. However, broad-based acceptance of perfluorodecalin as a temporary oxygen carrier has not occurred because of several limitations, including difficulty of use, limited oxygen-carrying capacity (only 7% vol of O_2 at a PO_2 of 760 mm Hg [101.31 kilopascals]), long retention in the reticuloendothelial system, complement activation, and temperature instability.[98–101] As a result of these disadvantages, perfluorodecalin has been removed from the market.

In 1986, a change in the manufacturing process allowed the production of more stable, highly concentrated perfluorocarbons that exhibited a higher oxygen-carrying capacity. These new perfluorocarbons were termed second generation to distinguish them from the first-generation products, which also were associated with numerous side effects.

Perflubron emulsion (Oxygent; Alliance Pharmaceutical, San Diego, CA), a second-generation perfluorocarbon, lacks many of the limitations observed with the first-generation agents. It is stable at room temperature, is highly concentrated, and appears to be well tolerated by hu-

Table 2
Investigational options for blood management

Product	Type	Clinical Status	Indication
Oxygent (Alliance Pharmaceutical, San Diego, CA)	Perfluorocarbon	Phase II	Hemodilution, cardiopulmonary bypass, cerebral hypoxia
PHP (pyridoxalated and conjugated hemoglobin) (Apex Bioscience, Research Triangle Park, NC)	Human hemoglobin	Phase I/II	Septic shock
HemAssist (Baxter Healthcare, Deerfield, IL)	Human hemoglobin	Phase III	Trauma, surgery, dialysis, stroke, shock
Hemopure (Biopure Pharmaceuticals, Cambridge, MA)	Bovine hemoglobin	Phase I/II	Surgery, hemodilution, sickle-cell disease
PEG-Hemoglobin (Enzon, Piscataway, NJ)	Bovine hemoglobin	Phase II	Radiation-therapy sensitization
Oxyfluor (Hemagen/PFC, St. Louis, MO)	Perfluorocarbon	Phase II	Cardiopulmonary bypass
Hemolink (Hemosol, Etobicoke, Ontario, Canada)	Human hemoglobin	Phase II	Surgery, hemodilution
PolyHeme (Northfield, Chicago, IL)	Human hemoglobin	Phase II/III	Trauma, surgery
Optro (Somatogen, Boulder, CO)	Recombinant hemoglobin	Phase II	Hemodilution, erythropoiesis

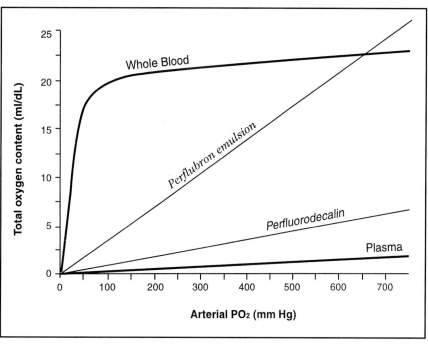

Fig. 1 Graph demonstrating the total oxygen-carrying capacity of 90% (weight per volume) perflubron emulsion compared with that of whole blood, 20% (weight per volume) perfluorodecalin, and plasma. The solubility of perfluorocarbons obeys Henry's law; therefore, perfluorocarbons are particularly effective oxygen carriers at higher ambient partial pressures of oxygen. (Reproduced with permission from Keipert PE, Faithfull NS, Bradley JD, et al: Oxygen delivery augmentation by low-dose perfluorochemical emulsion during profound normovolemic hemodilution, in Vaupel P, Zander RN, Bruley DF (eds): *Oxygen Transport to Tissue XV*. New York, NY, Plenum Press, 1994, pp 197–204.)

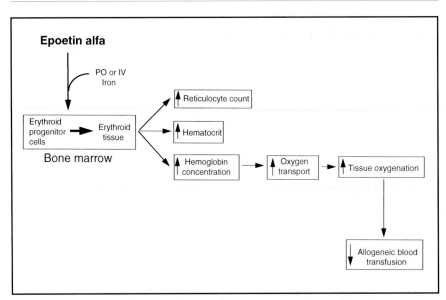

Epoetin alfa

PO or IV
Iron

Erythroid progenitor cells → Erythroid tissue

Bone marrow

↑ Reticulocyte count

↑ Hematocrit

↑ Hemoglobin concentration → ↑ Oxygen transport → ↑ Tissue oxygenation

↓ Allogeneic blood transfusion

Fig. 2 Schematic overview showing the physiologic effects of pharmacological doses of epoetin alfa. In the perioperative setting, epoetin alfa is administered 2 to 3 weeks preoperatively, to accelerate erythropoiesis, and once on the day of surgery, to increase both tissue oxygenation during surgery and the rate at which hemostasis is reestablished and the patient recovers after the procedure. PO = by mouth and IV = intravenous.

mans.[102] This agent is currently under investigation in phase II trials. The enhancement of oxygen delivery by synthetic perfluorocarbon emulsions gives these agents a wide range of potential clinical applications as temporary oxygen carriers in orthopaedic surgery; these uses include support of tissue oxygenation during ongoing blood loss and avoidance of the need for allogeneic blood transfusion.

Epoetin Alfa

Recombinant human erythropoietin (epoetin alfa), a secretory glycoprotein of 165 amino acids that is identical in sequence to endogenous human urinary erythropoietin,[103] is indicated for facilitating preoperative autologous blood donation by anemic patients (those with a hemoglobin level > 100 and ≤ 130 g/l) who are scheduled to have major elective surgery. The physiologic implications of epoetin alfa-accelerated erythropoiesis include improved tissue oxygenation and re-

duced need for allogeneic blood transfusion, secondary to increased concentrations of hemoglobin. Each g/dl increase of blood hemoglobin concentration results in an increase in oxygen-carrying capacity of approximately 1.39 ml O_2/dl[104] and a decrease in the need for allogeneic blood transfusion of approximately 15% (no numbers were reported).[17,19] Epoetin alfa is ideal for procedures in which a large amount of blood loss and associated tissue hypoxia are expected.

Patients undergoing orthopaedic surgery may require as many as 4 to 6 units of blood perioperatively.[57,58,105] The effectiveness of perioperative use of epoetin alfa in stimulating erythropoiesis in these patients has been established in clinical studies[6,7,17,19,21,106-120] (Table 3). The preoperative administration of epoetin alfa was found to increase the preoperative hemoglobin concentration,[6,7,17,19] hematocrit,[6,19,107,113,120] and reticulocyte

count[6,17,19,21,107,113,120] (Fig. 2). It also was found to facilitate preoperative autologous blood donation by patients scheduled for elective orthopaedic surgery.[21,105,108-111,113,114,116,117,119,120]

In several large clinical studies, perioperative use of epoetin alfa (without PAD) markedly decreased the requirements for allogeneic blood transfusion compared with those for the placebo group, and it was particularly effective in patients who had hemoglobin concentrations of > 100 to ≤ 130 g/l[6,7,17,19] (Fig. 3). As many as 78% (21) of 27 anemic patients who had received a placebo required a transfusion[19] compared with only 14% (3 of 21) to 32% (8 of 25) of the patients who were managed with epoetin alfa at daily doses of 300 IU/kg of body weight.[6,7,17,19] The need for allogeneic blood transfusion was similarly reduced in patients who were managed with a weekly regimen of 600 IU of epoetin alfa per kg of body weight, for a total of 4 doses, beginning 3 weeks preoperatively compared with those who were managed with a daily regimen of 300 IU/kg of body weight for 15 days, beginning 10 days before surgery.[7]

Epoetin alfa is well tolerated by orthopaedic patients and has an adverse-event profile similar to that of a placebo. Because Epoetin alfa-accelerated erythropoiesis increases red blood-cell mass and blood viscosity, clinicians have been particularly concerned about the potential for deep venous thrombosis. However, in several major clinical studies, the prevalence of deep venous thrombosis in patients who had been managed with epoetin alfa was similar to that in patients who had received a placebo;[6,17,19] it also was similar to the range of prevalences of deep venous thrombosis 3% (60) of 203 patients[121] to 37% (231) of 617 patients[122] reported in the literature.[123-129]

Table 3
Efficacy of epoetin alfa in major orthopaedic surgery

Reference	No. of Patients	Procedure	Treatment, Dose	Key Findings in Patients Managed With Epoetin Alfa
Cazenave et al[106]	80	Orthopaedic or cardiovascular	Epoetin alfa, 600 or 300 IU/kg of body weight intravenously, or placebo, ×3/wk for 1 wk beginning 18 to 21 days preoperatively; iron orally	Increased predonation of ≥ 4 units of of blood; dose-related increase in red blood-cell volume and production
Tryba[107]	125	Orthopaedic	Epoetin alfa, 150, 100, or 50 IU/kg of body weight intravenously, or placebo, ×2/wk for 3 wk beginning 18 to 21 days preoperatively; iron intravenously	Increased reticulocyte count; increased predonation of ≥ 4 units of blood; reduced risk of exposure to allogeneic blood
de Andrade et al[6]	290	Hip and knee arthroplasty	Epoetin alfa, 300 or 100 IU/kg of body weight subcutaneously, or placebo, daily for 15 days beginning 10 days preoperatively; iron orally	Dose-related increase in reticulocyte count and hematocrit; reduced risk of exposure to allogeneic blood
Faris et al[19]	185	Hip and knee arthroplasty	Epoetin alfa, 300 or 100 IU/kg of body weight subcutaneously, or placebo, daily for 15 days beginning 10 days preoperatively; iron orally	Dose-related increase in reticulocyte count, hemoglobin concentration, and hematocrit; reduced risk of exposure to allogeneic blood
Goldberg et al[7]	140	Hip and knee arthroplasty	Epoetin alfa, 600 IU/kg of body weight subcutaneously for 4 doses beginning 21 days preoperative, or 300 IU/kg of body weight intravenously daily for 15 days beginning 10 days preoperative; iron orally	Increased hemoglobin concentration from baseline to preoperatively; weekly subcutaneous regimen equivalent to daily intravenous regimen in terms of transfusion needs
Cazenave et al[108]	103	Orthopaedic or vascular	Epoetin alfa, 600 or 300 IU/kg of body weight, or placebo, intravenously, ×3/wk for 1 wk beginning 18 to 21 days preoperatively; iron orally	Increased predonation of ≥ 4 units of blood; dose-related increase in red blood-cell volume and production
Lefevre et al[109]	112	Orthopaedic or vascular	Epoetin alfa, 600 or 300 IU/kg of body weight, or placebo, intravenously, ×3/wk beginning 11 to 13 days preoperatively; iron orally	Increased predonation of ≥ 4 units of blood; minimized decrease in hematocrit
Mercuriali et al[110]	38	Total hip arthroplasty	Epoetin alfa, 300, 150, or 75IU/kg of body weight, or placebo, intravenously, ×2/wk; for 3 wk; iron intravenously	Increased predonation of ≥ 4 units of blood; dose-related increase in red blood-cell volume and production and in units donated
Price et al[111]	102	Orthopaedic	Epoetin alfa, 600 IU/kg of body weight intravenously, or placebo, ×2/wk for 3 wk; iron orally	Increased predonation of blood; reduced risk of exposure to allogeneic blood
Tryba et al[112]	124	Orthopaedic	Epoetin alfa, 150, 100, or 50 IU/kg of body weight, or placebo, subcutaneously, ×2/wk for 3 wk; iron intravenously	Dose-related increase in red blood-cell volume and production and in units donated
Goodnough et al[113]	116	Orthopaedic	Epoetin alfa, 600, 300, or 150 IU/kg of body weight, or placebo, intravenously, ×2/wk for 3 wk; iron orally	Increased reticulocyte count and red blood-cell volume
Mercuriali et al[114]	23	Total hip arthroplasty	Epoetin alfa, 300 IU/kg of body weight, or placebo, intravenously, ×2/wk for 3 wk; iron intravenously	Increased predonation of ≥ 2 units of blood; reduced risk of exposure to allogeneic blood
Beris et al[115]	101	Orthopaedic	Epoetin alfa, 150 to 180 IU/kg of body weight, subcutaneously, 6 × in 3 wk, or placebo; iron orally	Increased reticulocyte count; minimized decrease in hemoglobin concentration
COPESG[17]	198	Hip arthroplasty	Epoetin alfa, 300 IU/kg of body weight daily for 14 days beginning 10 days preoperatively; placebo for 5 days, beginning 10 days preoperatively and then Epoetin alfa, 300 IU/kg of body weight, for next 9 days; or placebo	Dose-related increase in reticulocyte count and hemoglobin concentration; reduced risk of exposure to allogeneic blood
Mercuriali et al[21]	50	Total hip arthroplasty	Epoetin alfa, 600 or 300 IU/kg of body weight, or placebo, intravenously, ×2/wk for 3 wk; iron orally and intravenously	Increased predonation of blood; reduced risk of exposure to allogeneic blood
Goodnough et al[116]	44	Orthopaedic	Epoetin alfa, 600 IU/kg of body weight, or placebo, intravenously, ×2/wk for 3 wk; iron orally	Increased predonation of blood; increased red blood-cell production
Hochreiter et al[117]	82	Total hip arthroplasty	Epoetin alfa, 200 or 100 IU/kg of body weight, or placebo, intravenously, ×2/wk for 3 wk, Increased predonation of blood by mildly anemic patients	Increased predonation of blood by mildly anemic patients
Tasaki et al[118]	25	Orthopaedic	Epoetin alfa, 9000, 6000, or 3000 IU, intravenously, ×2/wk for 3 wk; iron orally and intravenously daily ×2/wk.	Dose-related increase in red blood-cell volume
Graf et al[119]	10	Total hip arthroplasty	Epoetin alfa, 150 to 200 IU/kg of body weight intravenously, 3/wk for 2 to 6 wk (6 to 18 doses)	Predonation of a mean of 4.4 units of blood; no safety concerns
Goodnough et al[120]	47	Orthopaedic	Epoetin alfa, 600 IU/kg of body weight, or placebo, intravenously, ×2/wk for 3 wk; iron orally, blood-cell volume	Minimized decrease in hematocrite caused by phlebotomy; increased red blood-cell volume

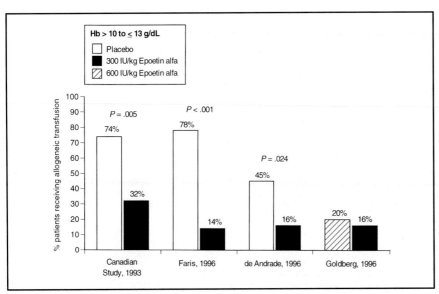

Fig. 3 Graph demonstrating the prevalence of allogeneic blood transfusion in orthopaedic patients who had a baseline hemoglobin concentration of > 100 to ≤ 130 g/l. The patients received a placebo or epoetin alfa at a dose of 300 IU/kg of body weight daily for 10 days before the procedure[6,17,19] or at a dose of 600 IU/kg of body weight once a week for 3 weeks (a total of 4 doses).[7] The p values denote the level of significance of the difference between the patients who were managed with epoetin alfa and those who received the placebo.

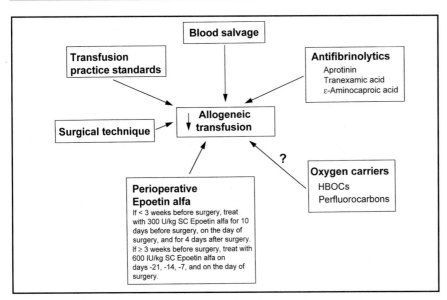

Fig. 4 Chart summarizing the options for blood management in the orthopaedic setting. Measures that have been taken to eliminate patient exposure to the risks associated with allogeneic blood transfusion include the development and promotion of transfusion standards, improvements in surgical technique, autotransfusion of blood that has been salvaged perioperatively, use of antifibrinolytics to reduce blood loss, and perioperative administration of Epoetin alfa to accelerate erythropoiesis and the preoperative buildup of red blood-cell volume. Oxygen carriers, including those that are hemoglobin-based (HBOCs) and perfluorocarbons, are currently under investigation to determine their potential role in orthopaedic procedures. SC = subcutaneous.

Overview

In summary, the ultimate goal of blood management by orthopaedic surgeons is to eliminate the need for allogeneic blood transfusion. Despite numerous important advances in surgical procedures, including changes in transfusion practices, improvements in surgical technique, and the use of intraoperative and postoperative blood salvage, patients still receive transfusions of allogeneic blood. The risks associated with such transfusions are well known. Because approximately two thirds of blood transfusions in the United States are related to surgical procedures, all clinicians working in the orthopaedic setting should be aware of the blood-conservation strategies currently available and should be cognizant of the potentially clinically relevant agents that are under development. These pharmaceutical agents include hemoglobin-based oxygen carriers and second-generation perfluorocarbons. To date, however, epoetin alfa is the only agent available for the treatment of perioperative anemia. Besides being a powerful tool for the clinical management of this condition, it also reduces the need for allogeneic blood transfusion.

Blood management has advanced to the point where the need for allogeneic blood transfusion can be eliminated or markedly reduced (Fig. 4). In the surgical setting, it is likely that combinations of blood-management options will be employed to make the possibility of allogeneic blood transfusion remote. The relative cost-effectiveness of these options, used either alone or in conjunction with other techniques, is a subject of ongoing investigation and debate.

References

1. Mezrow CK, Bergstein I, Tartter PI: Postoperative infections following autologous and homologous blood transfusions. *Transfusion* 1992;32:27–30.

2. Murphy P, Heal JM, Blumberg N: Infection or suspected infection after hip replacement surgery with autologous or homologous blood transfusions. *Transfusion* 1991;31:212–217.

3. Triulzi DJ, Vanek K, Ryan DH, Blumberg N: A clinical and immunologic study of blood transfusion and postoperative bacterial infection in spinal surgery. *Transfusion* 1992;32:517–524.

4. Fernandez MC, Gottlieb M, Menitove JE: Blood transfusion and postoperative infection in orthopedic patients. *Transfusion* 1992;32: 318–322.

5. Vamvakas EC, Moore SB: Blood transfusion and postoperative septic complications. *Transfusion* 1994;34:714–727.

6. de Andrade JR, Jove M, Landon G, Frei D, Guilfoyle, Young DC: Baseline hemoglobin as a predictor of risk of transfusion and response to epoetin alfa in orthopedic surgery patients. *Am J Orthop* 1996;25:533–542.

7. Goldberg MA, McCutchen JW, Jove M, et al: A safety and efficacy comparison study of 2 dosing regimens of epoetin alfa in patients undergoing major orthopedic surgery. *Am J Orthop* 1996;25:544–552.

8. Blumberg N, Heal JM: Immunomodulation by blood transfusion: An evolving scientific and clinical challenge. *Am J Med* 1996;101:299–308.

9. Schreiber S, Howaldt S, Schnoor M, et al: Recombinant erythropoietin for the treatment of anemia in inflammatory bowel disease. *N Engl J Med* 334:619–623.

10. Dodd RY: The risk of transfusion-transmitted infection. *N Engl J Med* 1992;327:419–421.

11. Zuckerman AJ: The new GB hepatitis viruses. *Lancet* 1995;345:1453–1454.

12. Klein HG: Allogeneic transfusion risks in the surgical patient. *Am J Surg* 1995; 170(suppl 6A):21S–26S.

13. Strang TI, Whitaker DK: Blood conservation strategies. *Curr Opin Anesthes* 1994;7:53–58.

14. Biro GP: Perfluorocarbon-based red blood cell substitutes. *Transfus Med Rev* 1993;7:84–95.

15. Dietz NM, Joyner MJ, Warner MA: Blood substitutes: Fluids, drugs, or miracle solutions? *Anesth Analg* 1996;82:390–405.

16. Scott MG, Kucik DF, Goodnough LT, Monk TG: Blood substitutes: Evolution and future applications. *Clin Chem* 1997;43:1724–1731.

17. Canadian Orthopedic Perioperative Erythropoietin Study Group: Effectiveness of perioperative recombinant human erythropoietin in elective hip replacement. *Lancet* 1993;341: 1227–1232.

18. Eschbach JW, Egrie JC, Downing MR, Browne JK, Adamson JW: Correction of the anemia of end-stage renal disease with recombinant human erythropoietin: Results of a combined phase I and II clinical trial. *N Engl J Med* 1987; 316:73–78.

19. Faris PM, Ritter MA, Abels RI: The effects of recombinant human erythropoietin on perioperative transfusion requirements in patients having a major orthopaedic operation: The American Erythropoietin Study Group. *J Bone Joint Surg* 1996;78A:62–72.

20. Lamm DL, Crawford ED, Blumenstein B, Crissman J, deVere White R: Abstract: SWOG 8795:A randomized comparison of bacillus Calmette-Gu,rin and mitomycin C prophylaxis in stage TA and T1 transitional cell carcinoma of the bladder. *J Urol* 1993;149:282A.

21. Mercuriali F, Zanella A, Barosi G, et al: Use of erythropoietin to increase the volume of autologous blood donated by orthopedic patients. *Transfusion* 1993;33:55–60.

22. Winearls, CG, Oliver DO, Pippard M.J, Reid C, Downing MR, Cotes PM: Effect of human erythropoietin derived from recombinant DNA on the anaemia of patients maintained by chronic haemodialysis. *Lancet* 1986;2:1175–1178.

23. Goodnough LT, Despotis GJ: Establishing practice guidelines for surgical blood management. *Am J Surg* 1995;170(suppl 6A):16S–20S.

24. American College of Physicians: Practice strategies for elective red blood cell transfusion. *Ann Intern Med* 1992;116:403–406.

25. Carson JL, Willett LR: Is a hemoglobin of 10g/dL required for surgery? *Med Clin North Am* 1993;77:335–347.

26. Nelson CL, Bowen WS: Total hip arthroplasty in Jehovah's Witnesses without blood transfusion. *J Bone Joint Surg* 1986;68A:350–353.

27. Nelson CL, Fontenot HJ: Ten strategies to reduce blood loss in orthopedic surgery. *Am J Surg* 1995;170(suppl 6A):64S–68S.

28. Spence RK: Surgical red blood cell transfusion practice policies: Blood Management Practice Guidelines Conference. *Am J Surg* 1995; 70(suppl 6A):3S–15S.

29. Spence RK, Carson JA, Poses R, et al: Elective surgery without transfusion: Influence of preoperative hemoglobin level and blood loss on mortality. *Am J Surg* 1990;159:320–324.

30. Viele MK, Weiskopf RB: What can we learn about the need for transfusion from patients who refuse blood? The experience with Jehovah's Witnesses. *Transfusion* 1994;34: 396–401.

31. Consensus Conference: Perioperative red blood cell transfusion. *JAMA* 1988;260: 2700–2703.

32. Fasulo F, Giori A, Fissi S, Bozzetti F, Doci R, Gennari L: Cavitron Ultrasonic Surgical Aspirator (CUSA) in liver resection. *Int Surg* 1992;77:64–66.

33. Miller E, Paull DE, Morrissey K, Cortese A, Nowak E: Scalpel versus electrocautery in modified radical mastectomy. *Am J Surg* 1988; 54:284–286.

34. Wyman A, Rogers K: Randomized trial of laser scalpel for modified radical mastectomy. *Br J Surg* 1993;80:871–873.

35. Shah DM, Chang BB, Paty PS, Kaufman JL, Koslow AR, Leather RP: Treatment of abdominal aortic aneurysm by exclusion and bypass: An analysis of outcome. *J Vasc Surg* 1991;13: 15–20.

36. Terblanche J, Krige JE, Bornman PC: Simplified hepatic resection with the use of prolonged vascular inflow occlusion. *Arch Surg* 1991;126:298–301.

37. Sharrock NE, Mineo R, Urquhart B, Salvati EA: The effect of two levels of hypotension on intraoperative blood loss during total hip arthroplasty performed under lumbar epidural anesthesia. *Anesth Analg* 1993;76:580–584.

38. Kram HB, Nathan RC, Stafford FJ, Fleming AW, Shoemaker WC: Fibrin glue achieves hemostasis in patients with coagulation disorders. *Arch Surg* 1989;124:385–387.

39. Hayes A, Murphy DB, McCarroll M: The efficacy of single-dose aprotinin 2 million KIU in reducing blood loss and its impact on the incidence of deep venous thrombosis in patients undergoing total hip replacement surgery. *J Clin Anesth* 1996;8:357–360.

40. Janssens M, Joris J, David JL, Lemaire R, Lamy M: High-dose aprotinin reduces blood loss in patients undergoing total hip replacement surgery. *Anesthesiology* 1994;80:23–29.

41. Llau JV, Hoyas L, Higueras J, Ezpeleta J, Garcia-Polit J: Letter: Aprotinin reduces intraoperative bleeding during spinal arthrodesis interventions (Spanish). *Rev Esp Anestesiol Reanim* 1996;43:118.

42. Murkin JM, Shannon NA, Bourne RB, Rorabeck CH, Cruickshank M, Wyile G: Aprotinin decreases blood loss in patients undergoing revision or bilateral total hip arthroplasty. *Anesth Analg* 1995;80:343–348.

43. Parodi JC, Criado FJ, Barone HD, Schonholz C, Queral L: Endoluminal aortic aneurysm repair using a balloon-expandable stent-graft device: A progress report. *Ann Vasc Surg* 1994;8: 523–529.

44. Utada K, Matayoshi Y, Sumi C, et al: Aprotinin 2 million KIU reduces perioperative blood loss in patients undergoing primary total hip replacement (Japanese). *Masui* 1997;46:77–82.

45. Yusuf SW, Baker DM, Chuter TA Whitaker SC, Wenham PW, Hopkinson BR: Transfemoral endoluminal repair of abdominal aortic aneurysm with bifurcated graft. *Lancet* 1994; 344:650–651.

46. Benoni G, Fredin H: Fibrinolytic inhibition with tranexamic acid reduces blood loss and blood transfusion after knee arthroplasty: A prospective, randomised, double-blind study of 86 patients. *J Bone Joint Surg* 1996;78B:434–440.

47. Benoni G, Lethagen S, Fredin H: The effect of tranexamic acid on local and plasma fibrinolysis during total knee arthroplasty. *Thromb Res* 1997; 85:195–206.

48. Benoni G, Carlsson A, Petersson C, Fredin H: Does tranexamic acid reduce blood loss in knee arthroplasty? *Am J Knee Surg* 1995;8:88–92.

49. Hiippala ST, Strid LJ, Wennerstrand MI, et al: Tranexamic acid radically decreases blood loss and transfusions associated with total knee arthroplasty. *Anesth Analg* 1997;84:839-844.

50. Howes JP, Sharma V, Cohen AT: Tranexamic acid reduces blood loss after knee arthroplasty. *J Bone Joint Surg* 1996;78B:995–996.

51. Chen RH, Frazier OH, Cooley DA: Anti-fibrinolytic therapy in cardiac surgery. *Tex Heart Inst J* 1995;22:211–215.

52. Landymore RW, Murphy JT, Lummis H, Carter C: The use of low-dose aprotinin, epsilon-aminocaproic acid or tranexamic acid for prevention of mediastinal bleeding in patients receiving aspirin before coronary artery bypass operations. *Eur J Cardiothorac Surg* 1997; 11:798–800.

53. Penta de Peppo A, Pierri MD, Scafuri A, et al: Intraoperative antifibrinolysis and blood-saving techniques in cardiac surgery: Prospective trial of 3 antifibrinolytic drugs. *Tex Heart Inst J* 1995;22:231–236.

54. Karnezis TA, Stulberg SD, Wixson RL, Reilly P: The hemostatic effects of desmopressin on patients who had total joint arthroplasty: A double-blind randomized trial. *J Bone Joint Surg* 1994;76A:1545–1550.

55. Schott U, Sollen C, Axelsson K, Rugarn P, Allvin I: Desmopressin acetate does not reduce blood loss during total hip replacement in patients receiving dextran. *Acta Anaesthesiol Scand* 1995;39:592–598.

56. Theroux MC, Corddry DH, Tietz AE, Miller F, Peoples JD, Kettrick R G: A study of desmopressin and blood loss during spinal fusion for neuromuscular scoliosis: A randomized, controlled, doubleblinded study. *Anesthesiology* 1997; 87:260–267.

57. Goodnough LT, Vizmeg K, Sobecks R, Schwarz A, Soegiarso W: Prevalence and classification of anemia in elective orthopedic surgery patients: Implications for blood conservation programs. *Vox Sang* 1992;63:90–95.

58. Toy PT, Kaplan EB, McVay PA, Lee SJ, Strauss RG, Stehling LC: Blood loss and replacement in total hip arthroplasty: A multicenter study. The Preoperative Autologous Blood Donation Study Group. *Transfusion* 1992;32:63–67.

59. Arnestad JP, Bengtsson A, Bengtson JP, Tylman M, Redl H, Schlag G: Formation of cytokines by retransfusion of shed whole blood. *Br J Anaesth* 1994;72:422–425.

60. Sculco TP: Blood management in orthopedic surgery. *Am J Surg* 1995;170(suppl6A):60S–63S.

61. Han CD, Shin DE: Postoperative blood salvage and reinfusion after total joint arthroplasty. *J Arthroplasty* 1997;12:511–516.

62. Simpson MB, Murphy KP, Chambers HG, Bucknell AL: The effect of postoperative wound drainage reinfusion in reducing the need for blood transfusions in elective total joint arthroplasty: A prospective, randomized study. *Orthopedics* 1994;17:133–137.

63. Slagis SV, Benjamin JB, Volz RG, Giordano GF: Postoperative blood salvage in total hip and knee arthroplasty: A randomised controlled trial. *J Bone Joint Surg* 1991;73B:591–594.

64. Gannon DM, Lombardi AV Jr, Mallory TH, Vaughn BK, Finney CR, Niemcryk S: An evaluation of the efficacy of postoperative blood salvage after total joint arthroplasty: A prospective randomized trial. *J Arthroplasty* 1991;6:109–114.

65. Faris PM, Ritter MA, Keating EM, Valeri CR: Unwashed filtered shed blood collected after knee and hip arthroplasties: A source of autologous red blood cells. *J Bone Joint Surg* 1991;73A: 1169–1178.

66. Ayers DC, Murray DG, Duerr DM: Blood salvage after total hip arthroplasty. *J Bone Joint Surg* 1995;77A:1347–1351.

67. Goodnough LT, Verbruuge D, Marcus RE: The relationship between hematocrit, blood lost, and blood transfused in total knee replacement: Implications for postoperative blood salvage and reinfusion. *Am J Knee Surg* 1995;8:83–87.

68. Huo MH, Paly WL, Keggi KJ: Effect of preoperative autologous blood donation and intraoperative and postoperative blood recovery on homologous blood transfusion requirement in cementless total hip replacement operation. *J Am Coll Surg* 1995;180:561–567.

69. Marks RM, Vaccaro AR, Balderston RA, Hozack WJ, Booth RE Jr, Rothman RH: Postoperative blood salvage in total knee arthroplasty using the Solcotrans autotransfusion system. *J Arthroplasty* 1995;10:433–437.

70. Law JK, Wiedel JD: Autotransfusion in revision total hip arthroplasties using uncemented prostheses. *Clin Orthop* 1989;245:145–149.

71. Council on Scientific Affairs: Autologous blood transfusions. *JAMA* 1986;256:2378–2380.

72. Devine P, Postoway N, Hoffstadter L, et al: Blood donation and transfusion practices: The 1990 American Association of Blood Banks Institutional Membership Questionnaire. *Transfusion* 1992;32:683–687.

73. Surgenor DM, Wallace EL, Hao SH, Chapman RH: Collection and transfusion of blood in the United States, 1982-1988. *N Engl J Med* 1990; 322:1646–1651.

74. Wasman J, Goodnough LT: Autologous blood donation for elective surgery: Effect on physician transfusion behavior. *JAMA* 1987;258: 3135–3137.

75. Goodnough LT, Shafron D, Marcus RE: The impact of preoperative autologous blood donation on orthopaedic surgical practice. *Vox Sang* 1990;59:65–69.

76. Woolson ST, Watt JM: Use of autologous blood in total hip replacement: A comprehensive program. *J Bone Joint Surg* 1991;73A:76–80.

77. Cohen JA, Brecher ME: Preoperative autologous blood donation: Benefit or detriment? A mathematical analysis. *Transfusion* 1995;35: 640–644.

78. Goodnough LT, Brittenham GM: Limitations of the erythropoietic response to serial phlebotomy: Implications for autologous blood donor programs. *J Lab Clin Med* 1990;115: 28–35.

79. Kickler TS, Spivak JL: Effect of repeated whole blood donations on serum immunoreactive erythropoietin levels in autologous donors. *JAMA* 1988;260:65–67.

80. Holland PV, Schmidt PH (eds): *Standards for Blood Banks and Transfusion Services*, ed 12.

Arlington, VA, American Association of Blood Banks, 1987.

81. AuBuchon JP: Cost-effectiveness of preoperative autologous blood donation for orthopedic and cardiac surgeries. *Am J Med* 1996;101: 38S–42S.

82. Domen RE: Preoperative autologous blood donation: Clinical, economic, and ethical issues. *Cleve Clin J Med* 1996;63:295–300.

83. Rosenblatt MA, Cantos EM Jr, Mohandas K: Intraoperative hemodilution is more cost-effective than preoperative autologous donation for patients undergoing procedures associated with a low risk for transfusion. *J Clin Anesth* 1997;9:26–29.

84. Mott LS, Jones MJ: Autologous blood donation in a small general acute-care hospital. *J Nat Med Assoc* 1995;87:549–552.

85. Messmer K, Kreimeier U, Intaglietta M: Present state of intentional hemodilution. *Eur Surg Res* 1996;18:254–263.

86. D'Ambra MN, Kaplan DK: Alternatives to allogeneic blood use in surgery: Acute normovolemic hemodilution and preoperative autologous donation. *Am J Surg* 1995;170 (suppl 6A): 49S–52S.

87. Oishi CS, D'Lima DD, Morris BA, Hardwick ME, Berkowitz SD, Colwell CW Jr: Hemodilution with other blood reinfusion techniques in total hip arthroplasty. *Clin Orthop* 1997;339:132–139.

88. Vamvakas EC, Taswell HF: Epidemiology of blood transfusion. *Transfusion* 1994;34:464–470.

89. Cumming PD, Wallace EL, Schorr JB, Dodd RY: Exposure of patients to human immunodeficiency virus through the transfusion of blood components that test antibody-negative. *N Engl J Med* 1989;321:941–946.

90. Donahue JG, Muñoz A, Ness PM, et al: The declining risk of post-transfusion hepatitis C virus infection. *N Engl J Med* 1992;327:369–373.

91. Schriemer PA, Longnecker DE, Mintz PD: The possible inmmunosuppressive effects of perioperative blood transfusion in cancer patients. *Anesthesiology* 1998;68:422–428.

92. Amberson WR, Jennings JJ, Rhode CM: Clinical experience with hemoglobin-saline solutions. *J Appl Physiol* 1949;1:469–489.

93. Bunn HF, Esham WT, Bull RW: The renal handling of hemoglobin: I. Glomerular filtration. *J Exp Med* 1969;129:909–923.

94. Fratantoni JC: Blood substitutes: Problems and prospects, in AuBuchon JP, Issitt LA (eds): *Limiting Donor Exposure in Hemotherapy*. Bethesda, MD, American Association of Blood Banks, 1994 pp 61–73.

95. Roberge JQ: Search narrows for "blood substitutes." *Biotech Lab Inst* 1996;6.

96. Faithfull NS, Keipert PE, Rhoades GE, Bradley JD, Trouwborst A: Development and validation of a computer model for evaluation of efficacy of perfluorochemical emulsions. *Artif Cells Blood Substit Immobil Biotechnol* 1994;22:A96.

97. Keipert PE, Faithfull NS, Bradley JD, et al: Oxygen delivery augmentation by low-dose perfluorochemical emulsion during profound normovolemic hemodilution, in Vaupel P, Zander R, Bruley DF (eds): *Oxygen Transport to Tissue XV*. New York, NY, Plenum Press, 1994, pp 197–204.

98. Biro GP, Blais, P: Perfluorocarbon blood substitutes. *Crit Rev Oncol Hematol* 1987;6:311–374.

99. Hong F, Shastri KA, Logue GL, Spaulding MB: Complement activation by artificial blood substitute Fluosol: In vitro and in vivo studies. *Transfusion* 1991;31:642–647.

100. Hubmayr RD, Rodarte JR: Acute and long-term effects of Fluosol-DA 20% on respiratory system mechanics and diffusion capacity in dogs. *J Crit Care* 1988;3232–239.

101. Riess JG: Fluorocarbon-based in vivo oxygen transport and delivery systems. *Vox Sang* 1991; 61:225–239.

102. Keipert PE: Use of Oxygent, a perfluorochemical-based oxygen carrier, as an alternative to intraoperative blood transfusion. *Artif Cells Blood Substit Immobil Biotechnol* 1995;23: 381–394.

103. Storring PL, Gaines Das RE: The International Standard for Recombinant DNA-derived Erythropoietin: Collaborative study of 4 recombinant DNA-derived erythropoietins and two highly purified human urinary erythropoietins. *J Endocrinol* 1992;134:459–484.

104. West JB (ed): *Respiratory Physiology: The Essentials*, ed 3. Baltimore, MD, Williams & Wilkins, 1985.

105. Goodnough LT, Soegiarso RW, Geha AS: Blood lost and blood transfused in coronary artery bypass graft operation as implications for blood transfusion and blood conservation strategies. *Surg Gynecol Obstet* 1993;177:345–351.

106. Cazenave JP, Irrmann C, Waller C, et al: Epoetin alfa facilitates presurgical autologous blood donation in nonanaemic patients scheduled for orthopaedic or cardiovascular surgery. *Eur J Anaesthesiol* 1997;14:432–442.

107. Tryba M: Epoetin alfa plus autologous blood donation in patients with a low hematocrit scheduled to undergo orthopedic surgery. *Semin Hematol* 1997;33(suppl 2):22–24.

108. Cazenave JP, Sondag D, Genetet B, et al: Abstract: Recombinant human erythropoietin in nonanaemic patients scheduled for orthopaedic or cardiovascular surgery, to facilitate perisurgical autologous blood donation. *Br J Anaesth* 1995;74(suppl 1):64.

109. Lefevre P, Tryba M, Fournel JJ, et al: Abstract: Recombinant human erythropoietin in nonanaemic patients scheduled for elective surgery to facilitate presurgical autologous blood donation combined with normovolaemic haemodilution. *Br J Anaesth* 1995;74(suppl 1):64.

110. Mercuriali F, Gualtieri G, Biffi E, et al: Abstract: Randomized, double-blind, placebo-controlled dose-finding study with recombinant human erythropoietin to facilitate autologous blood donation in low haematocrit patients undergoing total hip replacement. *Br J Anaesth* 1995;74(suppl 1):63.

111. Price TH, Goodnough LT, Vogler W, et al: Abstract: Effect of recombinant human erythropoietin (epoetin alfa) administration on allogenic blood use during orthopaedic surgery. *Br J Anaesth* 1995;74(suppl 1):64.

112. Tryba M, Kindler D, Schulte-Tamburen A: Abstract: Preoperative use of recombinant human erythropoietin (epoetin alfa) in patients scheduled for orthopaedic surgery to facilitate autologous blood donation. *Br J Anaesth* 1995; 74(suppl 1):63.

113. Goodnough LT, Price TH, Friedman KD, et al: A phase III trial of recombinant human erythropoietin therapy in nonanemic orthopedic patients subjected to aggressive removal of blood for autologous use: Dose, response, toxicity, and efficacy. *Transfusion* 1994;34:66–71.

114. Mercuriali F, Gualtieri G, Sinigaglia L, et al: Use of recombinant human erythropoietin to assist autologous blood donation by anemic rheumatoid arthritis patients undergoing major orthopedic surgery. *Transfusion* 1994;34:501–506.

115. Beris P, Mermillod B, Levy G, et al: Recombinant human erythropoietin as adjuvant treatment for autologous blood donation: A prospective study. *Vox Sang* 1993;65:212–218.

116. Goodnough LT, Price TH, Rudnick S, Soegiarso RW: Preoperative red cell production in patients undergoing aggressive autologous blood phlebotomy with and without erythropoietin therapy. *Transfusion* 1992;32:441–445.

117. Hochreiter J, Nietsche D, Oswald J, Jakubek H, Michlmayr G, Hohenwallner W: Preoperative autologous blood collection under erythropoietin stimulation: Preliminary results in patient selection, erythropoietin dosage and administration (German). *Z Orthop Ihre Grenzgeb* 1992;130:519–523.

118. Tasaki T, Ohto H, Hashimoto C, Abe R, Saitoh A, Kikuchi S: Recombinant human erythropoietin for autologous blood donation: Effects on

119. perioperative red-blood-cell and serum erythropoietin production. *Lancet* 1992;339:773–775.

119. Graf H, Watzinger U, Ludvik B, Wagner A, Hocker P, Zweymuller KK: Recombinant human erythropoietin as adjuvant treatment for autologous blood donation. *Br Med J* 1990;300: 1627–1628.

120. Goodnough LT, Rudnick S, Price TH, et al: Increased preoperative collection of autologous blood with recombinant human erythropoietin therapy. *N Engl J Med* 1989;321:1163–1168.

121. Kraay MJ, Goldberg VM, Herbener TE: Vascular ultrasonography for deep venous thrombosis after total knee arthroplasty. *Clin Orthop* 1993;286:18–26.

122. Hull R, Raskob G, Pineo G, et al: A comparison of subcutaneous low-molecular-weight heparin with warfarin sodium for prophylaxis against deep-vein thrombosis after hip or knee implantation. *N Engl J Med* 1993;329:1370–1376.

123. Bursten S, Weeks R, West J, et al: Potential role for phosphatidic acid in mediating the inflammatory responses to TNF alpha and IL-1 beta. *Circ Shock* 1994;44:14–29.

124. Davidson BL, Elliott CG, Lensing AW: Low accuracy of color Doppler ultrasound in the detection of proximal leg vein thrombosis in asymptomatic high-risk patients: The RD Heparin Arthroplasty Group. *Ann Intern Med* 1992;117:735–738.

125. Imperiale TF, Speroff T: A meta-analysis of methods to prevent venous thromboembolism following total hip replacement. *JAMA* 1994; 271:1780–1785.

126. Isaacs C, Paltiel O, Blake G, Beaudet M, Conochie L, Leclerc J: Age-associated risks of prophylactic anticoagulation in the setting of hip fracture. *Am J Med* 1994;96:487–491.

127. Mohr DN, Silverstein MD, Murtaugh PA, Harrison JM: Prophylactic agents for venous thrombosis in elective hip surgery: Meta-analysis of studies using venographic assessment. *Arch Intern Med* 1993;153:2221–2228.

128. O'Brien BJ, Anderson DR, Goeree R: Cost-effectiveness of enoxaparin versus warfarin prophylaxis against deep-vein thrombosis after total hip replacement. *Can Med Assoc J* 1994; 150:1083–1090.

129. Pellegrini VD Jr, Langhans MJ, Totterman S, Marder VJ, Francis CW: Embolic complications of calf thrombosis following total hip arthroplasty. *J Arthroplasty* 1993;8:449–457.

Outcomes Assessment in the Information Age: Available Instruments, Data Collection, and Utilization of Data

Barry P. Simmons, MD
Mark F. Swiontkowski, MD
Roger W. Evans, PhD
Peter C. Amadio, MD
Willie Cats-Baril, PhD

Introduction

The purpose of this chapter is to introduce the reader to the concept of outcomes research, to explain how it differs from traditional research, and to describe how the information can be collected and used.

What is outcomes research? It is a wide spectrum of research activities that include assessment of treatment, measurement of treatment, and, when that data is gathered, management of the treatment. However, the single easiest way to differentiate outcomes research from traditional research is that it is patient based rather than process based. Outcomes research covers what the patient thinks of the results of the medical care he or she has been given; traditional research covers the standard evaluation of range of motion, strength, radiographs, etc. Outcomes research is in no way meant to replace the usual methods of research in the evaluation of treatment for musculoskeletal disease; it is meant to add another dimension for evaluation.

Medical care has entered an era of critical assessment and accountability,[1-4] as health care providers, patients, insurers, government agencies, and employers seek to determine whether specific interventions satisfy the needs of patients. The general medical and orthopaedic communities have responded to this mandate by calling for studies of the outcomes of treatment of common conditions. This research requires measures of outcome that address patients' principal concerns,[1,4] which, in orthopaedic conditions, include relief of symptoms and functional improvement.[5]

John E. Wennberg has been a major figure in the development of outcomes research. In his index paper in 1973,[6] he states that "Experience with a population based health data system in Vermont reveals that there are wide variations of resource input, utilization of services, and expenditures among neighboring communities. Variations in utilization indicate that there is considerable uncertainty about the effectiveness of different levels of aggregate as well as specific kinds of health services." An example is in Table 1, which is an analysis of carpal tunnel releases for the year 1990 to 1991 in different counties within the state of Maine. For no apparent reason, there is a considerable variation in carpal tunnel releases from York County (0.7 per thousand people) to Dover/Greenville County (2.1 per thousand people). This table is not meant to imply which of the rates is correct. Perhaps the citizens of

Table 1
Area specific annual rates of carpal tunnel release: 1990–1991*

Area	Population	Cases/1,000	WC Cases/1,000
York	18,570	0.7	0.1
Sanford	28,899	0.8	0.3
Biddeford	62,296	1.0	0.4
Portland	212,830	1.1	0.3
Bangor	110,585	1.2	0.5
Augusta	76,673	1.2	0.5
Rockland	51,970	1.6	0.5
Bath	27,947	1.8	0.7
Dover/Greenville	25,119	2.1	1.2
Total	1,227,926	1.2	0.4

*Select Maine hospital service areas; rates unadjusted; WC, Workers' Compensation

York County are getting less good results because they are not having higher rates of carpal tunnel release. Unpublished data that we have gathered suggest that, depending on the severity of symptoms, carpal tunnel release is the best treatment for carpal tunnel syndrome when compared to nonsurgical measures.

A good example of the "patient satisfaction" factor is an analysis of total hip replacement.[5] When the results are evaluated by the usual criteria, as interpreted by the surgeon, the success rate is 86%. However, when an independent health researcher surveyed the patients, only 55% had their "expectations" fulfilled.

Obviously, outcomes research is not confined to the area of musculoskeletal disease. In an evaluation of a prostatectomy for benign prostatic hypertrophy, despite the fact that the procedure was effective in reducing symptoms in 93% of severely and 79% of moderately symptomatic patients, there was no statistically significant improvement in indices of quality of life in any patients except those with severe symptoms or acute retention.[7] Furthermore, postprostatectomy patients had a 4% incidence of incontinence and a 5% incidence of impedance, which made both patients and urologists examine the indications for the procedure.

Outcomes research involves a broad spectrum of input, from not only physicians, but also from statisticians and health care researchers. Retrospective methodologies are available using the Medicare statistical file system, claims data systems, or meta-analysis, but all of these are expensive and have serious drawbacks because of the initial intent of the information entered, which was not for outcomes research.[8] Meta-analysis has played a significant role in clinical research. Meta-analysis is a research

tool in which multiple articles involving small series of patients can be combined to produce statistically significant data. However, for the articles to be included, they have to conform to a rather rigorous protocol. Unfortunately, most articles in the orthopaedic literature do not satisfy the protocols of well-controlled, prospective studies.

Instruments and Techniques for Orthopaedic Outcomes Assessment

This section describes the currently available questionnaires for use in orthopaedic practice and the process used to develop them. More detail on the development of the MFA (Musculoskeletal Functional Assessment) Index is provided. The section will also provide suggestions on how to use these tools in orthopaedic practice.

Health-Related Quality of Life (HRQL) Instruments in Common Use for Musculoskeletal Problems

Questionnaires should not be derived by aggregating questions that seem important based on a clinician's experience. Questions that are reflective of patient function cannot simply be developed based on clinical opinion, because physicians' perceptions of functional issues may be inaccurate. Guyatt and associates[9] have described the steps in the development of a functional assessment questionnaire.

Item Development The patient population to be evaluated must be described, and functional issues of concern to this group must be derived from interviewing patients and clinicians, or alternatively, selected from literature and validated questionnaire review.

Item Reduction This is determined by frequency and importance

of item endorsement in a sample patient cohort or by statistical methods, such as factor analysis.

Format Selection Scaled responses (Likert Scales) are compared with endorsed statements. The former yield better discrimination but are more difficult for patients. An endorsed statement format is much easier for patients.

Pretesting The questionnaire is administered with an interviewer present to discover poorly worded or confusing items.

Reproducibility and Responsiveness Reproducibility is first evaluated by reviewing the variability in responses in relation to the variability in clinical status. It then is evaluated by a "test-retest" exercise in which the same patients complete the questionnaire twice in a short interval during which no clinical change has taken place. Responsiveness is the measure of the questionnaire's ability to detect clinically important changes even if they are small. Responsiveness analysis involves administering the questionnaire twice at a minimum 3-month interval after a clinical intervention of known efficacy.

Validity Face validity is assessed by clinician review. Construct validity is assessed by developing hypotheses about how the scores should change between and within subjects and by comparison with already validated instruments. Criterion validity is addressed by comparing scores with objective tests (range of motion, self-selected walking speed, etc) and by clinician evaluations of the same group of patients.

Several health status instruments have been developed and validated and are available for use in assessing patient function following musculoskeletal injury. The 4 most widely used and evaluated scales that are appropriate for use in musculoskeletal disease/injury are the Short Form-36 (SF-36), the Sickness Impact Profile (SIP), the Nottingham Health Profile, and the Quality of Well Being Scale (QWB), which forms the backbone of the Quality Adjusted Life Years (QALYs) methodology.[10] These scales share the common characteristic of assessing all "domains" of human activity, including physical, psychological, social, and role functioning. In addition, they share the characteristic of assessing the patient as a whole (from the patient's perspective) and not as an organ system, disease, procedure, or limb. They are internally consistent, reproducible, can discriminate between clinical conditions of different severity, and are sensitive to change in health status over time.[11] There are added benefits derived from the fact that they are not physician administered, which increases their reliability; patients will frequently underreport functional disability to their physicians. Brief descriptions of these instruments follow.

The SF-36 was developed by Ware and associates[12–16] and the Rand Corporation as a part of the Medical Outcomes Study. It is the most widely applied general health status instrument and has certain features that make it the most appealing for studying musculoskeletal disease. Its 36 scaled questions relate to 6 different functional subscales: bodily pain, role function (physical and mental health), social function, physical function, energy/fatigue, and general health perceptions. The scales are scored separately, and there is no aggregate scale, a feature that seems to limit its utility somewhat. The SF-36 has been validated to be a reliable and reproducible questionnaire that has been applied to numerous health conditions. Furthermore, it has been validated to be reliable whether ad-

ministered by the patient, by an interviewer, by telephone, or by mail, and it only takes 5 to 7 minutes to complete. These features make its use appealing; the SF-36 is the most practical for use in a busy office or clinic setting. This instrument, however, may well have a "floor effect" for musculoskeletal conditions; that is, clinically important functional problems may not be adequately characterized by this scale because the disability is too minimal to be picked up by the questions in the scale. This scale is more often recommended to researchers who wish to study musculoskeletal injury than the other scales discussed here. Our experience in administering the SF-36 shows that patients with musculoskeletal disease or injury tend to misinterpret the questions on general health as being exclusive of their musculoskeletal disease.[17,18] It has relative weakness in assessing upper extremity function.

The SIP is a 136-item questionnaire developed by Bergner and associates[19–21] at the University of Washington that is best administered by trained interviewers and takes 25 to 35 minutes to complete. It has 12 different domains, which are addressed by the endorsable statements; the patient simply affirms "yes" or "no" if the statement of function applies to their current situation. These 12 areas are scored independently and aggregated into physical and psychosocial subscales, as well as 1 aggregate score. The scale is 0 to 100 points; the higher the score, the worse the disability. Scores in excess of the mid 30s bring serious quality of life issues into question. The SIP has also been used in multiple health conditions, which make comparisons of impact of disease on health possible. It has been used in musculoskeletal trauma with good

success.[22,23] Because of the difficulty and length of administration it may be most useful for well-funded outcome studies or controlled trials. It is likely that it also suffers from the "floor effect," in which lesser degrees of musculoskeletal function are not detected.

The Nottingham Health Profile is interviewer administered and has been successfully used to assess functional outcomes of limb salvage versus early amputation.[24–26] It has been shown to be valid in trials in Great Britain and Sweden. Part I of the profile measures subjective health status through a series of 38 weighted questions that assess impairments in the categories of sleep, emotional reaction, mobility, energy level, pain, and social isolation. In each category, 100 points represents maximal disability and 0 represents no limitations. Part II consists of 7 statements that require yes or no responses. These assess the influence of health problems on job, home, family life, sexual function, recreation, and enjoyment of the holidays. The responses to both parts of the profile can be compared to the average scores for the population as a whole with similar age and sex distributions.

The QWB is the foundation for QALYs and was designed to be a commonly used effectiveness measure for policy analysis and resource allocation. Patients are asked to respond to questions regarding their level of physical activity (3 levels), mobility (3 levels), social activity (5 levels), and according to the 1 symptom or problem that bothers them the most on the day the questionnaire is administered (choice of 22 symptom complexes). The QWB is calculated by combining preference weights that were derived from responses to a household survey that asked respondents to rate their preferences for various health states on a 1 to 10 scale ranging from death to perfect health. The methodology for using the quiz is somewhat complex. Multiple QWB scores are calculated separately for each of 6 days preceding the interview and the final score is taken as the average of the 6 scores. The scale ranges from 0 equals death to 1 equals perfect health. The QWB is interviewer administered. Using data from large populations, and multiplying the data times years of life expectancy and cost per intervention gives the QALY; cost per year of well life expectancy. QALYs provide a methodology for making difficult decisions regarding resource allocation. When orthopaedic interventions, such as hip arthroplasty and hip fracture fixation, have been studied using this methodology they have fared well.[10,27] The QWB physical function scale also likely suffers from the "floor effect."

The above examples are general health status instruments that have broad acceptance and lend the ability to compare the functional impact of various diseases. Disease- or condition-specific instruments, such as the carpal tunnel syndrome instrument, offer increased sensitivity and maximum limitation of floor and ceiling effects.[28] Table 2 lists the general health status instruments individually with their attributes and identifies a source for the reader.

Development of a Musculoskeletal Outcomes Research Tool

In response to the need for a validated instrument that would allow clinicians to determine the functional outcome of patients with musculoskeletal disease or injury (extremity trauma, overuse syndromes, osteoarthritis, or rheumatoid arthritis), the MFA was recently developed under National Institutes of Health/

National Institute of Child Health and Human Development (NIH/NICHHD) funding.[17,18,29] This 100-item instrument allows clinicians to assess patients' function in 10 distinct domains (self-care, emotional, recreation, household work, employment, sleep and rest, relationships, thinking, activities using arms and legs, and activities using hands). The MFA long form requires 15 to 17 minutes to complete and can be either self or interviewer administered. When used by members of the medical community who treat musculoskeletal disease, it will allow for analyses of the effectiveness of treatment and comparisons of the functional impact of various diseases and injuries. The floor effect that other general health status instruments suffer from has been significantly improved upon.[18,29]

The MFA was field tested on the populations of extremity trauma, overuse syndrome, osteoarthritis, and rheumatoid arthritis. These specific populations were chosen because they account for significant costs, both to the patient and to society. Extremity trauma costs range from $75 to $150 billion annually.[30–32] Overuse injuries accounted for 48% of the reported occupational injuries in 1988. Surgical procedures related to carpal tunnel syndrome alone add medical costs of over $1 billion.[33] Arthritis and related diseases have associated costs due to resultant morbidity, estimated to be as high as $41.6 billion.[33] Numerous joint- and procedure-specific evaluation scales are currently in use (Harris Hip Score, Indiana Knee Scale, etc) but these arbitrarily mix clinical and functional outcomes, and few have been subjected to rigorous statistical validation.

The MFA is a quality of life instrument, with an emphasis on the musculoskeletal system and muscu-

loskeletal disease. Its domains are designed to give treating physicians categories they can identify with and use to help target treatment for individual patients. Because it is a single instrument dealing with all extremity disorders, it alleviates the need for community practices to have multiple outcome tools available for patient use and different skills to interpret them.

The MFA was developed using unstructured open-ended patient interviews with 136 patients and 12 clinicians, resulting in 6,800 statements in 25 domains. These items, using the patients' own wording whenever possible, were reduced into a 12-domain, 177-item questionnaire. Three hundred and twenty-seven patients from the Seattle Hand Clinic, Valley Medical Center (level 2 trauma center), Northwest Foot and Ankle Clinic, and Harborview Medical Center (level 1 trauma center) participated in the first field trial of the MFA. Reliability was between 72.6% and 100% for all items. Internal consistency was 0.85 based on Cronbach's alpha. Validity was assessed by comparing objective measures (eg, range of motion, self-selected walking speed, grip dynamometer, isokinetic testing) on 119 patients to relevant domains. Significant relationships ($r > 0.33$) were found between objective measure scores and category scores in mobility, housework, fine motor, self-care, and confinement.[23] Physician assessment based on medical record and radiograph review on a sample of 24 patients demonstrated correlations between 0.04 and 0.50. Significant relationships were also found by comparing survey scores with the presence of comorbidities, complications, gender, joint degeneration (arthritis), functional level (overuse), and injury severity scale. The survey was then reduced to its final 100-item format

Table 2
HRQOL Instruments and Scoring Resources

	Method of Administration	Training Time Required	Length of Time to Complete	Populations Designed For	Conditions Used On	Where/How to Get It
SF-36	Self or interviewer	2 hours	5 to 10 minutes	All	General health status/quality of life measures	Medical Outcomes Trust 20 Park Plaza, Suite 1014 Boston, MA 02116-4313
SIP	Self or interviewer	1 week	30 minutes	All	General health status/quality of life measures	Ann Skinne 624 N Broadway, Rm 647 Baltimore, MD 21205
WOMAC	Self	1 week	10 minutes	Arthritis patient	Arthritis	Jane Campbell London Health Science Center, Suite 303 South Campus 375 South St London, Ontario N6A 4G5 CANADA
Nottingham Health Profile	Self	1 week	10 minutes	All	General health status/quality of life measures	Jim McEwan Department of Public Health University of Glasgow
QWB	Trained interviewer	2 weeks	12 minutes	All	General health status/quality of life measures	Holly Teetzel Department of Family & Preventive Medicine, Box 0622 UCSD 9500 Gilman Drive La Jolla, CA 92093
AAOS Instruments Upper extremity, lower extremity, spine and pediatrics	Self or interviewer	1 week	Variable, depending on which modules used; 10 to 40 minutes	Patients with specific regions of disease/injury or specific age	Quality of life measure applied to regional (or age) musculoskeletal populations	Department of Research and Scientific Affairs American Academy of Orthopaedic Surgeons 6300 N. River Road Rosemont, IL 60018
MFA	Self or interviewer	2 hours	15 minutes	Patients with musculoskeletal disease	Quality of life measure applied to musculoskeletal disease	Julie Agel Dept Orthopaedics Box 359798 325 Ninth Avenue Seattle, WA 98104

by removing items that were more unstable, unclear, unresponsive, significantly intercorrelated, or internally inconsistent.

The MFA has been given to 557 patients to evaluate its responsiveness, validity, and reliability.[29] The long-term MFA was developed as a tool useful for funded outcome research projects and randomized control trials. The MFA may provide the community clinician with more detail and be more demanding on staff and patients than is necessary for routine use or for participation in regional outcome assessments. As

such, the SMFA (Short Musculoskeletal Functional Assessment) has been developed. Clinicians trying to routinely and quantitatively compare patient progress over time, as well as against patients from other settings, need a self-administered instrument that requires no lengthy explanations to the patient and does not disrupt the daily flow of the office or create an excessive cost. The SMFA is designed to meet those needs and to be a stand-alone tool for the routine assessment of orthopaedic outcomes, regardless of the disease or injury being evaluated. The investigators

have selected 32 questions from the longer instrument based on universality and applicability, uniqueness, reliability, and validity, as demonstrated by the MFA data, to formulate the SMFA. The responses have been scaled to add discriminating capability, and a 10-item patient utility section has been added.

Recommendations for Clinical Outcomes Research and Outcomes Assessment

Keller and associates[34,35] are responsible for making the important differentiation between outcomes research and outcomes assessment for the orthopaedic community. Outcomes research involves the systematic study of an individual disease process or injury. The development of such projects generally involves individuals who are trained in research methodology (often health services researchers). The projects are frequently multicenter trials, in order to satisfy patient accrual targets, and most often they require outside sources of funding to pay individuals responsible for data collection, monitoring of the study, and analysis of data. Results from these studies frequently result in changes in practice informally and through the modification of existing practice guidelines. The procedure for initiation of such a study involves first identifying a condition that has substantial impact on patient function or longevity and then analyzing retrospective data to identify key elements in the process of treatment that need further study. This is one of the major uses of data from trauma registries, such as the one developed by the Orthopaedic Trauma Association.

Once the clinical issues are identified, a study design must be developed and based on the data reviewed, and a power calculation must be performed to determine how many patients need to be enrolled in order to detect a clinically important difference in patient outcome. A trial enrollment period of 1 to 2 months at each potential site will give the investigators a good idea as to whether there are sufficient patients to complete the study. As a part of the study design phase, it will be determined which assessment questionnaires are optimum for the study and the intervals at which the patient should complete them. It is also determined in this phase which clinical data will be collected and which, if any, physical measurements (such as strength, range of motion, self-selected walking speed, handheld dynamometer, etc) should be collected at follow-up intervals. Practicality in terms of staffing for patient enrollment, tracking and data management, patient transportation needs, cultural and language issues (different from site to site based on the local population), and institutional cooperation must be considered in the study planning phase for each potential site. These types of studies generally require external funding to allow more rapid accrual of patients, appropriate data collection and analysis, and clear definition of responsibility.

These studies are constructed to address specific hypotheses, and attention must be directed to collecting the data necessary to address those hypotheses. The tendency is often to collect data hoping to find some interesting use for it later. This approach is resource intensive, frustrating for individuals collecting the data, and should be avoided.

The process described above is to be contrasted with outcomes assessment. This type of patient assessment involves the collection of health-related quality-of-life (HRQOL) data on patient samples to evaluate effectiveness of care. It is often done at the office, group, or health plan level and provides the type of data that payers are interested in. The collection of patient satisfaction data and HRQOL data is done on a preidentified segment of a practice at predetermined intervals, before and after treatment, forming the basis of outcome assessment. A common approach is to begin such a process by collecting these data on all patients within a practice. This approach should be discouraged. It results in accumulation of large volumes of data, which can be time consuming if not impossible to analyze. The collection process quickly leads to frustration of the office staff responsible for form administration and collection. Patient cooperation and support of these projects is rarely a problem. Patients have been found to be most receptive to completing these types of questionnaires, and they feel that this process, as well as satisfaction surveys, represents an effort on behalf of the practice to meet their needs and the needs of future patients.

The best approach in beginning outcomes assessment within a practice or trauma group is to select as a target condition a musculoskeletal condition or injury that is frequently seen within the practice. Each patient selected should be approached and asked to complete an HRQOL questionnaire and notified that he or she will be contacted at predetermined intervals to complete the same survey. The decision as to which HRQOL questionnaire to use depends on the clinical issue under review and the structure of the practice in which the data collection is taking place. The physicians responsible for the project should decide before enrolling patients which clinical data they will need to collect to properly analyze the HRQOL data. These data points involving clinical, demographic, or radiographic assessments should be collected prior to treatment and at select intervals. A minimalist approach, in terms of the number of conditions studied, is the most fruitful when starting to assess outcomes in clinical practice. Identifying a condition that is common to the practice, (and thus important to the success of the practice) and collecting data on patients with this condition will lead to a product that will be useful for evaluating current practice and planning for changes in the process of care.

What Do Purchasers Expect?

Over the past several years, the merits of health care reform have been subject to unproductive debate. Attempts at forceful leadership have given way to significant compromise. Politicians have failed, as business leaders have achieved a modest level of success. Thus, we are now in an era of private sector initiatives. Individual employers have decided the context within which our health care system will evolve.[36–48] Broad-based public reforms appear unlikely as incremental changes have gathered momentum.

It is now clear that our health care system must respond to a heretofore unobtrusive economic mandate. At the same time, medical care organizations are being asked to deliver high quality services in a publicly accountable manner. Finally, the consumers of medical care are no longer passive participants in a complex system that is widely regarded as providing too few benefits at too high a price. Medical providers are being asked to demonstrate the value of the services they offer relative to the expense borne by purchasers. In short, social accountability is no longer assumed; it must be documented. Consumers, whether they are patients or purchasers, believe they have a "right" to know what they have rarely asked. How accessible and of what quality are the services for which they believe they have been paid dearly?

National Health Care Expenditures

In 1940, the United States devoted 4.0% of its gross domestic product (GDP) to health, increasing to 7.1% in 1970[49–53] (Fig. 1). By 1995, nearly 14% of the GDP was spent on health care. Debate continues as to how much we can afford to spend. In 1940, $4.0 billion seemed like a siz-

able amount; however, this pales in comparison with the nearly $1.0 trillion we spend today (Fig. 2). Likewise, per capita expenditures for health care have increased at a remarkable pace, from $26 per capita in 1940 to $3,621 per capita in 1995 (Fig. 3).

National projections for health care expenditures are startling. By the year 2000, we are expected to spend $1.8 trillion on health care; by 2010, $3.8 trillion; by 2020, $7.8 trillion; and by 2030, $16.0 trillion[49–53] (Fig. 4). Thus, per capita expenditures will be approximately $6,555 in the year 2000; $12,765 in 2010; $24,171 in 2020; and $46,122 in 2030 (Fig. 5).

As these data suggest, both as a society and as individuals, we continue to have good reason to be concerned about health care expenditures. Whether we realize it or not, we are collectively responsible for paying the health care bill for the United States. As employees, we earn salaries and are provided benefits, including private health insurance coverage. As taxpayers we subsidize public health insurance programs such as Medicare and Medicaid. Thus, it behooves all of us to be ever mindful of the cost of health care because, in one way or another, we are both consumers and payers.

Employers

As noted, employers remain major "players" in the private health insurance market.[36–48] Not surprisingly, therefore, they have done more than the federal and state governments to provide incentives for health care reform. Admittedly, their interest has been somewhat self-serving; health care benefits constitute a major expense in the cost of doing business. Thus, in their efforts to remain competitive, business leaders continue to look for ways to cut health care costs.

Unfortunately, in many instances, cutting costs has entailed shifting expenses to employees through reducing benefits, eliminating insurance coverage, and increasing deductibles and copayments.[54] As a result, workers are beginning to realize that health care is not "free" and that they, not just their employer, are a major payer.

Of the $950 billion spent on health care in the United States in 1994, private health insurance accounted for about one third ($313 billion).[47,48] Businesses were responsible for over 40% of total spending on private health insurance.

As shown in Figure 6, there have been some significant changes in health care expenditures from 1980 to 1994 for different categories of spending.[47,48] In 1980, private health insurance covered 28.2% of national health care expenditures, compared with 33.0% in 1994.

Unfortunately, since 1980, the percentage of the nonelderly population with private health insurance has continued to decline, from 79.5% to 70.5% in 1995.[48] Meanwhile, the percentage of individuals covered by Medicaid increased from 8.2% in 1980 to 12.5% in 1995. Likewise, the percentage of uninsured persons increased from 11.8% in 1980 to 17.3% in 1995.

Employers continue to grapple with the cost of health care insurance. Increases in employer-based health insurance premiums far exceeded the general price inflation rate in the late 1980s, but premium growth rates have declined in the 1990s[54] (Fig. 7). For example, the average annual premium for employer-based family health insurance increased by 111%, from $2,530 to $5,349, between 1988 and 1996, while general prices rose by 33% during this period. Similarly, the average

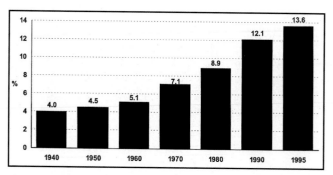

Fig. 1 Percentage of the gross domestic product devoted to health care, 1940-1995. (Reproduced with permission from The Mayo Foundation.)

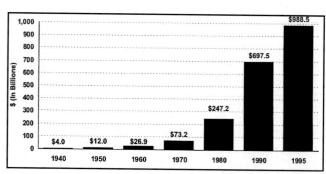

Fig. 2 Total national health care expenditures, 1940-1995. (Reproduced with permission from The Mayo Foundation.)

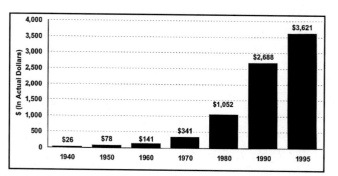

Fig. 3 Per capita national health care expenditures, 1940-1995. (Reproduced with permission from The Mayo Foundation.)

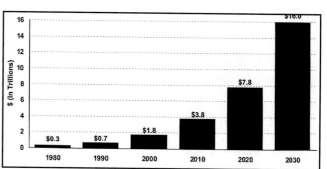

Fig. 4 National health care expenditures projected to 2030. (Reproduced with permission from The Mayo Foundation.)

annual premium for employer-based single coverage increased by 79%, from $1,153 to $2,059, between 1988 and 1996.[48]

Despite the foregoing data, the General Accounting Office (GAO) reports that the real annual rate of increase in health insurance premiums has slowed across all employer-based health plan types in the past 7 years.[47,48] Real premium growth rates of indemnity, preferred provider organization (PPO), and health maintenance organization (HMO) plans peaked in 1989 at rates of 15%, 13%, and 11% respectively. Real premium growth rates slowed to an average of about 5% across all plan types in 1993, whereas over the past 2 years premiums experienced near-zero growth. In 1996, premiums increased at lower rates than the consumer price index and the medical cost index.

As noted above, the relationship between wages, salaries, and benefits serves to underscore the significant contributions that employees make to their health care. In 1980, employer private health insurance spending amounted to 3.4% of an employee's total compensation.[47,48] However, as shown in Figure 8, this amount has increased to 5.6% of total compensation. Not surprisingly, for many years, the rate of increase in health insurance premiums far outstripped the annual increase in workers' earnings (Fig. 9). However, since 1995, annual increases in workers' earnings have exceeded the percentage increase in health insurance plan premiums. Thus, it is possible to argue that there has been a tradeoff between benefits and earnings.

Managed Care

Many analysts have attributed the slowdown in annual insurance premium growth to several causes, including the increased use of managed care and a downward trend in what is often referred to as the health insurance underwriting cycle, in which premiums decline when health insurers' profits are high[55-64] (Fig. 10). However, as the GAO has noted, no studies have comprehensively examined the reasons for the recent 7-year decline in premium increases.[47,48]

Although the effect of managed care remains a matter of debate, some observers contend that managed care has contributed to the slowdown in premium increases because HMO plans generally cost less than other health plans, and many managed care organizations control the use of

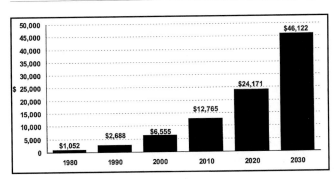

Fig. 5 Per capita national health expenditures projected to 2030. (Reproduced with permission from The Mayo Foundation.)

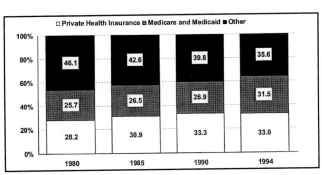

Fig. 6 Private health insurance and national health expenditures, 1980-1994. (Reproduced with permission from *Private Health Insurance Coverage: Continued Erosion of Coverage Linked to Cost Pressures.* Washington DC, U.S. General Accounting Office, 1997, p 14.)

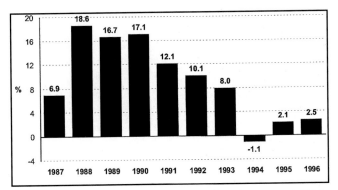

Fig. 7 Annual change in average total health benefit cost, 1987-1996. (Reproduced with permission from *National Survey of Employer-Sponsored Health Plans/1996: Report.* New York, NY, Foster Higgins, 1997, p 8.)

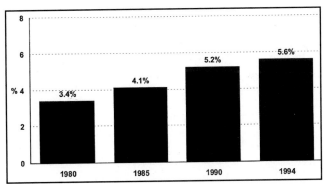

Fig. 8 Employer private health insurance spending as a percentage of total compensation, 1980-1994. (Adapted with permission from *Private Health Insurance Coverage: Continued Erosion of Coverage Linked to Cost Pressures.* Washington DC, U.S. General Accounting Office, 1997, p 33.)

health care services.[47,48] As a result, the savings actually occur as consumers move from indemnity plans to HMO plans. In contrast, other research attributes the savings from managed care to changes in the operation of the health insurance market when managed care penetration rates reach a critical threshold.[65]

Reasonable observers must be wary of attributing too much to managed care. As already noted, workers have seen their benefits decrease, which, in turn, has contributed to behavior modification.[54] In other words, in the absence of managed care, higher deductibles and copay-

ments are likely to result in a significant reduction in the use of health care services. Moreover, it is conceivable that people have not accessed health care services from which they might have benefited over the past several years. As a result, when the economic implications of this "period effect" are considered, the benefits of managed care may be found to have been grossly exaggerated. After all, health care policymakers have been frantically searching for a "magic bullet" to ease the health care controversy.

Therefore, it should come as no surprise that many analysts now pro-

ject a significant increase in the costs of health care coverage.[66,67] The reasons industry experts cite for the market's turn are numerous and varied (Outline 1), including an inevitable rebound from years of artificially low pricing by HMOs eager to gain market share, an "HMO backlash" by consumers and legislators, savvier contracting by physicians and hospitals, and a general return of health care cost inflation that reflects a lack of any structural change in the nation's health care system. In short, the rhetoric of managed care has done little to change the constellation of the problem.

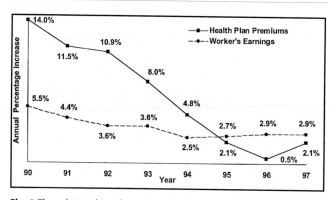

Fig. 9 The relationship of wages to health insurance premiums, 1990-1997. (Reproduced with permission from The Mayo Foundation.)

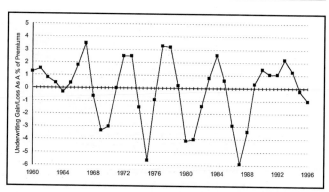

Fig. 10 Blue Cross/Blue Shield underwriting results, 1960-1996. (Adapted with permission from Reilly PK: *Forecasting Health Insurer Profitability: 1997–1999*. Philadelphia, PA, Milliman & Robertson, 1997, p 3.)

Outline 1

Factors likely to contribute to health insurance premium increases in 1998

Many HMOs increased premiums in 1997 to cover sagging profits in 1996

Health care providers are consolidating and gaining more bargaining clout with managed care plans

State and federal laws are requiring health insurance plans to expand the benefits covered

There is little room for additional savings in costs from shifting employees to managed care plans, because more than 75% of active employees are already in managed care plans

With low unemployment, the prospects of a tight labor market could reverse the low, overall inflation rate of the past several years

---

Outline 2

Value in health care

Value—the combined product of quality and cost-effectiveness

Optimum value—the best attainable quality at the lowest justifiable cost

---

Value in Health Care

As is true of any fad, managed care has nearly run its course. As a conceptual chameleon, managed care has exhibited remarkable survivability. However, as is usually the case, one fad is readily replaced with another. As a result, we have now entered the era of value in health care.[68] Value has been defined by employers as the "best quality at the lowest justifiable price." Unfortunately, we have yet another situation where an old concept is described by a new word (Outline 2). Within their limited means, prudent shoppers have always attempted to get the best deal at the lowest price. As a commodity, health care is also expected to subject itself to market forces.

A variety of health care consulting firms continue to survey employers concerning their expectations of the health care system. In this context, employers are referred to as purchasers, and their expectations appear to be very similar to those of traditional public and private third party payers.[68]

As shown in Figure 11, of many factors presented to employers as the basis for selecting a health plan, 93% considered "cost" to be important, followed by member services, employee access, customer service, and utilization data.[68] In another survey (Fig. 12), access, member satisfaction, cost, outcomes, and National Committee for Quality Assurance

accreditation were ranked with respect to the evaluation and selection of an HMO by purchasers.[69] According to this survey, access was considered to be "extremely important" by 71% of the purchasers, and "cost" by only 41%.

Data such as these underscore the significance of cost in purchaser decisions; however, they clearly indicate that it is not the only consideration. In yet another survey of 384 United States companies, 51% indicated that health care costs were a primary factor when contracting with health plans, and that 34% of the employers viewed quality of care as a primary concern.[70] The survey also showed that an increasing number of employers view quality of care as important. In effect, employers seeking a combination of low costs and high quality are trying to determine which plans can deliver the best value for the employers' health care dollars.

In the spring of 1997, the Washington Business Group of Health (WBGH) and the health care consulting firm Watson Wyatt Worldwide conducted a follow-up survey of 325 United States employers.[70] Employers were specifically asked to weigh the importance of 4 key fac-

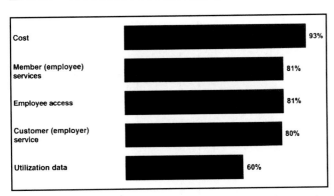

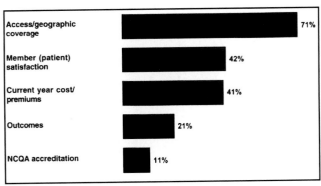

Fig. 11 Factors employers are most likely to consider in selection of a health plan, 1997. (Adapted with permission from *Getting What You Pay For: Purchasing Value in Health Care,* 1997. Bethesda, MD, Watson Wyatt Worldwide, 1997.)

Fig. 12 Ranking of various criteria in selecting and evaluating HMOs, 1997. Bars indicate the number of respondents rating the attribute extremely important. (Adapted with permission from *Mercer's FAX Facts Surveys: HMOs.* New York, NY, William M Mercer, 1997, p 4.)

tors—cost, access, quality, and employee satisfaction—they use to evaluate health plans. Thirty-one percent of the employers place the greatest weight on cost, 26% on access, and 20% on employee satisfaction.

Other aspects of the WBGH-Watson Wyatt Worldwide survey are noteworthy as follows:[70] One third of employers (33%) believe cost pressures are hurting the quality of health care being provided, up from 28% a year ago. Sixty-three percent say they are effective or very effective when buying health care value, up slightly from 59% a year ago. Some type of long-term partnership with health plans has been established by 44% of the respondents to better ensure consistent, value-based health care delivery. Sixty-two percent of large employers now use data from the Health Plan Employer Data and Information Set (HEDIS) to help with purchasing decisions. However, HEDIS is used by only 7% of small employers. Accreditation status has become more common as an evaluation tool. Seventy-nine percent of large employers and 48% of small employers now use such information. More than half of the employers surveyed now offer incentives to

employees to influence plan choice. Large employers are much more likely than small employers to provide quality- and outcome-related information to employees to help them make informed plan choices.

Although survey data such as these often provide useful insight, they rarely yield a complete picture. Information is not always available to understand costs or quality. Although cost data are routinely collected, information on quality is not as readily available. Moreover, when available, quality data are rarely straightforward. Their interpretation is often contingent on many factors.

Accreditation Efforts

Because of the cost and quality concerns, the demand for accountability on behalf of health care providers and plans is significant. Increasingly, payers want to know what they are getting for their money, while the general public is rightfully concerned about managed care constraints.

In general, accountability for quality has followed two paths: the accreditation process and performance measurement. The Joint Commission on Accreditation of Healthcare Organizations (JCAHO) has accredited hos-

pitals and other providers since 1951.[71,72] More recently, the National Committee for Quality Assurance (NCQA) was formed to ensure quality of care rendered to persons enrolled in HMOs through a set of measures known as the Health Plan Employer Data and Information Set (HEDIS).[72] Finally, and still more recently, the Foundation for Accountability (FACCT) was formed, not as an accrediting body, but as a resource for identifying and endorsing consumer-related measures of quality, encouraging the adoption of these measures in the field, and striving to ensure that their information is effectively communicated and used by consumers.[73] FACCT's goal is to have its performance measures incorporated into JCAHO and NCQA accreditation efforts.

As might be expected, health care providers, as well as health plans, must be prepared to report on various quality or performance measures. This information is then used by employers and patients alike to make informed decisions about health plans and providers. In principle, the goal is worthy but, in practice, a variety of problems have been encountered. For example, as shown

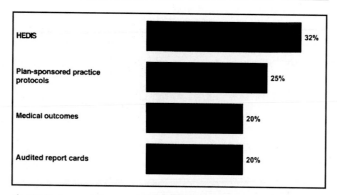

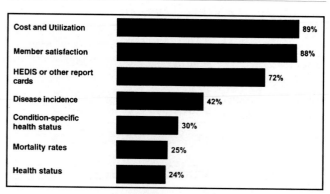

Fig. 13 Factors employers are least likely to consider in selecting a health plan, 1997. (Adapted with permission from *Getting What You Pay For: Purchasing Value in Health Care, 1997*. Bethesda, MD, Watson Wyatt Worldwide, 1997.)

Fig. 14 Percentage of HMOs reporting specific quality measures to employers. (Adapted with permission from *The InterStudy Competitive Edge, Part II: Industry Report 5.1*. Minneapolis, MN, InterStudy, 1995, p 77.)

in Figure 13, employers seem less than enthusiastic about various activities associated with the aforementioned organizations. Only 32% use HEDIS, 20% consider outcomes, and 20% have found value in audited report cards.[68] Nonetheless, as is apparent from Figure 14, many HMOs indicate that they now report a variety of cost and quality indicators to employers.[74] Fully 88% provide satisfaction data and 72% HEDIS information.

Finally, despite the enthusiasm associated with cost and quality assessment, some health plans are still unable to provide data on a variety of critical indicators, including patient satisfaction, NCQA accreditation, and outcomes. Thus, although accreditation is a reality with which we must all deal in both the short- and the long-term, it is evident the ideal is inconsistent with reality. This is, perhaps, best exemplified by the excessive emphasis on outcomes as an indicator of the quality of health care.

Outcomes and Quality

Needless to say, for centuries physicians and surgeons have had an acute interest in the outcomes of the services they provide. However, as now construed, the concept of "outcomes management," as envisioned by Ellwood, is naïve, misleading, and hardly heuristic.[75-79] Quality, effectiveness, and efficiency, as Codman, Cochrane, and Donabedian have made clear, is a combination of many factors, including medical care structure, process, and outcomes.[80-84] As such, we do not, nor will we ever, "manage" outcomes per se. Outcomes merely tell us where we have been, not where we are going.

Not surprisingly, therefore, as now contrived, outcomes exist as an abstract concept in search of substance. Moreover, when properly conceived, it is clear, even to the casual observer, that both clinical and nonclinical outcomes are significantly impacted by factors over which the medical profession exercises limited, if any, control.[85,86] Thus, outcomes "managers" are inclined to become social "messiahs" when they realize their clinical deeds have been undone by social circumstances.[77] Such is the basis for the renewed interest in public health.[87-90]

Ellwood[75] (as well as the constituency he apparently represents) is little more than an opportunist promoting conceptual hyperbole. In the absence of structure and process, we are left to ponder a house of cards. Indeed, too much has been made of nothing. Sociologically speaking, outcomes management is little more than a social movement intent on creating expectations it will never fulfill. Nevertheless, the literature is now replete with 1 dubious misadventure after another, wherein concepts such as health status, functional ability, and quality of life are used interchangeably to describe distinctly different features of Ellwood's nightmare—that is, the so-called "technology of patient experience."[91-93]

Unfortunately, to his dismay, Ellwood has already been left holding the bag, managed care; he has yet to realize he has another in hand, outcomes management. Like the now infamous chameleons in a popular beer commercial, Ellwood might well speculate as to what his future might be if his misleading ideas were consistent with reality.

Discussion

Although annual increases have moderated, national health care expenditures remain a serious concern. Employers have seen these increases reflected in the premiums they pay for insurance benefits. Unhappy with the efforts of the federal government to control national health care expenditures, employers have a variety of initiatives intended to enhance the value of health care services. Managed care has served as a cornerstone in these efforts. As a result, proponents argue that, for the past 2 years, premiums have exhibited near-zero growth.

The actual impact of managed care is probably overstated. At the same time employers have introduced managed care, they have reduced employee benefits and cost-shifted through higher deductibles and copayments. Moreover, the insurance underwriting cycle has been positioned favorably in time.[55] Thus, there is considerable evidence suggesting that insurance premiums will begin to increase in 1997. This unfavorable situation is likely to add fuel to an emerging fad, value in health care. This, in turn, may stimulate, still further, various accreditation efforts directed at measuring the performance of health care providers and health insurance plans.

The National Committee for Quality Assurance, the Joint Commission on Accreditation of Healthcare Organizations, and the Foundation for Accountability are remarkably redundant with those of other organizations, including the Medical Outcomes Trust and the Health Outcomes Institute.

Although all the aforementioned organizations provide a range of useful services, the hype they generate is often disproportionate to their accomplishments. For example, performance measurement systems endorsed by the JCAHO leave a lot to be desired from the perspective of cost, utility, and, to the point in question, value. Likewise, NCQA accreditation efforts are, at the very least,

subject to controversy, and, at times questionable in the absence of audit. More pointedly, the Foundation for Accountability has yet to demonstrate its worth.

Finally, the rhetoric of outcomes at least matches that associated with managed care. As described above, when it comes to outcomes, too much is being made of too little. Outcomes are a critical part of the health care quality equation, and, potentially, they have something to contribute to the debate concerning value. However, a great deal of work remains to be done with respect to the conceptualization, measurement, assessment, and use of outcomes data. In this regard, we are clearly in need of information, not data.

Current Status of AAOS-Sponsored Outcome Instrument Development

In 1994, American Academy of Orthopaedic Surgeons (AAOS), through its Council of Musculoskeletal Specialty Societies (COMSS), began the process of developing a basic set of outcome assessment questionnaires for the musculoskeletal practitioner. This effort was motivated by a desire to provide a greater level of detail for functional status assessment, beyond that provided by general health status questionnaires like the SF-36, while trying to avoid the necessity of developing individual questionnaires for individual conditions. Representatives from all the specialty societies within COMSS met for an intensive 3-day session to determine whether such a project is feasible, what the scope of the project should be, and how the work should be organized.

It was determined that the project was both possible and necessary. Existing questionnaires addressed either general health status or specific

problems, such as rheumatoid arthritis, and were not applicable to general musculoskeletal problems. There were problems of both scope and what are called ceiling and floor effects: either the questionnaire was designed primarily for survey among very ill patients (like those with rheumatoid arthritis) so that a large number of people with less severe but still important pathology scored as normal, or the questionnaire was designed for individuals functioning at a very high level (like a professional athlete), with most of the general population scoring at the low end of the scale. There were also problems of scope: some questionnaires focused purely on function, others on symptoms, and others included various social and emotional parameters. Few considered the issue of cosmesis or self-image, both of which appeared to be important issues for patients with musculoskeletal problems.

A consensus panel approach was used to determine what the scope of the AAOS project should be. It was generally agreed that the SF-36 questionnaire was an excellent overall health status tool, and that there was no need to reproduce its functionality with regard to the assessment of overall impact on the patient, general burden of pain, and the impact of the disease on social and emotional function. It was elected instead to focus on musculoskeletal function and symptoms on a more specific level than that captured by the SF-36 and, specifically, to emphasize attribution of symptoms. For example, the SF-36 asks for the total burden of pain; an AAOS instrument might ask how much pain a person has in their hip or knee or hand. Attribution is very important if an intervention is directed only at a part of the global problem; it is unlikely that a total knee arthroplasty will significantly improve total body pain or pain from a migraine headache, for example, but it might significantly improve knee pain and knee function.

A series of task forces were established to create function and symptom questionnaires in 4 general clusters: upper extremity, lower extremity, spine, and pediatrics. Questions were modified from existing questionnaires, where possible, and added where no suitable questionnaire existed. The goal was to create questionnaires that were relatively brief, yet comprehensive enough to cover the broad spectrum of orthopaedic pathology. Once the questionnaires were designed, they were field tested to be sure that they adequately captured the symptoms in patients with a broad range of musculoskeletal pathology, as seen in a general or subspecialty orthopaedic practice. Statistical analyses were then used to eliminate redundant questions and to cluster the questions into relevant subscales. Focus groups were used in some cases to identify additional questions, such as those related to cosmesis and self image.

The initial process is now completed and a complete set of questionnaires is available. In addition to the basic upper extremity module, there is an additional upper limb optional set of questions that address specific work and sports (high performance) issues. The lower limb module has a 7-question core, with optional add-on modules, which capture attributed function and symptom data for hip and knee arthritis, sports, and foot problems. The spine module comes in 3 versions: 1 each for neck, back, and scoliosis. The pediatric module also has 3 versions: 1 for children, to be completed by parents; 1 for teens, to be completed by the patient; and 1 for teens, to be completed by the parents.

To make these questionnaires easier to use, they have been clustered with a set of additional basic questions regarding patient demographics (age, gender, occupation, handedness, etc) and comorbidities (presence or absence of a variety of conditions such as hypertension, diabetes, cigarette smoking, etc). For initial assessment, a series of questions probes a patient's expectations with regard to treatment. For follow-up assessment, a series of questions probes the patient's satisfaction with the results of treatment. A physician module captures information about diagnosis, treatment, injury or disease severity, and complications. Finally, an additional optional module captures information on patient satisfaction with the process of care. Process, a frequent concern of managed care organizations, includes satisfaction with access, promptness of service, and the like.

This information is useful not only for research purposes but for the management of everyday clinical practice. To make it easier for clinicians to collect and use this information, the Academy has sponsored the development of a database and reporting project, entitled MODEMS.™ The details of the MODEMS™ project follow.

An Introduction to the MODEMS™ Program

The mission of the Musculoskeletal Outcomes Data Evaluation and Management System (MODEMS) Program is to improve the care of patients with musculoskeletal complaints by critically analyzing medical and surgical treatment using validated patient-based outcomes instruments.

Program Definition

The MODEMS™ Program consists of: (1) a set of 4 generic, anatomic-re-

gion based, patient-based instruments to collect outcomes data; (2) a series of specialized modules to customize the generic instruments to more specific needs; (3) a patient satisfaction questionnaire; (4) a series of certified vendors who will provide practices with the means of collecting and transmitting outcomes data; (5) a national repository of outcomes data; and (6) a series of reports detailing national norms and best practices.

The 4 generic, anatomic-region based, patient-based questionnaires are the Spine Instrument; the Lower Limb Instrument; the Disability of the Arm, Shoulder, and Hand (DASH) Instrument; and the Pediatrics Instrument. These outcomes instruments have been thoroughly validated and tested. They represent the consensus of a broad cross-section of surgeons as to what constitutes the minimum data set to define quality of care in musculoskeletal conditions. Each questionnaire takes no more than 15 minutes to complete. A series of more specific modules have also been developed to address special needs. The patient satisfaction questionnaire is a 9-item instrument designed to assess the satisfaction of your patients with the process of care, which is designed to be administered to just a sample of your patients twice a year.

To participate in MODEMS™, surgeons are required to use the outcomes instruments to evaluate their patients. The use of the specialized modules and the patient satisfaction questionnaire is optional. The required instruments all have a baseline and follow-up versions. Follow-up data must be collected at 3, 6, 12, and 24 months.

Entering data into the database requires medical practices to subscribe to MODEMS™, to use the outcomes instruments, and to transmit the data through a MODEMS™ certified vendor. A MODEMS™ certified vendor is a vendor of data collection and transmission systems who has successfully completed a comprehensive quality control process administered by the MODEMS™ staff. Several vendors offer a wide range of technologies from paper-and-pencil forms and manual entry to touchscreen, patient-driven software.

The national repository is a highly secure database that allows comparisons between individual practices and national statistics. Reports from the national repository will be produced at least once a year. These reports will present national statistics and allow for comparisons of your practice with similar practices treating similar patients across the country.

MODEMS™ Development

MODEMS™ is a project of the AAOS, COMSS of the AAOS, and the Council of Spine Societies (COSS). The project has been developed and is being overseen by the MODEMS™ Task Force on Data Management, which includes representatives from the AAOS and the organizations that belong to COMSS and COSS. The project started formally in Spring 1995 at a meeting in Tarpon Springs, Florida jointly organized and sponsored by the AAOS Committee on Outcome Studies and COMSS. More than 150 surgeons from all specialties in orthopaedic surgery were involved in developing the program.

MODEMS™ Purpose

MODEMS™ provides participants with the process and the necessary instruments to measure, record, store, and analyze information about the outcomes of the musculoskeletal care they provide. The instruments have been designed to allow simple, consistent, and scientifically sound measurement of important outcomes of musculoskeletal care delivered by a variety of caregivers. This information is collected and stored locally for use by the participants and is also transmitted to a national database overseen by the MODEMS™ Task Force on Data Management. Once in the database, the data will contribute to the development of national norms and guidelines for treatment of a broad range of musculoskeletal conditions.

Instrument Reliability

The 4 MODEMS™ instruments and the optional modules have gone through extensive testing and revision since version 1.0 was created in 1995. Version 2.0 of the instruments, released in Fall 1997, has been thoroughly tested for validity, reliability, and sensitivity. These instruments have been shown to perform as well as or better than SF-36 in describing and classifying patients with musculoskeletal complaints. Version 2.0 will remain unchanged until at least Spring 2000.

A report describing the testing process and results of all 4 instruments is now available. Specific questions on the development of the instruments can be directed to the address and numbers provided at the end of the section. A list of studies, publications, and professional presentations that have used these instruments is available on the MODEMS™ web site www.modems.org or by request at the address provided.

Data Ownership

You own the data that you have collected in your office. The data that you submit to the national repository (stripped of all surgeons' and patients' personal identifiers) is owned by AAOS, COMSS, and COSS. Access to the national repository is strictly limited to the MODEMS™ Task Force on Data Management. The Task Force is the only body that decides what analyses are run, what comparisons are made, and how the data are reported.

Data Confidentiality

To ensure confidentiality, the Task Force has established a technologically "bullet-proof" data management system. This data management system has several levels of security to insure (1) the confidentiality of the patient and the surgeon; (2) the quality and integrity of the incoming data; (3) that there is absolutely no unauthorized access; (4) that there are regular and frequent back-ups and a secure archival system; and (5) that there is constant and ongoing electronic quality checking of the collected data.

When a physician subscribes to MODEMS™, his or her practice is given a unique identifier, a password, and a number of surgeon identifier numbers equal to the number of participating surgeons. The surgeon identifier number is assigned by the practice to each surgeon. At this point, the practice is the only body that knows which number is identified with which surgeon. All patient records are given a unique identifier number made of a combination of social security number, gender, and birth date, and are stripped of other personal information before they are transmitted to the national repository.

To ensure confidentiality, the data transmitted to the MODEMS™ database are automatically encrypted several times. First, the data are encrypted using a single use Digital Encryption Standard (DES) secret key, and then the secret key used to encrypt the data is itself encrypted using the central repository database's key just before the data are transferred to the central database.

For the data transmission to be accepted, the receiving computer must recognize the practice's user-name and password. Once the user-name and password are authenticated, the data being transferred are permitted to enter the receiving computer. The data are then tested for authentication, completeness, and adherence to file specifications before being admitted into the database. After the data have been authenticated and tested, they are imported through a 1-way "firewall" stand-alone computer into the database. This "firewall" computer insulates the computer where the national database resides and makes the database totally inaccessible from the outside. As the data are entered into the database, they are encrypted 1 final time. The database is regularly and frequently backed-up. Archival tapes of the database are stored in a bank security vault for safe-keeping.

If you are interested in the technical details of the encryption system and/or the database please let the MODEMS™ staff know and they will be pleased to send you an in-depth description of the security system and the database management system.

Analysis and dissemination of the data contained within the database are the sole responsibility of the Task Force. They have instituted the following guidelines: (1) all reporting and analysis will include and take place on aggregate data only; (2) routine database reports and analyses will be available only to participating MODEMS™ practitioners; (3) surgeons or other organizations that do not contribute to the MODEMS™ database will not be permitted to purchase these reports or analyses;

and (4) requests for special analyses of the aggregate data will be decided upon by the Task Force.

Reasons for Participating

The data collection instruments have been developed by your peers and are simple, short, and practical. Moreover, a physician who is interested only in collecting outcomes data on the musculoskeletal care that he or she delivers can use the MODEMS™ instruments without joining the program. That is, a physician collects data on his or her own practice without sending it to the national repository. However, for those who are interested in collecting outcomes data on the musculoskeletal care that they deliver and who want to compare their results with national norms, MODEMS™ is the only truly national outcomes data program. MODEMS™ practitioners receive: (1) training on collecting data and implementing outcomes-based continuous improvement programs; (2) reports describing national norms of practices like theirs treating patients like theirs; (3) participation in discussion groups (of both surgeons and practice staff) made of practices that have similar interests and are faced with similar challenges; (4) support in analyzing their own "outcomes" data; (5) a quarterly newsletter, describing interesting results, showcasing specific practices, and reporting on outcomes-related issues and events; and (6) invitations to symposia. MODEMS™ practitioners receive training on the operation of the data collection and transmission system they choose to purchase. They also receive instruction on the selection of patients to follow, administration of the questionnaires, transmission of data, and analysis of the data they collect and of the reports interpreting the data from the national database.

The vendor of the data collection and transmission system whose product the subscriber has purchased will administer most of the training. The MODEMS™ Task Force on Data Management has established guidelines for training that each vendor must follow. The Task Force has also provided each vendor with materials specific to the program to be incorporated into the vendor's training program. From time to time, the MODEMS™ staff will provide training sessions as well. These sessions are free of charge to the MODEMS™ practitioners and their staffs.

At least once a year, MODEMS™ practitioners receive reports of the contents of the database on computer diskette. These reports will vary in content and format as the database grows. Participating practitioners have input into the content and format of these reports.

Each MODEMS™ practitioner also becomes a member of at least 1 MODEMS™ user group. These groups bring together participants, vendors, and Task Force members to share information about their experiences with data collection, use of software, and interpretation and use of local and national data. In addition, MODEMS™ user groups will serve as a feedback mechanism to the MODEMS™ Task Force on Data Management.

Modems™ Reports

The Task Force on Data Management has created the format of the first set of reports. These reports will vary in content and format as the database grows. Every subscriber will receive a copy of the reports on disk. These routine reports will be generated once a year. Requests for special reports can be submitted to the Task Force on Data Management.

Uses for MODEMS™ Data

Some of the benefits of collecting outcomes data include having data comparing patient performance, developing targets for continuous improvement, documenting quality, and developing algorithms and guidelines. The MODEMS™ data can be helpful for internal review of current practices (comparing across surgeons in practice for example). The data can also affect a practice's revenue by improving the ability to retain or increase existing contracts from managed care organizations and by improving chances to get new contracts.

Certified MODEMS™ Vendors

MODEMS™ does not sell data collection systems or services. The data collection and transmission system is purchased directly through a MODEMS™ certified vendor. The MODEMS™ certification process is a series of quality checks. A vendor submits a product for certification to the Task Force on Data Management. MODEMS™ staff then tests the products, making sure that the exact version of the MODEMS™ instruments is being used to insure that the vendor can provide reliable and knowledgeable support. The vendor is certified only after all quality checks have been passed. Vendors are recertified every year. Part of the recertification process involves surveying clients of that vendor to check on its performance.

Not all certified vendors offer computer-based data entry. MODEMS™ offers a certified paper-form data entry. With this service, the physician only needs to have the patients complete the questionnaires and send them to the vendor for data entry and transmission. A physician can use the data entry service while deciding whether to purchase a computerized system or for as long as is desired.

Subscribers and Practitioners

A MODEMS™ subscriber can be a single practicing physician, a physician group, a hospital, a health care facility, a health maintenance organization, or any other entity in which an individual practitioner delivers care. Only practitioners who are represented by a MODEMS™ subscriber may participate in the program.

If a subscriber has more than 1 office, it is up to the subscriber to decide whether to be treated as just 1 subscriber or to maintain a separate subscription for each participating office site. Each location must have its own Clinic ID number.

To participate in the MODEMS™ program, a practitioner must be a resident member, candidate member, fellow, or emeritus fellow of the AAOS or be in an equivalent category in any member society of COMSS or COSS. If a practitioner is currently a participant in another database and would like to submit data to that database and to MODEMS™ simultaneously, he or she should contact the MODEMS™ staff to discuss this possibility. If a MODEMS™ practitioner is affiliated with more than 1 subscriber, he or she may choose to participate with just 1 subscriber or through each subscriber separately.

Subscriber Responsibilities and Fees

A MODEMS™ subscriber is the only entity through which individual practitioners may participate in the program. A subscriber is required to pay a 1-time $500 fee to initialize the database. In addition, the subscriber will be responsible for paying an annual fee of $500 for each participating practitioner who is affiliated with that subscriber.

Practitioner Responsibilities

MODEMS™ practitioners have a number of responsibilities, each of which is intended to help ensure the quality, security, and utility of the data being collected and shared. The practitioner is responsible for obtaining patient responses to the outcomes data collection instruments developed by the Task Force on Data Management. A practitioner can administer these questionnaires to the patient populations that are most relevant to his or her own practice, but must administer them in accordance with the guidelines received during training.

Practitioners are required to transmit copies of their data to the national database at regular intervals via a transmission interface sold by a vendor certified by the MODEMS™ Task Force on Data Management. The MODEMS™ logo will be indicated on the packaging and advertising of the product. Practitioners are responsible for monitoring the quality and completeness of data they submit and for ensuring that the data are a consistent and accurate recording of information collected from patients on the MODEMS™ questionnaires.

Communication With the MODEMS™ Program

The MODEMS™ Program has a toll free telephone number, (800) 288-0018. This number is available to subscribers and practitioners during regular business hours (8AM to 5PM central time on weekdays). The staff may be reached by e-mail at MODEMS@AAOS.org. Subscribers and practitioners will also receive and contribute to a quarterly newsletter and have access to on-line help and news of training sessions and the latest developments through the MODEMS™ internet homepage at www.modems.org.

Any written correspondence may be sent by first-class mail to:

MODEMS
P.O. Box 2354
Des Plaines, IL 60017-2354

References

1. Epstein AM: The outcomes movement: Will it get us where we want to go? *N Engl J Med* 1990;323:266–270.

2. Relman AS: Editorial: Assessment and accountability: The third revolution in medical care. *N Engl J Med* 1988;319:1220–1222.

3. Sarmiento A: Staying the course. *J Bone Joint Surg* 1991;73A:479–483.

4. Rineberg BA: Editorial: A call to leadership: The role of orthopaedic surgeons in musculoskeletal outcomes research. *J Bone Joint Surg* 1990;72A:1439–1440.

5. Burton KE, Wright V, Richards J: Patients' expectations in relation to outcome of total hip replacement surgery. *Ann Rheum Dis* 1979;38:471–474.

6. Wennberg J, Gittelsohn A: Small area variations in health care delivery. *Science* 1973;182:1102–1108.

7. Fowler FJ Jr, Wennberg JE, Timothy RP, Barry MJ, Mulley AG Jr, Hanley D: Symptom status and quality of life following prostatectomy. *JAMA* 1988;259:3018–3022.

8. L'Abbe KA, Detsky AS, O'Rourke K: Meta-analysis in clinical research. *Ann Intern Med* 1987;107:224–233.

9. Guyatt GH, Kirshner B, Jaeschke R: Measuring health status: What are the necessary measurement properties? *J Clin Epidemiol* 1992;45:1341–1345.

10. Williams A: Setting priorities in health care: An economist's view. *J Bone Joint Surg* 1991;73B:365–367.

11. Liang MH, Fossel AH, Larson MG: Comparisons of five health status instruments for orthopaedic evaluation. *Med Care* 1990;28:632–642.

12. Ware JE Jr, Sherbourne CD, Davies AR: Developing and testing the MOS 20-item short-form health survey: A general population application, in Stewart AL, Ware JE Jr (eds): *Measuring Functioning and Well-Being: The Medical Outcomes Study Approach.* Durham, NC, Duke University Press, 1992, pp 277–290.

13. Stewart AL, Ware JE, Brook RH, Davies-Avery A: *Conceptualization and Measurement of Health for Adults in the Health Insurance Study: Volume II, Physical Health in Terms of Functioning.* Santa Monica, CA, Rand Corp, 1978.

14. Tarlov AR, Ware JE Jr, Greenfield S, Nelson EC, Perrin E, Zubkoff M: The Medical Outcomes Study: An application of methods for monitoring the results of medical care. *JAMA* 1989;262:925–930.

15. Ware JE, Johnston SA, Davies-Avery A, Brook RH: *Conceptualization and Measurement of Health for Adults in the Health Insurance Study: Volume III, Mental Health.* Santa Monica, CA, The Rand Corp, 1979.

16. Ware JE Jr, Sherbourne CD: The MOS 36-item short-form health survey (SF-36): I. Conceptual framework and item selection. *Med Care* 1992;30:473–483.

17. Engelberg R, Martin DP, Agel J, Obremsky W, Coronado G, Swiontkowski MF: Musculoskeletal Function Assessment instrument: Criterion and construct validity. *J Orthop Res* 1996;14:182–192.

18. Martin DP, Engelberg R, Agel J, Snapp D, Swiontkowski MF: Development of a musculoskeletal extremity health status instrument: The Musculoskeletal Function Assessment instrument. *J Orthop Res* 1996;14:173–181.

19. Bergner M, Bobbitt RA, Carter WB, Gilson BS: The Sickness Impact Profile: Development and final revision of a health status measure. *Med Care* 1981;19:787–805.

20. Bergner M, Bobbitt RA, Kressel S, Pollard WE, Gilson BS, Morris JR: The Sickness Impact Profile: Conceptual formulation and methodology for the development of a health status measure. *Int J Health Serv* 1976;6:393–415.

21. Bergner M, Bobbitt RA, Pollard WE, Martin DP, Gilson BS: The Sickness Impact Profile: Validation of a health status measure. *Med Care* 1976;14:57–67.

22. MacKenzie EJ, Burgess AR, McAndrew MP, et al: Patient-oriented functional outcome after unilateral lower extremity fracture. *J Orthop Trauma* 1993;7:393–401.

23. MacKenzie EJ, Cushing BM, Jurkovich GJ, et al: Physical impairment and functional outcomes six months after severe lower extremity fractures. *J Trauma* 1993;34:528–539.

24. Georgiadis GM, Behrens FF, Joyce MJ, Earle AS, Simmons AL: Open tibial fractures with severe soft-tissue loss: Limb salvage compared with below-the-knee amputation. *J Bone Joint Surg* 1993;75A:1431–1441.

25. McDowell I, Newell C (eds): *Measuring Health: A Guide to Rating Scales and Questionnaires.* New York, NY, Oxford University press, 1987, pp 104–151.

26. Meek RN, Vivoda EE, Pirani S: Comparison of mortality of patients with multiple injuries according to type of fracture treatment: A retrospective age- and injury-matched series. *Injury* 1986;17:2–4.

27. Parker MJ, Myles JW, Anand JK, Drewett R: Cost-benefit analysis of hip fracture treatment. *J Bone Joint Surg* 1992;74B:261–264.

28. Levine DW, Simmons BP, Koris MJ, et al: A self-administered questionnaire for the assessment of severity of symptoms and functional status in carpal tunnel syndrome. *J Bone Joint Surg* 1993;75A:1585–1592.

29. Martin DP, Engelberg R, Agel J, Swiontkowski MF: Comparison of the musculoskeletal Function Assessment questionnaire with the Short Form-36, the Western Ontario and McMaster Universities Osteoarthritis Index, and the Sickness Impact Profile health-status measures. *J Bone Joint Surg* 1997;79A:1323–1335.

30. MacKenzie EJ, Siegel JH, Shapiro S, Moody M, Smith RT: Functional recovery and medical costs of trauma: An analysis by type and severity of injury. *J Trauma* 1988;28:281–297.

31. Morris JA Jr, Sanchez AA, Bass SM, MacKenzie EJ: Trauma patients return to productivity. *J Trauma* 1991;31:827–834.

32. National Safety Council: *Accident Facts.* Chicago, IL, National Safety Council, 1990.

33. Praemer A, Furner S, Rice DP (eds): *Musculoskeletal Conditions in the United States.* Park Ridge, IL, American Academy of Orthopaedic Surgeons, 1992.

34. Keller RB, Soule DN, Wennberg JE, Hanley DF: Dealing with geographic variations in the use of hospitals: The experience of the Maine Medical Assessment Foundation Orthopaedic Study Group. *J Bone Joint Surg* 1990;72A:1286–1293.

35. Keller RB, Rudicel SA, Liang MH: Outcomes research in orthopaedics. *J Bone Joint Surg* 1993;75A:1562–1574.

36. *Community-Based Healthcare Reform Through Employer Group Purchasing: An Assessment of Select Initiatives.* Solon, OH, Health Action Council of Northeast Ohio, 1994.

37. Torchia M: How Twin Cities employers are re-shaping health care. *Business Health* 1994;12:30–36.

38. United States General Accounting Office: *Access to Health Insurance: Public and Private Employers' Experience with Purchasing Cooperatives.* Washington, DC, United States General Accounting Office, 1994.

39. United States General Accounting Office: *Health Care: Employers and Individual Consumers Want Additional Information on Quality.* Washington, DC, United States General Accounting Office, 1995.

40. Kotin AM, Kuhlman TJ: The employer's view of managed health care: From a passive to an aggressive role, in Kongstvedt PR (ed): *The Managed Health Care Handbook,* ed 3. Gaithersburg, MD, Aspen Publishers, 1996, pp 580–592.

41. Rybowski L: Coalition close-ups. *Business Health* 1996;14:41–45.

42. Meyer JA, Naughton DH, Perry MJ (eds): *Assessing Business Attitudes on Health Care.* Washington, DC, Economic and Social Research Institute, 1996.

43. United States General Accounting Office: *Employment-Based Health Insurance: Costs Increase and Family Coverage Decreases.* Washington, DC, United States General Accounting Office, 1997.

44. Shiels JF, Haught RA: *Managed Care Savings for Employers and Households: 1990 Through 2000.* Washington, DC, American Association of Health Plans, 1997.

45. Smith BM: Trends in health care coverage and financing and their implications for policy. *N Engl J Med* 1997;337:1000–1003.

46. Gabel JR, Ginsburg PB, Hunt KA: Small employers and their health benefits, 1988–1996: An awkward adolescence. *Health Aff* (Millwood) 1997;16:103–110.

47. United States General Accounting Office: *Health Insurance: Management Strategies Used by Large Employers to Control Costs.* Washington, DC, United States General Accounting Office, 1997.

48. United States General Accounting Office: *Private Health Insurance Coverage: Continued*

Erosion of Coverage Linked to Cost Pressures.
Washington, DC, United States General
Accounting Office, 1997.

49. Burner ST, Waldo DR: National health expenditure projections, 1994–2005. *Healthc Financ Rev* 1995;16:221–242.

50. Levit KR, Lazenby HC, Braden BR, et al: National health expenditures, 1995. *Health Care Financ Rev* 1996;18:175–214.

51. Levit KR, Lazenby HC, Sivarajan L: Health care spending in 1994: Slowest in decades. *Health Aff* (Millwood): 1996;15:130–144.

52. Levit KR, Lazenby HC, Sivarajan L, et al: National health expenditures, 1994. *Health Financ Rev* 1996;17:205–242.

53. Vincenzino JV: Trends in medical care cost: Revisited. *Stat Bull Metrop Insur Co* 1997;78: 10–16.

54. *National Survey of Employer-Sponsored Health Plans/1996: Tables.* New York, NY, Foster Higgins, 1997.

55. Reilly PK: *Forecasting Health Insurer Profitability: 1997–1999.* Philadelphia, PA, Milliman & Robertson, 1997.

56. Greene J: Has managed care lost its soul? *Hosp Health Netw* 1997;71:36–38.

57. Fuchs VR: Managed care and merger mania. *JAMA* 1997;277:920–921.

58. Kassirer JP: Editorial: Managing managed care's tarnished image. *N Engl J Med* 1997;337: 338–339.

59. Philadelphia HMOs post losses on Medicaid managed care. *Am Med News* 1997;40:43.

60. Jacob JA: HMO profits plunge in '96: Premium hikes likely result. *Am Med News* 1997; 40:11–12.

61. Miller TE: Managed care regulation: In the laboratory of the states. *JAMA* 1997;278: 1102–1109.

62. Remler DK, Donelan K, Blendon RJ, et al: What do managed care plans do to affect care? Results from a survey of physicians. *Inquiry* 1997;34:196–204.

63. Kertesz L: Oxford expects $68 million loss. *Mod Healthcare* 1997;27:8.

64. Morgan RO, Virnig BA, DeVito CA, Persily NA: The Medicare-HMO revolving door: The healthy go in and the sick go out. *N Engl J Med* 1997;337:169–175.

65. Lippman H: Another health cost explosion: It's not inevitable. *Business Health* 1997;15:27–32.

66. Rovner J: U.S. health-care costs likely to rise. *Lancet* 1997;349:336.

67. Thorpe KE: Why health care costs are rising–again, in Burns J, Sipkoff M (eds): *Guide to Managed Care Strategies 1998: An Annual Report of the Latest Practices and Policies in the New Managed Care Environment.* New York, NY, Faulkner & Gray's Healthcare Information Center, 1997, pp 28–38.

68. *Getting What You Pay For: Purchasing Value in Health Care, 1997.* Bethesda, MD, Watson Wyatt Worldwide, 1997.

69. *Mercer's FAX Facts Surveys: HMOs.* New York, NY, William M Mercer, 1997.

70. Watson Wyatt Worldwide, Washington Business Group on Health: Getting what you pay for: Quality, access, value–purchasing value in health care, in Burns J, Sipkoff M (eds): *Guide to Managed Care Strategies 1998: An Annual Report of the Latest Practices and Policies in the New Managed Care Environment.* New York, NY, Faulkner & Gray's Healthcare Information Center, 1997, pp 312–317.

71. Praeger LO: Joint Commission to require outcomes data reports, in Segre G, Loughran K, Rosenthal B, Cooper B, Beck D (eds): *1998 Comparative Performance Data Sourcebook.* New York, NY, Faulkner & Gray, 1998, pp 367–368.

72. Mangano JJ: New performance standards and their marketplace impact, in Segre G, Loughran K, Rosenthal B, Cooper B, Beck D (eds): *1998 Comparative Performance Data Sourcebook.* New York, NY, Faulkner & Gray, 1998, pp 361–365.

73. Bethell C, Lansky D: Framework for accountability, in Segre G, Loughran K, Rosenthal B, Cooper B, Beck D (eds): *1998 Comparative Performance Data Sourcebook.* New York, NY, Faulkner & Gray, 1998, pp 145–164.

74. InterStudy: *The InterStudy Competitive Edge 5 (vol 2) Part II: Industry Report.* St. Paul, MN, InterStudy, 1995.

75. Ellwood PM: Shattuck lecture: Outcomes management: A technology of patient experience. *N Engl J Med* 1988;318:1549–1556.

76. Johnson LA: Outcomes management a decade out: An interview with Paul Ellwood. *Group Pract J* 1997;46:12–15.

77. Evans RW: Focus on structure and process rather than managing outcomes. *Group Pract J* 1997;46:5–6.

78. Codman EA, Mayo WJ, Chipman WW, Clarke JG, Kanavel AB: Report of Committee on Hospital Standardization. *Surg-Gynecol-Obstet* 1916;22:119–120.

79. Bloom BS: Does it work? The outcomes of medical interventions. *Int J Technol Assess Health-Care* 1990;6:326–332.

80. Donabedian A: Evaluating the quality of medical care. *Milbank Mem Fund Q* 1966;44(Suppl 3):166–206.

81. Cochrane AL (ed): *Effectiveness and Efficiency: Random Reflections on Health Services.* London, England, Nuffield Provincial Hospitals Trust, 1972.

82. Donabedian A: The end results of health care: Ernest Codman's contribution to quality assessment and beyond. *Milbank Q* 1989;67: 233–256.

83. Neuhauser D: Ernest Amory Codman, MD, and end results of medical care. *Int J Technol-Assess Health Care* 1990;6:307–325.

84. Editorial: Cochrane's legacy. *Lancet* 1992;340: 1131–1132.

85. Evans RW: Editorial: Socio-economic explanations for medical failure. *Gastroenterol Int* 1993; 6:123–125.

86. Evans RW: Outcomes measurement and continuous quality improvement: A health services research perspective, in Morrey BF, An KN, Cabanela ME, Cofield RH, Cooney WP III, Kitaoka HB, et al (eds): *Reconstructive Surgery of the Joints,* ed 2. New York, NY, Churchill Livingstone, 1996, 217–224.

87. Pearson M, Wistow G: Editorial: The boundary between health care and social care. *BMJ* 1995; 311:208–209.

88. Blane D: Editorial: Social determinants of health: Socioeconomic status, social class, and ethnicity. *Am J Public Health* 1995;85:903–905.

89. Reiser SJ: Medicine and public health: Pursuing a common destiny. *JAMA* 1996;276: 1429–1430.

90. Editorial: The moral maze of public health. *Lancet* 1997;349:583.

91. Evans RW, Manninen DL, Garrison LP Jr, et al: The quality of life of patients with end-stage renal disease. *N Engl J Med* 1985;312:553–559.

92. Hart LG, Evans RW: The functional status of ESRD patients as measured by the Sickness Impact Profile. *J Chronic Dis* 1987;40(suppl 1):117S–136S.

93. Leplege A, Hunt S: The problem of quality of life in medicine. *JAMA* 1997;278:47–50.

Amputation Surgery in Peripheral Vascular Disease

Michael S. Pinzur, MD
John H. Bowker, MD
Douglas G. Smith, MD
Frank Gottschalk, MD

Burgess[1] focused on amputation surgery as reconstructive, not destructive, surgery; the first step in the rehabilitation of a patient with a nonfunctionally salvageable limb. The metabolic cost of walking is increased with proximal level amputations, being inversely proportional to the length of the residual limb and the number of joints preserved. In dysvascular transfemoral amputees, this cost becomes so severe that they use virtually maximum energy expenditure during normal walking.[2–4] Not only is the energy cost of walking related to amputation, the functional independence of the individual also appears to be correlated with the length of the residual limb.

Prior to surgical decision making, rehabilitation potential and wound healing ability should be assessed. To enable them to become proficient with a prosthesis, patients must possess the cognitive capacities of memory, attention, concentration, and organization.[5] Wound healing rates are dependent on vascular inflow, total body nutrition, and immunocompetence. In patients with peripheral vascular disease, amputation wounds generally heal by collateral blood flow; therefore, arteriography is rarely useful. Vascular inflow is

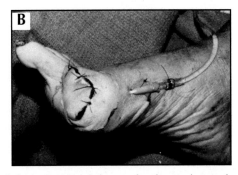

Fig. 1 A, Wet gangrene of the great toe in a diabetic. **B,** Wound closure after disarticulation of the great toe using skin salvaged from the lateral aspect. Features of the Kritter flow-through irrigation system include widely spaced sutures to permit egress of the irrigation fluid and fixation of the catheter to the skin. (Reproduced with permission from Bowker JH, Michael JW (eds): American Academy of Orthopaedic Surgeons *Atlas of Limb Prosthetics: Surgical, Prosthetic, and Rehabilitation Principles,* ed 2. St. Louis, MO, Mosby-Year Book, 1992, p 41.)

determined by ultrasound Doppler or transcutaneous oximetry. An ultrasound Doppler ischemic index (ratio of Doppler pressure at the level in question to the brachial pressure) of 0.5, or a transcutaneous oxygen pressure ($TCPo_2$) of between 20 and 30 mm Hg, are minimum measures of vascular inflow. Patients are malnourished when their serum albumin is below 3.5 g/dl and immune deficient when their total (absolute) lymphocyte count is below 1,500, conditions often present in the dysvascular population. In such patients, surgery can be delayed until these

values are improved, usually by oral hyperalimentation, to support wound healing. When infection or gangrene dictates urgent surgery, drainage of the infection or open amputation at the most distal viable level, followed by open wound care, culture-specific antibiotic therapy, and metabolic support, can be accomplished until wound healing potential can be optimized.[6–11]

Foot and Ankle Amputation

Foot and ankle amputations are most frequently performed in ambulatory diabetics. Surgery can be performed

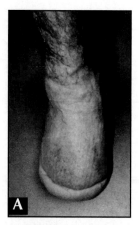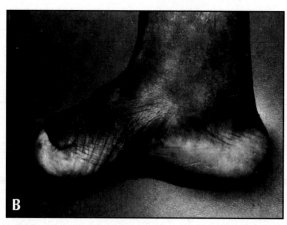

Fig. 2 A, Ideal transmetatarsal amputation. Dorsal view. B, Medial view. Note placement of the distal plantar flap, overall length of the residual forefoot, maintenance of the medial arch, and absence of ankle equinus. (Reproduced with permission from Bowker JH: Role of lower limb amputation in diabetes mellitus, in Levin ME, O'Neal LW, Bowker JH (ed): *The Diabetic Foot*, ed 5. St. Louis, MO, Mosby-Year Book, 1993.)

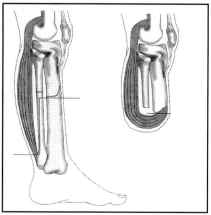

Fig. 3 Schematic drawing of a long posterior flap technique for transtibial amputation. The posterior flap length is equal to the diameter of the limb at the level of the bone transection plus 1 cm. (Rotation of the flap occurs posteriorly, not at the midpoint of the anteroposterior plane.) The fibula is divided 1 to 2 cm shorter than the tibia to avoid distal fibular pain in the prosthesis. A bevel is placed on the anterior tibia to minimize distal tibial pain. The fascia of the posterior flap is secured up over the tibia with myoplasty or myodesis techniques, to prevent loss of distal padding. (Reproduced with permission from Prosthetics Research Study.)

for neuropathic ulceration leading to deep infection/osteomyelitis, gangrene, or a combination. Partial foot amputation or ankle disarticulation preserves the weightbearing tissues of the foot, as well as proprioception not possible with transtibial amputation and prosthetic fitting. Preservation of a durable weightbearing soft-tissue envelope requires avoiding split-thickness skin grafting except over the dorsum of the residual foot. Aggressive removal of all infected or necrotic tissue is essential. If bone is contacted on probe through an ulcer or open wound, a presumptive diagnosis of osteomyelitis can be made.[12] Primary wound closure can be used for clean, noncontaminated wounds. When there is a question of contamination, or a large "dead space" volume, loose wound closure and inflow drainage can be used[13,14] (Fig. 1).

In toe amputations, long plantar flaps are preferred. Preservation of the base of the great toe proximal phalanx (insertion of the flexor hallucis brevis) will prevent retraction of the sesamoid bones proximally, thus preventing prominence of the lateral 4 metatarsal heads. If this is not feasible due to soft-tissue constraints or bone infection, the sesamoids should be removed. Removal of the second toe may lead to a problematic hallux valgus, which can be avoided by preserving the base of the proximal phalanx, or by second ray resection. When the fifth toe is removed, the metatarsal head should be removed in order to retain a smooth contour to the lateral foot, decreasing the risk for late breakdown. The first ray is important in push-off; therefore, length preservation is much more crucial here than in the fourth and fifth rays.

Transmetatarsal amputation should be considered in the following situations: the entire first ray needs to be resected, 2 or more rays need to be resected, or more than 1 central ray needs to be resected. Residual metatarsal length is valuable as a lever arm during the terminal stance phase of gait. Retained metatarsal length should parallel the 15° transverse metatarsal angle of the tarsometatarsal joint and the normal "toe break" of the shoe. When the available soft-tissue envelope dictates, a tarsometatarsal (Lisfranc) amputation can be performed. To avoid the risk of late equinus, a percutaneous Achilles tendon lengthening should be performed. Bony prominences should be beveled prior to wound closure. Both midfoot levels should be managed postoperatively in a well-molded short leg walking cast for 3 to 4 weeks[8] (Fig. 2).

Hindfoot amputations at the Boyd and Chopart levels should be avoided, because they provide an insufficient lever arm for push-off, and are often complicated by severe equinus that cannot be well compensated in shoes.

Ankle disarticulation (Syme's) preserves the normal heel pad for normal proprioceptive end bearing. There is little energy cost in walking with a prosthesis, and patients rarely require more than minimal physical

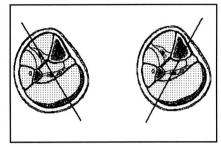

Fig. 4 Schematic of the skew and sagittal flap techniques. (Reproduced with permission from Prosthetics Research Study.)

therapy. It can be performed in 1 stage, removing the malleoli and contouring the metaphyseal flares of the tibia and fibula to provide a durable residual limb. The heel pad is best secured through drill holes in the anterior tibia. A modified Foley catheter or Shirley drain can be used to reduce hematoma collection. At 3 days, a well-fitted cast can be applied to decrease swelling and centralize the heel pad. The cast should be changed weekly for 4 to 5 weeks, at which time a walking cast can be applied until prosthetic fitting can be initiated.[15–17]

Transtibial (Below Knee) Amputation

The goals of transtibial amputation are to obtain primary wound healing, avoid infection, and create a well-padded residual limb that can easily tolerate the stresses of prosthetic fitting and full weightbearing. The long posterior myocutaneous flap, with no dissection between skin and muscle layers, is generally favored in the United States.[18] The level of tibial transection should be as long as possible between the tibial tubercle and the mid/distal third junction, based on the available soft-tissue envelope. The fibula should be transected just proximal to the tibia to create a cylindrical, not conical, residual limb. The

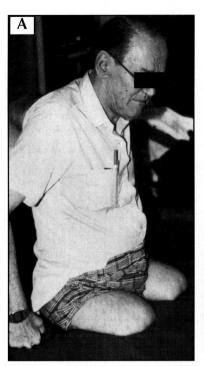

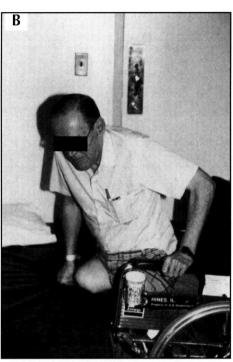

Fig. 5 A, Nonambulatory transfemoral amputees have a small surface area to use as a sitting platform, and (**B**) a short lever arm to assist in transfer. (Reproduced with permission from Pinzur MS: Knee disarticulation: Surgical procedures, in Bowker JH, Michael JW (eds): American Academy of Orthopaedic Surgeons *Atlas of Limb Prosthetics: Surgical, Prosthetic, and Rehabilitation Principles,* ed 2. St. Louis, MO, Mosby-Year Book, 1992, pp 479–486.)

gastrocnemius is secured to the anterior tibia by suture to the periosteum and anterior compartment fascia, or through drill holes in the anterior tibia. The exact placement of surgical scars is not as important as the avoidance of scars adherent to bone (Fig. 3). Both the skew and sagittal flap techniques are variations with slightly oblique equal-length flaps, with an axis offset from the anteroposterior plane[19–21] (Fig.4).

Knee Disarticulation (Through Knee Amputation)

Knee disarticulation is generally performed in the nonambulatory patient, for whom it provides a muscle-balanced residual limb that will not develop hip or knee joint contracture. Functionally, it provides an excellent platform for sitting, and lever arm for

transfer[22] (Fig. 5). In the ambulatory patient, it allows end bearing, with a long femoral lever arm and ease of prosthetic suspension, due to the bulbous end. A four-bar linkage prosthetic polycentric knee joint allows stable walking. Recent experience with a posterior myofasciocutaneous flap, similar to that used in transtibial amputation, has simplified the technique[23] (Fig. 6).

Transfemoral (Above Knee) Amputation

Patients with diabetes and peripheral vascular disease who undergo transfemoral amputation are generally sicker, at greater risk for perioperative morbidity, and are very unlikely to become prosthetic limb users.[2–4,24,25] Conventional transfemoral amputation uses "fish-mouth" flaps, in

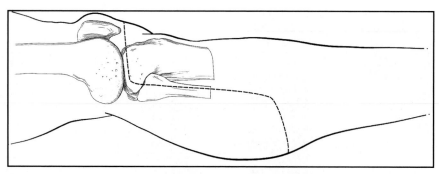

Fig. 6 Posterior myocutaneous flap technique now used in knee disarticulation. (Reproduced with permission from Pinzur MS: Current concepts: Amputation surgery in peripheral vascular disease, in Springfield DS (ed): *Instructional Course Lectures 47*. Rosemont, IL, American Academy of Orthopaedic Surgeons, 1997, pp 501–509.)

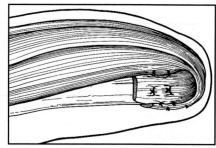

Fig. 9 Diagram depicting attachment of the quadriceps over the adductor magnus. (Reproduced with permission from Gottschalk F: Transfemoral amputation: Surgical procedures, in Bowker JH, Michael JW (eds): American Academy of Orthopaedic Surgeons *Atlas of Limb Prosthetics: Surgical, Prosthetic, and Rehabilitation Principles*, ed 2. St. Louis, MO, Mosby-Year Book, 1992, pp 501–507.)

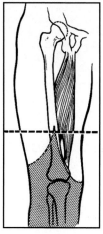

Fig. 7 Diagram depicting proposed skin flaps and level of bone transection in transfemoral amputation. (Reproduced with permission from Gottschalk F: Transfemoral amputation: Surgical procedures, in Bowker JH, Michael JW (eds): American Academy of Orthopaedic Surgeons *Atlas of Limb Prosthetics: Surgical, Prosthetic, and Rehabilitation Principles*, ed 2. St. Louis, MO, Mosby-Year Book, 1992, pp 501–507.)

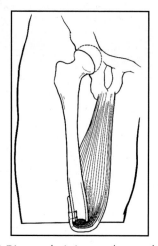

Fig. 8 Diagram depicting attachment of adductor magnus to the lateral residual femur. (Reproduced with permission from Gottschalk F: Transfemoral amputation: Surgical procedures, in Bowker JH, Michael JW (eds): American Academy of Orthopaedic Surgeons *Atlas of Limb Prosthetics: Surgical, Prosthetic, and Rehabilitation Principles*, ed 2. St. Louis, MO, Mosby-Year Book, 1992, pp 501–507.)

which the hamstring and adductor muscles are severed, which reduces their ability to extend and adduct the hip. Ischial containment prosthetic sockets attempt to control the femur in a more physiologic adducted position.[26,27] Weightbearing radiographs revealed that prosthetic socket configuration does not influence the position of the residual femur and

that dynamic alignment depends on surgical technique.[28] Adductor myodesis anchors the adductor muscles and eliminates the abductor lurch seen with transfemoral amputee gait.

A long medially based myocutaneous flap is used with this currently accepted method (Fig. 7). The quadriceps tendon is transected just proximal to the patella. The adductor mag-

nus is detached from the femur by sharp dissection, exposing the femoral shaft. The femur is transected approximately 14-cm proximal to the joint. The adductor magnus tension is retained by repairing the remaining tendon to drill holes in the lateral cortex of the residual femur, with the femur positioned in maximal adduction (Fig. 8). The quadriceps tendon is secured to the posterior residual femur through drill holes, being careful not to create an iatrogenic hip flexion contracture by accomplishing the repair with the hip in flexion (Fig. 9). The remaining posterior muscles are secured to the adductor magnus prior to skin closure.[29]

Phantom Limb Pain

Phantom limb sensation following amputation in the adult is common but is not usually bothersome. True phantom limb pain, a sensation of burning, or searing pain in the amputated part is fortunately rare. New studies indicate that mechanisms designed to block the pain pathways around the time of surgery reduce perioperative pain, as well as chronic phantom pain. This can be accomplished by various techniques of continuous regional anesthesia initiated before, during, or after surgery. It appears that pretreatment, or continuous neural blockade following surgery can be successful in altering pain following amputation.[30-33]

References

1. Burgess EM: General principles of amputation surgery, in American Academy of Orthopaedic Surgeons *Atlas Limb Prosthetics*. St. Louis, MO, CV Mosby, 1981, p 160.

2. Fisher SV, Gullickson G Jr: Energy cost of ambulation in health and disability: A literature review. *Arch Phys Med Rehabil* 1978;59:124–133.

3. Pinzur MS, Gold J, Schwartz D, Gross N: Energy demands for walking in dysvascular amputees as related to the level of amputation. *Orthopaedics* 1992;15:1033–1037.

4. Waters RL, Perry J, Antonelli D, Hislop H: Energy cost of walking of amputees: The influence of level of amputation. *J Bone Joint Surg* 1976;58A:42–46.

5. Pinzur MS, Graham G, Osterman H: Psychologic testing in amputation rehabilitation. *Clin Orthop* 1988;229:236–240.

6. Pinzur MS: New concepts in lower-limb amputation and prosthetic management, in Greene WB (ed): *Instructional Course Lectures XXXIX*. Park Ridge, IL, American Academy of Orthopaedic Surgeons, 1990, pp 361–366.

7. Dickhaut SC, DeLee JC, Page CP: Nutritional status: Importance in predicting wound-healing after amputation. *J Bone Joint Surg* 1984;66A: 71–75.

8. Pinzur M, Kaminsky M, Sage R, Cronin R, Osterman H: Amputations at the middle level of the foot: A retrospective and prospective review. *J Bone Joint Surg* 1986;68A:1061–1064.

9. Pinzur MS, Sage R, Stuck R, Ketner L, Osterman H: Transcutaneous oxygen as a predictor of wound healing in amputations of the foot and ankle *Foot Ankle* 1992;13:271–272.

10. Wyss CR, Harrington RM, Burgess EM, Matsen FA III: Transcutaneous oxygen tension as a predictor of success after an amputation. *J Bone Joint Surg* 1988;70A:203–207.

11. Pinzur MS: Amputation surgery in peripheral vascular disease, in Springfield DS (ed): *Instructional Course Lectures 46*. Rosemont, IL, American Academy of Orthopaedic Surgeons, 1997, pp 501–509.

12. Grayson ML, Gibbons GW, Balogh K, Levin E, Karchmer AW: Probing to bone in infected pedal ulcers: A clinical sign of underlying osteomyelitis in diabetic patients. *JAMA* 1995;273:721–723.

13. Kritter AE: A technique for salvage of the infected diabetic gangrenous foot. *Orthop Clin North Am* 1973;4:21–30.

14. Bowker JH: The choice between limb salvage and amputation: Infection, in Bowker JH, Michael JW (eds): American Academy of Orthopaedic Surgeons *Atlas of Limb Prosthetics: Surgical, Prosthetic, and Rehabilitation Principles*, ed 2. St. Louis, MO, Mosby-Year Book, 1992, pp 39–43.

15. Pinzur MS, Smith D, Osterman H: Syme ankle disarticulation in peripheral vascular disease and diabetic foot infection: The one-stage versus two-stage procedure. *Foot Ankle Int* 1995;16:124–127.

16. Wagner FW Jr: Management of the diabetic-neurotrophic foot: Part II. A classification and treatment program for diabetic, neuropathic, and dysvascular foot problems, in Cooper RR (ed): American Academy of Orthopaedic Surgeons *Instructional Course Lectures XXVIII*. St. Louis, MO, CV Mosby, 1979, pp 143–165.

17. Wagner FW Jr: The Syme ankle disarticulation, in Bowker JH, Michael JW (eds): American Academy of Orthopaedic Surgeons *Atlas of Limb Prosthetics: Surgical, Prosthetic, and Rehabilitation Principles*, ed 2. St. Louis, MO, Mosby-Year Book, 1992, pp 413–422.

18. Pinzur MS, Gottschalk F, Smith D, et al: Functional outcome of below-knee amputation in peripheral vascular insufficiency: A multicenter review. *Clin Orthop* 1993;286:247–249.

19. Robinson KP, Hoile R, Coddington T: Skew flap myoplastic below-knee amputation: A preliminary report. *Br J Surg* 1982;69:554–557.

20. Alter AH, Moshein J, Elconin KB, Cohen MJ: Below-knee amputation using the sagittal technique: A comparison with the coronal amputation. *Clin Orthop* 1978;131:195–201.

21. Persson BM: Sagittal incision for below-knee amputation in ischaemic gangrene. *J Bone Joint Surg* 1974;56B:110–114.

22. Pinzur MS, Smith DG, Daluga DJ, Osterman H: Selection of patients for through-the-knee amputation. *J Bone Joint Surg* 1988;70A: 746–750.

23. Bowker JH, Pinzur: Knee disarticulation with a posterior myofasciocutaneous flap. *Clin Orthop*, in press.

24. Gonzalez EG, Corcoran PJ, Reyes RL: Energy expenditure in below-knee amputees: Correlation with stump length. *Arch Phys Med Rehabil* 1974:55:111–119.

25. Volpicelli LJ, Chambers RB, Wagner FW Jr: Ambulation levels of bilateral lower-extremity amputees: Analysis of one hundred and three cases. *J Bone Joint Surg* 1982;65A:599–605.

26. Long IA: Normal shape-normal alignment (NSNA) above-knee prosthesis. *Clin Prosthet Orthot* 1985;9:9–14.

27. Sabolich J: Contoured adducted trochanteric-controlled alignment method (CAT-CAM): Introduction and basic principles. *Clin Prosthet Orthot* 1985;9:15–26.

28. Gottschalk FA, Kourosh S, Stills M, McClellan B, Roberts J: Does socket configuration influence the position of the femur in above-knee amputation? *J Prosthet Orthot* 1989;2:94–102.

29. Gottschalk F: Transfemoral amputation: Surgical procedures, in Bowker JH, Michael JW (eds): American Academy of Orthopaedic Surgeons *Atlas of Limb Prosthetics: Surgical, Prosthetic, and Rehabilitation Principles*, ed 2. St. Louis, MO, Mosby-Year Book, 1992, pp 501–507.

30. Bach S, Noreng MF, Tjellden NU: Phantom limb pain in amputees during the first 12 months following limb amputation, after pre-operative lumbar epidural blockade. *Pain* 1988; 33:297–301.

31. Malawer MM, Buch R, Khurana JS, Garvey T, Rice L: Postoperative infusional continuous regional analgesia: A technique for relief of postoperative pain following major extremity surgery. *Clin Orthop* 1991;266:227–237.

32. Melzack R: Phantom limbs. *Sci Am* 1992;266: 120–126.

33. Pinzur MS, Garla PG, Pulth T, Vrbos L: Continuous postoperative infusion of a regional anesthetic after an amputation of the lower extremity: A randomized clinical trial. *J Bone Joint Surg* 1996;78A:1501–1505.

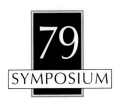

Work-Related Upper Extremity Complaints

Michael Vender, MD
Morton L. Kasdan, MD, FACS

Review of the Literature

Physicians process patients' allegations of "disorders" (symptoms) related to performing their work activities. The lay press describes the crippling effects of various work activities and product utilization (for example, computer keyboards). In legal proceedings, determining causal relationship is a primary issue. Our personal review of medical records and proceedings of legal cases indicates physicians often state that in their opinion and based on the literature there is causal relationship of work activities to disease.

How does one determine if an illness is related to work activities? The National Institute of Occupational Safety and Health (NIOSH) set out 6 criteria for determining if a disease is causally related to work activities.[1] One of these criteria is consideration of epidemiologic data, with experimental and matched control cohorts.

What scientific evidence exists that demonstrates a relationship of work to disease? Why is it that only persons who are employed are crippled by keyboards, yet persons who use home computers are not crippled? Why is the performance of physical activities at work deleterious, yet persons who are active in nonwork-related activities do not present to the office with the same frequency, severity of complaints, refractoriness to treatment, and reported impairment and disability? These are some of the questions that led to a review of the literature reporting a relationship of work activities to development of upper extremity work-related complaints.[2]

Do these articles indicate disease processes identified only in persons who work? Are there specific job activities with specific risk factors? Is there correlation between work activities and the development of specific disorders? How consistent are the opinions throughout the literature? Are there articles that indicate that carpal tunnel syndrome (CTS), for example, can be prevented by avoiding work? Do ergonomic changes affect incidence of disease?

One of the more striking findings of this literature review is that many of these studies that so definitively state the causal relationship of work to disorders did not even study objective upper extremity diagnoses. Many simply recorded subjective complaints and did not identify a specific disease process. Many studies that attempted to look at a condition, such as CTS, did not use adequate definition or criteria to identify such a condition. For example, it was common to survey a place of employment using questionnaires to determine the presence of a disease or injury. At times this may be coupled with a very cursory physical examination, relying on findings such as Tinel's and Phalen's signs. Are these adequate diagnostic criteria? The lack of reliability of these signs is well demonstrated.[3] These tests are subjective in that they depend on patient cooperation for a response and the physician's subjective interpretation of the evaluation. These tests are not performed or interpreted the same among physicians. Patient education and the examiners' experience are confounding factors that eliminate Tinel's and Phalen's signs as diagnostic indicators of CTS.

To determine adequacy of data collection, or diagnostic criteria, it is necessary to understand the purpose and method for the data collection. To screen for all persons with a diagnosis, the screening process must have a high degree of sensitivity. As there is an inverse relationship of sensitivity and specificity, a method with high sensitivity will have low specificity. High sensitivity increases the true positive rate but also increases the false positive rate. While sensitivity is important for surveillance, it is not appropriate for trying to determine causal relationship, implicating and altering job activities, or for determining treatment. Before performing surgery on a patient, a surgeon would have information that is objective and reliable.[4] In spite of unsatisfactorily low specificity surveillance, information gathering is used by researchers and government agencies to make profound judgments that affect employers by forcing work place changes and levying fines.

Although many articles were found to be inadequate simply on the basis of examining subjective complaints and demonstrating poor definition of disease and injury, there were a few remaining articles that examined specific conditions and employed adequate definitions. However, these articles demonstrated major design flaws. The information contained would be of use for academic discussion and to serve as a springboard for further study. The information is far from definitive, and no conclusions should be drawn.[5]

Upper Extremity Diseases

Numerous conditions that occur in the hand and upper extremity are seen in both work and nonwork environments. As mentioned previously, NIOSH's criteria to determine work relatedness includes as the very first criterion "evidence of disease." While this may seem obvious, reviews of patients' medical records frequently lack substantiation of reported diagnoses. Before determining whether a problem is related to work activities, it is necessary to arrive at an appropriate and reliable diagnosis. Numerous possible diagnoses (and labels) that are not always appropriate can be placed after evaluating patients with subjective complaints.

Neck and Shoulder Girdle Area

Neck and shoulder complaints are very common in the general population. They can be secondary to something as routine as excessive tension from static muscle positioning or anxiety. Conditions such as

shoulder impingement and rotator cuff pathology should be diagnosed by focused and consistent symptoms of localized pain in the shoulder[6] and substantiated by appropriate provocative maneuvers on physical examination. There is frequently a therapeutic and diagnostic response to local anesthetic and steroid injections. When present, rotator cuff injury can be diagnosed by both shoulder arthrograms and magnetic resonance imaging (MRI) scans.

Thoracic outlet syndrome is a condition frequently diagnosed without adequate objective findings.[7] Appropriate diagnostic indicators have shown that this condition is rare. Even when thoracic outlet-like symptoms are present, they are not necessarily abnormal. Many of the changes associated with thoracic outlet syndrome, such as the hands falling asleep or becoming weak and tired with certain maneuvers, especially when working with the arms overhead, fall within the spectrum of normal.

Elbow Region

Although many conditions occur around the distal arm, elbow, and proximal forearm region, the great majority of these are represented by only a few diagnoses.[8] Most elbow complaints are related to "lateral/medial epicondylitis" and/or ulnar nerve irritation. In these conditions, focused, consistent, and reproducible symptoms and findings are important, because diagnostic evaluation (for example, electromyography or nerve conduction velocity) is less reliable.

Hand and Wrist

Common conditions include digital flexor tendon entrapment (trigger finger), deQuervain's disease, and CTS. We believe that deQuervain's disease is a commonly overdiagnosed

condition. Symptoms involve localized radial wrist pain. Tenderness is specifically over the first extensor compartment and not in adjacent areas. Provocative testing includes Finkelstein's test. However, for control purposes, the tests should be performed and compared with other provocative maneuvers that should not cause pain. If patients have positive response to these other provocative maneuvers, the reliability of the diagnosis should be questioned.[9]

Probably the most common diagnosis about the hand and wrist and even the upper extremity involves the nerve compression syndrome of CTS. Symptoms can be vague and nonspecific, but the great majority of cases have a specific and predictable set of complaints. Physical examination is frequently not helpful in verifying the diagnosis but is useful in identifying coexistent or confounding conditions. If the condition has progressed significantly, examination may document any neurologic change in the way of abnormal sensation or loss of muscle strength or bulk.[10]

Tinel's sign and Phalen's tests are not objective tests because they are influenced by the examiner and involve the patient's input. The tests are not performed in a consistent manner. The false positive and negative rates are unacceptably high to allow use of these tests for diagnostic purposes.[3]

The diagnosis of CTS should be made only when the appropriate history is correlated with positive findings on electrodiagnostic studies. Numerous changes are described as being possibly indicative of CTS. However, absolute prolongation of distal sensory and/or motor latencies of the median nerve as it crosses through the carpal tunnel is most reliable. At times this change will be noted only in orthodromic sensory testing. With improved technology and guideline standards for performing the test, the electromyographic nerve compression study has a negligible rate of false negatives, when performed by an appropriate tester.[11]

Many diagnoses are made without appropriate history, physical examination, and objective documentation on laboratory testing. Physicians may use these premature diagnoses as "working diagnoses." While it may be reasonable to consider certain diagnoses as possibilities, there can be significant negative effects when a diagnosis/label is placed prematurely. Labeling a patient with a specific diagnosis creates potential psychological impairment, because the patient believes he or she is diseased or injured. It leads to treatment expectations. When early treatment fails to relieve mislabeled symptoms, the next step can be unnecessary surgery. When patients have subjective complaints that cannot be reliably diagnosed, a better label would be that of pain in the upper extremity (ICD-9 code 729.5). Patients may find this less satisfactory, but it avoids the dangerous effects of premature and erroneous diagnoses.

Cumulative Trauma Disorders

Several terms have been used interchangeably to describe the various symptoms developed by patients. Many patients are inappropriately labeled with diagnostic entities, such as tendinitis or CTS, when no reliable objective evidence exists. Other patients are provided the generic diagnostic label of cumulative trauma disorder, repetitive motion disorder, repetitive motion injury, overuse syndrome, cervical brachial disorder, or repetitive strain injury to explain subjective complaints.[12] Symptoms do not mean a disease is present. These labels are of limited usefulness in evaluating and treating patients and when used with occupational illnesses they are harmful.

Some health care providers consider cumulative trauma disorder as being an umbrella label for specific diagnoses, such as CTS or deQuervain's disease. The term is also used to mean a specific disease entity. The concept of cumulative trauma is based on engineering principles. The concept of structural fatigue states that an inert material, such as metal, will eventually break after being subjected to repeated stress. It was assumed that the body would respond in a similar manner. The main flaw in this reasoning is that metal is inert while the body is a dynamic living tissue that not only is able to heal itself, but actually responds in a positive manner to physical stress. A theme common to these terms is that forceful and repetitive occupational activities (overuse, repetitive) are followed by disease (syndrome, disorder, injury). At best, these terms are used to explain symptoms. At worst, it is a category of disease used to justify prolonged, frequently unnecessary, and inappropriate medical treatment.

Epidemiology

From earlier days, when work-related injuries were loss of limb and loss of life, we have moved to an era of less clearly defined injuries. To better understand the relationship of various complaints or disease processes to work activities requires an adequate understanding of epidemiology.

Epidemiology is "the study of distribution and determination of health-related states or events in specified populations, and the application of the study to control of health problems."[13] It allows a differentiation between the terms association and causation. Association is the extent to which the occurrence of 2 or more characteristics is linked either through a causal or noncausal relationship in a statistically significant manner. Causality is the extent to which the occurrence of a risk factor is responsible for the subsequent occurrence of a disease.

To better understand epidemiology and causation, certain terms must be defined. In 1951, Sir Bradford Hill[14] described how to analyze an association of 2 occurrences (eg, work and disease) to see if one (work) is causing the other (disease). The most important factor is the strength of association. Next in importance is consistency—observed by different persons, in different places, circumstances, and time. The third major factor is specificity. The fourth characteristic is temporality. Do people have the disease prior to the exposure? The fifth major characteristic is biologic gradient. Is there a certain amount of exposure needed to get the disease? Is there a dose-response relationship?

Influences on the Reporting of Work-Related Upper Extremity Disorders
Background Stimulus

A person who has a somatic experience will interpret it as being pleasurable or unpleasurable based on the background stimulus he or she is experiencing at that time. Muscle discomfort in the context of a health club or sports activity is frequently interpreted as being positive and beneficial, whereas the same discomfort experienced while performing an ungratifying job under poor working conditions will be experienced as being unpleasurable. The latter is likely to lead to medical intervention; the former is not. Psychosocial influences play a major role in perception of disease process, utilization of medical services, and impairment and disability.[15]

Job Dissatisfaction

A major determinate in reporting work-related injuries is job dissatisfaction. Persons who reported that they hardly ever enjoyed their jobs were 2.5 times more likely to report back symptoms than persons who reported being generally or almost always happy with their jobs.[16]

Somatization

The term somatization refers to the reporting of symptoms that have no pathophysiologic explanation. Somatic refers to complaints referable to the body. Somatization is the propensity to report somatic symptoms that have no basis in actual pathology and to wrongly attribute these symptoms to a disease or injury.[17]

It is a fact of normal life that all persons experience subjective symptoms throughout their body. These include symptoms as diverse as headache, neck pain, muscle pain, trigger points, abdominal pain, chest pain, diarrhea, constipation, fatigue, memory loss, and joint pain. Focusing on bodily complaints is a universal phenomenon. However, it becomes a significant problem when it occurs in the context of a psychiatric disorder, stressful life experiences, or major emotional turmoil. The person who is a somatosizer may actually be experiencing discomfort. It becomes problematic when these complaints make the patient preoccupied and dysfunctional.

Medicalization

It is clear we are experiencing an increased prevalence of persons with refractory upper extremity complaints. They do not fit into the various diagnostic categories physicians have been trained to understand and diagnose. They do not respond to treatment. Physicians are unable to classify these into true disease categories, and, in a benevolently misinformed way, they diagnose these patients as having cumulative trauma disorder and repetitive strain injuries. Medicalization is taking various symptoms in persons without objective disease (somatisizers) and classifying these symptoms as a real disease or injury.

Cost Shifting in Workers' Compensation

Research demonstrates that workers respond to economic incentives as they relate to workers' compensation. Workers' compensation as a disability system "becomes not just a rehabilitation experience when health conditions, objectively defined, are serious enough, but can become an alternative to working itself."[18] Doctors in health maintenance organizations (HMOs) are more likely to classify claims as compensable under worker's compensation than are other physicians. While managed care severely limits income from patient evaluations either by capitation or by significant discounts on fee for service, workers' compensation typically has a more generous reimbursement schedule. This represents a strong incentive to attribute vague soft-tissue complaints and disorders to work activities.

Iatrogenesis

In July of 1989 the Hazard Evaluations and Technical Assistance branch of the National Institute for Occupational Safety and Health (NIOSH) received a request from U.S. West Communications and the Communication Workers of America Union to evaluate how video display terminals affect the health of directory assistance operators. They studied 5 different job titles in 3 different locations of U.S. West Communications. Directory assistance did not appear to have a higher prevalence of job disorders as compared to industry standards. One of the most striking findings was the number of diagnoses and surgical procedures performed in 1 specific location.[15] NIOSH concluded that "almost all of the physical workstations observed in the study were of high ergonomic quality, therefore we cannot evaluate its contribution to work related upper extremity disorders and upper extremity musculoskeletal symptoms."[15] This leads to the important point that ergonomics is frequently not the issue in determining upper extremity complaints and disease, which correlates with findings in the scientific literature. There is little to substantiate that disease processes are altered by major ergonomic changes.

Nocebo

To many, physical disease is thought to originate solely in the body itself. However, the brain affects the body in many ways. The mind affects the body's major hormones and also influences the immune system. A placebo is a positive effect from an interaction that would not be expected to have an influence on a particular outcome or experience. A less appreciated concept is that of nocebo, that is the opposite of placebo.[19] Nocebo is an intervention that has a negative effect on a person's well-being or outcome, where such an effect would not be expected. In a group of psychology students participating in an experiment who are told they are going to have an electric current pass through their head by electrodes, a significant number will have complaints of pain or headache even if no such current is actually passed.

Media/Legal System

One effective source of the nocebo effect is the media. If a person experiencing normal upper extremity musculoskeletal symptoms reads that work or product (for example computers or breast implants) causes an illness or injury, it is not unexpected that this would exacerbate the individual's perception of and concerns about these symptoms. We believe that it will likely increase the reporting of these symptoms to a health care provider. Legal advice for a possible work- or product-related condition could have further negative effect on a patient's perception of well-being and also affect satisfactory resolution and outcome. Some people believe that the media benefits from portraying American society as victims. It is not uncommon to see newspaper and magazine articles that portray workers as victims of their workplace activities. Sensational articles that make allegations that are not scientifically substantiated can create a dramatic effect on the public consciousness.[20] A pointed example is that of Dow Corning and its reported liability in the alleged relationship of silicone breast implants and the development of systemic disease in women. With no scientific substantiation, billions of dollars have been placed in settlements. This debacle continues in spite of multiple substantive scientific reports that have demonstrated no association or causal relationship of silicone breast implants to systemic disease.

Some investigators feel a growing number of conditions that stem from somatization have created disease syndromes that have little scientific substantiation. These include chronic fatigue syndrome, food hypersensitivity, reactive hypoglycemia, systemic yeast infection, Gulf War syndrome, fibromyalgia, sick-building syndrome, and cumulative trauma disorder. Many of these conditions have been prominently discussed in newspapers, trade magazines, and news shows, leading to a heightened public consciousness. A balanced presentation, indicating that science does not support many of the theories and allegations, is lacking. In spite of the lack of scientific corroboration, support groups, national organizations, and litigation develop. This heightened awareness causes patients to consult their physicians. It is easy to see how the media can exacerbate and feed into the somatization experienced by the average person. Bringing these patients with their heightened awareness into the physician's office leads to medicalization.

References

1. Kusnetz, Hutchinson (ed): *A Guide to Work-Relatedness of Disease.* NIOSH Publication No. 79-116; 1979.

2. Vender MI, Kasdan ML, Truppa KL: Upper extremity disorders: A literature review to determine work-relatedness. *Hand Surg* 1995;20A:534–541.

3. Katz JN, Larson MG, Fossel AH, Liang MH: Validation of a surveillance case definition of carpal tunnel syndrome. *Am J Public Health* 1991;81:189–193.

4. Szabo RM: Occupational carpal tunnel syndrome, in Kasdan ML (ed): *Occupational Hand and Upper Extremity Injuries and Diseases,* ed 2. Philadelphia, PA, Hanley and Belfus, 1998, pp 113–128.

5. Vender MI, Truppa KT: How meaningful is the literature? *Tech Hand Upper Extrem Surg* 1997;1:273–276.

6. Sagerman SD, Truppa KT: Diagnosis and management of occupational disorders of the shoulder, in Kasdan ML (ed): *Occupational Hand and Upper Extremity Injuries and Diseases,* ed 2. Philadelphia, PA, Hanley and Belfus, 1998, pp 277–286.

7. Wilbourn AJ: Thoracic outlet syndromes: A plea for conservatism. *Neurosurg Clin N Am* 1991:2:235–245.

8. Burgess RC: Diagnosis and management of occupational disorders of the elbow, in Kasdan ML (ed): *Occupational Hand and Upper Extremity Injuries and Diseases,* ed 2. Philadelphia, PA, Hanley and Belfus, 1998, pp 269–276.

9. Vender MI, Pomerance JF, Kasdan ML: Tendon entrapment of the hand and wrist, in Kasdan ML (ed): *Occupational Hand and Upper Extremity Injuries and Diseases,* ed 2. Philadelphia, PA, Hanley and Belfus, 1998, pp 183–190.

10. Vender MI, Ruder JR, Pomerance JF, Truppa KL: Upper extremity compressive neuropathies, in Kasdan ML (ed): *Occupational Hand and Upper Extremity Injuries and Diseases,* ed 2. Philadelphia, PA, Hanley and Belfus, 1998, pp 83–96.

11. Corwin HM, Kasdan ML: Electrodiagnostic reports of median neuropathy at the wrist. *J Hand Surg* 1998;23A:55–57.

12. Weiland AJ: Repetitive strain injuries and cumulative trauma disorders. *J Hand Surg* 1996;21A:337.

13. Last JM: *A Dictionary of Epidemiology.* New York, NY, Oxford University Press, 1988.

14. Hill AB: The environment and disease: Association or causation. *Proc Roy Soc Med* 1965;J8:295–300.

15. Hadler NM: Arm pain in the workplace: A small area analysis. *J Occup Med* 1992;34: 113–119.

16. Bigos SJ, Battie MC, Spengler DM, et al: A prospective study of work perceptions and psychosocial factors affecting the report of back injury. *Spine* 1991;16:1–6.

17. Barsky AJ, Borus JF: Somatization and medicalization in the era of managed care. *JAMA* 1995;274:1931–1934.

18. Butler RJ, Hartwig RP, Gardner H: HMOs: Moral hazard and cost shifting in worker's compensation. *J Health Economics* 1997;16:191–206.

19. Wade N: The Spin doctors. *New York Times Magazine* 1996.

20. Elmer-Dewitt P: A royal pain in the wrist. *Time* 1994, October 24:60–62.

Medical Malpractice: Defending Yourself

Isadore G. Yablon, MD

The Trauma of Litigation for Yourself and Others

It is unsettling to anyone to have a deputy sheriff or process server show up at your office or home with a complaint and summons containing exaggerated allegations of wrongdoing, stated in the vaguest of terms. Although no documented clinical studies have been done, there is no doubt that a malpractice suit causes significant emotional trauma to a physician and the physician's family. The most appropriate way to respond to this initial bad news is to contact your insurer immediately. A claim representative will be assigned to the case, who will interview you and then make arrangements for the appointment of an attorney to represent your interests. One should never under any circumstances attempt to contact the patient or the lawyer who has brought suit against you. Any such attempt will be guaranteed to return to haunt you at future times during the course of litigation. You should also not feel that you are an inferior physician merely because of these allegations. The vast majority of medical malpractice cases that are tried to conclusion are resolved in favor of the physician.[1]

The attorney appointed by your insurer will arrange to have expert review done to determine the nature and extent of your treatment of the patient and whether it complied with the standards of care of the average qualified physician in your type of practice. It is important not to change title to any significant assets such as a home purely for the purpose of protecting your property from potential personal liability, because to do so could be construed as an admission of guilt or liability on your part. If you have a legitimate real estate or other financial transaction in the offing, discuss that with your defense attorney to make sure that he or she is aware of it and that it is clearly not meant to put assets out of the reach of a potential plaintiff.

Your cooperation with your attorney is an essential part of the case as you pass through the litigation process. It is most frustrating to defense attorneys to have an uncooperative physician as a client. They can only do their best when they have your best assistance. That means that you may have to interrupt your regular schedule to accommodate your attorney, who will do his or her best to cause minimal disruption of your regular routine. You must somehow learn to trust and place your reliance in your defense attorney. You should not discuss the nature of the case with any other treating physicians without the approval of your defense attorney. These are matters that will be brought up later on during the course of discovery when you are asked questions relative to conversations you had with any caregivers.

Physician support groups are being formed across the country,[2] in which individuals who have difficulty in coping with litigation can meet with others who have gone through the process or are in the midst of the process to help you deal with this upset in your life. Contact your insurance carrier or attorney for the location of such groups.

The Defendant Doctor in Court

Once you have notified your insurance carrier that you have been sued, your carrier will send a representative to take a recorded statement from you.[3] This statement will assist your insurance company in determining how defensible your case is. This interview occurs in your office and is usually quite informal.

Following this, your carrier will select an attorney to defend you. A meeting will be arranged subsequently, at which time your attorney will sound you out and get the facts of the case as you see them. Do not be surprised if you detect a lack of urgency in your lawyer. While being sued is understandably a traumatic event in your life, this is what he or she does every day for a living. Furthermore, the actual trial may not take place until anywhere from 3 to 7 years later, and much will happen in the interim, as will be subsequently explained. It is important to stress again that you cooperate fully with your attorney. Although it may interfere with your practice, bear in mind that it is your trial and it is you who is being sued. The more help you give your attorney, the better he or she will serve you.

There are rare instances in which the relationship between you and your lawyer deteriorates and for whatever reasons you either have lost confidence or don't seem to be getting along with him or her. Under these circumstances, call your insurance carrier and ask them to select another attorney to represent you. The insurance company will almost always comply with your request because it is in its best interest to have a well-coordinated team as the trial goes forward.

Once the patient's complaint has been filed and your attorneys have been selected, the next event to occur will be the interrogatory. This consists of a number of questions that the plaintiff asks you. Each state has a set limit to the number of questions permitted. Be aware that the patient's husband or wife will join the suit claiming a loss of consortium because of your supposed error. In the case of a child, 1 of the parents will join the suit claiming the same loss of consortium. This serves to increase the dollar amount of the suit. You will therefore be served with 2 sets of interrogatories, 1 by each plaintiff. Obviously, you as a defendant, through your attorney, have the right to serve 2 sets of interrogatories on the plaintiffs.

Your attorney will review the interrogatories submitted by the plaintiffs and select portions which he or she will answer and some to which an objection will be raised. The rest of the questions in the interrogatory will be forwarded to you for you to

answer. Your attorney will then put all of these answers into legal format and submit the finished product for your review and signature. Bear in mind that you are signing these interrogatories under oath so that if you have any questions or are uncertain about any answers discuss them with your attorney before signing. Once you have signed the interrogatories you must stick with your answers, because any departure will be construed as an inconsistency on your part. At a later date, and prior to your trial, you will be deposed by the plaintiff's attorney. This will be discussed in the subsequent section.

There have been numerous occasions when, on the night before a trial, a physician would call his defense attorney at home to tell him that he has discovered a completely new theory for the defense of this case and that a continuance must be requested in order to obtain the services of an expert from a totally unrelated field to deal with some obscure point which has come to the attention of the defendant at the eleventh hour. You must learn that your role at the trial stage is that of a witness who should be able to make a good impression on the jury, but you are not the "expert." You do not need to provide all or even a significant part of the defense of your conduct in the case.[4] It is more important that a jury likes you and feels that you are a caring, concerned doctor. You need not be involved with doing literature searches and the like. Leave these matters to the experts who are going to testify on your behalf and concentrate more on being natural and acting as yourself in court and even following the advice of your defense attorney down to the issue of how to dress appropriately for a trial. Much as a patient who reaches an operating room has matters basically taken from his or her hands, you must

learn that in a malpractice case you are there to act in a relatively limited capacity, but will always be called on for input from those defending you.

Avoid being argumentative with the plaintiff's attorney during the trial.[5] He or she will attempt to portray you as an insensitive, mistake-prone individual. The plaintiff's attorney will almost certainly take certain passages from your notes or from your patient's hospital record and exaggerate them to give them a significance out of proportion to what really happened. For example, you may have performed a total hip replacement on a patient who 2 or 3 weeks later developed a postoperative infection. This patient may have had a low grade fever for the first 4 or 5 days after surgery, which subsequently returned to normal only to reappear at a later time. The white count and sedimentation rate, may also have been elevated during the patient's postoperative stay in hospital. The plaintiff's attorney will try to show that the elevated temperature, white count, and sedimentation rate, which occurred early in the postoperative period, were a precursor to the infection and, much to your dismay, will request that you answer with a simple yes or no. The natural response on your part is to want to explain that these changes in the early postoperative period may have been secondary to the stress of the surgery and to other factors unrelated to the infection. If you attempt to do this you will become argumentative and the plaintiff's attorney will certainly try to goad you into fighting with him, but to do so will only affect the jury in a negative way. It is best to answer the questions put to you by the plaintiff's attorney as simply and respectfully as possible without attempting to explain or defend your position. You will be given ample opportunity to explain your position when your attorney has his chance on his redirect examination of you. Again, it must be emphasized that your role as a defendant in a malpractice suit is not a major one. If you can avoid being argumentative, and if you can convey to the jury that you are a caring and compassionate individual, you will have gone a long way in helping to secure a verdict in your favor.

The same philosophy should also guide you through the deposition, which will be discussed subsequently. Bear in mind that a courteous individual makes a far better impression on a lay jury than one who is combative.

Avoid making statements that could malign your patient even though you may harbor hostile feelings, which are understandable under the circumstances. Statements such as "I can't understand why I am being sued after all I have done for my patient," or "I can't understand why my patient doesn't appreciate what I have done for him" should be avoided.

Physician Liability Under Managed Care Programs

Managed care programs now play a major role in patient care. The participating physician is under contract to provide medical care and very often the terms of this agreement favor the managed care facility and place the physician at risk.[6]

Contractual Agreements

The contract between a managed care facility and the physician outlines the obligations and responsibilities between the 2 parties. The contract should be fully understood by the physician and, if necessary, should be reviewed by an attorney. Liability suits have arisen in situations in which these obligations and responsibilities were absent or left ambiguous. The contract should also contain a provision as to how a dis-

pute that arises between the managed care facility and the physician should be resolved.

Third Party Liability

An increasing number of health care facilities are inserting hold-harmless clauses into their contracts. These require physicians to indemnify the health care facility not only for negligence on the part of the physician but also for breaches in patient care including the denial of care by the health care facility. Consult your attorney before signing such a contract and follow his or her advice regarding the appropriate response.

Practice Responsibility

This is closely related to the hold-harmless concepts. Health care facilities may deny a request for admission or consultation and may insist on a premature discharge of the patient. The courts have held the physician responsible if the patient suffers adversely from such actions. Some states are now offering malpractice policy protection against such an occurrence for a higher premium. Notwithstanding, a patient who in the opinion of the doctor requires admission to a hospital should be admitted even if permission was denied by the health care facility.

Administrative Responsibility

The managed care entity frequently requires the participating physician to conduct peer review activities, and these, too, can expose the physician to a potential lawsuit. Some states do provide statutory immunity under such circumstances, but where this is not the case, the physician should obtain legal advice before agreeing to serve on a committee that could expose the doctor to a lawsuit.

Recent Developments in Health and Hospital Law

In the past few years,[7] significant changes have been made in both state and national laws that affect medical practitioners. COBRA, the appropriate acronym for the Comprehensive Omnibus Budget Reconciliation Act of 1986, contains provisions whereby a physician may be strictly liable under federal law for inappropriate transfers of patients without first stabilizing the patients. At least 1 physician has been fined for transferring a patient who was in an unstable condition. One of the other consequences of a violation of this federal law is that you lose your Medicare/Medicaid billing rights for up to 5 years. On-call physicians are subject to the provisions of COBRA in that they must respond to the request for a consultation from the emergency room within a "reasonable time." The courts are still trying to determine what a "reasonable time" is. Once the on-call expert or specialist is notified of a patient who needs his services, he or she becomes the physician responsible under these federal provisions and the emergency room doctor is relieved of liability.

At least 2 recent cases have led to decisions by the highest court in Massachusetts and the United States Court of Appeals for the First Circuit that a physician may be liable for failure to follow up a no-show patient. In 1 case, Gray versus Kieger, 27 Mass. App. Ct. 583 (1989), an orthopaedic surgeon was found liable for not following up with a young man who turned out to have an adamantinoma of the tibia. This case said that because there was a very serious potential for the undiagnosed lesion in the patient's leg that the doctor was "bound to pursue the no-show and to continue the investigation until the scope and true nature of the lesion were determined." The Court presumed that the patient would permit this further investigation. In the case of Dunning versus Kerzner, the United States Court of Appeals for the First Circuit held that a Rhode Island physician could be found negligent for failing to follow up with a patient who did not obtain medical records and information as the doctor directed. This was a case in which the patient had told his treating physicians that he had studies done at a Veteran Administration Hospital for blood in stools. The doctor told the patient to get those records and come back to see him, but the patient returned a few years later with a bowel malignancy that proved to be incurable. As these cases illustrate, COBRA may impose liability on you even though you never established a traditional physician-patient relationship with the patient. The no-show cases obviously call for some adjustment to your customary practice so that a chart should be at least reviewed by someone in your office when a patient fails to keep an appointment, and, if there is any potential for a serious condition, the patient should be notified by certified mail and a copy kept in the patient's chart.

The Expert Witness

The institution of a malpractice action against any physician is always a frustrating experience, because in most instances the physician has done his utmost for the patient and is naturally hostile and hurt when his patient brings a lawsuit against him. The physician may question his own abilities and may harbor feelings of guilt, reasoning that if he had done a better job, the suit would not have originated.

The vast majority of negligence suits involve maloccurrences rather than malpractice. It is in this specific area that the expert witness can be of greatest assistance to the defendant, because, if there has been no breach in orthopaedic standards of care, the witness will be prepared to support the defendant doctor in court.

Contrary to popular belief, malpractice suits have proliferated not so much because of greedy patients or because of ambulance-chasing lawyers, but due to the fact that qualified physicians are becoming more and more willing to appear as plaintiff's expert witnesses. Indeed some of these doctors advertise their services in legal journals and work for medicolegal corporations that specialize in providing expert witnesses for plaintiffs.[8-13] Once the plaintiff's attorney has a report from another physician that a breach in the standard of care has occurred, that case will go to court because the plaintiff's attorney is not required to decide on the merit of the case but will leave this to a jury. Because a jury will determine whether a malpractice case has merit, the defendant requires an expert witness who will champion his cause against the testimony of the plaintiff's expert witness. In the final analysis, it really comes down to a battle between the expert witnesses and opposing attorneys, and the case will be decided on which expert witness the jury believes.

Although the attorney generally selects the expert witness, he or she will welcome your input. If you know of an expert physician in your particular field who has experience in the matter on which you are being sued, your attorneys will listen to your suggestions and will contact that expert. Bear in mind, however, that not all experts are willing to testify in a court of law or are willing to travel in order to appear personally. If the expert refuses to come to court, his assistance will be of little help to you. It is far better to accept the testimony of a less famous individual who is willing to personally represent you than that of a distinguished professor who is unwilling to do so.

In order to be maximally effective, the expert must have evidence to show that there was no departure from accepted orthopaedic standards. Well-kept records are the best assurance that such evidence will be available. It goes without saying that records should never be altered. Should it be necessary to make changes, the defendant should consult with his attorney prior to making any alterations in the records.

The area in which the defendant has the most difficulty is the deposition. A deposition is a question-and-answer period in which the plaintiff's attorney attempts to obtain as much pretrial information as possible from the defendant. This session can be quite prolonged and may last the entire day. In some instances, the plaintiff's attorney may call you back for more questioning if he feels that additional inquiry is indicated. This deposition usually takes place in the plaintiff's attorney's office and you as the defendant are accompanied by your attorney. If other doctors or institutions are involved in the suit, their respective attorneys may be present in order to protect the interests of their client. The deposition is a legal document and is used in court during your trial. A court stenographer swears you in and takes down every word that you say. Obviously, if anything you say is untrue or is inconsistent with your later trial testimony, it can devastate your defense.

Do not provide gratuitous information beyond what appears in your patient's hospital record and in your office file. Most defendants say too much in their deposition in an attempt to convince the opposition that they are innocent of any wrong doing. They feel that if they explain in great detail what transpired and that they acted in accordance with good medical practice, the plaintiff's attorney or the patient will realize the error of their ways and drop the suit. Nothing can be further from the truth. Once you have been called to a deposition, it is almost certain that a trial will go forward unless a last-minute settlement occurs, because the plaintiff already has an expert witness who will testify in court that you have breached the standard of care. It is therefore essential that you do not educate the opposition during this deposition, because whatever you say will be subsequently given to the plaintiff's expert witness, who will use your deposition testimony to discredit you during the trial. It has happened on more than 1 occasion that an otherwise perfectly good and defensible case was lost because the defendant either said too much at his deposition or, by saying too much, incriminated himself in such a way that it made it difficult to defend him. A good rule to follow, therefore, is tell the truth but avoid engaging in long lectures and dissertations that could come back to haunt you. Questions should be answered whenever possible with 1 word, yes or no. If it is not possible to answer with 1 word, answer with 1 sentence. If you find that it is taking you more than 3 sentences to respond to a question, then you are in trouble; stop, rethink your answer and start again. The only exception to this rule should be if you are asked to read something from your notes or from the hospital chart. Because these records will become exhibits and will be used during the trial, it is quite permissible to read whatever the plain-tiff's attorney wants you to.

It is also important not to speculate during your deposition. Responses such as "I don't know," or "I don't remember" are perfectly good and concise answers, if that is the truth. You may well be asked about minute details that occurred 4 or 5 years ago, and it is quite natural to have forgotten these occurrences. If that is the case, say so. You might be asked where certain hospital records are kept or where a former associate of yours who may have been peripherally associated with the case is living or practicing at present. If you know this for a fact, answer accordingly. But if you are not certain where that record is or where that person may be then you should indicate that you do not know. Avoid answers such as "I think the record may be in the hospital record room," or "I am not sure but I think that Dr. X may be living in such and such a place." That is speculation and should be avoided. Bear in mind that the deposition becomes a record that the plaintiff's attorney will use to his advantage to discredit you during the trial. The less you say, the better off you are.

Promises to patients assuring a quick recovery or describing a surgical procedure in an oversimplified form should not be made.[14] Statements such as "I'll have you walking within a week" or "this operation is a simple procedure" should be avoided. Patients tend to take such assurances literally, and if the results are not as expected, the expert witness will find it difficult to support such comments on cross-examination.

After all is said and done, the final outcome of any medical malpractice suit rests with a lay jury. Unfortunately, we physicians are judged not by our peers, but by 12 individuals who have no understanding of the complexities and the events surrounding the malpractice action. That being the case, in some instances a perfectly defensible case can be lost because the jury was swayed by emotion rather than by fact.

Nevertheless, by following these relatively simple suggestions you will be helping your expert witness and attorney to better represent you and, hopefully, you will strengthen your chances of obtaining a verdict in your favor.

References

1. Taragin MI, Martin K, Shapiro S, Trout R, Carson JL: Physician malpractice: Does the past predict the future? *J Gen Intern Med* 1995;10:550–556.
2. Carter R: The subpoena: Coping with the anxiety and stress. *N Y State Dent J* 1997;63:16–17.
3. Plunkett LR: Anatomy of a dental malpractice case: The trial. *N Y State Dent J* 1997;63:10–14.
4. Leonard JJ: The key to successful litigation: A strong defense team. *J Med Assoc G* 1993;82:399–400.
5. Lisko KO: Testifying strategies: Telling the truth as effectively as possible. *Natl Med Leg J* 1996;7:1.
6. Manuel BM: Physician liability under managed care. *J Am Coll Surg* 1996;182:537–546.
7. Levine RJ, Guisto JA, Meislin HW, Spaite DW: Analysis of federally imposed penalties for violations of the Consolidated Omnibus Reconciliation Act. *Ann Emerg Med* 1996;28:45–50.
8. Beck M: The hired gun expert witness. *Mo Med* 1994;91:179–182.
9. Brahams D: Expert witnesses under scrutiny. *Lancet* 1997;349:896.
10. Habal MB: Responsibility, integrity, and clinical experts. *Plast Reconstr Surg* 1997;99:1134–1135.
11. Harty-Golder B: The physician as expert. *J Fla Med Assoc* 1994;81:361–363.
12. Morris WO: An expert witness should tell it as it is: Not as he would wish it. *J NJ Dent Assoc* 1993;64:29.
13. Schrager GO: Medical "experts" for hire! *Pediatrics* 1995;95:320–321.
14. Hyams AL, Shapiro DW, Brennan TA: Medical practice guidelines in malpractice litigation: An early retrospective. *J Health Polit Policy Law* 1996;21:289–313.

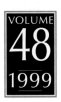

Cumulative Index
1997-1999

Please note: Page numbers in bold refer to information in this volume, ICL Volume 48, published in 1999. All other page numbers refer to Volumes 46 and 47 published in 1997 and 1998. Page numbers in italic/bold italic refer to figures or figure legends.

A

G

Gait, abnormalities in diabetic neuropathy, **48: 294**
Gait cycle, 47: 398, *399*
Gait training, pediatric thoracic myelomeningocele, **48: 564-566**
Gallium-67 citrate, 47: 288
Galveston technique, segmental spinal fusion, **48: 556,** *558*
Gamekeeper's thumb, 47: 184-*185*
Gamma irradiation, 47: 380, 382-385
Ganglion, distinguished from sarcoma, **48: 584**
Ganglion cysts, denervation caused by, 47: *12*
Gangrene, wet, **48:** *687*
Gastrocnemius, transfer of medial head, for reconstruction of posterior cruciate ligament, **48: 205**
Gastrocnemius muscle anatomy, 47: 419
Gastronemius soleus, strength of complex, **48: 225**
Gaucher's disease, osteonecrosis of the humeral head, **48: 350**
General Accounting Office (GAO), on health insurance premiums, **48: 674**
General health assessment instruments for use after fractures in elderly, 46: 441-442
Gentamicin, antibiotic-impregnated cement, **48: 117**
Gentamicin-impregnated beads, and serum bactericidal titer testing, **48: 116**
Gerber retractor, 47: 81
Gerber test for subscapularis function, 46: *58,* 47: 137, 144
Gerdy's tubercle, 47: *373, 374*
    in iliotibial band syndrome, 47: 413
Geriatrics for orthopaedists, 46: 409-416
    changes in focus of medical care, 46: 410-414
    ethical dilemmas, 46: 415
    iatrogenic conditions, 46: 415
    medical conditions, 46: 414-415
    pharmacology and aging, 46: 415
    reasons for change in demographics, 46: *409*
    theories of aging, 46: 410
Geyser sign, 47: 79
Giant cell tumors
    differentiation from metaphyseal fibrous defect, **48:** *615*
    treatment of, **48: 595-596**
Girdlestone arthroplasty, 47: 301
    and total knee arthroplasty, **48: 161**
Glenohumeral joint
    arthroscopy, 47: 59. *See also* Shoulder arthroscopy
    evaluation of, 46: 44
    instability, 47: 97-110
        biomechanical considerations, 47: 98-101
        failed repairs for, 113-125
        multidirectional, 47: 101-109
        and posterior capsular contracture, 46: 571
        reconstruction for severe glenoid loss, 47: 109-110
    loss of motion with arthrosis, after surgery for shoulder instability, **48: 360**
    osteoarthritis, 47: 129, *130*
    septic arthritis of, 46: *33*
Glenohumeral ligaments/labrum, imaging of, 46: 521-522
Glenohumeral proprioceptive neuromuscular facilitation patterns, 46: 47
Glenohumeral stability, provocative tests for, 46: 44
Glenohumeral strength, estimation of, 46: 44
Glenoid arthritis as complication in humeral head replacement, 46: 20
Glenoid bone, loss of, 47: *108,* 110
Glenoid labrum, function of, 47: 97, *98*
Glenoid loosening, after total shoulder arthroplasty, **48: 364**
Gloves, perforations of, and infection at arthroplasty sites, **48: 113**
Glucocorticoids in osteoporosis, 46: 447
Glycocalyx slime
    and antibiotics, **48: 116**

and infection at arthroplasty sites, **48: 114**
Glycosaminoglycans, 47: 480
GM-1 gangliosides in treating spinal cord injuries, 46: 118
Gold compounds in treating rheumatoid arthritis, 46: 78
Gonarthrosis
    unicompartmental, arthroscopic treatment of, **48: 139**
    unicondylar knee arthroplasty for, **48: 143-148**
Gore-Tex grafts, 47: 365
Gout, 46: 75-76
    and Achilles tendon rupture, **48: 220**
    and posterior heel pain, **48: 213**
Gouty arthritis, 46: 75
Grafts. *See also* Allografts; Autografts; Bone grafting
    bone
        biology of, **48: 645-651**
        classification of, **48: 58**
        donors of, **48: 58**
        dynamic bone turnover in, **48: 84-85**
        history of, **48: 79-80**
        incorporation of, **48: 86-87**
        and infection of arthroplasty sites, **48: 119-120**
        principles of, **48: 58-59**
        revitalization of, **48: 80**
        surgical technique, **48: 70-73**
    and bone loss, total knee arthroplasty, **48: 179**
    impaction, histologic analysis, **48: 84-86**
    ligament, selection of, **48: 520**
    morcellized bone, **48: 58-59**
    preparation and placement, total knee arthroplasty, **48: 180-181**
Gram stain, 47: 291
Graspers, 46: 131-132, 135
Great toe. *See* Metatarsophalangeal (MTP) joint, first
    amputation of, 46: 505-508
Greater trochanter
    fractures of, 47: 252
    longitudinal split, **48: 77**
Greater tuberosity nonunions, 46: 26
Gross classification, of acetabular deficiencies, for total hip arthroplasty, **48:** *50*
Gross domestic profit, health care percentage, **48:** *674*
Ground reaction force (GRF), 47: 399, *401*
Growth factor receptors, 46: 474-475
Growth factors
    articular cartilage restoration, **48: 624**
    effect on cartilage repair, 46: 488-490
        acute mechanical damage, 46: 487-488
        as agents of healing, 46: 490-491
        carriers, 46: 491-492
        inflammatory disease, 46: 488
        and repair capacity, 47: 498-*499*
    for fracture healing, 46: 483-486, 47: 530-532
        bone morphogenetic proteins, 46: 484, 47: 530-531
        fibroblast growth factors, 46: 484, 47: 530
        insulin-like growth factors, 46: 485
        platelet-derived growth factor, 46: 485, 47: 531-532
        transforming growth factor-ß, 46: 483-484, 47: 531
    and joint degeneration, 47: 472-473
    and regulation of cartilage proliferation, 47: 464-466, 469-473
        bone morphogenetic proteins, 47: 471-472
        fibroblast growth factor, 47: 465, 471
        insulin-like growth factors, 47: 465, 470
        parathyroid hormone related protein (PTHrP), 47: 465
        transforming growth factor-ß, 47: 465, 470-471
    as therapeutic agents, 46: 473-474
        challenges to clinical application, 46: 475-476
        in osteoporosis, 46: 495-497

P